Decision Making in Medicine

An Algorithmic Approach

Decision Making in Medicine

An Algorithmic Approach

Third Edition

Stuart B. Mushlin, MD, FACP, FACR
Assistant Professor of Medicine
Harvard Medical School
Master Clinician
Brigham and Women's Hospital
Julian Cohen Teaching Scholar
Brigham and Women's Hospital
Director of Primary Care, ad interim, Department of Medicine
Brigham and Women's Hospital
Boston, Massachusetts

Harry L. Greene II, MD, FACP
Former Executive Vice President
Massachusetts Medical Society
Waltham, Massachusetts
Instructor in Medicine
Harvard Medical School
Boston, Massachusetts

MOSBY

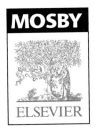

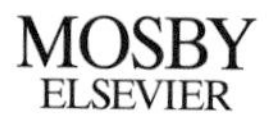

1600 John F. Kennedy Blvd.
Ste 1800
Philadelphia, PA 19103-2899

DECISION MAKING IN MEDICINE: AN ALGORITHMIC APPROACH, THIRD EDITION   ISBN: 978-0-323-04107-2

Notice

Knowledge and best practice in this field are constantly changing. As new research and experience broaden our understanding, changes in research methods, professional practices, or medical treatment may become necessary.

Practitioners and researchers must always rely on their own experience and knowledge in evaluating and using any information, methods, compounds, or experiments described herein. In using such information or methods they should be mindful of their own safety and the safety of others, including parties for whom they have a professional responsibility.

With respect to any drug or pharmaceutical products identified, readers are advised to check the most current information provided (i) on procedures featured or (ii) by the manufacturer of each product to be administered, to verify the recommended dose or formula, the method and duration of administration, and contraindications. It is the responsibility of practitioners, relying on their own experience and knowledge of their patients, to make diagnoses, to determine dosages and the best treatment for each individual patient, and to take all appropriate safety precautions.

To the fullest extent of the law, neither the Publisher nor the authors, contributors, or editors assume any liability for any injury and/or damage to persons or property as a matter of products liability, negligence or otherwise, or from any use or operation of any methods, products, instructions, or ideas contained in the material herein.

Previous editions copyrighted 1998, 1992

Library of Congress Cataloging-in-Publication Data
Decision making in medicine : an algorithmic approach / [edited by]
Stuart B. Mushlin, Harry L. Greene II. -- 3rd ed.
p. ; cm.
Includes bibliographical references and index.
ISBN 978-0-323-04107-2
1. Medical protocols. 2. Medicine--Decision making. I. Mushlin, Stuart B. II. Greene, Harry L. (Harry Lemoine), 1942-
[DNLM: 1. Diagnosis. 2. Algorithms. 3. Decision Making. 4. Therapeutics. WB 141 D294 2009]
RC64.D43 2009
616--dc22

2009036313

Acquisitions Editor: Druanne Martin
Developmental Editor: Agnes Byrne
Publishing Services Manager: Mary Stermel
Design Direction: Steven Stave

Printed in the United States of America

Last digit is the print number: 9 8 7 6 5 4 3 2 1

To my wonderful wife, Francine. She is generous, wise, witty, literate, constructive, and patient. There are many events we have forgone so that I may work on "the book." I thank her for believing in me and embracing the concept that every day we should strive to do more than we thought we could do.

SBM

To my family: Linda Clark Greene, Harry L. Greene III, Evelyn Lockwood Greene, Michele Greene Moynihan, Chris Moynihan, Hayden Moynihan, Jennifer Greene Reynoso, and David Reynoso.

HLG

SECTION EDITORS

Sherleen Chen, MD, FACS
Instructor in Ophthalmology, Harvard Medical School; Director, Comprehensive Ophthalmology Service, Boston, Massachusetts
Ocular

Bradford C. Dickerson, MD
Instructor in Neurology, Harvard Medical School; Assistant in Neurology, Department of Neurology, Massachusetts General Hospital; Associate Neurologist, Division of Cognitive and Behavioral Neurology, Brigham and Women's Hospital, Boston, Massachusetts
Neurology

M. Brian Fennerty, MD
Professor of Medicine, Division of Gastroenterology and Hepatology, Health and Science University, Portland, Oregon
Gastroenterology

John A. Fromson, MD
Assistant Clinical Professor of Psychiatry, Harvard Medical School; Chairman, Department of Psychiatry, Metro West Medical Center, Boston, Massachusetts
Behavioral Medicine

Barbara A. Gilchrest, MD
Professor and Chair, Department of Dermatology, Boston University School of Medicine; Chief of Dermatology, Boston Medical Center, Boston, Massachusetts
Dermatology

Michael D. Katz, PharmD
Associate Professor, Department of Pharmacy Practice and Service, University of Arizona, College of Pharmacy, Tucson, Arizona
Pharmacology

Lisa Kaufmann, MD
Professor of Medicine, SUNY Upstate Medical University, Syracuse, New York
General Medicine

Michael Klompas, MD, MPH, FRCPC
Associate Hospital Epidemiologist, Brigham and Women's Hospital, Boston, Massachusetts
Infectious Diseases

Patricia Kritek, MD
Pulmonary and Critical Care Medicine, Brigham and Women's Hospital, Boston, Massachusetts
Pulmonary Disease

Ana Maria López, MD, MPH, FACP
Associate Dean for Outreach and Multicultural Affairs, Professor of Medicine and Pathology, Medical Director, Arizona Telemedicine Program, University of Arizona, Tucson, Arizona
Hematology/Oncology

Graham T. McMahon, MD, MMSc
Department of Endocrinology, Brigham and Women's Hospital, Boston, Massachusetts
Endocrinology

Paul A. Monach, MD, PhD
Assistant Professor of Medicine, Section of Rheumatology, Boston University School of Medicine, Boston, Massachusetts
Rheumatology

Stuart B. Mushlin, MD, FACP, FACR
Assistant Professor of Medicine, Harvard Medical School; Master Clinician, Brigham and Women's Hospital; Julian Cohen Teaching Scholar, Brigham and Women's Hospital; Director of Primary Care, ad interim, Department of Medicine, Brigham and Women's Hospital, Boston Massachusetts
Women's Health

Ajay K. Singh, MBBS, FRCP
Associate Professor of Medicine, Harvard Medical School; Renal Division, Brigham and Women's Hospital, Boston, Massachusetts
Nephrology

Graeme Steele, MD, FCS, FACS
Division of Urologic Surgery, Brigham and Women's Hospital, Boston, Massachusetts
Urology

Stephen D. Wiviott, MD
Assistant Professor of Medicine, Cardiovascular Division, Department of Medicine, Harvard Medical School; Investigator, TIMI Study Group, Brigham and Women's Hospital, Boston, Massachusetts
Cardiology

Richard D. Zane, MD, FAAEM
Assistant Professor of Medicine, Harvard Medical School; Vice Chair, Department of Emergency Medicine, Brigham and Women's Hospital, Boston, Massachusetts
Emergency Medicine

CONTRIBUTORS

Sandeep K. Agarwal, MD, PhD
Assistant Professor, Division of Rheumatology and Immunogenetics, University of Texas Medical School at Houston, Houston, Texas
Scleroderma; Elevated Creatine Kinase Level

Frederick R. Ahmann, MD
Professor of Medicine and Surgery, University of Arizona, Arizona Cancer Center, Tucson, Arizona
Superior Vena Caval Syndrome

Essam Al-Ansari, MD
Pulmonary Specialists-Northern, Florence, Kentucky
Dyspnea

Erik K. Alexander, MD
Assistant Professor of Medicine, Harvard Medical School; Department of Endocrinology, Brigham and Women's Hospital, Boston, Massachusetts
Tests of Thyroid Function; Goiter; Thyroid Function Tests in Nonthyroidal Illness

Elaine J. Alpert, MD
Formerly Associate Professor of Medicine, Boston University, Boston, Massachusetts
Domestic Violence

Nenad Antic, MD
Arizona Center for Hematology and Oncology, Glendale, Arizona
Polycythemia

Elliott M. Antman, MD
Professor of Medicine, Harvard Medical School; Department of Medicine, Brigham and Women's Hospital, Boston, Massachusetts
Assessment and Initial Management of ST-Segment Elevation Myocardial Infarction

Mohammed Asmal, MD, PhD
Division of Infectious Diseases, Brigham and Women's Hospital, Boston, Massachusetts
Encephalitis

Usman Baber, MD
Department of Medicine, University of Texas Southwestern Medical School, Dallas, Texas
Hypertension

Aaron L. Baggish, MD
Division of Cardiology, Massachusetts General Hospital, Boston, Massachusetts
Systolic Murmurs; Diastolic Murmurs; Cardiac Dyspnea

Homeira Baghdadi, MD
Clinical Associate in Medicine, University of Arizona College of Medicine, Tucson, Arizona
Nipple Discharge

Juan Diego Baltodano, MD
Assistant Professor of Medicine, Virginia Commonwealth University, Division of Gastroenterology, Hepatology, and Nutrition, Richmond, Virginia
Acute Abdominal Pain; Chronic Abdominal Pain; Nausea and Vomiting; Dyspepsia; Jaundice; Ascites; Rectal Bleeding; Chronic Diarrhea; Asymptomatic Abnormal Liver Aminotransferases

Glen W. Barrisford, MD
Department of Urology, National Naval Medical Center, Bethesda, Maryland
Urinary Retention

Iris R. Bell, MD, PhD
Associate Professor, Department of Psychiatry, University of Arizona College of Medicine; Director, Program in Geriatric Psychiatry, Tucson VA Medical Center, Tucson, Arizona
Depression

Jeanne E. Bishop, MD
Associate Professor of Medicine, SUNY Upstate Medical University, Syracuse, New York
Falls in Geriatric Patients

Marc P. Bonaca, MD
Division of Cardiovascular Medicine, Brigham and Women's Hospital, Boston, Massachusetts
Stable Angina; Post–Myocardial Infarction Care and Counseling

Yvette M. Bordelon, MD, PhD
Assistant Professor, Department of Neurology, University of California Medical School, Los Angeles, California
Tremor; Hyperkinesias

Jessica Byron, MD
Clinical Assistant Professor, Department of Obstetrics and Gynecology, University of Arizona College of Medicine, Tucson, Arizona
Premenstrual Dysphoric Disorder

Christopher P. Cannon, MD
Associate Professor of Medicine, Harvard Medical School; TIMI Study Group, Brigham and Women's Hospital, Boston, Massachusetts
Unstable Angina/Non-ST-Elevation Myocardial Infarction

Shari Carney, MD
Clinical Instructor of Ophthalmology, SUNY Upstate Medical University, Syracuse, New York
The Red Eye

Daniela Carusi, MD, MSc
Instructor of Obstetrics, Gynecology and Reproductive Biology, Harvard Medical School; Director of Ambulatory General Gynecology, Department of Obstetrics and Gynecology, Brigham and Women's Hospital, Boston, Massachusetts
Ectopic Pregnancy

Sherleen Chen, MD, FACS
Instructor in Ophthalmology, Harvard Medical School; Director, Comprehensive Ophthalmology Service, Boston, Massachusetts
Dilated Pupil; Corneal Abrasion; Conjunctivitis; Acute Visual Loss

Michael Cho, MD
Channing Laboratory, Brigham and Women's Hospital, Boston, Massachusetts
Solitary Pulmonary Nodule

Sherry Chou, MD
Stroke and Neurological Critical Care Fellow, Massachusetts General Hospital, Boston, Massachusetts
Transient Ischemic Attack and Stroke Evaluation; Stroke Treatment and Prophylaxis

Lynn Cleary, MD
Professor of Medicine, SUNY Upstate Medical University, Syracuse, New York
Involuntary Weight Loss

Nancy A. Curosh, MD
Private Practice, Endocrinologist, Portland, Oregon
Secondary Amenorrhea

Paul Currier, MD
Pulmonary Unit, Massachusetts General Hospital, Boston, Massachusetts
Diffuse Interstitial Lung Disease

James A. De Lemos, MD
Department of Cardiology, University of Texas Southwestern Medical School, Dallas, Texas
Hypertension; Hypotension; Syncope

Ashwin Dharmadhikari, MD
Pulmonary and Critical Care Medicine, Massachusetts General Hospital, Boston, Massachusetts
Positive Tuberculin Skin Test (PPD)

Allitia B. DiBernardo, MD
Instructor in Neurology, Harvard Medical School; Assistant in Neurology, Massachusetts General Hospital; Boston, Massachusetts
Weakness

Bradford C. Dickerson, MD
Instructor in Neurology, Harvard Medical School; Assistant in Neurology, Department of Neurology, Massachusetts General Hospital; Associate Neurologist, Division of Cognitive and Behavioral Neurology, Brigham and Women's Hospital, Boston, Massachusetts
Memory Loss; Acute Confusional State; Chronic Behavior Change

Gregory L. Eastwood, MD
Professor of Bioethics and Humanities, SUNY Upstate Medical University, Syracuse, New York
Belching; Gastrointestinal Bleeding; Flatulence

Robert E. Eckart, DO
Cardiovascular Division, Brigham and Women's Hospital, Boston, Massachusetts
Bradycardia

Brian L. Erstad, PharmD
Professor and Assistant Department Head, Department of Pharmacy Practice and Science, University of Arizona College of Pharmacy, Tucson, Arizona
Antimicrobial Prophylaxis in Surgical Patients; Use and Monitoring of Aminoglycoside Antibiotics; Use and Evaluation of Serum Drug Levels

Laurie L. Fajardo, MD
Professor and Head, Department of Radiology, University of Iowa, Iowa City, Iowa
Breast Mass

James C. Fang, MD
Professor of Medicine, Case Western Reserve University, School of Medicine, Cleveland, Ohio
Evaluation of a New Diagnosis of Congestive Heart Failure; Diagnosis and Treatment of Acute Pulmonary Edema

John J. W. Fangman, MD
Assistant Professor of Medicine, Medical College of Wisconsin, Milwaukee, Wisconsin
Respiratory Symptoms in HIV-Infected Patients

M. Brian Fennerty, MD
Professor of Medicine, Division of Gastroenterology and Hepatology, Oregon Health and Science University, Portland, Oregon
Noncardiac Chest Pain; Acute Diarrhea; Irritable Bowel Syndrome; Positive Fecal Occult Blood Test (FOBT); Elevated Serum Iron

John A. Fromson, MD
Assistant Clinical Professor of Psychiatry, Harvard Medical School; Chairman, Department of Psychiatry, Metro West Medical Center, Boston, Massachusetts
Alcoholism; Anxiety; Depression; Emotional Disorders with Somatic Expression; Grief; Psychosis; Suicidal Patient

Deborah Fuchs, MD
Anatomic and Clinical Pathology, Hematology, University Medical Center, Tucson, Arizona
Coagulation Abnormalities

Diana Gallagher, MD
Pulmonary, Critical Care, and Sleep Medicine, Beth Israel Deaconess Medical Center, Boston, Massachusetts
Hemoptysis; Stridor

Alan J. Gelenberg, MD
Professor and Head, Department of Psychiatry, University of Arizona College of Medicine, Tucson, Arizona
Psychosis

David W. Gibson, MD
Henry County Medical Center, Paris, Tennessee
Edema

Barbara A. Gilchrest, MD
Professor and Chair, Department of Dermatology, Boston University School of Medicine; Chief of Dermatology, Boston Medical Center, Boston, Massachusetts
Leg Ulcer; Generalized Pruritus

Guillermo Gonzales-Osete, MD
Arizona Oncology Associates, Tucson, Arizona
Deep Venous Thrombosis; Lymphadenopathy; Spinal Cord Compression

Heather L. Gornik, MD
Staff Physician and Medical Director, Noninvasive Vascular Laboratory, Department of Cardiovascular Medicine, Cleveland Clinic, Cleveland, Ohio
Claudication

Harry L. Greene II, MD, FACP
Former Executive Vice President, Massachusetts Medical Society, Waltham; Instructor in Medicine, Harvard Medical School, Boston, Massachusetts
Edema; Smoking Cessation

David M. Greer, MD
Assistant Professor in Neurology, Harvard Medical School; Assistant in Neurology, Massachusetts General Hospital, Boston, Massachusetts
Coma; Brain Death

Kristyn M. Greifer, MD
Associate Medical Director for Ambulatory and Hospital Medicine, The Southeast Permanente Group, Inc., Atlanta, Georgia
Sexual Dysfunction

Sarah P. Hammond, MD
Instructor in Medicine, Harvard Medical School; Division of Infectious Diseases, Brigham and Women's Hospital, Boston, Massachusetts
The Acutely Ill Patient with HIV

Simon Helfgott, MD
Division of Rheumatology, Immunology, and Allergy, Brigham and Women's Hospital, Boston, Massachusetts
Neck Pain; Low Back Pain

Leigh R. Hochberg, MD
Instructor in Neurology, Harvard Medical School; Acute Stroke and Neurocritical Care Service, Massachusetts General Hospital and Brigham and Women's Hospital, Boston, Massachusetts
Acute Stroke

Risa Hoffman, MD, MPH
Clinical Instructor, Department of Medicine, Division of Infectious Diseases, David Geffen School of Medicine, University of California, Los Angeles, Los Angeles, California
Postexposure Prophylaxis for HIV and Hepatitis B and C

Maria K. Houtchens, MD
Instructor in Neurology, Harvard Medical School; Associate Neurologist, Multiple Sclerosis Program, Brigham and Women's Hospital, Boston, Massachusetts
Transient Monocular Visual Loss; Dizziness

Tomaz Hruczkowski, MD
Assistant Professor of Medicine, Cardiology Arrhythmia Services, University of Alberta, Edmonton, Alberta, Canada
Sudden Cardiac Death

Philip E. Jaffe, MD
Private Practice, New Haven, Connecticut
Dysphagia; Biliary Colic; Constipation; Fecal Incontinence

Alyssa Johnsen, MD, PhD
Division of Rheumatology, Immunology, and Allergy, Brigham and Women's Hospital, Boston, Massachusetts
Raynaud's Phenomenon; Low Bone Density; Antinuclear Antibody Test

William P. Johnson, MD
Associate Professor of Medicine, University of Arizona, College of Medicine, Tucson, Arizona
Chronic Pain

Anthony Karabanow, MD
Director, Section of Hospital Medicine, Assistant Professor of Medicine, SUNY Upstate Medical University, Syracuse, New York
Preoperative Evaluation

Banu A. Karimi-Shah, MD
Critical Care Practitioner, Internist, Pulmonologist, Solver Springs, Maryland
Pleural Effusion

Michael D. Katz, PharmD
Associate Professor, Department of Pharmacy Practice and Service, University of Arizona College of Pharmacy, Tucson, Arizona
Urinary Tract Infection in Women; Acute Anticoagulation; Long-Term Anticoagulation; Anaphylaxis; Evaluation of Adverse Drug Reactions; Choosing Appropriate Antimicrobial Therapy

Richard M. Kaufman, MD
Assistant Professor of Pathology, Harvard Medical School; Medical Director, Adult Transfusion Service; Brigham and Women's Hospital, Boston, Massachusetts
Transfusion Therapy: Fresh Frozen Plasma and Cryoprecipitate; Transfusion Therapy: Platelets; Transfusion Therapy: Red Blood Cells; Transfusion Therapy: Granulocytes; Transfusion Reactions

Lisa Kaufmann, MD
Professor of Medicine, SUNY Upstate Medical University, Syracuse, New York
Fatigue; Persistent Excessive Sweating

Santosh Kesari, MD
Instructor in Neurology, Harvard Medical School; Associate Neurologist, Center for Neuro-Oncology, Dana-Farber/Brigham and Women's Cancer Center, Division of Cancer Neurology, Department of Neurology, Brigham and Women's Hospital, Boston, Massachusetts
Acute Headache; Chronic Headache; Disturbances of Smell and Taste

Megan Tamburini Khosla, MD
SUNY Upstate Medical University, Syracuse, New York
Prevention and Screening

Peter Kim, MD
Division of Rheumatology and Immunology, David Geffen School of Medicine, University of California, Los Angeles, Los Angeles, California
Polyarticular Arthritis; Hyperuricemia and Gout; Diffuse Muscle Pain and Stiffness: Polymyalgia Rheumatica and Giant Cell Arteritis

Michael Klompas, MD, MPH, FRCPC
Associate Hospital Epidemiologist, Brigham and Women's Hospital, Boston, Massachusetts
Chronic Meningitis; Toxic Shock Syndromes

William H. Kreisle, MD
Mountain State Tumor Institute, Boise, Idaho
Leukopenia

Patricia Kritek, MD
Pulmonary and Critical Care Medicine, Brigham and Women's Hospital, Boston, Massachusetts
Cough; Mediastinal Lymphadenopathy; Multiple Pulmonary Nodules; Respiratory Symptoms and Occupational Exposure to Asbestos; Asthma

Dawn Lemcke, MD
Assistant Professor of Clinical Medicine, University of Arizona College of Medicine, Tucson, Arizona
Chest Pain in Women

Norman Levine, MD
Professor of Medicine, Department of Dermatology, University of Arizona College of Medicine, Tucson, Arizona
Pigmented Lesions; Urticaria; Generalized Pruritus; Palpable Purpura

Ana Maria López, MD, MPH, FACP
Associate Dean for Outreach and Multicultural Affairs, Professor of Medicine and Pathology, Medical Director, Arizona Telemedicine Program, University of Arizona, Tucson, Arizona
Coagulation Abnormalities; Neutropenia and Fever; Pathologic Fractures; Contraceptive Choices

Philip A. Lowry, MD
Medical Director, Simonds-Simon Regional Cancer Center, Fitchburg, Massachusetts
Clinical Considerations for Stem Cell Transplantation; Late Issues for Patients Who Survive the Initial Diagnosis and Treatment of Cancer

Colm C. Magee, MD
Renal Unit, Beaumont Hospital, Dublin, Ireland
Selection of Patients for Transplantation; Fever in the Transplant Recipient

Daruka Mahadevan, MD, PhD
Associate Professor of Medicine, Department of Medicine, Hematology/Oncology, University of Arizona College of Medicine, Arizona Cancer Center, Tucson, Arizona
Carcinoma of Unknown Primary Site (CUPS)

Lorna A. Marshall, MD
Associate Clinical Professor, Department of Obstetrics and Gynecology, University of Washington; Pacific Northwest Fertility and IVF Specialists, Seattle, Washington
Female Infertility

Kathryn R. Matthias, PharmD
Clinical Assistant Professor, Department of Pharmacy Practice and Science, University of Arizona College of Pharmacy, Tucson, Arizona
Use and Evaluation of Serum Drug Levels; Use and Evaluation of Vancomycin Serum Drug Level

David McDermott, MD
Division of Urologic Surgery, Brigham and Women's Hospital, Boston, Massachusetts
Scrotal Mass

Graham T. McMahon, MD, MMSc
Department of Endocrinology, Brigham and Women's Hospital, Boston, Massachusetts
Hypoglycemia; Hyperglycemia; Hypocalcemia; Hypercalcemia; Hypothyroidism; Hyperthyroidism; Thyroid Nodule; Sick Euthyroid Syndrome; Adrenal Incidentaloma; Cushing's Syndrome; Pituitary Tumor; Hirsutism; Gynecomastia

Lisa M. Mielniczuk, MD
Cardiology Director, Ottawa PH Program, University of Ottawa Heart Institute, Ottawa, Ontario, Canada
Evaluation of a New Diagnosis of Congestive Heart Failure; Diagnosis and Treatment of Acute Pulmonary Edema

Hugh S. Miller, MD
Clinical Associate Professor, Department of Obstetrics and Gynecology, University of Arizona College of Medicine, Tucson, Arizona
Cervicitis; Abnormal Vaginal Bleeding; Abnormal Pap Smear

Tracey A. Milligan, MD
Instructor in Neurology, Harvard Medical School; Associate Neurologist, Brigham and Women's and Faulkner Hospitals; Director of EEG/Epilepsy at Faulkner Hospital, Boston, Massachusetts
Seizures; Status Epilepticus

John Misiaszek, MD
Professor of Clinical Psychiatry, University of Arizona College of Medicine; Medical Director, Psychiatric Outpatient Clinic, University of Arizona Health Sciences Center, Tucson, Arizona
Emotional Disorders with Somatic Expression

Manuel Modiano, MD
Medical Director and Chairman, Arizona Clinical Research Center, Tucson, Arizona
Leukopenia; Deep Venous Thrombosis; Coagulation Abnormalities; Lymphadenopathy; Spinal Cord Compression

Paul A. Monach, MD, PhD
Assistant Professor of Medicine, Section of Rheumatology, Boston University School of Medicine, Boston, Massachusetts
Seronegative Arthritis; Soft-Tissue Pain; Shoulder Pain; Hip Pain; Hand and Wrist Pain; Knee Pain; Foot Pain; Dry Eyes and Dry Mouth (Sjögren's Syndrome); Temporomandibular Pain; Elevated Serum Alkaline Phosphatase Level

Janet Moore, MD
Private Practice, Obstetrics and Gynecology, Scottsdale and Phoenix, Arizona
Vaginal Bleeding in Pregnancy

David A. Morrow, MD, MPH
Division of Cardiovascular Medicine, Brigham and Women's Hospital, Boston, Massachusetts
Stable Angina; Post–Myocardial Infarction Care and Counseling

Myra L. Muramoto, MD
Assistant Professor, Department of Family and Community Medicine, University of Arizona College of Medicine, Tucson, Arizona
Alcoholism

Stuart B. Mushlin, MD, FACP, FACR
Assistant Professor of Medicine, Harvard Medical School; Master Clinician, Brigham and Women's Hospital; Julian Cohen Teaching Scholar, Brigham and Women's Hospital; Director of Primary Care, ad interim, Department of Medicine, Brigham and Women's Hospital, Boston, Massachusetts
Obesity; Joint Hypermobility

Amir Nasseri, MD
Private Practice, Obstetrics and Gynecology, Las Vegas, Nevada
Vaginal Discharge

William H. Nesbitt, MD
HeartPlace, Arlington, Texas
Syncope

MingMing Ning, MD
Instructor in Neurology, Harvard Medical School; Assistant in Neurology, Stroke Service, Massachusetts General Hospital, Boston, Massachusetts
Transient Ischemic Attack and Stroke Evaluation; Stroke Treatment and Prophylaxis

Erika Noss, MD, PhD
Division of Rheumatology, Immunology, and Allergy, Brigham and Women's Hospital, Boston, Massachusetts
Monoarticular Arthritis

Bisola Ojikutu, MD, MPH
Clinical Instructor in Medicine, Harvard Medical School, Infectious Disease Associates, Massachusetts General Hospital, Boston, Massachusetts
Sexually Transmitted Diseases; Approach to the Newly Diagnosed HIV-Positive Patient

Cynthia A. O'Neil, MD
355th Medical Group, Tucson, Arizona
Leg Ulcer

Steven Palley, MD
Private Practice, Gastroenterology and Internal Medicine, Flagstaff, Arizona
Acute Abdominal Pain

Lamioko Shika Pappoe, MD
Department of Medicine-Nephrology and Internal Medicine, Pomona Valley Hospital Medical Center, Pomona, California
Hypophosphatemia

Mahesh J. Patel, MD
Private Practice, Cardiology, Durham, North Carolina
Hypotension

Daniel O. Persky, MD
Assistant Professor of Clinical Medicine, Arizona Cancer Center, University of Arizona, Tucson, Arizona
Classical Hodgkin's Lymphoma

Christopher Pickett, MD
Assistant Professor of Medicine, Co-director, Heart Rhythm Program, Cardiac Electrophysiology Laboratory, University of Connecticut Health Center, Farmington, Connecticut
Wide-Complex Tachycardia; Palpitations

Rebeca M. Plank, MD
Instructor in Medicine, Harvard Medical School; Division of Infectious Diseases, Brigham and Women's Hospital, Boston, Massachusetts
Foreign Travel: Immunizations and Infections; Aseptic Meningitis; Central Nervous System Infection in the Patient with HIV

Ann Partridge, MD, MPH
Assistant Professor of Medicine, Harvard Medical School, Dana Farber Cancer Center, Boston, Massachusetts
Adjuvant Therapy Choices in Breast Cancer

Carol S. Portlock, MD
Professor of Clinical Medicine, New York Weill Cornell University Medical College, Attending Physician, Department of Medicine/Lymphoma Service, Memorial Sloan-Kettering Cancer Center, New York, New York
Classical Hodgkin's Lymphoma

Rebecca L. Potter, MD
Professor of Clinical Psychiatry, University of Arizona College of Medicine, Tucson, Arizona
Suicidal Patient

Caitlin Reed, MD
Research Associate, Johns Hopkins Center for Tuberculosis Research, Johns Hopkins Bloomberg School of Public Health, Baltimore, Maryland
Staphylococcus aureus *Bacteremia, Fever of Unknown Origin*

Eric M. Reiman, MD
Professor of Psychiatry, University of Arizona College of Medicine, Tucson; Scientific Director, Samaritan PET Center, Good Samaritan Regional Medical Center, Phoenix, Arizona
Anxiety

Robert M. Rifkin, MD, FACP
Director of Cellular Therapeutics, Rocky Mountain Cancer Center, Denver, Colorado
Neutrophilia; Chronic Myelogenous Leukemia

Terra A. Robles, PharmD
Director, US Medical, Pfizer Inc., New York, New York
Use of Oral Contraceptives

Theresa Rohr-Kirchgraber, MD
SUNY Upstate Medical University, Syracuse, New York
Tinnitus; Hearing Loss

Jason M. Rominski, PharmD
University of Arizona Health Sciences Center, Tucson, Arizona
Use and Evaluation of Serum Drug Levels; Use and Evaluation of Vancomycin Serum Drug Level

Anastasia Rowland-Seymour, MD
SUNY Upstate Medical University, Syracuse, New York
Rhinitis

Alison C. Roxby, MD, MSc
Infectious Disease Fellow, University of Washington, Seattle, Washington
Acute and Subacute Meningitis; Sepsis

George Ruiz, MD
Medicine/Cardiovascular Disease, Washington Hospital Center, Washington, DC
Right Ventricular Failure

Marc S. Sabatine, MD
Division of Cardiovascular Medicine, Brigham and Women's Hospital, Boston, Massachusetts
Systolic Murmurs; Diastolic Murmurs; Cardiac Dyspnea

Richard E. Sampliner, MD
Southern Arizona VA Health Care System, Tucson, Arizona
Heartburn

Robert N. Samuelson, MD
Private Practice, Obstetrics and Gynecology, Waterbury, Connecticut
Acute Abdominal Pain in Women

Susan Fisk Sander, MD
SUNY Upstate Medical University, Syracuse, New York
Tinnitus; Hearing Loss

Bipin Saud, MD
Assistant Professor of Medicine, SUNY Upstate Medical University, Syracuse, New York
Acute Abdominal Pain; Chronic Abdominal Pain; Nausea and Vomiting; Dyspepsia; Jaundice; Ascites; Rectal Bleeding; Chronic Diarrhea; Asymptomatic Abnormal Liver Aminotransferases

Mark J. Scharf, MD
University of Arizona Health Science Center, Tucson, Arizona
Pigmented Lesions

Gail L. Schwartz, MD
Housestaff Counselor, University of Arizona College of Medicine, Tucson, Arizona
Grief

Benjamin M. Scirica, MD
Brigham/Faulkner Cardiology Associates, Boston, Massachusetts
Unstable Angina/Non-ST-Elevation Myocardial Infarction

Michael E. Scott, MD
Clinical Assistant Professor, Department of Psychiatry, University of Arizona College of Medicine; Medical Director, Clinical Psychiatry, Sierra Tucson Hospital, Tucson, Arizona
Alcoholism

Sunita Sharma, MD
Channing Laboratory, Brigham and Women's Hospital, Boston, Massachusetts
Wheezing

Ajay K. Singh, MBBS, FRCP
Associate Professor of Medicine, Harvard Medical School; Renal Division, Brigham and Women's Hospital, Boston, Massachusetts
Chronic Kidney Disease; Acute Renal Failure; Proteinuria; Hematuria; Kidney Stones; Renal Cysts and Masses; Metabolic Acidosis; Metabolic Alkalosis; Hyponatremia; Hypernatremia; Hypomagnesemia; Hypermagnesemia; Hypophosphatemia

Micheal Singh, MD
Children's Hospital Boston, BACH Group, Boston, Massachusetts
Right Ventricular Failure

Marsha Smith, MD
Atlanta Neurological Associates, PC; Rockdale Medical Center, Conyers, Georgia
Gait Disturbances; Parkinson's Disease

Ana R. Stankovic, MD
Renal Division, Brigham and Women's Hospital, Boston, Massachusetts
Renal Cysts and Masses

Graeme Steele, MD, FCS, FACS
Division of Urologic Surgery, Brigham and Women's Hospital, Boston, Massachusetts
Scrotal Mass; Benign Prostatic Hypertrophy; Prostatitis; Urinary Incontinence; Urinary Retention

Khatuna Stepkovitch, MD
SUNY Upstate Medical University, Syracuse, New York
Geriatric Functional Assessment

Emily Deborah Szmuilowicz, MD
Fellow in Endocrinology, Diabetes and Metabolism, Harvard Medical School, Endocrine Division, Brigham and Women's Hospital, Boston, Massachusetts
Thyroid Pain

Raymond Taetle, MD
Clinical Professor of Medicine and Pathology, University of Arizona College of Medicine, Tucson, Arizona
Anemia

Usha B. Tedrow, MD, MS
Cardiovascular Division, Brigham and Women's Hospital, Boston, Massachusetts
Bradycardia; Sudden Cardiac Death

Sheeba K. Thomas, MD
Assistant Professor, Department of Lymphoma/Myeloma, Division of Cancer Medicine, University of Texas M. D. Anderson Cancer Center, Houston, Texas
Abnormal Serum Protein Electrophoresis

M. Angelo Trujillo, MD
Flagstaff Medical Center, Flagstaff, Arizona
Anorexia; Anorectal Pain; Elevated Serum Amylase

J. Kevin Tucker, MD
Renal Division, Brigham and Women's Hospital, Boston, Massachusetts
Choosing a Chronic Dialysis Modality

Ronan J. Walsh, MD

Instructor in Neurology, Harvard Medical School; Associate Neurologist, Division of Neuromuscular Disease, Department of Neurology, Brigham and Women's Hospital; Boston, Massachusetts

Peripheral Neuropathy; Muscle Cramps and Aches

Michael Wang, MD

Assistant Professor, Department of Lymphoma and Myeloma, University of Texas M. D. Anderson Cancer Center, Houston, Texas

Abnormal Serum Protein Electrophoresis

Donna M. Weber, MD

Associate Professor, Department of Lymphoma/Myeloma, University of Texas M. D. Anderson Cancer Center, Houston, Texas

Abnormal Serum Protein Electrophoresis

Robert W. Weisenthal, MD

Clinical Professor of Ophthalmology, SUNY Upstate Medical University, Syracuse, New York

The Red Eye

Steven B. Williams, MD

Division of Urologic Surgery, Brigham and Women's Hospital, Boston, Massachusetts

Urinary Incontinence

Stephen D. Wiviott, MD

Assistant Professor of Medicine, Cardiovascular Division, Department of Medicine, Harvard Medical School; Investigator, TIMI Study Group, Brigham and Women's Hospital, Boston, Massachusetts

Assessment and Initial Management of ST-Segment Elevation Myocardial Infarction

Cynthia Cooper Worobey, MD

Department of Medicine, Massachusetts General Hospital, Boston, Massachusetts

Proteinuria; Hematuria

Alexi Wright, MD

Hematology/Oncology Fellow, Dana-Farber Cancer Institute /Partners Cancer Care, Boston, Massachusetts

Adjuvant Therapy Choices in Breast Cancer

David Yeo, MD

Division of Urologic Surgery, Brigham and Women's Hospital, Boston, Massachusetts

Benign Prostatic Hypertrophy; Prostatitis

Maria A. Yialamas, MD

Instructor in Medicine, Harvard Medical School; Associate Program Director, Internal Medicine Residency, Brigham and Women's Hospital, Boston, Massachusetts

Osteoporosis and Osteopenia

Kambiz Zandi-Nejad, MD

Renal Division, Brigham and Women's Hospital, Boston, Massachusetts

Hypokalemia; Hyperkalemia

Richard D. Zane, MD, FAAEM

Assistant Professor of Medicine, Harvard Medical School; Vice Chair, Department of Emergency Medicine, Brigham and Women's Hospital, Boston, Massachusetts

Acute Pulseless Extremity; Foreign Body Ingestion; Caustic Ingestion and Exposure; Mammal Bites; Snake Venom Poisoning; Hypothermia; Submersion

Paul C. Zei, MD, PhD

Instructor in Medicine, Cardiac Electrophysiology, Stanford University School of Medicine, Stanford, California

Narrow-Complex Tachycardia

Peter Zimetbaum, MD

Clinical Director of Cardiovascular Division, Director of the Cardiac Intensive Care Unit, Beth Israel Deaconess Medical Center, Boston, Massachusetts

Wide-Complex Tachycardia; Palpitations

PREFACE

Decision Making in Medicine is a book for the practitioner, resident physician, medical student, nurse practitioner, and physician assistant seeking guidelines for diagnosis. Where available it uses evidence-based medicine tempered by the experience of expert clinicians. This edition has been expanded based on feedback from readers of the two earlier editions and on progress in the diagnostic armamentarium.

The topics are brief and are organized by sign, symptom, problem, or abnormal laboratory finding. For the majority of topics, the left-hand page carries the explanatory material to describe the algorithm that appears on the right-hand page. Following this decision-tree approach one arrives at the appropriate diagnosis, family of diagnoses, or appropriate therapy for the problem under concern.

This book assumes orderliness to diagnosis in medicine. The approach offers a template that can minimize unnecessary testing, control medical costs, and provide uniform quality care in the patient's evaluation.

Medicine cannot be taught by "cookbooks." Much of the art of medicine comes from the interplay between physician style and patient preferences. The dialogue between them is occurring in an environment increasingly controlled by outside forces. The approaches presented here reflect the expertise and preferences of the individual authors, but there is still latitude for the reader's art of medicine.

Since I (SBM) returned to the full-time academic environment from many years as a community practitioner, I have wanted to write a textbook of medicine. When my friend, colleague, and teacher, Harry Greene II, MD, invited me to participate in the third edition of *Decision Making in Medicine,* I was very enthused. Our collaboration has been stimulating and free of stress. It has been fun every step of the way.

We would like to thank the section editors and contributing authors who have successfully put their daily practice and evidence-based best practices into a systematic form, providing a solid path to follow. We would like to acknowledge Mike Maricic, William P. Johnson, and Dawn Lemcke, who served as senior editors for the earlier editions. Their hard work helped set a high standard for those to follow.

We would also like to thank our colleagues at Elsevier: Druanne Martin, Acquisitions Editor; Agnes Byrne, Developmental Editor; and Mary Stermel, Project Manager, for their support, encouragement, and publishing expertise.

Marshall Wolf, my practice partner and teacher, deserves special thanks, as he always saw more in me than I did. Joseph Loscalzo, Chairman of the Department of Medicine, has created an environment that fosters clinical medicine as well as bench research. I (SBM) am very grateful to you both. The medical house staff of the Brigham and Women's Hospital teach me, inspire me, and challenge me on a daily basis. It is a privilege to work with them so closely.

Special thanks go to Rachel Willis, administrative assistant to Dr. Mushlin, and Carla Perez, editorial assistant to Dr. Greene.

Stuart B. Mushlin
Harry L. Greene II

CONTENTS

NEPHROLOGY

NEUROLOGY

Urology

Women's Health

Emergency Medicine

Behavioral Medicine

Pharmacology

General Medicine

Lisa Kaufmann, MD
Section Editor

PREVENTION AND SCREENING

Megan Tamburini Khosla, MD

A. *Screening* is defined as the examination of a group of asymptomatic individuals to detect those with a given disease or risk factor. This is typically done by the means of an inexpensive diagnostic service. The service can take many forms, including history taking, physical examination, laboratory testing, and other procedures. The discussion that follows applies to a patient at average risk. Different sets of recommendations apply to those who are at higher-than-average risk for a selected disease or risk factor.

B. The United States Preventive Services Task Force (USPSTF) has created a grading system for its recommendations. The grading system is based on the strength of the supporting evidence and the size of the net benefit (benefits minus harms).
   - **Grade A.** The USPSTF strongly recommends that clinicians provide [the service] to eligible patients. The UPSTF found good evidence that [the service] improves important health outcomes and concludes that benefits substantially outweigh harms.
   - **Grade B.** The USPSTF recommends that clinicians provide [the service] to eligible patients. The UPSTF found at least fair evidence that [the service] improves important health outcomes and concludes that benefits outweigh harms.
   - **Grade C.** The USPSTF makes no recommendations for or against routine provision of [the service]. The UPSTF found at least fair evidence that [the service] can improve health outcomes but concludes that the balance of benefits and harms is too close to justify a general recommendation.
   - **Grade D.** The USPSTF recommends against routinely providing [the service] to asymptomatic patients. The UPSTF found at least fair evidence that [the service] is ineffective or that harm outweighs benefits.
   - **Grade I.** The USPSTF concludes that the evidence is insufficient to recommend for or against routinely providing [the service]. Evidence that [the service] is effective is lacking, of poor quality, or conflicting, and the balance of benefits and harms cannot be determined.

   The Canadian Task Force for Preventive Health Care (CTFPHC) has also created a grading system for its recommendations. Grades A and B are similar to the USPSTF grading system. Grade C states that there is insufficient evidence regarding inclusion or exclusion of the condition or maneuver in a periodic health examination, but recommendations may be made on other grounds. Grade D states that there is fair evidence to support the recommendation that the condition or maneuver be specifically excluded from a periodic health examination. Grade E states that there is good evidence to support the recommendation that the condition or maneuver be specifically excluded from a periodic health examination.

   The remainder of this discussion will focus on the details of the recommended preventive services (i.e., those that have been given Grade A or B recommendations by the UPSTF) along with the more controversial prostate cancer screening service.

C. *Alcohol misuse screening:* The USPSTF and the CTFPHC both recommend screening and behavioral counseling interventions to reduce alcohol misuse by adults in the primary care setting (Grade B). The term *alcohol misuse* refers to "risky/hazardous" and "harmful" drinking. "Risky" or "hazardous" drinking has been defined in the United States, for women, as >7 drinks per week or >3 drinks per occasion and, for men, as >14 drinks per week or >4 drinks per occasion. "Harmful" drinking is used to describe persons who are currently experiencing physical, social, or psychological harm from alcohol use but who do not meet dependence criteria. Screening and interventions for alcohol dependence were not evaluated by the USPSTF because these benefits have already been well established. The Alcohol Use Disorders Identification Test (AUDIT) is the most studied screening tool for detecting alcohol-related problems in primary care settings. The CAGE questionnaire is the most popular screening test used to detect alcohol abuse or dependence in the primary care setting. The optimal interval for screening and intervention is uncertain, but should probably be based at least in part on previous responses.

   Breast cancer screening: The USPSTF recommends screening mammography, with or without clinical breast examination, every 1–2 years for women aged ≥40 (Grade B). Controversy exists over the appropriate interval for screening, especially in women in the 40- to 49-year age group. The American College of Obstetricians and Gynecologists (ACOG) recommends screening every 1–2 years in this age group and annually in women aged ≥50. The American Cancer Society (ACS) recommends annual mammography in women >40 years of age. The Canadian guidelines state that there is good evidence for screening women aged 50–69 years by clinical examination and mammography (Grade A) and that the best available data support screening every 1–2 years. They also state that current evidence does not support the recommendation that screening mammography be included in or excluded from the periodic health examination or women aged 40–49 years at average risk of breast cancer (Grade C). The precise age to discontinue screening is not known, mostly because controlled trials have not enrolled older females and, consequently, there are no data available. Most organizations agree that older women are as likely to benefit from screening as younger women, provided that they have no comorbid conditions that limit their life expectancy. The USPSTF concludes that the evidence is insufficient to recommend for or against teaching or performing routine breast self-examination (BSE or CBE) (Grade I). The ACS recommends CBE at least every 3 years in young women and annually in women >40 years. They also suggest that from the 20s, women should be offered instruction in BSE but that it is acceptable for patients to choose not to perform them.

Cervical cancer screening: The USPSTF strongly recommends screening women for cervical cancer if they have a cervix and have been sexually active (Grade A). The optimal age to begin screening is unknown, but the ACS guidelines suggest that age 21 years or 3 years after the onset of sexual activity may be appropriate. Most U.S. organizations agree that cervical cancer screening can be discontinued safely in the elderly population; however, the appropriate age is again uncertain. The USPSTF recommends against screening women >65 years of age if they have had adequate recent screening with normal results and are not otherwise at high risk (Grade D). The ACS suggests that it may be appropriate to stop at age 70 years, but they suggest that women should have at least 3 consecutive, documented normal results and no abnormal test results within the past 10 years. The USPSTF also found no direct evidence to support that annual screening leads to better outcomes than does screening every 3 years. However, most organizations recommend that annual screening be continued until a certain number (usually 2–3) test results are normal before the interval is lengthened. Additionally, the ACS recommends waiting until at least age 30 before increasing the interval. Most organizations agree that it is safe to discontinue screening after hysterectomy for benign disease. At this point, the USPSTF concludes that there is insufficient evidence to recommend for or against the routine use of human papillomavirus testing as a method for cervical cancer screening (Grade I). The CTFPHC agrees that there is fair evidence to include Pap smears in the periodic health examination of sexually active women (Grade B).

Colorectal cancer screening: The USPSTF strongly recommends that clinicians screen men and women ≥50 years for colorectal cancer (Grade A), although they do not specify the acceptable methods. The ACS suggests that the following are acceptable potential screening options: (1) annual home fecal occult blood testing (FOBT), three specimens; (2) flexible sigmoidoscopy every 5 years; (3) annual FOBT plus flexible sigmoidoscopy every 5 years; (4) double contrast barium enema every 5 years; and (5) colonoscopy every 10 years. It should be mentioned that a stool sample collected in the office by digital rectal examination is not an acceptable substitute for home FOBT. In addition, the combination of FOBT and flexible sigmoidoscopy is preferable to either of these tests alone. The age of discontinuation is again not clear, but most organizations agree that it should be decided based on comorbid conditions that limit life expectancy. The Canadian guidelines recommend including annual or biennial FOBT (Grade A) and flexible sigmoidoscopy (Grade B) in the periodic health examination of patients >50 years. They do report that there is insufficient evidence to make recommendations about the combination of these screening tests or about the use of colonoscopy (Grade C).

Chlamydial and gonorrhea infection screening: The USPSTF strongly recommends that clinicians routinely screen all sexually active women ≤25 years for chlamydial infection (Grade A) and gonorrheal infection (Grade B). This assumes that women in this age group are at higher risk because of their young age. They also state that there is insufficient evidence to recommend for or against routinely screening asymptomatic men for chlamydial or gonorrheal infection even if they are at increased risk (Grade I). They make no recommendations for or against screening for chlamydia in women who are at low risk for infection (Grade C), and they recommend against routine screening for gonorrheal infections in men or women who are at low risk for infection (Grade D). Screening intervals should depend on previous results and changes in sexual behaviors. The Canadian guidelines state that there is fair evidence to support annual screening of this group (Grade B) and fair evidence to exclude routine screening of the general population (Grade D).

Depression screening: The USPSTF and the CTFPHC both recommend screening adults for depression in clinical practices that have systems in place to ensure accurate diagnosis, effective treatment, and follow-up (Grade B). Several formal screening tools are available, including the Zung Self-Assessment Depression Scale, the Beck Depression Inventory, the General Health Questionnaire, and the Center for Epidemiologic Study Depression Scale. There is little evidence to recommend one screening tool over another, so practitioners should choose the one that fits best with their personal preference, the patient population they serve, and their practice setting. Again, the ideal interval for screening is not known but should probably be based at least in part on previous responses.

High blood pressure screening: The USPSTF strongly recommends that clinicians screen adults ≥18 years for high blood pressure (Grade A). The CTFPHC also concludes that there is fair evidence to include measurement of blood pressure in periodic health examinations (Grade B). Evidence is lacking for the appropriate interval for screening but the seventh report of the Joint National Committee on Prevention, Detection, Evaluation, and Treatment of High Blood Pressure (JNC 7) suggests that every 2 years for those with systolic blood pressure <130 mm Hg and diastolic blood pressure <85 mm Hg may be appropriate.

Lipid disorder screening: The USPSTF strongly recommends that clinicians routinely screen men ≥35 years and women ≥45 years for lipid disorders and treat abnormal lipids in people who are at increased risk for coronary heart disease (Grade A). It makes no recommendation for or against routine screening in younger adults (men aged 20–35 years or women aged 20–45 years) in the absence of known risk factors for coronary heart disease (Grade C). It recommends that screening for lipid disorders include measurement of total cholesterol and high-density lipoprotein (Grade B) but concludes that there is insufficient evidence to recommend for or against the inclusion of triglyceride measurement for routine screening(Grade I). The optimal interval for screening is unknown, but on the basis of expert opinion and other guidelines, every 5 years is believed to be a reasonable option. The ATP III (Adult Treatment Panel), the expert panel created by the National Cholesterol Education Program (NCEP), suggests that all adults ≥20 years have a fasting lipid panel once every 5 years. However, the CTFPHC reports that there is insufficient evidence that the measurement of blood total cholesterol should be included in or excluded from the periodic health examination (Grade C). They do, however, suggest that although it has not evaluated for its effectiveness, screening should be considered in all men aged 30–59 years and that individual clinical judgment should be exercised in all other cases.

Immunizations: The Centers for Disease Control and Prevention (CDC) recommends annual influenza vaccine for all persons ≥50 years and persons in selected high-risk groups. Pneumococcal vaccine is recommended for all immunocompetent individuals who are ≥65 years or otherwise at increased risk for pneumococcal disease. A revaccination with MMR (measles, mumps, rubella) is also recommended for those students entering a postsecondary educational institution. Additionally, a one-dose booster of the tetanus vaccination is recommended for adults every 10 years.

Obesity screening: The USPSTF recommends that clinicians screen all adult patients for obesity and offer intensive counseling and behavioral interventions to promote sustained weight loss for adults who are obese (Grade B). They state that there is insufficient evidence to recommend for or against behavioral counseling to promote a healthy diet or physical activity in unselected patients in the primary care setting (Grade I). Clinicians may use waist circumference or body mass index (BMI) as measure of obesity. The CTFPHC states that there is fair evidence to support providing general dietary advice and recommending that individuals engage in the regular practice of moderate-intensity physical activity (Grade B). However, it also states that because of the lack of evidence supporting long-term effectiveness of weight-reduction interventions, there is insufficient evidence to recommend for or against BMI measurement as part of the periodic health examination (Grade C).

Osteoporosis screening: The USPSTF recommends that women ≥65 years be screened routinely for osteoporosis and that routine screening begin at age 60 years in women who are at increased risk for osteoporotic fractures (Grade B). They make no recommendations for or against osteoporosis screening in postmenopausal women who are <60 years or in women aged 60–64 years who are not at increased risk for osteoporotic fractures (Grade C). The ACOG recommends that clinicians offer bone mineral density (BMD) testing to women ≥65 years and younger postmenopausal women with one or more risk factors (except being white, postmenopausal, and female). Lower body weight (<70 kg) is the single best predictor of low bone mineral density. Additional risk factors that are commonly considered (although with less supporting evidence) include smoking, weight loss, family history, decreased physical activity, alcohol or caffeine use, and low calcium and vitamin D intake. Bone density measured at the femoral neck by dual-energy x-ray absorptiometry (DEXA) is the best predictor of hip fracture and is comparable to forearm measurements for predicting fractures at other sites. No studies have evaluated the optimal interval to repeat screening. Two years is often thought of as the minimum appropriate interval based on the limitations in the precision of testing and the fact that at least that long is needed to reliably measure a change in BMD. There are no data regarding the appropriate age to stop screening. The CTFPHC agrees that there is fair evidence supporting screening postmenopausal women with a history of previous fracture, those who are ≥65 years, and women who have risk factors (as measured by high scores on the Osteoporosis Risk Assessment Instrument [ORAI]) to prevent fragility fractures (Grade B). The ORAI incorporates low weight, no current use of estrogen, and age into a three-item score. The CTFPHC found that there is good evidence to recommend using the ORAI to predict low BMD (Grade A) and fair evidence to recommend using BMD testing to predict fractures (Grade B).

Tobacco use screening: The USPSTF and CTFPHC both strongly recommend that clinicians screen all adults for tobacco use and provide tobacco cessation interventions for those who use tobacco products (Grade A).

Prostate cancer screening: The USPSTF concludes that the evidence is insufficient to recommend for or against routine screening for prostate cancer using prostate-specific antigen (PSA) testing or digital rectal

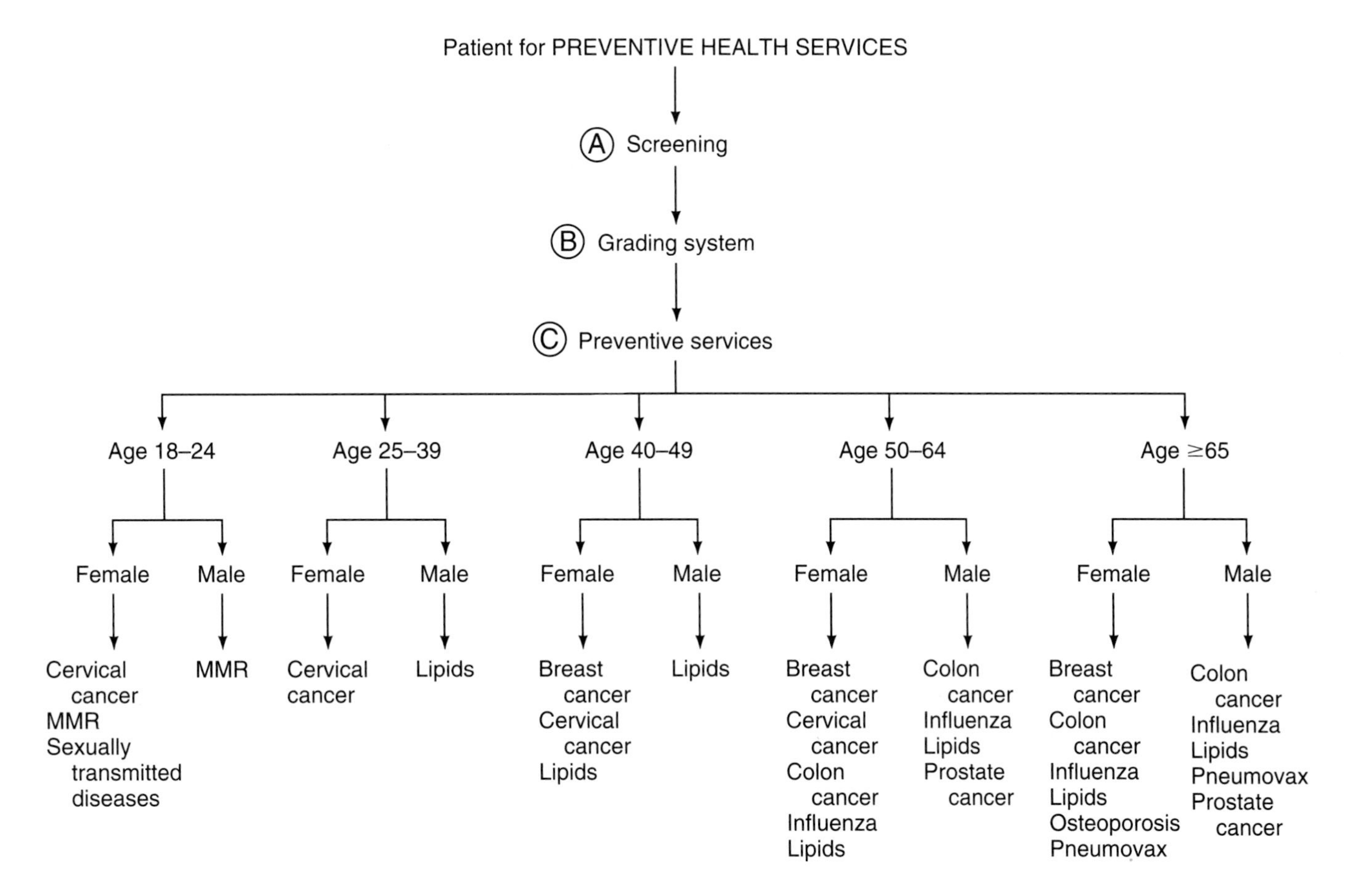

examination (DRE) (Grade I). There is good evidence that PSA can detect early prostate cancer but inconclusive evidence that the currently available treatments decrease morbidity and mortality from early prostate cancer. PSA screening is more sensitive than DRE for the detection of early prostate cancer. Clinicians are advised that they should not order a PSA without first discussing with the patient the potential but uncertain benefits and the possible harms. If it is true that early detection improves health outcomes, then those most likely to benefit are men aged 50–70 who are at average risk. The CTFPHC found poor evidence to include or exclude DRE (Grade C) and fair evidence to exclude PSA screening (Grade D) from the periodic health examination of asymptomatic men >50 years of age. They state that this recommendation is made based on the poor positive predictive value and the known risk of adverse effects associated with therapies of unproved effectiveness.

For access to the most recent recommendations from various organizations, please go to www.guidelines.gov. This is the website for the National Guideline Clearinghouse (NGC), a public resource for evidence-based clinical practice guidelines. NGC is an initiative of the Agency for Healthcare Research and Quality (AHRQ) of the U.S. Department of Health and Human Services.

References

Advisory Committee on Immunization Practice, American Academy of Family Physicians. General recommendations on immunization. MMWR Recomm Rep 2002;51(RR-2):1–36.

American College of Obstetricians and Gynecologists (ACOG). Breast cancer screening. Washington, DC: ACOG 2003 (ACOG practice bulletin; no. 42).

Canadian Task Force on Preventive Health Care. www.ctfphc.org

Guide to Clinical Preventive Services, 2005. AHRQ Publication No. 05-0570, June 2005. Agency for Healthcare Research and Quality, Rockville, MD. http://www.ahrq.gov/clinic/pocketgd.htm.

Harper SA, Fukuda K, Uyeki TM, et al. Prevention and control of influenza. Recommendations of the Advisory Committee on Immunization Practices (ACIP). MMWR Recomm Rep 2005;54(RR-8):1–40.

National Osteoporosis Foundation. Physician's guide to prevention and treatment of osteoporosis. Washington, DC: National Osteoporosis Foundation, 2003.

Smith RA, Cokkinides V, Eyre HJ. American Cancer Society guidelines for the early detection of cancer, 2003. CA Cancer J Clin 2003;53(1):27–43.

Smith RA, Saslow D, Sawyer LA, et al. American Cancer Society guidelines for breast cancer screening: update 2003. CA Cancer J Clin 2003;53(3):141–169.

FATIGUE

Lisa Kaufmann, MD

Acute (<6 months' duration) and chronic (>6 months' duration) fatigue are associated with many diseases, but most patients have signs and symptoms of the primary disease process. In a large urban internal medicine practice, 25% of patients admitted to at least 1 month of fatigue that interfered with their daily activities and 11%–12% of patients in two other series had chronic fatigue. Fatigue is the chief complaint in 1%–7% of office visits by adults. Acute fatigue is more likely than chronic fatigue to be associated with a clear-cut cause or to resolve spontaneously.

A. Although 75% of patients with a chief complaint of chronic fatigue have a psychiatric diagnosis and 20% have no definable diagnosis, about 7% have significant physical disease (4% have both medical and psychiatric disease, and 3% have only a medical diagnosis). Because fatigue is so nonspecific, a careful history and physical are essential and should include a description of the fatigue (e.g., is it exhaustion, breathlessness, lack of interest?), precipitating and palliative factors (is it related to work, less on vacations or weekends, affected by bed rest, onset, relationship to activities?), and any associated physical or psychological symptoms.

B. Physiologic fatigue results from a situation that would cause most people to become fatigued. It is common in sleep-deprived new parents, working mothers of toddlers, and workers doing rotating shifts or overtime, but it also can result from overtraining in athletes, malnutrition, and exposure to high noise levels. Rest, improved scheduling, and/or ear protection usually resolve the fatigue. Boring, low-paying jobs are more likely to be experienced as fatiguing than are more stimulating jobs, especially if they involve low levels of physical activity (perhaps they fall below the level needed to maintain arousal).

C. Consider drugs or toxins (alcohol, illicit drugs, sedating medications such as antihistamines, beta blockers, or nonsteroidals, including over-the-counter and herbal medications, and occupational toxin exposures). Neurologic disease (e.g., multiple sclerosis, Parkinson's disease, postpolio, seizures), and medical disease can cause fatigue. Adrenal insufficiency may present as fatigue but usually is associated with orthostatic hypotension. Hypothyroidism, hypopituitarism, asthma, sarcoidosis, anemia, lupus, hepatitis, chronic infections, and malignancy have all been identified in case series. Many illnesses produce severe fatigue, but usually other symptoms are more prominent (e.g., heart failure, tuberculosis).

D. Unless another cause of the fatigue is obvious on initial evaluation, carefully question all patients with fatigue for risk factors for HIV, syphilis, and hepatitis B and C, all of which can present as isolated fatigue.

E. Lyme disease occurs in temperate wooded climates. Coccidioidomycosis is caused by a fungus endemic in the desert southwest and can be acquired with brief exposure, such as driving through the area. Both illnesses may present as isolated fatigue.

F. Fibromyalgia affects about 3% of adult women in the general population and is characterized by aching muscles both above and below the waist, multiple tender points, and the absence of other disease to explain the symptoms. Although the American Rheumatologic Association criteria require 11 tender points of 18 tested, population studies show a spectrum of symptoms with aching muscles and increasing numbers of tender points being correlated with sleep disturbance, fatigue, and depression. Up to 70% of patients who meet criteria for chronic fatigue syndrome (Figure 1) also meet criteria for fibromyalgia. Because other rheumatologic conditions may cause similar symptoms, add a careful joint and skin examination as well as screening rheumatologic laboratory testing (creatine phosphokinase [CPK], C-reactive protein [CRP], ANA, and rheumatoid factor [RF]) to the usual laboratory evaluation of fatigue when fibromyalgia is suspected.

G. Because most patients with a presenting symptom of fatigue have a psychiatric diagnosis, perform a careful psychosocial assessment (Table 1). Because few of these patients think that their symptoms are psychiatric

Table 1 **Areas of Psychosocial Assessment for Symptoms of Fatigue**

Historical data	Current functioning
Work history	Current work experience
Past or current substance abuse	Quality of relationships or support networks
Addictive behavior patterns	Sexual activity and function
Depression, anxiety, or other psychiatric diagnosis	Appetite and diet
	Life goals
Abuse (physical, sexual, emotional)	Self-esteem
Family history of chronic health problems	Exercise or recreational activities
	Coping skills
Significant life changes or losses	Relaxation techniques

From Ruffin MT, Cohen M. Evaluation and management of fatigue. Am Fam Physician 1994;50:625, as adapted from Holmes GP. Defining the chronic fatigue syndrome. Rev Infect Dis 1991;13(Suppl 1):S53.

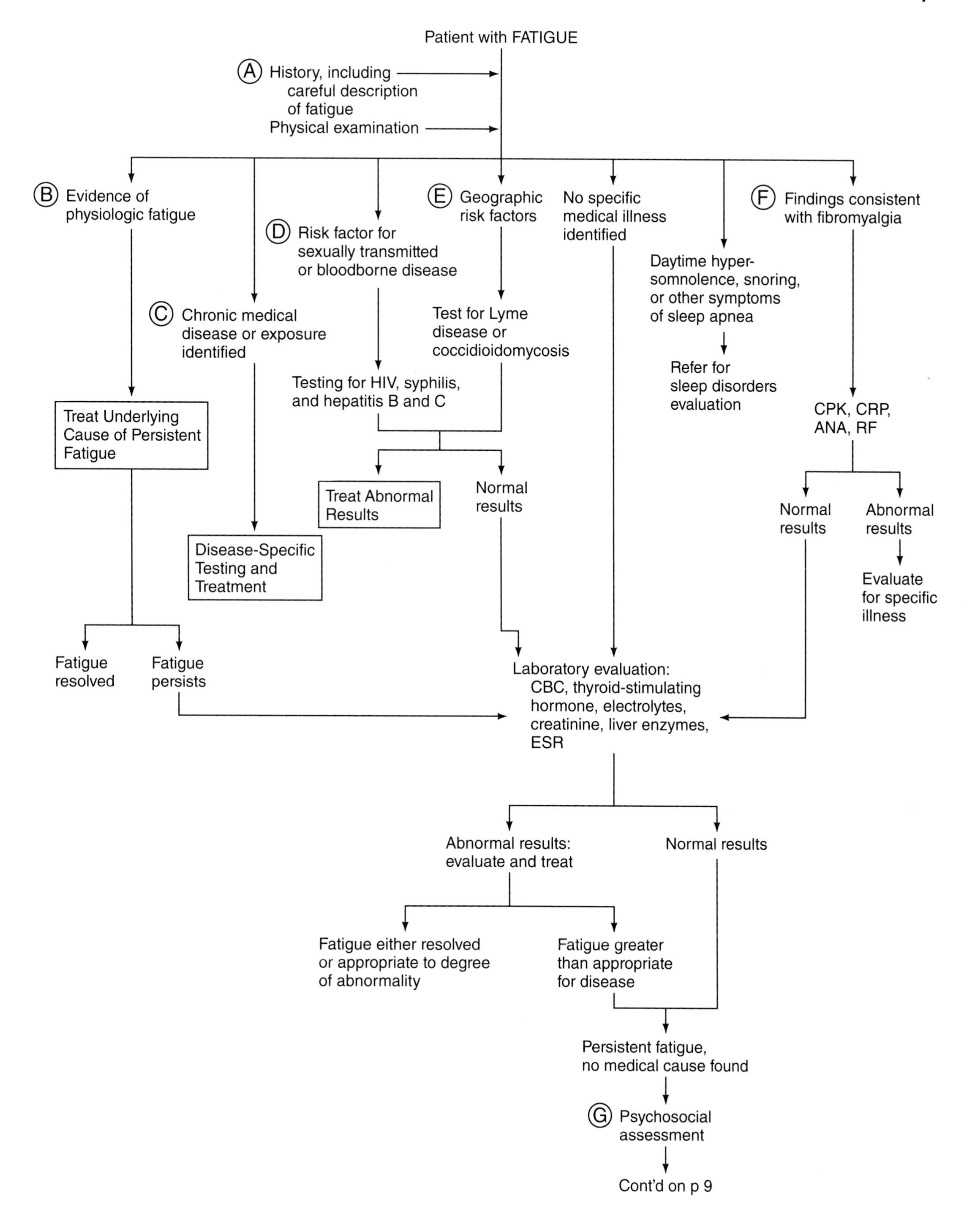
Patient with FATIGUE
Ⓐ History, including careful description of fatigue
Physical examination
Ⓑ Evidence of physiologic fatigue
Treat Underlying Cause of Persistent Fatigue
Fatigue resolved
Fatigue persists
Ⓒ Chronic medical disease or exposure identified
Disease-Specific Testing and Treatment
Ⓓ Risk factor for sexually transmitted or bloodborne disease
Testing for HIV, syphilis, and hepatitis B and C
Ⓔ Geographic risk factors
Test for Lyme disease or coccidioidomycosis
Treat Abnormal Results
Normal results
No specific medical illness identified
Daytime hypersomnolence, snoring, or other symptoms of sleep apnea
Refer for sleep disorders evaluation
Ⓕ Findings consistent with fibromyalgia
CPK, CRP, ANA, RF
Normal results
Abnormal results
Evaluate for specific illness
Laboratory evaluation: CBC, thyroid-stimulating hormone, electrolytes, creatinine, liver enzymes, ESR
Abnormal results: evaluate and treat
Normal results
Fatigue either resolved or appropriate to degree of abnormality
Fatigue greater than appropriate for disease
Persistent fatigue, no medical cause found
Ⓖ Psychosocial assessment
Cont'd on p 9

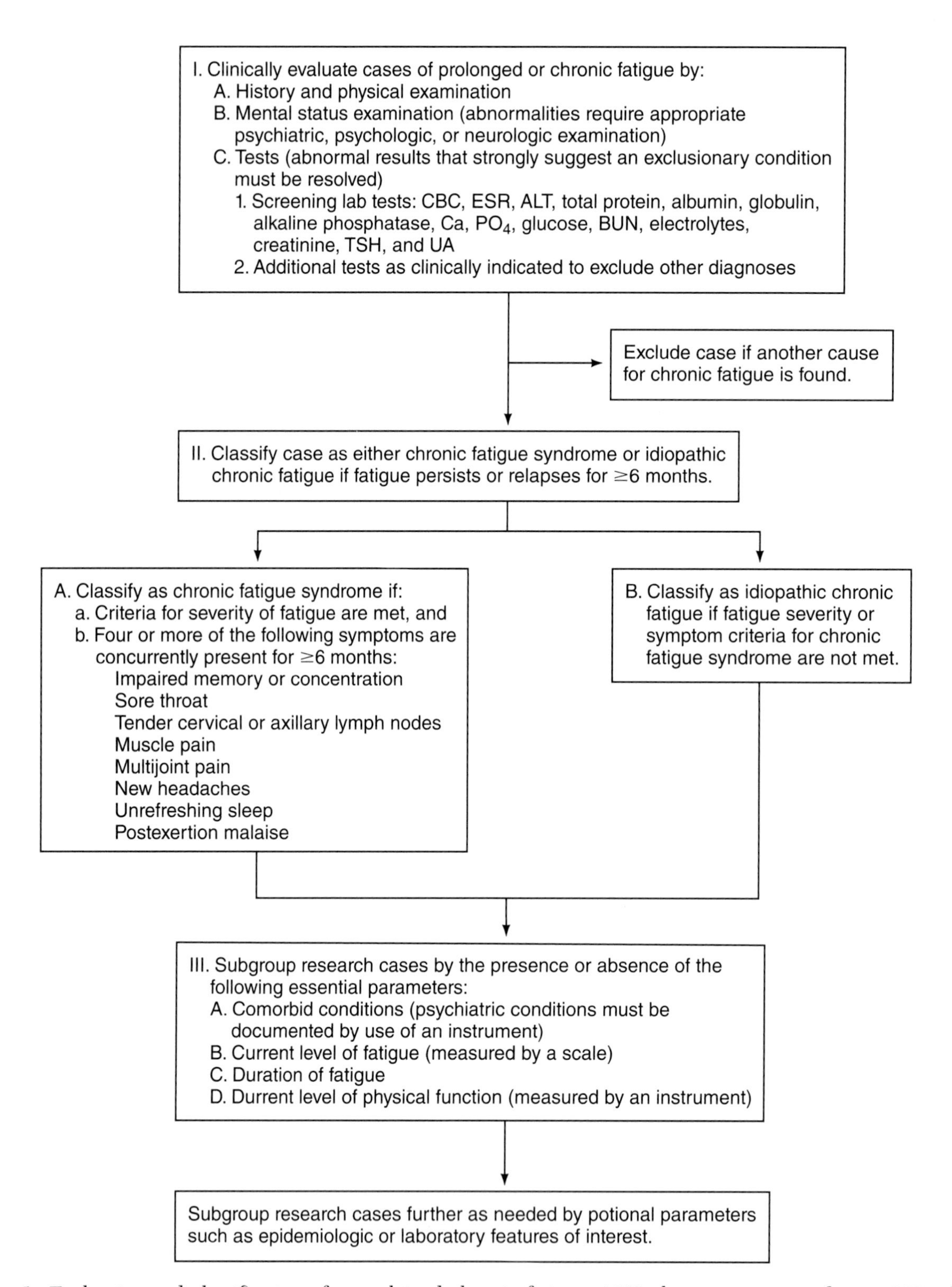

Figure 1. Evaluation and classification of unexplained chronic fatigue. ALT, alanine aminotransferase; BUN, blood urea nitrogen; CBC, complete blood count; ESR, erythrocyte sedimentation rate; PO4, phosphorus; TSH, thyroid-stimulating hormone; UA, urinalysis. (From Fukuda K, Strauss SE, Hickie I, et al: The chronic fatigue syndrome: a comprehensive approach to its definition and study. International Chronic Fatigue Syndrome Study Group. Ann Intern Med 1994;121:953–959.

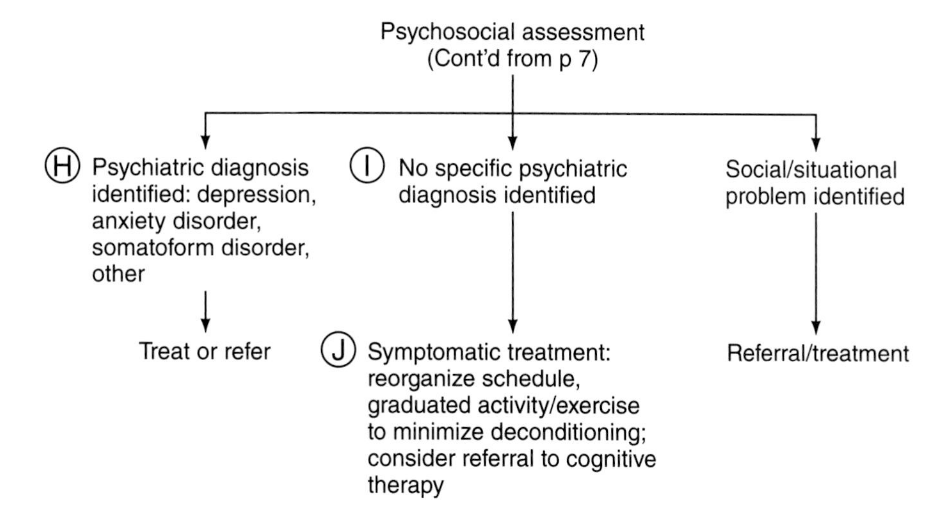

in origin, it is helpful to the maintenance of a strong therapeutic relationship for the primary physician to do the assessment if possible.

H. The most common cause of chronic fatigue is major depression, followed by anxiety disorders and somatoform disorders. Treatment of these conditions is described elsewhere in this book. Many patients in this group with fatigue rather than complaints of depressed or anxious mood prefer to conceptualize their illness as physical and may be more willing to take appropriate medications if possible improvements of the physical symptoms such as insomnia and fatigue are emphasized. Sometimes presenting a psychiatric referral as helping with coping with an overall difficult life situation may make it more acceptable.

I. Patients who are chronically fatigued for >6 months with no specific cause identified may meet criteria for the chronic fatigue syndrome (see Figure 1). These criteria are useful for research purposes, but because there is no specific cause or treatment associated with the criteria, these patients should be treated like any other patients with chronic fatigue of unknown cause.

J. About 20% of patients with chronic fatigue have no identifiable medical or psychiatric cause, a situation frustrating to both the patient and the physician. Encourage patients to remain as active as possible because excessive rest results in deconditioning, which exacerbates the fatigue. This can be accomplished by scheduling important activities when fatigue is least severe (a symptom diary is helpful) and encouraging regular mild exercise (graded by the patient to avoid severe exhaustion). For patients with fibromyalgia, stretching and swimming are useful. Chronic fatigue and the inability to perform activities previously taken for granted cause major social stress and grief. Brief cognitive therapy geared toward refocusing goals and expectations has proved useful. Patient support groups are less helpful. These modalities also can help patients with chronic fatigue of a known cause.

References

Bates DW, Schmitt W, Buchwald D, et al. Prevalence of fatigue and chronic fatigue syndrome in a primary care practice. Arch Intern Med 1993;153:2759.

Manu P, Lane TJ, Matthews DA. Chronic fatigue and chronic fatigue syndrome: clinical epidemiology and aetiological classification. CIBA Foundation Symposium 1993;173:23.

Patel V, Kirkwood BR, Weiss H, et al. Chronic fatigue in developing countries: populations-based survey of women in India. BMJ 2005;330:1990.

Ruffin MT, Cohen M. Evaluation and management of fatigue. Am Fam Physician 1994;50:625.

Wessely S, Chalder T, Hirsh S, et al. The prevalence and morbidity of chronic fatigue and chronic fatigue syndrome: a prospective primary care study. Am J Public Health 1997;87:1449.

Whiting P, Bagnall AM, Sowden A, et al. Interventions for the treatment and management of chronic fatigue syndrome: a systematic review. JAMA 2001;286:1360.

INVOLUNTARY WEIGHT LOSS

Lynn Cleary, MD

Involuntary weight loss (IWL) is defined as >5% loss of usual body weight within 6 months. It is significantly associated with older age; poorer health status; smoking; lower body mass index; and, in men, widowhood and less education. It is also associated with higher mortality rates in patients with and without established disease and merits diagnostic and therapeutic intervention.

Clinical studies looking at underlying causes have studied small numbers of patients with wide variability in their demographic characteristics (e.g., age, inpatients vs. outpatients, long-term care residents, veterans). Generalization in the diagnostic approach to IWL is therefore limited in its applicability to different populations.

Diagnostic causes are found in 65%–90% of cases. Inpatients on medical service have a high proportion of physical causes, whereas ambulatory patients are found to have psychiatric disease almost as often as physical causes. Geriatrics studies have shown a high prevalence of both. In 10%–35% of cases, no cause can be found.

A. It is important to document the complaint of weight loss or to look for indirect evidence of weight loss if documentation is unavailable. Many patients complaining of weight loss do not in fact have any documented loss.

B. Common underlying causes include neoplasm, primary gastroenterologic disease, chronic underlying illness (cardiovascular, metabolic, pulmonary), poor nutrition, hyperthyroidism, dementia, depression, and anxiety. Weight loss may precede the diagnosis of dementia. The prevalence of each diagnosis greatly depends on the group being studied.

C. Review risks, symptoms, and examination results for evidence of cancer, diabetes, heart/lung disease, oral/dental disease, GI pathology, hyperthyroidism, infection (including AIDS), alcoholism or other substance abuse, dementia, and psychiatric illness.

D. Physical causes often are apparent early in the investigation. This may not be as applicable to the elderly, in whom disease often presents in nonspecific ways and IWL is more prevalent. Although there are no data to support more aggressive testing in the elderly, it may be reasonable to focus more attention on the oral/dental, gastroenterologic, cognitive, and psychosocial contributions to IWL if the initial evaluation is unrevealing.

E. Whether or not a diagnostic cause is confirmed, the patient with IWL should be followed closely because there is an association with higher mortality and lower health status regardless of specific cause.

References

Alibhai SM, Greenwood C, Payette H. An approach to the management of unintentional weight loss in elderly people. CMAJ 2005;172(6):773–780.

Meltzer AA, Everhart JE. Unintentional weight loss in the United States. Am J Epidemiol 1995;142:10.

Sahyoun NR, Serdula MK, Galuska DA, et al. The epidemiology of recent involuntary weight loss in the United States population. J Nutr Health Aging 2004;8(6):510–517.

Wise GR, Craig D. Evaluation of involuntary weight loss. Where do you start? Postgrad Med 1994;95:4.

Yaari S, Goldbourt U. Voluntary and involuntary weight loss: associations with long term mortality in 9,228 middle-aged and elderly men. Am J Epidemiol 1998;148(6):546–555.

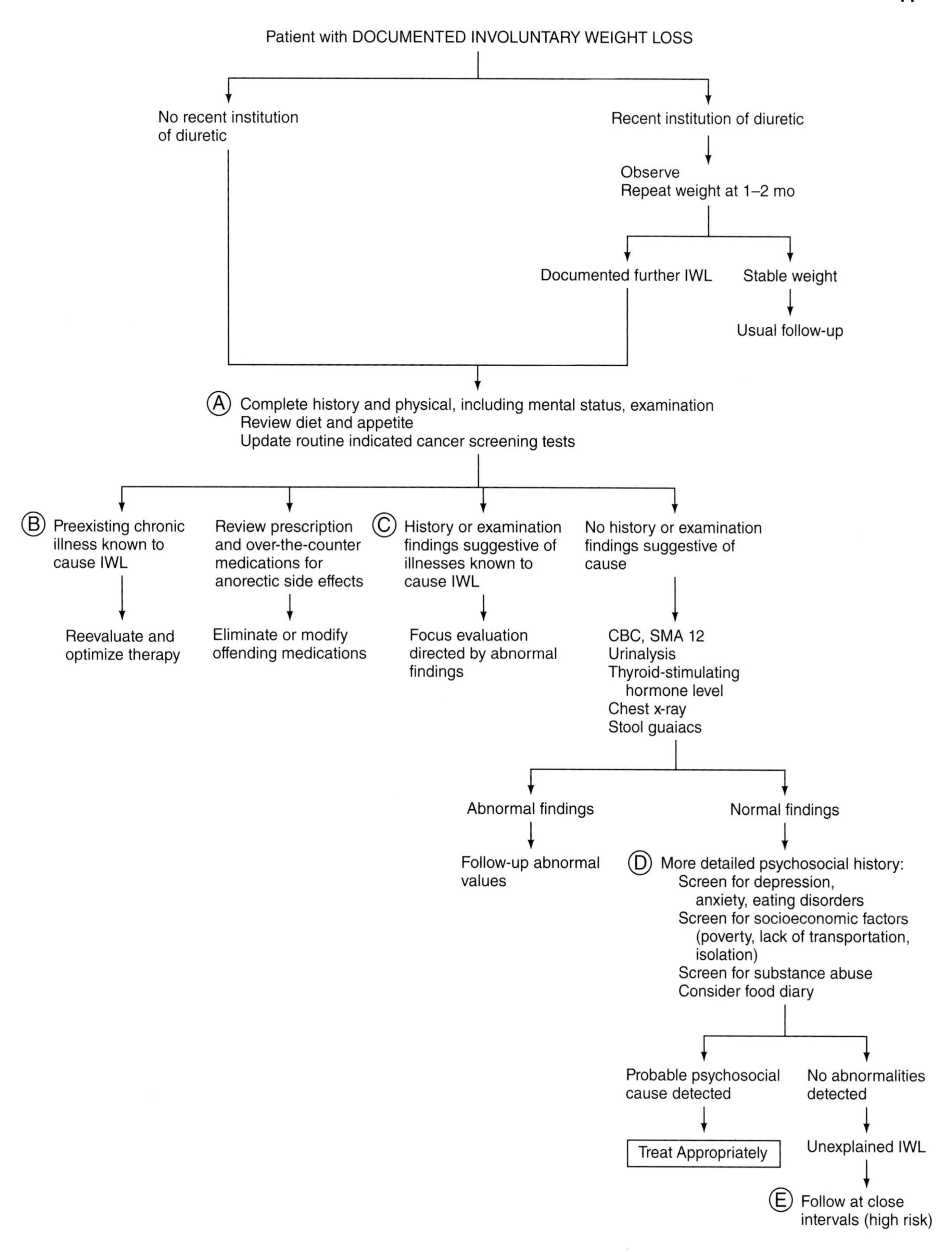
Patient with DOCUMENTED INVOLUNTARY WEIGHT LOSS
No recent institution of diuretic
Recent institution of diuretic
Observe
Repeat weight at 1–2 mo
Documented further IWL
Stable weight
Usual follow-up
Ⓐ Complete history and physical, including mental status, examination
Review diet and appetite
Update routine indicated cancer screening tests
Ⓑ Preexisting chronic illness known to cause IWL
Reevaluate and optimize therapy
Review prescription and over-the-counter medications for anorectic side effects
Eliminate or modify offending medications
Ⓒ History or examination findings suggestive of illnesses known to cause IWL
Focus evaluation directed by abnormal findings
No history or examination findings suggestive of cause
CBC, SMA 12
Urinalysis
Thyroid-stimulating hormone level
Chest x-ray
Stool guaiacs
Abnormal findings
Follow-up abnormal values
Normal findings
Ⓓ More detailed psychosocial history:
Screen for depression, anxiety, eating disorders
Screen for socioeconomic factors (poverty, lack of transportation, isolation)
Screen for substance abuse
Consider food diary
Probable psychosocial cause detected
Treat Appropriately
No abnormalities detected
Unexplained IWL
Ⓔ Follow at close intervals (high risk)

OBESITY

Stuart B. Mushlin, MD, FACP, FACR

A. Obesity is epidemic throughout the world. Current estimates in the United States are that 32.2% of adults are obese, and that number has been steadily increasing since the 1980s. Obesity is prevalent in Western Europe and Asia and much of the Third World. In England, it is estimated that 23% of men and women over 50 years of age are obese; in Pakistan 13% of men and 8% of women are obese.

The etiology of obesity is part of the initial evaluation of the patient. A dietary and caloric expenditure history is important. So too is family history and exploration of socioeconomic factors and medications. Many medications cause weight gain (including many antipsychotic and antidepressant medications, insulin, sulfonylureas, anticonvulsants, beta blockers, and cyproheptadine). Endocrine causes are rare and include Cushing's disease, hypothyroidism, or hypothalamic disorders. Routine testing for endocrine causes is not recommended unless the history, physical examination, and distribution of adipose tissue support the endocrine diagnosis.

Obesity may be multifactorial, but the major cause in both Western and non-Western society is diet. Many patients prefer to believe that their obesity is determined by an endocrine or neuroendocrine cause. However, this is rare indeed. It has been well studied that sedentary subjects in a metabolic chamber over time expend a baseline of about 1150 calories per day for maintenance. When patients claim they are not losing weight on a diet below 1200 calories per day, it almost invariably means they are not keeping an accurate record of their caloric intake

B. Obesity is generally defined as a body mass index (BMI) >30. Morbid obesity is generally accepted as a BMI >40, and the morbidity of obesity increases with other comorbid variables such as diabetes. The BMI has been a well-validated measure of total body fat and is computed as

Body weight (in kg) / height (in meters) squared.

Another measure of obesity is the waist circumference (as measured parallel to the floor at the superior iliac crest or umbilicus) or the ratio of waist circumference to hip circumference. In men with a waist circumference over 40 inches or in women with a waist circumference over 34.5 inches and a BMI of 24–34.9, there is a greater risk of type 2 diabetes, coronary heart disease, dyslipidemia, and hypertension. At BMIs ≥35 there is less correlation with waist circumference and disease.

In general, overweight is broken down by BMI to stratify risk. The best ideal BMI is 22 (levels above and below confer risk for increased mortality). BMIs <25 are considered nil to low risk; 25–30, mild risk; 30–35, moderate risk; 35–40, very significant risk; and >40, severe risk.

Obesity has been correlated with the following morbid or comorbid conditions: osteoarthritis, cholelithiasis, diabetes mellitus, coronary artery disease, sleep apnea, and social stigmatization. There is also a generalized reduction in quality of life in patient surveys.

C. Management of obesity is most successful over both long and short terms if the patient endorses the plan, has frequent follow-up (such as in a group experience), is educated about caloric intake, and exercises for additional caloric expenditure. Many dietary approaches work, and no single approach is successful for all people. Long-term, recidivism is extremely common (as high as 85%) and long-term commitment to exercise is one documented factor that is useful in mitigating recidivism. Extremely–low-fat diets may predispose to cholelithiasis, and there is evidence suggesting either the addition of 10% fat to a diet or the use of chenodeoxycholic acid to prophylax this possibility. There is no proof of a linear increase in weight loss with diets below 800 calories, so it is not necessary to ingest less than that amount in order to lose a maximal amount of weight. As well as empowering the patient with knowledge about diet, exercise, recidivism, and impulse control, realistic expectations about weight loss are important. Patients should not expect to lose more than 5% of their weight in 6 months, though many who adhere to a program lose twice that much in 6 months time.

Other approaches to weight-loss management may involve pharmacologic therapy and bariatric surgery. The American College of Physicians guidelines outline their recommendations for when these modalities should be used, but a brief summary is that if comorbidities (e.g., coronary artery disease and dyslipidemia) are present, the threshold is lower. There are a number of drugs currently approved by the FDA, and they involve differing mechanisms of action. They include: orlistat, sibutramine, diethylpropion, phentermine, benzphetamine, and phendimetrazine. All but orlistat are class III or IV drugs. Newer drugs are available in Europe or in Phase III FDA trials (rimonabant, lorcaserin, and others). Bariatric surgery is reserved for

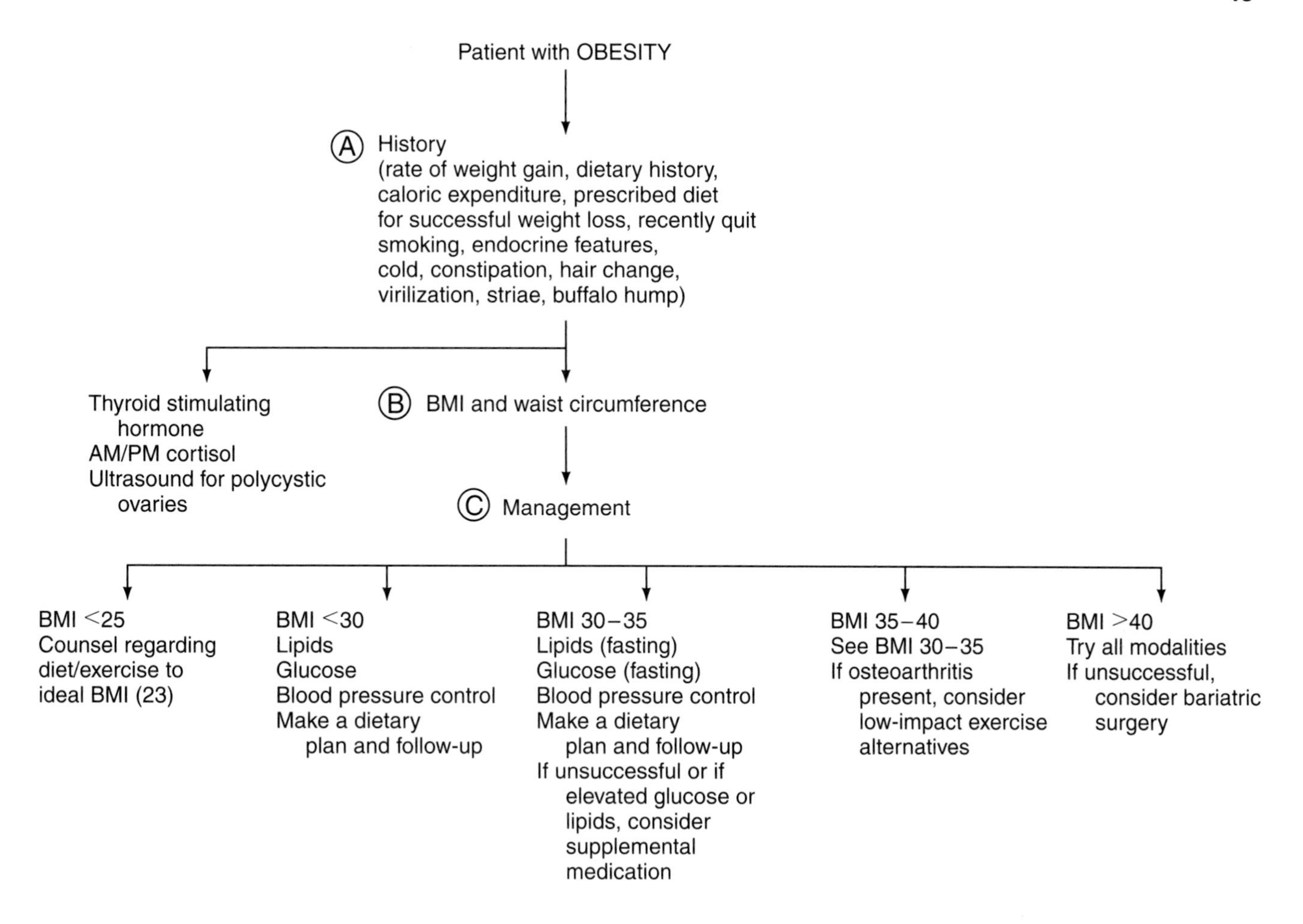

patients with a BMI ≥40 or greater or with significant comorbidities. It is not recommended unless previous, more conservative modalities have been unsuccessful. Mortality is high (about 2% in most studies), even with minimally invasive gastric lap banding, and long-term results are not available. It should be noted that liposuction, in a number of studies, has not been shown to cause improvement in insulin resistance or long-term weight loss.

References

Bardia A, Holtan SG, Slezak JM, et al. Diagnosis of obesity by primary care physicians and impact on obesity management. Mayo Clinic Proc 2007;82:927.

Bray GA. Medical consequences of obesity. J Clin Endoc Metab 2004;89:2583.

Snow V, Barry P, Fitterman N, et al. Pharmacologic and surgical management of obesity in primary care: a clinical practice guideline from the American College of Physicians. Ann Int Med 2005;142:525.

SEXUAL DYSFUNCTION

Kristyn M. Greifer, MD

A. Although a few patients will volunteer sexual difficulties, most will not. A detailed medical history should include a sexual history to elicit complaints. Ask general, nonjudgmental questions, including effects on current relationships, to open the discussion. Make no assumptions about a patient's sexual preferences or experiences.

B. Decreased libido can be associated with depression, other psychiatric disorders, or their medical treatment. Stress in relationships or work can also contribute. Psychiatric evaluation and counseling can help. Medical causes of decreased sexual desire include medications (e.g., antihypertensives or selective serotonin reuptake inhibitors [SSRIs], substance abuse, and acute and chronic illness. Hypogonadism is treatable with testosterone replacement therapy. Sex and/or marital therapy should be considered for patients with significant relationship problems (as either a cause or a result of decreased libido).

C. Erectile dysfunction, or impotence, can be classified as organic or psychogenic, although many men have a mixture of both. The presence of morning erections is highly specific for psychogenic impotence, although not very sensitive. There are a number of organic causes for erectile dysfunction, including endocrine, vascular, and neurologic disorders. Surgical procedures such as radical prostatectomy may result in erectile dysfunction as well. A careful history and physical will help elicit organic etiologies. Check testosterone level in organic impotence. Routine serologic screening for other endocrine disorders is not warranted in the absence of other indicators found in the history and physical. Medications (e.g., antihypertensives and SSRIs) have been implicated. Acute and chronic illness can contribute to organic and psychological erectile dysfunction. A nocturnal penile tumescence test using stamps or an inexpensive strain gauge will more reliably differentiate one from the other. However, in either case first-line therapy should be PDE5 inhibitors such as sildenafil, vardenafil, or tadalafil (with others on the way) unless contraindicated. PDE5 inhibitors must be avoided in patients taking oral or topical nitrates. Other options for treatment include injection therapies, prostaglandin agents such as alprostadil, or external devices that enhance erections (e.g., penile rings or vacuum pumps). Sex therapy can also be useful for patients with a psychological component. Referral to urology is appropriate in refractory cases.

D. Premature ejaculation is a common complaint among men who are young and sexually inexperienced. It is also seen in patients having relationship or situational stresses and is well known to occur with fatigue. Therapy was once limited to the pause (or hold) and squeeze technique in addition to increased sexual stimulation, which is thought to increase the latency period. SSRIs have shown efficacy in delaying ejaculation, and PDE5 inhibitors are now being studied as well. Sex therapy can be helpful in some cases. Absent ejaculation may be organic and a result of hypogonadism or a complication of prostate surgery. Retrograde ejaculation requires referral to urology. Rarely, anorgasmia occurs in the absence of hypogonadism and is best addressed by sex therapy.

(Continued on page 16)

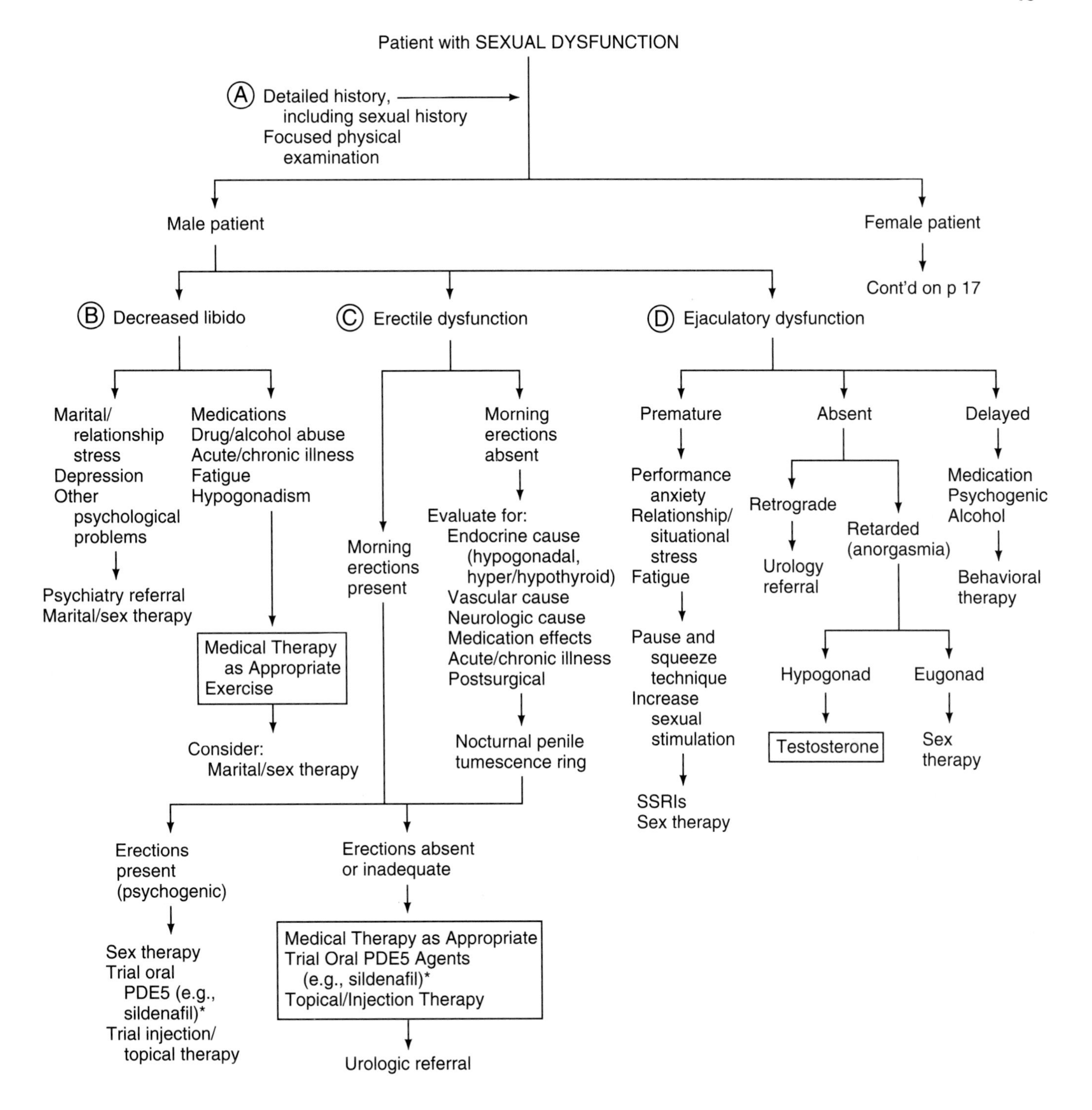

*Note: PDE5 inhibitors are contraindicated in patients taking nitrates.

E. Hypoactive sexual desire in women, as in men, can be associated with medications (e.g., antihypertensives, SSRIs), substance abuse, and chronic illness. It can accompany menopause (natural or surgical). Appropriate hormone replacement therapy (HRT) can improve sexual desire, especially if lack of desire is related to dyspareunia (painful intercourse) resulting from inadequate lubrication. Given the newly recognized risks of HRT, a physician must weigh the benefit against the risk. Women who have had bilateral oophorectomy or who suffer from severe androgen deficiency as in Addison's disease may benefit from androgen replacement therapy. Depression, difficulties with body image, and the maternal role also can decrease female desire. Reducing fatigue with the addition of regular exercise often is accompanied by an increase in sexual desire. A history of sexual abuse or domestic violence may present as hypoactive sexual desire and avoidance of sexual contact. Depression can be treated medically, although many antidepressants have decreased sexual desire as a prominent side effect (studies using PDE5 inhibitors to overcome this are under way). Psychiatric referral is appropriate for all women with a history of sexual abuse and may be appropriate for treatment of hypoactive sexual desire regardless of cause.

F. Anorgasmia is much more common in women than in men. Often it is a combination of inhibition relating to sex itself and a lack of knowledge about female sexual arousal. Education about anatomy and use of self-stimulation coupled with erotic materials may enhance a woman's sexual experience. Sex therapy can also be useful in these cases. Medications such as SSRIs or pelvic trauma also can lead to reduced ability to achieve orgasm.

G. Dyspareunia is a common sexual complaint of women. It is important to distinguish between insertional (just before or during penile penetration) and deep thrust dyspareunia. Insertional pain has a number of easily reversed causes such as vulvovaginitis, urethritis, and inadequate lubrication. Treatment with antibiotics when indicated and the use of topical estrogens in perimenopausal or postmenopausal women can eliminate the problem. Atrophic vaginitis often responds to estrogen replacement as well. Vulvar dystrophies, vulvar vestibulitis, and urethral syndromes require gynecologic referral. Pelvic inflammatory disease can be treated with antibiotics. Most other causes of deep thrust dyspareunia require gynecologic evaluation.

H. Vaginismus is a severe type of insertional dyspareunia. The patient complains of inability to achieve penetration—she may be unable to insert a tampon or tolerate a speculum examination—secondary to involuntary muscle contraction. If there is no history of sexual abuse, it may be related to fear and inhibition surrounding sex. Education about anatomy and sexual response coupled with insertion of progressively larger vaginal dilators may allow receptive penetration. Botulinum toxin is being studied as a potential medical therapy for severe cases. Sex therapy, psychiatric evaluation, or both may also be required. A history of sexual abuse demands psychiatric referral.

References

Arlt W. Androgen therapy in women. Eur J Endocrinol 2006;154(1):1–11.

Lightner D. Female sexual dysfunction. Mayo Clin Proc 2002;77(7): 698–702.

Montague DK, Jarow JP, Broderick GA, et al. Chapter 1: the management of erectile dysfunction: an AUA update. J Urol 2005; 174(1):230–239.

Ralph DJ, Wylie KR. Ejaculatory disorders and sexual function. BJU Int 2005;95:1181–1186.

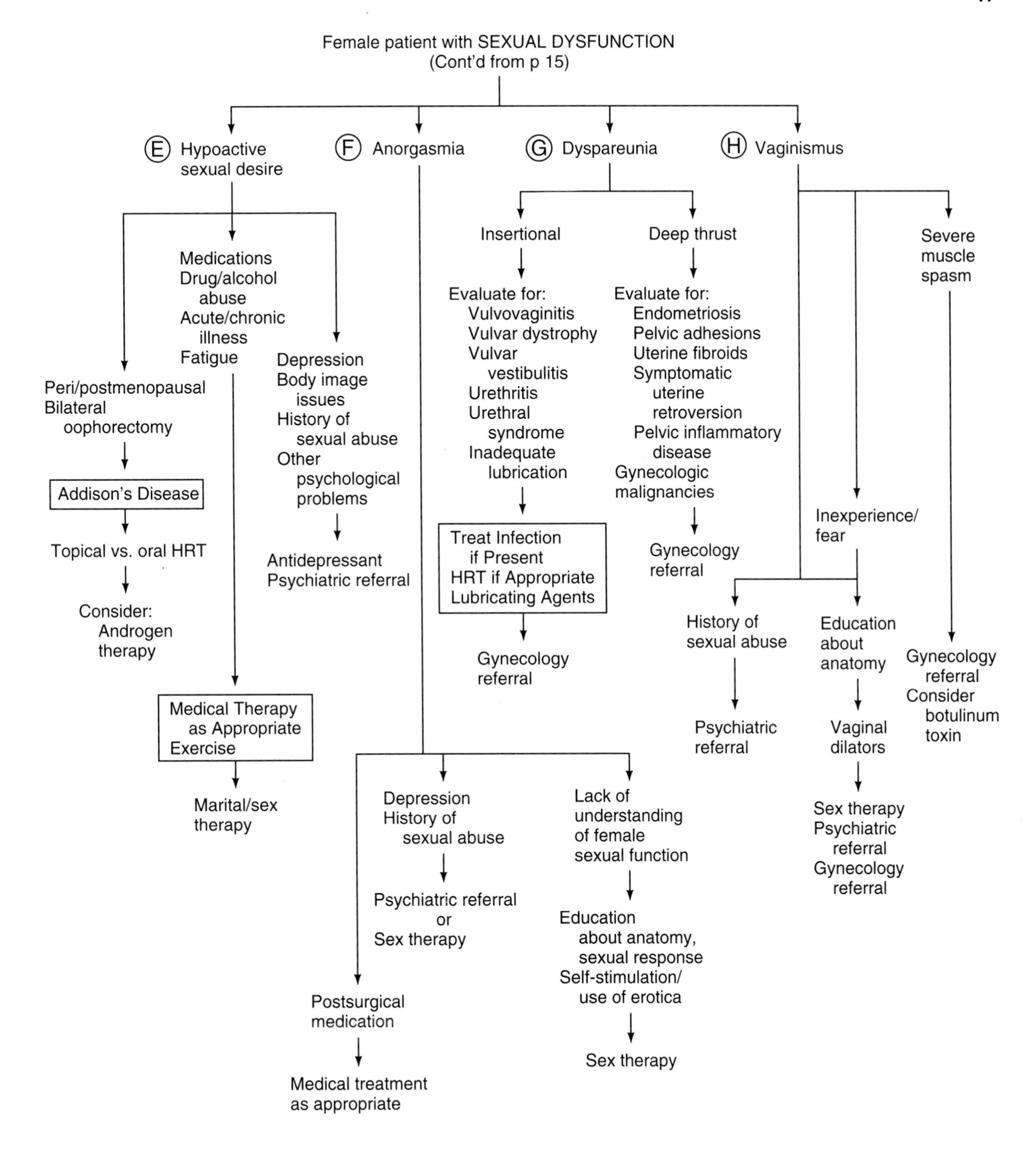

Female patient with SEXUAL DYSFUNCTION
(Cont'd from p 15)
E Hypoactive sexual desire
F Anorgasmia
G Dyspareunia
H Vaginismus
Medications
Drug/alcohol abuse
Acute/chronic illness
Fatigue
Peri/postmenopausal
Bilateral oophorectomy
Addison's Disease
Topical vs. oral HRT
Consider: Androgen therapy
Depression
Body image issues
History of sexual abuse
Other psychological problems
Antidepressant
Psychiatric referral
Medical Therapy as Appropriate
Exercise
Marital/sex therapy
Insertional
Evaluate for:
Vulvovaginitis
Vulvar dystrophy
Vulvar vestibulitis
Urethritis
Urethral syndrome
Inadequate lubrication
Treat Infection if Present
HRT if Appropriate
Lubricating Agents
Gynecology referral
Deep thrust
Evaluate for:
Endometriosis
Pelvic adhesions
Uterine fibroids
Symptomatic uterine retroversion
Pelvic inflammatory disease
Gynecologic malignancies
Gynecology referral
Depression
History of sexual abuse
Psychiatric referral
or
Sex therapy
Lack of understanding of female sexual function
Education about anatomy, sexual response
Self-stimulation/ use of erotica
Sex therapy
Postsurgical medication
Medical treatment as appropriate
Severe muscle spasm
Gynecology referral
Consider botulinum toxin
Inexperience/ fear
History of sexual abuse
Psychiatric referral
Education about anatomy
Vaginal dilators
Sex therapy
Psychiatric referral
Gynecology referral

EDEMA

David W. Gibson, MD, and Harry L. Greene II, MD, FACP

Edema is an abnormal collection of fluid in the interstitial space that may be localized or generalized. Fluid movement between the intravascular and extravascular space is related to the interacting forces of hydrostatic pressure, colloid oncotic pressure, and capillary permeability and to the effects of lymphatic drainage. Normally there exists an equilibrium among these forces, and no net fluid accumulation takes place. Edema occurs when there is a decrease in plasma oncotic pressure, an increase in hydrostatic pressure, an increase in capillary permeability, or a combination of these factors. Edema also can be present when lymphatic flow is obstructed.

A. The history and physical examination focus on the causes of edema and seek to ascertain whether it is generalized or localized.

B. Generalized edema can be documented by weight gain and often is associated with increased capillary hydrostatic pressure as seen in congestive heart failure (CHF), in renal failure with increased sodium and water load, after expansion of the intravascular volume from IV fluids, or in conditions of sodium retention. Edema may occur after corticosteroid therapy or with estrogens or other medications. Edema involving the whole body (e.g., anasarca) may extend to involve the peritoneal cavity (e.g., ascites) or the pleural space (e.g., hydrothorax). In patients with generalized edema the first step is to estimate central venous pressure by determining jugular venous pressure (JVP). The distance from the manubrium sterni to the fluid meniscus in the jugular vein should be ≤2 cm at 45 degrees or 5 cm from the left atrium.

C. Determine serum albumin and urinary protein in patients with generalized edema and normal JVP.

D. If serum albumin is normal, perform urinalysis, looking for abnormal urinary sediment, and check BUN and creatinine to evaluate the possibility of renal pathology. If urinalysis findings are normal, order thyroid function tests (TFTs) to look for myxedema. Remaining patients should be considered as possibly having idiopathic edema or drug-induced edema.

E. If serum albumin is decreased, perform urinalysis to check for proteinuria. More than 3.5 g protein suggests nephrotic syndrome; <3.5 g in a normal urinalysis suggests another cause, such as hepatitis or hepatic infiltration disease. Order liver function tests (LFTs); if results are abnormal, evaluate for liver pathology. If LFT results are normal, check prealbumin and cholesterol to evaluate for malnutrition. If the prealbumin is <20 mg/dl and the cholesterol level is low, malnutrition is suggested. If the prealbumin is >20 mg/dl, a capillary leak, abnormal protein synthesis, and protein-losing enteropathy are all possibilities.

F. In patients with an elevated JVP and generalized edema, order chest radiographs to look for cardiomegaly.

G. If cardiomegaly is found, order an echocardiogram to look for pericardial effusion; pericardial thickening, as in acute or chronic pericarditis; abnormal contractility of the heart, as might be seen in CHF; or signs of infiltrative cardiac problems, such as hypertrophic obstructive cardiomyopathy, amyloid, or neoplasm.

H. If cardiac size is normal on the chest film, evaluate the lung fields for pulmonary hypertension. Such a finding should lead to evaluation for cor pulmonale. Clear lung fields should prompt echocardiography to seek pericardial constriction.

I. Regional edema or localized edema often is caused by increased capillary pressure. Some causes include chronic venous insufficiency; incompetent venous valves; vascular obstructions, either extrinsic because of neoplasm, lymph nodes, surgery, fibrosis, or radiation, or intrinsic because of deep venous thrombosis, surgery, infection, immobility, trauma, or a hypercoagulable state (e.g., protein C deficiency, protein S deficiency, antithrombin 3 deficiency, the presence of neoplasms, or secondary to the venodilating effects of drugs such as calcium channel blockers).

(Continued on page 20)

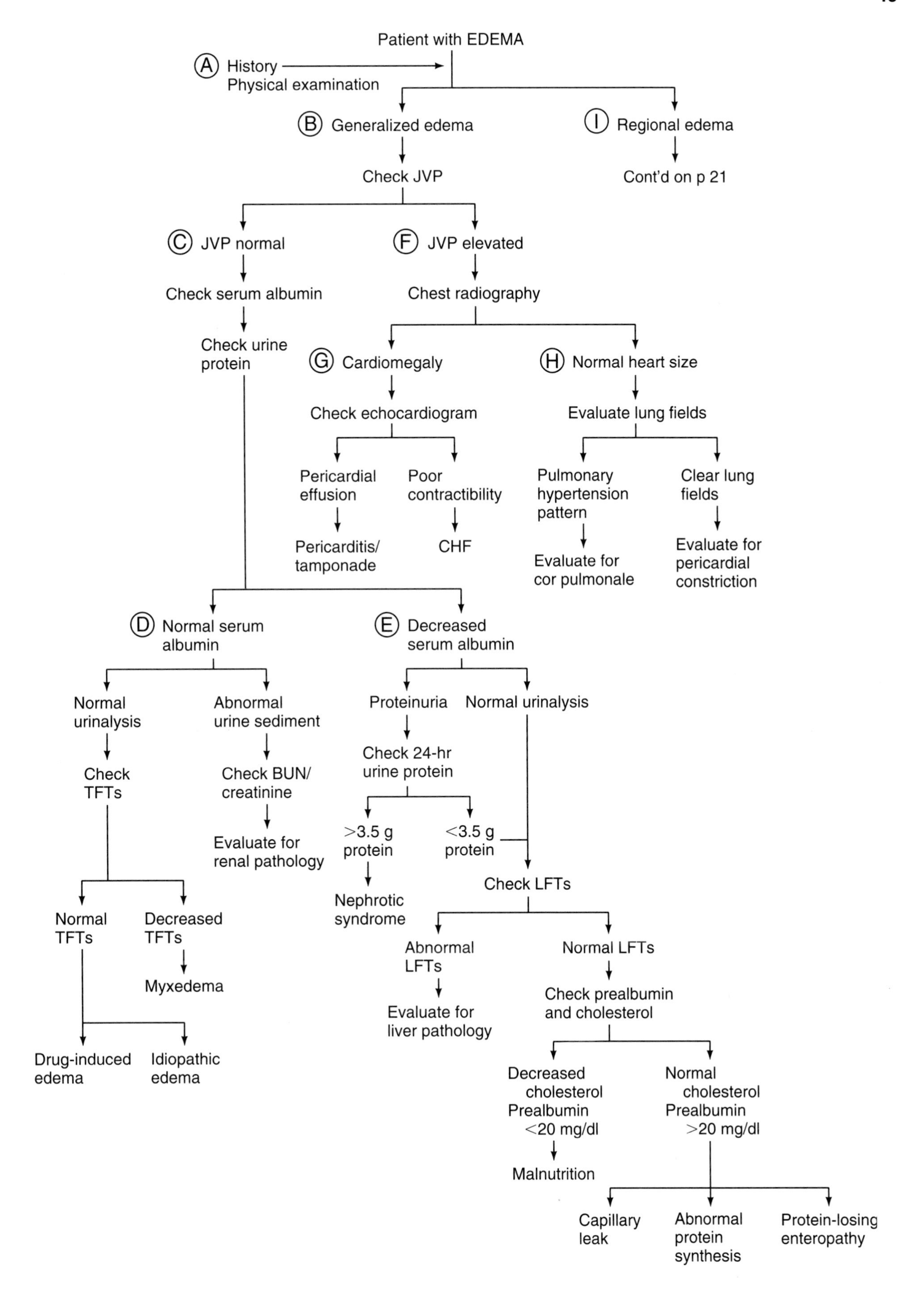

Patient with EDEMA
(A) History
Physical examination
(B) Generalized edema
(I) Regional edema
Check JVP
Cont'd on p 21
(C) JVP normal
(F) JVP elevated
Check serum albumin
Chest radiography
Check urine protein
(G) Cardiomegaly
(H) Normal heart size
Check echocardiogram
Evaluate lung fields
Pericardial effusion
Poor contractibility
Pulmonary hypertension pattern
Clear lung fields
Pericarditis/ tamponade
CHF
Evaluate for cor pulmonale
Evaluate for pericardial constriction
(D) Normal serum albumin
(E) Decreased serum albumin
Normal urinalysis
Abnormal urine sediment
Proteinuria
Normal urinalysis
Check TFTs
Check BUN/ creatinine
Check 24-hr urine protein
Evaluate for renal pathology
>3.5 g protein
<3.5 g protein
Nephrotic syndrome
Check LFTs
Normal TFTs
Decreased TFTs
Myxedema
Abnormal LFTs
Normal LFTs
Evaluate for liver pathology
Check prealbumin and cholesterol
Drug-induced edema
Idiopathic edema
Decreased cholesterol Prealbumin <20 mg/dl
Normal cholesterol Prealbumin >20 mg/dl
Malnutrition
Capillary leak
Abnormal protein synthesis
Protein-losing enteropathy

J. When regional edema is present, note its location. If it is in one or both upper extremities, determine JVP.

K. Patients with upper extremity edema and normal JVP should undergo a Doppler study, impedance plethysmography (IPG), venography, or color flow duplex scanning to look for venous obstruction from either intrinsic or extrinsic causes. A negative study suggests lymphatic obstruction.

L. Evaluate patients with upper extremity edema and elevated JVP for superior vena cava syndrome with a chest radiograph, CT scan, or MRI of the chest.

M. If the regional edema is confined to the lower extremities, note whether it is unilateral or bilateral. Seek historical features specifically directed toward trauma, a hypercoagulable state, history of neoplasm, or conditions that might cause lymphatic or venous obstruction.

N. If the history is negative, order a Doppler study or IPG. If this study is positive, venography may be indicated to evaluate venous thrombosis versus extrinsic compression. If the Doppler study is negative, rhabdomyolysis, musculoskeletal edema, or localized vascular defects may be present.

O. Patients with a positive history of lower extremity edema should undergo IPG, Doppler study, or venography of the lower extremity. Again, a positive study result may suggest venous thrombosis, with treatment for this. A negative study result may suggest lymphatic obstruction. This can be evaluated with lymphangiography.

References

Berczeller PH. Idiopathic edema. Hosp Pract (Off Ed) 1994;29:115.

Braunwald E. Edema. In Fauci AS, Braunwald E, Isselbacher KJ, et al, eds. Harrison's Principles of Internal Medicine, 14th ed. New York: McGraw-Hill, 1997:210.

Ciocon JO, Fernandez BB, Ciocon DG. Leg edema: clinical clues to the differential diagnosis. Geriatrics 1993;48:34.

Goroll AH, May LA, Mulley AG. Primary Care Medicine, 3rd ed. Philadelphia: Lippincott-Raven, 1995:105.

Greene HL, Kreis SR, Kahn KL. Edema. In Greene HL, ed. Clinical Medicine. 2nd ed. St. Louis: Mosby, 1996:138.

Rogers RL, Feller ED, Gottlieb SS. Acute congestive heart failure in the emergency department. Cardiol Clin 2006;24(1):115–123, vii.

Schmittling ZC, McLafferty RB, Bohannon WT, et al. Characterization and probability of upper extremity deep venous thrombosis. Ann Vasc Surg 2004;18:552–557.

Ware LB, Matthay MA. Clinical practice. Acute pulmonary edema. N Engl J Med 2005;353:2788–2796.

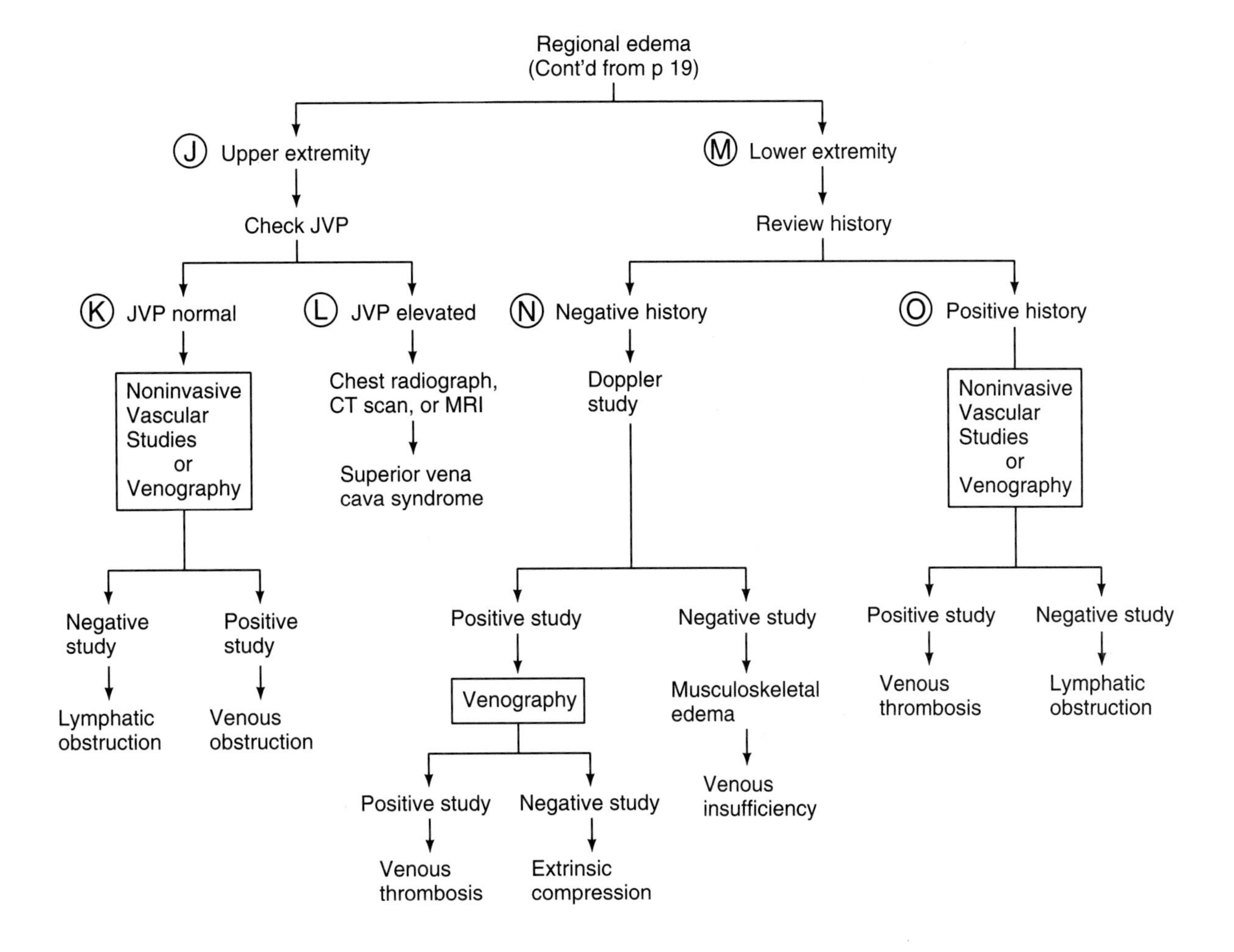
Regional edema
(Cont'd from p 19)
J Upper extremity
Check JVP
K JVP normal
Noninvasive Vascular Studies or Venography
Negative study
Lymphatic obstruction
Positive study
Venous obstruction
L JVP elevated
Chest radiograph, CT scan, or MRI
Superior vena cava syndrome
M Lower extremity
Review history
N Negative history
Doppler study
Positive study
Venography
Positive study
Venous thrombosis
Negative study
Extrinsic compression
Negative study
Musculoskeletal edema
Venous insufficiency
O Positive history
Noninvasive Vascular Studies or Venography
Positive study
Venous thrombosis
Negative study
Lymphatic obstruction

CHRONIC PAIN

William P. Johnson, MD

A. The information needed to evaluate the patient includes a detailed history of the pain complaint(s), an understanding of pain characteristics, response to past treatments, a thorough understanding of the patient's history (i.e., a review of the often voluminous medical records and psychosocial history), and the temporal relationship of all these factors to the onset and exacerbation of pain.

B. Acute pain often is associated with an increase in circulation, ventilation, and metabolism and a decrease in urinary and GI function. Patients are in obvious pain, and often there are associated findings of pallor, diaphoresis, and nausea.

C. Chronic pain is defined as any pain continuing beyond the usual course of an acute injury process. It can be dangerous to place an arbitrary time limit, such as 6 months, on this definition. For example, the pain of a broken wrist should last, at most, 2 weeks. Any continuing pain may indicate a reflex sympathetic dystrophy. This is a cause of chronic pain in which early recognition and treatment lead to complete recovery. Waiting 6 months to consider this pain chronic could leave the patient with a permanent disability. Patients with constant pain develop vegetative signs: disturbances in sleep and appetite, constipation, increased irritability, decreased libido, psychomotor retardation, and lowered pain tolerance. Patients with intermittent chronic pain (e.g., those with recurrent bouts of neuralgia, headaches, or angina) may have responses similar to those with acute pain.

D. Chronic benign pain is a diagnostic and management challenge. If possible, it sometimes is useful to localize the pain to the target organ most affected.

E. Some patients do not fit nicely into any of the usual chronic benign pain subcategories. The approach to this group of patients needs to be individualized.

F. All patients with chronic pain go through proven psychological changes while coping with their pain. Psychological and environmental factors play a great role in chronic pain, with 30% of patients becoming clinically depressed. However, psychogenic pain occurs when the pain is a result of psychological mechanisms. The fact that a physician cannot find a specific organic cause for the pain is insufficient, by itself, to warrant a psychiatric diagnosis. Positive evidence for a psychiatric diagnosis must be found. (DSM-IV criteria should be applied.)

G. A multidisciplinary pain center (MPC) should have on its staff a variety of health care providers capable of assessing and treating physical, psychosocial, medical, vocational, and social aspects of chronic pain. A multidisciplinary pain team may include an internist, pschiatrist, physiatrist, pharmacist, anesthesiologist, neurosurgeon, nurse, dentist, psychologist, physical therapist, and occupational therapist. At least three medical specialties should be represented on the staff of an MPC. If one of the physicians is not a psychiatrist, physicians from two specialties and a clinical psychologist are the minimum required. The MPC may exist in either an inpatient or outpatient setting. An MPC should establish protocols for patient management and assess their efficiency periodically. With benign pain the emphasis should be on pain management and rehabilitation, with little or no use of controlled medications. Many anesthesiologists specialize in chronic pain; however, do not expect a comprehensive approach by these practitioners. They may be useful for some procedures such as epidurals, but their approach is usually too focused.

H. Effective pain management requires consistent strategies: (1) establishing treatment goals in terms of outcomes with a definite timeline, (2) regularly scheduling follow-up appointments, (3) establishing medication refill guidelines, and (4) establishing patient behavior guidelines. You need to be familiar with your state board of medical examiners regulations. If your state board does not have explicit regulations, you can find explicit regulations and useful forms at the Arizona Board of Medical Examiners website (www.azmd.gov—click on the Physician Center drop down and go to guidelines for opioid prescribing).

I. This group of patients may cause licensing and legal headaches unless certain guidelines are followed.
   - Do an initial comprehensive clinical examination, which results in an explicit working diagnosis.
   - Call the last treating physician and discuss the case.
   - Review all outside records.
   - Establish a written treatment plan with recorded measurable objectives.
   - If habituating medications are used, informed consent must be given and the physician must make explicit the material risks of treatment, including alternative treatments, treatment side effects and potential interactions, risk of tolerance, how to withdraw treatment, risk of addiction, and risk of impaired judgment.
   - Review current treatment and modify as indicated.
   - Consult as indicated.
   - Be comprehensive and compulsive in record keeping.

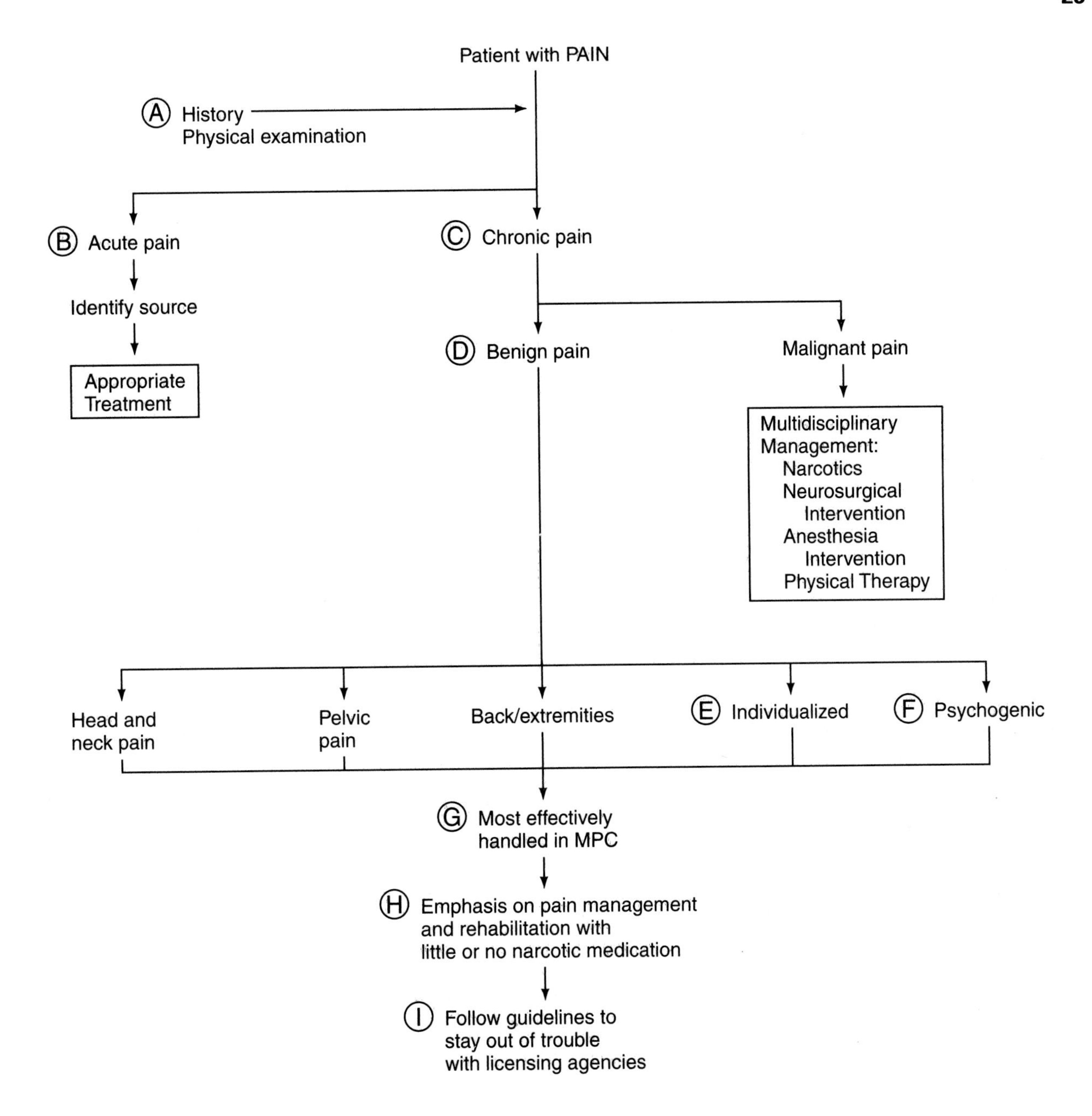

References

Arnold RM, Han PK, Seltzer D. Opioid contracts in chronic nonmalignant pain management: objectives and uncertainties. Am J Med 2006;119:292.

Ballantye JC, Mad J. Opioid therapy for chronic pain. N Engl J Med 2003;349:1943–1953.

Godfrey RG. A guide to the understanding and use of tricyclic antidepressants in the overall management of fibromyalgia and other chronic pain syndromes. Arch Intern Med 1996;156:1047.

Levy MH. Pharmacologic treatment of cancer pain. N Engl J Med 1996;335:1124.

Portenoy RK. Opioid therapy for chronic nonmalignant pain: a review of the critical issues. J Pain Symptom Manage 1996;11:203.

Vasudevan SV, Lynch NT. Pain centers: organization and outcome. In Rehabilitation medicine—adding life to years (special issue). West J Med 1991;154:532.

PERSISTENT EXCESSIVE SWEATING

Lisa Kaufmann, MD

A. Several dermatologic conditions are associated with localized hyperhidrosis: increased sweating in areas of vitiligo, granulosis, rubra nasi, dyshidrotic eczema, pachydermoperiostosis, epidermolysis, bullosa, pachyonychia congenita, nail-patella syndrome, palmoplantar keratodermas, and others. These conditions should be detectable on physical examination.

B. Anxiety or stimulants may increase sweating, but some people have severe hyperhidrosis without an obvious precipitating event. Such patients often have a family history of hyperhidrosis. Severe hyperhidrosis may cause difficulty with hand work, infection caused by the moist environment (especially in the feet), and considerable social distress. Topical treatments have varying success. Treatment with botulinum toxin A, iontophoresis, sympathectomy, or removal of the axillary sweat glands gives good results in severe cases (see references).

C. A structural lesion in the sympathetic nervous system may cause abnormalities in sweating. Cerebrocortical tumors, stroke, or infection may cause contralateral hyperhidrosis through release of inhibition. When injured sympathetic nerves regrow, connections may develop between the parasympathetic and sympathetic nerves. This can result in sweating of the innervated skin, as seen with gustatory sweating. Spinal cord disease (including syringomyelia, spinal cord injury, tabes dorsalis) may cause segmental areas of hyperhidrosis. Thoracic sympathetic nerve trunk injury may also cause localized hyperhidrosis. A large area of anhidrosis, as in severe diabetic autonomic neuropathy or after a sympathectomy involving more than one limb, may result in compensatory hyperhidrosis of other areas.

D. Many chemicals may cause sweating, either during withdrawal states (as from alcohol or opiates) or with use (e.g., alcohol, antidepressants, some antipsychotics, "triptans," theophylline, sildenafil, opiates, cholinergic and adrenergic agents, acetylcholinesterase inhibitors, and others). Chronic ingestion of mercury or arsenic can cause excessive sweating.

E. Malaria, tuberculosis, HIV, brucellosis, abdominal abscesses, rheumatic fever, and endocarditis are commonly seen with fevers and sweats as the predominant symptoms, but any infection producing a fever may cause sweating through the hypothalamic temperature regulatory centers as the fever falls. Even after a severe febrile illness resolves, patients may continue to have sweats for days to months.

F. Certain malignant conditions, including lymphoma, monocytic leukemia, and renal carcinoma, classically cause fevers, but fever with associated sweats also may be found in other malignancies. Carcinoid syndrome may cause excessive sweating. Rheumatologic diseases associated with excessive sweating include rheumatoid arthritis and Raynaud's phenomenon.

G. Other endocrine causes of hyperhidrosis include menopause, pregnancy, diabetes mellitus, gout, obesity, porphyria, rickets, and hyperpituitarism. In some cases of hypoglycemia, CNS dysfunction and sweat may occur in the absence of other adrenergic symptoms.

References

Champion RH. Disorders of the sweat glands. In Champion RH, Burton JL, Ebling FJG, eds. Rook/Wilkinson/Ebling Text-book of Dermatology. London: Blackwell Scientific, 1992:1745.

Eisenbach JH, Atkinson JLD, Fealy RD. Hyperhidrosis: evolving therapies for a well established phenomenon. Mayo Clin Proc 2005;80:657.

Haider A, Nowell S. Focal hyperhidrosis: diagnosis and management. CMAJ 2005;172:69.

Viera AJ, Bond MM, Yates SW. Diagnosing night sweats. Am Fam Physician 2003;67:1019.

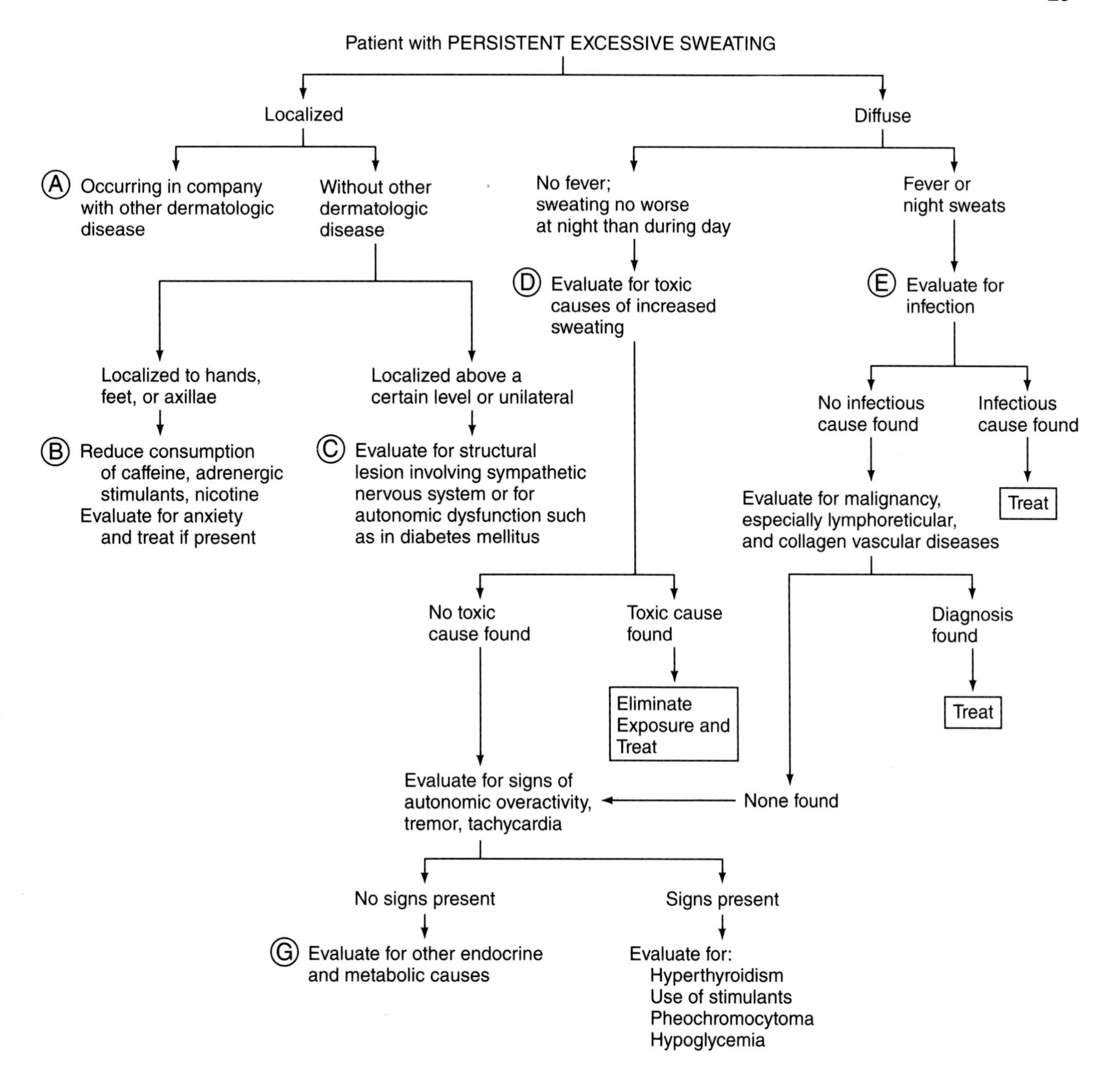
Patient with PERSISTENT EXCESSIVE SWEATING
Localized
Diffuse
(A) Occurring in company with other dermatologic disease
Without other dermatologic disease
No fever; sweating no worse at night than during day
Fever or night sweats
(D) Evaluate for toxic causes of increased sweating
(E) Evaluate for infection
Localized to hands, feet, or axillae
Localized above a certain level or unilateral
No infectious cause found
Infectious cause found
(B) Reduce consumption of caffeine, adrenergic stimulants, nicotine
Evaluate for anxiety and treat if present
(C) Evaluate for structural lesion involving sympathetic nervous system or for autonomic dysfunction such as in diabetes mellitus
Evaluate for malignancy, especially lymphoreticular, and collagen vascular diseases
Treat
No toxic cause found
Toxic cause found
Diagnosis found
Eliminate Exposure and Treat
Treat
Evaluate for signs of autonomic overactivity, tremor, tachycardia
None found
No signs present
Signs present
(G) Evaluate for other endocrine and metabolic causes
Evaluate for:
Hyperthyroidism
Use of stimulants
Pheochromocytoma
Hypoglycemia

THE RED EYE

Shari Carney, MD, and Robert W. Weisenthal, MD

Many patients present with a red eye to an emergency department or their primary care physician. It is important to determine which cases need ophthalmology referral and which cases can be managed by the primary care physician. A thorough ocular and systemic history is extremely helpful in making this decision. Key questions include loss of vision, presence of deep versus superficial pain, trauma, history of angle-closure glaucoma, uveitis or systemic illness, and recent ocular history such as surgery. Physical examination also is important. It is essential in all patients with ocular complaints to check visual acuity. Many patients with tearing or discharge note blurred vision, but they can improve it by blinking. If patients have forgotten their glasses, using a pinhole to check vision will compensate for uncorrected refractive error. Patients with deep pain, truly decreased vision, severe perilimbal injection, corneal opacification, and recent ocular surgery all need ophthalmology evaluation. See the algorithm for details on timing.

A. Orbital cellulitis presents with lid erythema, proptosis, and restricted eye movements. The lid may look ptotic (pseudoptosis) secondary to the swelling. The patient also may give a history of sinusitis. In children orbital cellulitis may easily spread from nasal preseptal cellulitis. These patients need to be admitted for IV antibiotics. Some patients may have a real ptosis and a red eye. The examiner needs to look further for cranial nerve palsies. Orbital congestion secondary to a cavernous sinus thrombosis will present with a red, congested eye and an isolated or combined III, IV, or VI nerve palsy. A VII nerve palsy may cause a red eye secondary to poor lid function causing chronic exposure.

B. A history of thyroid abnormalities, lid retraction, proptosis, and injection over the rectus muscles may indicate Graves' orbitopathy. These patients require a thyroid workup and an ophthalmic evaluation to determine optic nerve involvement on a semiurgent basis.

C. Scleritis presents as a severe, deep pain similar to a toothache. If left undiagnosed and untreated, it can have significant visual morbidity. The globe is tender to touch. The sclera appears violaceous in sunlight because of involvement of the deep episcleral vessels. The redness may be either focal or diffuse. It often is associated with systemic immunologic disease. Semiurgent referral is required.

(Continued on page 28)

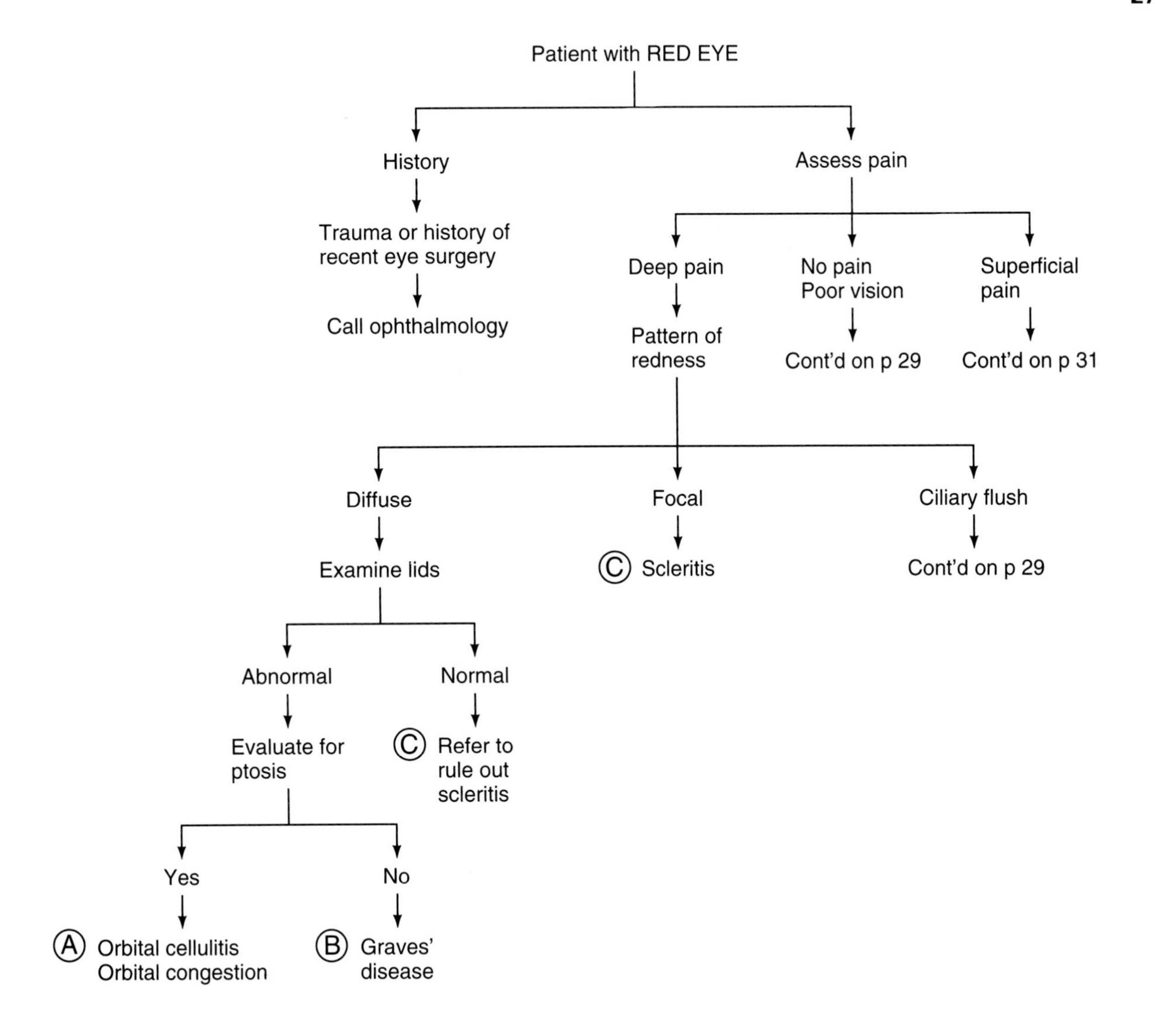
Patient with RED EYE
History
Trauma or history of recent eye surgery
Call ophthalmology
Assess pain
Deep pain
No pain
Poor vision
Superficial pain
Pattern of redness
Cont'd on p 29
Cont'd on p 31
Diffuse
Focal
Ciliary flush
Examine lids
(C) Scleritis
Cont'd on p 29
Abnormal
Normal
Evaluate for ptosis
(C) Refer to rule out scleritis
Yes
No
(A) Orbital cellulitis
Orbital congestion
(B) Graves' disease

D. Acute angle-closure glaucoma presents with a red eye, decreased vision, eye pain, headache, a mid-dilated pupil, and corneal edema. The patient may be able to give a history of prior episodes. Immediate (within 1–2 hours) referral to an ophthalmologist is indicated.

E. If the patient has injection primarily around the cornea (ciliary flush), decreased vision, and a small pupil compared with the contralateral eye, the patient may have an anterior uveitis (iritis). Inquire about other systemic symptoms such as arthritis, back pain, and coexisting medical conditions such as ulcerative colitis. These patients need referral for proper diagnosis and treatment on a semiurgent basis (within 24 hours).

F. If the cornea has a white opacity, the patient may have a corneal ulcer, which should be referred to an ophthalmologist urgently for cultures and intensive treatment. Herpes simplex keratitis also may present with a dendritic figure that will highlight with fluorescein, with an underlying clear cornea.

G. A hypopyon is layered WBCs in the anterior chamber and may indicate an infection throughout the eye (endophthalmitis) or may be secondary to a corneal ulcer. The patient may give a history of recent ophthalmic surgery or trauma. This requires immediate referral for cultures and proper treatment.

H. It is essential to examine the anterior chamber in a patient with a red eye. Layered blood in the anterior chamber (hyphema) may also be associated with a flat or shallow anterior chamber, a possible sign of a ruptured globe, requiring immediate referral. A hyphema with a well-formed chamber and no other signs of a ruptured globe should be referred that day.

I. A patient with a red eye, decreased vision, and no other obvious signs may have a retinitis, vitreitis, or posterior scleritis. These are rare causes of a red eye. Refer these patients to an ophthalmologist on a semiurgent basis.

(Continued on page 30)

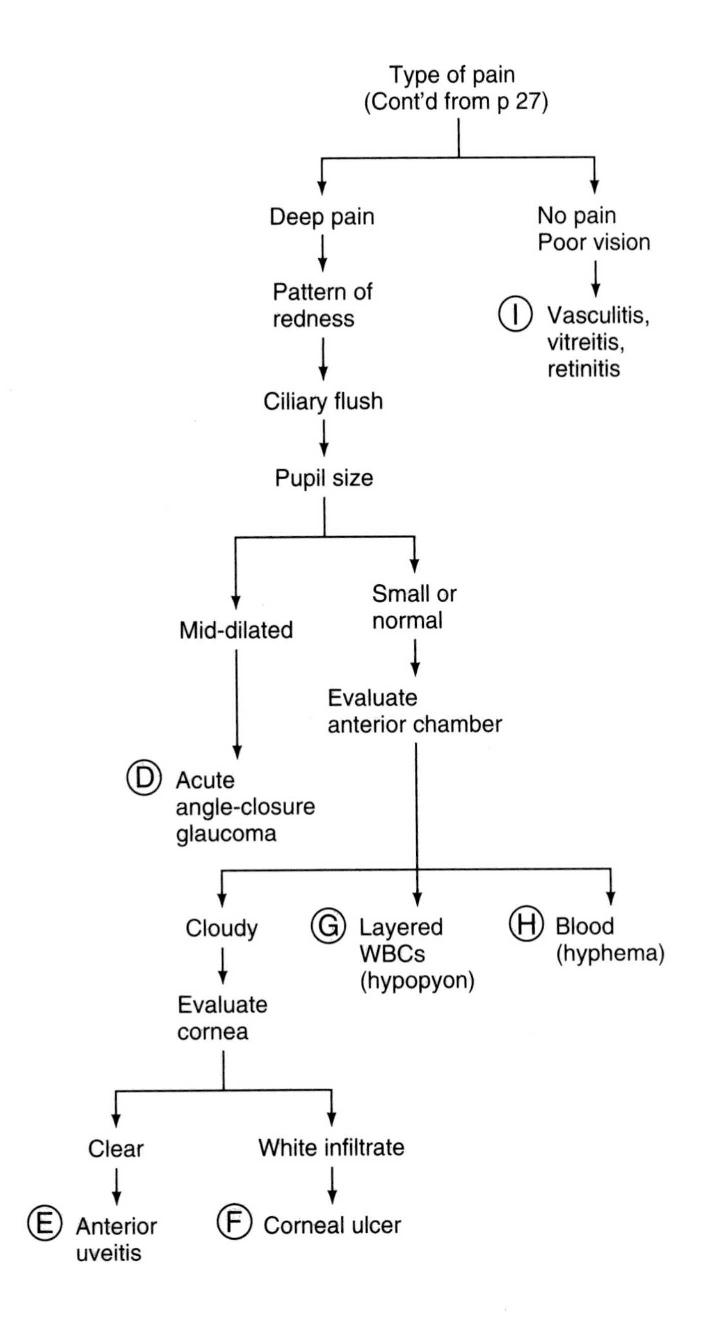
Type of pain
(Cont'd from p 27)
Deep pain
No pain
Poor vision
Pattern of
redness
Ⓘ Vasculitis,
vitreitis,
retinitis
Ciliary flush
Pupil size
Mid-dilated
Small or
normal
Evaluate
anterior chamber
Ⓓ Acute
angle-closure
glaucoma
Cloudy
Ⓖ Layered
WBCs
(hypopyon)
Ⓗ Blood
(hyphema)
Evaluate
cornea
Clear
White infiltrate
Ⓔ Anterior
uveitis
Ⓕ Corneal ulcer

J. If the patient was working with metal or wood, inspect the eye for a foreign body. Irrigating the eye with normal saline may help remove a foreign body. Removal of a conjunctival foreign body may be attempted by rolling a cotton swab over it. A patient with an embedded corneal foreign body that does not irrigate out should be referred to an ophthalmologist within 24 hours for removal. Start the patient on topical antibiotics to prevent infection. If there is a residual rust ring, the patient should follow up with an ophthalmologist in 24–48 hours for removal. If the vision is significantly decreased or there is a question of a globe laceration from the foreign body, urgent referral is necessary.

K. Exposure to chemicals warrants immediate copious saline irrigation (500 ml). If the chemical injury is mild and characterized by mild injection without fluorescein uptake, start topical antibiotics and follow up in 1–2 days. If the chemical injury is severe with corneal clouding and loss of conjunctival blood vessels (porcelain sclera), the patient should be seen by an ophthalmologist immediately.

L. Corneal abrasions present with a severe foreign body sensation, and on Wood's lamp examination they show fluorescein uptake in an otherwise clear cornea. Treatment consists of topical antibiotic ointment and patching. Recheck these patients in 24 hours; if not dramatically improved, refer them to an ophthalmologist.

M. Blepharitis is an inflammation of the eyelids characterized by redness of the eyelids, crusting, and foreign body sensation. The treatment is warm compresses and lid hygiene. Acne rosacea can cause a secondary blepharitis, which should be treated with oral tetracycline or doxycycline. A hordeolum (stye) or chalazion should also be treated with warm compresses and topical antibiotic ointment. Chalazia need to be incised and drained only if they do not respond to a 2-week course of medical therapy.

N. The most common cause of conjunctivitis is a viral infection. The eyes are diffusely red with a watery discharge. Many patients have a preauricular lymph node on the affected side. Treatment is palliative; cool compresses and astringent drops are used because the condition is self-limited. The patient should follow up on a routine basis if the condition does not resolve in 1 week to 10 days.

O. Allergic conjunctivitis is typically seasonal and always presents with itching and occasionally with mild foreign body sensation. Topical antihistamine and/or mast cell stabilizing drops relieve the symptoms. Follow-up is indicated only if symptomatic treatment is ineffective.

P. Bacterial conjunctivitis comprises <5% of all conjunctivitis. Sight-threatening disease can occur with a virulent bacterial species such as gonococcus. Usually the onset is hyperacute (<24 hours) with a fulminant mucopurulent discharge and requires urgent workup with cultures/Gram stain. *Streptococcus pneumoniae*, *Haemophilus influenzae*, and *Chlamydia* are other common pathogens and present as a less purulent conjunctivitis. The appropriate topical and, in severe cases, systemic antibiotic is based on results of the Gram stain/culture. Initially, use a broad-spectrum antibiotic, altering therapy according to culture results if the conjunctivitis does not respond to initial therapy. Patients who develop corneal or scleral thinning require urgent referral to an ophthalmologist.

Q. Nonspecific conjunctivitis results from mild inflammation of the ocular surface and can be treated with a topical antihistamine or mild topical antibiotic.

R. A pterygium is a fibrovascular growth that extends onto the nasal portion of the cornea. It can sometimes become inflamed or may grow slowly over the pupil (taking months to years). If it extends into the central cornea, reducing the patient's vision, excision is necessary. Pingueculae are degenerative lesions of the bulbar conjunctiva that do not extend onto the cornea. They occur secondary to ultraviolet light exposure. They usually are nasal in location and are yellow-white in appearance. They are benign. If they become inflamed, artificial tears are helpful. Routine follow-up is indicated only if symptoms persist.

S. A subconjunctival hemorrhage consists of blood trapped under the conjunctiva. It can occur with any injury to the globe or with Valsalva's maneuvers. It usually is benign; however, a history of trauma with a flat anterior chamber requires an ophthalmic evaluation on an urgent basis. If a patient has recurring subconjunctival hemorrhage with no known cause, a workup for a hematologic disorder is indicated. Episcleritis is localized inflammation of the episcleral blood vessels that responds to topical steroids. Be certain that the patient does not have herpetic keratitis before starting treatment.

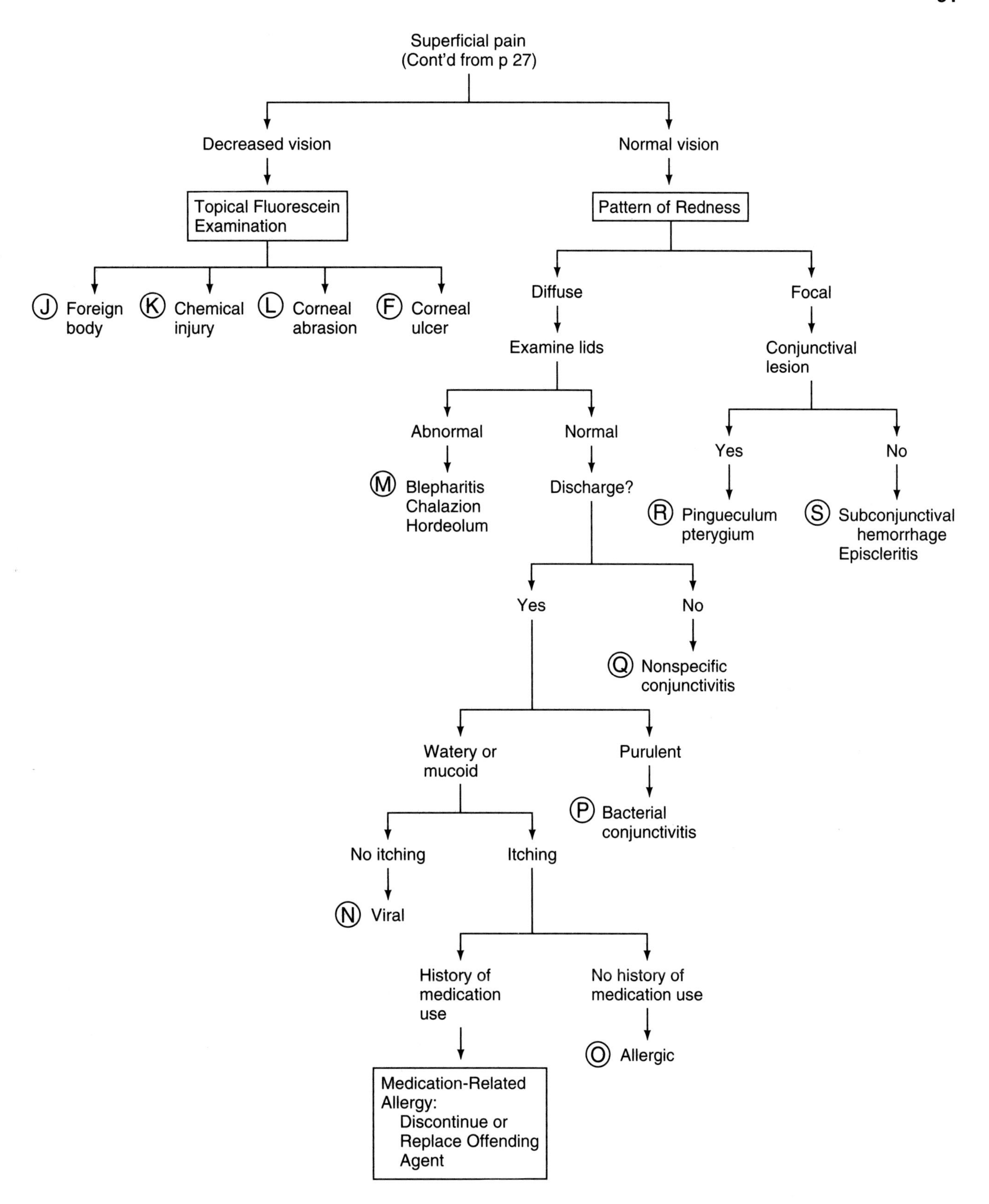
Superficial pain
(Cont'd from p 27)
Decreased vision
Normal vision
Topical Fluorescein Examination
Pattern of Redness
J Foreign body
K Chemical injury
L Corneal abrasion
F Corneal ulcer
Diffuse
Focal
Examine lids
Conjunctival lesion
Abnormal
Normal
Yes
No
M Blepharitis
Chalazion
Hordeolum
Discharge?
R Pingueculum pterygium
S Subconjunctival hemorrhage
Episcleritis
Yes
No
Q Nonspecific conjunctivitis
Watery or mucoid
Purulent
P Bacterial conjunctivitis
No itching
Itching
N Viral
History of medication use
No history of medication use
O Allergic
Medication-Related Allergy:
Discontinue or Replace Offending Agent

RHINITIS

Anastasia Rowland-Seymour, MD

Rhinitis is described as inflammation of the nasal mucosa and is characterized by the constellation of symptoms, including nasal congestion, rhinorrhea, sneezing, and itching of the eyes and/or nose. The sinuses, ears, and throat may also be involved. Allergic rhinitis is by far the most common type of rhinitis. Types of rhinitis include allergic rhinitis, infectious rhinitis (viral and bacterial), and nonallergic rhinitis. Nonallergic rhinitis includes nonallergic rhinitis with eosinophilia syndrome (NARES), vasomotor rhinitis, gustatory rhinitis (vagally mediated), hormonal rhinitis (e.g., related to pregnancy and hypothyroidism), rhinitis medicamentosa (e.g., topical decongestants; antihypertensives and oral contraceptives), anatomic rhinitis (e.g., deviated septum, choanal atresia, adenoid hypertrophy, foreign body, nasal tumor), immotile cilia syndrome (ciliary dyskinesis), granulomatous rhinitis (e.g., Wegener's granulomatosis, sarcoidosis), and atrophic rhinitis (colonization with *Klebsiella ozaenae*).

One must also consider cerebrospinal fluid leak or nasal polyps. Nasal polyps often occur in common with allergic rhinitis, but not necessarily a causal relationship, and may not respond to medications.

A careful history and physical examination usually can determine the cause of the rhinitis. Historical clues to diagnosis include environmental exposures, occupational exposure, personal and family history of allergies, additional past medical history (hypothyroidism, pregnancy, sarcoidosis), recent sick contacts, and medication usage (>5 days of taking nasal sympathomimetics). Physical clues may include "allergic shiners" (dark circles under eyes); pale, bluish boggy turbinates; and cobblestoning in posterior pharynx (allergic rhinitis) versus erythematous turbinates (rhinitis medicamentosa, infectious, or vasomotor rhinitis).

A. Allergic rhinitis is by far the most common type of rhinitis. Estimates suggest 9%–40% of the U.S. population have some degree of allergic rhinitis. In 80% of cases, allergic rhinitis develops by age 20 years. Incidence wanes as we age, and it is much less common in the geriatric population. History of eczema and family history of atopy may help in the diagnosis. Symptoms occur in individuals who produce an immunoglobulin E (IgE)–mediated response to particular allergens. Allergens may be one or many, seasonal or perennial. Common seasonal allergens are trees, grasses, and weeds. Common perennial allergens include dust mites, cockroaches, animal proteins, dander, and molds. Diagnosing occupational rhinitis can be challenging because symptoms may occur several hours after exposure. Additionally, with chronic exposure, symptoms may not improve on weekends, requiring longer periods of avoidance. With occupational rhinitis, patients typically present with concomitant occupational asthma. Physical examination may reveal allergic shiners; injected conjunctivae; clear nasal discharge; pale, bluish boggy turbinates; and cobblestoning in the posterior pharynx. Allergen avoidance is of utmost importance. Maintaining indoor humidity to ≤50% to limit house dust mite and mold growth may be helpful. First-line treatment of allergic rhinitis is topical intranasal steroids. Additional treatment choices include oral or intranasal antihistamines as a good second choice. Intranasal cromolyn started several weeks prior to allergy season may be effective, leukotriene inhibitors alone or in conjunction with antihistamines are useful, and oral decongestants can be effective. Topical decongestants must be used sparingly because of the development of tachyphylaxis after 3–7 days of use. With prolonged use a resulting rebound nasal congestion and rhinitis medicamentosa develop. Hypertonic saline rinsing of the nares can be used for additional benefit in both acute and chronic rhinosinusitis. If medical maneuvers fail, skin testing and immunotherapy remain an option. Perennial allergic rhinitis appears to be a predisposing factor for acute bacterial rhinosinusitis by causing ostial obstruction.

B. NARES accounts for 15%–20% of patients with rhinitis. It is characterized by perennial symptoms of nasal congestion, nasal itching, rhinorrhea, hyposmia, and sneezing. These symptoms are milder than in patients with perennial allergic rhinitis, but they are still bothersome. Nasal secretions contain 25% eosinophils on smear. IgE antibodies to inhalant allergens are usually absent. Some researchers believe this is a precursor to the triad of asthma, nasal polyposis, and aspirin allergy. The most useful medications have proved to be topical nasal steroids, and if polyps are present, leukotriene inhibitors have also been shown to be helpful.

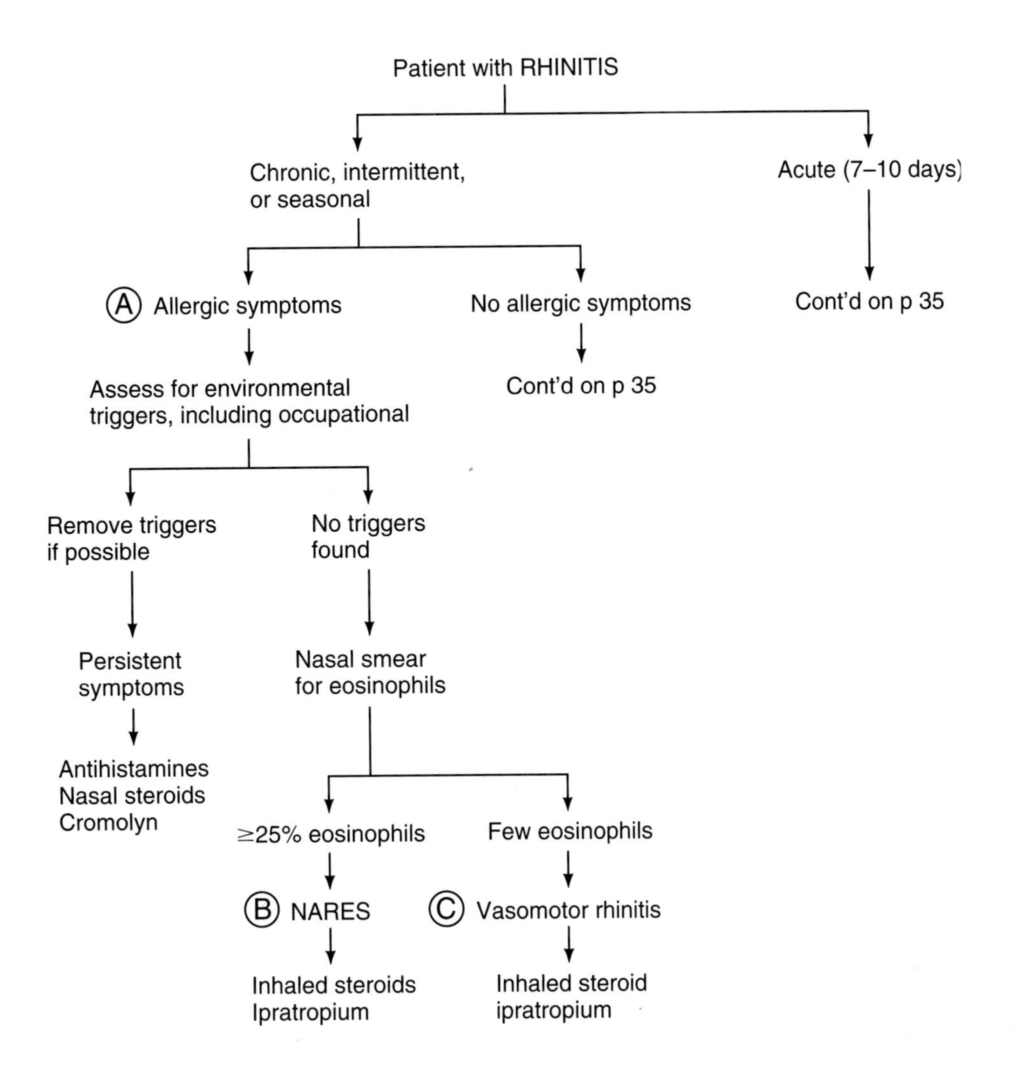

C. *Vasomotor rhinitis* (idiopathic rhinitis) is an umbrella term for many types of nonallergic rhinitis, including gustatory and hormonal rhinitis. Patients with vasomotor rhinitis complain of chronic nasal congestion with or without persistent rhinorrhea, exacerbated by cold air, strong odors, stress, or inhaled irritants. For the most part, vasomotor rhinitis is believed to result from autonomic dysfunction in the nose where the parasympathetic system dominates, resulting in vasodilation and edema of the nasal vasculature. Idiopathic rhinitis is a diagnosis of exclusion. Allergy skin testing is negative. Nasal steroids are useful, and if rhinorrhea is a major factor, ipratropium can be effective.

(Continued on p 34)

D. Imaging (CT scan of sinuses) should be limited to those patients who have persistent symptoms or if symptoms recur. Recurrent rhinosinusitis may also indicate an underlying process such as nasal polyps, other anatomic abnormalities, ciliary dysfunction, cystic fibrosis, immune deficiency, sarcoidosis, Wegener's granulomatosis, or relapsing polychondritis. Last, atrophic rhinitis is a syndrome of progressive atrophy of the nasal mucosa in the elderly debilitated population. Patients report a persistent foul odor that is a result of nasal mucosal colonization with *Klebsiella ozaenae*. These patients respond best to nasal irrigation.

E. Prolonged use of intranasal decongestants can result in rebound congestion (rhinitis medicamentosa). The restoration of normal nasal function may take up to 21 days after withdrawal of the sympathomimetics. Additionally, numerous medications can cause rhinitis, including antihypertensives such as angiotensin-converting enzyme inhibitors, reserpine, phentolamine, methyldopa, and beta blockers; chlorpromazine; gabapentin; penicillamine; aspirin; NSAIDs; exogenous estrogens; and oral contraceptives. The use of intranasal cocaine can cause these symptoms as well.

F. Infectious rhinitis can be caused by both viruses and bacteria (bacterial rhinitis), with the common cold being the most common cause of infectious rhinitis. Acute infectious rhinitis is often considered in conjunction with acute sinusitis. Symptoms statistically associated with culture-proven acute bacterial sinusitis include nasal congestion, purulent rhinorrhea, postnasal drip, facial or dental pain, and cough. The guidelines recommend that a diagnosis of acute bacterial rhinosinusitis (ABRS) is appropriate in patients who have had symptoms of a viral upper respiratory infection who have not improved after 10 days or worsen after 5–7 days. *Streptococcus pneumoniae* and *Haemophilus influenzae* account for 50% of rhinosinusitis bacterial isolates. *Moraxella catarrhalis*, other streptococcal species, *Staphylococcus aureus*, and anaerobic bacteria each account for a small proportion of cases. Of symptomatic patients, 30% have negative bacterial cultures, suggesting either viral or allergic disease. Because it is not possible to predict which cases of ABRS will resolve spontaneously, the use of an antimicrobial is recommended.

Prior antibiotic use is a major risk factor for infection with antimicrobial-resistant strains. For patients with mild disease who have not received antibiotics in the prior 4–6 weeks, initial therapy should include amoxicillin-clavulanate, amoxicillin, cefpodoxime, cefuroxime, or cefdinir. Fluoroquinolones or high-dose amoxicillin-clavulanate is recommended as first-line therapy for patients with mild disease who have had recent antibiotics or for patients with moderate disease. Treatment with a macrolide after treatment failure with amoxicillin or a cephalosporin will result in a second treatment failure in about 60% of cases as a result of high rates of resistance to macrolides in penicillin-resistant *S. pneumoniae* and *H. influenzae*.

References

Becker B, Borum S, Nielsen K, et al. A time-dose study of the effect of topical ipratropium bromide on methacholine-induced rhinorrhoea in patients with perennial non-allergic rhinitis. Clin Otolaryngol 1997;22(2):132–134.

deShazo RD, Kemp SF. Rhinosinusitis. South Med J 2003;96(11): 1055–1060.

Dykewicz MS, Fineman S. Executive Summary of Joint Task Force Practice Parameters on Diagnosis and Management of Rhinitis. Ann Allergy Asthma Immunol 1998;81(5 Pt 2):463–468.

Dykewicz MS, Fineman S, Skoner DP, et al. Diagnosis and management of rhinitis: complete guidelines of the Joint Task Force on Practice Parameters in Allergy, Asthma and Immunology. American Academy of Allergy, Asthma, and Immunology. Ann Allergy Asthma Immunol 1998;81(5 Pt 2):478–518.

Meltzer EO, Hamilos DL, Hadley JA, et al. Rhinosinusitis: establishing definitions for clinical research and patient care. Otolarygol Head Neck Surg 2004;131(6):S1–62.

Poole MD, Portugal LG. Treatment of rhinosinusitis in the outpatient setting. Am J Med 2005;118(7A):455–505.

Tomooka LT, Murphy C, Davidson TM. Clinical study and literature review of nasal irrigation. Laryngoscope 2000;110(7):1189–1193.

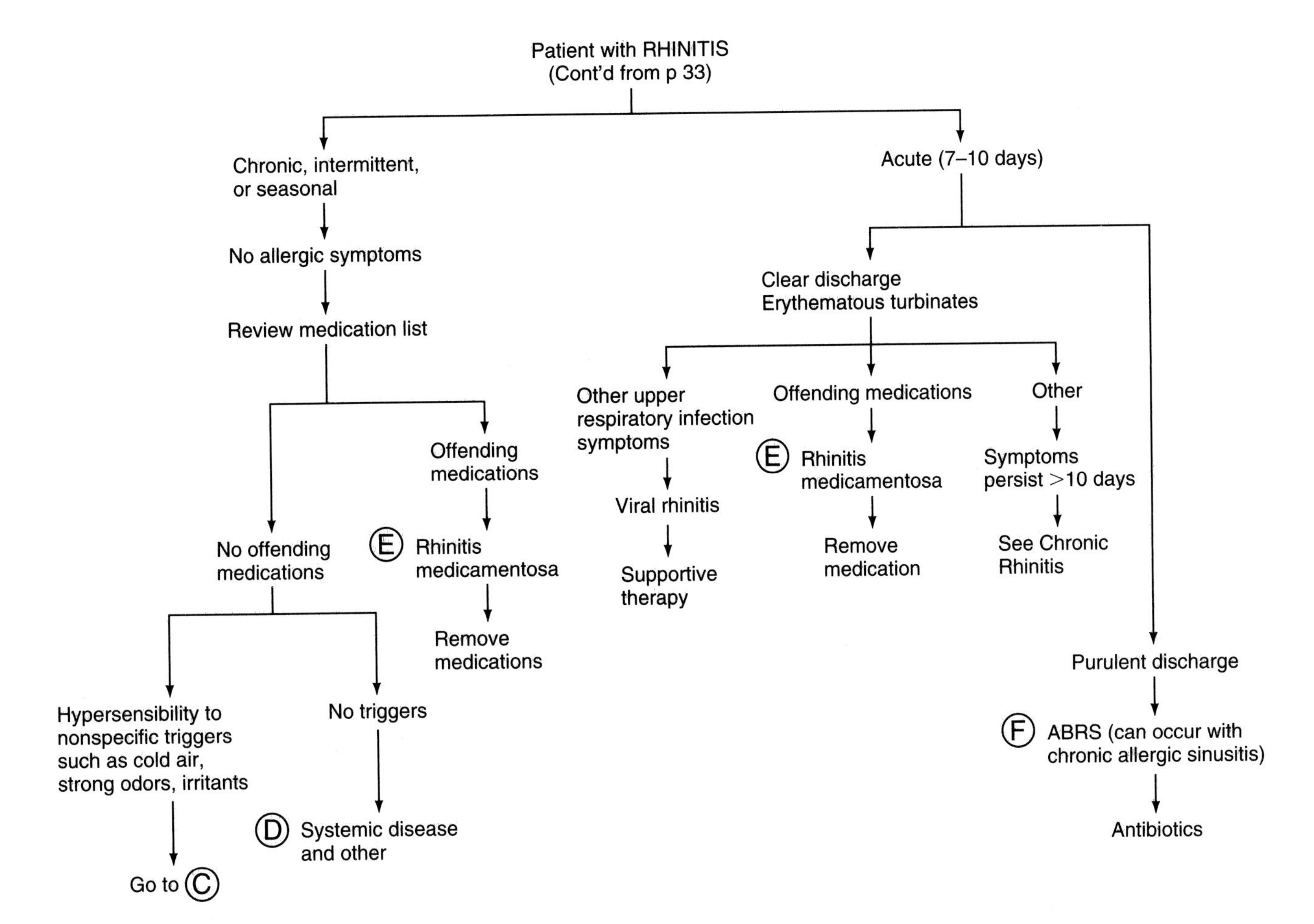
Patient with RHINITIS
(Cont'd from p 33)
Chronic, intermittent, or seasonal
No allergic symptoms
Review medication list
No offending medications
Offending medications
E Rhinitis medicamentosa
Remove medications
Hypersensibility to nonspecific triggers such as cold air, strong odors, irritants
Go to C
No triggers
D Systemic disease and other
Acute (7–10 days)
Clear discharge
Erythematous turbinates
Other upper respiratory infection symptoms
Viral rhinitis
Supportive therapy
Offending medications
E Rhinitis medicamentosa
Remove medication
Other
Symptoms persist >10 days
See Chronic Rhinitis
Purulent discharge
F ABRS (can occur with chronic allergic sinusitis)
Antibiotics

TINNITUS

Susan Fisk Sander, MD, and Theresa Rohr-Kirchgraber, MD

Tinnitus is a perceived sound that is not related to an external source. It usually is described by patients as a ringing, clicking, humming, or blowing sound. Most patients with tinnitus have an underlying otologic problem, most commonly hearing loss. It is postulated that tinnitus is the result of an imbalance between excitation and inhibition of auditory pathways. The imbalance may occur at any level, including cochlear hair cells, midbrain, and cortical central auditory pathways.

A. Diagnosing the cause of tinnitus requires a detailed history. Onset, duration, frequency, and localization are helpful in the evaluation for the underlying cause. Tinnitus may be caused by systemic disease, infection, metabolic abnormalities, medication exposure, or inflammatory conditions. Review exposure to aminoglycosides, loop diuretics, salicylates, quinine, antimalarials, NSAIDs, and any history of toxic exposure to heavy metals with the patient.

B. The physical examination should include a check of the blood pressure, a head and neck examination, and an auscultation for vascular bruits and heart murmurs.

C. If tinnitus is diffuse and not localized to either ear, consider encephalitis of the temporal lobe and psychiatric illnesses. Auditory hallucinations are noted primarily in patients with psychosis.

D. It occurs in objective (perceived by the examiner and patient) and subjective (heard only by the patient) forms.

E. Subjective tinnitus is more common than objective tinnitus, but diagnosis of the underlying cause is more difficult. The differential diagnoses of subjective tinnitus are medication and toxic exposure, metabolic abnormalities, pathologic condition in the peripheral (cochlear) or central (retrocochlear) pathways, anxiety, depression, and dental disorders. Metabolic abnormalities include hypothyroidism, hyperthyroidism, hyperlipidemia, anemia, and zinc deficiency. The initial workup of a patient should include a CBC, fasting glucose, triglycerides, cholesterol, and thyroid-stimulating hormone. Pathologic conditions of the ear associated with subjective tinnitus include otosclerosis, chronic suppurative otitis media, Meniere's disease, presbycusis, and noise-induced hearing loss.

F. Objective tinnitus is rare. Causes include acquired and congenital vascular malformations, neuromuscular disorders (palatal myoclonus, stapedius muscle spasm, and temporomandibular disorders), intracranial tumors, and structural defects of the ear. Objective tinnitus is of two types: vascular and mechanical.

G. Pulsatile tinnitus refers to nonexternal sounds that are amplified and synchronous with the patient's pulse. Benign intracranial hypertension, jugular bulb abnormalities, and aberrant carotid artery are included in the differential diagnoses. High-resolution CT of the temporal bones is needed when a retrotympanic mass is noted on examination. MRI and angiography are indicated for patients with normal otoscopic examination to evaluate for dural venous thromboses and to look for the empty sella and small ventricles associated with benign intracranial hypertension. Angiography is used when atherosclerotic carotid artery disease, fibromuscular dysplasia, and small dural arteriovenous (AV) malformations are suspected and the patient is a surgical candidate.

H. Stapedial muscle spasm–induced tinnitus is amplified with external noise and is intermittent. Stapedial muscle spasm is associated with facial nerve palsies, although it can occur without them. Division of the stapedius muscle and tensor tympani tendons is reserved for severe cases. Long-term use of benzodiazepines for stapedial muscle spasm is not recommended.

I. Palatal myoclonus is apparent on examination of the oral cavity. The tinnitus is thought to be generated from the opening and closing of the eustachian tube and the rubbing of mucosal surfaces. Electromyography (EMG) of the palatal muscles confirms the diagnosis. Treatment with benzodiazepines results in a decrease in anxiety.

J. Tinnitus associated with the patulous eustachian tube is synchronous with breathing. The patient may experience autophony (hearing of his or her own voice or breathing). Rapid weight loss and high estrogen states (e.g., use of birth control pills, postpartum) are associated with patulous eustachian tubes.

(Continued on page 38)

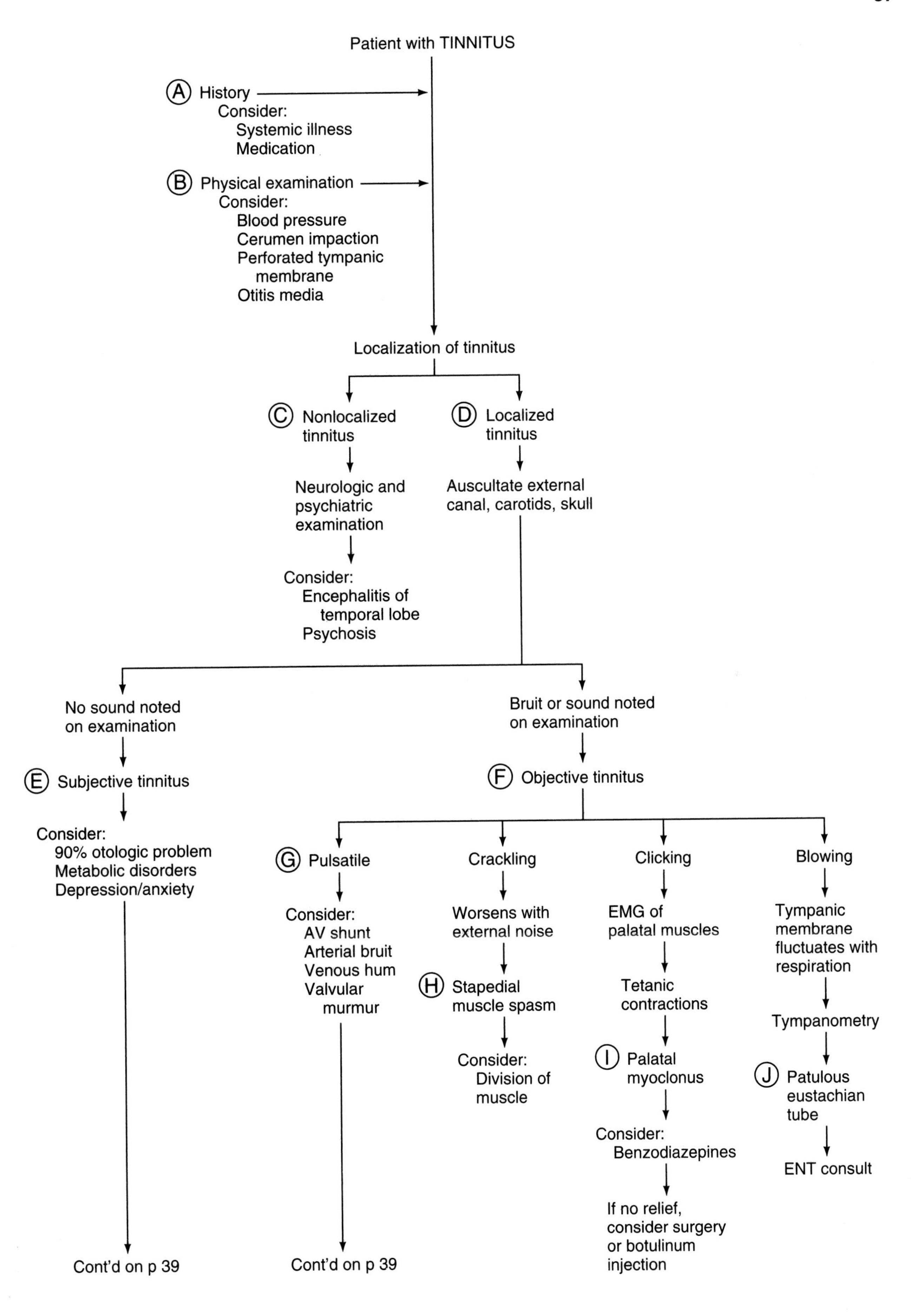
Patient with TINNITUS
(A) History
Consider:
Systemic illness
Medication
(B) Physical examination
Consider:
Blood pressure
Cerumen impaction
Perforated tympanic membrane
Otitis media
Localization of tinnitus
(C) Nonlocalized tinnitus
Neurologic and psychiatric examination
Consider:
Encephalitis of temporal lobe
Psychosis
(D) Localized tinnitus
Auscultate external canal, carotids, skull
No sound noted on examination
(E) Subjective tinnitus
Consider:
90% otologic problem
Metabolic disorders
Depression/anxiety
Cont'd on p 39
Bruit or sound noted on examination
(F) Objective tinnitus
(G) Pulsatile
Consider:
AV shunt
Arterial bruit
Venous hum
Valvular murmur
Cont'd on p 39
Crackling
Worsens with external noise
(H) Stapedial muscle spasm
Consider:
Division of muscle
Clicking
EMG of palatal muscles
Tetanic contractions
(I) Palatal myoclonus
Consider:
Benzodiazepines
If no relief, consider surgery or botulinum injection
Blowing
Tympanic membrane fluctuates with respiration
Tympanometry
(J) Patulous eustachian tube
ENT consult

K. Hearing evaluations include assessment of sensorineural hearing impedance testing and speech discrimination. These tests assist in localizing the otologic deficit. Nonvibratory tinnitus lesions can be attributed to defects in the cochlea (75%), CNS (18%), and middle ear (4%).

L. Peripheral tinnitus is associated with symmetric hearing loss, usually gradual in onset. Presbycusis is common with this condition. As hearing loss increases, tinnitus increases. Treating the hearing loss may result in a decrease in tinnitus because ambient background noise is amplified. In patients with hearing loss that is not treatable by a surgical procedure, a hearing aid may improve the tinnitus. Hearing aids and masking devices may be used together in patients who do not respond to hearing aids alone. Medications should be given to patients with severe disability.

M. Central tinnitus requires an evaluation for posterior fossa problems, including cerebellopontine angle tumors. The most common cerebellopontine tumor is the acoustic neuroma. Symptoms of an acoustic neuroma include unilateral hearing loss, tinnitus, and disequilibrium. Distinguishing Meniere's disease from acoustic neuromas is difficult clinically. Meniere's tinnitus is intermittent, whereas the tinnitus of acoustic neuroma is constant. Meniere's disease is associated with vertigo as distinguished from the disequilibrium of an acoustic neuroma. MRI with gadolinium contrast to assess for posterior masses is indicated for abnormal auditory brainstem response (ABR) tests. The sensitivity for acoustic neuromas <15 mm is greater with MRI with gadolinium contrast than with high-resolution CT. In patients with unilateral hearing loss and normal ABR tests, surveillance is required at 6 months and 1 year to assess for progression of symptoms. ENT referrals are indicated for all patients with asymmetric hearing loss. Treatment for tumors depends on the size, location, and the patient's preoperative state.

N. Conductive hearing loss requires evaluation for a pathologic condition of the external and middle ear, malignancy, glomus tumor, and cholesteatoma. Early referral to ENT is recommended.

References

Crummer RW, Hassan GA. Diagnostic approach to tinnitus. Am J Family Physician 2004;69:120.

Dinces EA. Tinnitus UpToDate 206. www.uptodate.com.

Dobie RA, Sakai CS, Sullivan MD, et al. Antidepressant treatment of tinnitus patients: report of a randomized clinical trial and clinical prediction of benefit. Am Otol 1993;14:18.

House JW. Tinnitus. In Rakel RE, Bope ET, eds. Conn's Current Therapy.Philadelphia: WB Saunders, 2005:45.

Johnson RM, Brummett R, Scheuning A. Use of alprazolam for relief of tinnitus. Arch Otolaryngol Head Neck Surg 1993;119:842.

Marai K, Tyler RS, Harker LA, Stouffer JL. Review of pharmacologic treatment of tinnitus. Am J Otol 1992;13:454.

Schleuning AJ II. Management of the patient with tinnitus. Med Clin North Am 1991;75:1225.

Sismanis A, Smoker WRK. Pulsatile tinnitus: recent advances in diagnosis. Laryngoscope 1994;104:681.

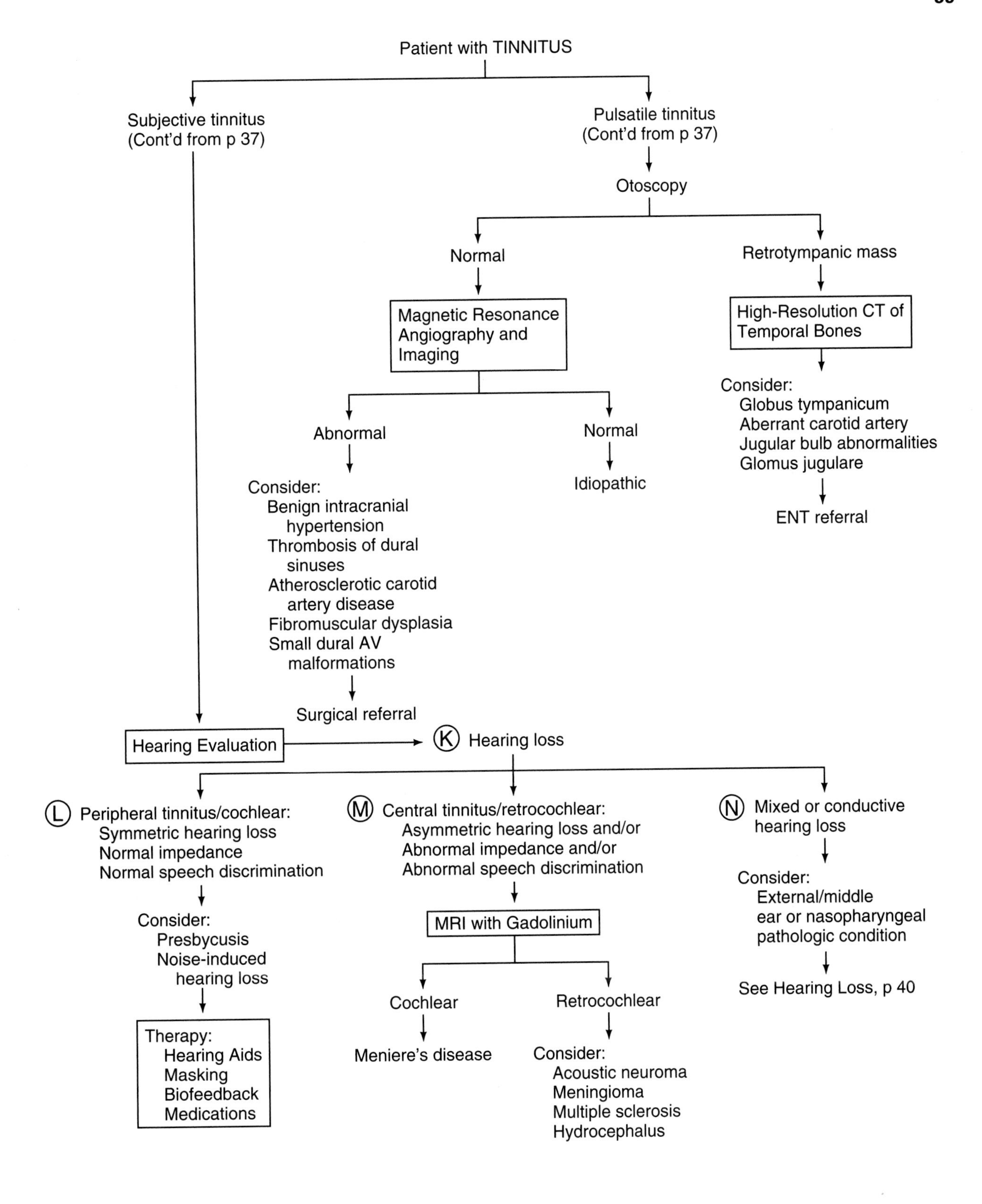
Patient with TINNITUS
Subjective tinnitus
(Cont'd from p 37)
Pulsatile tinnitus
(Cont'd from p 37)
Otoscopy
Normal
Retrotympanic mass
Magnetic Resonance Angiography and Imaging
High-Resolution CT of Temporal Bones
Abnormal
Normal
Consider:
Globus tympanicum
Aberrant carotid artery
Jugular bulb abnormalities
Glomus jugulare
ENT referral
Idiopathic
Consider:
Benign intracranial hypertension
Thrombosis of dural sinuses
Atherosclerotic carotid artery disease
Fibromuscular dysplasia
Small dural AV malformations
Surgical referral
Hearing Evaluation
K Hearing loss
L Peripheral tinnitus/cochlear:
Symmetric hearing loss
Normal impedance
Normal speech discrimination
Consider:
Presbycusis
Noise-induced hearing loss
Therapy:
Hearing Aids
Masking
Biofeedback
Medications
M Central tinnitus/retrocochlear:
Asymmetric hearing loss and/or
Abnormal impedance and/or
Abnormal speech discrimination
MRI with Gadolinium
Cochlear
Meniere's disease
Retrocochlear
Consider:
Acoustic neuroma
Meningioma
Multiple sclerosis
Hydrocephalus
N Mixed or conductive hearing loss
Consider:
External/middle ear or nasopharyngeal pathologic condition
See Hearing Loss, p 40

HEARING LOSS

Susan Fisk Sander, MD, and Theresa Rohr-Kirchgraber, MD

More than 28 million Americans have some form of hearing loss. Approximately 50% of the 16 million Americans who are hearing impaired are >65 years old. Hearing loss can be acute, gradual, permanent, or temporary and requires a thorough history and physical examination. Hearing loss can be conductive when sound is impeded through the external ear, middle ear, or both; sensorineural with problems in the cochlea or neural pathway to the auditory cortex; or mixed.

A. History should include questions regarding physical trauma; barotrauma; deafness; exposure to ototoxins; medications; recent upper respiratory infection; and associated symptoms such as otalgia, tinnitus, or vertigo.

B. Examination of the ear includes otoscopy to look for otitis externa, foreign body, cerumen impaction, canal cholesteatoma, exostosis (osteochondroma), tympanic membrane perforation, and effusions (hemorrhagic, purulent, or serous). Perform Weber's test by placing a tuning fork on the central forehead. Lateralization of the sound to one ear is consistent with either a conductive defect of the affected ear or a sensorineural defect of the opposite ear. No lateralization indicates either a normal result or bilaterally symmetric sensorineural or conductive defects. Perform Rinne's test by placing the handle of a vibrating tuning fork against the mastoid process and having the patient signal when he or she can no longer hear it. Then hold the vibrating tines near the ear and have the patient signal when sound is no longer audible. Normally air conduction persists twice as long as bone conduction but not in a conductive hearing loss.

C. Hearing evaluation includes audiography (pure tone testing of air and bone thresholds), speech reception and discrimination, and acoustic impedance. In sensorineural hearing loss (SNHL) both air and bone thresholds are depressed compared with normal. In conductive hearing loss the bone conduction threshold is greater than air conduction thresholds. In mixed deficits air conduction, both are depressed.

D. SNHL is a lesion in the organ of Corti or in the central pathways, including the eighth nerve and auditory cortex. It may be the result of an inherited disorder or congenital abnormality, or it may be an acquired deficit.

E. Hereditary loss can be present at birth or can present when the patient is a young adult. Family history is key.

F. Congenital hearing loss occurs at or shortly after birth. It may result from viral infections during pregnancy (e.g., cytomegalovirus [CMV], rubella, and mumps), maternal hypothyroidism, birth anoxia, exposure to fetal ototoxins, Rh incompatibility, or other causes. It also may occur as a hereditary autosomal disorder.

G. Sudden-onset SNHL is of variable severity and develops in <3 days. Profound loss is associated with poor prognosis for recovery.

H. Trauma and sudden loss suggest a temporal fracture. A longitudinal fracture results in middle ear damage and is associated with a conductive hearing loss. Transverse fracture may damage the facial nerve and labyrinth and result in a sensorineural deficit. Both require a referral to ENT (an ear, nose, and throat specialist). Concussion alone may result in a temporary SNHL as a result of acoustic trauma.

I. Treatment of sudden-onset SNHL is directed at the underlying disorder. In the past when the cause was not found, bed rest, head elevation, avoidance of loud noise, and steroids were prescribed. Controlled studies of steroid therapy for idiopathic sudden-onset hearing loss show a statistically significant improvement in hearing with steroids (up to 44% response). Sudden idiopathic sensorineural hearing loss is an urgent situation and requires consultation. Heavy lifting may result in a leak of inner ear fluid from a membranous rupture at the oval or round windows, leading to hearing loss and vestibular symptoms. Refer to ENT for repair.

J. Infectious causes for sudden onset of SNHL include suppurative labyrinthitis from otitis media or mastoiditis and viral infections (mumps, CMV, Epstein-Barr virus, rubella, rubeola, herpes zoster, and herpes simplex).

K. Vascular causes include vertebrobasilar insufficiency, embolism, hypercoagulable states, and basilar migraines.

L. Some medications cause sudden-onset hearing loss. Hearing loss from loop diuretics and aminoglycosides is usually reversible. Salicylate withdrawal results in improved hearing in most patients.

(Continued on page 42)

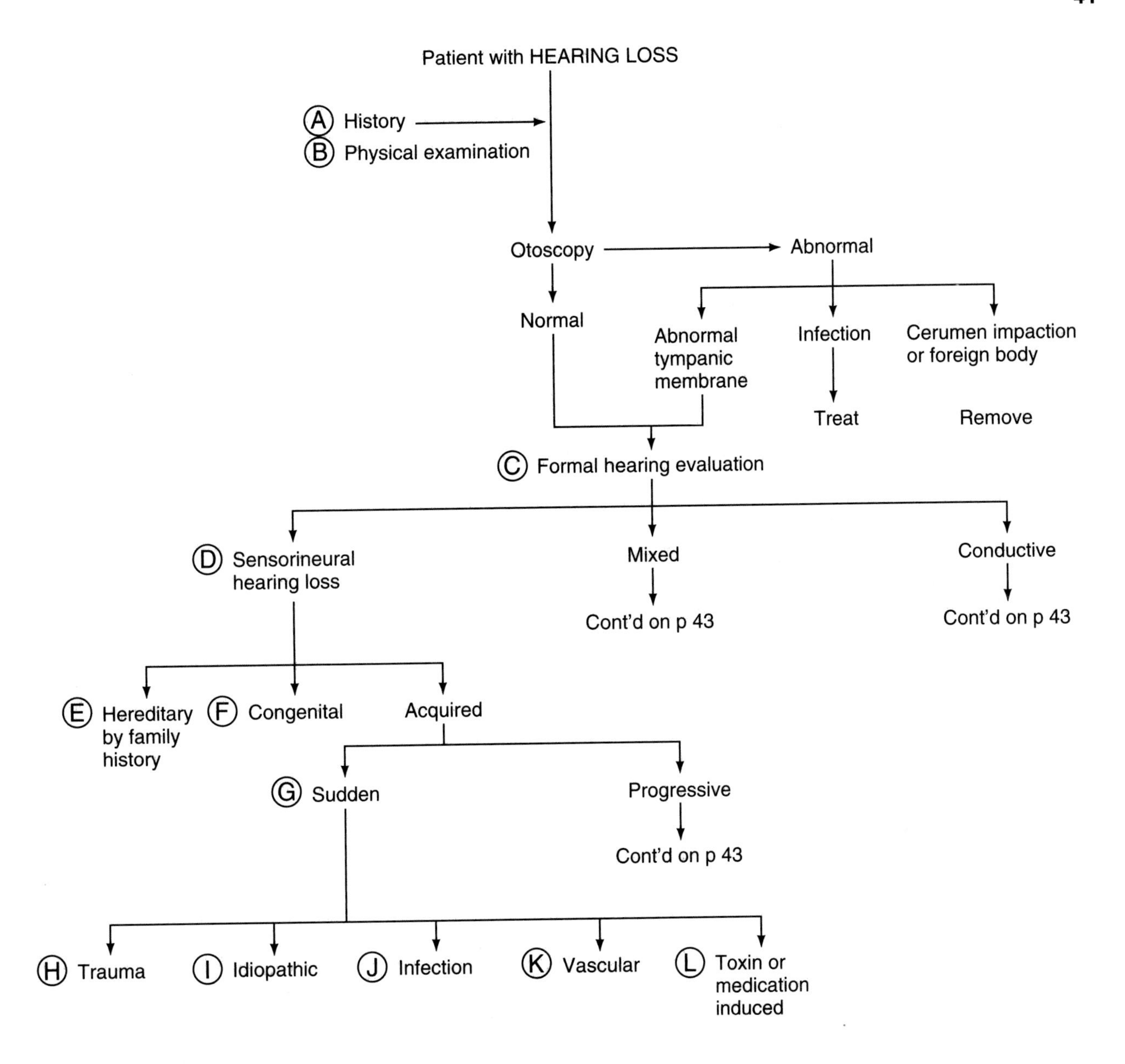
Patient with HEARING LOSS
(A) History
(B) Physical examination
Otoscopy
Abnormal
Normal
Abnormal tympanic membrane
Infection
Cerumen impaction or foreign body
Treat
Remove
(C) Formal hearing evaluation
(D) Sensorineural hearing loss
Mixed
Conductive
Cont'd on p 43
Cont'd on p 43
(E) Hereditary by family history
(F) Congenital
Acquired
(G) Sudden
Progressive
Cont'd on p 43
(H) Trauma
(I) Idiopathic
(J) Infection
(K) Vascular
(L) Toxin or medication induced

M. Acquired causes include metabolic disorders, vascular insufficiency, autoimmune disease, infection, degenerative disorder, and neoplasm. Although the most common cause of hearing loss in the elderly is presbycusis, a symmetric, progressive decrease in hearing, it is a diagnosis of exclusion. Workup for bilateral progressive SNHL includes an evaluation for diabetes mellitus, hyperthyroidism and hypothyroidism, anemia, hyperlipidemia, renal disease, infection, and syphilis. Review exposures to medications that are commonly known to cause hearing loss such as aminoglycosides, loop diuretics, and salicylates and others such as quinine, chloroquine, and antineoplastics such as cisplatinum. Autoimmune SNHL without systemic symptoms has occurred and the evaluation should include ANCA (antineutrophil cytoplasmic antibody); ANA; RF (rheumatoid factor); antibodies to cyclic citrullinated peptides (anti-CCP); antibodies to-double-stranded DNA; antibodies to extractable nuclear antigens (i.e., anti-Smith, anti-Ro/SSA, anti-La/SSB, and anti-RNP); cryoglobulins; and complement components (C3 and C4) to look for Cogan's syndrome, giant cell arteritis, systemic lupus erythematosus (SLE), polyarteritis nodosum, and Wegner's granulomatosis. Neoplasms such as acoustic neuromas and metastatic carcinoma of the breast, prostate, and kidney can result in SNHL. Acoustic neuromas can present with bilateral hearing loss in up to 22% of the cases. Diagnosis is by MRI with contrast. Degenerative disorders include presbycusis, noise-induced hearing loss, and Meniere's disease.

Therapy is aimed at the underlying cause: removal of the offending drug; treatment of the autoimmune disorder; a trial of steroids of idiopathic sudden SNHL; surgery, radiation, or chemotherapy for a neoplasm; surgical repair of a membrane rupture; and antibiotics and steroids for syphilis. Acoustic trauma requires surgical evaluation, whereas hearing aids are the treatment of choice for presbycusis and disorders not improved by medical or surgical intervention.

N. Unilateral hearing loss is more commonly associated with trauma, which may result from temporal bone injuries or rupture of the membranes with perilymph leaking into the middle ear. The trauma may be as mild as a sneeze, straining, or lifting. Meniere's disease may also cause a unilateral hearing loss. Progressive SNHL that is unilateral or asymmetric requires auditory brainstem response (ABR) testing to localize abnormalities in the retro cochlear lesion. MRI has a higher sensitivity of acoustic neuromas <15 mm than does a high-resolution CT scan. Posterior fossa meningioma and primary cholesteatoma are other masses that cause progressive SNHL in the retrocochlear area. Treatment of acoustic neuromas depends on the size of the tumor, cranial nerve involvement, and the patient's preoperative state. Radiation therapy is used for patients who are not surgical candidates. If ABR testing does not reveal an abnormality, continue surveillance of patients with asymmetric SNHL. Consider MRI.

O. Patients with chronic otitis media, tuberculosis, otosclerosis, skull fractures, and penetrating injury of the ear; Wegener's granulomatosis; and squamous cell carcinoma all have been observed to have a mixed conductive and sensorineural deficit in advanced disease.

P. Conductive hearing loss, defined as a lesion involving the outer and middle ear to the level of the oval window, results from mechanical disruption of the transmitted sound through the external auditory canal, tympanic membrane, and ossicle.

Q. Direct observation of the external canal during the examination allows evaluation of conditions causing mechanical disruption: atresias of the external canal, cerumen impaction, exostosis, foreign bodies, canal cholesteatoma, external otitis, tympanic membrane perforation or sclerosis, effusions, and ossicular damage. Multiple perforations of the tympanic membrane suggest tuberculous infection of the middle ear. Barotrauma resulting from unequal air pressure in the external auditory canal can result in an effusion and a temporary conductive loss.

R. Acoustic stapedius reflex testing for fixation of the stapedius is part of the evaluation of conductive hearing loss. Otosclerosis, the most common congenital form of conductive hearing loss, is diagnosed with this test and treated with stapedectomy.

S. Cholesteatoma, glomus tumor, and nasopharyngeal malignancies (squamous cell carcinoma, adenocarcinomas, and basal cell carcinomas) can produce conductive hearing loss. High-resolution CT of the temporal bones is the study of choice to evaluate masses in the middle ear. Therapy of the underlying problem may improve the conductive hearing loss: removal of the foreign body or cerumen, antituberculous drugs, tympanoplasty, ossiculoplasty, stapedectomy, and removal of excessive cartilage (exostosis). Treatments of masses within the middle ear depend on the site, pathologic condition, and preoperative evaluation of the patient. Referral to ENT is required.

References

Arts HA. Differential diagnosis of sensorineural hearing loss. In Cummings CW, Fredrickson JM, Harker LA, et al, eds. Otolaryngology: Head and Neck Surgery, 4th ed. St. Louis: Mosby, 1998.

Backous D, Niparko J. Differential diagnosis of conductive hearing loss. In Cummings CW, Fredrickson JM, Harker LA, et al, eds. Otolaryngology: Head and Neck Surgery, 4th ed. St. Louis: Mosby, 1998.

Grandis JR, Hirsch BE, Wagener MM. Treatment of idiopathic sudden sensorineural hearing loss. Am J Otol 1993;1:183.

Isaacson JE, Vora NM. Differential diagnosis of hearing loss. Am Fam Physician 2003;68:1125.

Nadol JB. Hearing loss. N Engl J Med 1993;329:1092.

Shikowitz MJ. Sudden sensorineural hearing loss. Med Clin North Am 1991;75:1239.

Weber PC. Etiology of hearing loss in adults. Up-To-Date 2006;13:3.

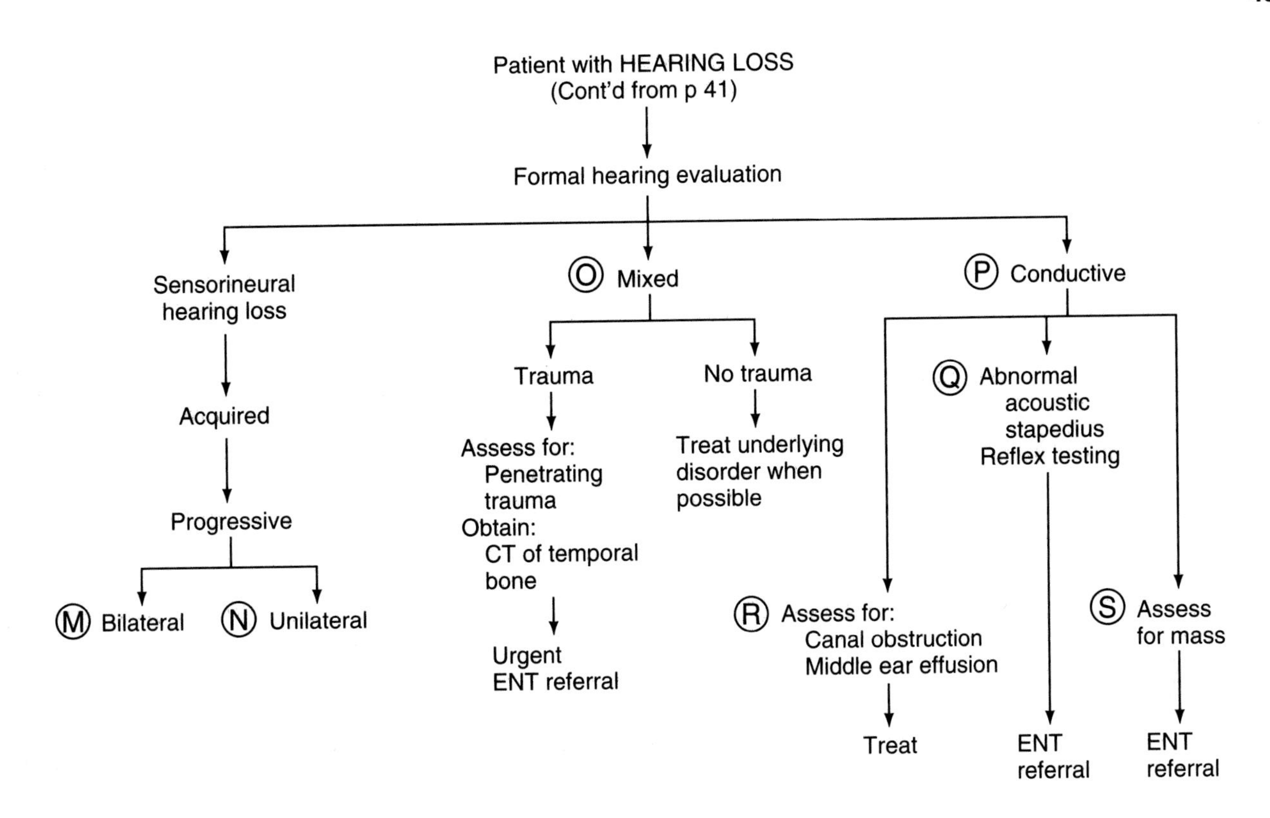
Patient with HEARING LOSS
(Cont'd from p 41)
Formal hearing evaluation
Sensorineural hearing loss
Acquired
Progressive
M Bilateral
N Unilateral
O Mixed
Trauma
Assess for: Penetrating trauma
Obtain: CT of temporal bone
Urgent ENT referral
No trauma
Treat underlying disorder when possible
P Conductive
Q Abnormal acoustic stapedius Reflex testing
ENT referral
R Assess for: Canal obstruction Middle ear effusion
Treat
S Assess for mass
ENT referral

PREOPERATIVE EVALUATION

Anthony Karabanow, MD

Several points deserve immediate mention. First, patients who require emergent surgery clearly do not benefit from the delay necessary for preoperative evaluation. Second, preoperative evaluation does not "clear" a patient for surgery and such terminology should be avoided. Preoperative evaluation provides an assessment of medical risk and the identification of measures to reduce that risk. Third, consultants need to have a clear understanding of their role in patient care. Formally speaking, consultants generate suggestions only and do not write orders. However, it is not uncommon for surgeons to expect "co-management" rather than formal consultation. In the latter, medical consultants are expected to assume responsibility for all nonsurgical matters relating to patient care.

A. Preoperative evaluation means an assessment of cardiac risk. The goal of perioperative cardiac risk assessment is to identify those patients with unstable cardiac disease for whom further study and treatment warrants the risk of surgical delay. The newest guidelines from the American College of Cardiology are summarized in the algorithm. Stress testing is unnecessary in patients with adequate functional capacity (e.g., can walk up a flight of stairs). Moreover, such testing should not be recommended unless patients are willing to postpone surgery so as to proceed with cardiac revascularization. Such delay may itself be harmful in the patient who is bedridden and thus at risk for decubitus ulcers, aspiration pneumonia, deep vein thrombosis (DVT), and functional decline. The use of coronary stents mandates postoperative use of antiplatelet agents. Cessation of these agents risks in-stent restenosis. Continuation of these agents risks perioperative bleeding. Discuss these issues with patients and their families before ordering a stress test. The same American College of Cardiology guidelines also state that there is no indication for routine preoperative echocardiography. An echocardiogram is reserved for patients whose clinical presentation is worrisome for undiagnosed heart failure.

   Recent data help guide the consultant when faced with a positive stress test result in the preoperative period. The Coronary Artery Revascularization Prophylaxis (CARP) trial indicated that patients with stable coronary disease do not benefit from preoperative revascularization. Exclusion criteria to this study included those with >50% left main disease, an ejection fraction <20%, and severe aortic stenosis. This study reinforces the concept that preoperative patients fall under the same guidelines for cardiac revascularization as do all other patients.

   Beta blockers are often routinely prescribed to reduce perioperative cardiac risk. However, a 2005 study suggests that only those at high risk benefit from beta blockers. Those at moderate risk did not benefit, and those at low risk actually experienced increased mortality. Thus, beta blockers are recommended only in patients with established coronary artery disease (CAD) or two or more of the following risk factors: congestive heart failure (CHF), CAD, cardiovascular accident (CVA), diastolic murmur (DM), or Cardiac Risk Index (CRI) (Cr >2) who are undergoing vascular or intermediate-risk (intrathoracic, intraperitoneal, orthopedic) surgery.

B. Postoperative pulmonary complications may occur more frequently than cardiac events. Such events include atelectasis, bronchospasm, pneumonia, prolonged mechanical ventilation, and exacerbation of underlying lung disease. Arozullah and colleagues have published a respiratory failure index that predicts the risk of respiratory failure based on the type of surgery, patient risk factors, and functional status. However, it is not surprising that patients with established lung disease are at higher risk for perioperative pulmonary complications. The role of the consultant is to identify patients with reversible pulmonary pathology who would benefit from preoperative intervention. Such patients may require pulmonary evaluation via chest x-ray, pulmonary function testing, and possibly ABG assessment. The results of such testing can then be used to determine disease-specific therapy, which, in turn, minimizes postoperative complications. Those with previously identified pulmonary pathology and baseline symptomatology do not require investigation or change in management. Patients undergoing lung resection or who are likely to have a prolonged period of mechanical ventilation benefit from early pulmonology input. All current smokers should be advised to discontinue tobacco use (preferably at least 2 months prior to surgery).

   Endocrine disorders that are frequently encountered during preoperative evaluation include diabetes, thyroid disease, and adrenal insufficiency. The American Diabetes Association has endorsed the following goals for glycemic control in hospitalized patients: 90 to 130 preprandial blood sugars and <180 postprandial blood sugars. However, the bulk of the data in favor of tight blood sugar control in hospitalized patients comes from studies performed in the intensive

(Continued on page 46)

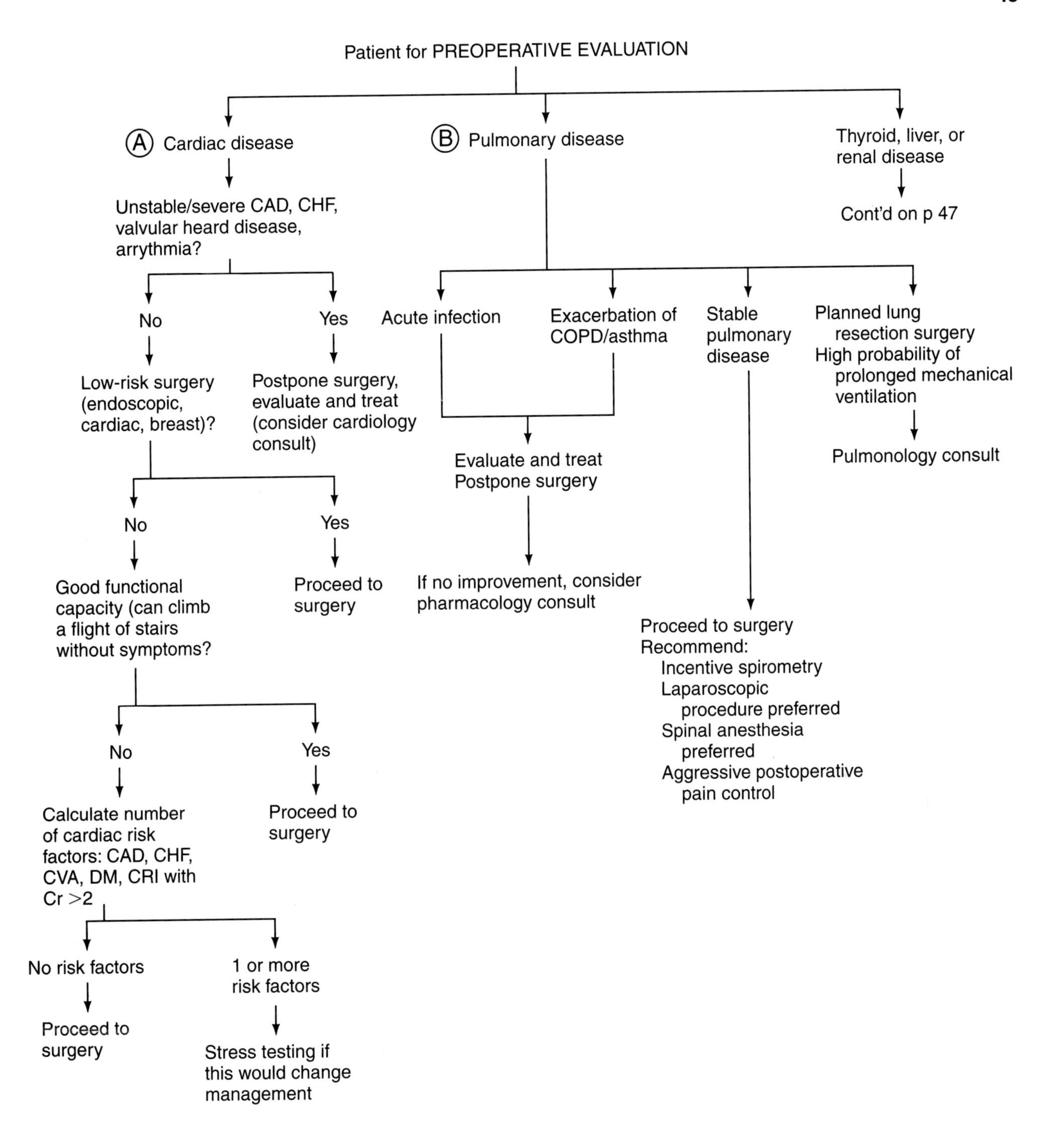

Patient for PREOPERATIVE EVALUATION
A Cardiac disease
B Pulmonary disease
Thyroid, liver, or renal disease
Cont'd on p 47
Unstable/severe CAD, CHF, valvular heard disease, arrythmia?
No
Yes
Low-risk surgery (endoscopic, cardiac, breast)?
Postpone surgery, evaluate and treat (consider cardiology consult)
No
Yes
Good functional capacity (can climb a flight of stairs without symptoms?
Proceed to surgery
No
Yes
Calculate number of cardiac risk factors: CAD, CHF, CVA, DM, CRI with Cr >2
Proceed to surgery
No risk factors
1 or more risk factors
Proceed to surgery
Stress testing if this would change management
Acute infection
Exacerbation of COPD/asthma
Stable pulmonary disease
Planned lung resection surgery
High probability of prolonged mechanical ventilation
Pulmonology consult
Evaluate and treat
Postpone surgery
If no improvement, consider pharmacology consult
Proceed to surgery
Recommend:
Incentive spirometry
Laparoscopic procedure preferred
Spinal anesthesia preferred
Aggressive postoperative pain control

care and critical care unit settings. Consultants need to be aware that hypoglycemia may be a greater threat than hyperglycemia in the acute setting of hospitalization. Nonetheless, there are convincing data that random blood sugars should be maintained at <200. Metformin should be discontinued in all hospitalized patients because of the increased risk of hypovolemia, hypoxia, and acute renal failure–induced lactic acidosis in this setting.

C. The interpretation of thyroid tests is problematic in acutely ill, hospitalized patients. Thus, such testing is discouraged unless there is a high suspicion of thyroid disease. The available data suggest that there is minimal additional surgical risk in those with mild or moderate hypothyroidism. Surgery in those with severe hypothyroidism (i.e., thyroxine level <1 μg/dl) risks precipitating myxedema coma. Unmanaged hyperthyroidism carries a theoretical risk of thyroid storm during surgery. Surgery should be postponed in such patients. If surgery must be performed, then early endocrinology input is advised.

Patients with known adrenal insufficiency and those taking chronic high-dose steroids (i.e., >20 mg of prednisone daily for >3 weeks) are at risk of adrenal crisis during the perioperative period. Such patients should receive stress dose steroids (i.e., 100 mg hydrocortisone IV every 8 hours). This regimen should be initiated prior to surgery and as soon as possible in patients with significant surgical illness.

D. Patients with liver disease are at risk both from surgical procedures and from anesthesia. Elective surgery is considered contraindicated in those with acute hepatitis (both viral and alcoholic), severe chronic hepatitis, and advanced cirrhosis (i.e., Child-Pugh class C) as a result of unacceptably high rates of perioperative mortality. Patients with stable liver disease may proceed to surgery after careful assessment for coagulopathy, electrolyte abnormalities, and encephalopathy.

E. When managing patients with renal failure, because thromboembolism is a significant cause of avoidable hospital morbidity and mortality, consultants should routinely recommend DVT prophylaxis with a heparinoid agent (i.e., unfractionated or low molecular weight heparin). Those at particularly high risk for DVT (e.g., spinal cord injury or general surgery in those with multiple risk factors) benefit from both pharmacologic and nonpharmacologic measures. Nonpharmacologic measures to reduce the incidence of DVT include graduated compression stockings and intermittent pneumatic compression. Note that aspirin alone is considered insufficient thromboprophylaxis for any category of surgical patient.

Patients should be routinely asked about alcohol intake and any prior symptoms of alcohol withdrawal. Those deemed at risk should be placed on an alcohol withdrawal pathway. Such pathways use either symptom-driven scales or fixed-schedule dosing for benzodiazepine administration.

References

Arozullah AM, Daley J, Henderson WG, et al. Multifactorial risk index for predicting postoperative respiratory failure in men after major noncardiac surgery. The National Veterans Administration Surgical Quality Improvement Program. Ann Surg 2000;232:242.

Clement S, Braithwaite SS, Magee MF, et al. Management of diabetes and hyperglycemia in hospitals. Diabetes Care 2004;27(2):553–591.

Fleisher LA, Beckman JA, Brown KA. ACC/AHA 2007 Guidelines on Perioperative Cardiovascular Evaluation and Care for Noncardiac Surgery: Executive Summary. A Report of the American College of Cardiology/American Heart Association Task Force on Practice Guidelines. J Am Coll Cardiol 2007;50:e159–241.

Geerts WH, Pineo GF, Heit JA, et al. Prevention of venous thromboembolism: the Seventh ACCP Conference on Antithrombotic and Thrombolytic Therapy. Chest 2004;126:338S–400S.

Lindenauer PK, Pekow P, Wang K, et al. Perioperative beta-blocker therapy and mortality after major noncardiac surgery. N Engl J Med 2005;353:349–361.

McFalls EO, Ward HB, Moritz TE, et al. Coronary-artery revascularization before elective major vascular surgery. N Engl J Med 2004;351: 2795–2804.

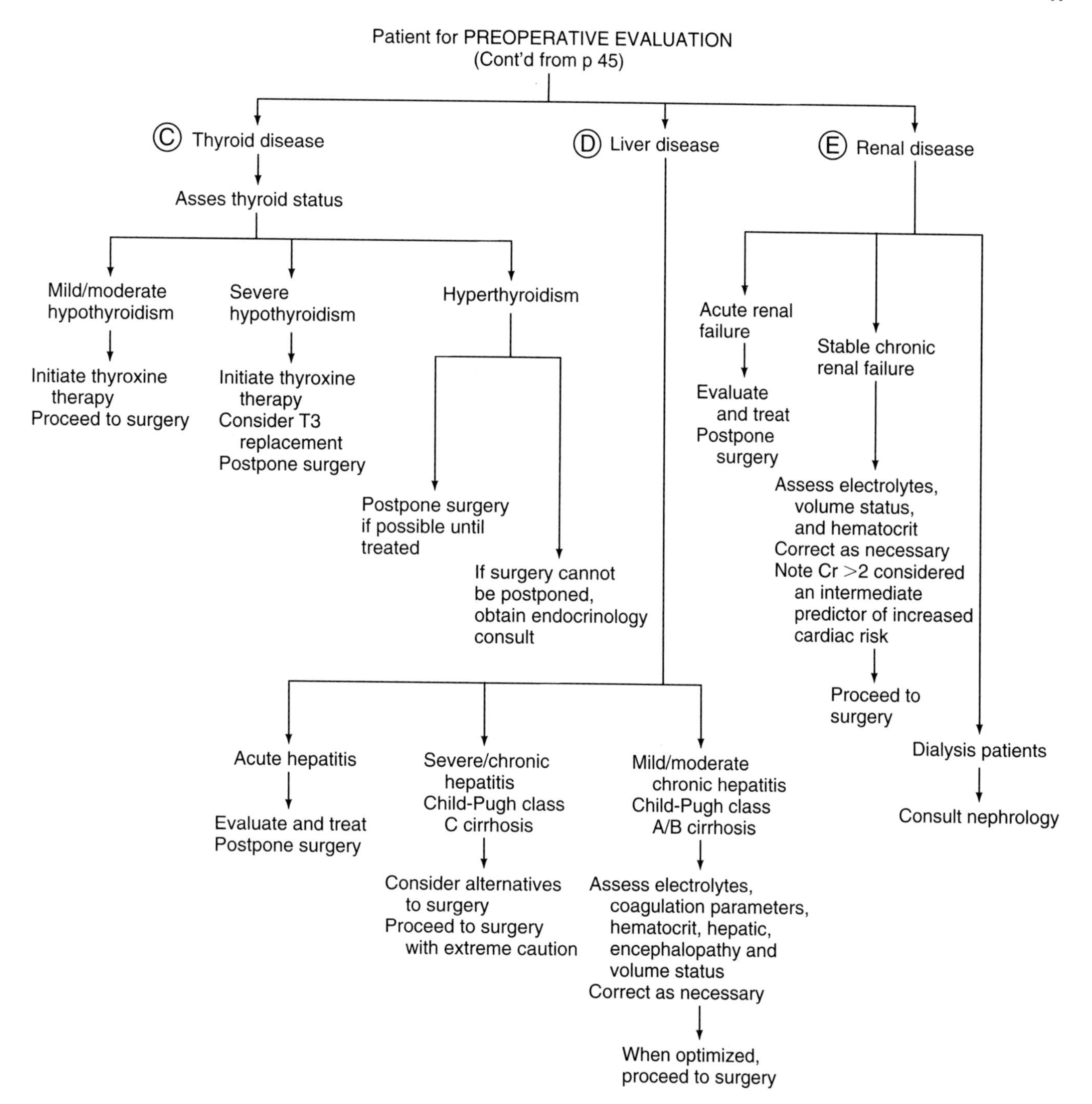
Patient for PREOPERATIVE EVALUATION
(Cont'd from p 45)
C Thyroid disease
Asses thyroid status
Mild/moderate hypothyroidism
Initiate thyroxine therapy
Proceed to surgery
Severe hypothyroidism
Initiate thyroxine therapy
Consider T3 replacement
Postpone surgery
Hyperthyroidism
Postpone surgery if possible until treated
If surgery cannot be postponed, obtain endocrinology consult
D Liver disease
Acute hepatitis
Evaluate and treat
Postpone surgery
Severe/chronic hepatitis
Child-Pugh class C cirrhosis
Consider alternatives to surgery
Proceed to surgery with extreme caution
Mild/moderate chronic hepatitis
Child-Pugh class A/B cirrhosis
Assess electrolytes, coagulation parameters, hematocrit, hepatic, encephalopathy and volume status
Correct as necessary
When optimized, proceed to surgery
E Renal disease
Acute renal failure
Evaluate and treat
Postpone surgery
Stable chronic renal failure
Assess electrolytes, volume status, and hematocrit
Correct as necessary
Note Cr >2 considered an intermediate predictor of increased cardiac risk
Proceed to surgery
Dialysis patients
Consult nephrology

FALLS IN GERIATRIC PATIENTS

Jeanne E. Bishop, MD

Traditional medicine has viewed falls as the functional outcome of a primary medical condition. Medical conditions are worked up and ruled out; however, the reason for the fall often remains unexplained. With the aging of the population and the increased risk of falls with aging, geriatric medicine has embraced falls as a geriatric syndrome with a multiplicity of causes warranting careful analysis. With the cause suspected, therapeutic and preventive measures can be undertaken to prevent recurrence. Falls are associated with a subsequent decline in functional status, greater likelihood of nursing home placement, increased use of medical services, and a fear of falling in the individual.

The fall evaluation demands diligence and attention to detail, lending itself to an algorithmic approach. It includes a comprehensive history and physical examination, which can lead to a differential of causes, commonly multifactorial. Management interventions are then possible.

A. The fall history takes into account that falls are underreported. Knowing this, clinicians should ask about falls annually in the context of functional assessment and should establish the individual's baseline level of gait, balance, and use of assistive walking devices. Reported falls should be explored more fully by determining frequency (single or recurrent) and severity (minor injury such as soft tissue injury/sprain or major injury such as laceration requiring sutures, fractures, or head strike). The detail of the fall should be elicited in a systematic way from the faller or a witness. Distinguishing loss of consciousness, or not, is a critical feature, and the former should lead to a syncope workup. With no loss of consciousness there should be further differentiation into dizziness, or not, similarly leading to a "dizziness" workup where appropriate. Medication history, including over-the-counter and herbal medicines, and a history for environmental hazards, such as throw rugs, are key. Remember that most falls are multifactorial in origin.

B. A comprehensive physical examination includes vision, HEENT (head, eyes, ears, nose, and throat), cardiovascular, neurologic, musculoskeletal, gait/balance, and a heightened focus on any other areas suggested by the history. Vital signs should include orthostatic measurements of pulse and blood pressure, and pain should be assessed as the "fifth vital sign." The systematic traditional examination should include an assessment of ambulation using a functional status tool such as the "Tinetti Gait and Balance" test or the timed "Get Up and Go" test.

C. There are many causes for falls, and usually many factors play a role.
   1. Normal age-related changes, including declines in the following:
      a. Visual, proprioceptive, and vestibular systems, which are necessary to maintain upright posture
      b. Postural control manifested by increased postural sway
      c. Autoregulatory mechanisms, which help to maintain blood pressure
      d. Total body water, increasing the risk of dehydration and hypotension
   2. Acute medical conditions, which undermine any already-compromised reserve
   3. Lifetime accumulation of chronic medical conditions, especially ophthalmologic, ENT (ear, nose, and throat), cardiovascular, neurologic, rheumatologic, and orthopedic
   4. Medications, including cardiac drugs, psychotropics, hypoglycemic agents, alcohol, and anticholinergics/antihistamines
   5. Environmental hazards
   6. Risk-taking behavior
   7. Trip, slip, stumble, or loss-of-balance accident

D. Management interventions address likely reasons for the fall. These include treatment of acute and chronic medical conditions, medication modification, environmental hazard modification, risk-taking behavior modification, and gait/balance/exercise programs (which additionally address the need for proper footwear and assistive walking devices).

References

Kiel DP. Falls. In Cobbs EL, Duthie EH, Murphy JB, eds. Geriatrics Review Syllabus, 5th ed. New York: Blackwell Publishing, 2002–2004.

Podiasdlo D, Richardson S. The timed "Up & Go": a test of basic functional mobility for frail elderly persons. J Am Geriatr Soc 1991;39:142–148.

Tinetti M. Performance oriented assessment of mobility problems in elderly patients. J Am Geriatr Soc 1986;14:61–65.

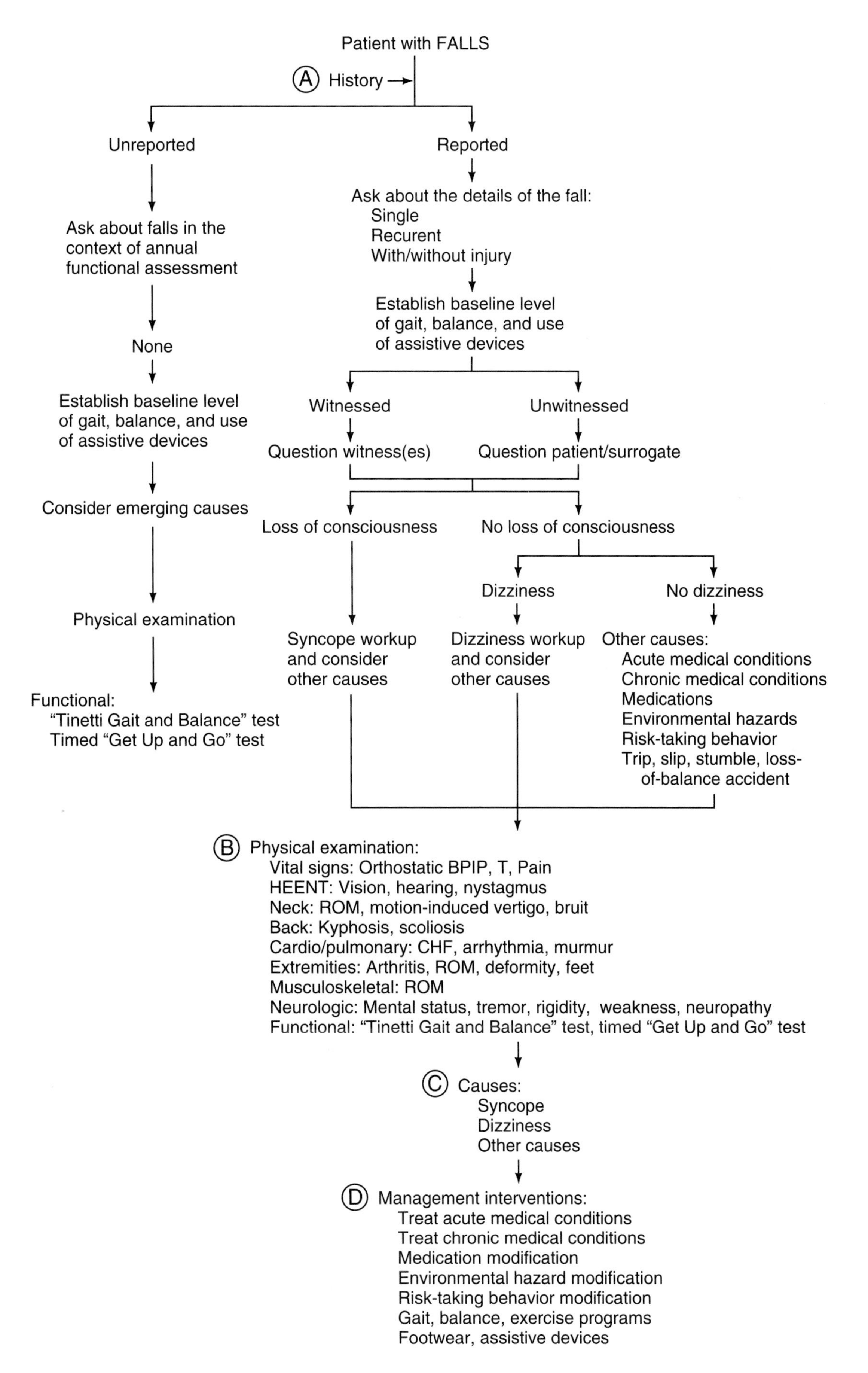
Patient with FALLS
(A) History
Unreported
Reported
Ask about falls in the context of annual functional assessment
None
Establish baseline level of gait, balance, and use of assistive devices
Consider emerging causes
Physical examination
Functional:
"Tinetti Gait and Balance" test
Timed "Get Up and Go" test
Ask about the details of the fall:
Single
Recurent
With/without injury
Establish baseline level of gait, balance, and use of assistive devices
Witnessed
Unwitnessed
Question witness(es)
Question patient/surrogate
Loss of consciousness
No loss of consciousness
Dizziness
No dizziness
Syncope workup and consider other causes
Dizziness workup and consider other causes
Other causes:
Acute medical conditions
Chronic medical conditions
Medications
Environmental hazards
Risk-taking behavior
Trip, slip, stumble, loss-of-balance accident
(B) Physical examination:
Vital signs: Orthostatic BPIP, T, Pain
HEENT: Vision, hearing, nystagmus
Neck: ROM, motion-induced vertigo, bruit
Back: Kyphosis, scoliosis
Cardio/pulmonary: CHF, arrhythmia, murmur
Extremities: Arthritis, ROM, deformity, feet
Musculoskeletal: ROM
Neurologic: Mental status, tremor, rigidity, weakness, neuropathy
Functional: "Tinetti Gait and Balance" test, timed "Get Up and Go" test
(C) Causes:
Syncope
Dizziness
Other causes
(D) Management interventions:
Treat acute medical conditions
Treat chronic medical conditions
Medication modification
Environmental hazard modification
Risk-taking behavior modification
Gait, balance, exercise programs
Footwear, assistive devices

ROM, range of motion

GERIATRIC FUNCTIONAL ASSESSMENT

Khatuna Stepkovitch, MD

The functional assessment is an integral part of a comprehensive geriatric assessment, the purpose of which is to promote wellness and independence and to improve the quality of life. A correct assessment of level of care and adequate assistance plays an integral part in decreasing, or preventing, admissions to the hospital; improving the quality of care for the elderly; and delaying, or even avoiding, unnecessary nursing home placement.

A. **Physical Assessment**

Nutritional Assessment: The nutritional assessment starts with a visual inspection of the patient, a calculation of body mass index (BMI), and a careful history to rule out weight loss. A BMI of <20 and a history of significant weight loss warrant further evaluation (see the chapter Involuntary Weight Loss). The differential of the geriatric patient who is malnourished should include not only medical etiologies but also depression or other psychiatric disorders, financial problems, or impairment in activities of daily living (ADLs), such as an inability to cook for oneself.

Visual Assessment: Often patients are unaware that they are experiencing deficits in vision, and, as such, a quick visual assessment should be performed on every patient. An easy way to assess vision is to have a patient read a paragraph from a newspaper or periodical. The patient can be evaluated further by the Snellen chart or Jaeger card. The cause for visual impairment should be found and treated accordingly. Cataracts, glaucoma, macular degeneration. and abnormalities of accommodation worsen with age.

Hearing Assessment: Hearing loss is common in older adults and is often overlooked. If left untreated, it can cause social withdrawal and depression. As such, a hearing assessment is an integral part of the physical assessment. Before a quick hearing evaluation, otoscopic examination should be done to rule out cerumen impaction. The examiner should then whisper a short, easily answered question in each ear while the examiner's face is out of direct view. Not acknowledging the question warrants further evaluation. The majority of hearing loss is categorized as presbycusis ("older hearing")—sensorineural, usually symmetric hearing loss. Many persons with presbycusis can be helped by amplification, usually hearing aids.

Functional Status Assessment: An assessment of functional status includes an evaluation of ADLs and mobility, which are a direct reflection of a geriatric patient's capacity to live independently. ADLs are characterized as basic or instrumental. Examples of basic ADLs include bathing, dressing, grooming, feeding, transferring from bed to chair, and toileting. Instrumental ADLs include using the telephone, preparing meals, managing household finances, taking medications properly, shopping, managing transportation, doing laundry, and doing housework. A cognitively impaired patient and with impairment in instrumental ADLs may require supervision of only medication intake and finances. Impairment in multiple basic ADLs requires more assistance, either through family/financial supports or through placement to a skilled nursing facility. If there is a deficit in bathing alone, a home health aid may suffice.

The information about basic and instrumental ADLs is usually provided by the patient or an informant (especially in the case of a patient who is cognitively impaired), so a thorough history is imperative. Questions about mobility should be asked, including the patient's ability to climb stairs, walk from room to room, and walk outside of the house. A great amount of information can also be gleaned by simply observing the patient during the office visit. A patient's capacity to unbutton and button a shirt or blouse, write a sentence with a pen, or take off and put on shoes are simple actions that give the physician a wealth of information. When searching for indications that the patient may have some impairment in mobility, look to see whether the patient has difficulty touching the back of the head with both hands or struggles to climb up and down from the examination table.

If impairment in mobility is suspected, the physician can further explore by conducting performance-based testing of functional status, which, in the outpatient setting, is focused on gait, balance, and transfers. The patient is asked to stand from the seated position in a hard-backed chair while keeping his or her arms folded. An inability to complete this task suggests a lower extremity (quadriceps) weakness and is highly predictive of future disability. Once standing, the patient should be observed to walk back and forth over a short distance with his or her usual walking aid. Abnormalities of gait include path deviation; diminished step height or length; trips, slips, or near falls; and difficulty with turning.

Fall risk can be evaluated quickly by the "Get Up and Go" test. The test is performed by asking the patient to rise from a chair; walk 10 feet 3 meters; turn around; and, on returning to the chair, turn and sit

(Continued on page 52)

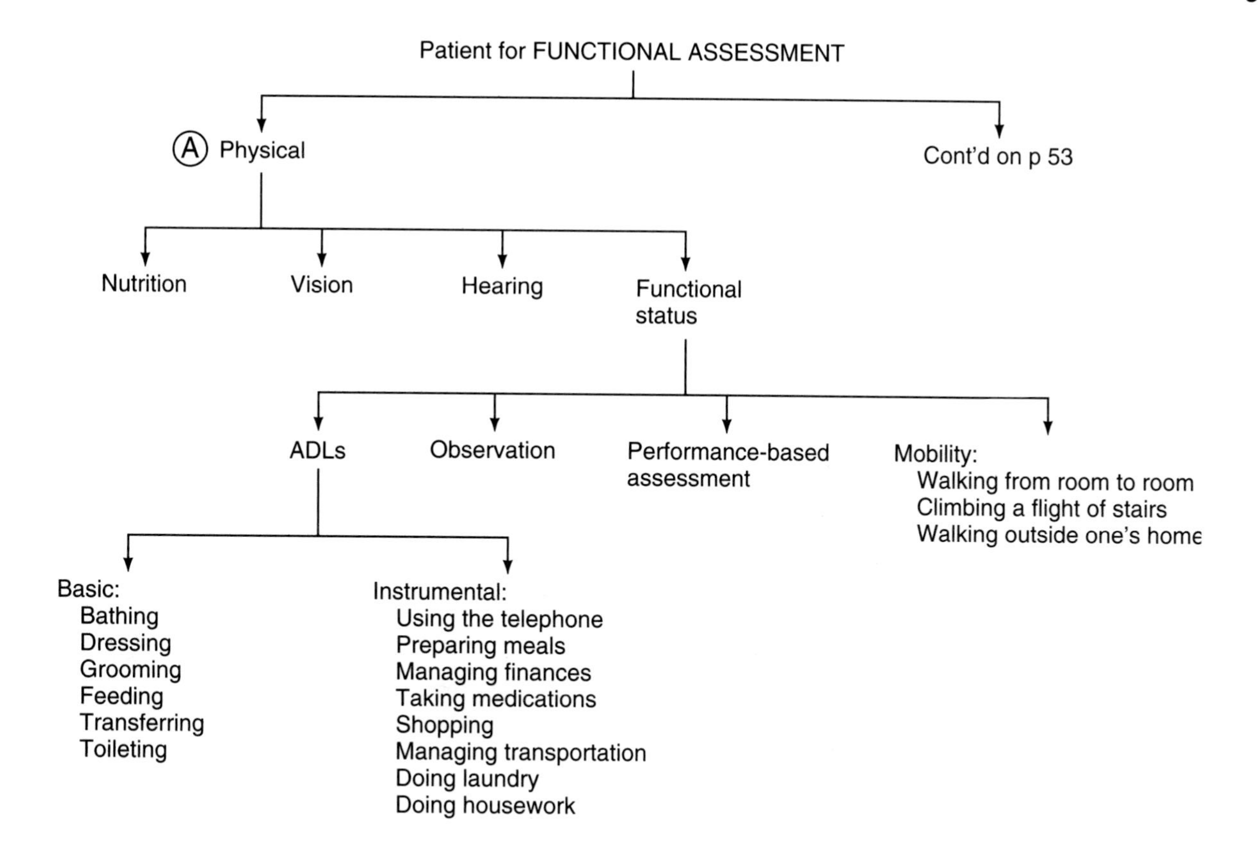
Patient for FUNCTIONAL ASSESSMENT
Ⓐ Physical
Cont'd on p 53
Nutrition
Vision
Hearing
Functional status
ADLs
Observation
Performance-based assessment
Mobility:
Walking from room to room
Climbing a flight of stairs
Walking outside one's home
Basic:
Bathing
Dressing
Grooming
Feeding
Transferring
Toileting
Instrumental:
Using the telephone
Preparing meals
Managing finances
Taking medications
Shopping
Managing transportation
Doing laundry
Doing housework

back down in the chair. Patients who take >10 seconds to complete this sequence have increased risk for falls. Those taking 10–19 seconds are considered to be fairly mobile; those taking 20–29 seconds are considered to have variable mobility; and those taking ≥30 seconds are considered to be dependent in balance and mobility. Patients with impaired gait and balance should be evaluated further to determine the cause and should be referred for gait evaluation and training to a physical therapist.

B. **Cognitive Assessment**

Because of the high prevalence of dementia, screening for cognitive impairment is very important. Cognitive impairment should always be explored in the functionally impaired geriatric patient with or without abnormalities in physical functioning. Because a comprehensive cognitive evaluation is time consuming, it should be reserved for patients who are at risk or show any signs of dementia.

A quick assessment such as three-word recall after 1 minute should be done to assess the need for further evaluation. If recall is impaired, then the patient should be scheduled for comprehensive evaluation to rule out dementia (see Chronic Behavior Change).

C. **Psychological Assessment**

Depression is known to be underdiagnosed. If left untreated, it can cause significant impairment in functional abilities, including cognitive abilities (pseudodementia), and thus needs to be differentiated from dementia. A positive answer to the question, "Do you often feel sad and depressed?" warrants further exploration (a geriatric depression scale can be used).

D. **Social Assessment**

An assessment of the patient's living environment, family and social supports, and financial well-being is an integral part of formulating a comprehensive treatment plan in the geriatric patient. The physician will need the help of social workers in providing information about available resources to the family, such as adult day care centers or assisted-living/skilled nursing facilities, especially if significant functional impairment is found. In cases of suspected elder mistreatment or caregivers being overburdened, social workers prove to be invaluable. Visiting nurses may be helpful in assessing home safety. Advance directives should be clarified.

E. **Evaluation of Driving Skills**

Cessation of driving is often perceived as a loss of independence, and many patients are reluctant to make this decision. The accident rates in older drivers are equivalent to those of drivers between the ages of 16 and 24 years. Risk factors for impaired driving include reduced vision; dementia; impaired neck and truck rotation; limitations in shoulders, hips, or ankles; foot abnormalities; poor motor coordination; medications; and alcohol abuse or dependence.

Effectively communicating with the patient and the family, by explaining risk factors, providing statistics, and helping to find alternative means of transportation, can often avert conflict.

For those geriatric patients who are capable of driving, it is appropriate to recommend against driving on highways, especially during busy periods; driving at night; and driving in poor weather. The clock drawing test appears to be a useful tool to screen for driving performance and to support the recommendation for a formal driving assessment.

The physician has an ethical obligation to notify the Department of Motor Vehicles when a patient who is clearly impaired insists on continuing to drive. The practitioner should be familiar with license renewal laws, mandatory physician reporting laws, and voluntary reporting laws. These vary from state to state.

References

Comprehensive Geriatric Assessment. The Merck Manual of Geriatrics, 2005. Section 1. Chapter 4. Accessed September 24, 2007 at http://www.merck.com/mkgr/mmg/sec2/ch20/ch20a.jsp.

Freund B. Clock drawing test tracks progression of driving performance in cognitively impaired older adults. Case comparisons. Clin Geriatr 2004;12(7):33–36.

Gill TM. Assessment. In Cobbs EL, Duthie EH, Murphy JB, eds. Geriatrics Review Syllabus, 5th ed. New York: Blackwell Publishing, 2002–2004:49–54.

Reuben DB. Comprehensive geriatric assessment and systems approaches to geriatric care. In Cassel CK, Leipzig RM, Cohen HJ, et al eds. Geriatric Medicine, 4th ed. New York: Springer-Verlag, 2003:195–203.

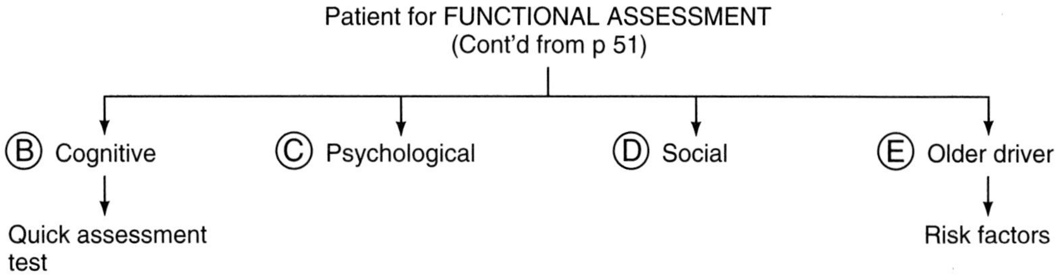

Patient for FUNCTIONAL ASSESSMENT
(Cont'd from p 51)

- (B) Cognitive
  - Quick assessment test
- (C) Psychological
- (D) Social
- (E) Older driver
  - Risk factors

CARDIOLOGY

Stephen D. Wiviott, MD
Section Editor

BRADYCARDIA

Robert E. Eckart, DO, and Usha B. Tedrow, MD, MS

Bradycardia can be physiologic, pathologic, or pharmacologic in origin. Alteration of either the sinoatrial (SA) or atrioventricular (AV) conduction system may play a role. Symptoms of bradyarrhythmias include fatigue, dizziness or syncope, and dyspnea and angina.

A. In the general population, heart rates in approximately 25% of men and 10% of women drop below 50 beats per minute (bpm) during sleep as a result of enhanced nocturnal parasympathetic tone. Sinus pauses up to 2 seconds in asymptomatic individuals can be considered normal. Conditioned athletes often can have high resting vagal tone during the day. During periods of heightened vagal tone, sinus bradycardia, sinus pauses, and first- and second-degree Mobitz type I (Wenckebach) AV block are commonly reported and generally have a benign prognosis. The identification of sinus slowing with AV block in the appropriate setting is characteristic of vagal hypersensitivity.

B. Degenerative disease of the AV node is one of the leading causes of progressive AV block. This degenerative process of the conduction system may be primary (Lenègre's disease) or secondary as a result of impingement by surrounding fibrosis or calcification (Lev's disease).

A large number of systemic diseases are associated with bradyarrhythmias. Hypothermia, hypoglycemia, hypercarbia, and hypothyroidism produce slow heart rhythms because of metabolic alteration. Electrolyte disorders (e.g., hyperkalemia) can result in both SA and AV node disorders. Myocarditis can be associated with both SA and AV node disease and generally portends a poor prognosis. Lyme myocarditis associated with conduction system disease, however, often resolves in the acute setting with appropriate antibiotic therapy. Endocarditis with complicating annular abscess may lead to AV block. Accelerated conduction system disease may also result from infiltrative diseases such as amyloidosis and hemochromatosis.

With inferior myocardial infarction (MI), sinus bradycardia and second-degree Mobitz type I (Wenckebach) AV block are not uncommon. Vagal tone is often high, and heart block is generally located at the level of the AV node because of the anatomy of the AV nodal artery. Consequently, the block tends to be reversible, with a narrow escape (QRS <120 msec). In contrast, the infranodal conduction system gets its blood supply from the septal branches of the left anterior descending artery. AV block with an anterior MI tends to be infranodal and may be associated with bundle branch block. The escape rhythm is often wide (QRS >120 msec) and unreliable, and permanent pacing is generally required.

Postoperative aortic or mitral valve replacement is associated with both mechanical disruption and inflammation that may cause AV block. Because heart block may result from edema, implementation of permanent pacing should be delayed for a minimum of 4 days to allow for any recovery of conduction that may occur.

The finding of atrial fibrillation with a slow ventricular response in the absence of drug therapy may be indicative of SA node dysfunction and susceptibility for offset pauses.

C. Diltiazem and verapamil slow conduction of the AV node. Both blockade and withdrawal of sympathetic tone with beta blockers slow AV nodal conduction via a vagotonic effect. Digoxin increases vagal tone and has a direct effect on AV nodal physiology. Amiodarone and propafenone act through antagonism of $[Ca^{2+}]$ channels and beta receptors. Alternatively, quinidine, procainamide, and disopyramide act via $[Na^{+}]$ channels and thereby can affect the infranodal conducting system.

(Continued on page 58)

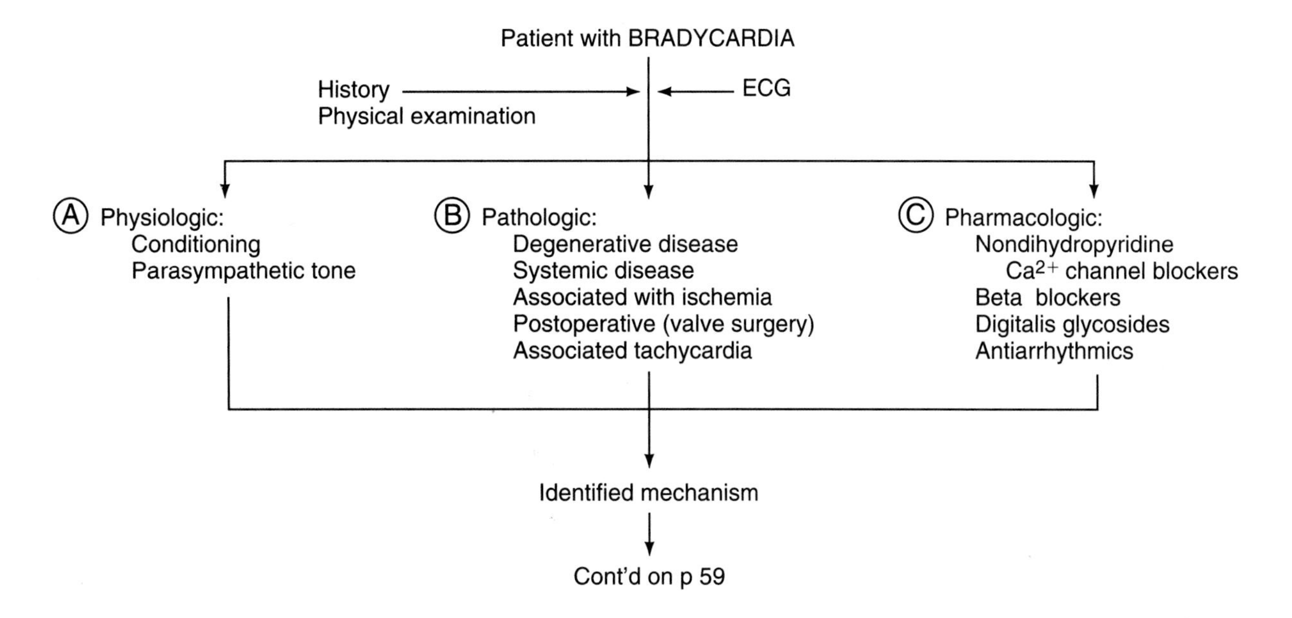
Patient with BRADYCARDIA
History
Physical examination
ECG
Ⓐ Physiologic:
Conditioning
Parasympathetic tone
Ⓑ Pathologic:
Degenerative disease
Systemic disease
Associated with ischemia
Postoperative (valve surgery)
Associated tachycardia
Ⓒ Pharmacologic:
Nondihydropyridine
Ca^{2+} channel blockers
Beta blockers
Digitalis glycosides
Antiarrhythmics
Identified mechanism
Cont'd on p 59

D. The presence of symptoms often guides the workup. It is important to identify patients at high risk based on acuity of onset and potential for comorbidities. Evaluation should include a full 12-lead ECG; a baseline echocardiogram; and stress testing to identify baseline conduction system disease, structural heart disease, and potential for myocardial ischemia. For those with suspected chronotropic incompetence, a treadmill ECG may be of additional diagnostic value. For evaluation of suspected vagally mediated conduction disorders, carotid sinus massage (CSM), used judiciously in the elderly, may reproduce findings. Ambulatory ECG recording may be necessary, either 24-hour continuous Holter monitoring for those with frequent symptoms or triggered loop recording for 2–4 weeks for those with less frequent symptoms. One clinical trial suggests that empiric pacemaker implantation may be of value in elderly patients with carotid sinus hypersensitivity and a history of nonmechanical fall. In the absence of documented carotid sinus hypersensitivity, the evidence for empiric permanent pacing is less clear.

Electrophysiology testing can be used to determine the intrinsic heart rate, measure SA node automaticity (corrected sinus node recovery time, or cSNRT), sinoatrial conduction time (SACT), AV node conduction, and refractoriness. Invasive testing for bradyarrhythmias has a low diagnostic yield, with a sensitivity of 20%–75%, and therapies should be guided by patient symptoms.

E. In general, asymptomatic sinus bradycardia, sinus pauses, and first-degree AV block require no treatment. An exception is made to allow medical therapy for coexistent tachyarrhythmias. Second-degree Mobitz type I (Wenckebach) AV block often involves the AV node and carries a benign prognosis. Mobitz type II AV block is most often infranodal (within the bundle of His or the fascicles), is associated with fixed distal conduction system disease, and is likely to progress to complete heart block. Temporary followed by permanent pacing is recommended.

A 2:1 AV block can be in the AV node or in the distal conduction system. Prolongation of the PR interval with a narrow QRS complex suggests AV nodal block, whereas a wide complex QRS suggests distal conduction system disease. Third-degree AV block can be either congenital or acquired. A narrow escape can suggest that the location of the block is at the AV node (~50%) or the bundle of His (~50%). In cases with a wide escape, the block is usually infranodal (~80%), less stable, and in the rate of 30–45 bpm. Treatment with permanent pacemaker placement is recommended for patients with all forms of infranodal block, regardless of symptom status.

F. Management of bradycardia involves not only identification of symptoms and etiology but also the acuity of presentation.

Acutely, in cases of suspected AV node involvement, treat with atropine. Be aware that atropine may appear to worsen conduction in infranodal block. Temporary transvenous pacing can be performed using a balloon-tipped catheter at the bedside or using a fixed catheter under fluoroscopic guidance. The indications for temporary pacing include both temporary treatment of reversible causes of symptomatic bradycardia and backup availability in those cases with high risk for development of complete heart block. Similarly, transcutaneous pacing may be used as an emergency method of pacing for symptomatic bradycardia. Early conversion to a transvenous system should be considered given discomfort of transcutaneous pacing and risk of intermittent noncapture. Note that temporary pacing has been shown to be ineffective in asystolic cardiac arrest and is not indicated.

In some patients, a beta blocker with intrinsic sympathomimetic activity (e.g., acebutolol, pindolol) may be of value in treating tachyarrhythmia with less bradyarrhythmia side effects. Because pharmacologic therapy for chronic conduction defects does not exist, the treatment of choice is either a temporary pacemaker for reversible causes or permanent pacemaker placement.

In many cases, permanent pacemaker implantation is considered for irreversible conditions, independent of the etiology. The serious risks of contemporary pacemaker implantation, a minor surgical procedure, are <1%. Because the endocardial leads are placed in the central venous circulation, it is critical that the patient be free of infection (e.g., urinary tract infections) prior to implantation because extraction of infected devices can have significant morbidity. At the time of consideration of pacing, thought must be given to the role of biventricular pacing (to improve symptoms with heart failure). A defibrillator (to reduce mortality) may be advisable if the patient has a depressed ejection fraction. Consultation with an electrophysiologist, implanting cardiologist, or surgeon familiar with current methodology is encouraged.

References

Brodsky M, Wu D, Denes P, et al. Arrhythmias documented by 24 hour continuous electrocardiographic monitoring in 50 male medical students without apparent heart disease. Am J Cardiol 1977;39:390–395.

Cummins RO, Graves JR, Larsen MP, et al. Out-of-hospital transcutaneous pacing by emergency medical technicians in patients with asystolic cardiac arrest. N Engl J Med 1993;328:1377–1382.

Johnson RL, Averill KH, Lamb LE. Electrocardiographic findings in 67,375 asymptomatic subjects. VII. Atrioventricular block. Am J Cardiol 1960;6:153–177.

Kenny RA, Richardson DA, Steen N, et al. Carotid sinus syndrome: a modifiable risk factor for nonaccidental falls in older adults (SAFE PACE). J Am Coll Cardiol 2001;38:1491–1496.

Koplan BA, Stevenson WG, Epstein LM, et al. Development and validation of a simple risk score to predict the need for permanent pacing after cardiac valve surgery. J Am Coll Cardiol 2003;41:795–801.

Reiffel JA, Schwarzberg R, Murry M. Comparison of autotriggered memory loop recorders versus standard loop recorders versus 24-hour Holter monitors for arrhythmia detection. Am J Cardiol 2005;95: 1055–1059.

Strickberger SA, Fish RD, Lamas GA, et al. Comparison of effects of propranolol versus pindolol on sinus rate and pacing frequency in sick sinus syndrome. Am J Cardiol 1993;71:53–56.

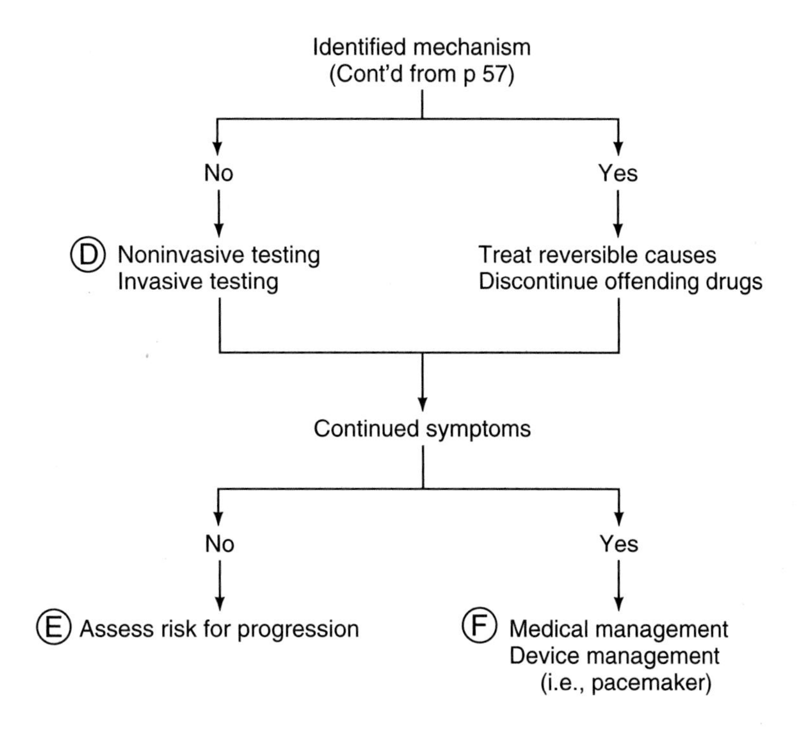
Identified mechanism
(Cont'd from p 57)
No
Yes
(D) Noninvasive testing
Invasive testing
Treat reversible causes
Discontinue offending drugs
Continued symptoms
No
Yes
(E) Assess risk for progression
(F) Medical management
Device management
(i.e., pacemaker)

NARROW-COMPLEX TACHYCARDIA

Paul C. Zei, MD, PhD

Clinical Evaluation of the Patient with NARROW-COMPLEX TACHYCARDIA

A. The patient presenting to the clinician with narrow-complex tachycardia should be immediately assessed for hemodynamic compromise and treated according to Advanced Cardiac Life Support (ACLS) guidelines. After stabilization, evaluation and therapy can ensue. Narrow-complex tachycardia is almost always a result of supraventricular tachycardias (SVTs), particularly if the QRS complex in tachycardia is identical to that in sinus rhythm.

B. The history and physical examination should be directed toward the search for underlying structural heart disease. Evidence of hemodynamic compromise during tachycardia, including syncope, presyncope, chest discomfort, or dyspnea, should be ascertained. Evaluation of the ECG in sinus rhythm should focus on the presence or absence of preexcitation. Echocardiography should be strongly considered in patients with narrow-complex tachycardia to assess the presence of underlying structural heart disease.

C. The presence of preexcitation warrants referral to an electrophysiologist for evaluation of the appropriateness of diagnostic electrophysiologic study (EPS) and possible catheter ablation in the setting of preexcitation and potential atrioventricular reciprocating tachycardia (AVRT). If preexcitation is not clearly manifest, significant symptoms, particularly syncope, also warrant evaluation by an electrophysiologist.

D. If the SVT is sustained and symptomatic, particularly if medical therapy has failed to suppress episodes, the patient should be referred to an electrophysiologist for possible EPS and catheter ablation. The differential diagnosis includes atrioventicular nodal reentrant tachycardia (AVNRT), AVRT, atrial tachycardia, PJRT (so-called permanent junctional reciprocating tachycardia), and atrial flutter with regular ventricular response.

E. If atrial fibrillation, multifocal atrial tachycardia (MAT), or atrial flutter are diagnosed, medical therapy may be initiated. The goals of medical therapy include symptom relief, rate control during tachycardia, and consideration of anticoagulation. Failure of medical therapy to relieve symptoms or control ventricular rate warrants consideration of catheter ablation.

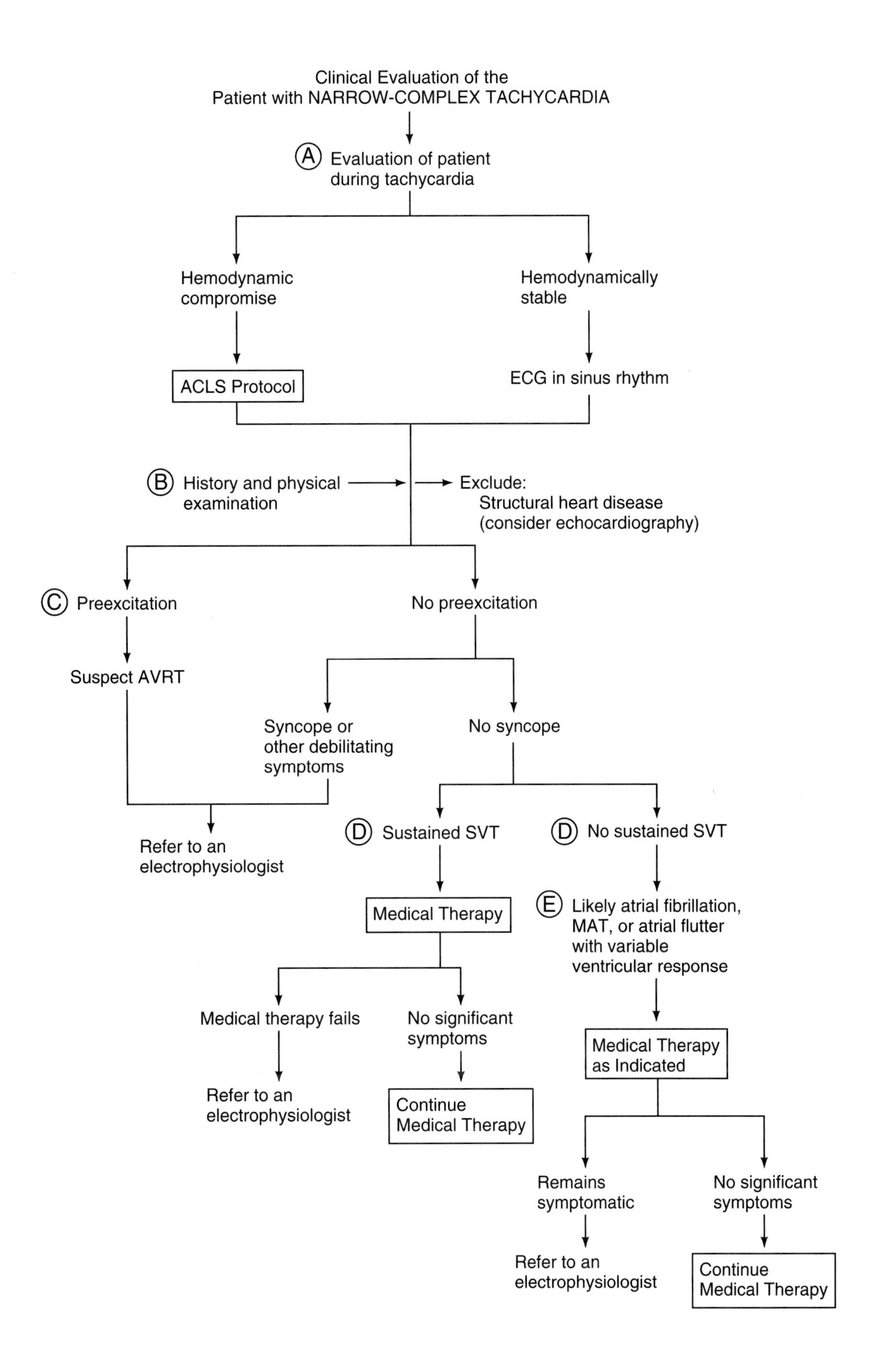
Clinical Evaluation of the
Patient with NARROW-COMPLEX TACHYCARDIA
(A) Evaluation of patient
during tachycardia
Hemodynamic
compromise
Hemodynamically
stable
ACLS Protocol
ECG in sinus rhythm
(B) History and physical
examination
Exclude:
Structural heart disease
(consider echocardiography)
(C) Preexcitation
No preexcitation
Suspect AVRT
Syncope or
other debilitating
symptoms
No syncope
Refer to an
electrophysiologist
(D) Sustained SVT
(D) No sustained SVT
Medical Therapy
(E) Likely atrial fibrillation,
MAT, or atrial flutter
with variable
ventricular response
Medical therapy fails
No significant
symptoms
Medical Therapy
as Indicated
Refer to an
electrophysiologist
Continue
Medical Therapy
Remains
symptomatic
No significant
symptoms
Refer to an
electrophysiologist
Continue
Medical Therapy

Electrocardiographic Evaluation of the Patient with NARROW-COMPLEX TACHYCARDIA

A. Electrocardiographic evaluation of narrow-complex tachycardia should always begin with evaluation of the ECG in sinus rhythm, if available. Evidence of preexcitation should be sought, and if it is found, AVRT should be suspected.

B. If no preexcitation is seen, evaluation of the ECG in tachycardia should begin with determining whether the RR interval is regular and constant or variable. A variable RR interval suggests atrial fibrillation, atrial tachycardia with variable ventricular response, atrial flutter with variable ventricular response, or MAT. If the RR interval is regular and fixed, the differential diagnosis remains broad. Evaluation should then proceed to searching for visible P waves.

C. If P waves are not clearly visible during tachycardia, AVNRT is likely because typical AVNRT using antegrade slow pathway conduction and retrograde fast pathway conduction usually results in P waves "buried" in the QRS complex. If more P waves than R waves are present (i.e., the atrial rate exceeds the ventricular rate), atrial tachycardia or atrial flutter are likely because this finding demonstrates that the AV node is not necessary to maintain the tachycardia circuit. If there is a 1:1 relationship between P and R waves, analysis should then proceed to the RP interval.

D. A long RP interval is defined as an RP interval *greater than* the PR interval. A short RP interval is the opposite, with an RP interval *less than* the PR interval. A long RP interval suggests tachycardias with rapid antegrade AV nodal conduction. This includes atrial tachycardia, PJRT, inappropriate sinus tachycardia, sinus reentry, and atypical AVNRT (fast pathway antegrade limb, slow pathway retrograde limb). A short RP interval suggests rapid retrograde limb conduction of the tachycardia circuit, including typical AVNRT and AVRT using an accessory pathway.

E. In short RP tachycardias, an RP interval <70 ms is consistent with AVNRT, whereas an RP interval >70 ms cannot distinguish between AVNRT and AVRT using an accessory pathway. Because retrograde atrial activation during AVRT follows antegrade AV nodal, His-Purkinje, and ventricular depolarization leading to retrograde accessory pathway depolarization, the resultant RP (ventricular to atrial depolarization) interval is almost never <70 ms.

References

Blomström-Lundqvist C, Scheinman MM, Aliot EM, et al. CC/AHA/ESC guidelines for the management of patients with supraventricular arrhythmias—executive summary. A report of the American College of Cardiology/American Heart Association Task Force on Practice Guidelines and the European Society of Cardiology Committee for Practice Guidelines (Writing Committee to Develop Guidelines for the Management of Patients with Supraventricular Arrhythmias) developed in collaboration with NASPE-Heart Rhythm Society. J Am Coll Cardiol 2003;42(8):1493–1531.

Josephson ME. Clinical Cardiac Electrophysiology: Techniques and Interpretations, 3rd ed. Philadelphia: Lippincott, 2001.

Morady F. Catheter ablation of supraventricular arrhythmias. J Cardiovasc Electrophysiol 2004;15(1):124–129.

Wellens HJJ. Twenty-five years of insights into the mechanisms of supraventricular arrhythmias. J Cardiovasc Electrophysiol 2003; 14:1–6.

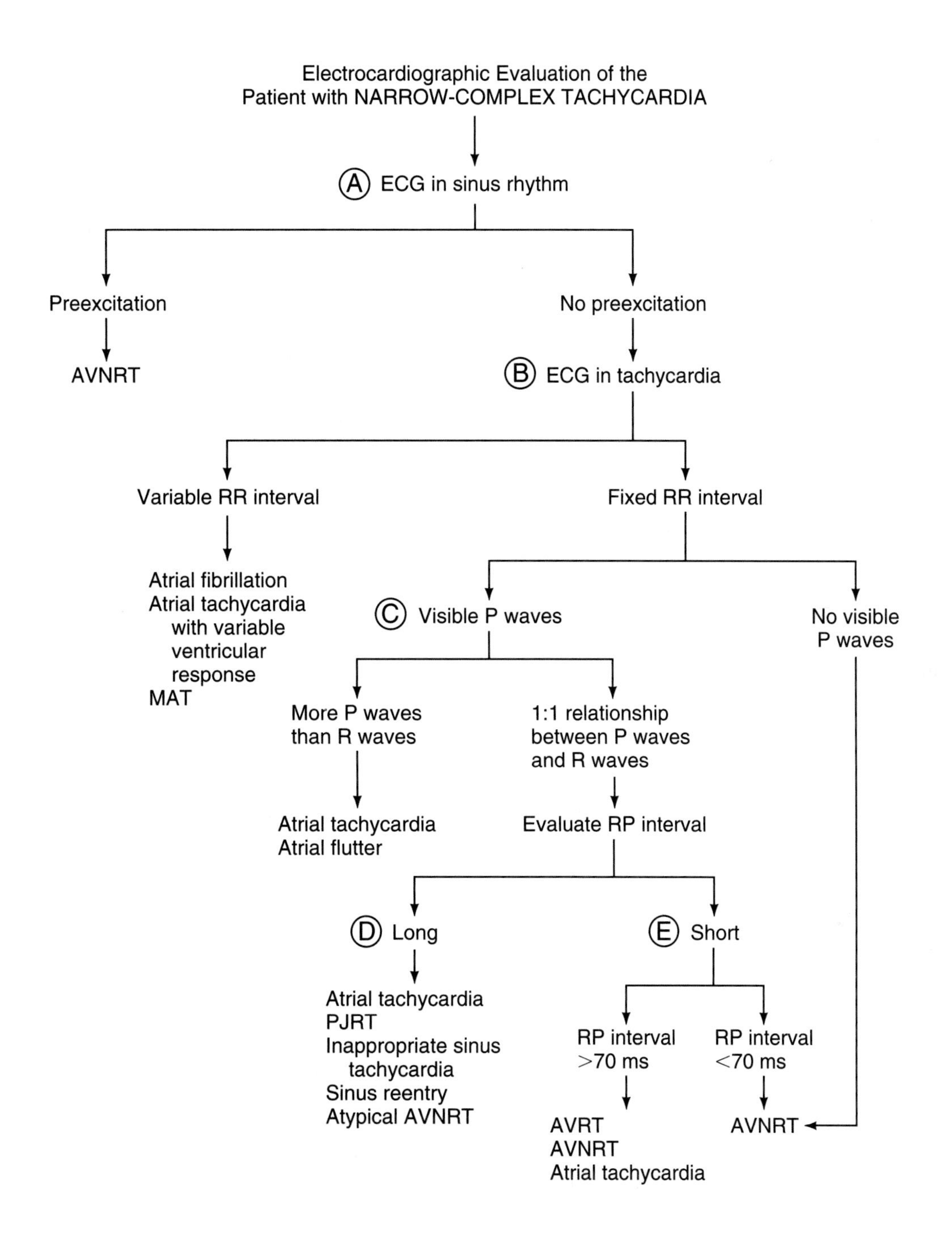
Electrocardiographic Evaluation of the
Patient with NARROW-COMPLEX TACHYCARDIA
(A) ECG in sinus rhythm
Preexcitation
AVNRT
No preexcitation
(B) ECG in tachycardia
Variable RR interval
Atrial fibrillation
Atrial tachycardia with variable ventricular response
MAT
Fixed RR interval
(C) Visible P waves
No visible P waves
More P waves than R waves
Atrial tachycardia
Atrial flutter
1:1 relationship between P waves and R waves
Evaluate RP interval
(D) Long
Atrial tachycardia
PJRT
Inappropriate sinus tachycardia
Sinus reentry
Atypical AVNRT
(E) Short
RP interval >70 ms
AVRT
AVNRT
Atrial tachycardia
RP interval <70 ms
AVNRT

WIDE-COMPLEX TACHYCARDIA

Christopher Pickett, MD, and Peter Zimetbaum, MD

Wide QRS complex tachycardia (WCT), defined as heart rate (HR) >100 beats per minute (bpm) with a QRS duration >120 ms, is a common arrhythmia with potentially life-threatening consequences, making rapid and accurate diagnosis with initiation of appropriate therapy essential.

A. After recognition of this arrhythmia, the clinician must immediately evaluate the patient for hemodynamic stability. If the patient is unstable, then Advanced Cardiac Life Support (ACLS) protocol should be initiated with direct current (DC) cardioversion of the patient.

   If the rhythm is sustained but tolerated or if it is not sustained, then the clinician should perform an evaluation with the goal of differentiation between ventricular tachycardia (VT) and supraventricular tachycardia (SVT) with aberrant conduction. Prognosis and therapy of these two conditions differ considerably.

B. The clinical history can be helpful in suggesting a diagnosis. Presence of prior myocardial infarction (MI) and structural heart disease is the strongest clinical predictor of VT. Patients with ischemic cardiomyopathy and WCT will have VT >98% of the time. Advanced age and presence of congestive heart failure (CHF) also favor VT. Younger patients or adults with a history of recurrent tachycardia since a young age or for >3 years are more likely to have SVT with aberrancy.

   Symptoms during tachycardia may be far ranging, from malaise to syncope. It is a common misconception that WCT is less likely to be VT if it is hemodynamically stable. Many VTs are hemodynamically tolerated and dismissing this diagnosis can lead to inappropriate triage and therapy, with subsequent cardiovascular collapse.

   After assessment of vital signs, the physical examination should be directed toward noting evidence of atrioventricular (AV) dissociation, which is frequently seen in VT but rarely in SVT. Beat-to-beat change in blood pressure, variability in S_1, and cannon A waves are all signs of AV dissociation. Carotid massage that terminates the arrhythmia indicates that the AV node was involved in the tachycardia circuit and that the mechanism is an SVT.

C. A 12-lead electrocardiogram (ECG) offers a great deal more information than a rhythm strip and should be obtained promptly. A prior ECG can also offer helpful clues. If there is evidence of ventricular pre-excitation or previous bundle branch block with similar morphology to the WCT, then it suggests SVT with aberrancy. If there are Q waves or other evidence of prior MI, the case for VT is supported.

D. Initial evaluation of the ECG should begin with the search for P waves and their relationship to the QRS. Dissociation of the P from the QRS or other evidence of AV dissociation, such as fusion or capture beats, is diagnostic of VT. It should be noted that the rate of the WCT does not reliably differentiate VT from SVT and that, although irregularity suggests atrial fibrillation, it can also be seen at the onset and termination of VT.

E. If the initial assessment fails to yield a diagnosis, more detailed analysis is necessary. This is done by identifying the WCT as right bundle branch block (RBBB)-type (V1 positive) or left bundle branch block (LBBB)-type (V1 negative) and applying specific morphologic criteria.

F. In RBBB-type WCT, a ventricular origin is suggested by QRS complex duration >140 ms, left axis deviation, a single (R) or biphasic (QR or RS) R wave in lead V1, or a triphasic R wave in lead V1 with the initial R wave taller than the secondary R wave, R:S ratio of <1 in V6, positive concordance.

G. In LBBB-type WCT, a ventricular origin is suggested by QRS complex >160 ms, a broad (>40 ms) R in V1, notching of the QRS and/or delayed downstroke with R to S interval >100 ms in V1, right axis deviation, a Q wave in V6, negative concordance.

   Unless there is definitive evidence that the WCT is SVT, one should never use adenosine or verapamil because it may lead to rapid hemodynamic collapse. Procainamide is the preferred agent for pharmacologic control of WCT.

References

Brugada P, Brugada J, Mont L, et al. A new approach to the differential diagnosis of a regular tachycardia with a wide QRS complex. Circulation 1991;83:1649–1659.

Buxton AE, Marchlinski FE, Doherty JU. Hazards of intravenous verapamil for sustained ventricular tachycardia. Am J Cardiol 1987;59:1107–1110.

Kindwall E, Brown J, Josephson ME. Electrocardiographic criteria for ventricular tachycardia in wide QRS complex left bundle-branch block morphology tachycardia. Am J Cardiol 1988;61:1279–1283.

Stewart RB, Bardy GH, Greene HL. Wide complex tachycardia: misdiagnosis and outcome after emergent therapy. Ann Intern Med 1986;104:766–771.

Wellens HJJ. Ventricular tachycardia: diagnosis of broad QRS complex tachycardia. Heart 2001;86:579–585.

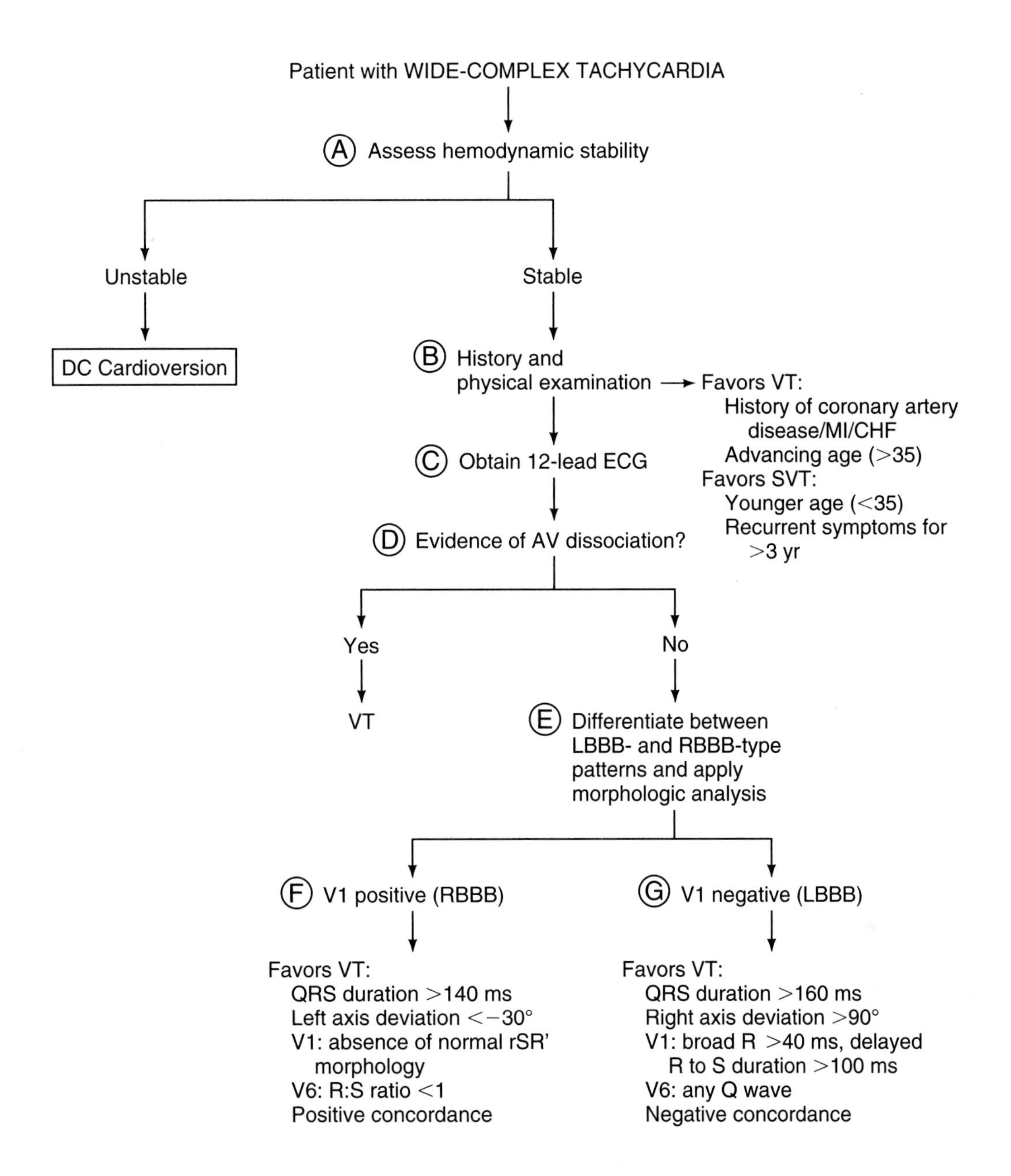
Patient with WIDE-COMPLEX TACHYCARDIA
(A) Assess hemodynamic stability
Unstable
Stable
DC Cardioversion
(B) History and physical examination
Favors VT:
History of coronary artery disease/MI/CHF
Advancing age (>35)
Favors SVT:
Younger age (<35)
Recurrent symptoms for >3 yr
(C) Obtain 12-lead ECG
(D) Evidence of AV dissociation?
Yes
No
VT
(E) Differentiate between LBBB- and RBBB-type patterns and apply morphologic analysis
(F) V1 positive (RBBB)
(G) V1 negative (LBBB)
Favors VT:
QRS duration >140 ms
Left axis deviation <−30°
V1: absence of normal rSR' morphology
V6: R:S ratio <1
Positive concordance
Favors VT:
QRS duration >160 ms
Right axis deviation >90°
V1: broad R >40 ms, delayed R to S duration >100 ms
V6: any Q wave
Negative concordance

STABLE ANGINA

Marc P. Bonaca, MD, and David A. Morrow, MD, MPH

Chronic stable angina is most commonly a manifestation of progressive obstruction of the coronary arteries by atheromatous plaque. Management of stable angina can be approached through lifestyle, pharmacologic, and invasive means aimed at reducing the imbalance of myocardial oxygen supply versus demand, delaying the progression of atherosclerosis, and stabilizing vulnerable coronary atheroma. Discussion among physicians and patients regarding the goals and risks of therapy is essential in the management of this condition.

A. The history and physical examination should be targeted to determine the severity and pattern of symptoms, underlying risk factors, concomitant exacerbating diseases, and signs or symptoms of left ventricular (LV) dysfunction. A fasting lipid profile, blood glucose, and ECG should be obtained. When possible, correct exacerbating medications/conditions, including anemia, hyperthyroidism, and tachyarrhythmia.
B. Behavioral risk factor assessment and modifications are essential; this includes diet restrictions, exercise, weight loss, and smoking cessation.
C. Preventive pharmacologic therapies should be instituted in cases in which lifestyle modifications are not sufficient. All patients without contraindication should take aspirin for secondary prevention. Blood pressure and dyslipidemia should be controlled to target for those with coronary artery disease (CAD) (Joint National Committee on Prevention, Detection, Evaluation, and Treatment of High Blood Pressure [JNC 7] and National Cholesterol Education Program [NCEP]).
D. Risk assessment should be initiated. If evidence of LV dysfunction or high-risk CAD is present by history, examination, chest x-ray, or ECG, cardiac catheterization may be considered. If risk stratification is incomplete, assess LV function and perform stress testing (unless contraindications exist).
E. Stress testing is considered to confirm the diagnosis in those with intermediate probability of CAD, to provide additional prognostic information needed to guide management, and to aid in directing intervention in patients with prior revascularization. Exercise testing is preferred to pharmacologic stress testing because the former provides valuable functional data. Exercise ECG is the first line if the ECG is interpretable. Imaging enhances prognostic assessment by localizing and quantifying the extent of ischemia and prior infarction and is necessary if the ECG is uninterpretable.
F. Assessment of symptom severity (and responsiveness to therapy) along with prognosis guides therapy for stable angina.
G. Pharmacologic therapy should be instituted for persistent symptoms. A beta blocker is generally preferred as initial therapy unless contraindications exist. Calcium antagonists may be preferred in specific situations such as pulmonary disease (chronic obstructive pulmonary disease, asthma), conduction abnormality (dihydropyridine), and vasospastic angina. Long-acting nitrates may be added for persistent symptoms. Combined therapy with a beta blocker and long-acting nitrates is superior to use of either agent alone for symptom relief.
H. The method of revascularization (percutaneous coronary intervention [PCI] vs. coronary artery bypass grafting [CABG]) is addressed once significant coronary disease is identified by angiography. CABG is preferred for certain anatomic subsets, in particular in those with a large territory of jeopardized myocardium, in patients with diabetes mellitus, in those with LV dysfunction, and in patients with lesions not amenable to PCI. The patient's surgical risk must also be considered when deciding among methods of intervention.
I. The patient's clinical status and symptom severity should be reassessed after medical or mechanical intervention. Patients who experience significant symptoms after maximal medical therapy should be considered for angiography and intervention. For patients who have been revascularized to the extent possible and still have significant symptoms despite maximal medication, alternative approaches (spinal cord stimulation, etc.) can be considered.

References

The BARI Investigators. Seven-year outcome in the Bypass Angioplasty Revascularization Investigation (BARI) by treatment and diabetic status. J Am Coll Cardiol 2000;35:1122–1129.

Beller GA, Zaret BL. Contributions of nuclear cardiology to diagnosis and prognosis of patients with coronary artery disease. Circulation 2000;101:1465–1478.

Califf RM, Armstrong PW, Carver JR, et al. 27th Bethesda Conference: matching the intensity of risk factor management with the hazard for coronary disease events. Task Force 5. Stratification of patients into high, medium and low risk subgroups for purposes of risk factor management. J Am Coll Cardiol 1996;27:1007–1019.

Gibbons RJ, Abrams J, Chatterjee K, et al. ACC/AHA 2002 guideline update for the management of patients with chronic stable angina—summary article: a report of the American College of Cardiology/American Heart Association Task Force on practice guidelines (Committee on the Management of Patients With Chronic Stable Angina). J Am Coll Cardiol 2003;41:159–168.

Heidenreich PA, McDonald KM, Hastie T, et al. Meta-analysis of trials comparing beta-blockers, calcium antagonists, and nitrates for stable angina. JAMA 1999;281:1927–1936.

Lee TH, Boucher CA. Clinical practice. Noninvasive tests in patients with stable coronary artery disease. N Engl J Med 2001;344:1840–1845.

Yusuf S, Zucker D, Peduzzi P, et al. Effect of coronary artery bypass graft surgery on survival: overview of 10-year results from randomised trials by the Coronary Artery Bypass Graft Surgery Trialists Collaboration. Lancet 1994;344:563–570.

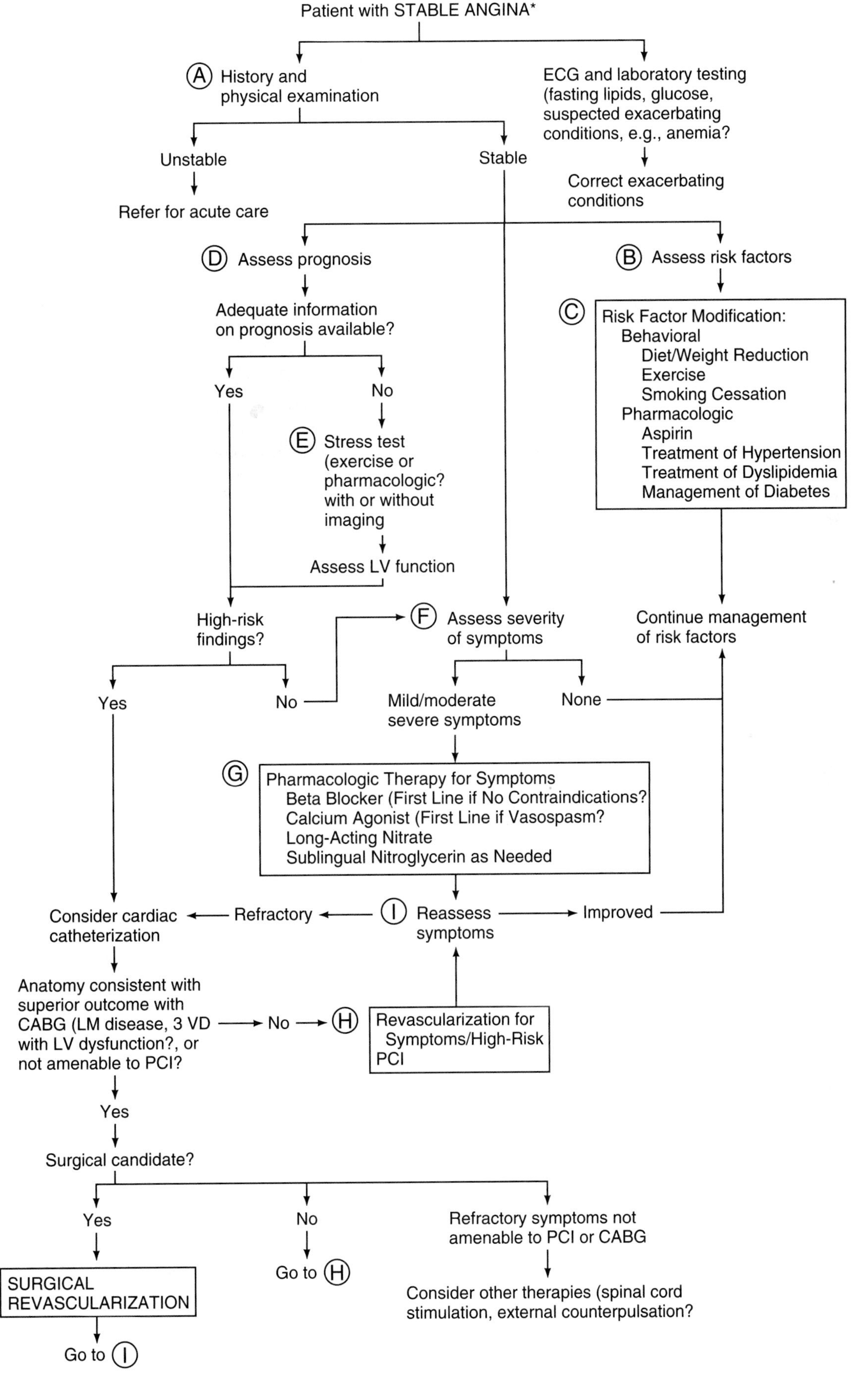

Patient with STABLE ANGINA*
(A) History and physical examination
ECG and laboratory testing (fasting lipids, glucose, suspected exacerbating conditions, e.g., anemia?
Unstable
Stable
Refer for acute care
Correct exacerbating conditions
(D) Assess prognosis
(B) Assess risk factors
Adequate information on prognosis available?
(C) Risk Factor Modification:
Behavioral
Diet/Weight Reduction
Exercise
Smoking Cessation
Pharmacologic
Aspirin
Treatment of Hypertension
Treatment of Dyslipidemia
Management of Diabetes
Yes
No
(E) Stress test (exercise or pharmacologic? with or without imaging
Assess LV function
High-risk findings?
(F) Assess severity of symptoms
Continue management of risk factors
Yes
No
Mild/moderate severe symptoms
None
(G) Pharmacologic Therapy for Symptoms
Beta Blocker (First Line if No Contraindications?
Calcium Agonist (First Line if Vasospasm?
Long-Acting Nitrate
Sublingual Nitroglycerin as Needed
Consider cardiac catheterization
Refractory
(I) Reassess symptoms
Improved
Anatomy consistent with superior outcome with CABG (LM disease, 3 VD with LV dysfunction?, or not amenable to PCI?
No
(H) Revascularization for Symptoms/High-Risk PCI
Yes
Surgical candidate?
Yes
No
Refractory symptoms not amenable to PCI or CABG
SURGICAL REVASCULARIZATION
Go to (H)
Consider other therapies (spinal cord stimulation, external counterpulsation?
Go to (I)

*Patients with moderate to high probability of coronary artery disease.

UNSTABLE ANGINA/NON-ST-ELEVATION MYOCARDIAL INFARCTION

Benjamin M. Scirica, MD, and Christopher P. Cannon, MD

Unstable angina (UA) and non-ST-elevation myocardial infarctions (NSTEMI) most commonly arise from nearly complete but not total occlusion of a coronary artery with a platelet- and fibrin-rich thrombus. Patients presenting with UA/NSTEMI represent a heterogeneous population, with the rate of death and recurrent myocardial infarction at 1 year ranging from <5% in patients at low risk to >20% in the patients at highest risk. The therapeutic options for patients with UA/NSTEMI have continued to increase to include more varied and potent antiplatelet and antithrombotic agents and improved percutaneous coronary interventional techniques. Thus, the clinician has many treatment options available and must effectively discriminate which patients are likely to benefit from the most aggressive treatment while balancing the risk of potential side effects or complications in those at lower risk. Effective risk stratification is critical to making appropriate decisions for therapeutic care.

A. The decision to hospitalize a patient with ischemic symptoms relies on a careful history, physical examination, a resting 12-lead ECG, and laboratory test for cardiac biomarkers (creatine kinase-MB [CKMB] or cardiac-specific troponins). Patients with intermediate to high likelihood of true ischemic disease should be hospitalized, whereas those without any of these features may be evaluated in an observation unit or as an outpatient.

B. Determining appropriate therapy for each patient admitted with presumed UA/NSTEMI requires an assessment of their clinical risk of recurrent ischemic events and death. Three easily obtained indicators of high risk for recurrent ischemic events—elevated levels of cardiac biomarkers (e.g., troponin), ST-segment deviation, and high clinical risk scores—identify those patients who are at highest risk and warrant the most aggressive medical and invasive therapy. One widely used clinical risk score is the TIMI Risk Score, which incorporates seven easily obtained clinical characteristics.

C. Patients with no ECG changes, normal levels of cardiac biomarkers, and low clinical risk factors can be managed conservatively with aspirin, heparin (unfractionated or low molecular weight heparin [UFH/LMWH]), beta blockers, clopidogrel, and nitrates as needed. If they do not develop recurrent ischemia or other clinical instability, they should undergo a stress test for further risk stratification.

D. Clinical trial evidence supports the use of more aggressive medical and invasive therapy in patients who are found to be at increased risk for death or recurrent ischemia. The benefit of glycoprotein IIb/IIIa inhibitors and an early invasive catheterization has been shown to be most beneficial in reducing both death and recurrent MI in patients with positive cardiac biomarkers, ST-segment changes, or a TIMI Risk Score ≥3.

E. Any patient who has recurrent ischemia, hemodynamic compromise or congestive heart failure (CHF), serious ventricular arrhythmia, reduced left ventricular function (ejection fraction <40%), or a strongly positive stress test should be considered for catheterization regardless of initial management strategy.

F. Long-term therapy for any patient with UA/NSTEMI includes risk factor modification together with aspirin, clopidogrel, beta blockers, high-dose statins, and angiotensin-converting enzyme (ACE) inhibitors/angiotensin receptor blockers (ARBs).

References

Antithrombotic Trialists' Collaboration. Collaborative meta-analysis of randomised trials of antiplatelet therapy for prevention of death, myocardial infarction, and stroke in high risk patients. BMJ 2002;324:71–86.

Antman EM, Cohen M, Bernink PJ, et al. The TIMI risk score for unstable angina/non-ST elevation MI: a method for prognostication and therapeutic decision making. JAMA 2000;284:835–842.

Braunwald E, Antman EM, Beasley JW, et al. ACC/AHA 2002 guideline update for the management of patients with unstable angina and non-ST-segment elevation myocardial infarction—summary article. A report of the American College of Cardiology/American Heart Association Task Force on Practice Guidelines (Committee on the Management of Patients with Unstable Angina). J Am Coll Cardiol 2002;40:1366–1374.

Cannon CP, Weintraub WS, Demopoulos LA, et al. Comparison of early invasive and conservative strategies in patients with unstable coronary syndromes treated with the glycoprotein IIb/IIIa inhibitor tirofiban (TACTICS-TIMI 18). N Engl J Med 2001;344:1879–1887.

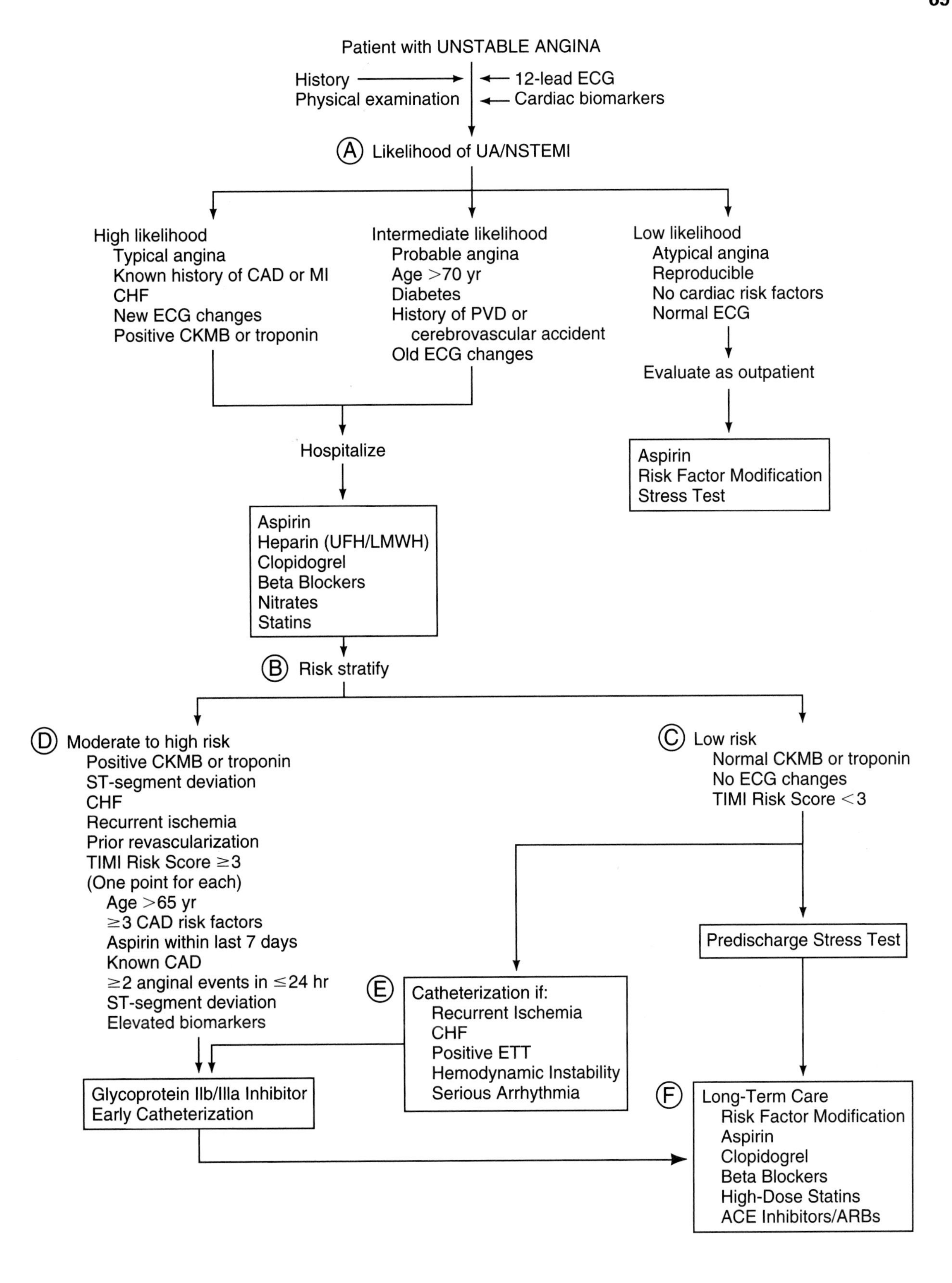
Patient with UNSTABLE ANGINA
History
Physical examination
12-lead ECG
Cardiac biomarkers
A Likelihood of UA/NSTEMI
High likelihood
Typical angina
Known history of CAD or MI
CHF
New ECG changes
Positive CKMB or troponin
Intermediate likelihood
Probable angina
Age >70 yr
Diabetes
History of PVD or cerebrovascular accident
Old ECG changes
Low likelihood
Atypical angina
Reproducible
No cardiac risk factors
Normal ECG
Evaluate as outpatient
Aspirin
Risk Factor Modification
Stress Test
Hospitalize
Aspirin
Heparin (UFH/LMWH)
Clopidogrel
Beta Blockers
Nitrates
Statins
B Risk stratify
D Moderate to high risk
Positive CKMB or troponin
ST-segment deviation
CHF
Recurrent ischemia
Prior revascularization
TIMI Risk Score ≥3
(One point for each)
Age >65 yr
≥3 CAD risk factors
Aspirin within last 7 days
Known CAD
≥2 anginal events in ≤24 hr
ST-segment deviation
Elevated biomarkers
C Low risk
Normal CKMB or troponin
No ECG changes
TIMI Risk Score <3
Predischarge Stress Test
E Catheterization if:
Recurrent Ischemia
CHF
Positive ETT
Hemodynamic Instability
Serious Arrhythmia
Glycoprotein IIb/IIIa Inhibitor
Early Catheterization
F Long-Term Care
Risk Factor Modification
Aspirin
Clopidogrel
Beta Blockers
High-Dose Statins
ACE Inhibitors/ARBs

CAD, Coronary artery disease.

SYSTOLIC MURMURS

Aaron L. Baggish, MD, and Marc S. Sabatine, MD

Cardiac murmurs are generated by turbulent blood flow and adjacent soft-tissue vibration. Turbulent or nonlaminar blood flow occurs in response to rapid acceleration or deceleration of flow such as that which occurs across a narrowed valve or vessel segment.

A. The initial goal after the detection of a murmur is to identify the portion(s) of the cardiac cycle at which the murmur can be heard. At slow heart rates (<80 beats per minute) systole can be identified by auscultation because it has a shorter duration than diastole. As heart rate increases, systole and diastole become more difficult to separate, and separation should be done by simultaneous palpation of the carotid arterial pulse.

   Murmurs in systole have several possible causes, including regurgitant flow across an atrioventricular (AV) valve (mitral or tricuspid), forward flow though a stenotic or abnormal semilunar valve (aortic or pulmonary), or flow through an anatomic defect (ventricular septum).

   Once a murmur has been determined to be systolic in timing, a series of steps can be undertaken to identify the exact cause. These include a determination of the murmur's location of optimal auscultation, configuration, quality, duration, and radiation. Provocative maneuvers can then be used to confirm the suspected pathology.

B. **Location:** Murmurs generated by flow across the semilunar valves are loudest in intensity at the left (pulmonic valve) and right (aortic valve) sternal border in the 2nd intercostal space (ICS). Those caused by AV valve pathology are heard lower on the chest wall at the left sternal border, 5th–6th ICS (tricuspid valve), and in the mid-clavicular line, 5th–6th ICS (mitral valve).

   Intensity: Murmur intensity is graded on a 6-point scale, with 1 being barely audible and 6 being audible without the assistance of a stethoscope. Intensity does not reliably correlate with the amount of turbulent blood flow or with the clinical relevance of the murmur. Intensity should be assessed primarily as a means of determining a baseline, which is helpful in the assessment of disease progression and response to therapy.

C. **Configuration:** The murmurs of systole either have a diamond-shaped crescendo-decrescendo or a uniform, holosystolic configuration. Murmurs caused by the forward ejection of blood through one of the semilunar valves are generally of the crescendo-decrescendo variety, whereas those generated by regurgitant flow through an AV valve are usually holosystolic.

   Quality: Several common systolic murmurs have distinct audible qualities that can be helpful in determining the etiology. The murmur of aortic stenosis tends to be a harsh, grating murmur, whereas that of mitral regurgitation has a gentle, blowing quality.

   Duration: Systolic murmurs can exist for the entire duration of the systolic period or can occur only early or late in the period. AV valve regurgitation without a prolapse etiology and ventricular septal defects can be confined to early systole or can persist for the entire ejection period. Murmurs beginning after the onset of systole (late systolic) are generally caused by AV valve prolapse and ensuing regurgitation.

D. **Provocative Maneuvers:** Several maneuvers that alter both cardiac blood flow and intracardiac volume can be used to clarify the cause of a systolic murmur. Abrupt standing and execution of the Valsalva maneuver reduce cardiac return, thereby diminishing preload, intracardiac volume, and transvalvular flow. These maneuvers decrease the intensity of all systolic murmurs other than the murmur of hypertrophic obstructive cardiomyopathy (HOCM). Passive leg raise, handgrip, standing and squatting, and inspiration are all maneuvers that can help to differentiate murmurs.

E. **Radiation:** Radiation of the murmur away from the point of loudest intensity can provide diagnostic clues. Mitral valve regurgitation murmurs can radiate to the axilla (anterior leaflet incompetence) or to the anterior chest wall (posterior leaflet incompetence). Aortic stenosis murmurs often radiate superiorly into the carotid arteries, while the otherwise-indistinguishable murmur of aortic valve sclerosis remains confined to the sternal border.

F. The management of systolic murmurs depends on the etiology, the acuity, and the hemodynamic significance of the underlying abnormality. Echocardiography can be used to confirm the cause of a systolic murmur and to determine the consequence of the structural abnormality. Both aortic stenosis and mitral regurgitation can exist for long periods without the presence of clinical symptoms or the need for treatment. The development of symptoms or objective evidence of left ventricular dysfunction is an indication for valve repair

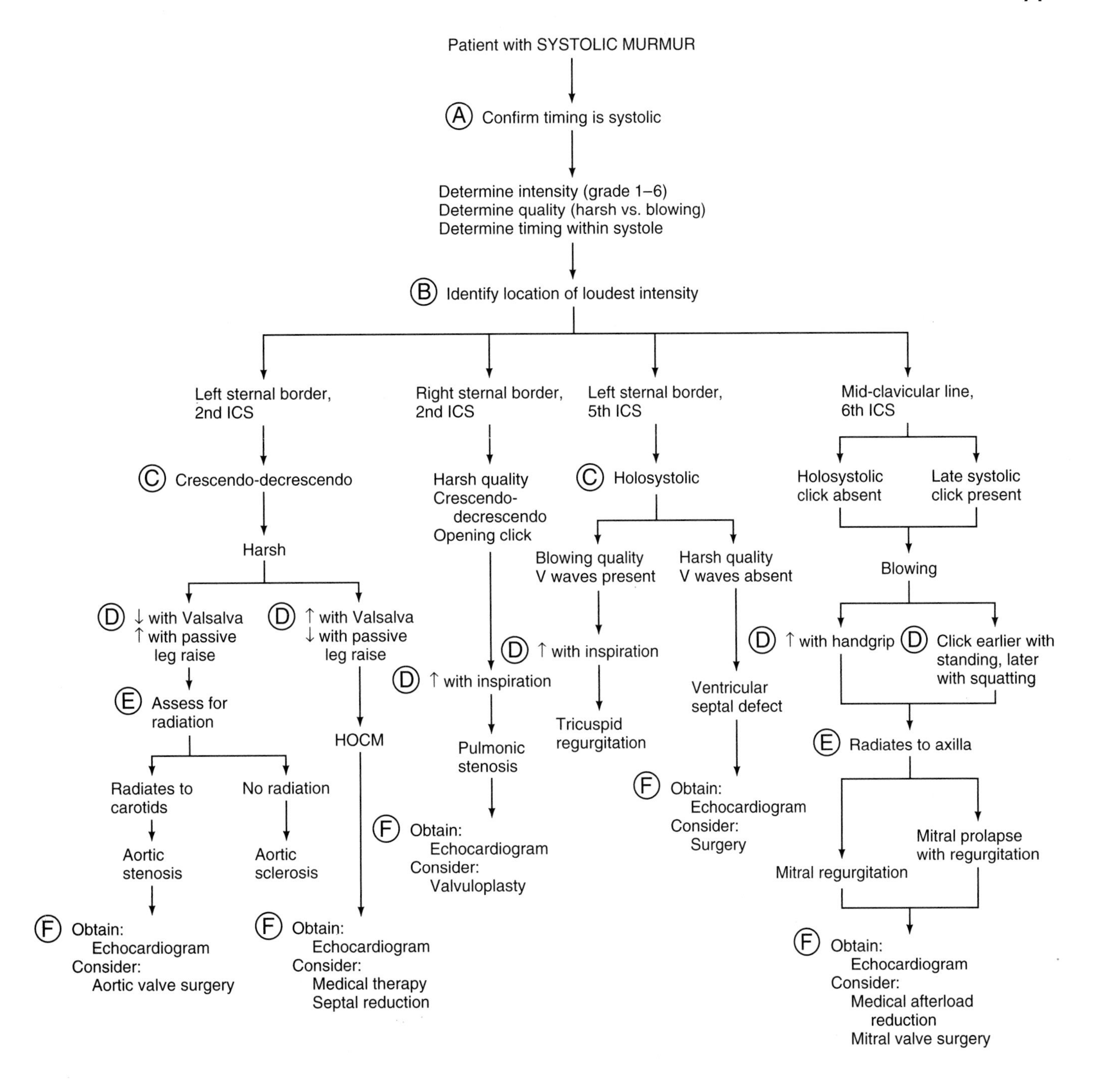

or replacement surgery. Tricuspid regurgitation is most often clinically benign but can be repaired if it is both severe and thought to be the cause of heart failure. Pulmonic stenosis is rare in adult patients because it is most frequently a congenital lesion. If detected in the adult, percutaneous valvuloplasty can be curative. Ventricular septal defects in the adult patient occur most commonly as a complication of myocardial infarction. Post–myocardial infarction ventricular septal defects carry a high short-term risk of mortality and should prompt urgent surgical repair.

References

ACC/AHA guidelines for the management of patients with valvular heart disease. J Am Coll Cardiol 1998;32(5):1486–1588.

Chen CR, Cheng TO, Huang T, et al. Percutaneous balloon valvuloplasty for pulmonic stenosis in adolescents and adults. N Engl J Med 1996;335(1):21–25.

Maron BJ, McKenna WJ, Danielson GK, et al. American College of Cardiology/European Society of Cardiology clinical expert consensus document on hypertrophic cardiomyopathy. A report of the American College of Cardiology Foundation Task Force on Clinical Expert Consensus Documents and the European Society of Cardiology Committee for Practice Guidelines. J Am Coll Cardiol 2003;42(9):1687–1713.

DIASTOLIC MURMURS

Aaron L. Baggish, MD, and Marc S. Sabatine, MD

Cardiac murmurs are generated by turbulent blood flow and adjacent soft-tissue vibration. Turbulent or nonlaminar blood flow occurs in response to rapid acceleration or deceleration of flow such as that which occurs across a narrowed valve or vessel segment.

A. Murmurs in diastole have several possible causes, including regurgitant flow across a semilunar valve (aortic or pulmonic), forward flow though a stenotic or abnormal atrioventricular (AV) valve (mitral or tricuspid), or flow through an anatomic defect (ventricular septum).

   Once a murmur has been determined to be diastolic in timing, a series of steps can be undertaken to identify the exact cause. The relative timing during diastole (early, middle, or late) and the location of optimal intensity are essential for determination of the underlying pathology.

B. **Timing:** Diastolic murmurs are characterized based on the part of the diastolic portion of the cardiac cycle during which they occur. Early diastolic murmurs begin with the aortic or pulmonic valve components of the second heart sound and have a steady decrescendo configuration. Mid-diastolic murmurs begin at the end of the silent interval following the second heart sound and terminate well before the first heart sound. The murmurs of late diastole (presystolic murmurs) occur immediately before the first heart sound and often obscure it.

C. **Early Diastolic Murmurs:** The murmurs of early diastole are most commonly caused by the regurgitant flow of blood across a semilunar valve. Aortic regurgitation produces a decrescendo murmur heard best at the superior right sternal border with radiation toward the apex. It is best heard with use of the diaphragm of the stethoscope in the patient who is seated and slightly bent forward. The duration of the murmur is useful in determining the acuity of aortic valve incompetence, with acute valve failure producing a brief murmur and chronic, compensated valve failure resulting in a more sustained murmur.

   The murmur of pulmonic valvular regurgitation is best heard in the left 2nd or 3rd intercostal space (ICS). Similar to aortic regurgitation, it has a decrescendo configuration. Pulmonic regurgitation in adults is most commonly seen in conjunction with pulmonary hypertension (Graham Steell's murmur) and is thus distinguishable from aortic regurgitation by the presence, of other signs of elevated pulmonary artery pressure, including an accentuated P_2 component of S_2 and right ventricular hypertrophy (RVH). Occasionally, pulmonary regurgitation results from congenital absence or abnormality of the pulmonic valve and is distinguished from that resulting from pulmonary hypertension by the absence of these signs.

   A rare cause of an early diastolic murmur is flow through a stenotic coronary artery, most often the proximal anterior descending artery that is in close proximity to the anterior chest wall.

D. **Mid-Diastolic Murmurs:** The murmurs of mid-diastole are generated by turbulent flow across one of the AV valves. They begin well after the second heart sound and tend to have a low-pitched rumbling quality. Mitral stenosis, most commonly a result of rheumatic heart disease, a low-pitched rumbling murmur initiated with an opening snap and heard best at the cardiac apex, is best heard with the patient in the left lateral decubitus position with use of the stethoscope bell. The duration of the murmur reflects the magnitude of the pressure gradient across the stenotic mitral valve and thus reflects the severity of mitral valve narrowing. Mitral stenosis murmurs that extend through until S_1 reflect severe disease.

   Tricuspid stenosis produces a murmur that is similar in timing and quality as that produced by mitral valve stenosis but is heard best at the left lower sternal border. The most characteristic element of the murmur of tricuspid stenosis is its increase in intensity with inspiration.

   Mid-diastolic murmurs can also occur with impediment of transatrioventricular valve flow by tumors such as an atrial myxoma, in conjunction with aortic regurgitation (Austin Flint murmur), and with conditions with supranormal cardiac flow (shunts and high-output physiology).

E. **Late Diastolic Murmurs:** The murmurs of late diastole are generated by the same underlying valve abnormalities that produce the aforementioned mid-systolic murmurs and are thus often more a late diastolic augmentation of a mid-diastolic murmur. This phenomenon results from a rapid increase in transvalvular flow from atrial contraction.

F. **Location:** Diastolic murmurs generated by regurgitant flow back through the semilunar valves are loudest in intensity at the left (pulmonic valve) and right (aortic valve) sternal border in the 2nd ICS. Those caused by turbulent flow across stenotic AV valves are heard lower on the chest wall at the left sternal border, in the 5th–6th ICS (tricuspid valve), and in the mid-clavicular line 5th–6th ICS (mitral valve).

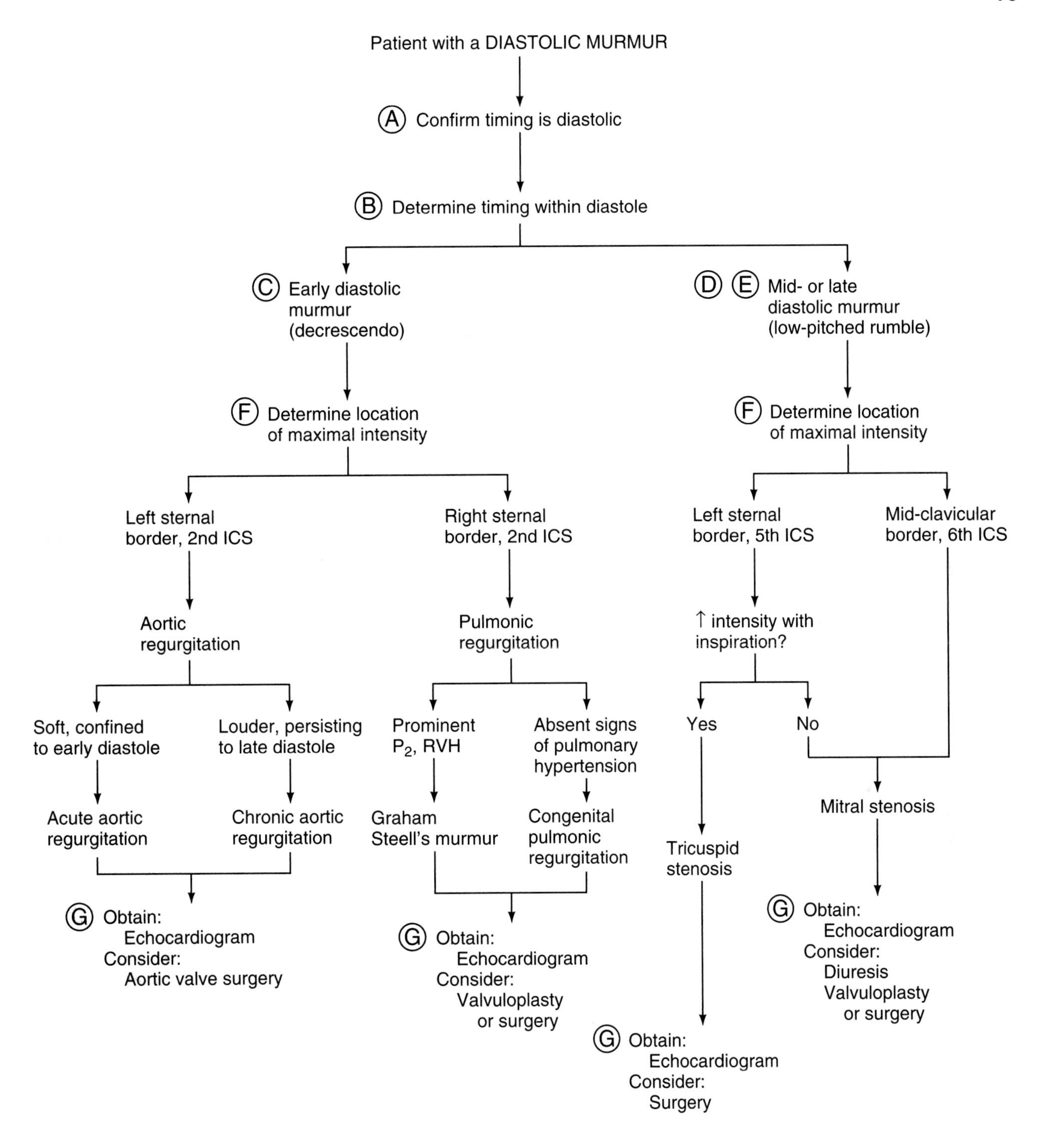

G. The management of diastolic murmurs depends on the etiology, the acuity, and the hemodynamic significance of the underlying abnormality. Echocardiography can be used to confirm the cause of a murmur. Aortic regurgitation and pulmonic regurgitation generally require surgical correction, though observation of the asymptomatic patient is a reasonable strategy. The optimal management of mitral stenosis is complicated. Options include medical management, mitral valve surgery, and percutaneous valvuloplasty.

Reference

Bonow RO, Carabello B, et al. ACC/AHA guidelines for the management of patients with valvular heart disease. J Am Coll Cardiol 1998; 32(5):1486–1588.

HYPERTENSION

Usman Baber, MD, and James A. De Lemos, MD

A. Appropriate and standard measurement of blood pressure (BP) is imperative to accurately diagnose, manage, and treat hypertension. Caffeine, exercise, and smoking should be avoided for at least 30 minutes prior to measurement and patients should be seated with the arm being measured at heart level. Indications for ambulatory BP monitoring include suspected "white coat" hypertension, hypotensive symptoms on therapy, episodic hypertension, and autonomic dysfunction.

B. Newer clinical guidelines for the management of hypertension stress the importance of treating all patients with hypertension (systolic BP [SBP] >140 mm Hg or diastolic BP [DBP] >90 mm Hg), rather than risk stratifying based on cardiovascular risk factors to determine who to treat. This is seen by the new designation of "prehypertension," which comprises those patients at high risk for the development of hypertension. In addition, those who present with markedly elevated BP (>180/120 mm Hg) must be assessed for end-organ damage to rule out hypertensive crisis (urgency or emergency) (see Table 2).

C. The initial evaluation of a patient with hypertension includes history, physical examination, laboratory tests (urinalysis [UA], glucose, chemistry, fasting lipids), and ECG. This allows for screening of identifiable causes of hypertension (e.g., hypokalemia → mineralocorticoid excess; elevated creatinine → kidney disease; striae → cushingoid state; age <30 and/or femoral bruit → renovascular disease; etc.).

D. The use of lifestyle modifications is a requisite component of hypertension management. Weight loss, physical activity, moderation of alcohol consumption, and the adoption of a low-salt diet can lower BP up to 20 mm Hg.

E. A large body of evidence from randomized controlled trials now supports the use of specific classes of antihypertensive medications based on underlying comorbid states (or compelling indications). Initial pharmacologic therapy should be guided based on such an indication (Table 1). When one is not present, a thiazide diuretic or angiotensin-converting enzyme (ACE) inhibitor (if risk for coronary artery disease is high) should be first-line therapy. If the target BP is not achieved, a different class of antihypertensive medication should be added rather than substituted because recent data indicate that most people will require multiple agents to achieve their target BP. As a result, two-drug combinations are reasonable first choices in those with stage 2 hypertension. In the event of a hypertensive crisis, the medications in Table 2 are indicated.

Table 1 Classes of Antihypertensive Medications Based on Compelling Indications

Drug Class	Compelling Indications	Adverse Effects
ACE inhibitor	Heart failure, post-MI, CKD, DM, high CAD risk	Cough, renal failure, hyperkalemia
ARB	Heart failure, DM, CKD, LVH	Hyperkalemia, renal failure
Beta blocker	Heart failure, post-MI, angina	Bronchospasm, heart block (2nd or 3rd), worsening peripheral vascular disease
Diuretic	Heart failure, elderly, African American	Gout, dyslipidemia
Calcium channel blocker	Angina, PSVT, Raynaud's disease	Heart block (2nd or 3rd degree), heart failure (systolic)

ACE, angiotensin-converting enzyme; ARB, adrenergic receptor binder; CAD, coronary artery disease; CKD, chronic kidney disease; DM, diabetes mellitus; LVH, left ventricular hypertrophy; MI, myocardial infarction; PSVT, paroxysmal supraventricular tachycardia.

Table 2 Hypertensive Crises

Drug	Mechanism	Indication
Nitroglycerin	Venodilator	Myocardial ischemia
Nitroprusside	Arteriolar/venous dilator	Aortic dissection (with concomitant beta blocker)
Nicardipine	Calcium channel blocker (dihydropyridine)	Most situations (caution in heart failure)
Labetalol	Alpha/beta blocker	Most situations
Hydralazine	Direct vasodilator	Pregnancy (preeclampsia)

If evidence of end-organ damage (Myocardial infarction, cerebrovascular accident, congestive heart failure, glomerulonephritis), must use parenteral agent to urgently lower BP. If asymptomatic, can use oral agents and follow up closely.

References

The ALLHAT Officers and Coordinators for the ALLHAT Collaborative Research Group. Major outcomes in high-risk hypertensive patients randomized to angiotensin-converting enzyme inhibitor or calcium channel blocker vs. diuretic: the Antihypertensive and Lipid-Lowering Treatment to Prevent Heart Attack Trial (ALLHAT). JAMA 2002;288:2981–2997.

August P. Initial treatment of hypertension. N Engl J Med 2003;348: 610-617.

Chobanian AV, Bakris GL, Black HR, et al. The seventh report of the Joint National Committee on Prevention, Detection, Evaluation, and Treatment of High Blood Pressure: the JNC 7 Report. JAMA 2003;289:2560–2572.

The Heart Outcomes Prevention Evaluation Study Investigators. Effects of an angiotensin-converting-enzyme inhibitor, ramipril, on cardiovascular events in high-risk patients. N Engl J Med 2000;342:145–153.

Kaplan N. Kaplan's Clinical Hypertension, 8th ed. Philadelphia: Lippincott Williams & Wilkins, 2002.

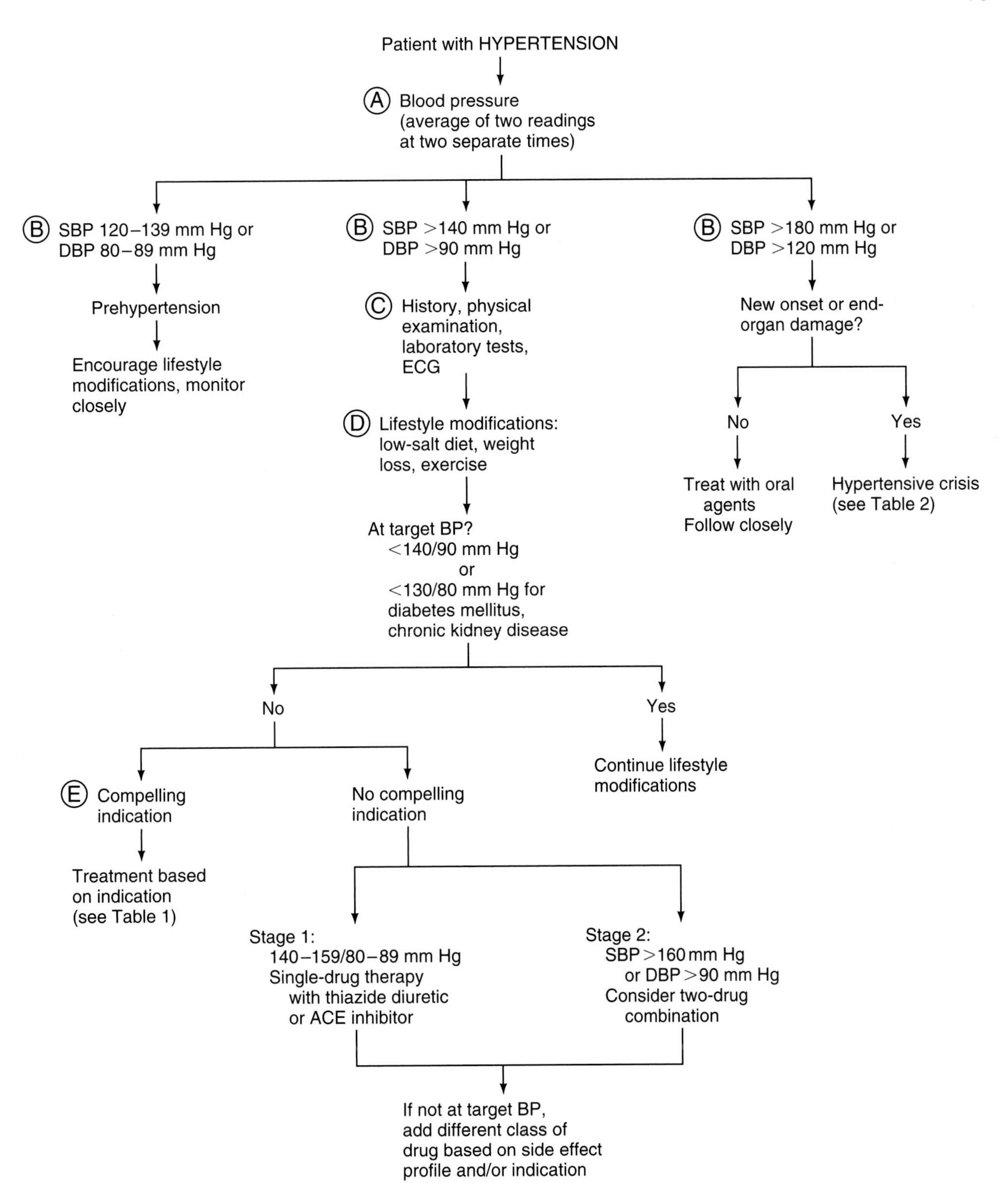
Patient with HYPERTENSION
A Blood pressure (average of two readings at two separate times)
B SBP 120–139 mm Hg or DBP 80–89 mm Hg
Prehypertension
Encourage lifestyle modifications, monitor closely
B SBP >140 mm Hg or DBP >90 mm Hg
C History, physical examination, laboratory tests, ECG
D Lifestyle modifications: low-salt diet, weight loss, exercise
At target BP? <140/90 mm Hg or <130/80 mm Hg for diabetes mellitus, chronic kidney disease
No
E Compelling indication
Treatment based on indication (see Table 1)
No compelling indication
Stage 1: 140–159/80–89 mm Hg Single-drug therapy with thiazide diuretic or ACE inhibitor
Stage 2: SBP >160 mm Hg or DBP >90 mm Hg Consider two-drug combination
If not at target BP, add different class of drug based on side effect profile and/or indication
Yes
Continue lifestyle modifications
B SBP >180 mm Hg or DBP >120 mm Hg
New onset or end-organ damage?
No
Treat with oral agents Follow closely
Yes
Hypertensive crisis (see Table 2)

HYPOTENSION

Mahesh J. Patel, MD, and James A. De Lemos, MD

Hypotension can result in multiorgan dysfunction if not treated immediately. As a result, diagnostic assessments and therapeutic maneuvers should occur rapidly and simultaneously.

A. Initially, a rapid assessment should be made to identify patients who are critically ill and unresponsive or who are clinically unstable. For these patients, Basic and Advanced Cardiac Life Support protocols should be immediately initiated.

B. Clinical examination, laboratory data, and noninvasive tests should be used to distinguish between cardiogenic and noncardiogenic causes of hypotension because the management of each one is markedly different. Careful attention to volume and perfusion status can help differentiate etiologies.

C. Invasive hemodynamic monitoring with pulmonary artery (PA) catheterization can help differentiate among different causes of hypotension. PA catheters should be used prudently because there is no indication from clinical trials that they provide clinical benefit when used routinely. (CO, cardiac output; PCWP, pulmonary capillary wedge pressure; SVR, systemic vascular resistance; PVR, pulmonary vascular resistance.)

D. Cardiogenic shock most commonly results from large myocardial infarctions (MIs; >40% of left ventricle) leading to pump failure. Mechanical complications of MI, including right ventricular dysfunction, acute mitral regurgitation, septal rupture, and free-wall rupture, can also lead to cardiogenic shock. In patients with mechanical complications, urgent surgical repair is needed. Other cardiac causes of cardiogenic hypotension include pericardial tamponade, severe obstructive valvular heart disease, and progression of a chronic cardiomyopathy. Urgent echocardiography is particularly helpful in delineating the causes of cardiogenic shock.

E. In cardiogenic shock from acute MI, urgent coronary revascularization is indicated, often with support of an intraaortic balloon pump (IABP). For initial stabilization and for treatment of ongoing cardiogenic shock, inotropic support may be initiated with dobutamine or dopamine (dobutamine is generally preferred because dopamine has significant chronotropic and vasoconstrictive properties that may worsen cardiac ischemia). If hypotension still persists, other drugs such as milrinone or norepinephrine may be tried.

F. Causes of vasodilatory hypotension include sepsis, adrenal crisis, drug effects, anaphylaxis, and neurogenic shock and require treatment of the underlying pathologic process and supportive treatment with volume resuscitation and IV vasopressors. Notably, volume resuscitation is the first-line supportive treatment for sepsis because sepsis is associated with hypovolemic hypotension. However, sepsis can also be associated with a cardiomyopathy, and this may limit the amount of volume resuscitation that can be administered.

G. Obstructive hypotension is most commonly caused by massive pulmonary thromboembolism. Treatment options include thrombolytic therapy or surgical embolectomy. Supportive measures involving volume resuscitation, vasopressors, and inotropes should be used cautiously because they may augment right ventricular strain.

H. The management of hypovolemic hypotension should involve volume resuscitation and treatment of the cause of intravascular volume loss (e.g., bleeding, diarrhea, third-space sequestration). Crystalloids, colloid-containing solutions, or blood products can be used for volume resuscitation; however, there is no clinical benefit to using colloid-containing solutions over crystalloids.

References

Connors AF Jr, Speroff T, Dawson NV, et al. The effectiveness of right heart catheterization in the initial care of critically ill patients. SUPPORT Investigators. JAMA 1996;276:889–897.

Finfer S, Bellomo R, Boyce N, et al. A comparison of albumin and saline for fluid resuscitation in the intensive care unit. N Engl J Med 2004;350:2247–2256.

Goldhaber SZ, Haire WD, Feldstein ML, et al. Alteplase versus heparin in acute pulmonary embolism: randomised trial assessing right-ventricular function and pulmonary perfusion. Lancet 1993;341:507–511.

Hochman JS, Sleeper LA, Webb JG, et al. Early revascularization in acute myocardial infarction complicated by cardiogenic shock. SHOCK Investigators. Should we emergently revascularize occluded coronaries for cardiogenic shock? N Engl J Med 1999;341:625–634.

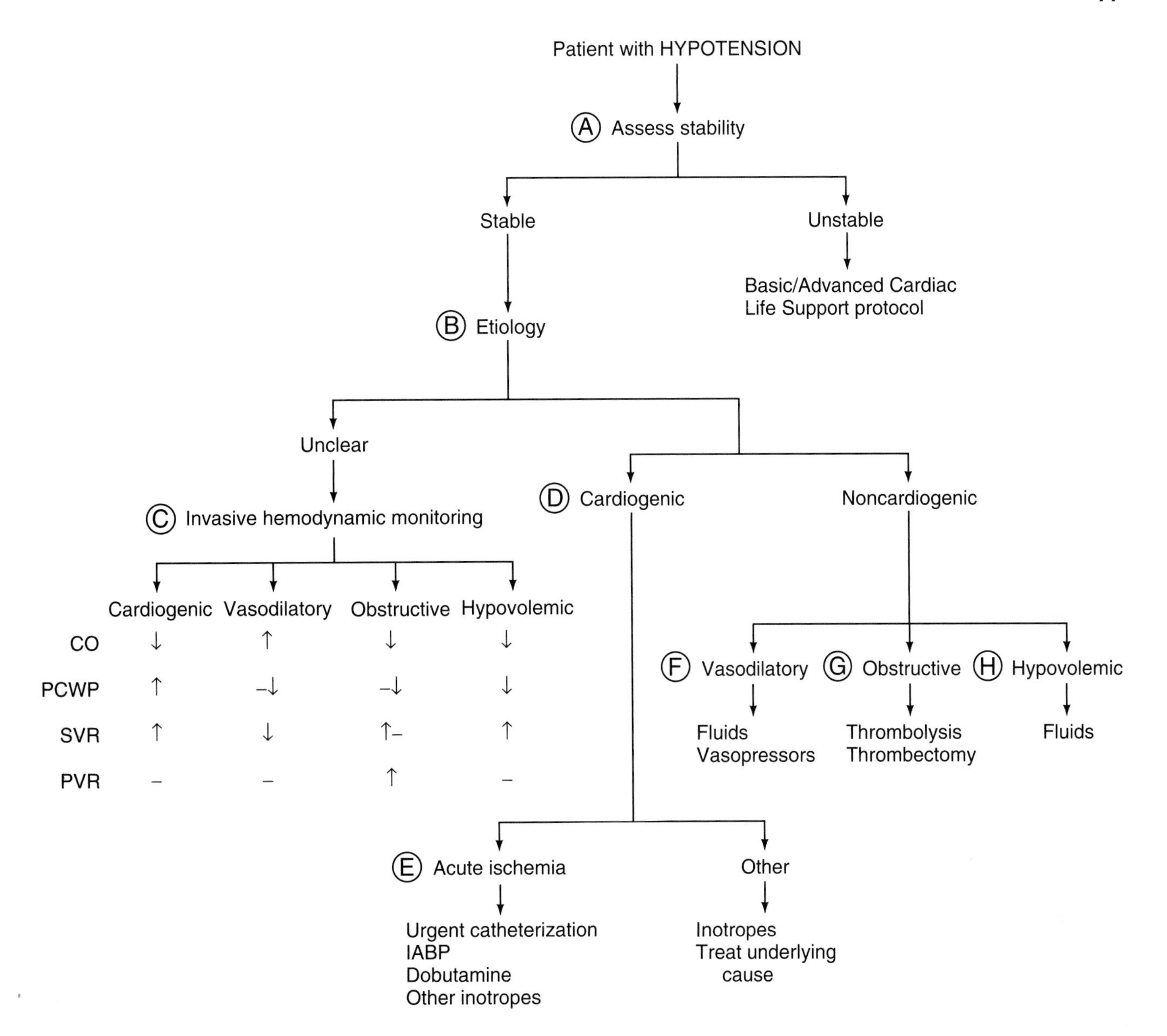

Patient with HYPOTENSION
(A) Assess stability
Stable
Unstable
Basic/Advanced Cardiac Life Support protocol
(B) Etiology
Unclear
(C) Invasive hemodynamic monitoring
Cardiogenic
Vasodilatory
Obstructive
Hypovolemic
CO
PCWP
SVR
PVR
(D) Cardiogenic
Noncardiogenic
(F) Vasodilatory
(G) Obstructive
(H) Hypovolemic
Fluids
Vasopressors
Thrombolysis
Thrombectomy
Fluids
(E) Acute ischemia
Other
Urgent catheterization
IABP
Dobutamine
Other inotropes
Inotropes
Treat underlying cause

PALPITATIONS

Christopher Pickett, MD and Peter Zimetbaum, MD

Palpitations are a common complaint. Although usually benign, they are occasionally a life-threatening condition. A stepwise approach is helpful in avoiding unnecessary workup yet still identifying patients at high risk.

A. The initial evaluation in all patients should include a directed history and physical examination and a 12-lead ECG. The initial history should be directed toward identifying patients at high risk for having a malignant etiology of their palpitations. This group includes those with prior myocardial infarction, especially with structural heart disease with an ejection fraction (EF) of <40% and congestive heart failure; those with palpitations associated with syncope; and patients with a family history of myopathy or sudden cardiac death. The patient's description of symptoms can be helpful in suggesting a diagnosis. A "flip-flopping" of the heart, especially when lying quietly in bed, suggests ventricular premature contractions (VPCs). Rapid irregular heartbeats suggest atrial fibrillation. A sensation of pounding in the chest suggests atrioventricular (AV) dissociation and is most often seen in AV nodal reentrant tachycardia (AVNRT).

   Palpitations in the setting of anxiety are often misdiagnosed as being psychiatric in origin, especially in young women. This diagnosis should not be accepted until true arrhythmic causes have been excluded.

   The 12-lead ECG can be helpful in certain circumstances: a short PR interval and delta waves suggest Wolf-Parkinson-White syndrome, marked left ventricular hypertrophy with deep septal Q waves in I, aVL, and V4-6 suggests hypertrophic cardiomyopathy; left atrial abnormalities are often seen in patients with atrial fibrillation; abnormal Q waves suggest prior MI leading to monomorphic ventricular tachycardia (VT); and a long QT interval can be seen in polymorphic VT.

B. If the patient does not have any high-risk features and the palpitations are not particularly bothersome, then reassurance can be offered. Otherwise, ambulatory cardiac monitoring should be performed using a patient-activated continuous loop monitor for up to 2 weeks or until a diagnosis is made. This approach is more cost-effective than using a Holter monitor, which is less likely to capture a significant event as a result of its shorter monitoring period.

C. If isolated ventricular or atrial ectopy is identified as the source of palpitations, then withdrawal of potential precipitants such as caffeine or alcohol is often helpful. Reassurance is often the best therapy; however, if the patient remains highly symptomatic, then a trial of beta blockade is reasonable.

D. Management of atrial fibrillation and flutter should focus on rate vs. rhythm control and stroke prevention with anticoagulation.

E. Sustained supraventricular tachycardia, when identified, are often amenable to curative therapy with an ablation. This is especially true of AVNRT, AV reentrant trachycardia (AVRT), atrial flutter, and increasingly atrial fibrillation. This option should be offered to patients whose symptoms are especially frequent or highly symptomatic, especially if associated with syncope or near-syncope.

F. Patients with sustained ventricular tachycardia or with high-risk features—family history of sudden cardiac death, or structural heart disease (EF <40%)—should be referred to an electrophysiologist for appropriate management, including possible electrophysiology study (EPS), antiarrhythmic therapy, and implantable cardiac defibrillator (ICD) implantation.

References

Josephson ME, Wellens HJJ. Differential diagnosis of supraventricular tachycardia. Cardiol Clin 1990;8:411–442.

Kennedy HL, Sprague MK, Kennedy LJ, et al. Long-term follow-up of asymptomatic healthy subjects with frequent and complex ventricular ectopy. N Engl J Med 1985;312:193–197.

Lessmeier TJ, Gamperling D, Johnson-Liddon V, et al. Unrecognized paroxysmal supraventricular tachycardia: potential for misdiagnosis as panic disorder. Arch Intern Med 1997;157:536–543.

Mayou R, Sprigings D, Birkhead J, Price J. Characteristics of patients presenting to a cardiac clinic with palpitation. QJM 2003;96(2):115–123.

Zimetbaum PJ, Kim KY, Josephson ME, et al. Diagnostic yield and optimal duration of continuous-loop event monitoring for the diagnosis of palpitations: a cost-effectiveness analysis. Ann Intern Med 1998;128(11):890–895.

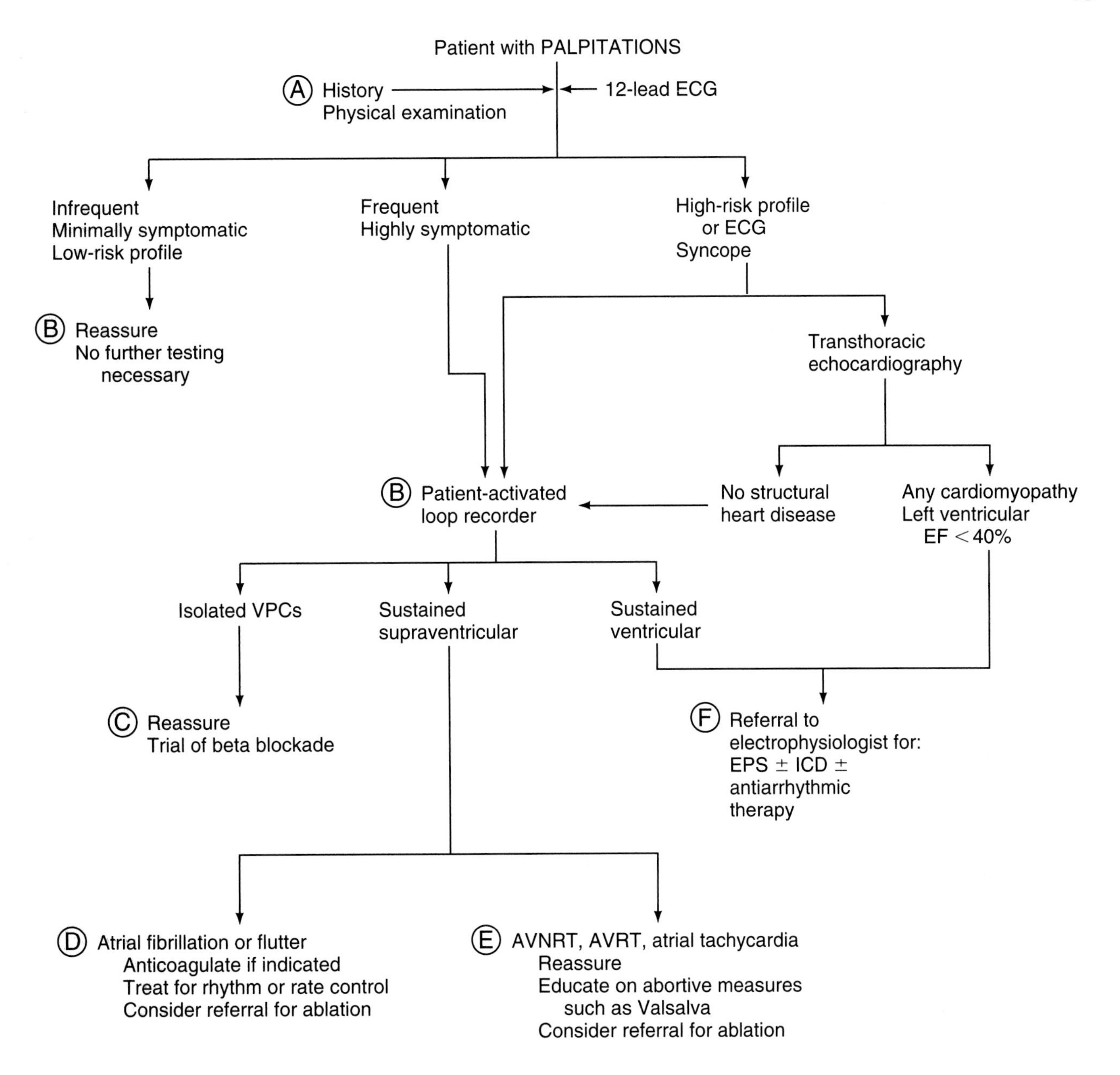
Patient with PALPITATIONS
A History
Physical examination
12-lead ECG
Infrequent
Minimally symptomatic
Low-risk profile
Frequent
Highly symptomatic
High-risk profile
or ECG
Syncope
B Reassure
No further testing
necessary
Transthoracic
echocardiography
B Patient-activated
loop recorder
No structural
heart disease
Any cardiomyopathy
Left ventricular
EF < 40%
Isolated VPCs
Sustained
supraventricular
Sustained
ventricular
C Reassure
Trial of beta blockade
F Referral to
electrophysiologist for:
EPS ± ICD ±
antiarrhythmic
therapy
D Atrial fibrillation or flutter
Anticoagulate if indicated
Treat for rhythm or rate control
Consider referral for ablation
E AVNRT, AVRT, atrial tachycardia
Reassure
Educate on abortive measures
such as Valsalva
Consider referral for ablation

SYNCOPE

William H. Nesbitt, MD, and James A. De Lemos, MD

Syncope is defined as a loss of consciousness resulting from decreased blood flow to the brain and is reported to occur in up to 3% of all people during their lifetime. The evaluation of syncope is centered on discriminating between cardiac and noncardiac causes, because a cardiac etiology has been associated with increased mortality.

A. The medical history, including family history, is an important tool in diagnosing the etiology of syncope. The patient's age can provide a framework because vasovagal syncope is common in younger individuals, whereas orthostatic hypotension, sick sinus syndrome, and heart block occur more commonly in the elderly.

B. The physical examination and ECG can yield important clues to the etiology. Examples include orthostatic blood pressures; cardiomegaly via palpation/percussion and chest x-ray; carotid sinus hypersensitivity; and ECG evidence of previous myocardial infarction, atrioventricular (AV) block, or long QT interval.

C. Studies have shown that the presence of structural heart disease is associated with an increased risk of a cardiac cause of syncope and is also associated with increased mortality. Imaging modalities, including echocardiogram, MRI, or contrast ventriculography, can provide insight to pathology such as impaired systolic function and wall motion abnormalities as well as high-risk diseases such as valvular heart disease, hypertrophic cardiomyopathy, cardiac sarcoidosis, and right ventricular dysplasia.

D. Supraventricular and ventricular tachyarrhythmias are common among patients with structural heart disease. Patients with syncope who have structural heart disease concomitant with coronary artery disease or a previous myocardial infarction may be considered for electrophysiologic evaluation because ventricular tachycardia is common in this group.

E. Electrophysiology testing consists of placing catheters that have the ability to both pace and sense in various sites within the heart. Commonly, electrograms are recorded from the high right atrium, anterior septum for bundle of His activation, and the right ventricle. Electrophysiologic properties of the heart are obtained, including refractory periods and AV nodal and His-Purkinje system conduction. In addition, programmed stimulation is used to pace the heart in an attempt to induce ventricular or supraventricular arrhythmias. Electrophysiology testing is sensitive for detecting ventricular tachycardia in the presence of an ischemic cardiomyopathy but lacks sensitivity for nonischemic cardiomyopathies. Patients with a left ventricular ejection fraction (LVEF) of <35% have a primary prevention indication for an implantable cardiac defibrillator (ICD); therefore, syncope in this population should lead to referral for an ICD with or without an electrophysiology study.

F. Bradyarrhythmias are common causes of syncope in the elderly. Electrophysiology testing for bradycardia is of more limited value in establishing the need for permanent pacing; therefore, noninvasive monitoring with a Holter monitor or event recorder can be used to correlate symptoms with slow heart rates.

G. Syncope in the absence of structural heart disease is often vasovagal in origin. This syndrome is characterized by the onset of prodromal symptoms such as yawning, nausea, or a feeling of warmth often provoked by noxious stimuli followed by bradycardia, hypotension, and syncope.

H. Tilt-table testing is a tool to aid in the diagnosis of vasovagal syncope as well as orthostatic hypotension, postural orthostatic tachycardia syndrome, and vasodepressor syncope. The patient is secured to a table that is tilted usually to 60 degrees in a quiet room while blood pressure and heart rate are monitored. Patients with vasovagal syncope will have variable responses, and most will develop their usual prodromal symptoms associated with a decrease in blood pressure and/or heart rate (sensitivity 70%). This is often associated with loss of consciousness that resolves with placing the patient back in the supine position.

I. Syncope in a patient with a normal heart and a negative tilt-table test result can safely be referred for a cardiac monitor to record heart rates and rhythm as an outpatient if an arrhythmia is suspected. A Holter monitor is a device the patient wears for 24 or 48 hours that records every beat. Continuous looping event monitors are worn by the patient and can record prospective and retrospective heart rhythms and can be patient activated with symptoms. A nonlooping event monitor records only when the patient activates the monitor. A continuous looping event monitor is preferable in a patient with syncope. Additionally, an implantable event monitor is a small device implanted just left of the sternum. It can be patient activated when symptoms occur or is automatically activated with slow or fast heart rates and can remain in place for 1–2 years.

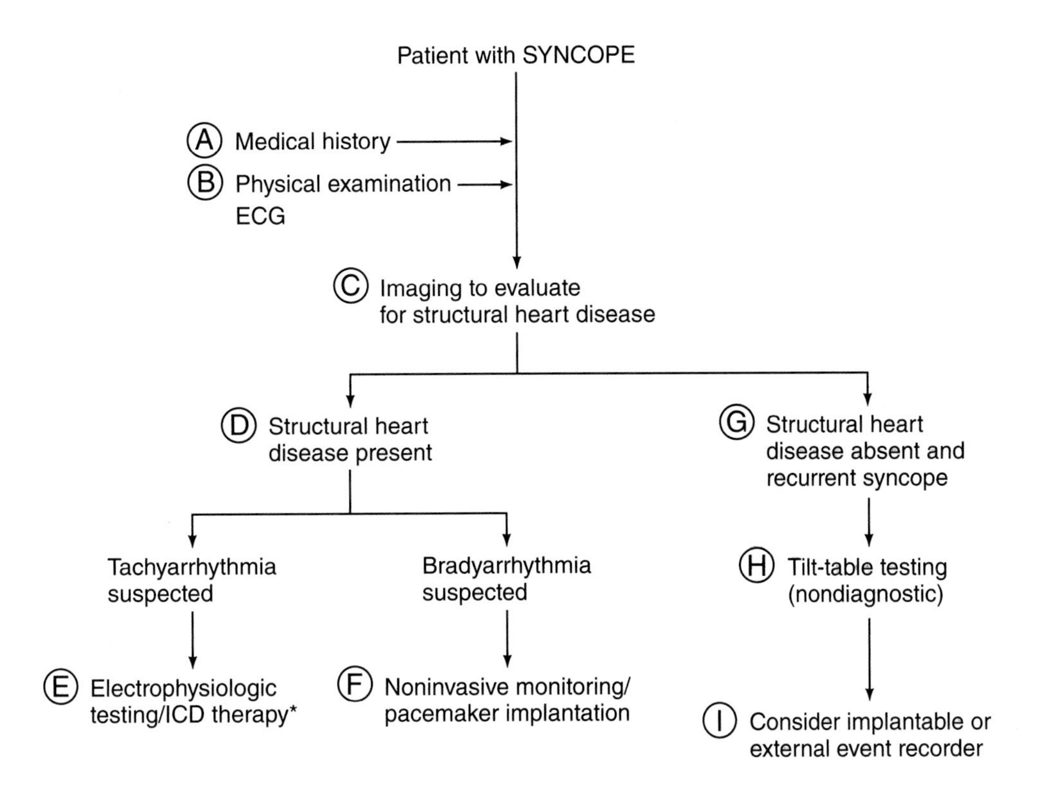

*ICD placement without EP testing is indicated if the LVEF is severely reduced.

References

Benditt DG. Pathophysiology and causes of syncope. In Cardiac Arrhythmia: Mechanisms, Diagnosis and Management. Baltimore: Williams & Wilkins, 1995:1073–1084.

Calkins H. Syncope. In Zipes D, Jalife J, eds. Cardiac Electrophysiology: From Cell to Bedside. Philadelphia: WB Saunders:, 2000:873–881.

Kapoor W. Evaluation and management of syncope. JAMA 1992;268: 2553–2560.

Kapoor W. Syncope. N Engl J Med 2000;343:1856–1862.

EVALUATION OF A NEW DIAGNOSIS OF CONGESTIVE HEART FAILURE

Lisa M. Mielniczuk, MD, and James C. Fang, MD

Heart failure (HF) is a significant cause of morbidity and mortality in the United States. It is estimated that 5 million patients currently have HF and approximately 550,000 patients are newly diagnosed each year. Early diagnosis and treatment of underlying and potentially reversible causes are essential to preventing the progression to more severe and debilitating symptoms.

A. The history and physical examination should focus on distinguishing between ischemic causes of HF (coronary artery disease [CAD]) and nonischemic causes of HF (valvular heart disease, diabetes, hypertension, alcohol abuse, neuromuscular disorders, and cardiomyopathies). The family history should be explored for premature CAD, HF, arrhythmias, and sudden cardiac death. The baseline ECG should be reviewed for evidence of myocardial infarction, conduction disturbances, and arrhythmias.
B. Approximately 40%–60% of patients with HF have evidence of CAD. Patients with angina and/or clinical suspicion for CAD should be referred for cardiac catheterization. Noninvasive testing for ischemia can also be considered, but cardiac catheterization should be performed in any patient in whom the diagnosis of CAD remains uncertain after noninvasive testing.
C. If CAD and ischemia are found, mechanical revascularization should be strongly considered. If left ventricular (LV) function is abnormal (i.e., ejection fraction [EF] <40%), then an assessment of myocardial viability should be performed. If viability is adequate, mechanical revascularization should be performed if the patient is otherwise a medically appropriate candidate.
D. Echocardiography is used to make the important clinical distinction between HF with either normal or abnormal systolic function and to assess valvular abnormalities, right-sided heart function, and chamber dimensions.
E. Primary anatomic abnormalities of valve structure (i.e., myxomatous mitral valve, bicuspid aortic valve) suggest HF is a result of valvular heart disease. Other causes include rheumatic heart disease, connective tissue disorders such as Marfan's syndrome, or calcific degeneration. When HF is secondary to significant primary valvular disease, referral for surgical intervention should be considered.
F. In patients with HF and nonischemic LV dysfunction, there are multiple other causes to consider. History should be specifically sought for drug and alcohol use, recent viral illness, and familial disorders. Systolic dysfunction can result from exposure to certain drugs (i.e., anthracyclines, trastuzumab, and cyclophosphamide) through hypersensitivity reactions by direct myocardial injury. Incessant atrial and ventricular tachycardias may also lead to nonischemic cardiomyopathies. Endomyocardial biopsy is required to establish the diagnosis of myocarditis. Many patients (20%–30%) will not have a definitive diagnosis despite extensive investigations and will be diagnosed with idiopathic cardiomyopathy. It is believed that many of these patients have either a familial disorder or a postviral etiology.
G. There are numerous causes of HF with preserved systolic function (also known as "diastolic heart failure"). This diagnosis is generally considered when the EF is >40%. Many of these patients will also exhibit abnormal diastolic function. Patients at risk for this type of HF are generally elderly females with diabetes and are hypertensive on presentation. In the absence of hypertension, restrictive cardiomyopathies should be considered. These disorders include infiltrative diseases (amyloid, sarcoid, and hemochromatosis), inherited myocardial diseases (hypertrophic cardiomyopathy), and radiation injury. Although the echocardiogram may have suggestive findings, cardiac biopsy is often necessary to diagnose infiltrative cardiomyopathies. Finally, constrictive pericardial disease should always be ruled out.
H. All patients with HF should have basic biochemical testing to look for renal dysfunction, anemia, electrolyte imbalances and thyroid dysfunction because these may contribute to HF symptoms and progression. Specific testing can assist in the diagnosis of hemochromatosis and amyloidosis. A cardiac biopsy may be useful in patients with acute myocarditis or if there is strong clinical suspicion of an infiltrative cardiomyopathy.

References

Chareonthaitawee P, Gersh BJ, Araoz PA, Gibbons RJ. Revascularization in severe left ventricular dysfunction: the role of viability testing. J Am Coll Cardiol 2005;46(4):567–574.

Fang J, Eisenhauer. Profiles in heart failure. In Baim DS, ed. Grossman's Cardiac Catheterization, Angiography, and Intervention. Philadelphia: Lippincott, Williams & Wilkins, 2005.

Felker GM, Thompson RE, Hare JM, et al. Underlying causes and long-term survival in patients with initially unexplained cardiomyopathy. N Engl J Med 2000;342(15):1077–1084.

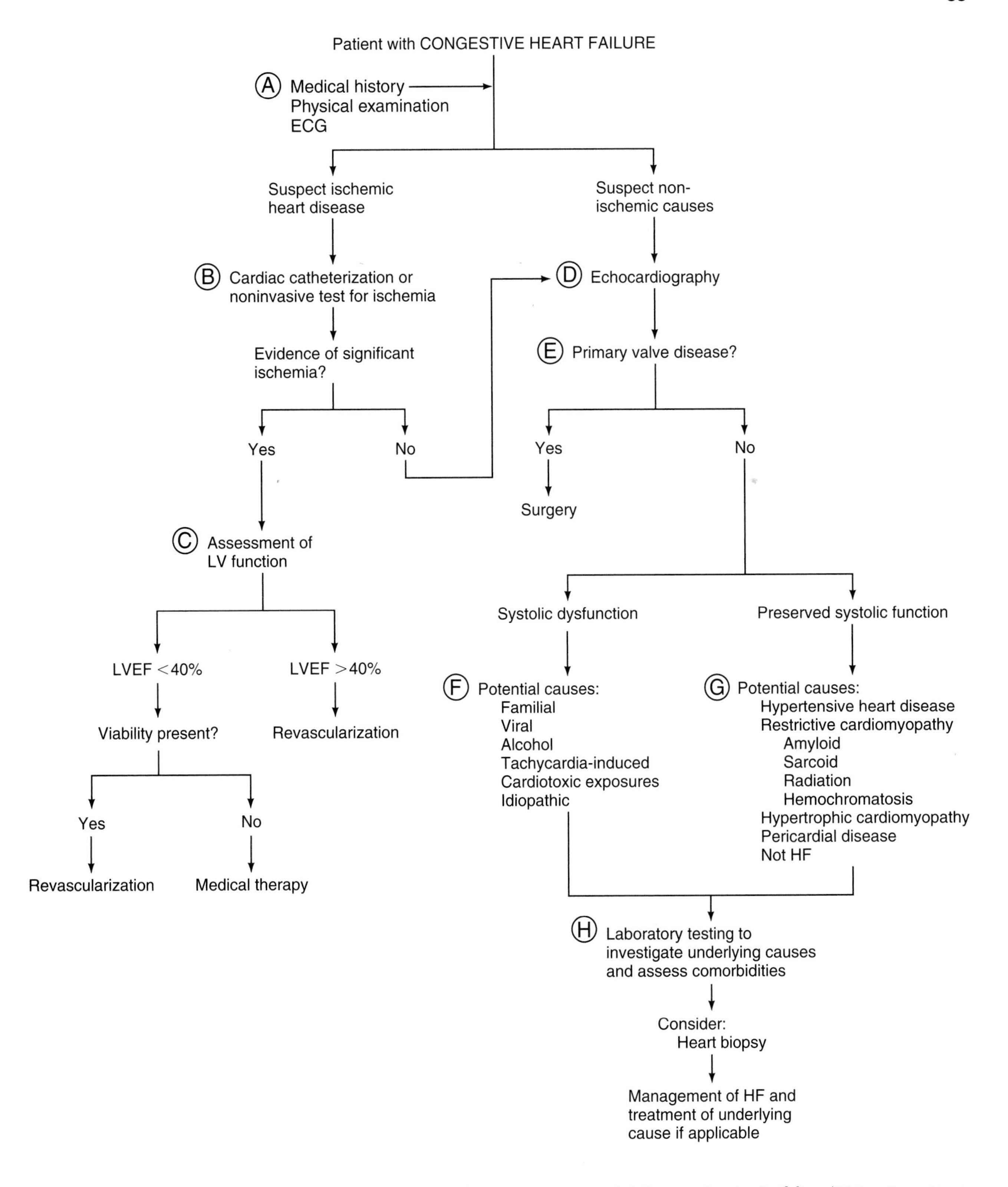

Fox KF, Cowie MR, Wood DA, et al. Coronary artery disease as the cause of incident heart failure in the population. Eur Heart J 2001;22(3):228–236.

Hunt SA, Abraham WT, Chin MH, et al. ACC/AHA 2005 guideline update for the diagnosis and management of chronic heart failure in the adult: a report of the American College of Cardiology/American Heart Association Task Force on Practice Guidelines (Writing Committee to Update the 2001 Guidelines for the Evaluation and Management of Heart Failure): developed in collaboration with the American College of Chest Physicians and the International Society for Heart and Lung Transplantation: endorsed by the Heart Rhythm Society. Circulation 2005;112(12):e154–235

DIAGNOSIS AND TREATMENT OF ACUTE PULMONARY EDEMA

Lisa M. Mielniczuk, MD, and James C. Fang, MD

Acute pulmonary edema is an emergency that necessitates admission to the hospital. Cardiogenic pulmonary edema results from an increase in left atrial pressure with a resultant increase in pulmonary venous and capillary pressure. This results in extravasation of fluid into the alveoli and impairment of gas exchange in the lungs.

A. The initial history and physical examination should be targeted toward confirming the diagnosis of pulmonary edema, assessing the severity, and identifying any immediate underlying precipitants. Symptoms may include acute or progressive shortness of breath, cough, orthopnea, paroxysmal nocturnal dyspnea, and occasionally hemoptysis. Clinical signs include tachypnea, tachycardia, an ausculatory S_3 or S_4, elevation in the jugular venous pressure, crackles, and hypoxia depending on the degree of alveolar edema.

B. Of significant importance to the initial patient assessment is the identification of patients with imminent respiratory failure who will require early and intensive therapy with either invasive or noninvasive ventilatory support. All patients should be provided with supplemental oxygen. ABGs may be required to assess adequacy of ventilation and oxygenation.

C. Patients with signs of hypoperfusion, including systolic blood pressure (SBP) of <90 mm Hg, cool extremities, altered mental status, and poor urine output, may be candidates for early hemodynamic support with inotropic therapy or intraaortic balloon counterpulsation. Urgent coronary angiography and revascularization should be performed if myocardial ischemia is suspected as the etiology of pulmonary edema and cardiovascular collapse.

D. The initial diagnostic workup should focus on the confirmation of pulmonary edema, identification of the severity, and investigation for an underlying cause. Chest radiograph may show bilateral perihilar edema and cephalization of pulmonary vascular markings. An ECG may identify any arrhythmias, ischemia, or injury. A serum brain natriuretic peptide (BNP) level of <100 pg/ml makes the diagnosis of heart failure (HF) very unlikely, whereas a BNP of >500 pg/ml increases the likelihood of HF. Occasionally, right-sided heart catheterization may be required to confirm the diagnosis and establish the hemodynamic profile. Baseline renal and electrolyte testing is critical to assess the contribution of renal insufficiency to the clinical picture. An echocardiogram will provide useful information about systolic, diastolic, and valvular function.

E. If the clinical assessment and supporting diagnostic evaluations do not support a diagnosis of pulmonary edema, other pulmonary conditions, including pneumonia, acute pulmonary embolism, and noncardiogenic pulmonary edema (i.e., acute respiratory distress syndrome [ARDS]), should be considered.

F. Therapy should be instituted immediately, often concurrently with diagnostic evaluation. Cardiogenic pulmonary edema is a manifestation of high left-sided filling pressures; thus investigation and management should be tailored to the specific causes:

- Acute ischemia—This is evidenced by history, ischemic ECG changes, and abnormal cardiac enzymes. Therapy will involve appropriate treatment for the acute coronary syndrome concurrent with HF therapy.
- Acute arrhythmia—HF can result from either tachyarrhythmias or bradyarrhythmias, and therapy will depend on the primary rhythm disturbance.
- Valvular—Acute mitral regurgitation and aortic insufficiency in particular may present in this fashion. Acute management involves hemodynamic stabilization with pharmacologic and/or mechanical afterload and preload reduction and surgical consultation.
- Hypertensive crisis—IV agents, such as nitroprusside or labetalol, should be used to acutely lower the mean arterial pressure by 25%–30%.
- Acutely decompensated chronic HF—Anemia, infection, dietary indiscretion, and medication noncompliance are all other potential causes precipitating pulmonary edema in those with chronic HF.

(Continued on page 86)

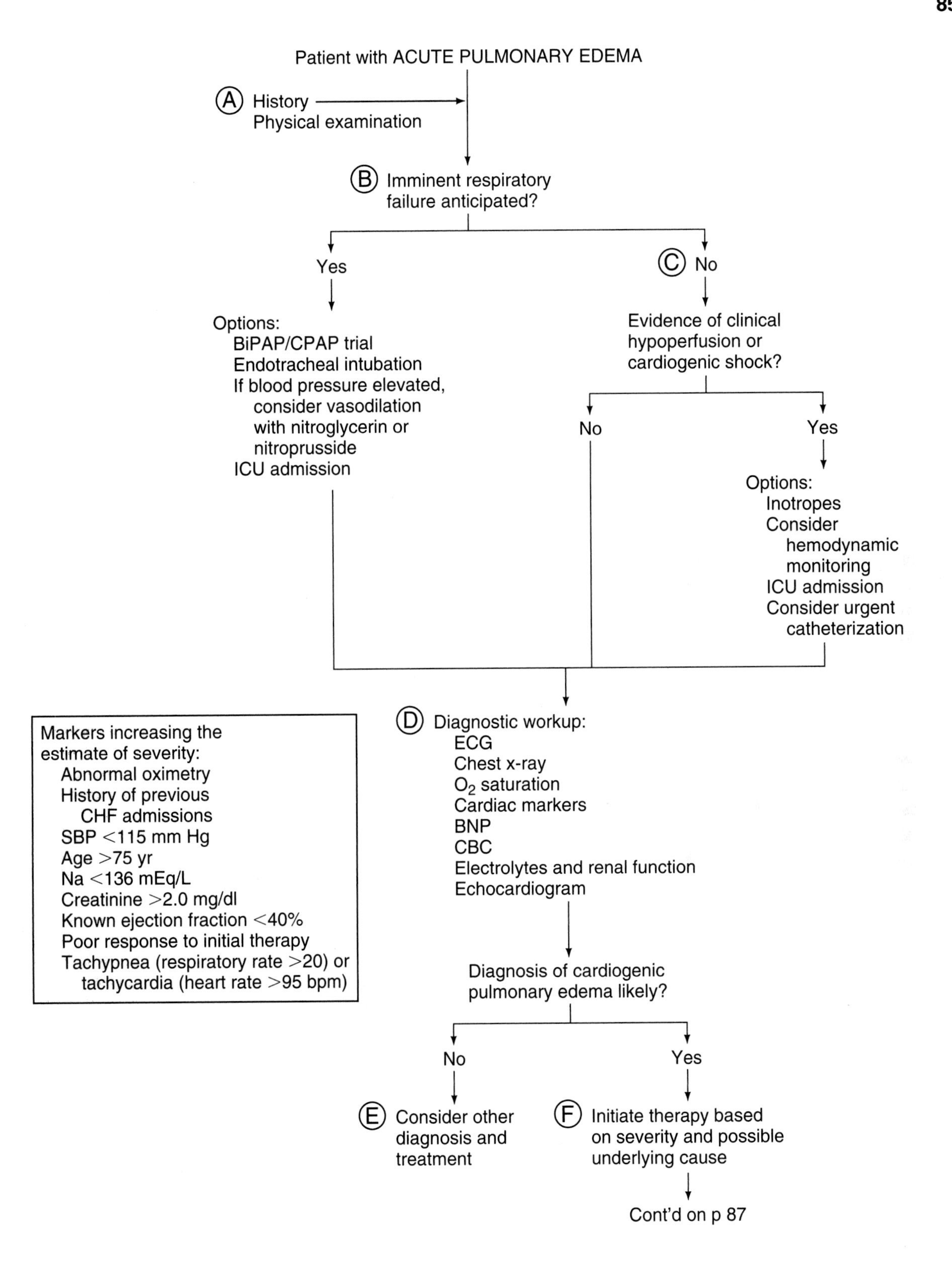

Patient with ACUTE PULMONARY EDEMA
(A) History
Physical examination
(B) Imminent respiratory failure anticipated?
Yes
Options:
BiPAP/CPAP trial
Endotracheal intubation
If blood pressure elevated, consider vasodilation with nitroglycerin or nitroprusside
ICU admission
(C) No
Evidence of clinical hypoperfusion or cardiogenic shock?
No
Yes
Options:
Inotropes
Consider hemodynamic monitoring
ICU admission
Consider urgent catheterization
Markers increasing the estimate of severity:
Abnormal oximetry
History of previous CHF admissions
SBP <115 mm Hg
Age >75 yr
Na <136 mEq/L
Creatinine >2.0 mg/dl
Known ejection fraction <40%
Poor response to initial therapy
Tachypnea (respiratory rate >20) or tachycardia (heart rate >95 bpm)
(D) Diagnostic workup:
ECG
Chest x-ray
O2 saturation
Cardiac markers
BNP
CBC
Electrolytes and renal function
Echocardiogram
Diagnosis of cardiogenic pulmonary edema likely?
No
Yes
(E) Consider other diagnosis and treatment
(F) Initiate therapy based on severity and possible underlying cause
Cont'd on p 87

BiPAP, Biphasic positive airway pressure; CPAP, continuous positive airway pressure.

G. The dose of diuretic will vary among individual patients. All patients with pulmonary edema should receive IV diuretics to ensure a quick response and assist with pulmonary venous dilation. In individuals taking chronic diuretics, an initial estimate is to administer an IV dose that is double the patient's baseline oral dose. In patients who are diuretic naïve, an initial IV dose of furosemide 0.5–1.0 mg/kg can be used. If an adequate response is not seen within 1 hour, the dose of diuretic should be doubled.

H. IV vasodilator therapy may have many beneficial effects in patients with acute pulmonary edema, including relief of cardiac ischemia (nitroglycerin), pulmonary vasodilation (nitroprusside, nesiritide, and itroglycerin), improvement in dyspnea (IV nesiritide, IV nitroglycerin), and reduction in afterload (nitroprusside).

I. The use of inotropic support in acute pulmonary edema should be reserved for patients presenting with advanced symptoms of congestion combined with evidence of hypoperfusion. When used, the dose of inotrope should be titrated slowly to a hemodynamic goal (dobutamine 2–10 μg/kg/min, dopamine 1–5 μg/kg/min, or milrinone 0.375–0.75 μg/kg/min), such as improvement in blood pressure or improved clinical perfusion manifest by an increase in pulse pressure, mental status, or increased urine output. Attempts should be made to wean inotropic therapy as soon as possible once the patient is stabilized.

References

1. Drazner MH, Rame JE, Stevenson LW, Dries SL. Prognostic importance of elevated jugular venous pressure and a third heart sound in patients with heart failure. N Engl J Med 2001;345:574–581.
2. Francis GS, Pierpont GL. Pathophysiology of congestive heart failure secondary to congestive and ischemic cardiomyopathy. In Shaver JA, ed. Cardiomyopathies: Clinical Presentation, Differential Diagnosis, and Management. Philadelphia: FA Davis, 1988:57–74.
3. Maisel A, Hollander JE, Guss D, et al. Primary results of the Rapid Emergency Department Heart Failure Outpatient Trial (REDHOT). A multicenter study of B-type natriuretic peptide levels, emergency department decision making, and outcomes in patients presenting with shortness of breath. J Am Coll Cardiol 2004;44:1328–1333.
4. Nohria, A, Lewis E, Stevenson LW. Medical management of advanced heart failure. JAMA 2002;287:628–640.

Patient with ACUTE PULMONARY EDEMA
(Cont'd from p 85)

(G) Low clinical severity (absence of any high-risk feature)
- O_2
- Loop diuretic
- Patient education
- Rule out reversible/precipitating causes
- Reevaluate response to therapy frequently to determine disposition

(H) Moderate clinical severity
- O_2
- IV diuretic
- Vasodilator therapy as needed
- Treat/investigate underlying causes
- In and out monitoring
- Admit to monitored bed

(I) Critical severity (any signs of impending respiratory failure or hypoperfusion)
- O_2
- IV diuretic bolus then infusion if needed
- Consider IV inotrope or vasodilator
- Continuous monitoring of urine output
- Critical care unit bed
- Treat/investigate underlying causes

RIGHT VENTRICULAR FAILURE

Michael Singh, MD, and George Ruiz, MD

Right ventricular (RV) failure is the final common path for several different clinical entities. RV function can be a useful clinical window into the state of the pulmonary vasculature and systemic circulation, including the left ventricle. Although in many cases the cause of RV failure is clear, the challenge is to discern if the underlying dysfunction is secondary to (1) "left-sided" or *systemic* cardiac dysfunction, (2) pathology in the lungs (either pulmonary vascular, parenchymal, or airway disease), (3) an issue isolated to the "right-sided" or *pulmonic* circulation, or (4) some combination of the general categories cited. Although classic conventions of *left*- and *right*-sided dysfunction are used, it is worth noting that such designations may be particularly confusing when addressing complex congenital heart abnormalities; therefore, *systemic* and *pulmonic* may prove to be more accurate descriptors. Because RV failure is a common final pathway, we advocate a systematic diagnostic and therapeutic approach.

A. A thorough history and physical examination are particularly useful in discerning the cause of RV failure.

The history should attempt to systematically exonerate or indict the broad categories depicted earlier, namely, systemic cardiac dysfunction, pulmonary pathology, isolated pulmonic cardiac dysfunction, or a combination of these factors. Interrogation about the systemic circulation includes any history of acquired ventricular or valvular dysfunction and contributing factors (coronary risk factors, history of myocardial infarction [MI], myocarditis, alcohol ingestion, and rheumatic fever). Paroxysmal nocturnal dyspnea and orthopnea may also be clues that RV failure may be present in the setting of left atrial (LA) hypertension. Any history or symptoms suggestive of pulmonary hypertension, interstitial lung disease (ILD), chronic airway issues, sleep apnea, kyphoscoliosis, pleural disease, or diaphragmatic dysfunction may be helpful and may point to the lungs as the primary pathologic focus. A family history of syncope, sudden death, or congenital heart abnormalities may also be useful. Symptoms of RV failure may include fatigue (from low cardiac output), nausea with or without vague right upper quadrant discomfort (from liver congestion), weight gain, increase in abdominal girth, lower extremity edema, and exertional symptoms (chest pain, dyspnea, decreased exercise tolerance). It is also very important to determine the chroniity of the patient's complaints (acute vs. chronic) to understand the rate at which the process is progressing.

The physical examination should focus on including/excluding diagnostic possibilities in addition to attempting to qualitatively discern the pressure/volume state of both the pulmonic and systemic ventricles. Vital signs (temperature, blood pressure, heart rate, peripheral O_2 saturation, and weight) not only may speak to level of decompensation but also may point to specific etiologies. Inspection of the chest wall and spine may be helpful, allowing visualization of the pattern of breathing and qualitative assessment of the tidal volume. Healed median sternotomy and thoracotomy scars can also provide useful clues (congenital heart disease [CHD], lung disease). Evaluation of the jugular venous pressure is essential because it can provide a window into the right ventricle's filling pressures and also into tricuspid valve function (prominent A waves—tricuspid stenosis; prominent V waves—tricuspid regurgitation). Kussmaul's sign should also be sought (constrictive pericarditis). In patients with RV failure on the basis of elevated pulmonary arterial pressures, pulmonic valve closure may be palpated left of the second intercostal space at end systole. Pulmonary arterial pulsations may be felt on either side of the sternum at the level of the second intercostal space. Placement of the examiner's hand on the patient's sternum may elicit the presence of an RV heave, and prominent RV pulsation may be felt just below the xiphoid. Percussion of the border on the right side of the heart may demonstrate an enlarged right atrium. Auscultation should focus on evaluation of valvular pathology, CHD, and the presence of right- and/or left-sided gallops (S_4 or S_3). Splitting of the second heart sound should also be noted (wide split is suggestive of a right bundle branch block; fixed split is suggestive of an atrial septal defect). Graham Steell's murmur (pulmonic regurgitation from pulmonary hypertension) may be present. Right-sided gallops are often heard at the lower-left sternal border or in the subxiphoid area with the bell of the stethoscope lightly held. The presence of gallops may speak to the presence of both pressure and volume overload in either ventricle. Hepatomegaly, ascites, and lower-extremity edema may also be present. Palpation of the proximal limbs may also be helpful indicators of systemic vascular resistance, with "cool" extremities suggestive of poor cardiac output with elevated systemic resistance.

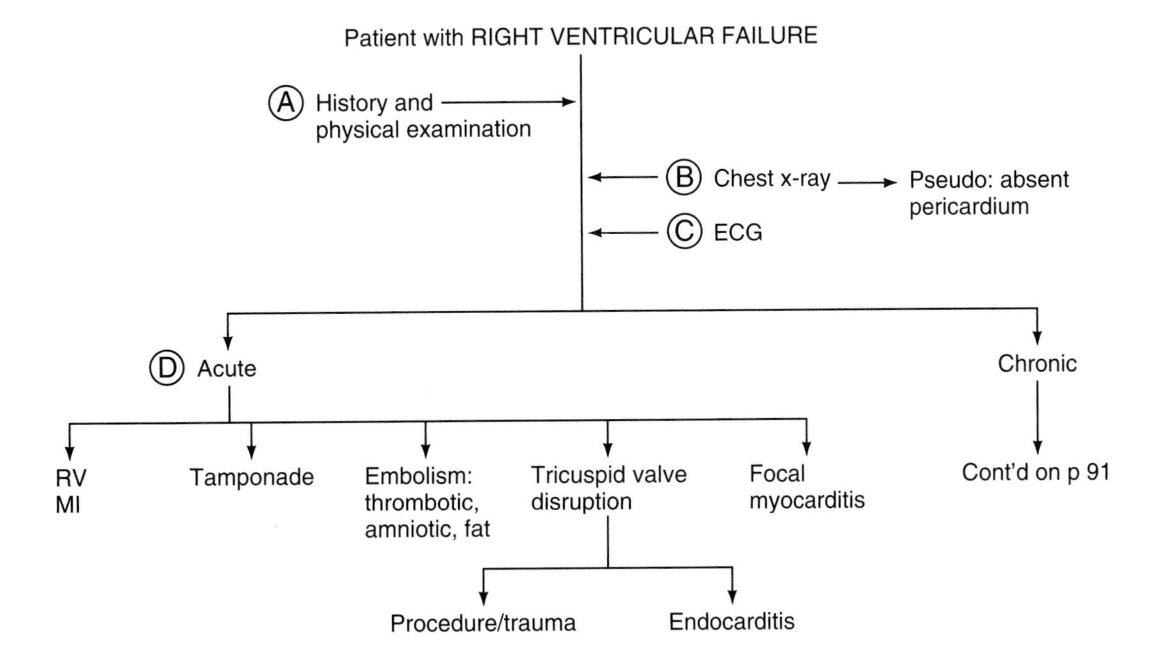

B. The chest x-ray can be a helpful diagnostic tool and can help confirm physical examination findings. It can be particularly useful as a preliminary screen for pulmonary parenchymal and pleural-based disease. It can also provide a gross estimate of heart size and particular chamber enlargement. Ideally, a lateral chest film should be included in addition to the traditional posteroanterior (PA) view. The lateral film can help with the diagnosis of rare issues, such as congenital absence of the pericardium (cardiomegaly present in the PA view, but not in the lateral) and Ebstein's anomaly. The extent and balance owf the pulmonary vascularity can also serve as important clues pointing not only to etiology but also to severity.

C. ECG is an essential part of the initial workup of right-sided heart failure. It is always valuable to look for evidence of chamber enlargement or hypertrophy, particularly of the right ventricle. The ECG may be particularly useful in the setting of acute RV decompensation, where RV infarction (ST elevation in V1 with inferior ST changes; ST elevation in V3 or V4R) and acute pulmonary embolism (sinus tachycardia, right bundle branch block, S1Q3T3, T-wave inversions across the precordium) may be prominent players. RV dysplasia may also be preliminarily diagnosed (epsilon wave).

(Continued on page 90)

D. Acute decompensation of RV function is almost always of great urgency and often requires equally rapid diagnosis and treatment. The right ventricle is designed to do primarily volume work; any acute increase in RV afterload (as is the case with a large pulmonary embolism) may lead to severe deterioration in cardiovascular status. A transthoracic echocardiogram may be particularly useful in discerning the underlying cause of acute RV failure and guiding therapeutic interventions. It is worth noting that many of the stigmata of chronic RV failure (i.e., peripheral edema, ascites, RV hypertrophy [RVH] on ECG, etc.) may not be present. This is also true of acute, massive pulmonary embolism, where the estimated PA pressures (based on tricuspid valve velocity) may be only slightly elevated. Systemic hypotension and cardiovascular collapse may be the only clues. A cardiology consultant and a cardiac surgeon may be extremely helpful in the diagnosis and management of acute RV decompensation.

E. Although potentially less dramatic, chronic failure of the right ventricle may lead to equally poor outcomes when compared with acute RV failure. Unlike a native right ventricle exposed to normal afterload, a chronically pressure-challenged right ventricle can become markedly hypertrophied and generate pressures in excess of the systemic ventricle ("suprasystemic RV"). As is the case with acute RV failure, a transthoracic echocardiogram can be a helpful first step in deciphering the etiology of RV dysfunction.

F. One of the most common causes of RV failure is left ventricular (LV), or systemic ventricular, failure. Before embarking on an expedition for the rare, it is worthwhile to exclude systemic ventricular or valvular dysfunction and rare causes of elevated LA pressure (cor triatriatum, supramitral ring, or LA myxoma). This is particularly true in older patients in whom left-sided heart disease is more prevalent. Other etiologies that affect the filling properties of both ventricles, such as constrictive pericarditis or restrictive cardiomyopathy, may also be present. Rarer causes of elevated RV afterload that are postcapillary include pulmonary venous stenosis from external compression (examples include granulomatous disease, such as sarcoid, or fibrosing mediastinitis from histoplasmosis) or internal obliteration of the pulmonary venous lumen after procedures such as pulmonary vein isolation for atrial fibrillation. Treating systemic ventricular failure aggressively can lead to simultaneous improvements in RV failure.

G. If LV failure has been largely excluded, the focus turns to the right ventricle and its interface with the pulmonary vasculature. The presence or absence of pulmonary hypertension is an important branch point in this evaluation. If pulmonary hypertension is present, the diagnostic evaluation is aimed at deciphering an underlying etiology.

H. If pulmonary hypertension is not present, consider inherent issues with RV function including arrhythmogenic RV dysplasia (ARVD), Ebstein's anomaly of the tricuspid valve, or other forms of congenital heart disease. CHD may be associated with both high and low pulmonary arterial pressures and RV dysfunction. The presence of CHD should prompt referral to a center skilled in the care of adults with CHD.

I. Most cases of chronic right-sided heart failure, particularly those with associated pulmonary hypertension, ultimately require evaluation via right-sided heart catheterization with the possibility of pulmonary vasodilator testing.

J. Over the past several years, the therapeutic armamentarium for the treatment of pulmonary hypertension has expanded to include continuous IV, SC, and inhaled prostacyclins in addition to oral endothelin antagonists, PDE5 inhibitors, and calcium channel blockers. Because the therapeutic algorithm is in flux, referral to centers specifically aimed at the treatment of pulmonary hypertension is recommended.

References

Cook AL, Hurwitz LM, Valente AM, Herlong JR. Right heart dilatation in adults: congenital causes. AJR AM J Roentgenol 2007;189(3): 592–560.

Farber HW, Loscalzo J. Pulmonary arterial hypertension. N Engl J Med 2004;351:1655–1665.

Haddad F, Hunt SA, Rosenthal DN, Murphy DJ. Right ventricular function in cardiovascular disease, part I: anatomy, physiology, aging, and functional assessment of the right ventricle. Circulation. 2008;117(11): 1436–1448.

McLaughlin VV, McGoon MD. Pulmonary arterial hypertension. Circulation 2006;114(13):1417–1431.

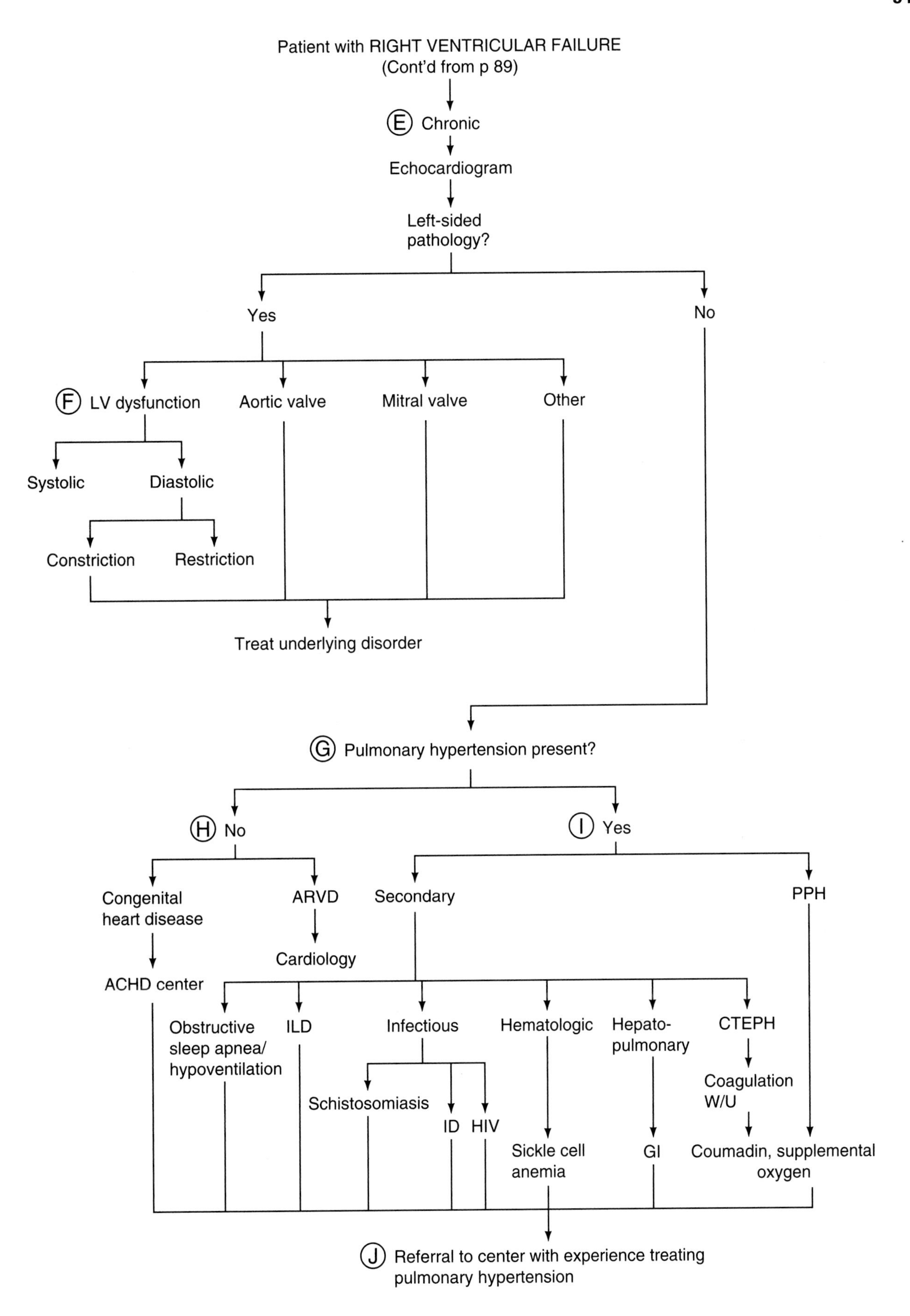
Patient with RIGHT VENTRICULAR FAILURE
(Cont'd from p 89)
E Chronic
Echocardiogram
Left-sided pathology?
Yes
No
F LV dysfunction
Aortic valve
Mitral valve
Other
Systolic
Diastolic
Constriction
Restriction
Treat underlying disorder
G Pulmonary hypertension present?
H No
I Yes
Congenital heart disease
ARVD
Secondary
PPH
ACHD center
Cardiology
Obstructive sleep apnea/ hypoventilation
ILD
Infectious
Hematologic
Hepato-pulmonary
CTEPH
Schistosomiasis
ID
HIV
Coagulation W/U
Sickle cell anemia
GI
Coumadin, supplemental oxygen
J Referral to center with experience treating pulmonary hypertension

SUDDEN CARDIAC DEATH

Tomaz Hruczkowski, MD, and Usha B. Tedrow, MD, MS

In the United States the total number of sudden cardiac death cases is estimated to exceed 300,000 annually. In the developing countries cardiovascular disease is the most common cause of natural death, with 50% of deaths occurring suddenly. Coronary artery disease is the most commonly documented etiology of events. Causative lesions have been demonstrated posthumously in up to 90% of victims of sudden cardiac death. Sudden cardiac death is the initial and only presentation in 20% of deaths related to coronary disease.

Other causes of sudden cardiac death include idiopathic-dilated cardiomyopathy, hypertrophic cardiomyopathy, left ventricular hypertrophy, long QT syndrome (congenital or acquired), arrhythmogenic right ventricular cardiomyopathy, Brugada syndrome, myocarditis, and congenital coronary artery anomalies. Nonarrhythmic and noncardiac causes simulating sudden cardiac death include rupture of aortic aneurysm, intracerebral hemorrhage, pulmonary embolism (PE), and prosthetic valve dysfunction.

The care of the patient successfully resuscitated after cardiac arrest should focus on timely evaluation for coronary artery disease with cardiac catheterization if there are no neurologic contraindications. ECG, echocardiography, and family history are essential adjuncts. Recognition of familial syndromes is essential, not only for the presenting patient, but also for screening of extended family. Survivors of sudden cardiac death should receive implantable defibrillator therapy for secondary prevention if no clear reversible cause is found, and selected patients with correctible ischemia should also receive implants for protection against future events.

The documented initial rhythm in sudden cardiac death is dependent on the time elapsed between the collapse and the first electrocardiographic recording. In a study that included patients wearing Holter monitors at the time of an arrest, the initial rhythm was ventricular fibrillation (VF) or ventricular tachycardia (VT) in 83% of cases, whereas bradyarrhythmias occurred in the remaining 17%. In another study, in which the time to evaluation was <4 minutes, VF was present in 95% of patients, with asystole in 5%. When the time to resuscitation was 12–15 minutes, VF was recorded in 71% and asystole in 21%.

Survival to hospital discharge following resuscitated sudden cardiac death is highly dependent on the initially documented rhythm. Survivor rates are highest for VT, with two thirds of patients surviving, followed closely by VF, but rates are close to zero when the presenting scenario is asystole or electromechanical dissociation. Thus a patient's chance of surviving cardiac arrest is related both to the presenting arrhythmia and to the time elapsed from the collapse to the initiation of resuscitation. For each minute of continued VF, the odds of survival decrease by 7%–10%.

Other factors that influence the likelihood of survival include the time of initiation of CPR and the time of initiation of Advanced Cardiac Life Support (ACLS) by trained personnel with defibrillation combined with drug therapy. Thus the Emergency Cardiovascular Care (ECC) guidelines published by the American Heart Association (AHA) stress the "chain of survival" concept to maximize the likelihood of successful resuscitation:

1. Early access: A bystander recognizes an arrest and alerts EMS
2. Early CPR: Initiation of effective CPR by a bystander
3. Early defibrillation: Ideally delivered within 1–2 minutes of VF onset to restore a perfusing rhythm by the emergency medical services (EMS) team or a bystander with an automated external defibrillator (AED)
4. Early ACLS: Trained personnel (physician in emergency department or in an ambulance or a paramedic) providing defibrillation, intubation, IV fluids, and antiarrhythmic medications

To maximize the likelihood of survival of a patient with sudden cardiac death, AHA promotes the awareness of cardiovascular health and provides the unified Basic Life Support (BLS) training protocols for the general public. Paramedics and medical personnel are further trained in ACLS delivery protocols adopted throughout North America. A summary of the AHA Emergency Cardiac Care algorithm follows. It is not intended as a replacement for the comprehensive ACLS training course, nor is it meant to replace the need for refresher courses. Our intention is to provide a quick memory guide for those already familiar with ACLS skills.

The algorithm illustrates the sequence that is appropriate in most instances of a cardiac arrest and is organized around the steps of the primary and secondary survey. Appropriate actions, ongoing information gathering, consideration of the possible underlying causes, and teamwork are key to the successful outcome of the resuscitation process.

References

1. American Heart Association Guidelines for Cardiopulmonary Resuscitation and Emergency Cardiovascular Care. Circulation 2005;24(Suppl I).
2. Cummins RO, Ornato JP, Thies WH, Pepe PE. Improving survival from sudden cardiac arrest: the "chain of survival" concept. A statement for health professionals from the Advanced Cardiac Life Support Subcommittee and the Emergency Cardiac Care Committee, American Heart Association. Circulation 1991;83(5):1832–1847.
3. de Luna AB, Coumel P, Leclercq JF. Ambulatory sudden cardiac death: mechanisms of production of fatal arrhythmias on the basis of data from 157 cases. Am Heart J 1989;117:151–159.
4. Deshpende SS, Akhtar M. Sudden cardiac death. In Topol EJ (ed). Textbook of Cardiovascular Medicine. 2nd ed. Philadelphia: Lippincott Williams & Wilkins, 2002.
5. Hallstrom AP, Eisenberg MS, Bergner L. The persistence of ventricular fibrillation and its implication for evaluating EMS. Emerg Health Serv Q 1983;1:42–47.
6. Mehta D, Curwin J, Gomesw A, Fuster V. Sudden death in coronary artery disease: acute ischemia versus myocardial substrate. Circulation 1997;96:3215–3223.
7. Myerburg R, Kessler KM, Castellanos A. Sudden cardiac death: epidemiology, transient risk, and intervention assessment. Ann Intern Med 1993;119:1187–1197.
8. Schatzkin A, Cupples LA, Heeren T, et al. Sudden death in the Framingham Heart Study. Differences in incidence and risk factors by sex and coronary disease status. Am J Epidemiol 1984;120:888–899.
9. Weaver WD, Hill D, Fahrenbruch CD, et al. Use of the automatic external defibrillator in the management of out-of-hospital cardiac arrest. N Engl J Med 1988;319:661–666.
10. Weaver WD, Cobb LA, Hallstrom AP, et al. Factors influencing survival after out-of-hospital cardiac arrest. J Am Coll Cardiol 1986;7:754.
11. Wyse DG, Friedman PL, Brodsky MA, et al. Life-threatening ventricular arrhythmias due to transient or correctable causes: high risk for death in follow up. J Am Coll Cardiol 2001;38(6):1718–1724.
12. Zheng ZJ, Croft JB, Giles WH, Mensah GA. Sudden cardiac death in the United States, 1989 to 1998. Circulation 2001;104:2158–2163.

1. Whether witnessing a collapse or being called to an unwitnessed event, assess the environment to allow delivery of care without putting the rescuers at risk. Assess (ask about) the circumstances to help narrow down the diagnostic possibilities. For example, a preceding chest pain versus an interrupted meal may point toward a cardiac or respiratory cause. Establish responsiveness by talking or shouting to the victim. On verification of unresponsiveness, call for help.
2. Activate EMS (911), call the code, and request bystander and/or paramedical/medical assistance. Request an AED or a code cart with a defibrillator, airway support equipment, and ACLS drugs. Begin the Primary Survey. Open/clear the airway, and "look, listen, feel" for spontaneous respirations.
3. Use one-way valve ventilation barrier device or bag-mask device and oropharyngeal airway if available, assess, and manage airway obstruction. Check carotid artery for pulse 5–10 seconds.
4. Full cardiac arrest confirmed, initiate adequate chest compressions and continue artificial respirations. Attach AED/defibrillator. Take charge or ask a more experienced rescuer; delegate tasks to bystanders/code team members.
5. Continue chest compressions, and monitor adequacy (carotid pulse). Assess rhythm.
6. If VF or pulseless VT.
7. Deliver three direct current (DC) shocks as needed (200 J, 300 J, 360 J—monophasic or equivalent biphasic). After three shocks, check pulse; if absent, resume CPR. Initiate secondary survey.
8. If asystole, recheck electrodes. Consider duration of the arrest and termination of efforts. If pulseless electrical activity (PEA), DO NOT SHOCK! Ascertain pulselessness versus low output state and consider typical causes of shock (differential diagnosis).
9. Consider transcutaneous pacing early, especially in a witnessed arrest. Monitor rhythm by differentiating pacing spikes from true QRS complexes. Monitor pulse by differentiating true pulse (carotid) from skeletal muscle twitches induced by electric current that may be observed in upper extremities.
10. Secondary survey and continuation of rescue protocol will generally require paramedical/medical (ACLS-trained) personnel. Delegate or assume predefined roles within the team. Intubate, confirm, and secure endotracheal tube placement and adequacy of ventilations (auscultation, pulse oximetry, end-tidal CO_2). Secure IV access. Monitor vital signs. If pulse is palpable, monitor blood pressure (BP). Administer adrenergic agents. Consider rhythm-appropriate antiarrhythmic medications:
    a. Amiodarone 300 mg IV push for persistent VF/VT; additional 150 mg IV for recurrent VF/VT. Maximum dose 2.2 g in 24 hr.
    b. Lidocaine 1–1.5 mg/kg IV push for persistent or recurrent VF/VT; may repeat in 3–5 minutes, maximum dose 3 mg/kg.
    c. Magnesium sulfate 1–2 g IV in torsades de pointes or if hypomagnesemia suspected.
    d. Procainamide up to 50 mg/min IV, maximum dose 17 mg/kg for recurrent VF/VT.

    Consider sodium bicarbonate 1 mEq/kg IV in known, preexisting hyperkalemia, acidosis, or tricyclic or aspirin overdose, after a long arrest interval.

11. Search for and treat reversible metabolic causes. Consider/memorize the list of typical causes of PEA and asystole.

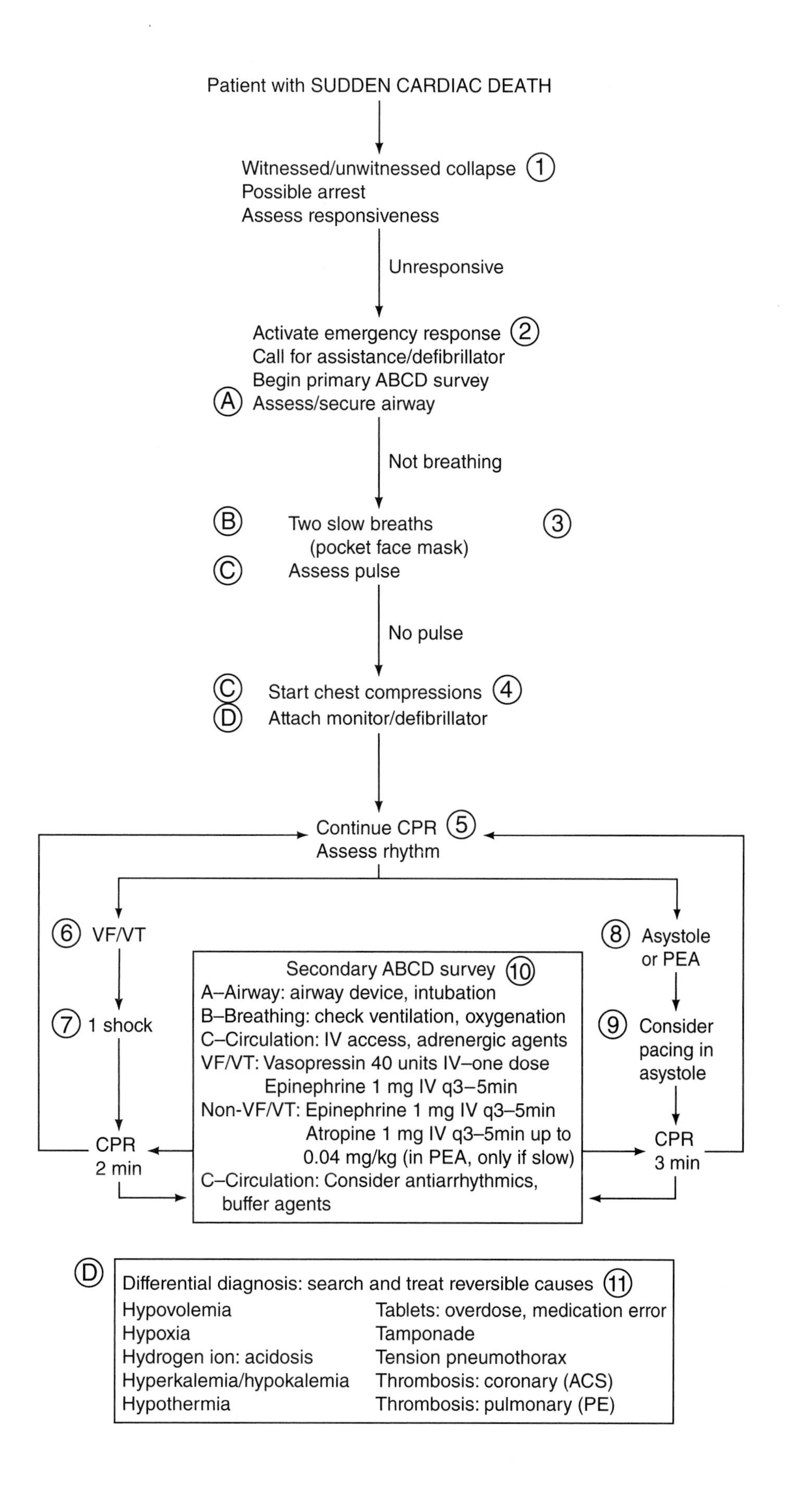
Patient with SUDDEN CARDIAC DEATH
Witnessed/unwitnessed collapse (1)
Possible arrest
Assess responsiveness
Unresponsive
Activate emergency response (2)
Call for assistance/defibrillator
Begin primary ABCD survey
(A) Assess/secure airway
Not breathing
(B) Two slow breaths (pocket face mask) (3)
(C) Assess pulse
No pulse
(C) Start chest compressions (4)
(D) Attach monitor/defibrillator
Continue CPR (5)
Assess rhythm
(6) VF/VT
(7) 1 shock
CPR
2 min
(8) Asystole or PEA
(9) Consider pacing in asystole
CPR
3 min
Secondary ABCD survey (10)
A–Airway: airway device, intubation
B–Breathing: check ventilation, oxygenation
C–Circulation: IV access, adrenergic agents
VF/VT: Vasopressin 40 units IV–one dose
Epinephrine 1 mg IV q3–5min
Non-VF/VT: Epinephrine 1 mg IV q3–5min
Atropine 1 mg IV q3–5min up to 0.04 mg/kg (in PEA, only if slow)
C–Circulation: Consider antiarrhythmics, buffer agents
(D)
Differential diagnosis: search and treat reversible causes (11)
Hypovolemia
Hypoxia
Hydrogen ion: acidosis
Hyperkalemia/hypokalemia
Hypothermia
Tablets: overdose, medication error
Tamponade
Tension pneumothorax
Thrombosis: coronary (ACS)
Thrombosis: pulmonary (PE)

CARDIAC DYSPNEA

Aaron L. Baggish, MD, and Marc S. Sabatine, MD

Dyspnea, the subjective sensation of breathlessness, is a common problem in patients with underlying cardiac disease. Because dyspnea has numerous cardiovascular and noncardiovascular causes, establishing a definitive diagnosis can be difficult. A thorough initial evaluation with emphasis on the history, examination, and several key tests is essential.

Although the pathophysiology responsible for dyspnea is complex and incompletely understood, most cardiac causes are attributable to elevations in intracardiac pressures, pulmonary vascular stretch, and activation of perivascular nerve fibers.

A. The history and physical examination should first be aimed at excluding noncardiac causes of dyspnea (pulmonary, musculoskeletal, and neurologic) and then on establishing the primary location of underlying cardiac dysfunction (right ventricular [RV] vs. left ventricular [LV]).

B. Cardiac causes of dyspnea can be conveniently dichotomized into processes with primary RV dysfunction and those with primary LV dysfuntion.

C. Physical examination findings suggestive of RV dysfunction include elevated jugular venous pressure (JVP), ascites, and lower extremity swelling. In contrast, LV dysfunction with resultant rise in pulmonary venous pressure is suggested by the presence of pulmonary rales.

D. RV failure can be divided on the basis of pathophysiology into three distinct categories. These include primary myocardial RV dysfunction, impairment of RV filling due to pericardial disease, and inadequate RV output due to increases in RV afterload.

E. The findings of an RV heave and right-sided extra heart sounds (S_3 or S_4) suggest intrinsic RV muscular dysfunction. Important causes include acute and chronic ischemia, restrictive cardiomyopathy, and pressure/volume overload due to intracardiac shunts from congenital and acquired causes.

F. Pericardial diseases resulting in clinical RV failure include pericardial tamponade and constrictive pericardial disease. Pericarditis, inflammation of the pericardium presenting with chest pain exacerbated by lying supine, pericardial friction rub, and diffuse ST-segment elevation on the ECG, can precipitate pericardial tamponade and set the stage for future constrictive disease. The presence of distant heart sounds, elevated neck veins, and systemic hypotension suggests the presence of a pericardial effusion with the resultant syndrome of tamponade. A history of pericardial injury with examination findings of RV failure and a pericardial knock suggest constrictive disease.

G. The findings of RV dysfunction associated with an increased P_2 component of the S_2 and a pulmonary artery (PA) tap suggest pulmonary arterial hypertension (PAH). Rare cases of pulmonary hypertension are attributable to primary disease (PPH), whereas most PAH is the result of an identifiable concomitant disease. Common causes of secondary PAH include thromboembolic disease, connective tissue diseases, HIV infection, and medication side effects.

H. Dyspnea attributable to primary LV dysfunction is caused by elevations in pulmonary venous pressures with resultant vascular stretch and extravascular fluid shifts impairing gas exchange. These processes are reflected by the physical examination finding of rales. Impairment of contraction, relaxation, and left cardiac valves can underlie this process.

I. A diffuse and laterally displaced left ventricle with an S_3 suggests decreased LV ejection fraction (LVEF) and dilation of the LV chamber. Dilated cardiomyopathy most often results from coronary artery disease, but other insults including toxin exposure, infection, endocrine disorders, long-standing arrhythmia, and chronic hypertension must be considered.

J. A normally located and focal point of maximal impluse (PMI) suggests preserved LVEF. Dyspnea from LV dysfunction with preserved LV function can result from intrinsic abnormalities in relaxation (acute ischemia, LV hypertrophy, and restrictive processes) and from processes that increase LV afterload (hypertensive urgency and aortic coarctation)

K. The presence of a murmur is often indicative of valvular pathology. In the dyspneic patient, the finding of a murmur may be explanatory and should be clarified with confirmatory examination maneuvers and echocardiography.

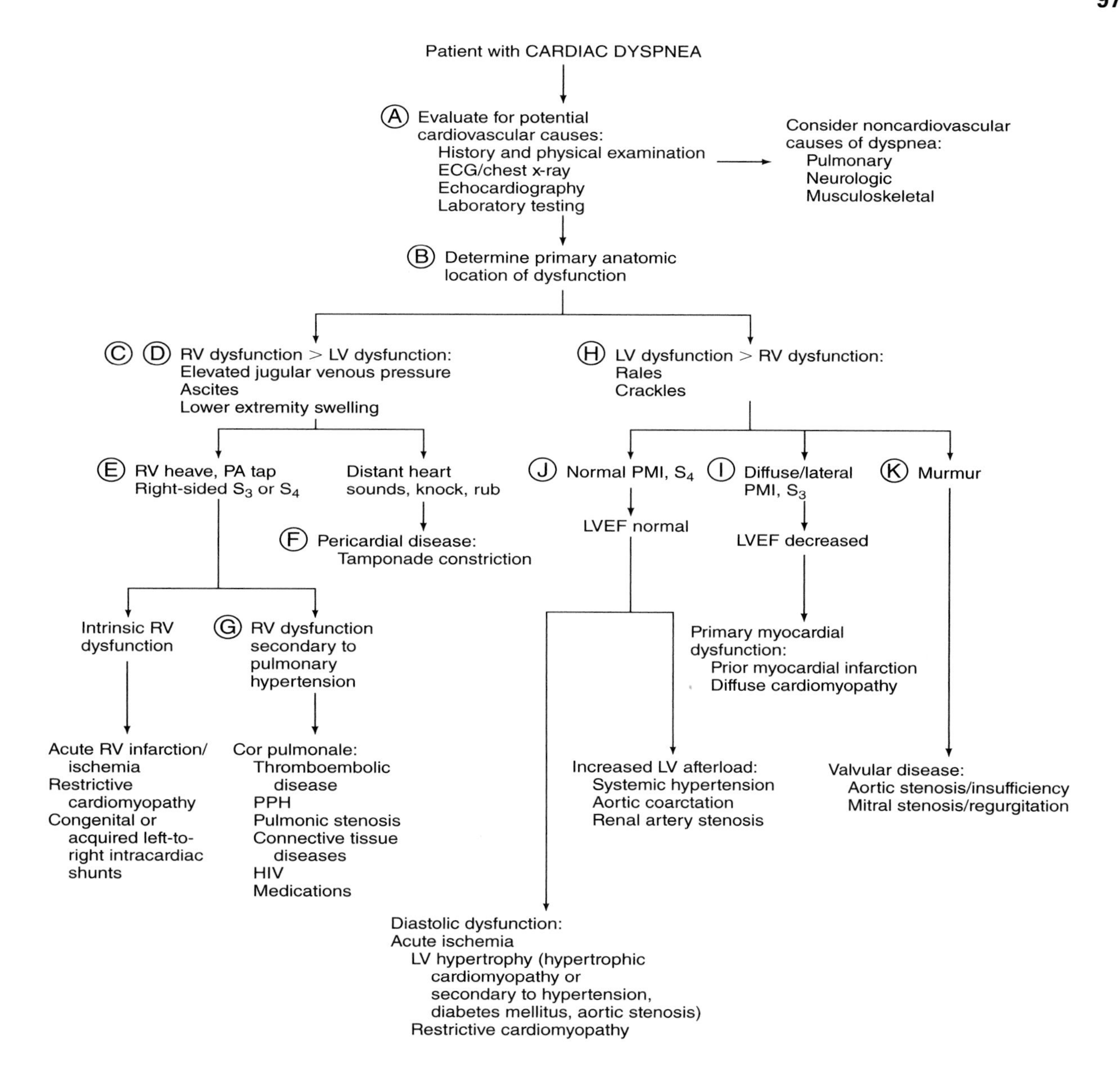

References

Antman EM, Anbe DT, Armstrong PW, et al. ACC/AHA guidelines for the management of patients with ST-elevation myocardial infarction: a report of the American College of Cardiology/American Heart Association Task Force on Practice Guidelines (Committee to Revise the 1999 Guidelines for the Management of patients with acute myocardial infarction). J Am Coll Cardiol 2004;44(3):E1–E211.

Braunwald E, Antman EM, Beasley JW, et al. ACC/AHA 2002 guideline update for the management of patients with unstable angina and non-ST-segment elevation myocardial infarction—summary article: a report of the American College of Cardiology/American Heart Association task force on practice guidelines (Committee on the Management of patients With Unstable Angina). J Am Coll Cardiol 2002;40(7):1366–1374.

Büller HR, Agnelli G, Hull RD, et al. Antithrombotic therapy for venous thromboembolic disease: the Seventh ACCP Conference on Antithrombotic and Thrombolytic Therapy. Chest 2004;126(3 Suppl):401S–428S.

Hunt SA, Abraham WT, Chin MH, et al. ACC/AHA 2005 guideline update for the diagnosis and management of chronic heart failure in the adult: a report of the American College of Cardiology/American Heart Association Task Force on Practice Guidelines (Writing Committee to Update the 2001 Guidelines for the Evaluation and Management of Heart Failure). Developed in collaboration with the American College of Chest Physicians and the International Society for Heart and Lung Transplantation: endorsed by the Heart Rhythm Society. Circulation 2005;112(12):e154–e235.

ASSESSMENT AND INITIAL MANAGEMENT OF ST-SEGMENT ELEVATION MYOCARDIAL INFARCTION

Stephen D. Wiviott, MD, and Elliott M. Antman, MD

Acute coronary syndromes (ACSs) are a major contributor to worldwide morbidity and mortality. In the subset of patients with ST-segment elevation myocardial infarction (STEMI), suggestive of complete coronary obstruction, the therapeutic principles favor prompt and early recognition of this condition and rapid restoration of coronary flow to reduce the likelihood of major sequelae of STEMI, including heart failure, arrhythmias, mechanical complications (ventricular rupture, ventricular septal defect, valvular dysfunction), and death. Early identification of symptoms suggestive of myocardial infarction (MI), including chest, back, neck, or jaw pain, and activation of medical services result in the most prompt treatment of this condition. Patients with suspected MI should receive 162–325 mg of aspirin, if available, prior to arrival of emergency medical personnel or on first medical contact. Prehospital management including fibrinolysis in appropriate settings is outside the scope of this textbook.

A. At initial hospital contact, an initial brief assessment by triage personnel should be targeted to rapidly identify patients with angina or anginal equivalent possibly suggestive of MI. All patients with suspected MI should have a 12-lead ECG performed and be evaluated by an experienced physician within 10 minutes of hospital presentation. Aspirin (162–325 mg) should be given if not previously received.

B. Initial physician contact should result in a targeted history and physical examination designed to assess the likelihood of MI or an alternative diagnosis, risks associated with MI, and possible therapies. History should include presence of cardiovascular risk factors, prior MI, ACSs, and cardiovascular procedures and should focus on symptoms related to ACSs, aortic dissection, risk of bleeding, and cerebrovascular disease (both acute and chronic). Physical examination should be performed to aid in the diagnosis of MI and assessment of possible complications, including mechanical complications, right ventricular (RV) infarction, and cardiogenic shock. A focused neurologic evaluation should be performed to assess for evidence of a prior stroke before initiation of fibrinolytic therapy. Laboratory evaluation including cardiac biomarkers should be performed but should not delay the initiation of reperfusion therapy. Similarly, chest radiography should be performed but should not delay initiation of reperfusion therapy unless it is used for the suspected identification of a contraindication to reperfusion such as aortic dissection.

Coincident with the initial history and physical evaluation, initial medical management should include the placement of a cardiac rhythm monitor, IV access, aspirin if not already received, supplemental oxygen, sublingual nitroglycerin in patients with chest discomfort (and systolic blood pressure [SBP] of >90 mm Hg, heart rate [HR] 50–100 beats per minute, and no suspected RV infarction).

C. If based on the initial evaluation STEMI is excluded, appropriate measures should be initiated for evaluation and treatment of alternative diagnoses.

D. For patients with confirmed STEMI, decision making regarding reperfusion strategy should be based on time since initial symptom onset, STEMI-related risk, risk of therapeutic options, and available resources. Uncomplicated presentations with very rapid presentations have favorable prognoses regardless of treatment strategy. Risk stratification for patients with STEMI includes infarct location (anterior vs. inferior), presence of cardiogenic shock, heart failure, hemodynamic compromise, or mechanical complications; the risk of complications associated with fibrinolysis; and the likely time to treatment dependent on strategy chosen. Contraindications to fibrinolysis are generally considered to include chest pain duration >12 hours, SBP >180 mm Hg, diastolic blood pressure [DBP] >110 mm Hg, blood pressure difference between arms of >15 mm Hg, known structural CNS disease, closed head/facial trauma within 3 months, major trauma or surgery within 6 weeks, GI or genitourinary bleeding, history of bleeding or clotting problems or current use of blood thinning agents, CPR >10 minutes, pregnancy, and serious systemic disease such as advanced cancer.

(Continued on page 100)

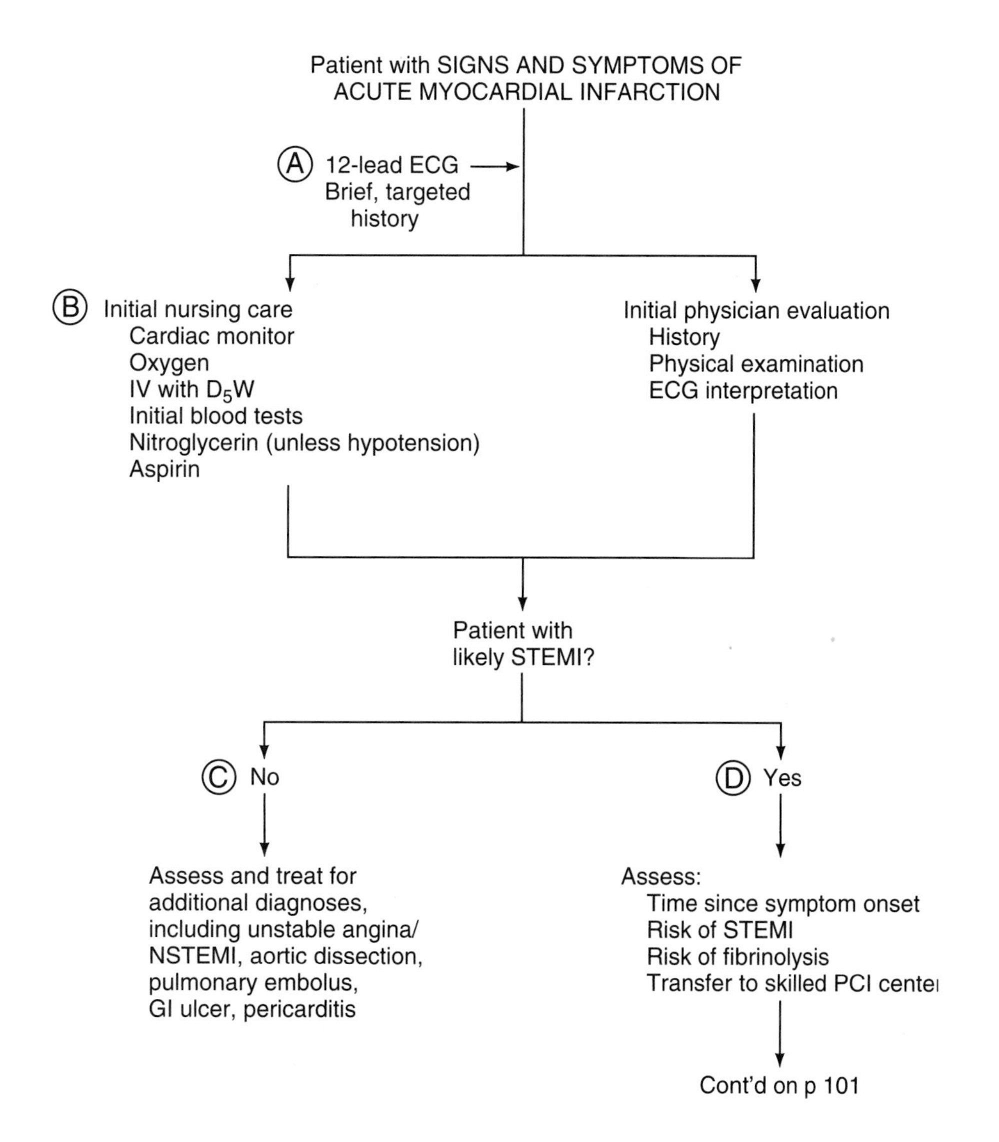
Patient with SIGNS AND SYMPTOMS OF
ACUTE MYOCARDIAL INFARCTION
(A) 12-lead ECG
Brief, targeted
history
(B) Initial nursing care
Cardiac monitor
Oxygen
IV with D5W
Initial blood tests
Nitroglycerin (unless hypotension)
Aspirin
Initial physician evaluation
History
Physical examination
ECG interpretation
Patient with
likely STEMI?
(C) No
(D) Yes
Assess and treat for
additional diagnoses,
including unstable angina/
NSTEMI, aortic dissection,
pulmonary embolus,
GI ulcer, pericarditis
Assess:
Time since symptom onset
Risk of STEMI
Risk of fibrinolysis
Transfer to skilled PCI center
Cont'd on p 101

E. Medical therapy coincident with planning for reperfusion includes IV and/or oral beta-adrenergic receptor antagonists (beta blockers) for patients without contraindication, morphine for patients with ongoing discomfort despite initial management, and antithrombotic therapy dependent of reperfusion strategy.

F. Choice of reperfusion strategy is dependent on factors noted in section D. An invasive cardiac catheterization strategy is generally preferred in patients for whom rapid treatment in an expert percutaneous coronary intervention (PCI) center (door to balloon time <60 minutes and medical contact to balloon time <90 minutes) is available. An invasive strategy is also preferred in patients who present late (beyond 12 hours), in those for whom fibrinolytic therapy is contraindicated, and in those with cardiogenic shock or Killip class ≥3. A fibrinolytic strategy is preferred if invasive therapy is not available or is likely to be delayed (door to needle time >60 minutes, medical contact to balloon time >90 minutes), especially if the patient presents within 3 hours of the onset of symptoms.

G. For those patients in whom an invasive strategy is selected, it is reasonable to begin treatment with an antithrombin (unfractionated heparin [UFH] or low molecular weight heparin [LMWH]), a glycoprotein IIb/IIIa inhibitor, and clopidogrel prior to cardiac catheterization. For patients receiving fibrin-specific thrombolytic therapy, antithrombotic therapy is indicated. For nonspecific fibrinolytic therapy, such as streptokinase, recent clinical trial evidence suggests that clopidogrel (300 mg in persons <75 years old, and 75 mg in patients >75 years old) improves clinical outcomes and long-term infarct-related artery patency and should be considered in the absence of contraindications.

H. In patients to whom fibrinolytics are administered, cardiac catheterization should be performed if there is evidence of failure of reperfusion manifest by ongoing anginal symptoms or failure of the ST-segment elevation to resolve. Among patients without these features, cardiac catheterization prior to discharge from the hospital is preferred in patients with evidence of congestive heart failure, significant left ventricular dysfunction, recurrent clinical ischemia, complex ventricular arrhythmias, or significant ischemia on a functional study.

I. Among patients who have either a primary invasive strategy for reperfusion or PCI or have cardiac catheterization following fibrinolysis, mechanical revascularization is based on coronary anatomy.

J. Post-MI management is described in an another chapter.

References

Antman EM, Anbe DT, Armstrong PW, et al. ACC/AHA guidelines for the management of patients with ST-elevation myocardial infarction: a report of the American College of Cardiology/American Heart Association Task Force on Practice Guidelines (Committee to Revise the 1999 Guidelines for the Management of patients with acute myocardial infarction). J Am Coll Cardiol 2004;44(3):E1–E211.

Antman EM, Anbe DT, Armstrong PW, et al. ACC/AHA guidelines for the management of patients with ST-elevation myocardial infarction—executive summary. A report of the American College of Cardiology/American Heart Association Task Force on Practice Guidelines (Writing Committee to revise the 1999 guidelines for the management of patients with acute myocardial infarction). J Am Coll Cardiol 2004;44(3):671–719.

Armstrong PW, Bogaty P, Buller CE, et al; Canadian Cardiovascular Society Working Group. The 2004 ACC/AHA Guidelines: a perspective and adaptation for Canada by the Canadian Cardiovascular Society Working Group. Can J Cardiol 2004;20(11):1075–1079.

Fox KA, Goodman SG, Anderson FA Jr, et al. From guidelines to clinical practice: the impact of hospital and geographical characteristics on temporal trends in the management of acute coronary syndromes. The Global Registry of Acute Coronary Events (GRACE). Eur Heart J 2003;24(15):1414–1424.

Giugliano RP, Braunwald E. 2004 ACC/AHA guideline for the management of patients with STEMI: the implications for clinicians. Nat Clin Pract Cardiovasc Med 2005;2(3):114–115.

Sabatine MS, Cannon CP, Gibson CM, et al. CLARITY-TIMI 28 Investigators. Addition of clopidogrel to aspirin and fibrinolytic therapy for myocardial infarction with ST-segment elevation. N Engl J Med 2005;352(12):1179–1189.

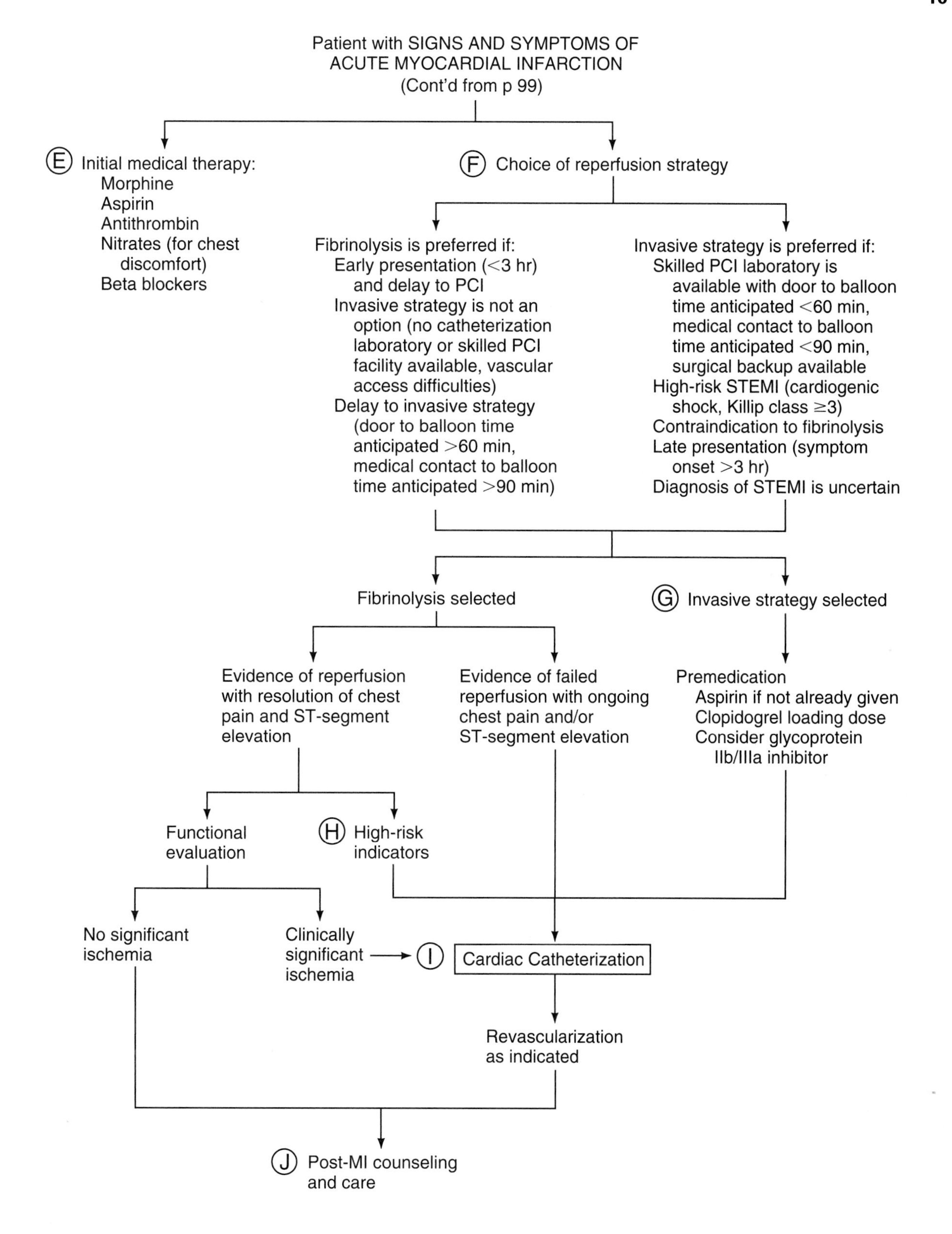
Patient with SIGNS AND SYMPTOMS OF
ACUTE MYOCARDIAL INFARCTION
(Cont'd from p 99)
(E) Initial medical therapy:
Morphine
Aspirin
Antithrombin
Nitrates (for chest discomfort)
Beta blockers
(F) Choice of reperfusion strategy
Fibrinolysis is preferred if:
Early presentation (<3 hr) and delay to PCI
Invasive strategy is not an option (no catheterization laboratory or skilled PCI facility available, vascular access difficulties)
Delay to invasive strategy (door to balloon time anticipated >60 min, medical contact to balloon time anticipated >90 min)
Invasive strategy is preferred if:
Skilled PCI laboratory is available with door to balloon time anticipated <60 min, medical contact to balloon time anticipated <90 min, surgical backup available
High-risk STEMI (cardiogenic shock, Killip class ≥3)
Contraindication to fibrinolysis
Late presentation (symptom onset >3 hr)
Diagnosis of STEMI is uncertain
Fibrinolysis selected
(G) Invasive strategy selected
Evidence of reperfusion with resolution of chest pain and ST-segment elevation
Evidence of failed reperfusion with ongoing chest pain and/or ST-segment elevation
Premedication
Aspirin if not already given
Clopidogrel loading dose
Consider glycoprotein IIb/IIIa inhibitor
Functional evaluation
(H) High-risk indicators
No significant ischemia
Clinically significant ischemia
(I) Cardiac Catheterization
Revascularization as indicated
(J) Post-MI counseling and care

POST–MYOCARDIAL INFARCTION CARE AND COUNSELING

Marc P. Bonaca, MD, and David A. Morrow, MD, MPH

Management and counseling of patients after myocardial infarction (MI) should be focused on the evaluation and modification of factors contributing to this disease process, treatment of complications such as heart failure and dysrhythmia, and control of recurrent angina. Interventions include education, behavioral modification, and pharmacologic secondary prevention. In some cases referral for further testing and invasive intervention may be required.

A. The history should include details of the patient's hospital course and general medical history. Details of the hospital course should include the extent of cardiac injury, treatment (percutaneous coronary intervention [PCI], coronary artery bypass graph [CABG], conservative therapy), complications (arrhythmia, heart failure), and any diagnostic studies performed prior to discharge (ECG, stress testing). Discharge medications and any adverse reactions to medications should be noted. General history should include symptoms of peripheral vascular disease (PVD) or cerebrovascular disease (CVD), tobacco use, dietary and exercise habits, diabetes, and drug use.

B. The examination should include evaluation for signs of ventricular dysfunction, valvular disease, or arrhythmia. Blood pressure, weight/body mass index (BMI), and waist circumference should be measured.

C. Laboratory testing should include creatinine; fasting lipids; fasting glucose; and, in the case of patients with diabetes, a hemoglobin A1c.

D. Testing of patients after MI should include a resting ECG and in most cases an echocardiogram. To accurately assess convalescent ventricular function, the echocardiogram should be performed after 6 weeks. However, earlier testing is warranted if it will be used for decision making. In patients managed without angiography or (in some cases) with incomplete revascularization, a submaximal stress test should be performed prior to hospital discharge. Exercise testing is preferred to pharmacologic stress.

E. Risk assessment should include evaluation for left ventricular (LV) dysfunction, high-risk indicators on stress testing, symptoms concerning for arrhythmia, or moderate to severe anginal symptoms. In some cases cardiac catheterization, electrophysiology evaluation, or additional revascularization may be indicated.

F. Education should be provided for both the patient and family. Emphasis is placed on the importance of lifestyle changes (tobacco cessation, exercise, weight loss, and dietary restrictions) and their impact on disease process. Acute cardiac symptoms should be reviewed along with the use of antianginal therapy (nitroglycorin [NIG]) and how to contact emergency medical services. Families may be given education and resources on CPR and automated external defibrillator (AED) use. Patients should be advised to avoid potentially harmful medications (e.g., sildenafil while using nitrates).

(Continued on page 104)

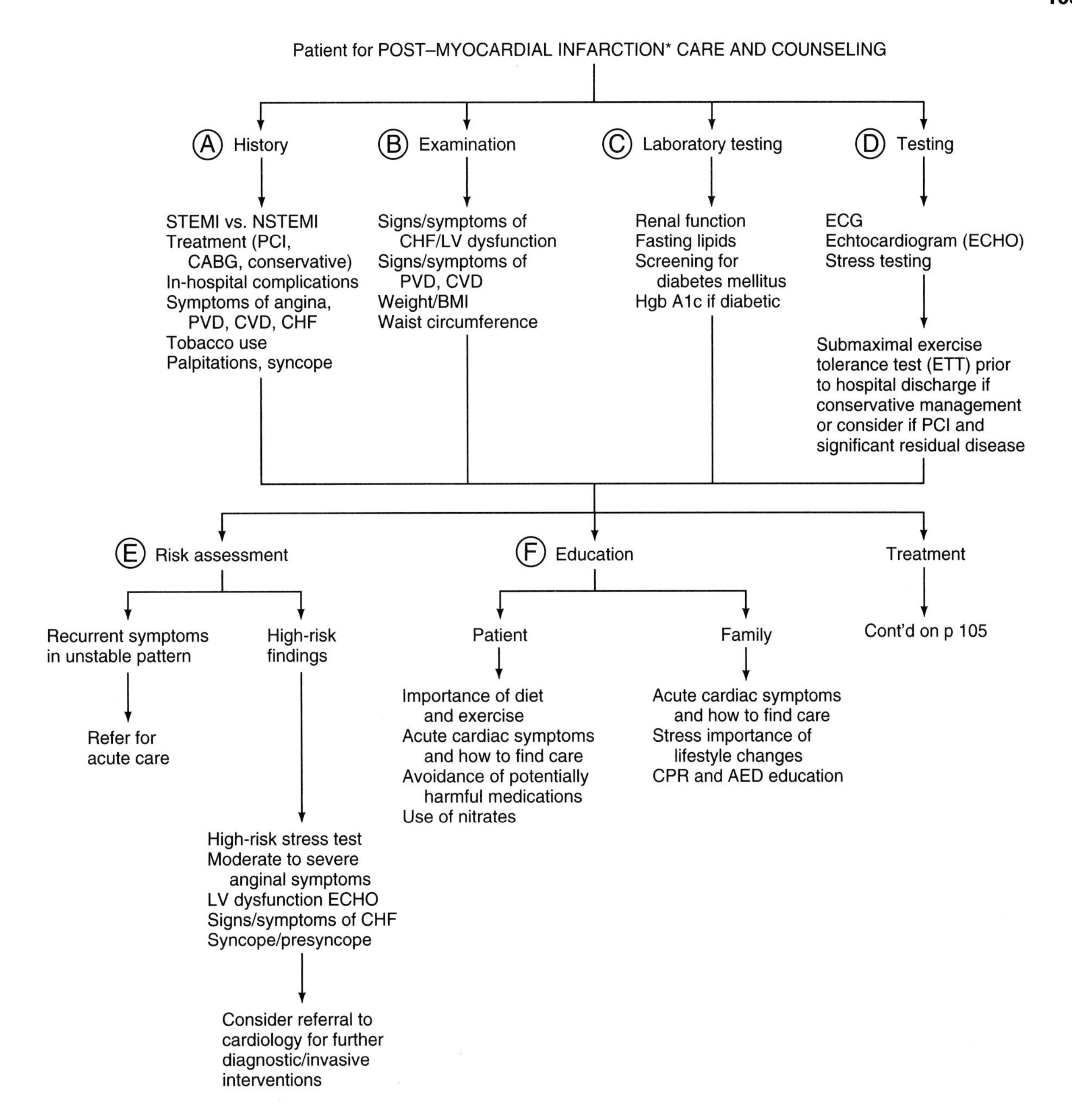

*Patients discharged from hospital after MI.
CHF, Congestive heart failure; NSTEMI, non-ST-segment elevation myocardial infarction; STEMI, ST-segment elevation myocardial infarction.

G. Pharmacologic secondary prevention aims to modify the principal risk factors of dyslipidemia and hypertension, in conjunction with antiplatelet, antiarrhythmic (beta blockers), and antiischemic therapy.

H. Psychosocial assessment should include evaluation for symptoms of depression or anxiety related to or contributing to the patient's symptoms with appropriate therapy when indicated. Coping mechanisms should be assessed, and referral for counseling should be made when indicated. In the case of patients with overall poor prognosis, discussion regarding values and overall goals of care is important.

I. Behavioral counseling is a critical intervention for secondary prevention and should be addressed at each office visit, including dietary/weight loss strategies, smoking cessation, and exercise. A low-fat and low-cholesterol diet is recommended as specified per American Hospital Association/American College of Cardiology (AHA/ACC) guidelines. Nutrition counseling should be considered for all patients after MI, especially in the case of diabetes and obesity. Education and information regarding available resources should be provided. After MI most patients may begin daily walking for 10–15 minutes with education regarding possible symptoms. This may be increased to 30 minutes of physical activity each day. Exercise treadmill testing (ETT) can be useful in assessing patient needs with regard to exercise, and symptom-limited testing should be performed in those managed without revascularization. In cases of patients with high-risk stress testing, poor functional capacity, or poor results with home rehabilitation, referral for supervised cardiac rehabilitation should be considered where available.

References

Antman EM, Anbe DT, Armstrong PW, et al. ACC/AHA guidelines for the management of patients with ST-elevation myocardial infarction: executive summary: a report of the ACC/AHA Task Force on Practice Guidelines (Committee to Revise the 1999 Guidelines on the Management of Patients With Acute Myocardial Infarction). J Am Coll Cardiol 2004;44:671–719.

Berkman LF, Blumenthal J, Burg M, et al., Enhancing Recovery in Coronary Heart Disease Patients Investigators (ENRICHD). Effects of treating depression and low perceived social support on the clinical events after myocardial infarction: the Enhancing Recovery in Coronary Heart Disease Patients (ENRICHD) Randomized Trial. JAMA 2003;289:3106–3116.

Dalal H, Evans PH, Campbell JL. Recent developments in secondary prevention and cardiac rehabilitation after acute myocardial infarction. BMJ 2004;328:693–697.

Daly LE, Mulcahy R, Graham IM, Hickey N. Long term effect on mortality of stopping smoking after unstable angina and myocardial infarction. BMJ (Clin Res Ed) 1982;287:324–326.

Froelicher ES, Kee LL, Newton KM, et al. Return to work, sexual activity, and other activities after acute myocardial infarction. Heart Lung 1994;23:423–435.

Krone RJ, Gillespie JA, Weld FM, et al. Low-level exercise testing after myocardial infarction: usefulness in enhancing clinical risk stratification. Circulation 1985;71:80–89.

O'Connor GT, Buring JE, Yusuf S, et al. An overview of randomized trials of rehabilitation with exercise after myocardial infarction. Circulation 1989;80:234–244.

Smith SC, Blair SN, Bonow RO, et al. AHA/ACC Scientific Statement: AHA/ACC Guidelines for Preventing Heart Attack and Death in Patients with Atherosclerotic Cardiovascular Disease: 2001 update: a statement for healthcare professionals from the American Heart Association and the American College of Cardiology. Circulation 2001;104:1577–1579.

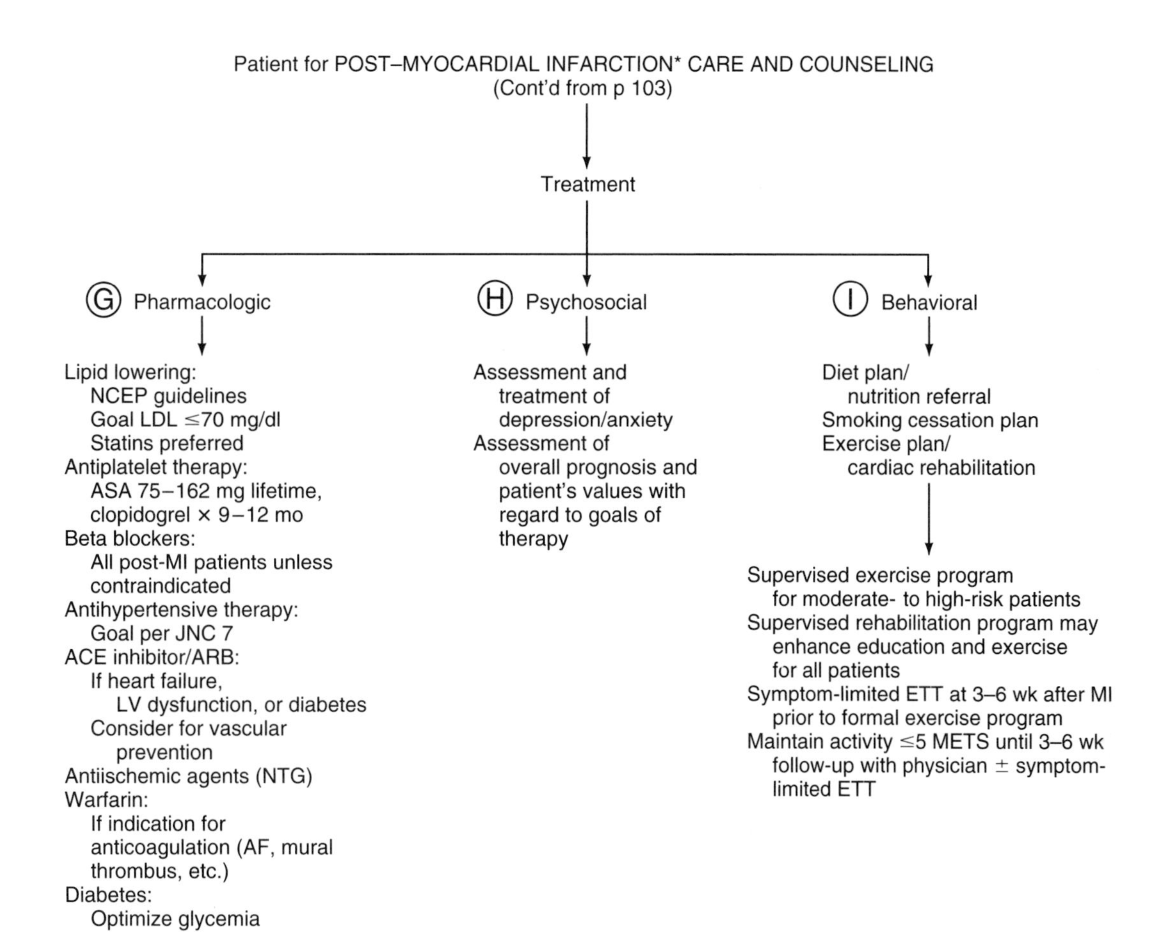

*Patients discharged from hospital after MI.

ACE, Angiotensin-converting enzyme; AF, atrial fibrillation; ARB, angiotensin receptor blocker; ASA, acetylsalicylic acid JNC, Joint National Committee; LDL, low-density lipoprotein; METS, metabolic equivalents (multiples of resting oxygen consumption); NCEP, National Cholesterol Education Program.

CLAUDICATION

Heather L. Gornik, MD

Claudication, the symptom of exertional (typically lower) limb discomfort that resolves with rest, is a common problem among elderly patients, estimated to involve up to 10% of patients >70 years. Claudication is generally caused by atherosclerotic blockages of the arteries of the limbs, termed *peripheral arterial disease* (PAD). Epidemiologic research has demonstrated that the prevalence of PAD goes far beyond patients with typical claudication to include patients with atypical leg symptoms, patients with abnormalities of gait, and patients with no leg symptoms at all. In fact, most patients with PAD do not have the classic symptom of claudication. Given the limited reliability of a history of claudication for diagnosing all patients with PAD, the ankle-brachial index (ABI) is a critical clinical tool to identify PAD. This review will focus on the approach to management of claudication. The management of the patient with asymptomatic PAD or with atypical leg symptoms is beyond the scope of this review, although general principles apply.

A. The history and physical examination are important components of the evaluation of the patient with suspected claudication. The history should focus on whether the leg symptoms are typical for claudication or whether they are more consistent with an alternative diagnosis. Claudication is a sensation of leg discomfort that comes on with a predictable amount of exertion and typically resolves within 5 minutes of rest. The discomfort may be unilateral or bilateral and may involve the buttocks, hips, thighs, or calves, depending on the anatomic location of arterial blockages. It is crucial to determine whether limb discomfort occurs at rest or only with exertion. Discomfort that occurs at rest may represent critical limb ischemia (CLI), a vascular urgency. A complete cardiovascular (CV) review of systems is important, because many patients with PAD also have occult coronary artery and cerebrovascular disease. Patients should also be asked about erectile dysfunction, neurologic symptoms, and postprandial abdominal pain (a symptom of mesenteric ischemia). A detailed smoking history must be obtained along with assessment of all other risk factors for atherosclerosis. The physical examination should include a comprehensive vascular examination, including measurement of blood pressures in both arms, palpation of the major pulses of the upper and lower extremities, and auscultation for bruits. The absence of a pedal pulse is suggestive of PAD in the patient who presents with exertional leg symptoms. The posterior tibial pulse is a more specific indicator of PAD, as the dorsalis pedis pulse is congenitally absent or anomalous in upward of 10% of patients. Careful inspection of the feet, with shoes and socks removed, is critical. Ischemic ulcers may occur on the foot or the heel or in between the toes ("kissing ulcers"). Other physical findings consistent with the presence of PAD include hair loss, diminished skin temperature, and elevation pallor of the symptomatic extremity.

B. The ABI is the cornerstone of diagnosis of PAD. The ABI should be measured with the patient in the supine position after a rest period of at least 5 minutes. A standard blood pressure cuff and handheld Doppler device are used to measure systolic blood pressure in both arms (brachial pressures) and at each ankle. The cuff is placed directly above the ankle. Systolic pressures are measured by listening over both the posterior tibial and dorsalis pedis arteries. The ABI for each leg is the ratio of the *higher* ankle pressure (dorsalis pedis or posterior tibial) over the *higher* of the two arm pressures. A normal resting ABI is generally defined as falling between 0.91 and 1.3, although a truly normal value should be ≥1.1. An ABI of ≤0.9 is diagnostic of PAD. An ABI >1.3 is also abnormal and is due to artifact from noncompressible vessels. This is a relatively common finding in diabetic patients and in patients with end-stage renal disease. An ABI of >1.3 is not interpretable, and an alternative diagnostic study should be obtained, such as measurement of the toe-brachial index, pulse volume recordings, or a magnetic resonance angiogram (MRA) or computed tomographic angiogram (CTA) of the lower extremities.

(Continued on page 108)

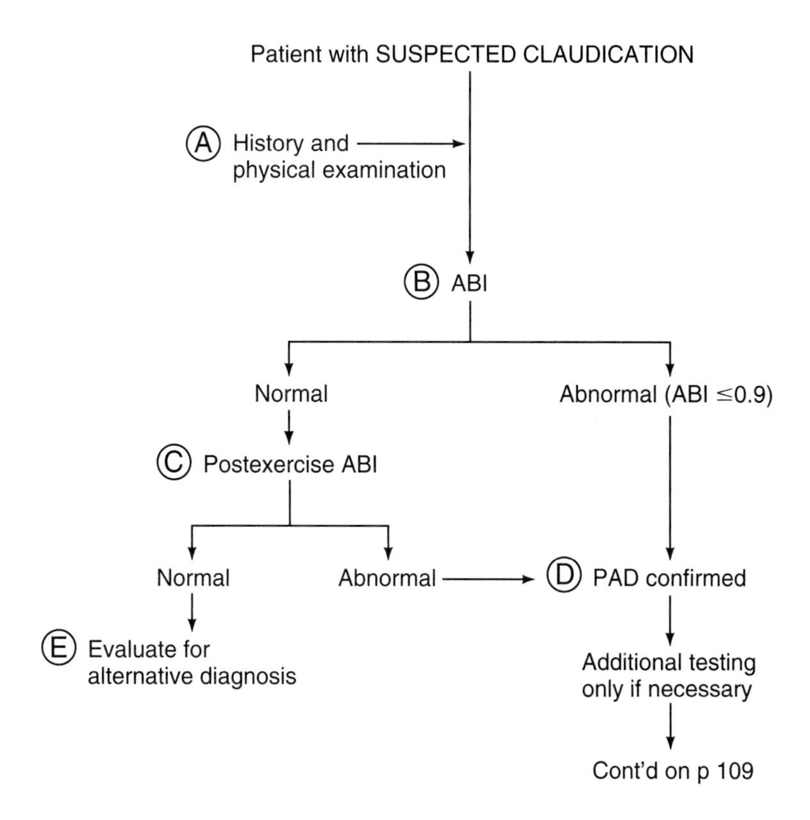

C. The presence of a normal ABI at rest, particularly if it is within the 0.91–1.1 range, does not exclude the possibility that a patient has PAD as the cause of his or her leg symptoms. In some patients with mild disease, or disease localized to the aortoiliac segment, the ABI may be normal at rest but may fall during exercise. Formal exercise testing protocols are in place in most vascular laboratories. A patient walks on a treadmill, using a standardized protocol, until the occurrence of leg symptoms or until the protocol has been completed. The ABI is remeasured with the patient in the supine position as soon as possible after exercise is completed. Any fall in ankle pressure after exercise is abnormal. The ABI will often fall by ≥20% in a patient with PAD who experiences claudication during the test. A simple bedside alternative to formal exercise testing is to measure the ABI at rest and then ask the patient to perform a series of standing calf raises until leg discomfort is provoked. The ABI in the symptomatic leg is then remeasured.

D. In most cases of claudication, the clinical evaluation and ABI complete the diagnostic workup for PAD. In the author's practice, an ABI along with measurement of segmental leg pressures and pulse volume recordings is routinely obtained in the vascular laboratory. In the author's practice, the use of additional diagnostic imaging, such as MRA, arterial duplex ultrasound, or CTA is limited to cases in which additional anatomic information is required. Settings in which additional imaging for claudication is obtained would include evaluation of PAD in a patient without risk factors for atherosclerosis when an unusual arterial disorder is suspected (e.g., Takayasu's arteritis, fibromuscular dysplasia, arterial entrapment syndrome), there is suspected aneurysmal disease, or arterial anatomy needs to be defined to delineate revascularization options, as well as for follow-up after lower extremity revascularization.

E. If PAD has been excluded as the cause of the patient's limb symptoms, a number of alternative diagnoses should be considered, depending upon the nature of the patient's symptoms. The differential diagnosis of leg pain is broad and includes lumbar canal stenosis (pseudoclaudication), osteoarthritis, venous disease, and painful peripheral neuropathy. Similarly,alternative diagnoses must be considered for a patient with a leg or foot ulcer and a normal resting ABI. The most common causes of nonischemic limb ulcers are venous insufficiency and diabetes mellitus–associated neuropathy.

F. Myocardial infarction and stroke are the leading causes of death among patients with PAD. As such, aggressive CV risk factor modification is critical for all patients with claudication, as well as for patients with PAD who have CLI, are asymptomatic, or have atypical leg symptoms. Specifically, patients should receive an antiplatelet drug (aspirin or clopidogrel), a statin, and rigorous blood pressure control. Smoking cessation is vital for improvement in limb-related outcomes and for the prevention of CV events. Diabetic patients with PAD should achieve appropriate glycemic control, often with the input of an endocrine specialist.

G. A patient with rest pain of an extremity, a nonhealing ulcer, or gangrene in the setting of an abnormal ABI has CLI. The ABI in these patients is typically <0.4. Patients with PAD and diabetes mellitus and those who continue to smoke are at particularly increased risk of developing CLI. CLI is a vascular urgency with the potential for loss of limb and a high rate of CV morbidity. The clinician must vigilantly follow all patients with claudication for the development of CLI. Deterioration to CLI can occur in previously stable patients, including those who had initially responded to conservative therapy. Although atypical, some patients with claudication may also present with a nonhealing ulcer in the absence of ischemic rest pain. All patients with CLI should be urgently referred to a vascular specialist for evaluation for revascularization.

H. For most patients, the initial management of claudication includes a trial of medical therapy. All patients should receive counseling regarding proper foot care. Supervised exercise training programs are highly successful at improving exercise capacity among claudicants, although they are not widely available. Patients with PAD should be advised to begin a walking program with a goal of walking for one-half hour (does not include rest periods) 5 times per week. Of the two FDA-approved medications available for the treatment of claudication (cilostazol and pentoxifylline), there is stronger efficacy data in support of the use of cilostazol. Cilostazol is contraindicated for use among patients with congestive heart failure.

I. If a patient with claudication does not experience improvement in leg symptoms with conservative therapy, particularly if there is substantial impairment of quality of life or functional capabilities, he or she should be referred to a vascular specialist for revascularization. During the past two decades, there have been great advances in catheter-based techniques, which allow for nonsurgical revascularization of many patients. Carefully selected patients with severely disabling symptoms or vocational disability caused by claudication may be considered for revascularization as first-line therapy, particularly if the patient has favorable anatomy for a catheter-based procedure. Patients with aortoiliac disease or short segment lesions of the femoral vessels are the most attractive candidates for catheter-based therapies.

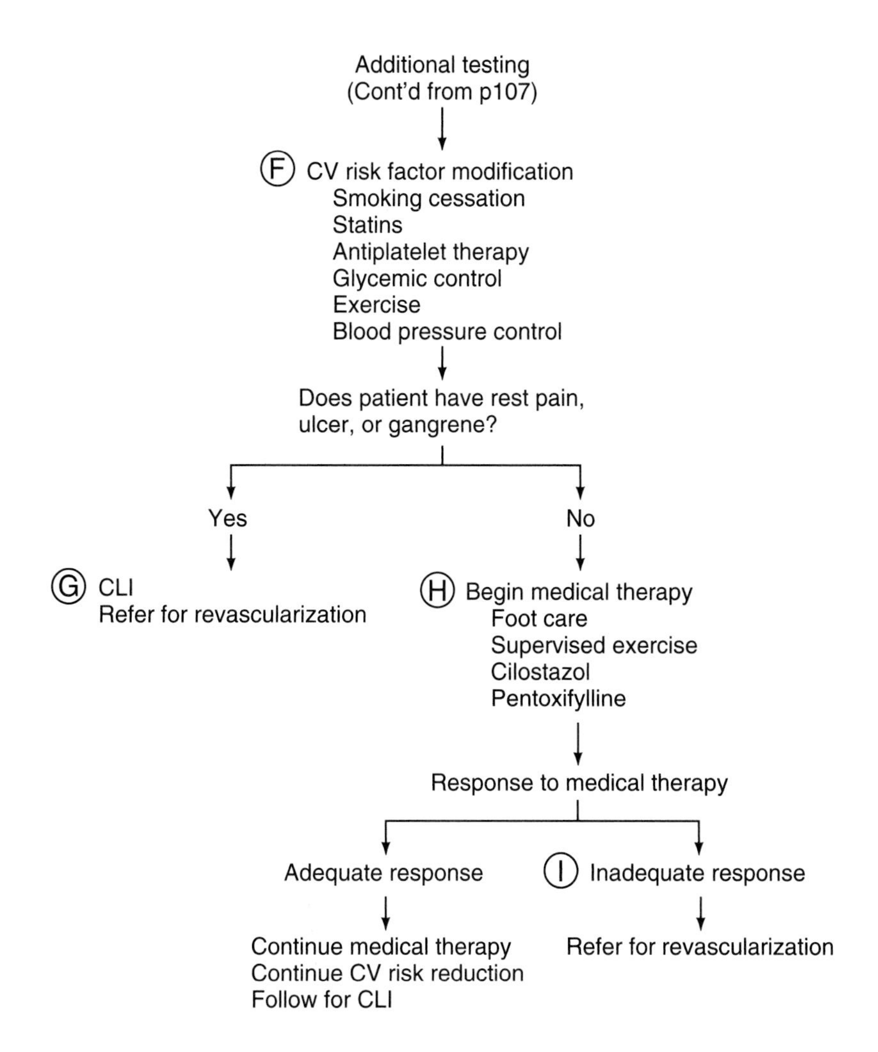

References

Creager MA, White CJ, Hiatt WR, et al. Atherosclerotic Peripheral Vascular Disease Symposium II: executive summary. Circulation 2008;118(25): 2811–2825.

Gornik HL, Creager MA. Contemporary management of peripheral arterial disease: I. Cardiovascular risk-factor modification. Cleve Clin J Med 2006;73(Suppl 4):S30–37.

Hirsch AT, Criqui MH, Treat-Jacobson D, et al. Peripheral arterial disease detection, awareness, and treatment in primary care. JAMA 2001;286(11):1317–1324.

Hirsch AT, Haskal ZJ, Hertzer NR, et al. ACC/AHA 2005 practice guidelines for the management of patients with peripheral arterial disease (lower extremity, renal, mesenteric, and abdominal aortic): a collaborative report from the American Association for Vascular Surgery/Society for Vascular Surgery, Society for Cardiovascular Angiography and Interventions, Society for Vascular Medicine and Biology, Society of Interventional Radiology, and the ACC/AHA Task Force on Practice Guidelines (Writing Committee to Develop Guidelines for the Management of Patients With Peripheral Arterial Disease): endorsed by the American Association of Cardiovascular and Pulmonary Rehabilitation; National Heart, Lung, and Blood Institute; Society for Vascular Nursing; TransAtlantic Inter-Society Consensus; and Vascular Disease Foundation. Circulation 2006;113(11):e463–654.

McDermott MM, Greenland P, Liu K, et al. Leg symptoms in peripheral arterial disease: associated clinical characteristics and functional impairment JAMA 2001;286(13):1599–1606.

Norgren L, Hiatt WR, Dormandy JA, et al. Inter-Society Consensus for the Management of Peripheral Arterial Disease (TASC II). J Vasc Surg 2007;45(Suppl S):S5–67.

Stewart KJ, Hiatt WR, Regensteiner JG, et al. Exercise training for claudication. N Engl J Med 2002;347(24):1941–1951.

DERMATOLOGY

Barbara A. Gilchrest, MD
Section Editor

PIGMENTED LESIONS

Mark J. Scharf, MD, and Norman Levine, MD

Skin color is determined mainly by the amount and distribution of melanin, a pigmented polymer produced by melanocytes. Hyperpigmentation is almost always the result of either production of too much melanin or abnormal distribution of pigment, although heavy metals or drug metabolites can change skin color.

A. Dermal melanosis/melanocytosis refers to a group of pigmentary skin conditions in which an increased number of melanocytes are producing melanin within the deeper levels of the dermis. The skin overlying these pigmented cells appears slate-blue to bluish-black. Mongolian spots are bluish macules presenting at or near birth that occur in 95% of black and 10% of white newborns. Of these lesions, 75% occur over the sacrum. They may be single or multiple and may be as large as 10 cm. They generally disappear by 5 years of age. Nevus of Ota is a form of dermal melanocytosis involving the distribution of the fifth cranial nerve. It is more common in Asians and also occurs in blacks. It is present at birth in 60% of those affected. Skin color is blue-gray to blue-brown. The sclera of the eye may also be involved.
B. Blue nevi are localized benign proliferations of melanocytes. They may be congenital or acquired. There are two types. Common blue nevi range in size from 2–10 mm. They present as small round to oval, smooth-surfaced, well-defined papules with a bluish-black pigmentation. Cellular blue nevi are less common and tend to be >1 cm. They are also bluish-black and may be mistaken for nodular melanoma. Rarely, cellular blue nevi can undergo malignant transformation.
C. When pigment derived from melanocytes is concentrated in the epidermis, the resulting skin color may range from tan to brown or even black. Freckles are an example of localized areas of increased pigment production caused by a normal concentration of melanocytes. They appear as small (2–5 mm) tan to brown macules on sun-exposed areas of skin and arise by age 2–4 years. They can be clinically differentiated from lentigos ("liver spots") or nevi by the fact that they darken with sun exposure in the summer and fade in the winter. Café-au-lait spots present at birth as well-marginated tan macules. Six or more lesions >1.5 cm in diameter are diagnostic of neurofibromatosis (NF). In these patients, take a history for any personal or family history of NF. In patients suspected of having NF, do a slit-lamp examination of their eyes to look for Lisch nodules, which are pathognomonic for NF and are present in all cases by age 5. Lentigos are well-demarcated tan to brown macules that may occur on any part of the skin, but particularly on sun-exposed areas of the face and dorsum of the hands. Unlike freckles, they do not fade over time. They are caused by an increased number of melanocytes with increased pigment production at the dermal-epidermal (DE) junction. Most lentigos are <5 mm. When lentigos are >5 mm and have irregular borders, perform a biopsy to determine whether the lesion is a lentigo maligna (LM). LMs are a form of melanoma in situ that can progress to invasive melanoma if not treated in time. If an LM is suspected, perform an incisional biopsy.
D. Congenital nevi are present from birth and range from 2 mm to >20 cm in diameter. They are typically deeply pigmented brown to black papules or plaques that may have verrucous surfaces and associated thick dark hairs. Giant congenital nevi (GCN) may involve an entire extremity or even large sections of the torso, scalp, or face. The risk of melanoma occurring in a GCN is estimated to be 5%. Although small and medium congenital nevi are associated with melanoma, the incidence of malignant transformation is far less than with GCNs; however, they should be followed with photographs and biopsied or excised if changes are seen.
E. Common acquired nevi (moles) appear during the first three decades of life and begin to regress after age 65. The average person has 40 nevi. Acquired nevi are divided into three categories depending on the localization of their melanocytes. In junctional nevi the melanocytes are present at the DE junction. These lesions are smooth-bordered macules <5 mm with uniform color ranging from light to dark brown or even black. Compound nevi are raised well-demarcated symmetric papules or thin plaques. They range from light to dark brown; some have a stippled appearance. Melanocytes are present at the DE junction and within the dermis. Dermal nevi present as flesh-colored or pink papules. All melanocytes are found within dermis. Compound nevi may progress to dermal nevi as the melanocytes lose their ability to produce pigment and melanocytes are lost from the DE junction.
F. A number of acquired pigmented lesions can mimic nevi. The most common of these are seborrheic keratoses (SKs) and dermatofibromas. SKs usually occur after age 35 and are well-defined, verrucous, usually hyperpigmented papules or plaques without surrounding pigment incontinence. They may become irritated by clothing or trauma, in which case they may show signs of inflammation or pruritus and require removal by cryotherapy, curettage, or shave excision. Occasionally, SKs

(Continued on page 114)

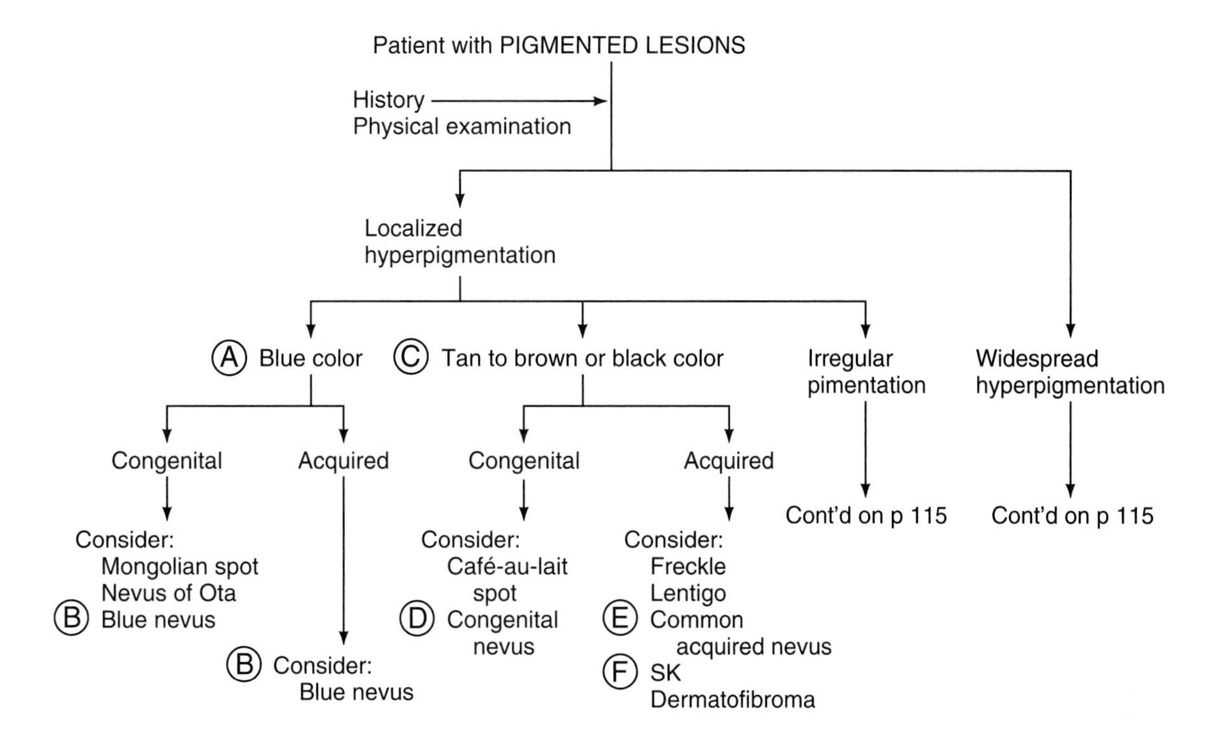
Patient with PIGMENTED LESIONS
History
Physical examination
Localized hyperpigmentation
(A) Blue color
(C) Tan to brown or black color
Irregular pimentation
Widespread hyperpigmentation
Congenital
Acquired
Congenital
Acquired
Consider:
Mongolian spot
Nevus of Ota
(B) Blue nevus
(B) Consider:
Blue nevus
Consider:
Café-au-lait spot
(D) Congenital nevus
Consider:
Freckle
Lentigo
(E) Common acquired nevus
(F) SK
Dermatofibroma
Cont'd on p 115
Cont'd on p 115

may be misdiagnosed as melanomas because of their dark color, and at times, melanomas may masquerade as SKs. When there is any doubt, a biopsy is indicated. Dermatofibromas are smooth, brown or pink papules that often pucker in the center when compressed from the edges (the "dimple sign" of Fitzpatrick). Although their cause is unclear, they may arise after minor trauma such as an insect bite or razor cut. Becker's nevus is a uniformly tan to brown plaque that occurs primarily on the upper trunk and shoulders. It is more common in males than in females. These lesions usually present in adolescents and may be confused with large congenital nevi as they mature and acquire coarse dark hairs. They are a form of connective tissue nevus and present no malignant potential.

G. Dysplastic or atypical nevi are acquired nevi that are >5 mm in diameter and have irregular or variegate pigmentation (blues, browns, black, red, or white) with poorly defined or irregular borders. Some of these lesions may be precursors for melanomas. Patients with atypical nevi who have two or more first-degree relatives with dysplastic nevi and a history of melanoma have nearly a 100% chance of developing melanomas. Follow these patients carefully for any signs of change in their nevi. These changes can best be assessed when baseline high-quality photographs have been taken so that the current findings can be compared with previous images.

H. Melanomas are skin cancers arising from the malignant transformation of melanocytes. As discussed, they may arise from precursor lesions such as atypical nevi, congenital nevi, and LM. They may also arise de novo from melanocytes within the skin. Suspect melanoma if a pigmented lesion displays any combination of asymmetry, border irregularity, variegate colors, or a diameter >5 mm. Other worrisome signs are pruritus, ulceration, bleeding, or change in color or size of the lesion.

I. Melasma is a form of hyperpigmentation characterized by mottled tan to brown macules coalescing into irregular patches on the face. The forehead, cheeks, and upper lip are often involved. Melasma is common in pregnancy, and the condition may also be triggered by oral contraceptive use. It may be idiopathic or familial and can also be seen in men. Postinflammatory hyperpigmentation is another form of localized macular hyperpigmentation that occurs after cutaneous trauma or inflammatory dermatoses. It is more common and may be more severe in darker-skinned individuals.

J. Pigmentary abnormalities of the skin can have both exogenous and endogenous causes. A number of medications can cause hyperpigmentation. Minocycline, if given in sufficient quantities for prolonged periods, can produce a gray-brown discoloration in old acne scars or a pattern of more diffuse hyperpigmentation over the anterior legs or trunk. Phenothiazines may cause a blue-gray color, particularly in sun-exposed skin. Hydroxychloroquine may produce irregular gray patches on the legs. Patients taking amiodarone may develop a slate-gray hyperpigmentation on the face, particularly after long-term sun exposure. Exposure to heavy metals such as gold or silver may result in a diffuse bluish-gray cast to the skin. Systemic disorders such as Addison's disease, uremia, and hemochromatosis can cause distinctive generalized patterns of hyperpigmentation.

References

Arndt KA, Leboit PE, Robinson JK, Wintroub BU, eds. Cutaneous Medicine and Surgery. Philadelphia: WB Saunders, 1996.

Bolognia J, Jorizza J, Rapine R. Dermatology, 2nd ed. Philadelphia: Elsevier, 2007.

Swerdlow AJ, English JS, Qiao Z. The risk of melanoma in patients with congenital nevi: a cohort study. J Am Acad Dermatol 1995;32:595.

Tucker MA, Halpern A, Holly EA, et al. Clinically recognized dysplastic nevi: a central risk factor for cutaneous melanoma. JAMA 1997;277:1439.

Wolff K, Goldsmith LA, Katz Sl, et al: Fitzpatrick's Dermatology in General Medicine, 7th ed. New York: McGraw-Hill, 2007.

Yohn J, Hoffman S, Norris D, Robinson W. Melanoma: diagnosis and treatment. Hosp Pract (Off Ed) 1994;29:27.

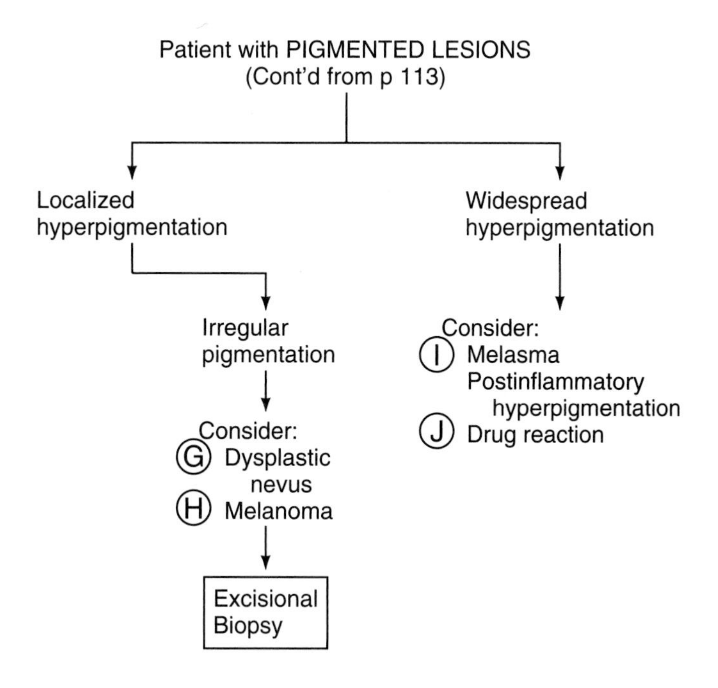

Patient with PIGMENTED LESIONS
(Cont'd from p 113)
Localized
hyperpigmentation
Widespread
hyperpigmentation
Irregular
pigmentation
Consider:
G Dysplastic
nevus
H Melanoma
Excisional
Biopsy
Consider:
I Melasma
Postinflammatory
hyperpigmentation
J Drug reaction

LEG ULCER

Cynthia A. O'Neil, MD, and Barbara A. Gilchrest, MD

A. The cause of a leg ulcer usually can be determined by history and physical examination alone. It is therefore important to ask the patient about trauma and any history of diseases such as coronary artery disease, deep venous thrombosis, and diabetes mellitus. Inquire about symptoms of vasculitis, chronic inflammatory disorders, and neoplasms. The physical examination should focus on evidence of edema, varicosities, arterial insufficiency, neuropathy, and infection.

B. Arterial ulcers account for 5% of all leg ulcers. They result from impairment of blood flow and have multiple causes, including emboli, thrombi, arteriosclerosis, Buerger's disease, hypertension, vasospasm, vasculitis, and hematologic disorders. Patients complain of pain at rest that is exacerbated with leg elevation and relieved with dependency. The ulcers are characterized by a pale or eschar-covered base with minimal granulation tissue, usually occurring on the distal foot. Other important signs of arterial involvement are coolness of the extremities, decreased pulses and slow capillary refill, a palpable or audible bruit over the femoral artery, and decreased hair on the distal legs. If arterial pulses are not palpable, use a Doppler flowmeter to hear the pulsations over the dorsalis pedis and posterior tibial arteries and calculate the ankle/brachial index (ABI) of systolic pressure. If the index is <0.7, moderate to severe disease is present and arteriography should be considered.

C. Chronic venous insufficiency accounts for about 90% of all leg ulcers. Venous stasis results from a dysfunction of venous outflow, most commonly caused by defective valves (usually secondary to deep venous thromboses or a congenital defect). Patients have edema and, in contrast to those with arterial disease, have relatively little pain. On physical examination an ulcer with exudate and granulation tissue often is seen over the medial malleolus. Varicosities, brown hemosiderin pigment, and stasis dermatitis support the diagnosis.

D. In the presence of normal vasculature and no obvious etiology, consider pyoderma gangrenosum (PG, which has a violaceous border that is undermined), inflammatory bowel disease, hematologic malignancies, or other systemic disease.

E. Neurotrophic ulcers are caused by the repeated trauma or pressure on weight-bearing areas where there is impaired cutaneous sensation. Diabetes mellitus accounts for most of these ulcers, but other causes include other forms of vascular disease (polyarteritis nodosa), lead/arsenic polyneuropathies, alcoholic polyneuropathy, sarcoidosis, leprosy, and syphilis.

F. Infection is another etiologic factor in leg ulcers. It occurs most commonly after primary inoculation of a pathogen, although dissemination from a primary focus elsewhere also is possible. Lesions are inflamed and purulent and may have draining sinuses. Perform a biopsy at the ulcer margin and send the tissue to be cultured for bacterial, fungal, mycobacterial, and viral pathogens, as well as for routine histology.

G. Lack of response of an ulcer to therapy or rapid growth of a lesion that was previously stable should lead one to suspect neoplasm. An elevated ulcer edge with central crust or granulation tissue is characteristic of many tumors. A biopsy of the ulcer margin should be performed.

H. Traumatic ulcers are diagnosed by history. Some patients with self-induced disease may be unwilling to divulge the cause and may, in fact, be inappropriately unconcerned. These ulcers are characterized by bizarre shapes that have minimal surrounding erythema.

References

Bolognia J, Jorizza J, Rapine R. Dermatology, 2nd ed. Philadelphia: Elsevier, 2007.

Burton CS III. Treatment of leg ulcers. Dermatol Clin 1993;11:315.

Douglas WS, Simpson NB. Guidelines for the management of chronic venous leg ulceration. Br J Dermatol 1995;132:446.

Krull EA. Chronic cutaneous ulcerations and impaired healing in the human skin. J Am Acad Dermatol 1995;12:394.

Phillips TJ, Dover JS. Leg ulcers. J Am Acad Dermatol 1991;25:965.

Wolff K, Goldsmith LA, Katz SI, et al: Fitzpatrick's Dermatology in General Medicine, 7th ed. New York: McGraw-Hill, 2007.

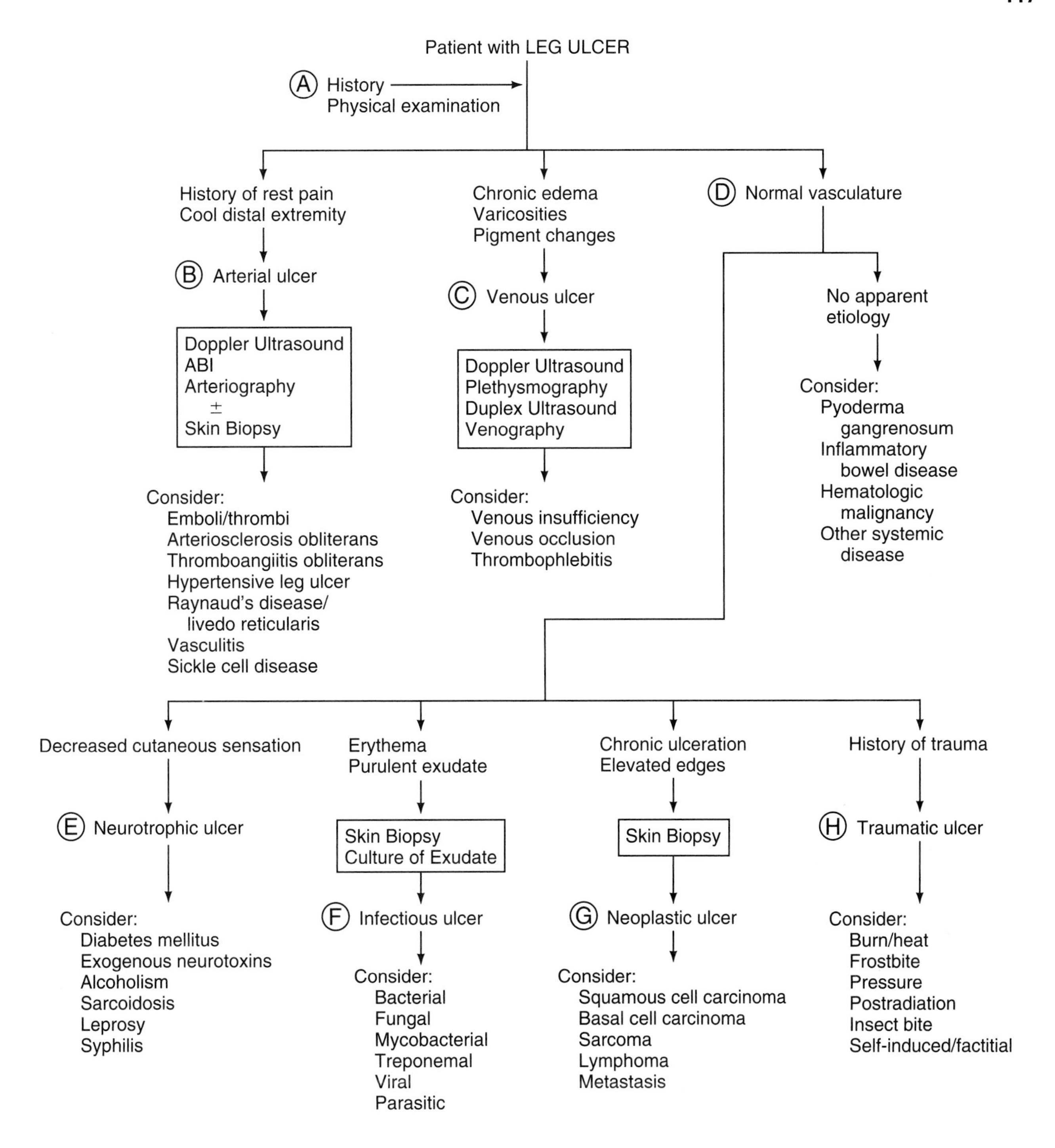
Patient with LEG ULCER
(A) History
Physical examination
History of rest pain
Cool distal extremity
(B) Arterial ulcer
Doppler Ultrasound
ABI
Arteriography
±
Skin Biopsy
Consider:
Emboli/thrombi
Arteriosclerosis obliterans
Thromboangiitis obliterans
Hypertensive leg ulcer
Raynaud's disease/
livedo reticularis
Vasculitis
Sickle cell disease
Chronic edema
Varicosities
Pigment changes
(C) Venous ulcer
Doppler Ultrasound
Plethysmography
Duplex Ultrasound
Venography
Consider:
Venous insufficiency
Venous occlusion
Thrombophlebitis
(D) Normal vasculature
No apparent
etiology
Consider:
Pyoderma
gangrenosum
Inflammatory
bowel disease
Hematologic
malignancy
Other systemic
disease
Decreased cutaneous sensation
(E) Neurotrophic ulcer
Consider:
Diabetes mellitus
Exogenous neurotoxins
Alcoholism
Sarcoidosis
Leprosy
Syphilis
Erythema
Purulent exudate
Skin Biopsy
Culture of Exudate
(F) Infectious ulcer
Consider:
Bacterial
Fungal
Mycobacterial
Treponemal
Viral
Parasitic
Chronic ulceration
Elevated edges
Skin Biopsy
(G) Neoplastic ulcer
Consider:
Squamous cell carcinoma
Basal cell carcinoma
Sarcoma
Lymphoma
Metastasis
History of trauma
(H) Traumatic ulcer
Consider:
Burn/heat
Frostbite
Pressure
Postradiation
Insect bite
Self-induced/factitial

URTICARIA

Norman Levine, MD

Urticaria is a vascular reaction of the skin characterized by evanescent edematous plaques (wheals, hives). Angioedema differs only in that the edema extends into the deep dermis and subcutaneous tissue. About 15% of the population develops this problem at some time in life. In about 60% of cases the lesions resolve in <6 weeks (acute urticaria); in the remaining patients the disease persists longer, usually in the form of recurrent episodes.

A. In about 25% of cases a definite cause can be uncovered, and in most of these patients the history and physical examination alone are sufficient to determine the cause.

B. The most common cause of acute urticaria is a drug reaction. The agents often implicated are sulfonamides, penicillin derivatives, barbiturates, diuretics, and anti-inflammatory agents. Medications taken within 14 days of the onset of the urticaria are the most likely offenders. Certain foods such as nuts, shellfish, and eggs may produce urticaria in susceptible individuals. Focal infections, such as sinusitis or genitourinary infections, and systemic infections, such as viral hepatitis or infectious mononucleosis, occasionally produce urticaria. In rare instances, patients may develop localized wheals after direct contact with an offending agent (contact urticaria).

C. Certain chronic skin diseases have lesions that appear urticarial and must be differentiated from urticaria. Urticaria pigmentosa (mastocytosis) presents with stable brown papules that urticate when rubbed. The lesions of urticarial vasculitis are wheals that persist for several days and often have a violaceous color. These diagnoses can be confirmed by a skin biopsy.

D. Many cases of chronic urticaria are secondary to physical stimuli that produce hives in susceptible patients. Dermographism occurs in 5% of the population and consists of wheals that develop 1–3 minutes after skin stroking. Stimuli as innocuous as toweling after bathing or rubbing one's eyes can produce hives. Less commonly, patients develop wheals after cold, heat, water, or sun exposure. Patients with cholinergic urticaria develop 2- to 4-mm wheals within 2–20 minutes after general overheating of the body, such as occurs after vigorous exercise.

E. In patients with chronic urticaria that is not secondary to physical stimuli, a routine noninvasive laboratory screen is indicated. However, abnormal laboratory test results rarely uncover an occult cause of urticaria in the face of a normal history and physical examination.

F. In many patients an identifiable cause of chronic urticaria is never uncovered. In some of these there may be psychogenic influences that exacerbate the urticarial episodes. Others may have a genetic tendency that makes them more prone to hives from a variety of stimuli. Some cases of chronic urticaria are caused by an autoimmune phenomenon in which autoantibodies bind to IgE receptors on the surface of mast cells, resulting in mast cell activation and degranulation.

References

Arndt KA, Leboit PE, Robinson JK, Wintroub BU, eds. Cutaneous Medicine and Surgery. Philadelphia: WB Saunders, 1996.

Bolognia J, Jorizza J, Rapine R. Dermatology, 2nd ed. Philadelphia: Elsevier, 2007.

Hirschmann JV, Lawlor F, English JSC, et al. Cholinergic urticaria: a clinical and histologic study. Arch Dermatol 1987;123:462.

Jacobson KW, Branch CB, Nelson HS. Laboratory tests in chronic urticaria. JAMA 1980;243:1644.

Kulp-Shorten CL, Callen JP. Urticaria, angioedema, and rheumatologic disease. Rheum Dis Clin North Am 1996;22:95.

Mahmood T. Urticaria. Am Fam Physician 1995;51:811.

Pollack CV Jr, Romano TJ. Outpatient management of acute urticaria: the role of prednisone. Ann Emerg Med 1995;26:547.

Sveum RJ. Urticaria: the diagnostic challenge of hives. Postgrad Med 1996;100:77.

Wolff K, Goldsmith LA, Katz SI, et al: Fitzpatrick's Dermatology in General Medicine, 7th ed. New York: McGraw-Hill, 2007.

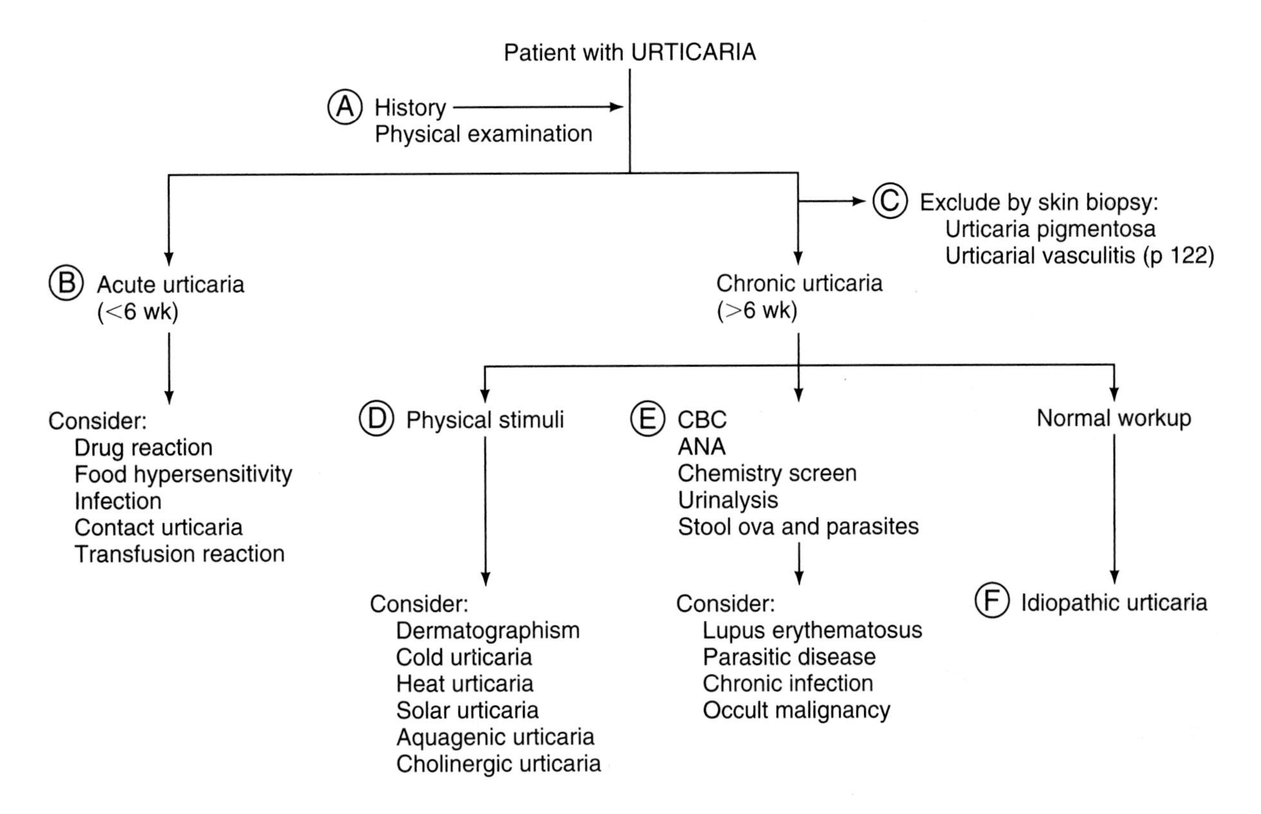
Patient with URTICARIA
(A) History
Physical examination
(C) Exclude by skin biopsy:
Urticaria pigmentosa
Urticarial vasculitis (p 122)
(B) Acute urticaria
(<6 wk)
Chronic urticaria
(>6 wk)
Consider:
Drug reaction
Food hypersensitivity
Infection
Contact urticaria
Transfusion reaction
(D) Physical stimuli
(E) CBC
ANA
Chemistry screen
Urinalysis
Stool ova and parasites
Normal workup
Consider:
Dermatographism
Cold urticaria
Heat urticaria
Solar urticaria
Aquagenic urticaria
Cholinergic urticaria
Consider:
Lupus erythematosus
Parasitic disease
Chronic infection
Occult malignancy
(F) Idiopathic urticaria

GENERALIZED PRURITUS

Norman Levine, MD, and Barbara A. Gilchrest, MD

Pruritus is an unpleasant sensation that provokes the desire to scratch. In at least half of cases when the workup is concluded, one is left with a diagnosis of idiopathic. It is frequently multifactorial. In the elderly, xerosis is common and careful attention to moisturization may reduce symptoms whether pruritus is idiopathic (common) or caused by systemic illness. Regardless of the underlying cause, most patients have maximal itching at bedtime. There are many pruritic dermatoses, but relatively few of these cause generalized itching. Generalized pruritus can be divided into conditions in which there is an associated dermatosis and those in which pruritus is a symptom of a noncutaneous disease.

A. Physical examination alone is sufficient to diagnose most primary cutaneous pruritic diseases. In the absence of an obvious primary lesion, a medical history may uncover occult dermatoses. For example, xerotic (dry) skin often itches just after bathing. Scabies may affect multiple household members and can be a venereally transmitted condition. Atopic dermatitis often appears in successive generations and is associated with asthma and allergic rhinitis.

B. The two most common causes of generalized pruritus are xerosis and atopic dermatitis. Xerosis is most prominent on the anterior legs and lateral arms. The plaques have fine fissures that look like a cracked pot ("erythema craquele"). The lesions of atopic dermatitis are thickened (lichenified) and excoriated. Occasionally patients with a psychosis will pick or scratch themselves and may bring a "sample" of "parasites" removed from the skin to the visit. On careful examination these are negative.

C. Diagnosis often can be confirmed by a skin biopsy. If scabies is suspected, examine the superficial contents of a burrow by performing a skin scraping.

D. Xerosis results in a dull appearance of the skin, with mild flakiness or scaling. It frequently coexists with other problems, particularly in the elderly. Also consider irritant or allergic contact dermatitis in this group. Causes include topical alcohol, harsh soap, wool clothing, detergent, and fabric softeners.

E. In the absence of an obvious cutaneous cause of generalized pruritus, empirically treat for xerosis with moisturizers. If the pruritus persists, a laboratory workup is indicated and should include a hemogram, serum chemistries, glucose tolerance test, thyroid function studies, urinalysis, and chest radiography.

F. Pruritus rarely predates the diagnosis of systemic malignancy, except in Hodgkin's disease, where 6% of cases present with pruritus alone. If after a routine workup there are no localizing signs of malignancy, further evaluation usually is not indicated.

G. Polycythemia vera is associated with pruritus after quick temperature change (e.g., bathing). Itching occurs commonly in leukemia and rarely in iron deficiency states, even in the absence of other signs and symptoms.

H. Pruritus often is the first symptom of biliary cirrhosis and extrahepatic biliary obstruction. An elevated serum alkaline phosphatase level is characteristic.

I. The pruritus of diabetes mellitus occurs in <5% of patients and is not correlated with disease severity.

J. Hyperthyroidism may produce generalized pruritus that improves when the patient becomes euthyroid. Most cases of pruritus with hypothyroidism are secondary to xerosis.

K. Chronic renal failure commonly produces generalized pruritus in patients with BUN >50 mg/dl. Dialysis may produce paroxysms of intense itching. Phototherapy with ultraviolet B (UVB) may relieve itching in these patients.

L. Although psychogenic pruritus is a common cause of itching, consider it only after all other causes have been ruled out.

References

Bergasa NV, Jones EA. The pruritus of cholestasis. Semin Liver Dis 1993; 13:319.

Bolognia J, Jorizza J, Rapine R. Dermatology, 2nd ed. Philadelphia: Elsevier, 2007.

Denman ST. A review of pruritus. J Am Acad Dermatol 1986;14:375.

Greaves MW. New pathophysiological and clinical insights into pruritus. J Dermatol 1993;29:735.

Kantor GR, Lookingbill DP. Generalized pruritus and systemic disease. J Am Acad Dermatol 1983;9:375.

Levine N. "Winter itch": what's causing this rash? Geriatrics 1996; 51:20.

Lober CW. Pruritus and malignancy. Clin Dermatol 1993;11:125.

Martin J. Pruritus. Int J Dermatol 1985;24:634.

Wolff K, Goldsmith LA, Katz SI, et al: Fitzpatrick's Dermatology in General Medicine, 7th ed. New York: McGraw-Hill, 2007.

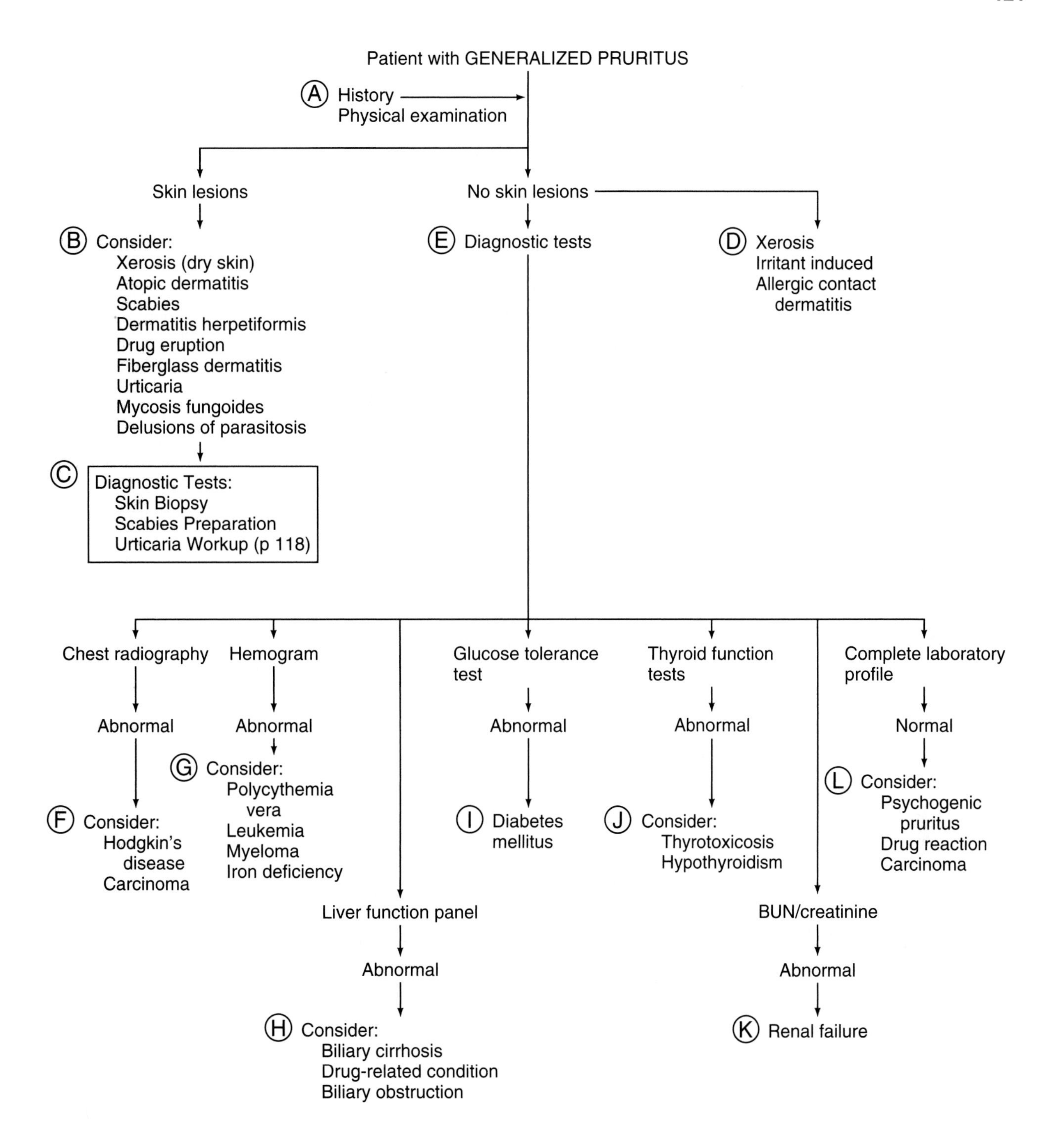
Patient with GENERALIZED PRURITUS
(A) History
Physical examination
Skin lesions
No skin lesions
(B) Consider:
Xerosis (dry skin)
Atopic dermatitis
Scabies
Dermatitis herpetiformis
Drug eruption
Fiberglass dermatitis
Urticaria
Mycosis fungoides
Delusions of parasitosis
(C) Diagnostic Tests:
Skin Biopsy
Scabies Preparation
Urticaria Workup (p 118)
(E) Diagnostic tests
(D) Xerosis
Irritant induced
Allergic contact dermatitis
Chest radiography
Abnormal
(F) Consider:
Hodgkin's disease
Carcinoma
Hemogram
Abnormal
(G) Consider:
Polycythemia vera
Leukemia
Myeloma
Iron deficiency
Liver function panel
Abnormal
(H) Consider:
Biliary cirrhosis
Drug-related condition
Biliary obstruction
Glucose tolerance test
Abnormal
(I) Diabetes mellitus
Thyroid function tests
Abnormal
(J) Consider:
Thyrotoxicosis
Hypothyroidism
BUN/creatinine
Abnormal
(K) Renal failure
Complete laboratory profile
Normal
(L) Consider:
Psychogenic pruritus
Drug reaction
Carcinoma

PALPABLE PURPURA

Norman Levine, MD

Palpable purpura is a skin lesion that is purpuric and has substance. It can be a papule, vesicle, or pustule. These lesions are highly indicative of inflammatory destruction of cutaneous blood vessel walls (vasculitis). Immune-mediated mechanisms of damage often are operative. Many clinically distinct disorders fall under the general heading of vasculitis, but the pathologic processes are similar in most of them.

A. The presence of palpable purpura is considered septic vasculitis until proved otherwise. Therefore, rule out underlying causes of sepsis before doing any other workup. Signs and symptoms of sepsis include fever, chills, mental status changes, tachycardia, tachypnea, and hypotension. In this clinical setting, several blood cultures and a skin biopsy of a purpuric lesion for light microscopy, bacterial smear, and culture are indicated.

B. Although there are few distinguishing clinical features of the skin lesions in septic vasculitis that would lead to the diagnosis of a specific infection, there occasionally are clues. In staphylococcal sepsis, showers of purpuric pustules appear. Gram stain reveals the offending organism. In gonococcemia, there are relatively few acral purpuric papules and vesicles that subsequently develop into pustules. Patients with meningococcemia have an explosive onset of hundreds of hemorrhagic macules and papules over the whole body. In Rocky Mountain spotted fever, palpable purpuric lesions occur after several days of illness, and only after the lesions have progressed from pink macules to red papules to purpuric papules.

C. In many cases, palpable purpura of the skin mirrors systemic vasculitides, most of which are immune mediated. Although laboratory abnormalities are common in systemic vasculitis, there are few abnormalities pathognomonic for given diseases. Therefore, the workup includes measurements of organ function and immune status along with the history and physical examination.

D. Henoch-Schönlein purpura is a small vessel vasculitis, usually occurring in children, that involves the skin (palpable purpura), joints, kidneys, and GI tract. In 90% of cases this follows an upper respiratory infection and lasts for 7–14 days. There may be recurrences. Several chronic disorders are characterized by granuloma formation involving blood vessels that can produce palpable purpuric lesions. Wegener's granulomatosis is a disease involving the skin, kidneys, and upper respiratory tract. Allergic granulomatosis (Churg-Strauss syndrome) occurs in asthmatic patients who develop palpable purpura, hypertension, chronic pneumonitis, and a neuropathy. Polyarteritis nodosa is a vasculitis of small- and medium-sized arteries with involvement of the skin, kidneys, pulmonary and nervous system, and joints. The skin lesions may be purpuric papules, subcutaneous nodules, and/or cutaneous ulcerations along with livedo reticularis. Urticarial vasculitis is a multisystem disorder with recurrent crops of purpuric wheals lasting several days. Some of these patients have associated hypocomplementemia. This is differentiated from other forms of vasculitis by the relatively evanescent nature of the lesions and by the fact that the lesions appear more urticarial.

E. In many cases, palpable purpura (vasculitis) occurs in an otherwise clinically healthy patient. A limited laboratory workup, including skin biopsy, is indicated to rule out occult immune complex diseases such as essential mixed cryoglobulinemia and hyperglobulinemic purpura, and purely cutaneous vasculitides such as erythema elevatum diutinum.

F. Hypersensitivity vasculitis does not have pathognomonic criteria but depends on a constellation of signs and symptoms. Most patients are >16 years of age and may have a history of intake of a medication that could be causative. They have palpable purpura and nonblanching red papules and macules, usually on the lower extremities.

References

Bolognia J, Jorizza J, Rapine R. Dermatology, 2nd ed. Philadelphia: Elsevier, 2007.

Calabrese LH, Michel BA, Bloch DA, et al. The American College of Rheumatology 1990 criteria for the classification of hypersensitivity vasculitis. Arthritis Rheum 1990;33:1108.

Lightfoot RW Jr, Michel BA, Bloch DA, et al. The American College of Rheumatology 1990 criteria for the classification of polyarteritis nodosa. Arthritis Rheum 1990;33:1088.

Manders SM. Serious and life-threatening drug eruptions. Am Fam Physician 1995;51:1805.

Mills JA, Michel BA, Bloch DA, et al. The American College of Rheumatology 1990 criteria for the classification of Henoch-Schönlein purpura. Arthritis Rheum 1990;33:1114.

Tapson KM. Henoch-Schönlein purpura. Am Fam Physician 1993;47:633.

Wolff K, Goldsmith LA, Katz SI, et al. Fitzpatrick's Dermatology in General Medicine, 7th ed. New York: McGraw-Hill, 2007.

ENDOCRINOLOGY

Graham T. McMahon, MD, MMSc
Section Editor

HYPOGLYCEMIA

Graham T. McMahon, MD, MMSc

A. Hypoglycemia is possibly the most common metabolic emergency because insulin-induced hypoglycemia is a common side effect of treatment of a common disease. Symptoms of hypoglycemia are partly sympathetic and related to the release of catecholamines. These symptoms develop as the plasma glucose falls below 55 mg/dl and include sweating, tremor, hunger, anxiety, fear, and palpitations. Other symptoms are caused by an insufficient supply of glucose to the brain, resulting in neuroglycopenia with symptoms such as slurred speech, blurred vision, weakness, and confusion. Neuroglycopenic symptoms, in general, occur when plasma glucose falls below 50 mg/dl. Symptoms should disappear with treatment.

   Treatment of mild episodes of hypoglycemia is intake of fast-absorbing carbohydrates. Severe episodes can be treated with either IV dextrose or glucagon injected intramuscularly or intravenously. The glycemic response and recovery of a normal level of consciousness is 1–2 minutes slower after glucagon than after glucose.

B. Patients receiving treatment for diabetes mellitus experience hypoglycemia when there is a mismatch between insulin levels (either exogenous insulin or as induced by sulfonylureas) and metabolic demands. Patients with hypoglycemia should have their records examined and insulin dosing and timing adjusted to reduce the risk of hypoglycemia without compromising overall glucose control. As targets for glycemic control have progressively declined, the incidence of hypoglycemia has increased. Patients with poor glucose control become symptomatic with adrenergic symptoms of hypoglycemia at progressively higher glucose thresholds, often when the plasma glucose is >100 mg/dl. When a sulfonylurea is implicated, its use should be reevaluated within the context of the patient's needs and alternative or shorter-acting agents should be considered. Because sulfonylureas have an extended half-life, patients with a sulfonylurea-induced symptomatic hypoglycemic event should not be discharged from the hospital until at least 24 hours have passed.

C. Ethanol is another common cause of hypoglycemia. In a nondiabetic person who has had an insufficient intake of food for 1 or 2 days, hypoglycemia will typically develop 6–24 hours after a moderate or heavy intake of ethanol. Drugs that are reported to induce hypoglycemia include salicylates in large doses, quinine, haloperidol, pentamidine, and trimethoprim-sulfamethoxazole.

D. Patients with hypoglycemic symptoms who are not known to have diabetes should be provided with a home glucometer and instructed in its use so that glucose measures can be taken at the time when symptoms are experienced. If hypoglycemia is confirmed by review of the glucometer data or clinical suspicion is high, a prolonged supervised fast is the most reliable test for establishing the diagnosis. Symptoms that occur in the presence of a normal glucose level eliminate the need for further evaluation for hypoglycemia.

   A supervised fast is performed to confirm that the symptoms result from hypoglycemia and that reversing it relieves the symptoms. The fast begins at the time of last food ingestion, which can be the evening meal on the previous day. Patients are provided with calorie-free and caffeine-free drinks and should remain active. Blood samples for plasma glucose, insulin, C-peptide, and proinsulin are drawn every 6 hours; these assays are not performed unless the glucose is <60 mg/dl. The testing frequency increases to hourly if any of these glucose levels drop below 60 mg/dl. The fast is ended when the plasma glucose drops below 45 mg/dl, if the patient has symptoms or signs of hypoglycemia, or when 72 hours have elapsed. Blood is drawn to test for the presence of sulfonylureas, IV glucose is given, and the patient is fed.

E. Insulin levels >6 μU/ml when the plasma glucose is <55 mg/dl are considered inappropriate insulin levels. Plasma C-peptide and proinsulin levels help distinguish exogenous from endogenous insulin sources: C-peptide and proinsulin levels should correlate with the insulin level when the insulin source is endogenous. Endogenous hyperinsulinemia can result from treatment with sulfonylureas; these can be detected in the plasma. Long-acting sulfonylureas are particularly high risk when prescribed to older patients.

F. Insulin-producing tumors, insulinomas, and non–islet cell tumors may be underlying causes of hypoglycemia in people without diabetes. When suggested by the results of a fast, insulinoma should be further investigated in consultation with an endocrinologist or endocrine surgeon. Endoscopic ultrasound is recommended for tumor identification. Intraoperative ultrasound or a selective arterial calcium-infusion test may be required to identify the source because these tumors are often extremely small.

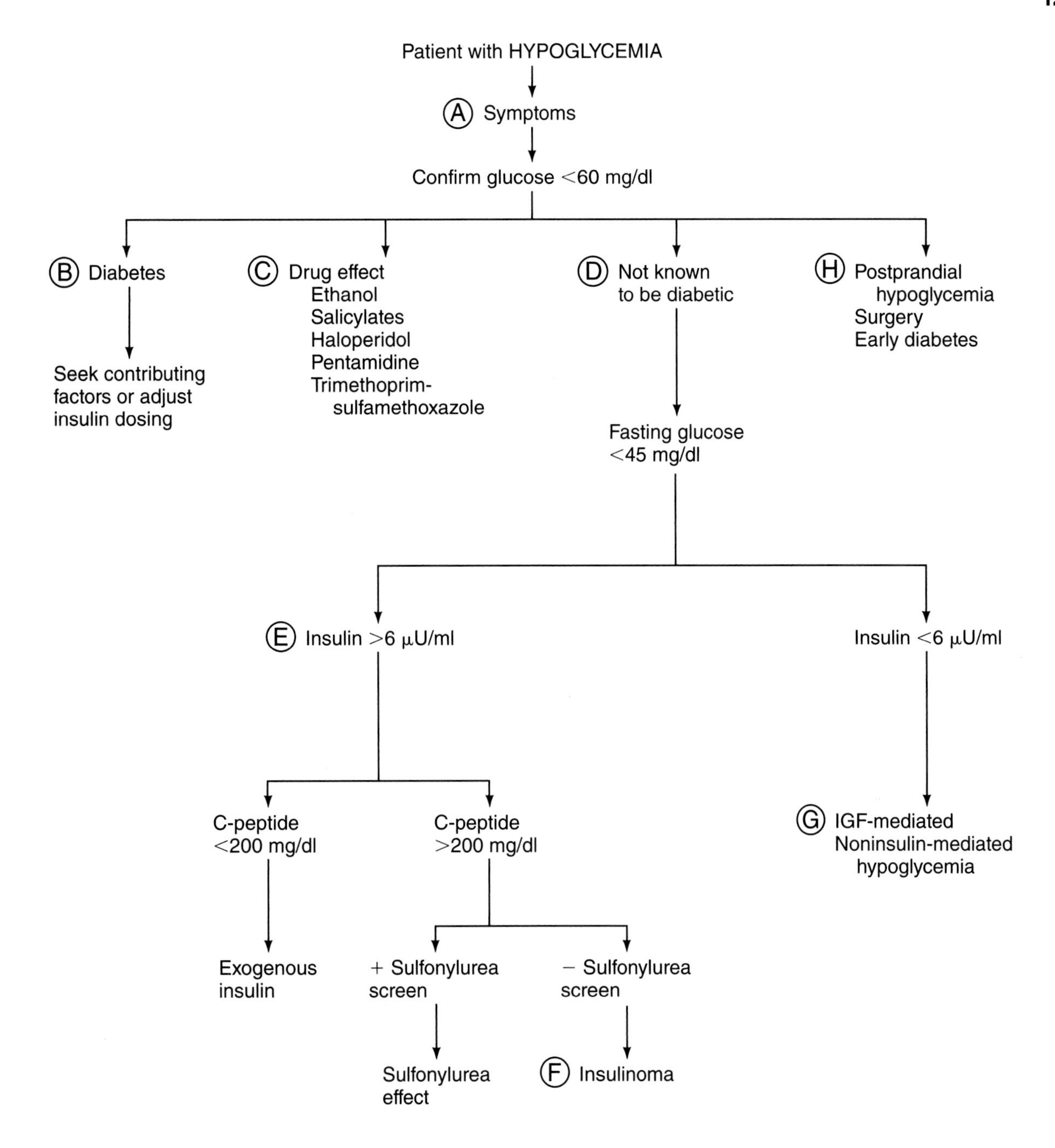

G. Fasting hypoglycemia that is not associated with hyperinsulinemia is most often found in the presence of advanced disease such as renal or liver failure or malnutrition. It may be a presentation of adrenal insufficiency. Nonpancreatic tumors may induce hypoglycemia through the paraneoplastic secretion of insulinlike growth factor-2 or its precursor.

H. Most patients with autonomic symptoms after eating do not have hypoglycemia, and normal individuals can develop glucose levels of <50 mg/dl after eating. Postprandial hypoglycemia can occur among patients who have undergone bariatric surgery and early in diabetes mellitus in which the insulin secretion becomes dysregulated.

References

Palardy J, Havrankova J, Lepage R, et al. Blood glucose measurements during symptomatic episodes in patients with suspected postprandial hypoglycemia. N Engl J Med 1989;321:1421.

Proye CA, Lokey JS. Current concepts in functioning endocrine tumors of the pancreas. World J Surg 2004;28(12):1231–1238.

Service FJ. Classification of hypoglycemic disorders. Endocrinol Metab Clin North Am 1999;28(3):501–517, vi.

Service FJ. Diagnostic approach to adults with hypoglycemic disorders. Endocrinol Metab Clin North Am 1999;28(3):519–532.

Thompson GB. Diagnosis and management of insulinomas. Endocr Pract 2002;8(5):385–386.

HYPERGLYCEMIA

Graham T. McMahon, MD, MMsc

The prevalence of diabetes mellitus is increasing exponentially in the United States and around the globe. The disease currently affects approximately 18 million Americans. Type 2 diabetes accounts for approximately 95% of all cases and is characterized by insulin resistance and hyperglycemia. Hyperinsulinemia occurs early in the disease but is not maintained indefinitely. Many patients ultimately require insulin to maintain glucose levels in the normal range. Because almost 90% of all patients with diabetes will die from cardiovascular complications, cardiovascular risk reduction is the primary target.

A. Diabetes is diagnosed if there are symptoms of diabetes (polyuria, polydipsia, unexplained weight loss) and a random glucose level of >200 mg/dl. A fasting glucose of >126 mg/dl or a glucose of >200 mg/dl 2 hours after a 75-g glucose load are also diagnostic. Diagnostic use of the hemoglobin A1c (HbA1c) is not recommended.

B. Hyperglycemia not sufficient to meet the diagnostic criteria for diabetes (prediabetes) is categorized as either impaired fasting glucose or impaired glucose tolerance. Diabetes can be prevented in patients with either of these conditions if patients lose weight and embark on an exercise program. Metformin can also be used to prevent the onset of diabetes in these patients at high risk.

C. Secondary causes of diabetes should be considered when evaluating any patient with diabetes. Drugs that cause diabetes such as glucocorticoids, thiazides, Dlantin, and protease inhibitors should have their doses reduced or replaced with alternative agents if possible. Genetic causes of diabetes should be excluded if a strong family history of diabetes or a phenotype (e.g., Down, Turner's, Klinefelter's syndromes) is noted. Endocrinopathies such as Cushing's syndrome, acromegaly, pheochromocytoma, hyperthyroidism, and others should be sought from the history and examination. Patients with diseases that affect the exocrine pancreas, such as hemochromatosis, chronic pancreatitis, pancreatic, malignancy, or cystic fibrosis, are at high risk for diabetes; treatment of the underlying disease is often critical to reduce the rate of progression to insulin deficiency and to managing the diabetes.

D. Patients with type 1 diabetes require lifelong insulin treatment. Typically basal insulin is used with ultra–short-acting insulins given before each meal or snack. Patients with type 1 diabetes should be taught to count carbohydrates and to calculate both correction and prandial insulin dosing. These patients should work with a diabetes team and be offered insulin-pump therapy. Blood pressure; lipid; and renal, eye, and foot care guidelines are similar to those for patients with type 2 diabetes.

E. Patients who are newly diagnosed with type 2 diabetes should be provided with a glucometer and testing instructions and referred for diabetes education and medical nutrition therapy. Smoking cessation and the benefits of exercise and weight loss should be emphasized.

(Continued on page 130)

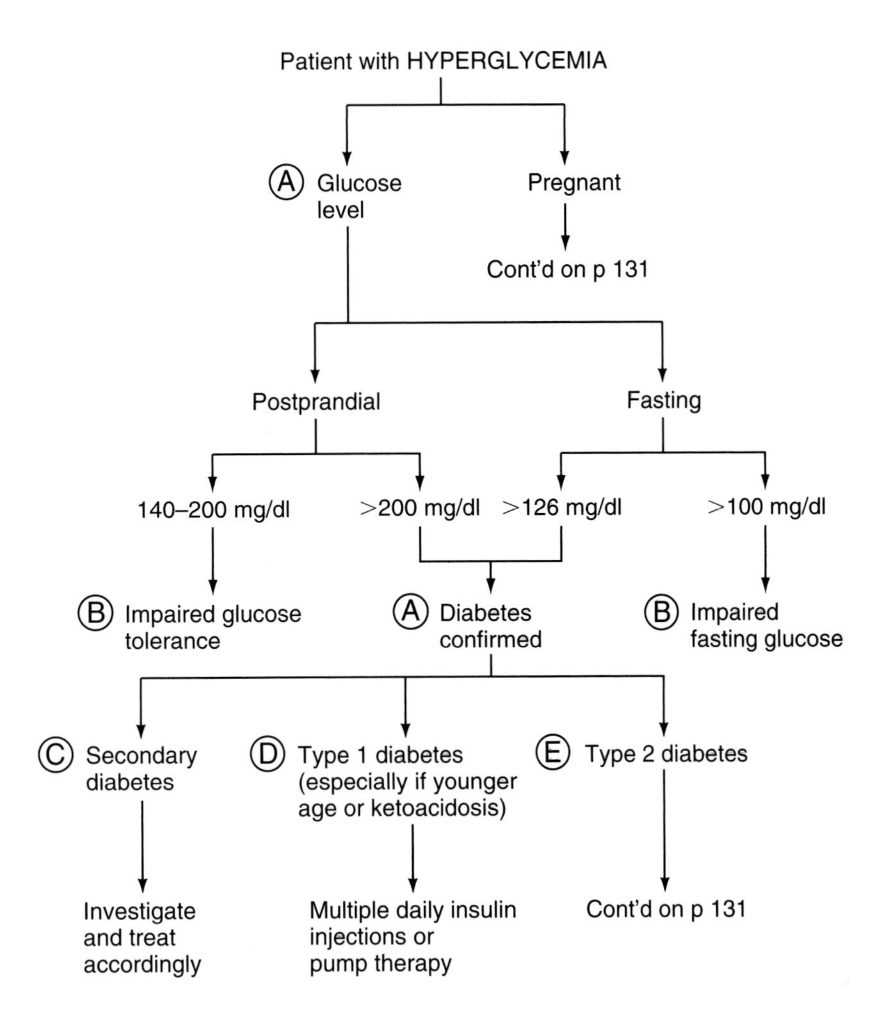
Patient with HYPERGLYCEMIA
(A) Glucose level
Pregnant
Cont'd on p 131
Postprandial
Fasting
140–200 mg/dl
>200 mg/dl
>126 mg/dl
>100 mg/dl
(B) Impaired glucose tolerance
(A) Diabetes confirmed
(B) Impaired fasting glucose
(C) Secondary diabetes
(D) Type 1 diabetes (especially if younger age or ketoacidosis)
(E) Type 2 diabetes
Investigate and treat accordingly
Multiple daily insulin injections or pump therapy
Cont'd on p 131

F. For patients requiring treatment, metformin remains the first-line agent of choice. Patients should be warned that early GI side effects are not uncommon and should be tolerated if possible; they usually abate within 2 weeks. Metformin use is associated with cardiovascular risk reduction but cannot be used in patients with creatinine levels >1.5 mg or in those who have severe chronic illnesses. Sulfonylureas are added as second-line agents because they are cost-effective. Short-acting sulfonylureas such as glipizide are preferred for their shorter half-life, especially among older patients. Thiazolidinediones such as pioglitazone are used as third-line therapy or among patients with contraindications to first- and second-line drugs; however, they have more limited efficacy and have been associated with cardiovascular risk and bone loss.

Gliptins have limited efficacy but are weight neutral and well tolerated. Exenatide has a high incidence of GI side effects and limited efficacy but can result in weight loss.

G. A typical starting dose of insulin is 0.3 U/kg. Insulin management should include a basal insulin (insulin glargine or neutral protamine Hagedorn [NPH]) with shorter-acting insulins added before meals in an incremental fashion. Doses are titrated to premeal and postprandial glucoses. Patients in need of insulin treatment should be warned to check their glucose before driving. Current approaches to glycemic management include the use of glucagon-like-peptide (GLP)-1 analogs, inhibitors of dipeptidyl-peptidase-4, and amylin analogs.

H. Blood pressure control is just as important as glycemic control. Treatment with an angiotensin-converting enzyme (ACE) inhibitor is typically used as a first line, with calcium channel blockers and thiazide diuretics added as necessary. Most patients require two to four antihypertensive agents to achieve a recommended blood pressure of <130/80 mm Hg.

I. Urinary microalbumin levels should be assessed yearly. The presence of >30 mg of microalbumin per gram of creatinine is a risk factor for nephropathy and cardiovascular disease. ACE inhibitors and angiotensin receptor blockers (ARBs) should be titrated until the microalbumin level is suppressed below 30 mg/g creatinine.

J. Hyperlipidemia in diabetes typically features hypertriglyceridemia and low levels of high-density lipoprotein (HDL). The latter can be treated with fibrates or niacin. Levels of low-density lipoprotein (LDL) >100 mg/dl are associated with increased cardiovascular risk. Statins should be offered to such patients.

K. *Gestational diabetes* refers to any diabetes that is diagnosed during pregnancy. Screening is optimally performed at 24–28 weeks of gestation or earlier in women at high risk (positive family history, obesity, prior macrosomia). Diagnosis is suggested by a fasting glucose >126 mg/dl, a random glucose >200 mg/dl, or a glucose >140 mg/dl 1 hour after a 50-g glucose load. Diagnosis during pregnancy is confirmed using a 3-hour oral glucose tolerance test (OGTT) using a 100-g glucose load. Criteria for a positive 3-hour glucose tolerance test include a fasting glucose >95 mg/dl, a 1-hour sample >180 mg/dl, a 2-hour sample >155 mg/dl, or a 3-hour sample >140 mg/dl. Patients with gestational diabetes should be provided with nutritional counseling and a glucometer. Fasting glucose readings should be kept at <90 mg/dl, and 1-hour postprandial levels should be <120 mg/dl. A minority of women with gestational diabetes will require insulin therapy; usually insulin NPH and ultra–short-acting insulins (lispro or aspart) are used. Oral agents are not routinely used to manage gestational diabetes. Sulfonylureas are contraindicated in pregnancy, and safety data for metformin use are very limited.

L. Hyperglycemia during hospitalization is associated with significant increases in morbidity and mortality. Normalization of glucose has been shown to be beneficial among patients in medical and surgical intensive care units. In intensive care unit settings, insulin should be infused intravenously if glucose is >120 mg/dl and titrated thereafter to a glucose level of <140 mg/dl. The patient can be transitioned to SC insulin when stable (e.g., extubated, off pressors) whether or not the patient is eating. If glucose control has been on target, many clinicians start with an insulin dose that is 80% of the previous day's total daily insulin use. Prescriptions should be written for basal, prandial, and correction doses.

Table 1 **Targets for Patients with Diabetes**

HbA1c	<7%
Fasting glucose	90–130 mg/dl
Peak postprandial glucose	<180 mg/dl
Blood pressure	<130/80 mm Hg
Urine microalbumin	<30 mg/day creatinine
Lipids	
LDL	<100 mg/dl (<70 mg/dl if additional risk factors are present)
HDL	>40 mg/dl

Daily low-dose aspirin therapy (age >40 or additional risk factors)
Annual foot examination
Yearly dilated eye examination by an ophthalmologist

References

American Diabetes Association. Clinical practice recommendations 2009. Diabetes Care 2009;28(Suppl 1):S1–79.

DeWitt DE, Hirsch IB. Outpatient insulin therapy in type 1 and type 2 diabetes mellitus: scientific review. JAMA 2003;289(17):2254–2264.

Galerneau F, Inzucchi SE. Diabetes mellitus in pregnancy. Obstet Gynecol Clin North Am 2004;31(4):907–933, xi–xii.

Moghissi ES, Hirsch IB. Hospital management of diabetes. Endocrinol Metab Clin North Am 2005;34(1):99–116.

Van den Berghe G, Wouters P, Weekers F, et al. Intensive insulin therapy in the critically ill patients. N Engl J Med 2001;345(19):1359–1367.

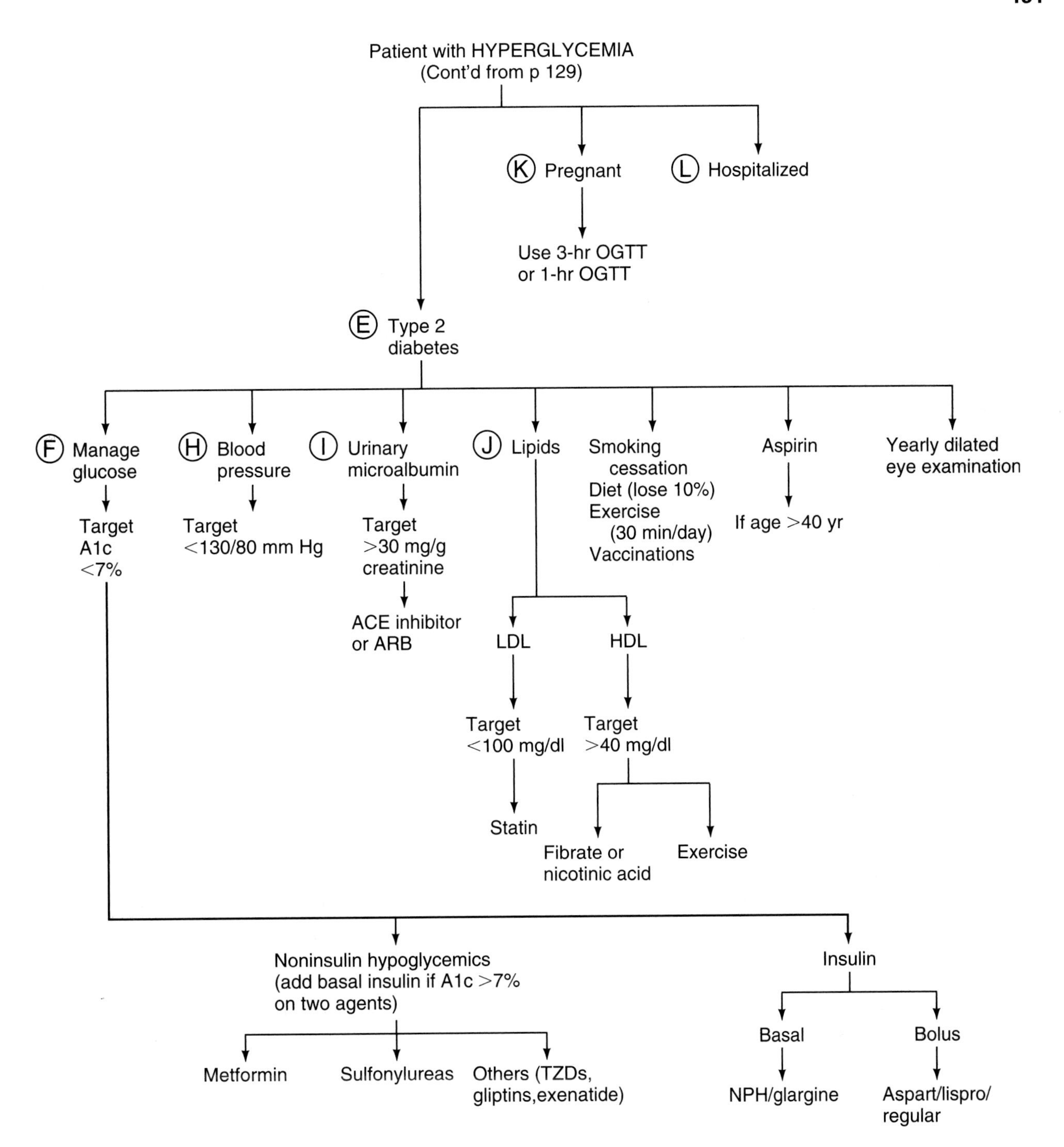

Patient with HYPERGLYCEMIA
(Cont'd from p 129)
K Pregnant
L Hospitalized
Use 3-hr OGTT
or 1-hr OGTT
E Type 2
diabetes
F Manage
glucose
H Blood
pressure
I Urinary
microalbumin
J Lipids
Smoking
cessation
Diet (lose 10%)
Exercise
(30 min/day)
Vaccinations
Aspirin
Yearly dilated
eye examination
Target
A1c
<7%
Target
<130/80 mm Hg
Target
>30 mg/g
creatinine
ACE inhibitor
or ARB
If age >40 yr
LDL
HDL
Target
<100 mg/dl
Target
>40 mg/dl
Statin
Fibrate or
nicotinic acid
Exercise
Noninsulin hypoglycemics
(add basal insulin if A1c >7%
on two agents)
Insulin
Metformin
Sulfonylureas
Others (TZDs,
gliptins,exenatide)
Basal
Bolus
NPH/glargine
Aspart/lispro/
regular

HYPOCALCEMIA

Graham T. McMahon, MD, MMSc

Hypocalcemia is a consequence of excess calcium loss (into tissue, urine, or bone) or binding, or a problem with a calcium source (GI or bone). Parathyroid hormone (PTH) works to maintain calcium levels by releasing calcium from bone and activates vitamin D to facilitate the absorption of calcium from the gut.

A. Calcium is necessary for normal neuromuscle activity, and hypocalcemia can be associated with paresthesias and carpopedal spasm. Latent tetany can be elucidated by tapping on the facial nerve (Chvostek's sign) or leaving a sphygmomanometer inflated to above the systolic pressure for 5 minutes on the arm and observing for hand and arm spasm (Trousseau's sign). The examination should look for signs of chronic hypocalcemia such as hypertension, dystonia, ataxia, dementia, malnutrition, dry skin, dermatitis, sparse and brittle hair, cataracts, and papilledema. With severe hypocalcemia, the ECG becomes abnormal, most typically with a prolonged QT interval.

B. Hypoalbuminemia is associated with lower serum calcium concentrations but normal ionized calcium levels. Simple correction formulas adjusting for the serum albumin (e.g., corrected calcium = serum calcium (mg/dl) + 0.8[4–serum albumin (g/dl)]) generally suffice in estimating ionized calcium if a direct measurement is not readily available. When possible, ionized calcium, phosphate, and 25-vitamin D levels should be measured.

C. In patients who are critically ill, the differential diagnosis of hypocalcemia narrows. Acute hyperphosphatemia (caused by acute renal failure, rhabdomyolysis, or tumor lysis, for example) causes acute hypocalcemia directly. Pancreatitis that is sufficiently severe to cause hypocalcemia (by forming soaps in the pancreatic bed) is usually obvious. Acute respiratory alkalosis, which increases calcium binding to albumin in the blood, reduces ionized calcium levels. Magnesium is critical for the efflux of PTH, and hypomagnesemia induces both a deficiency of and resistance to the effect of PTH. Hypomagnesemia is most commonly found in patients with a history of heavy alcohol abuse or malabsorption or in those receiving parenteral nutrition. Administer IV calcium to patients who are symptomatic and treat the underlying disease.

D. Renal disease is associated with hyperphosphatemia due to impaired glomerular filtration and reduced 1-alpha hydroxylase activity, which result in chronic hypocalcemia. This chronic hypocalcemia typically results in secondary or tertiary hyperparathyroidism, so PTH levels are high.

E. Persistent hypocalcemia and hyperphosphatemia is, in the absence of renal failure or increased tissue breakdown, virtually diagnostic of either postsurgical or idiopathic hypoparathyroidism. The PTH level in these patients is low. Idiopathic hypoparathyroidism is a rare condition that may be isolated or associated with familial polyglandular endocrinopathy type 2 (mucocutaneous candidiasis, Addison's disease, or hypoparathyroidism). It usually presents in childhood. Other rare causes of hypoparathyroidism include DiGeorge syndrome, Wilson's disease, and hemochromatosis. Head and neck surgery, primarily for thyroid or parathyroid diseases, and rarely radiation therapy, can result in transient or sometimes permanent PTH deficiency that may not develop immediately. Pseudohypoparathyroidism should be considered in patients with the appropriate phenotype (such as short metacarpals) and signs of resistance to other glycoprotein hormones.

F. Hypocalcemia associated with low phosphate and low 25-vitamin D usually indicates an absorptive problem. Differential diagnoses that should be considered include malabsorption states (sprue, short bowel, regional enteritis), hepatobiliary disease, anticonvulsant therapy, and vitamin D deficiency or resistance states. Bisphosphonates can induce hypocalcemia if vitamin D stores are low.

G. Treatment includes adequate replacement of calcium, magnesium, and vitamin D. In conditions in which conversion of vitamin D to 1,25-vitamin D is perturbed (i.e., renal disease, vitamin D–resistant rickets), replacement with calcitriol or a similar metabolite is necessary. Vitamin D deficiency syndromes can be treated with high-dose vitamin D (such as 50,000 U given orally once every 2 weeks).

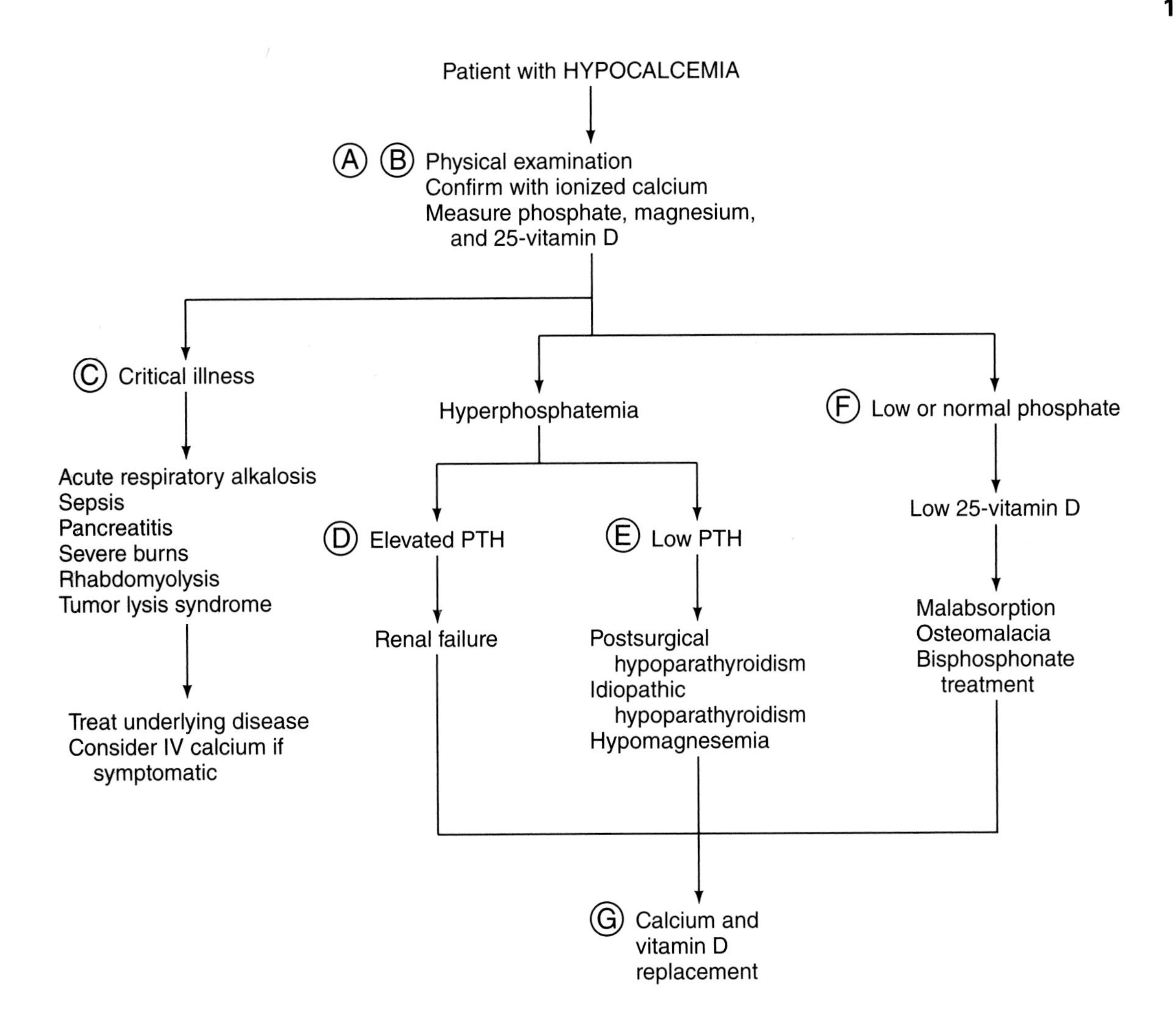

References

Akerström G, Hellman P, Hessman O, et al. Parathyroid glands in calcium regulation and human disease. Ann N Y Acad Sci 2005; 1040:53–58.

Brancaccio D, Cozzolino M, Galassi A, et al. Management of secondary hyperparathyroidism in uremic patients: the role of the new vitamin D analogs. J Nephrol 2007;20(1):3–9.

Carmeliet G, Van Cromphaut S, Daci E, et al. Disorders of calcium homeostasis. Best Pract Res Clin Endocrinol Metab 2003;17(4): 529–546.

Corrado A, Santoro N, Cantatore FP. Extra-skeletal effects of bisphosphonates. Joint Bone Spine 2007;74(1):32–38.

Friedman EA. Consequences and management of hyperphosphatemia in patients with renal insufficiency. Kidney Int Suppl 2005;(95):S1–7.

Potts JT. Parathyroid hormone: past and present. *J Endocrinol* 2005;187(3):311–325.

Sedlacek M, Schoolwerth AC, Remillard BD. Electrolyte disturbances in the intensive care unit. Semin Dial 2006;19(6):496–501.

Tong GM, Rude RK. Magnesium deficiency in critical illness. J Intensive Care Med 2005;20(1):3–17.

HYPERCALCEMIA

Graham T. McMahon, MD, MMSc

A. Hypercalcemia is frequently encountered by primary care physicians. Hypercalcemia is considered mild when the total serum calcium level is between 10.5 and 12 mg/dl. Levels >14 mg/dl are considered to be a hypercalcemic crisis and can be lethal. Patients with mild hypercalcemia are often asymptomatic. Patients with more severe hypercalcemia can present with nonspecific symptoms that include nausea, anorexia, constipation, abdominal pain, bone pain, fatigue, polydipsia, and confusion. Signs of hypercalcemia include dysrhythmias, hypertension, and short QT on an ECG. The two most common causes of hypercalcemia are primary hyperparathyroidism and neoplastic disease, accounting for >90% of cases, and these can be discriminated on the basis of the serum parathyroid hormone (PTH) level.

B. Primary hyperparathyroidism has a relatively benign course. Osteoporosis and renal impairment are two important long-term consequences that drive early intervention. Parathyroidectomy is recommended for patients with an elevated PTH level and hypercalcemia who are <50 years or if the calcium is >12.5 mg/dl, there are renal stones, there is evidence of renal insufficiency, the Z-score on bone densitometry is <2, or urinary calcium excretion is particularly high. A preoperative parathyroid sestamibi scan can assist the endocrine surgeon and limit the extent of surgery. Determining intraoperative PTH levels allows the surgeon to be confident of the procedure's success before surgical closure. Medical management of primary hyperparathyroidism with calcimimetics is currently limited to clinical trials.

Chronic renal failure generally causes hypocalcemia. If untreated, prolonged high phosphate and low vitamin D levels can lead to increased PTH secretion and subsequent hypercalcemia. This is termed *tertiary hyperparathyroidism* and can be managed surgically or medically.

C. Familial hypocalciuric hypercalcemia (FHH) is an autosomal-dominant condition caused by a mutation in the gene for the calcium receptor. Patients have an innocuous course characterized by mild to moderate hypercalcemia, normal or slightly elevated PTH levels, and low urinary calcium excretion. These patients do not benefit from parathyroidectomy.

D. Hypercalcemia of malignancy is usually symptomatic and can be severe. Solid tumors induce hypercalcemia by releasing parathyroid hormone–related protein (PTHrp), which mimics the action of endogenous PTH. Bone destruction by metastatic disease or myeloma can also induce hypercalcemia, often in association with an elevated alkaline phosphatase level.

E. Vitamin D can induce hypercalcemia if taken in overdose, or if there is excessive action of the 1-alpha-hydroxylase that creates the active form of vitamin D. This enzyme is hyperactive in patients with granulomatous disease such as sarcoidosis and responds well to treatment with glucocorticoids while the underlying disease is being treated. Consumption of large amounts of calcium or vitamin A can lead to hypercalcemia, but it is rare.

Treatment of severe hypercalcemia includes emergent fluid repletion with saline and IV administration of bisphosphonates. Initially saline is given at 200–300 ml/hr and is adjusted to maintain the urine output to 100–150 ml/hr. A loop diuretic can be added but is not always necessary and can lead to hypokalemia and hypomagnesemia. In the United States, pamidronate and zoledronate are bisphosphonates licensed for use in this indication. Zoledronate is preferred because it can be given over a shorter time (15 minutes as compared with 2 hours for pamidronate) and is more potent. Hypocalcemia occurs in up to 50% of patients treated with bisphosphonates for hypercalcemia of malignancy, although symptomatic hypocalcemia is rare. Calcitonin is characterized by good tolerability but poor efficacy in normalizing the serum calcium level. However, a major advantage of calcitonin is the acute onset of the hypocalcemic effect (reduction of 1–2 mg/dl within 6 hours), which contrasts with the delayed (approximately 2–4 days) but more pronounced effect of bisphosphonates. It is administered intramuscularly or subcutaneously every 12 hours at a dose of 4 IU/kg. Gallium nitrate is characterized by high efficacy and few adverse events apart from renal toxicity (10% of cases). However, data are limited, and further trials are necessary.

References

Jacobs TP, Bilezikian JP. Clinical review: rare causes of hypercalcemia. J Clin Endocrinol Metab 2005;90(11):6316–6322.

Mikhail N, Cope D. Evaluation and treatment of primary hyperparathyroidism. JAMA 2005;294(21):2700.

NIH conference. Diagnosis and management of asymptomatic primary hyperparathyroidism: consensus development conference statement. Ann Intern Med 1991;114:593–597.

Pecherstorfer M, Brenner K, Zojer N. Current management strategies for hypercalcemia. Treat Endocrinol 2003;2(4):273–292.

Saunders Y, Ross JR, Broadley KE, et al. Systematic review of bisphosphonates for hypercalcaemia of malignancy. Palliat Med 2004;18(5):418–431.

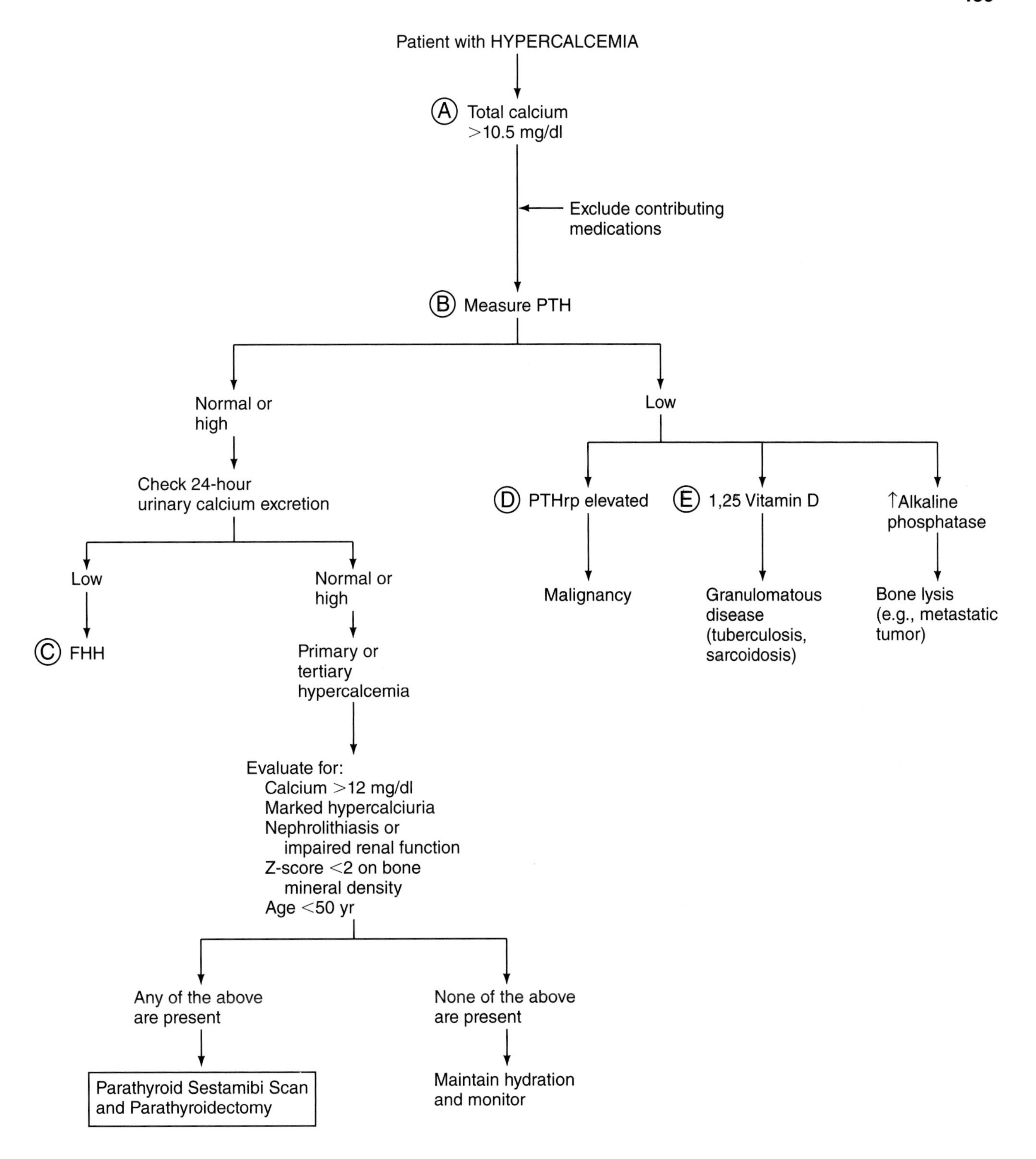

Patient with HYPERCALCEMIA
(A) Total calcium >10.5 mg/dl
Exclude contributing medications
(B) Measure PTH
Normal or high
Check 24-hour urinary calcium excretion
Low
(C) FHH
Normal or high
Primary or tertiary hypercalcemia
Evaluate for:
Calcium >12 mg/dl
Marked hypercalciuria
Nephrolithiasis or impaired renal function
Z-score <2 on bone mineral density
Age <50 yr
Any of the above are present
Parathyroid Sestamibi Scan and Parathyroidectomy
None of the above are present
Maintain hydration and monitor
Low
(D) PTHrp elevated
Malignancy
(E) 1,25 Vitamin D
Granulomatous disease (tuberculosis, sarcoidosis)
↑Alkaline phosphatase
Bone lysis (e.g., metastatic tumor)

TESTS OF THYROID FUNCTION

Erik K. Alexander, MD

The modern clinical laboratory offers several tests of thyroid function. The physician must be aware of the diagnostic accuracy and limitations of these tests. Abnormal test results must be interpreted with good clinical judgment. Thyroid function tests are probably not cost-effective as routine screens for thyroid disease.

Sensitive Thyroid-Stimulating Hormone (sTSH): A very useful test. Immunometric assays for TSH were introduced in the early 1980s. These assays generally make it possible to distinguish hyperthyroid from euthyroid patients. The sTSH is elevated in hypothyroidism. The sTSH assay has virtually no cross-reactivity with luteinizing hormone (LH), follicle-stimulating hormone (FSH), and human chorionic gonadotropin (hCG). The normal range for an sTSH assay is about 0.4–6.2 μU/ml.

Free Thyroxine Index (FTI): A useful calculation may soon be obsolete as new immunoassays for free thyroxine (FT_4) become available:

$$FTI = \text{total } T_4 \times T_3 \text{ Resin Uptake}$$

This calculation "corrects" the total T_4 for protein-binding abnormalities. In general, the FTI is a good estimate of free thyroid hormone concentration, although serum TSH is a better indicator of the total body thyroid status.

Free Thyroxine (FT_4): FT_4 is the amount of non–protein-bound circulating thyroxine (about 0.03%). Previously, measurement of FT_4 was difficult and time-consuming (equilibrium dialysis). Two-step immunoassays are now available to measure FT_4 quickly and accurately and probably will replace the calculated FTI.

Triiodothyronine by RIA (T_3 RIA): Measures total T_3. Useful only in diagnosing T_3 toxicosis.

Thyroid Antimicrosomal (TMab) and Antithyroglobulin (TgAb) Antibodies: These antibodies may be elevated in Graves' disease and Hashimoto's thyroiditis. A patient may have Hashimoto's thyroiditis and no circulating antibodies. Positive antibodies also are found in portions of the general population and in patients with nonthyroidal illness.

24-Hour Radioactive Iodine Uptake (RAIU): Measures the thyroid's ability to metabolize iodine. The test uses a tracer amount of ^{123}I or ^{131}I given orally. A gamma scintillation counter is used to measure the radioactivity over the thyroid at 4–6 hours and 24 hours after the dose. Normal percentage uptake varies widely. By itself, this test is not a very accurate test of thyroid function, but it is used frequently in the diagnostic evaluation of patients with hyperthyroidism.

Thyroid Imaging–Radionuclide Scan (^{123}I or ^{99m}Tc pertechnetate): Does not produce a picture like a CT or MRI scan. Can provide information about gland/lobe contour. Identifies thyroid nodules as "hot" (functioning), "cold" (nonfunctioning), or "warm."

References

Bauer DC, Brown AN. Sensitive thyrotropin and free thyroxine testing in outpatients: are both necessary? Arch Intern Med 1996;156:2333.

Behnia M, Gharib H. Primary care diagnosis of thyroid disease. Hosp Pract (Off Ed) 1996;31:121.

Bethune JE. Interpretation of thyroid function tests. Dis Mon 1989;35:543.

Kaye TB. Thyroid function tests: application of newer methods. Postgrad Med 1993;94:81.

Klee GG, Hay ID. Sensitive thyrotropin assays: analytical and clinical performance criteria. Mayo Clin Proc 1988;63:1123.

Santos ET, Mazzaferri EL. Thyroid function tests: guidelines for interpretation in common clinical disorders. Postgrad Med 1989;85:333.

Surks MI, Chopra IJ, Mariash CN, et al. American Thyroid Association guidelines for use of laboratory tests in thyroid disorders. JAMA 1990;263:1529.

HYPOTHYROIDISM

Graham T. McMahon, MD, MMSc

Clinically apparent hypothyroidism affects about 2% of adult women and about 0.2% of adult men. Primary hypothyroidism refers to intrinsic thyroid failure and accounts for 99% of cases; secondary hypothyroidism refers to hypothyroidism that results from pituitary dysfunction.

A. Patients with hypothyroidism may present with a variety of nonspecific symptoms. Some of the most common features include dry skin, cold intolerance, weight gain, constipation, and fatigue. The clinical picture of hypothyroidism is now a good deal milder because thyrotropin screening became more common. The most common signs in patients with moderate to severe hypothyroidism include bradycardia, delayed ankle reflexes, periorbital puffiness, and coarse hair. The term *myxedema* refers to the appearance of the skin and subcutaneous tissues in a patient with severe hypothyroidism.

B. The most common cause of primary hypothyroidism in iodine-sufficient areas is chronic autoimmune (Hashimoto's) thyroiditis. This is most common among older women and is generally permanent. Thyroidectomy, radioiodine treatment, and external radiation therapy are other frequent causes of hypothyroidism. Both iodine deficiency and excess can cause hypothyroidism. Iodine deficiency is a type of hypothyroidism associated with goiter. It is the most common cause of hypothyroidism worldwide but is uncommon in the United States, where iodine is added to salt. Acute administration of iodine suppresses thyroxine (T_4) synthesis; however, patients recover their thyroid function after just a few days of treatment. Other drugs that cause hypothyroidism include antithyroid medications (e.g., methimazole, propylthiouracil), amiodarone, lithium, and interferon-α.

C. Thyrotropin (or thyroid-stimulating hormone [TSH]) is the most sensitive marker of thyroid function. Patients with a TSH level of >10 μU/L should be treated with replacement T_4 with a target TSH of between 1 and 2 μU/L. Levothyroxine has a long half-life, and once-daily treatment results in a nearly constant serum T_4 level. As a result of variations in the T_4 content of individual formulations, reassessment of the adequacy of replacement is indicated if the formulation is changed. The mean replacement dose of T_4 is 1.6–1.8 μg/kg (75–112 μg/day in women and 125–200 μg/day in men). A lower dosage should be initiated in the elderly and titrated. Patients who are obese require doses that are approximately 20% higher. Drugs that interfere with the absorption of levothyroxine include cholestyramine, calcium carbonate, and ferrous sulfate. Patients receiving estrogen replacement also require a higher dosage of levothyroxine.

Combination replacement of liothyronine and levothyroxine is requested by some patients but is not supported by the balance of clinical trial data. If instituted, 25 μg of levothyroxine can be replaced with 5 μg of liothyronine. Desiccated thyroid, liothyronine alone, and other thyroid preparations are not recommended.

D. Patients with a TSH of 5–10 μU/L with a low free T_4 level should be treated with replacement levothyroxine. Patients with a TSH of 5–10 μU/L with a normal (T_4) level are most likely to have subclinical hypothyroidism. Testing for the presence of thyroid peroxidase antibody can be helpful in such patients because it predicts the progression to permanent hypothyroidism. These patients should be monitored for the development of more severe hypothyroidism, or levothyroxine can be initiated at the outset.

Hypothyroidism can be transient when related to thyroiditis. Inflammation of the thyroid gland can be painful or entirely painless. Hypothyroidism occurring postpartum is one of the most common presentations of thyroiditis. Transient hypothyroidism lasts as long as 6 months, but the hypothyroidism will have resolved in a significant majority of patients within 3 months. Transient hypothyroidism can be difficult to distinguish from Hashimoto's thyroiditis. It is reasonable to attempt to reduce the dosage of levothyroxine by 50% after approximately 3 months in patients who are suspected to have had transient hypothyroidism. If the TSH measured 6 weeks later rises, then the initial dosage is reinstated; if the TSH is stable, then T_4 can be withdrawn and the TSH checked again.

E. Central hypothyroidism should be suspected if the TSH is normal or low and the T_4 level is low. These patients should have their T_4 dose titrated to the level

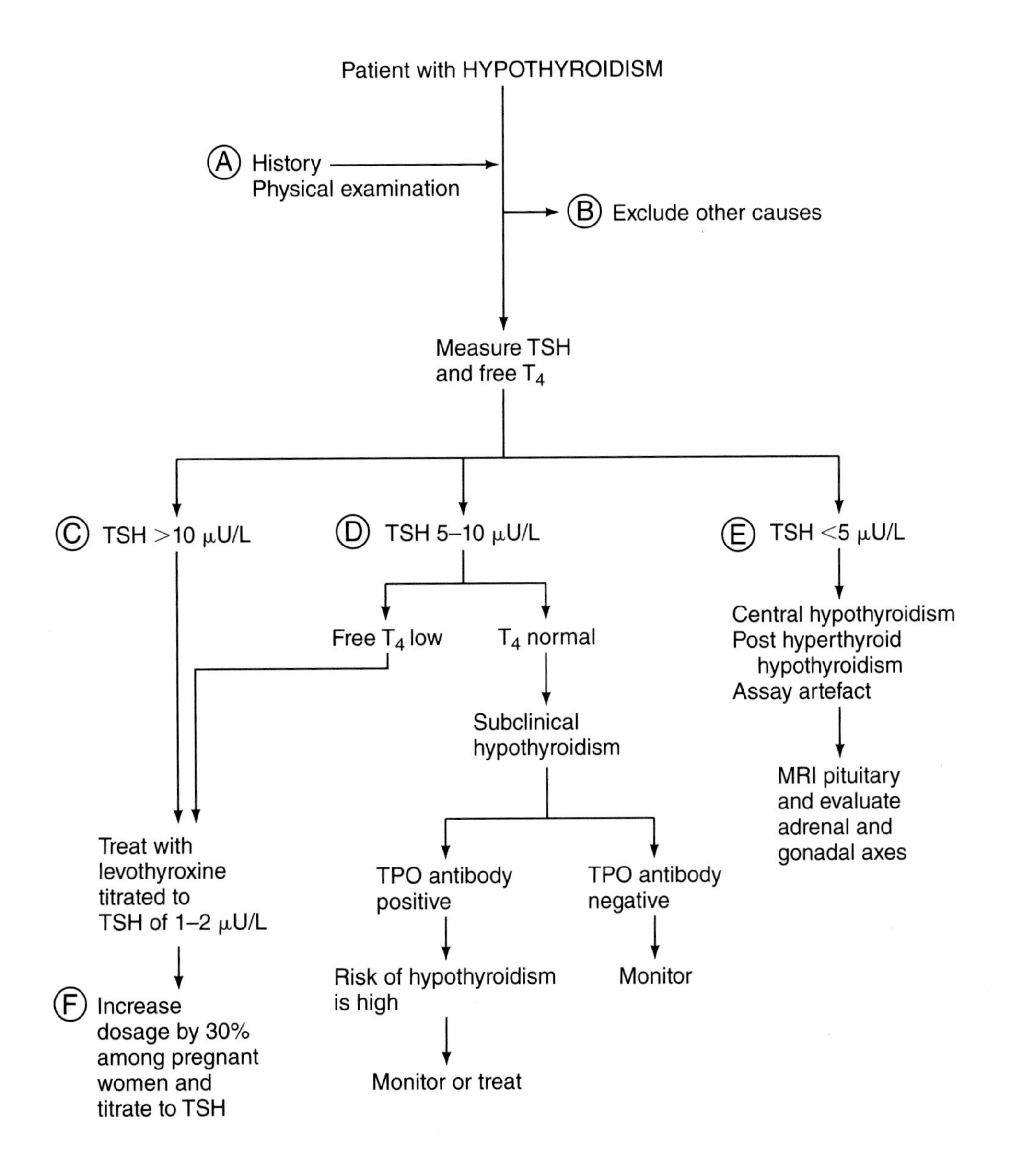

of free T_4. Patients receiving high-dose salicylates or phenytoin appear to have low TSH levels as a result of an assay artifact.

F. Levothyroxine requirements increase as early as the fifth week of gestation. Given the importance of maternal euthyroidism for normal fetal cognitive development, women with hypothyroidism should have their levothyroxine dosage increased by approximately 30% as soon as pregnancy is confirmed. Thereafter, serum thyrotropin levels should be monitored and the levothyroxine dosage should be adjusted accordingly.

References

Basaria S, Cooper DS. Amiodarone and the thyroid. Am J Med 2005;118(7):706–714.

Clarke N, Kabadi UM. Optimizing treatment of hypothyroidism. Treat Endocrinol 2004;3(4):217–221.

Cooper DS. Clinical practice. Subclinical hypothyroidism. N Engl J Med 2001;345(4):260–265.

Escobar-Morreale HF, Botella-Carretero JI, Escobar del Rey F, Morreale de Escobar G. Treatment of hypothyroidism with combinations of levothyroxine plus liothyronine. J Clin Endocrinol Metab 2005;90(8): 4946–4954.

Ibay AD, Bascelli LM, Nashelsky J. Management of subclinical hypothyroidism. Am Fam Physician 2005;71(9):1763–1764.

Pearce EN, Farwell AP, Braverman LE. Thyroiditis. N Engl J Med 2003;348(26):2646–2655.

HYPERTHYROIDISM

Graham T. McMahon, MD, MMSc

Hyperthyroidism can be caused by an increased production of thyroid hormone (as in Graves' disease or an autonomous nodule) or increased release of preformed thyroid hormone (as in thyroiditis). Hyperthyroidism can also be caused by overreplacement with exogenous thyroid hormone, ectopic hyperthyroidism, or unregulated stimulation of the thyroid-stimulating hormone (TSH) receptor (as in trophoblastic disease or a TSH-secreting pituitary adenoma).

A. The presentation of hyperthyroidism can range from asymptomatic to thyroid storm. In particular, the presentation in older patients can be highly variable. Characteristic symptoms include anxiety, tremor, palpitations, heat intolerance, insomnia, oligoamenorrhea, and weight loss despite an increased appetite. Typical signs include tachycardia, systolic hypertension, tremor, lid retraction, lid lag, warm skin, and hyperreflexia. The presence of a goiter will depend on the cause of the hyperthyroidism. A single palpable nodule or multiple nodules suggest an autonomous thyroid adenoma or a multinodular goiter as the source, respectively; a painful, tender thyroid gland suggests granulomatous thyroiditis. Signs that are suggestive of Graves' disease include goiter, thyroid bruit, exophthalmos, periorbital edema, and pretibial myxedema.

B. The diagnosis of hyperthyroidism is confirmed using biochemical testing of the thyroxine and TSH levels. An increased thyroxine level with a suppressed TSH level characterizes overt hyperthyroidism. Patients with subclinical hyperthyroidism may have a normal thyroxine level and a suppressed TSH level. Some patients demonstrate T_3 toxicosis with a normal thyroxine level and an elevated level of triiodothyronine. TSH-induced hyperthyroidism and thyroid hormone resistance, each characterized by an increased level of TSH, are very rare. An elevated thyroxine with a normal TSH level is usually attributed to abnormalities in thyroid-binding proteins in patients who are clinically euthyroid.

C. When the etiology of the hyperthyroidism is unclear, a thyroid radioiodine uptake study can be performed. Graves' disease is characterized by a high uptake; thyroiditis is characterized by a low uptake.

D. Propylthiouracil and methimazole are the antithyroid medications used in the United States. These agents are actively concentrated by the thyroid gland and their primary effect is to inhibit thyroid hormone synthesis by interfering with thyroid peroxidase–mediated iodination of tyrosine residues in thyroglobulin, a critical step in the synthesis of thyroxine and triiodothyronine. Propylthiouracil also blocks the conversion of thyroxine to triiodothyronine within the thyroid and peripheral tissues, although the clinical importance of this function is uncertain. No dosage adjustment is needed in patients with renal or liver failure or among children or the elderly.

The usual starting dosage of methimazole is 20 mg per day as a single daily dose, and the usual starting dosage of propylthiouracil is 100 mg given three times a day. Following initial dosing, follow-up testing of thyroid function is suggested for approximately every 6 weeks until the thyroid function tests normalize. Many patients can ultimately be controlled at a low dosage. Testing frequency can be reduced to every 6 months over time. Following a discussion about the risk of relapse, antithyroid drugs can be withdrawn after 12–18 months to determine whether ongoing treatment is required.

E. Cutaneous reactions to antithyroid drugs are not uncommon and are usually mild. The drug should be stopped in patients with arthralgias because this may be a presentation of a severe transient migratory polyarthritis associated with antithyroid drug use. Agranulocytosis, the most feared side effect, occurs in approximately 1 in 270 patients prescribed antithyroid medications. A baseline differential white cell count should be obtained before treatment is restarted, and retesting should be done if fever or sore throat develops. The medication should be discontinued if the granulocyte count is <1000 per cubic millimeter. Hepatotoxicity and vasculitis (drug-induced lupus) are rare but well described.

F. Current treatments for Graves' disease include antithyroid medications, radioiodine, and surgery. Initial treatment usually includes an antithyroid medication and a beta blocker for symptomatic relief. A typical starting combination would include methimazole 20 mg with atenolol 25 mg, both given once daily. For patients with more severe hyperthyroidism, iodine treatment can provide rapid relief of symptoms. A typical approach would be to prescribe 3 drops of saturated solution of potassium iodide 3 times daily for up to 10 days. Radioiodine can be given as primary treatment for patients with Graves' hyperthyroidism, although many clinicians will wait until the first relapse before offering this approach. Hyperthyroidism can be exacerbated for a short time by radioiodine treatment. In patients with cardiac disease or in the elderly, in whom such an exacerbation

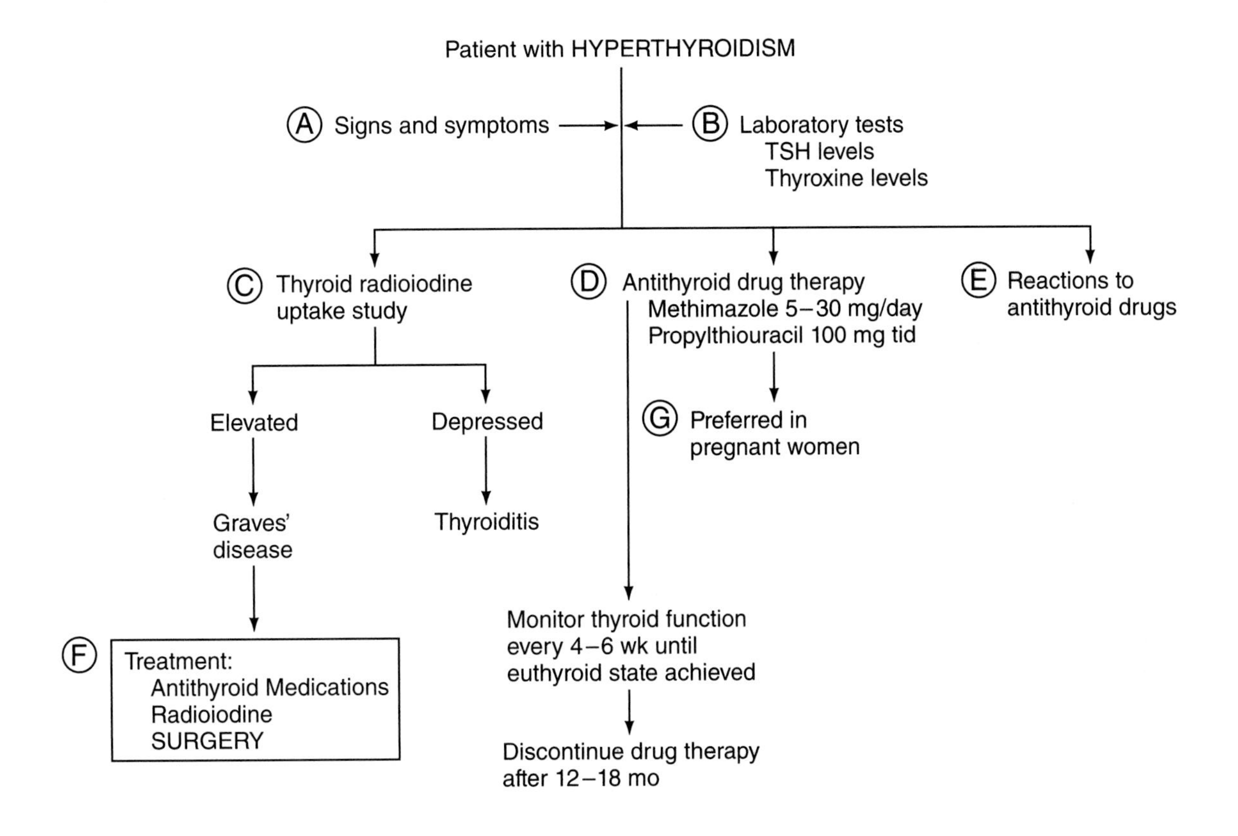

would be risky, pretreatment with antithyroid medications can be useful. Surgery is usually reserved for patients with an obstructing goiter.

Hyperthyroidism associated with a toxic thyroid adenoma can be treated with antithyroid medications and a beta blocker. Because these autonomous nodules do not resolve spontaneously, more definitive treatment is usually indicated after the initial symptoms have been controlled. Radioiodine is a preferred over surgery for most patients but is less likely to be effective in patients with large or multiple nodules.

G. Women who develop hyperthyroidism while pregnant are at increased risk of spontaneous abortion, premature labor, stillbirth, and preeclampsia. Changes in thyroid hormone–binding globulin (usually doubles), levels of human chorionic gonadotropin (that can mimic the actions of TSH), and endogenous physiology (altered TSH responsiveness) can complicate the biochemical assessment of thyroid function in pregnancy. Because radioiodine is absolutely contraindicated during pregnancy, antithyroid medications are the preferred treatment for pregnant women with hyperthyroidism. Propylthiouracil remains the preferred treatment for hyperthyroidism occurring during pregnancy. The dose should be minimized to prevent fetal hypothyroidism because the drug does cross the placenta. Methimazole may be associated with congenital anomalies, including aplasia cutis and choanal or esophageal atresia. Generally treatment is given to a point where mild hyperthyroidism is allowed to persist. Low thyroid function at birth is found in approximately half of neonates whose mothers received an antithyroid medication; ultimate intelligence has been demonstrated to be normal. Both methimazole and propylthiouracil are approved for nursing mothers by the American Academy of Pediatrics, although they do appear in breast milk in minute quantities.

References

Cooper DS. Drug therapy: antithyroid drugs. N Engl J Med 2005;352: 905–917.

Weetman AP. Graves' disease. N Engl J Med 2000;343:1236–1248.

GOITER

Erik K. Alexander, MD

Patients with goiters usually are euthyroid but can have significant hyperthyroidism or hypothyroidism, compressive symptoms of dysphagia or choking, and concerns about the appearance of the goiter. Common types of goiter include multinodular goiter (MNG) and those associated with hypothyroidism (Hashimoto's thyroiditis) or hyperthyroidism (Graves' disease). Less commonly, goiters are produced by consumption of goitrogens. Lithium commonly induces a modest goiter. Rarer goitrogens include kelp, the antithyroidal medications propylthiouracil and methimazole, and cassava root, rutabaga, and turnips in association with an iodine-deficient diet. Excess iodine, including iodine-containing medications (amiodarone), occasionally can cause significant goiters. Iodine treatment during pregnancy has been associated with goiter in newborns. Endemic goiter has essentially disappeared in the United States because of adequate iodine intake, but about 200 million people around the world have it. Rarely, thyroid cancer or metastasis from other malignancies can cause a goiter through nodule growth.

A. Physical examination of the thyroid starts with careful visual inspection while the patient is swallowing. Often the outline of the entire goiter can be seen because the thyroid gland moves with swallowing. Next, palpate the entire gland during repeated swallows to characterize the goiter as diffuse or nodular, and identify any dominant nodules. Nodules longer than 1 cm should have a fine needle aspiration (see the chapter Thyroid Nodule). If the inferior border of the goiter is not easily palpable, try palpation with the patient supine and the neck moderately extended. If the inferior border is still not palpable, the patient may have a substernal goiter.

B. Measure serum concentrations of thyroid-stimulating hormone (TSH) and free thyroxine (FT_4). If the TSH is completely suppressed ("undetectable"), the patient is hyperthyroid. If the TSH is >10 μU/ml, the patient is hypothyroid. If the TSH is normal, the patient typically is euthyroid. If the TSH is mildly but not completely suppressed, the thyroid gland is producing a slight excess of thyroid hormone. This typically occurs in patients with MNGs that develop autonomously functioning nodules and cause subclinical hyperthyroidism. Some of these patients may develop frank hyperthyroidism, but most remain with goiters that are autonomously functioning. All such patients should be treated.

C. Hypothyroidism with goiter usually is caused by the autoimmune disease lymphocytic (or Hashimoto's) thyroiditis. Autoantibodies destroy parts of the thyroid. The goiters typically are modest in size, 2–3 times normal, and slightly nodular (bosselated) and firmer than normal thyroid tissue because there are areas of fibrosis, inflammation, and active follicles. Treat with T_4 replacement.

D. Euthyroid patients with goiters usually are older adults with MNG. One theory on the formation of MNG (simple or nonimmunologic goiters) is that there is underproduction of thyroid hormone with a compensatory increase in TSH that stimulates goiter formation. Therefore a common, but now not commonly accepted, therapy is T_4 suppression to remove the TSH stimulation. However, T_4 therapy in older adults must be administered cautiously, starting at a low dosage, perhaps 0.05 mg/day, and keeping TSH within the normal range while increasing the dosage. MNG can slowly develop autonomous functioning nodules that produce enough hormone to cause hyperthyroidism in combination with exogenous T_4. Therefore patients should be aware of the symptoms of hyperthyroidism and have TSH monitored at least every year after achieving a steady dose of T_4. Substernal and large goiters may respond to radioactive ^{131}I, so surgical treatment for goiter rarely is necessary. Large substernal goiters can cause superior venocaval syndrome, and some patients have signs of obstruction if they raise their arms above their head (Pemberton's sign). Occasionally surgery is done because of a patient's concern about appearance, or persistent obstructive symptoms.

E. Hyperthyroid patients with diffuse goiters usually have autoimmune Graves' disease. Thyroid-stimulating antibodies typically cause a diffuse enlargement of the entire gland. A unilateral asymmetric goiter associated with hyperthyroidism can occur in patients with a large functioning adenoma (Plummer's disease). Treatment of hyperthyroidism usually decreases the size of these goiters (see section on Hyperthyroidism).

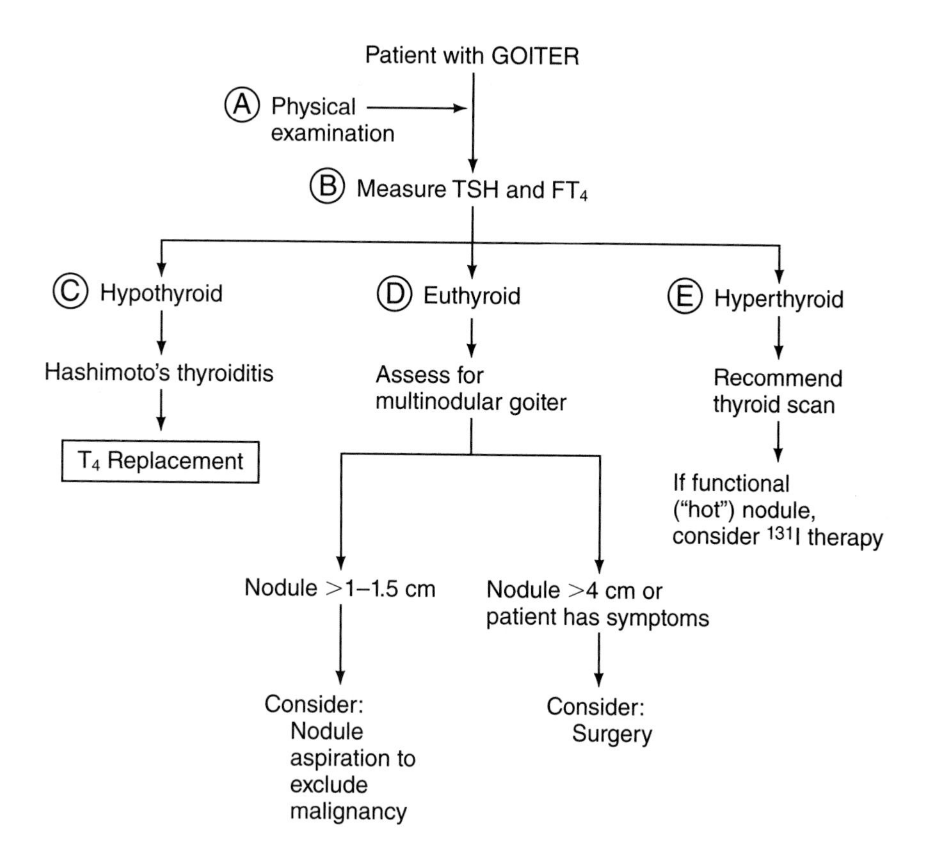
Patient with GOITER
(A) Physical examination
(B) Measure TSH and FT4
(C) Hypothyroid
Hashimoto's thyroiditis
T4 Replacement
(D) Euthyroid
Assess for multinodular goiter
Nodule >1–1.5 cm
Consider: Nodule aspiration to exclude malignancy
Nodule >4 cm or patient has symptoms
Consider: Surgery
(E) Hyperthyroid
Recommend thyroid scan
If functional ("hot") nodule, consider 131I therapy

THYROID NODULE

Graham T. McMahon, MD, MMSc

In the United States, between 4% and 7% of the adult population have a palpable thyroid nodule. Only 5% of these are malignant. Other causes of nodules include thyroid cyst, a colloid nodule, a focal area of thyroiditis, and a benign follicular neoplasm. Nodules can be solitary or multiple. The risk of cancer is not lower when nodules are multiple.

A. A thyroid-stimulating hormone (TSH) test is performed. A suppressed TSH level suggests a benign hyperfunctioning nodule. Hyperfunctioning nodules are so rarely malignant that if the TSH is suppressed, fine needle aspiration (FNA) can be deferred. A normal or high TSH level does not obviate the need for further investigation.

B. Perform clinical evaluation. High-risk features include rapid tumor growth, regional lymphadenopathy, a firm or hard nodule, and a family history of thyroid carcinoma or multiple endocrine neoplasia. Risk increases more moderately with the following features: age younger than 20 years or older than 70 years; male gender; a history of head and neck irradiation; a nodule >4 cm; or the presence of local symptoms such as dysphagia, hoarseness, or cough. Patients with at least two high-risk features should be referred for surgical management.

C. FNA with ultrasonography can be performed in the office and increases the sensitivity and specificity of the FNA result (Marqusee, 2000). Ultrasonography can detect high-risk features such as hypoechogenicity, microcalcifications, irregular margins, increased vascularity by Doppler, and evidence of local lymphadenopathy.

   Patients undergoing FNA do not typically need to stop taking aspirin or anticoagulants. The procedure is safe and well tolerated. Each lesion >1 cm in size should be sampled with two to four passes of the needle.

   Cystic nodules can be drained after any solid portion is aspirated, although most recur; use of sclerosants such as ethanol and tetracycline has been disappointing.

D. Radionucleotide scanning uses iodine-123, iodine-131, or technetium-99m-pertechnetate to detect whether a nodule is functioning. A scan can also determine whether a nodule is dominant within a multinodular gland or retrosternal. A scan cannot accurately determine the size of a thyroid nodule.

E. Benign nodules can remain in situ. Repeat ultrasonography after 9–12 months to ensure that there has been no significant change in size is suggested. Levothyroxine suppression is no longer recommended because TSH must be suppressed to <0.1 mU/L to effectively suppress nodular growth or formation and suppression to this level is associated with an increased risk of bone loss and atrial fibrillation.

F. Follicular neoplasm may be benign or malignant because cellular aspirates cannot distinguish these two. If the patient prefers, or if the nodule is cold on radionucleotide scanning, then excision is recommended.

G. Malignant nodules should be excised with a total thyroidectomy and usually require postoperative thyroid ablation with iodine-131. Disease recurrence can be screened for using thyroglobulin measurements.

H. Nondiagnostic aspirates occur about 10% of the time. If a second sample is again nondiagnostic, then referral for surgical excision is appropriate.

References

Castro MR, Gharib H. Continuing controversies in the management of thyroid nodules. Ann Intern Med 2005;142(11):926–931.

Hegedus L. Clinical practice. The thyroid nodule. N Engl J Med 2004;351(17):1764–1771.

Marqusee E, Benson CB, Frates MC, et al. Usefulness of ultrasonography in management of nodular thyroid disease. Ann Intern Med 2000;133(9):696-700.

Silver RJ, Parangi S. Management of thyroid incidentalomas. Surg Clin North Am 2004;84(3):907–919. Review.

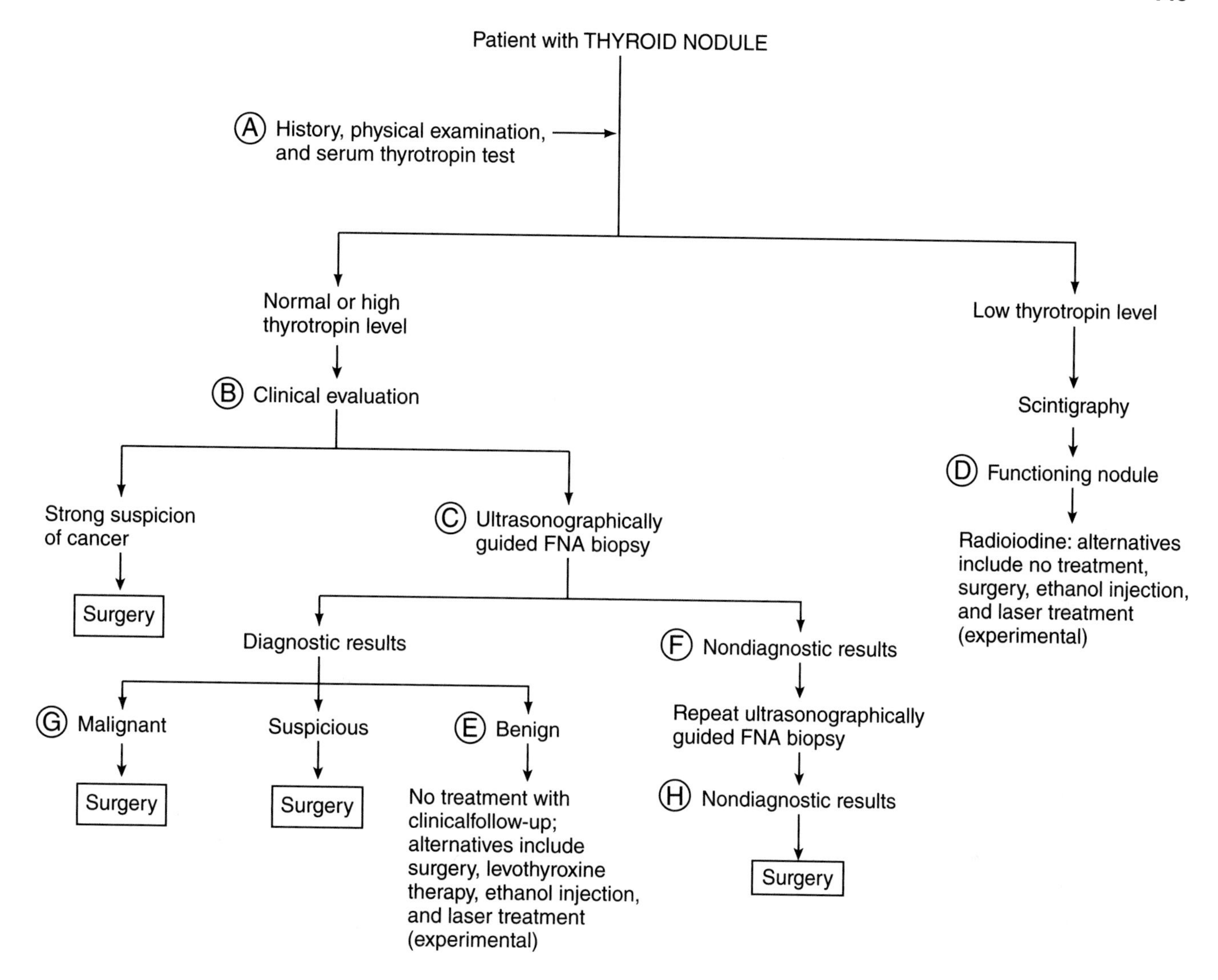
Patient with THYROID NODULE
A History, physical examination, and serum thyrotropin test
Normal or high thyrotropin level
B Clinical evaluation
Strong suspicion of cancer
Surgery
C Ultrasonographically guided FNA biopsy
Diagnostic results
G Malignant
Surgery
Suspicious
Surgery
E Benign
No treatment with clinicalfollow-up; alternatives include surgery, levothyroxine therapy, ethanol injection, and laser treatment (experimental)
F Nondiagnostic results
Repeat ultrasonographically guided FNA biopsy
H Nondiagnostic results
Surgery
Low thyrotropin level
Scintigraphy
D Functioning nodule
Radioiodine: alternatives include no treatment, surgery, ethanol injection, and laser treatment (experimental)

THYROID PAIN

Emily Deborah Szmuilowicz, MD

The four main causes of thyroid pain are painful subacute thyroiditis (PST), hemorrhage into a nodule, acute infectious thyroiditis (AIT), and radiation thyroiditis (RT). Extremely rare causes (including Hashimoto's thyroiditis, rapidly enlarging thyroid carcinoma, and palpation- or trauma-induced thyroiditis) are not discussed here.

A. PST (also known as de Quervain's thyroiditis and subacute granulomatous thyroiditis) is a self-limited inflammatory disorder. PST typically follows an upper respiratory tract infection. The pain is usually but not always bilateral. The onset of pain may be sudden or gradual, and it often radiates to the ear, jaw, or throat. Associated symptoms may include fever, myalgias, malaise, sore throat, and dysphagia. Hyperthyroidism is usually present at the time of diagnosis as a result of unregulated release of thyroid hormone from the inflamed thyroid follicles, but the dominant symptoms are thyroid pain and tenderness. Pain and hyperthyroidism typically last 2–6 weeks, followed by euthyroidism, and then transient hypothyroidism in up to half of patients (or, rarely, permanent hypothyroidism). Physical examination reveals a firm, tender, moderately enlarged thyroid. Ultrasonography (which need not be performed if the history and physical examination strongly suggest the diagnosis) reveals an enlarged and hypoechoic thyroid.

B. Hemorrhage into a nodule most commonly presents with sudden onset of unilateral neck pain associated with an increase in size of a preexisting nodule. Ultrasonography reveals a fluid-filled nodule. Thyroid function test results are usually normal.

C. AIT results from bacterial (most common), fungal, mycobacterial, or parasitic infection of the thyroid. Risk factors include immunosuppression, preexisting thyroid disorders, and pyriform sinus fistulas to the thyroid. Patients are typically acutely ill, with sudden onset of severe unilateral or bilateral thyroid pain and tenderness (which may radiate to the ipsilateral ear or jaw), fever, chills, dysphagia, and dysphonia. Thyroid function tests are usually normal. Ultrasonography reveals single or multiple discrete abscesses.

D. RT occurs rarely after radioactive iodine treatment of hyperthyroidism and even more rarely after radioactive iodine remnant ablation in thyroid cancer. Pain typically starts 5–10 days after treatment and resolves within a few weeks. RT may cause hyperthyroidism as a result of unregulated release of thyroid hormone from the inflamed thyroid follicular cells.

E. Typical findings early in the course of PST include elevations in ESR and serum C-reactive protein (CRP), increased or normal WBC count, and low (<5%) radioactive iodine uptake (RAIU).

F. Fine needle aspiration biopsy (FNAB) of a hemorrhagic nodule reveals bloody fluid containing few (if any) thyroid cells. Any solid component of the nodule should be biopsied.

G. ESR, serum CRP, and WBC count are typically elevated in AIT, as in PST. In contrast to PST, overall RAIU is usually normal (and abscesses appear hypofunctioning on thyroid scans). Samples obtained by FNAB for cytology, Gram stain, and culture are diagnostic. Neck imaging should be performed to evaluate for fistulas.

H. NSAIDs are usually given for pain relief, and oral glucocorticoids are given when NSAIDs are inadequate or contraindicated (prednisone 40 mg daily or equivalent for 1 week, followed by a taper over 2–6 weeks; the glucocorticoid can be increased and tapered more slowly if pain recurs during withdrawal). If pain is not relieved by NSAIDs, the diagnosis of PST should be questioned. Symptoms of hyperthyroidism can be treated with a beta blocker. Antithyroid drugs are not used because there is no excess thyroid hormone production.

I. Contents of the nodule should be aspirated. If hemorrhage recurs, surgical excision can be considered.

J. Treatment of AIT involves abscess drainage and targeted parenteral antibiotic therapy. Any predisposing fistulas must be corrected surgically to prevent recurrence.

K. As in PST, NSAIDs or oral glucocorticoids are given for pain relief, and a beta blocker can be given for symptoms of hyperthyroidism.

References

Farwell AP. Subacute thyroiditis and acute infectious thyroiditis. In Werner SC, Ingbar SH, Braverman LE, et al, eds. Werner & Ingbar's the Thyroid: A Fundamental and Clinical Text, 9th ed. Philadelphia: Lippincott Williams & Wilkins, 2005:536–547.

Pearce EN, Farwell AP, Braverman LE. Thyroiditis. N Engl J Med 2003;348(26):2646–2655.

The painful thyroid. Lancet 1986;1(8493):1308–1309.

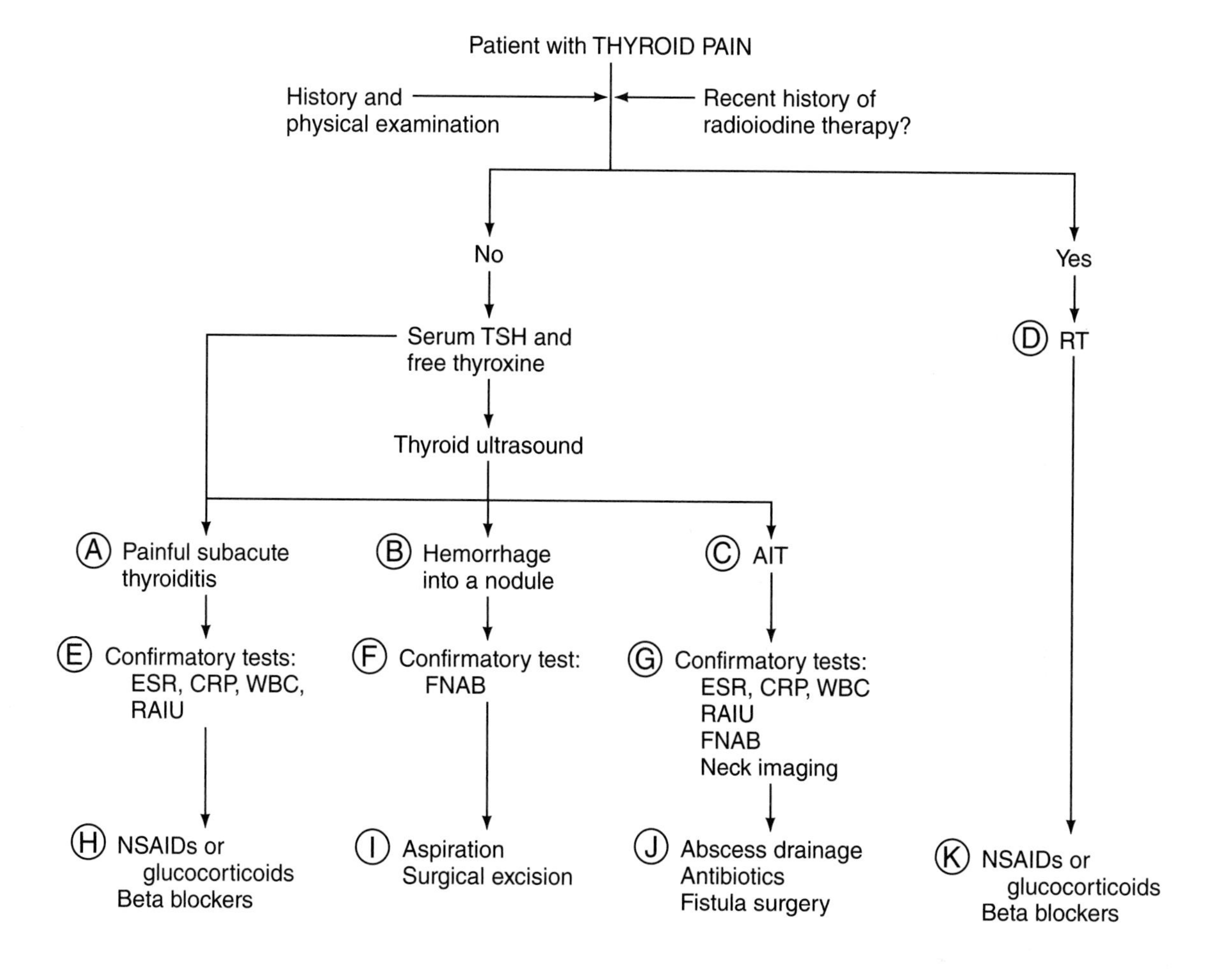
Patient with THYROID PAIN
History and physical examination
Recent history of radioiodine therapy?
No
Yes
Serum TSH and free thyroxine
Thyroid ultrasound
(D) RT
(A) Painful subacute thyroiditis
(B) Hemorrhage into a nodule
(C) AIT
(E) Confirmatory tests: ESR, CRP, WBC, RAIU
(F) Confirmatory test: FNAB
(G) Confirmatory tests: ESR, CRP, WBC
RAIU
FNAB
Neck imaging
(H) NSAIDs or glucocorticoids
Beta blockers
(I) Aspiration
Surgical excision
(J) Abscess drainage
Antibiotics
Fistula surgery
(K) NSAIDs or glucocorticoids
Beta blockers

SICK EUTHYROID SYNDROME

Graham T. McMahon, MD, MMSc

Changes in the function of the hypothalamic-pituitary-thyroid axis and in thyroid hormone transport and metabolism are common in patients with nonthyroidal illness. The magnitude of these changes usually correlates with the severity of the illness. Changes include reduced activity of the hypothalamic-pituitary axis and reduced extrathyroidal production of triiodothyronine (T_3).

A. The earliest physiologic change in thyroid function that occurs during illness is a decreased concentration of free T_3. Low free T_3 levels result from decreased concentrations of 5-monodeiodinase, the enzyme that catalyzes the conversion of thyroxine (T_4) to T_3. High concentrations of cortisol and free fatty acids, present during illness, inhibit the activity of this enzyme. Changes in the activity of the 5-monodeiodinase also result in higher levels of reverse T_3, which is used in research studies to help distinguish nonthyroidal illness from true central hypothyroidism. High reverse T_3 levels correlate with increased mortality in severe nonthyroidal illness.

B. Thyrotropin (or thyroid-stimulating hormone [TSH]) levels also may be normal to low. Low TSH occurs in patients with the most severe nonthyroidal illness. Although most of these patients have TSH levels at the low end of normal, TSH may be undetectable in some. This may be followed by low free T_4 and TSH concentrations, resulting in transient central hypothyroidism. The central and peripheral changes can occur independently of each other. Together these changes result in a reduction of the level of T_3 that is speculated to represent a beneficial adaptation to illness, conserving energy and limiting tissue catabolism.

The finding of very low TSH and low total T_4 and T_3 levels suggests altered pituitary or hypothalamic responsiveness to circulating thyroid hormone levels. TSH levels may also be low among patients treated with dopamine or corticosteroids. During the recovery period, TSH levels return to normal or may even increase transiently before returning to normal.

TSH levels can be mildly to moderately elevated during nonthyroidal illness, particularly during the recovery phase. In combination with very low serum free T_4 values, an elevated TSH level suggests primary hypothyroidism, as does finding an enlarged thyroid gland.

Normal changes in thyroid hormones that are common during illness must be distinguished from those resulting from thyroid disease, which are appropriately sought in patients for other reasons. Secondary (central) hypothyroidism can mimic the changes of nonthyroidal illness, but it is very rare. Additionally, an elevated TSH, particularly when $>20\ \mu U/ml$, may be considered indicative of underlying primary hypothyroidism unless the patient is in the recovery phase of his or her illness.

C. The diagnosis of secondary hypothyroidism during severe illness is challenging. In patients with severe illness, TSH and total T_4 and T_3 values are usually low. These patients are often given medications that inhibit TSH, such as dopamine and glucocorticoids. If the levels are very low, pituitary dysfunction should be considered more strongly and repletion with corticosteroid and thyroid hormone supplements may be indicated. Additional tests, including measurement of cortisol, gonadotropin, and prolactin levels, may clarify the cause of unusually low thyroid tests. If the cortisol and prolactin levels are high, as would be expected in stressful situations, no intervention is needed. T_3, T_4, and TSH levels should be tested again when the illness is resolved or improved.

D. Although severe nonthyroidal illness may become maladaptive, the limited data available suggest that administration of thyroid hormone to patients with nonthyroidal illness does not improve the outcome of their illness. In studies where supraphysiologic doses of T_3 were given for 1 day following bypass surgery, the cardiac index was slightly higher and systemic vascular resistance was slightly lower in patients given T_3 as compared with patients given a placebo; however, neither morbidity nor mortality differed between groups. Patients with primary hypothyroidism or very low thyroid hormone levels may benefit from replacement. However, evidence does not support the routine treatment of patients suspected to have sick euthyroidism with thyroid hormone.

References

Camacho PM, Dwarkanathan AA. Sick euthyroid syndrome. What to do when thyroid function tests are abnormal in critically ill patients. Postgrad Med 1999;105(4):215–219.

Chopra IJ. Euthyroid sick syndrome: is it a misnomer? J Clin Endocrinol Metab 1997;82:329.

Stathatos N, Wartofsky L. Perioperative management of patients with hypothyroidism. Endocrinol Metab Clin North Am 2003;32(2):503–518.

Utiger RD. Altered thyroid function in nonthyroidal illness and surgery—to treat or not to treat? N Engl J Med 1995;333:1562–1563.

Wartofsky L, Burman KD, Ringel MD. Trading one "dangerous dogma" for another? Thyroid hormone treatment of the "euthyroid sick syndrome." J Clin Endocrinol Metab 1999;84:1759–1760.

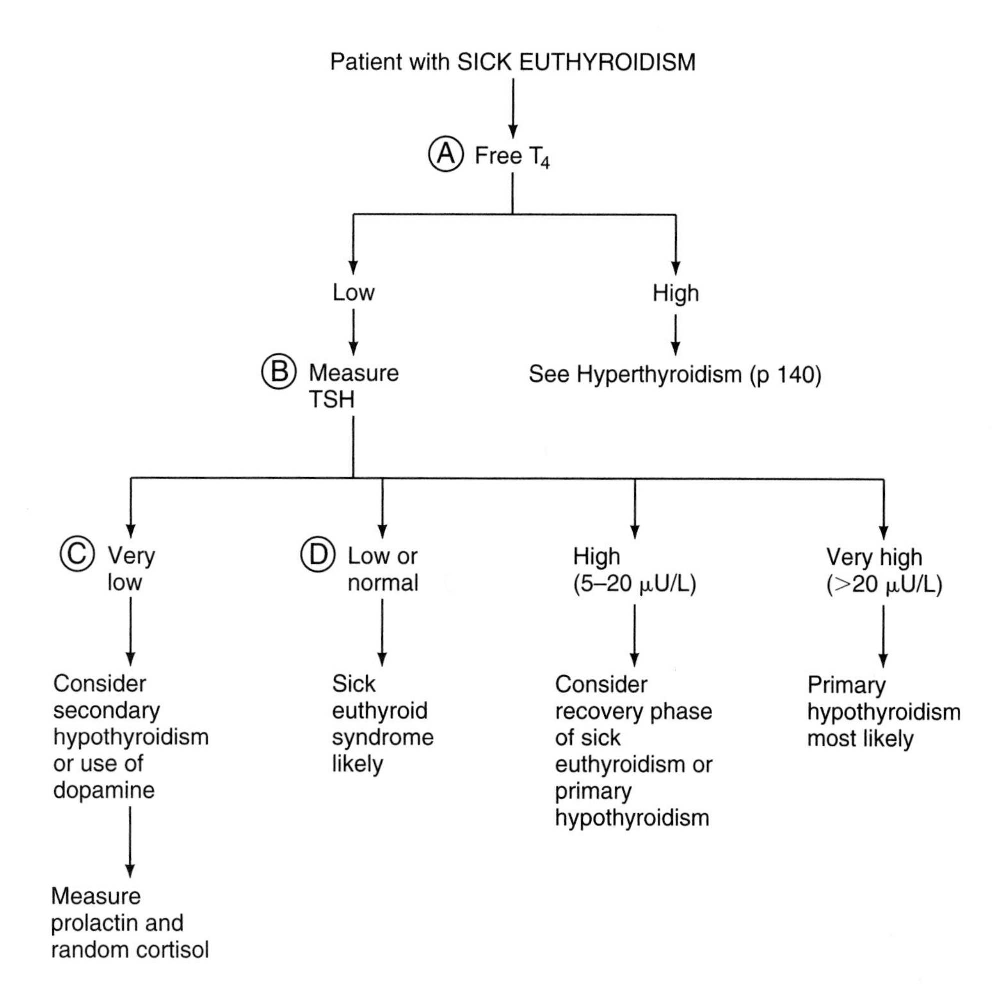
Patient with SICK EUTHYROIDISM
(A) Free T_4
Low
High
(B) Measure TSH
See Hyperthyroidism (p 140)
(C) Very low
(D) Low or normal
High (5–20 μU/L)
Very high (>20 μU/L)
Consider secondary hypothyroidism or use of dopamine
Sick euthyroid syndrome likely
Consider recovery phase of sick euthyroidism or primary hypothyroidism
Primary hypothyroidism most likely
Measure prolactin and random cortisol

THYROID FUNCTION TESTS IN NONTHYROIDAL ILLNESS

Erik K. Alexander, MD

In hospitalized patients the incidence of true hypothyroidism or hyperthyroidism is <1%. Clinical signs of thyroid disease may be masked in acutely ill patients. Conversely, some signs of severe illness mimic changes seen in thyroid diseases. Serum triiodothyronine (T_3) radioimmunoassay (RIA) usually is decreased in patients with acute illness. The thyroid-stimulating hormone (TSH) response to thyrotropin-releasing hormone (TRH) also usually is normal. It may be difficult to identify acutely ill patients with hypothalamic or pituitary disease. A sensitive TSH (sTSH) >10 μU/ml and low free thyroxine (T_4) (FT_4) are good evidence for primary thyroid failure.

A. The TSH and free thyroxine index (FTI) are the preferred tests for assessing the thyroxine level in this setting.

B. Up to 50% of acutely ill patients have a decrease in total T_4 and/or T_3. Both FT_4 and sTSH usually are normal, although they can be suppressed. The more severe the illness, the more likely TSH and FTI suppression will be noted.

In the setting of acute illness, repeating thyroid function tests is very useful every 7–10 days. Thyroid test abnormalities will improve in parallel with the patient's improving condition. The converse is true as well.

Numerous studies have documented that levothyroxine therapy does not improve the outcome of patient's with thyroid function abnormalities attributable to nonthyroidal illness.

C. Patients with nephrotic syndrome may have mildly depressed FT_4 and normal sTSH. Glucocorticoids in stress doses acutely inhibit TSH secretion, and a small decrement in both sTSH and FT_4 may be observed. Dopamine infusions also cause acute suppression of TSH. In a truly hypothyroid patient receiving a dopamine infusion and/or stress doses of glucocorticoids, the TSH may be suppressed into the normal range.

D. Elevation of sTSH with normal FT_4 is found in patients recovering from a nonthyroidal illness. sTSH usually is <20 μU/ml. Slight elevations of TSH commonly are found in patients with chronic renal failure. Although the pathophysiology is unknown, these patients have a blunted TSH response to TRH.

References

Burmeister LA. Reverse T_3 does not reliably differentiate hypothyroid sick syndrome from euthyroid sick syndrome. Thyroid 1995;5:435.

Cavaliere RR. The effects of nonthyroid disease and drugs on thyroid function tests. Med Clin North Am 1991;75:27.

Docter R, Krenning EP, dejong M, Henneman G. The sick euthyroid syndrome: changes in thyroid hormone serum parameters and hormone metabolism (review). Clin Endocrinol 1993;39:499.

Faber J, Kirkegaena C, Rasmassen B, et al. Pituitary-thyroid axis in critical illness. J Clin Endocrinol Metab 1987;65:315.

Lim S, Fang V, Katz A, et al. Thyroid dysfunction in chronic renal failure: a study of the pituitary-thyroid axis and peripheral turnover kinetics of thyroxine and triiodothyronine. J Clin Invest 1977;60:522.

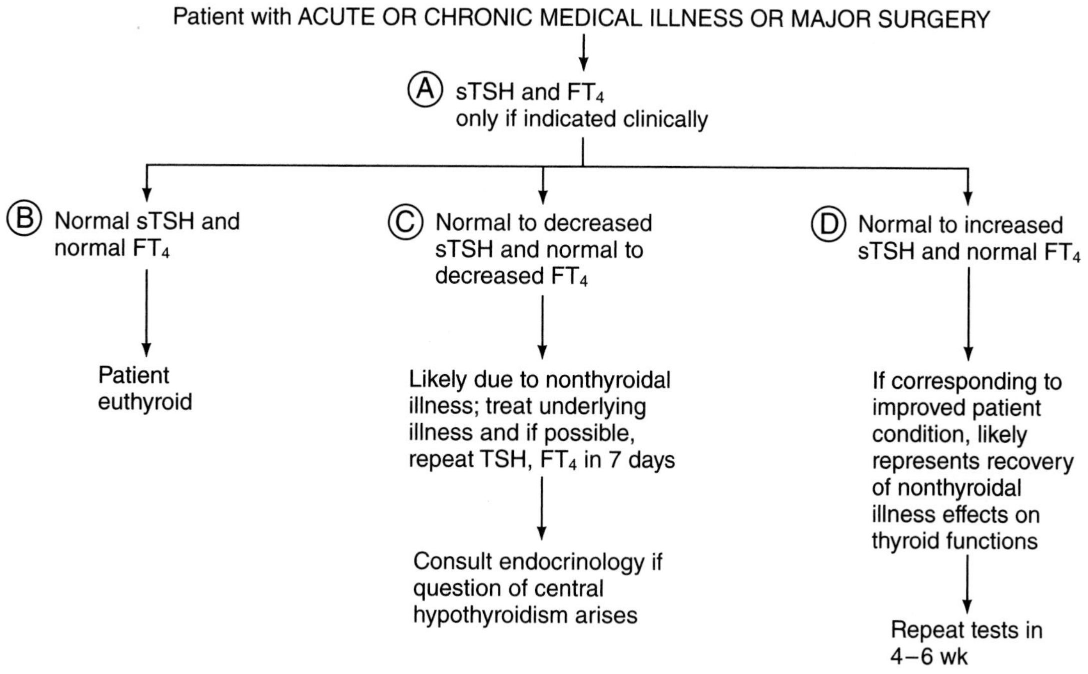

Patient with ACUTE OR CHRONIC MEDICAL ILLNESS OR MAJOR SURGERY

(A) sTSH and FT_4 only if indicated clinically

(B) Normal sTSH and normal FT_4

Patient euthyroid

(C) Normal to decreased sTSH and normal to decreased FT_4

Likely due to nonthyroidal illness; treat underlying illness and if possible, repeat TSH, FT_4 in 7 days

Consult endocrinology if question of central hypothyroidism arises

(D) Normal to increased sTSH and normal FT_4

If corresponding to improved patient condition, likely represents recovery of nonthyroidal illness effects on thyroid functions

Repeat tests in 4–6 wk

ADRENAL INCIDENTALOMA

Graham T. McMahon, MD, MMSc

Adrenal masses are detected in approximately 3% of all abdominal CT scans and in approximately 10% of all autopsies. The discovery of an adrenal mass raises two questions: Is it malignant, and is it functioning?

A. Imaging features can help to determine the malignancy risk. High-risk features include irregular shape, diameter >4 cm, high CT attenuation value (>10 Hounsfield units [HU]), and inhomogeneous enhancement after IV contrast. Metastatic disease from another source tends to cause bilateral disease and have a similar attenuation as the liver on T1 imaging and a high T2-signal intensity.

B. Benign nodules (that may be functional) tend to be round, homogenous, and smaller (<4 cm), with low CT attenuation (<10 HU), and are isointense with the liver on T1- and T2-weighted MRI.

   Adrenal cysts, myelolipoma, and adrenal hemorrhage are usually readily distinguishable by their unique imaging characteristics.

   The adrenal cortex can produce a variety of hormones and syndromes, including cortisol (Cushing's syndrome), aldosterone (Conn's syndrome), androgens (virilization), and estrogens (feminization); the adrenal medulla generates catecholamines (pheochromocytoma).

C. Pheochromocytoma can be suggested by the presence of hypertension (can be chronic or paroxysmal), a history of "spells," headache, palpitations, or pallor. Even in the absence of any symptoms, pheochromocytoma should always be excluded before proceeding to surgery because intraoperative risks of an unrecognized pheochromocytoma are high. Serum metanephrines are specific and sensitive, provided that the patient has not consumed acetaminophen in the prior 72 hours. Two consecutive 24-hour urinary collections for total metanephrines and catecholamines provide confirmatory evidence.

D. Cushing's syndrome can be suggested by the presence of truncal obesity, violaceous striae, proximal muscle weakness, hypertension, and insomnia. An 8-AM cortisol level should be <5 μg/dl after a midnight dose of 1 mg of dexamethasone. Two consecutive cortisol measurements more than three times the upper limit of normal in a 24-hour urinary collection with a creatinine of at least 1 g provide confirmatory evidence.

E. Primary aldosteronism is suggested by refractory hypertension and occasionally hypokalemia. An aldosterone-to-renin ratio >30 when the aldosterone is at least 10 ng/dl is suggestive. To obtain an interpretable result, patients must not be taking aldosterone-receptor antagonists (such as spironolactone or eplerenone) or beta blockers. A suppressed renin in a patient taking an angiotensin-converting enzyme inhibitor or angiotensin-receptor blocker is highly suggestive of hyperaldosteronism.

F. Measures of androgens and estrogens are not routinely performed in the absence of suggestive symptoms or signs. Virilization in women is suggested by male-pattern baldness, deepening of the voice, and clitoromegaly. Feminization in men is suggested by gynecomastia, decreased libido, and loss of muscle strength.

References

Kievit J, Haak HR. Diagnosis and treatment of adrenal incidentaloma. A cost-effectiveness analysis. Endocrinol Metab Clin North Am 2000;29(1):69–90.

Munver R, Fromer DL, Watson RA, Sawczuk IS. Evaluation of the incidentally discovered adrenal mass. Curr Urol Rep 2004;5(1):73–77.

NIH state-of-the-science statement on management of the clinically inapparent adrenal mass ("incidentaloma"). NIH Consens State Sci Statements 2002;19(2):1–25.

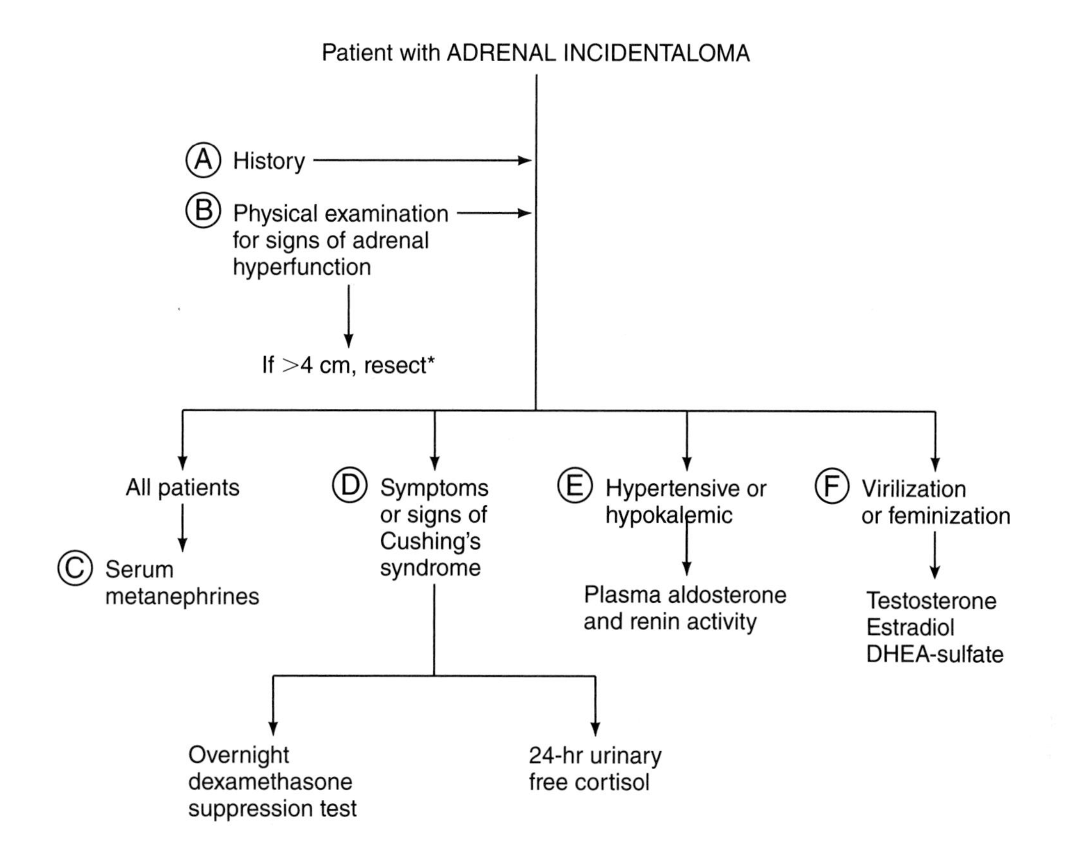

*Always exclude pheochromocytoma before operative intervention.

CUSHING'S SYNDROME

Graham T. McMahon, MD, MMSc

Cushing's syndrome is characterized by hypercortisolemia that can be adrenal in origin or can result from a pituitary adenoma secreting adrenocorticotropin. The clinical features are diverse and are related to the severity of the hypercortisolemia; no symptom or sign is specific. The most common presenting feature is obesity of the face, neck, and abdomen that spares the extremities. Facial fat deposition can result in a "moon" face exacerbated by deposition of fat in the supraclavicular fat pads, which makes the neck appear shortened. These patients develop skin thinning, atrophy, and easy bruising. Striae typical of Cushing's syndrome are typically purple in color, wide, and multiple, factors that help distinguish them from stretch marks associated with obesity. Women with Cushing's disease may have signs of hyperandrogenism such as hirsutism. Proximal myopathy (usually described as difficulty rising from a seated position), psychiatric change (emotional lability, depression, and mild paranoia are common), and hypertension are often at present. Other features associated with longer-standing or more severe hypercortisolemia include glucose intolerance, glaucoma, and osteopenia.

A. The first step in evaluating whether a patient may have Cushing's syndrome is to elucidate any history of exposure to corticosteroids, including potent inhaled, injected, or topical steroids, or medroxyprogesterone acetate (a progestin with intrinsic steroid activity). Factitious Cushing's syndrome accounts for <1% of all cases and is suggested by erratic and inconsistent results. In such cases, synthetic glucocorticoids can be assayed directly in the urine.

B. To establish hypercortisolemia, at least two 24-hour urine samples for free cortisol should be obtained. Patients whose levels are greater than three times higher than the upper reference range can be assumed to have Cushing's syndrome. Patients with equivocal values should be retested after a few weeks or evaluated with further testing according to the clinical suspicion.

C. An overnight dexamethasone suppression test is also used as a screening test to diagnose hypercortisolemia. In this test, an 8-AM serum cortisol level is drawn after a 1-mg dexamethasone dose at 11 PM–midnight. The sensitivity and specificity of the test for Cushing's syndrome varies widely depending on the threshold level chosen. Most normal patients should suppress their endogenous cortisol level to <2 μg/dl. Using a level of 6.3 μg/dl, the test has a sensitivity and a specificity of 91%. For a level of 1.2 μg/dl, the corresponding values were 100% and 41%.

A screening strategy that uses three consecutive late-evening salivary cortisols and may ultimately replace these aforementioned tests can be performed with minimal instruction by a patient who is ambulatory. Reference ranges are laboratory specific. The sensitivity may be as high as 100% and the specificity may be as high as 96% among patients with Cushing's syndrome.

D. Some conditions, such as severe obesity, severe depression, or chronic alcoholism, are associated with elevated cortisol levels, a circumstance labeled "pseudo-Cushing's." Among patients in whom a diagnosis of pseudo-Cushing's is suspected, a corticotropin-releasing hormone (CRH)–dexamethasone test can be preformed. This test capitalizes on the finding that the pituitary is less responsive to CRH among patients who are depressed than among patients with Cushing's disease or syndrome after dexamethasone suppression. Ovine CRH is usually infused 2 hours after the last dose of a series of 8 doses of 0.5 mg dexamethasone given every 6 hours. Serum cortisol is measured at 0, 15, and 30 minutes. In one series, all patients with a level <1.4 μg/dl in the 15-minute sample had pseudo-Cushing's; all other patients responded with higher cortisol levels.

Once the diagnosis of Cushing's syndrome is secure, a source for the hypercortisolemia should be sought. Determining whether Cushing's syndrome is adrenocorticotropic hormone (ACTH) dependent or adrenal in origin requires accurate measurement of ACTH levels. It is possible to expedite the evaluation process by measuring ACTH and cortisol levels on the morning following a dexamethasone-suppression test or on completion of one or more collections for urinary-free cortisol.

E. Cortisol secretion can be deemed ACTH independent if the ACTH is <5 pg/ml when the cortisol level is <15 μg/dl. Under the same circumstances, the syndrome is very likely to be ACTH dependent (Cushing's disease) if the ACTH level is >15 pg/ml when the cortisol is ≥15 μg/dl; ACTH levels of between 5 and 15 pg/ml are less specific but usually indicate ACTH dependency. Patients with equivocal values should be reinvestigated.

(Continued on page 156)

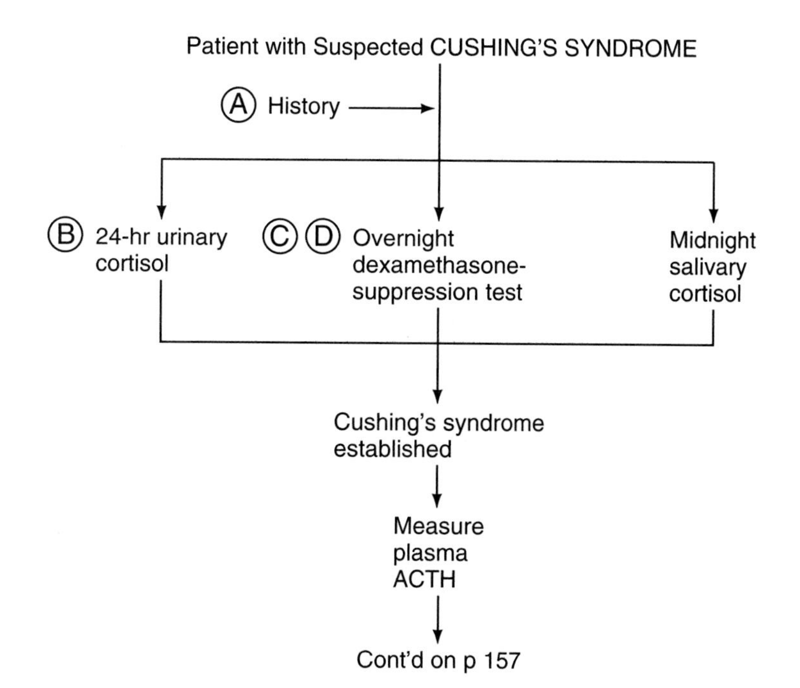

Patient with Suspected CUSHING'S SYNDROME
(A) History
(B) 24-hr urinary cortisol
(C) (D) Overnight dexamethasone-suppression test
Midnight salivary cortisol
Cushing's syndrome established
Measure plasma ACTH
Cont'd on p 157

F. Patients with ACTH-independent hypercortisolemia should undergo thin-slice CT of the adrenal glands to identify the responsible adenoma, carcinoma, or nodules.

G. Patients with ACTH-dependent hypercortisolemia should undergo further testing to discriminate between Cushing's disease related to a pituitary adenoma and that related to ectopic ACTH secretion. Tumors recognized to secrete ACTH include small cell cancer of the lung and bronchial and thymic carcinoids. Clinicians should resist the temptation to image the pituitary because 10% of the population have a structurally abnormal pituitary. Patients should instead undergo a high-dose dexamethasone-suppression test, where 2 mg of dexamethasone is given every 6 hours for 2 days. This test capitalizes on the fact that ACTH-pituitary adenomas retain some feedback responsiveness and often suppress their ACTH production when ambient glucocorticoid levels are high. Cortisol levels are reduced by >90% among 70% of those with Cushing's disease. In the same study, by contradistinction, no patients with ectopically derived ACTH suppressed their cortisol below 90% in response to this high-dose suppression test.

H. Petrosal sinus sampling using CRH stimulation is a final approach to confirming that ACTH is derived from the pituitary. Criteria for confirming the pituitary as the source of the ACTH include a ratio of ACTH between one side of the petrosal sinus and the peripheral plasma >2 or a ratio >3 during infusion of CRH as compared with the level before infusion is begun. If one side has an ACTH level that is a multiple $\geq$1.4 times the level on the opposite side, then the adenoma is highly likely to reside on that side.

I. Patients with suspected ectopic ACTH should have an octreotide imaging performed with chest plain and tomographic images obtained as indicated.

The goal of treatment of Cushing's syndrome is the eradication of any tumor, suppression of cortisol levels to as low as possible, and avoidance of permanent hormone dependency.

J. The treatment of choice for Cushing's disease is transsphenoidal pituitary resection, irrespective of the size of the pituitary tumor. The more extensive the resection, the greater the risk of permanent hypopituitarism. This may have particular implications for younger patients who plan to have children. Pituitary radiation can be provided to patients with unresectable or residual tumors, although this is associated with a high rate of hypopituitarism.

K. Adrenal tumors causing hypercortisolemia are best resected. Medical management of unresectable tumors, or patients with metastatic hormonally active adrenal cancer, is challenging because these malignancies are poorly responsive to adjuvant therapies. Patients may benefit from the use of mitotane, an adrenal poison. These patients must be given supplemental glucocorticoids in replacement doses to ensure that they do not develop adrenal insufficiency during treatment. Patients with uncontrollable hypercortisolemia can benefit from adrenal steroid enzyme inhibitors such as ketoconazole or metyrapone. Experimental chemoradiotherapy or additional agents may be available as part of a clinical trial.

References

Arnaldi G, Angeli A, Atkinson AB, et al. Diagnosis and complications of Cushing's syndrome: a consensus statement. J Clin Endocrinol Metab 2003;88(12):5593–5602.

Findling JW, Raff H. Screening and diagnosis of Cushing's syndrome. Endocrinol Metab Clin North Am 2005;34(2):385–402.

Lindsay JR, Nieman LK. Differential diagnosis and imaging in Cushing's syndrome. Endocrinol Metab Clin North Am 2005;34(2):403–421.

Raff H, Findling JW. A physiologic approach to diagnosis of the Cushing syndrome. Ann Intern Med 2003;138(12):980–991.

Sonino N, Boscaro M, Fallo F. Pharmacologic management of Cushing syndrome: new targets for therapy. Treat Endocrinol 2005;4(2):87–94. Review.

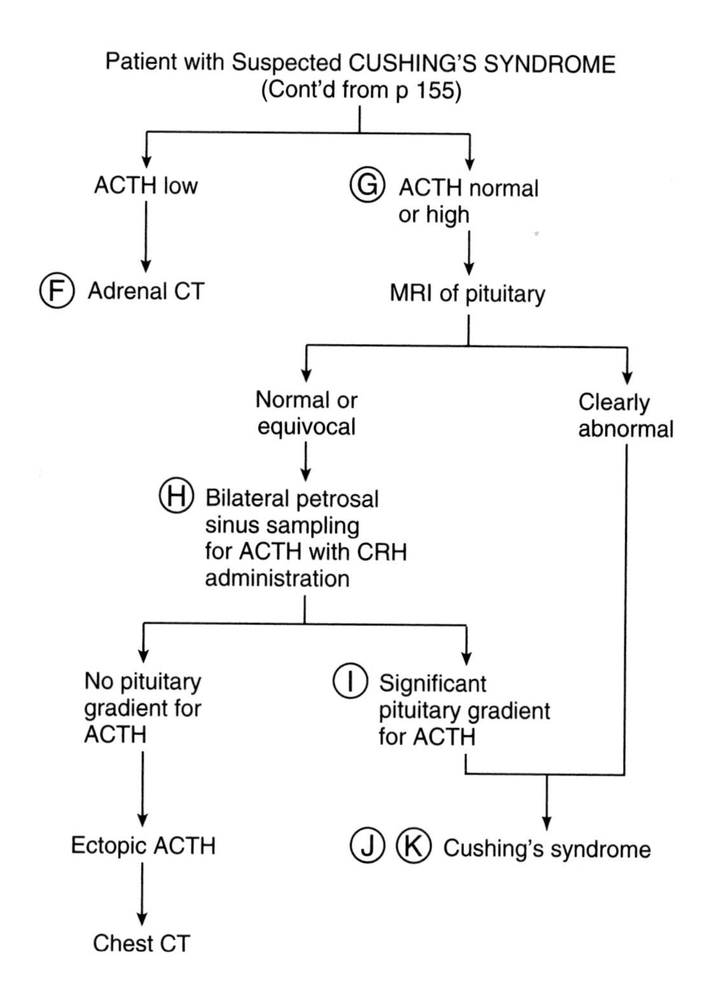
Patient with Suspected CUSHING'S SYNDROME
(Cont'd from p 155)
ACTH low
(F) Adrenal CT
(G) ACTH normal or high
MRI of pituitary
Normal or equivocal
Clearly abnormal
(H) Bilateral petrosal sinus sampling for ACTH with CRH administration
No pituitary gradient for ACTH
(I) Significant pituitary gradient for ACTH
Ectopic ACTH
Chest CT
(J) (K) Cushing's syndrome

PITUITARY TUMOR

Graham T. McMahon, MD, MMSc

A. Pituitary tumors present as incidentalomas following radiographic imaging for another reason, as a result of mass effect (typically visual impairment or headache), or because evidence emerges for either hypofunction or hyperfunction. Tumors can be divided into two groups: Microadenomas are up to 10 mm in size, and anything larger is classified as a macroadenoma. Tumors can be functional or nonfunctional. Clinicians should consider imaging the pituitary in patients who have hypothyroidism with a low or low-normal thyroid-stimulating hormone (TSH) level, are anovulatory with a low or low-normal follicle-stimulating hormone (FSH) level, have erectile dysfunction, or have symptoms of hypogonadism with a low or normal luteinizing hormone (LH) level.

B. Any patient with a recognized pituitary tumor should be evaluated with a serum prolactin level. Patients with a macroadenoma should be more carefully evaluated with an assessment of their growth hormone (GH), gonadotropin, thyrotropin, and corticotropin levels.

C. Pituitary hypofunction is suggested by low thyroxine levels with a low TSH. Patients with thyroxine levels below the normal range should be treated with exogenous levothyroxine. Patients with reduced gonadotropins should receive either androgens or estrogens as appropriate. Progesterone replacement should be provided to women with an intact uterus. Estrogen replacement doses do not need to be as high as the doses contained in the oral contraceptive pill. Patients with central hypoadrenalism should be treated with oral glucocorticoids; mineralocorticoid replacement is not necessary in these patients. GH replacement in adults with GH deficiency is controversial.

D. Clinicians should consider whether the pituitary tumor is an adenoma (most common), a meningioma, a metastatic tumor, or a craniopharyngioma, each of which has typical imaging characteristics. Other considerations are a physiologic pituitary enlargement during pregnancy, a pituitary cyst or abscess (often associated with a fluid level on imaging), arteriovenous fistula, or lymphocytic hypophysitis (a rare condition usually associated with late pregnancy and associated with a high incidence of adrenal insufficiency and diabetes insipidus).

E. A serum prolactin level of >200 ng/ml is diagnostic of a prolactinoma. Levels lower than this may be the result of a prolactinoma or any other sellar mass. Prolactin levels should be measured on a diluted sample if the tumor is large and the prolactin level is low. Prolactinomas of any size are best treated with cabergoline or bromocriptine, even when causing apoplexy.

F. Acromegaly is best excluded by measuring the level of serum insulinlike growth factor (IGF)-1. When the level is not diagnostic, GH levels can be measured 2 hours after a 75-g glucose load. Normally the level should fall to ≤1 ng/ml. Patients with acromegaly should be treated with transsphenoidal resection of the tumor. Medical treatment with cabergoline or long-acting somatostatin is first-line treatment for patients who have failed surgery. A GH receptor antagonist and/or radiotherapy may be useful when other medical treatments and surgery have failed.

G. Elevated adrenocorticotropic hormone (ACTH) levels in the presence of Cushing's syndrome suggest either ectopic production of ACTH or Cushing's disease. Inferior petrosal sinus sampling is often indicated to confirm Cushing's disease in such patients. Transsphenoidal resection is the best treatment for Cushing's disease. (See Cushing's Syndrome.)

H. Nonfunctioning pituitary adenomas that are not causing mass effect or pituitary hypofunction can be monitored carefully with repeat imaging every 12 months. Tumors causing mass effect or hypopituitarism should be resected.

References

Aron DC, Howlett TA. Pituitary incidentalomas. Endocrinol Metab Clin North Am 2000;29(1):205–221.

Chanson P, Salenave S. Diagnosis and treatment of pituitary adenomas. Minerva Endocrinol 2004;29(4):241–275.

Kreutzer J, Fahlbusch R. Diagnosis and treatment of pituitary tumors. Curr Opin Neurol 2004;17(6):693–703.

Verhelst J, Abs R. Hyperprolactinemia: pathophysiology and management. Treat Endocrinol 2003;2(1):23–32.

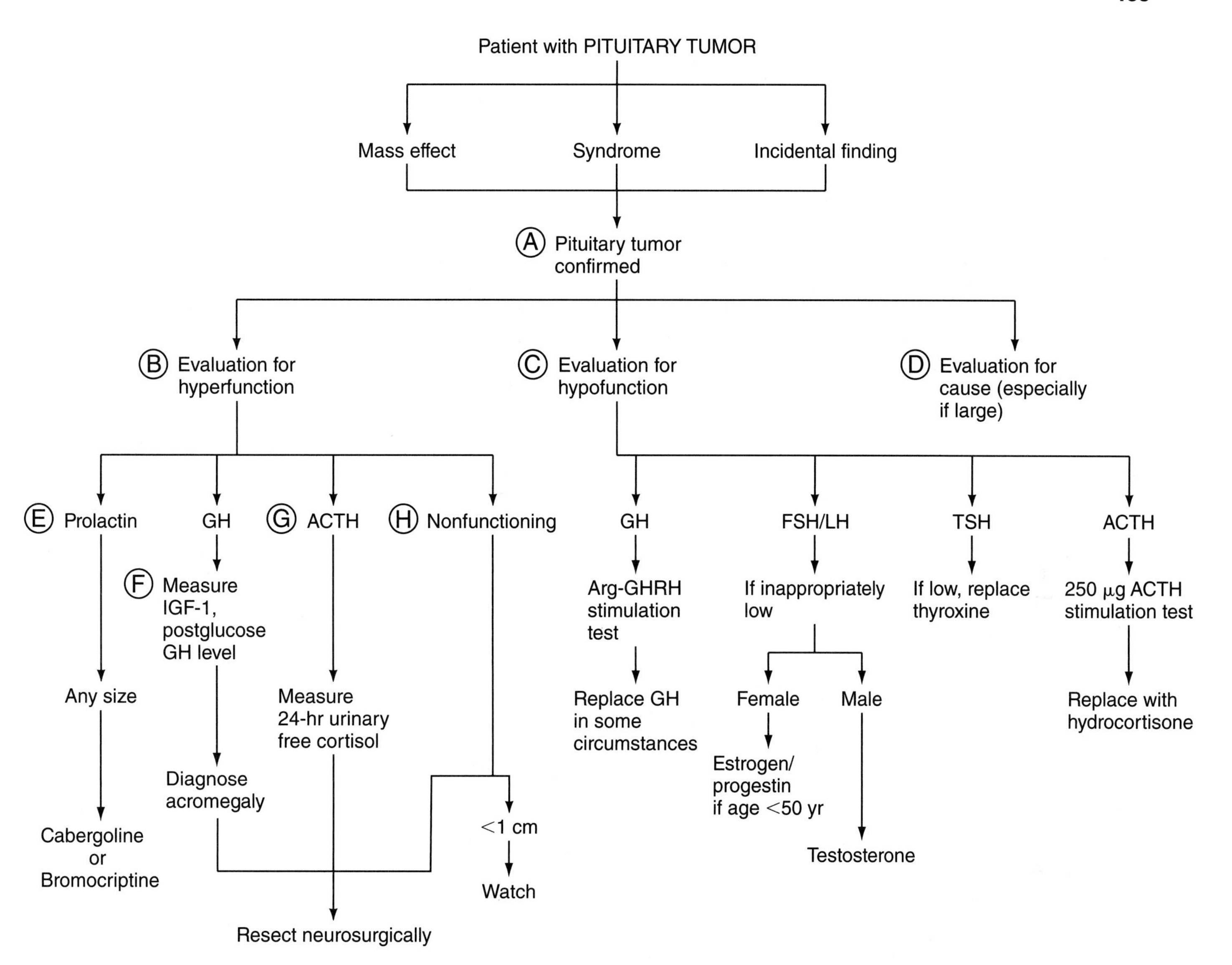

Patient with PITUITARY TUMOR
Mass effect
Syndrome
Incidental finding
(A) Pituitary tumor confirmed
(B) Evaluation for hyperfunction
(C) Evaluation for hypofunction
(D) Evaluation for cause (especially if large)
(E) Prolactin
GH
(G) ACTH
(H) Nonfunctioning
GH
FSH/LH
TSH
ACTH
(F) Measure IGF-1, postglucose GH level
Arg-GHRH stimulation test
If inappropriately low
If low, replace thyroxine
250 μg ACTH stimulation test
Any size
Measure 24-hr urinary free cortisol
Replace GH in some circumstances
Female
Male
Replace with hydrocortisone
Diagnose acromegaly
Estrogen/ progestin if age <50 yr
<1 cm
Cabergoline or Bromocriptine
Testosterone
Watch
Resect neurosurgically

HIRSUTISM

Graham T. McMahon, MD, MMSc

Hirsutism refers to the appearance of excessive terminal hair that appears in a male pattern in women. Approximately 5% of women are hirsute. Hirsutism results from an interaction between the androgen level and the sensitivity of the hair follicle to androgen; as a result, androgen levels do not correlate well with the degree of hirsutism. Approximately one half of women with hirsutism have the idiopathic condition.

A. Clinical features that suggest one of the rare or more serious causes of hirsutism include abrupt onset, a presentation later in life, and progressive worsening. Symptoms and signs of virilization include frontal balding, acne, clitoromegaly, and deepening of the voice. Hair growth on the upper lip, chin, chest, abdomen, back, pubis, and legs should be assessed. Hirsutism should be distinguished from hypertrichosis, the appearance of generalized excessive hair growth that is genetically determined or follows treatment with glucocorticoids, phenytoin, or cyclosporine.

B. If hirsutism is moderate or severe, the plasma testosterone and free testosterone should be measured in the early morning (ideally, on days 4–10 of the menstrual cycle in cycling women).

C. Hyperandrogenism is most frequently related to the polycystic ovary syndrome (PCOS), one of the most common hormonal disorders affecting women. The syndrome is diagnosed when the patient has at least two symptoms of chronic hyperandrogenism, oligo-ovulation or anovulation, and polycystic ovaries. Other diagnoses must have been excluded also. These patients often have menstrual irregularity, obesity, and evidence of insulin resistance (e.g., acanthosis nigricans). A pelvic ultrasound is not required for diagnosis. Additional testing may include a pregnancy test if the patient has amenorrhea. These patients should be evaluated for glucose intolerance and sleep apnea and often respond well to insulin sensitizers such as metformin or a thiazolidinedione. Spironolactone and oral contraceptives are often used to manage hirsutism in these patients.

D. Other causes of hyperandrogenism are unusual. Virilizing congenital adrenal hyperplasia is suggested by the premature growth of pubic hair and clitoromegaly and can be excluded by measuring the morning 17-alpha-hydroxyprogesterone level.

E. Cushing's syndrome is suggested by the development of truncal obesity, moon face, buffalo hump, purple striae, or proximal muscle weakness. (See the chapter on Cushing's syndrome.) Hyperprolactinemia is suggested by the presence of galactorrhea and an elevated prolactin level. Acromegaly is suggested by the coarsening of facial features or by hand enlargement and is confirmed by an elevated insulinlike growth factor-1 level.

F. Androgen-secreting tumors are rare but should be considered among women with an acute presentation or those who have very high levels of testosterone (>200 ng/dl). Such women should be evaluated with a level of dehydroepiandrosterone sulfate (DHEAS) and an abdominal and pelvic ultrasound.

G. Idiopathic hirsutism is the most common diagnosis after these other disorders are excluded by clinical or laboratory features. The hirsutism can be managed with cosmetic and hormonal therapy. It is useful to complete an objective assessment of the degree of hirsutism in advance of initiating treatment. The Ferriman-Gallwey score is one such scoring system.

H. Cosmetic approaches include bleaching, shaving, waxing, electrolysis, laser treatment, and the use of depilatory agents. Eflornithine hydrochloride cream can be used for facial hirsutism but must be used for approximately 8 weeks before its efficacy can be determined.

I. Estrogen-progestin contraceptives suppress plasma testosterone levels, can reduce the need for shaving, and slow the progression of hirsutism. Contraceptives with nonandrogenic progestins (e.g., Yasmin, Ortho-Cyclen, or Demulen 1-50) are preferred. Antiandrogens can be offered when hirsutism is moderate to severe. Spironolactone at high dosages (50–100 mg twice a day) is effective in reducing hirsutism. Patients must be informed that spironolactone may be teratogenic and is generally not prescribed to women who are sexually active and not using an oral contraceptive. Hyperkalemia is rarely associated with spironolactone among women with normal renal function. Flutamide is an antiandrogen that is associated with hepatotoxicity and is not generally recommended for managing hirsutism. Cyproterone acetate is an antiandrogen that is available in Canada, Mexico, and Europe but not in the United States.

References

Azziz R. The evaluation and management of hirsutism. Obstet Gynecol 2003;101(5 Pt 1):995–1007.

Ehrmann DA. Polycystic ovary syndrome. N Engl J Med 2005;352(12): 1223–1236.

Ferriman D, Gallwey J. Clinical assessment of body hair growth in women. J Clin Endocrinol Metab 1961;21:1440.

McKenna, TJ. Screening for sinister causes of hirsutism. N Engl J Med 1994;331:1015.

Rosenfield RL. Hirsutism. N Engl J Med 2005;353(24):2578–2588.

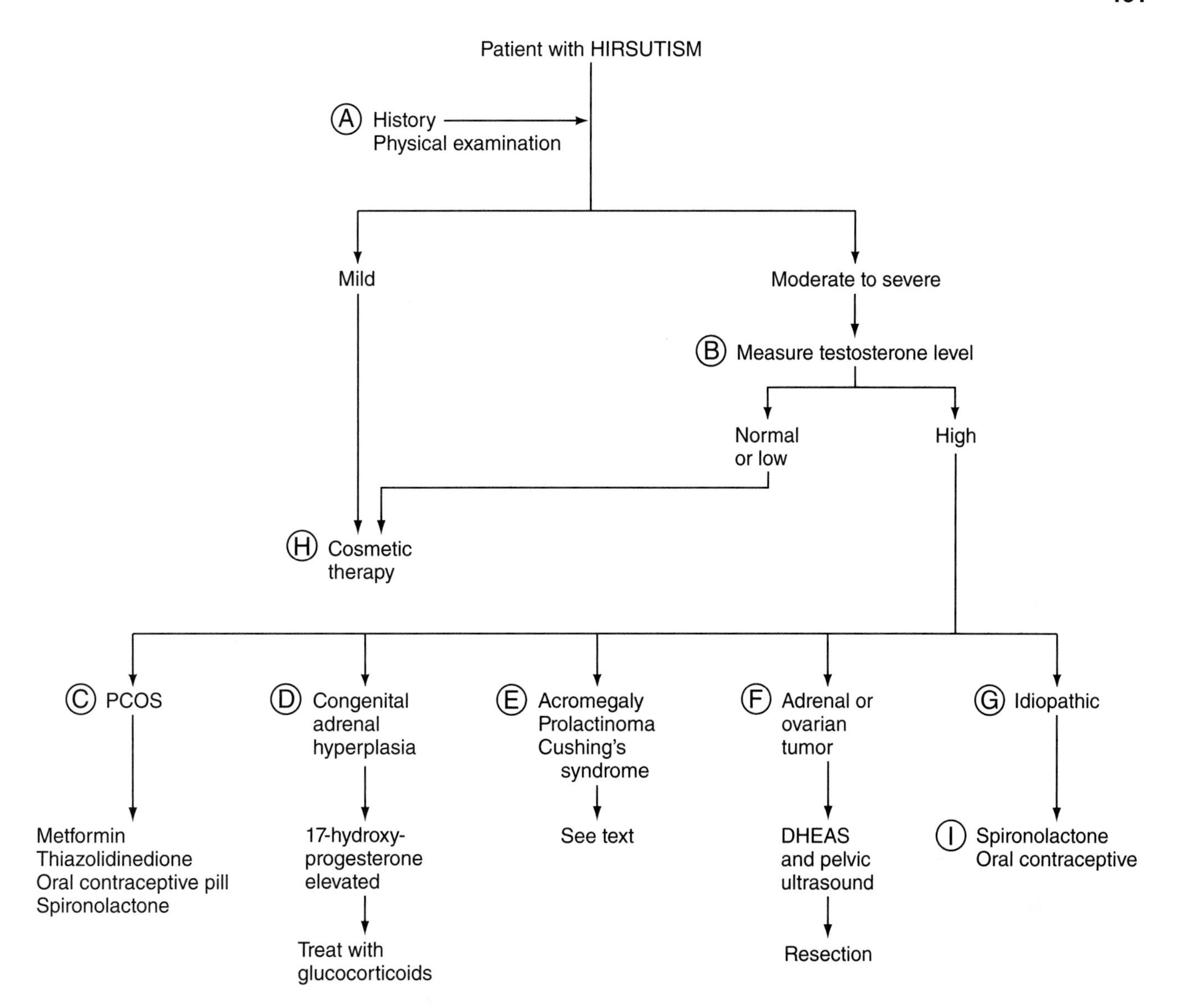

Patient with HIRSUTISM
A History
Physical examination
Mild
Moderate to severe
B Measure testosterone level
Normal
or low
High
H Cosmetic
therapy
C PCOS
D Congenital
adrenal
hyperplasia
E Acromegaly
Prolactinoma
Cushing's
syndrome
F Adrenal or
ovarian
tumor
G Idiopathic
Metformin
Thiazolidinedione
Oral contraceptive pill
Spironolactone
17-hydroxy-
progesterone
elevated
Treat with
glucocorticoids
See text
DHEAS
and pelvic
ultrasound
Resection
I Spironolactone
Oral contraceptive

GYNECOMASTIA

Graham T. McMahon, MD, MMSc

Gynecomastia refers to enlargement of glandular breast tissue behind the male nipple. The breast tissue usually hypertrophies in response to an absolute or apparent excess of estrogen or a deficiency of androgen. These levels may be affected by changes in the function of the adrenal gland or testes, conversion of estrogens in tissues such as adipose, the circulating level of sex-hormone–binding globulin, or tissue-specific sensitivity to hormonal stimulation.

A. If the patient is an adolescent or young adult, then pubertal gynecomastia is the most likely etiology. Transient imbalances in the ratio of estrogen to androgen during puberty can result in erratic and asymmetric breast development in boys. These changes may persist to adulthood. As the ratio of adipose to muscle increases with age, the increased peripheral conversion of androgens to estrogens may trigger the onset of gynecomastia de novo. Germ cell tumors of the testis, prevalent in this age group, should be excluded and the patients reexamined for stability in 6 months.

B. Testicular neoplasms often secrete human chorionic gonadotropin (hCG) that interferes with normal testicular androgen production and increases the conversion of androgen to estrogen. Gynecomastia in these patients is a poor prognostic sign. In patients in whom further investigation of gynecomastia is warranted, levels of luteinizing hormone (LH), testosterone (T), estradiol (E_2), and hCG should be determined.

C. Drugs are commonly implicated in the etiology of gynecomastia. Gynecomastia should not be unexpected when treating patients with antiandrogens or estrogens. Some drugs have an intrinsic estrogenic activity; others, such as chemotherapeutic agents and drugs of abuse (especially marijuana and heroin), interfere with normal androgen production in the testes or centrally. Spironolactone is an antiandrogen and increases the conversion of androgen to estrogen. Similar changes are not noted with eplerenone, a newer aldosterone antagonist. Alcohol, antituberculous agents, and H_2 receptor antagonists (such as cimetidine or ranitidine) have also been implicated as etiologic agents in causing gynecomastia.

D. Other systemic causes should be considered in patients not taking contributing drugs, who are beyond puberty, and have testicular neoplasm excluded. Malnutrition induces a central hypogonadism that does not affect adrenal estrogen production. Cirrhosis is associated with an increase in the adrenal production of estrogen precursors and increased conversion to estrogen.

E. Endocrine causes of gynecomastia include central hypogonadism, testicular failure, hyperthyroidism, feminizing adrenal tumors, and true hermaphroditism. The etiology and investigation of primary and secondary hypogonadism are presented in standard endocrinology texts. Hyperthyroidism is associated with an increase in the concentration of sex-hormone–binding globulin, and a shift in the androgen-to-estrogen ratio. A feminizing adrenal tumor-can produce large amounts of estrogen. Patients with true hermaphroditism who have functioning ovarian tissue may similarly present with gynecomastia.

F. Most patients with gynecomastia require no therapy other than the removal of the inciting cause, if identified. Even if the cause is not identified, spontaneous regression occurs in up to 85% of cases, particularly in younger men. Therapy is indicated in cases where the gynecomastia causes sufficient pain, embarrassment, or distress to interfere with daily life. Surgery remains the mainstay of treatment, because gynecomastia of long duration becomes fibrosed and unresponsive to medical treatment. When onset is recent, medical therapy may be useful. Several drugs have been tried for gynecomastia, including the antiestrogens tamoxifen and clomiphene, the aromatase inhibitor testolactone, and danazol, a weak androgen that inhibits gonadotropin secretion. Treatment with dihydrotestosterone, which cannot be aromatized to estrogen, is reported to provide symptomatic improvement. Prophylactic radiation to the breasts can be used where gynecomastia can be predicted, such as when treating prostate cancer patients with estrogens.

References

Bembo SA, Carlson HE. Gynecomastia: its features, and when and how to treat it. Cleve Clin J Med 2004;71(6):511–517.

Braunstein GD. Gynecomastia. N Engl J Med 1993;328:490–495.

Daniels IR, Layer GT. Gynaecomastia. Eur J Surg 2001;167(12): 885–892.

De Sanctis V, Bernasconi S, Bona G, et al. Pubertal gynecomastia. Minerva Pediatr 2002;54(4):357–361.

Glass AR. Gynecomastia. Endocrinol Metab Clin North Am 1994;23(4): 825–837.

Neuman JF. Evaluation and treatment of gynecomastia. Am Fam Physician 1997;55(5):1835–1844, 1849–1850.

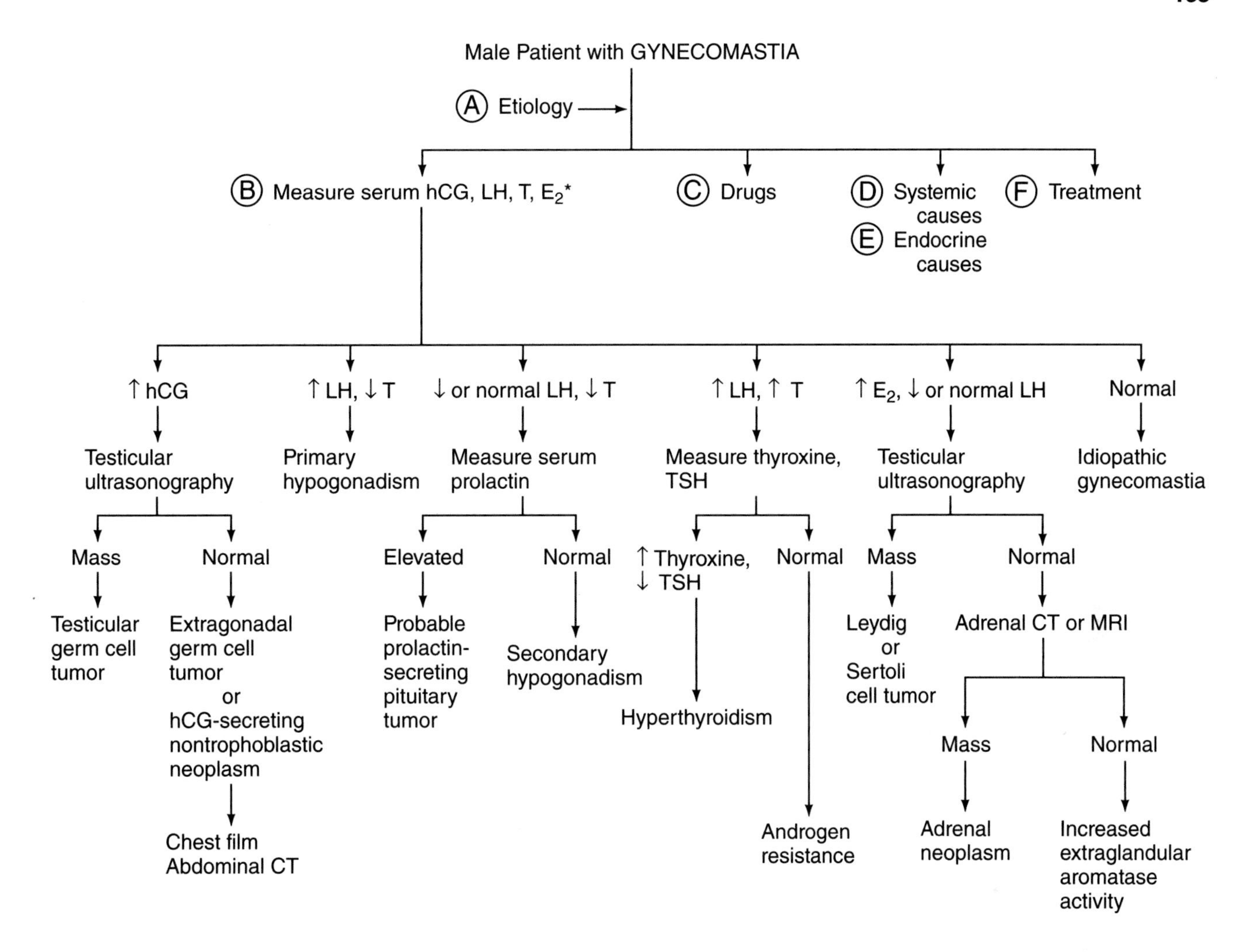
Male Patient with GYNECOMASTIA
(A) Etiology
(B) Measure serum hCG, LH, T, E2*
(C) Drugs
(D) Systemic causes
(E) Endocrine causes
(F) Treatment
↑ hCG
↑ LH, ↓ T
↓ or normal LH, ↓ T
↑ LH, ↑ T
↑ E2, ↓ or normal LH
Normal
Testicular ultrasonography
Primary hypogonadism
Measure serum prolactin
Measure thyroxine, TSH
Testicular ultrasonography
Idiopathic gynecomastia
Mass
Normal
Elevated
Normal
↑ Thyroxine, ↓ TSH
Normal
Mass
Normal
Testicular germ cell tumor
Extragonadal germ cell tumor or hCG-secreting nontrophoblastic neoplasm
Probable prolactin-secreting pituitary tumor
Secondary hypogonadism
Hyperthyroidism
Leydig or Sertoli cell tumor
Adrenal CT or MRI
Mass
Normal
Chest film
Abdominal CT
Androgen resistance
Adrenal neoplasm
Increased extraglandular aromatase activity

*Modified from Braunstein.

Gastroenterology

M. Brian Fennerty, MD
Section Editor

ACUTE ABDOMINAL PAIN

Bipin Saud, MD; Juan Diego Baltodano, MD; and Steven Palley, MD

Acute abdominal pain is a common clinical presentation in the emergency department and primary care setting. The clinician addressing the patient with acute abdominal pain ideally should eliminate acute medical causes of abdominal pain and recognize the proper setting for surgical consultation. There should be a low threshold for involving surgical expertise. History and physical examination are critical in evaluation. Admission for evaluation is common and should be considered for acute pain without obvious surgical indication that persists for 6 hours. Abdominal pain can be visceral, parietal, and referred. Noxious stimulation affecting abdominal viscera produces dull and usually poorly localized pain to the ventral midline of the abdomen. This can be explained by multisegmental innervation of the affected organs. Irritation of the parietal peritoneum produces more localized and often more severe pain. Finally, referred pain is experienced in remote areas from the site of injury because these areas share the same segmental innervation as the involved organ.

A. A careful history can narrow the differential diagnosis. Age and sex are important considerations. Mesenteric adenitis occurs in younger persons, whereas vascular and neoplastic disease occur in elderly persons. In a sexually active female, consider ectopic pregnancy or pelvic inflammatory disease. Medical history can reveal previous peptic ulcer disease, gallstones, diverticular disease, inflammatory bowel disease, and abdominal surgery. Medication history can disclose corticosteroid or immunosuppressant use. Coexisting medical conditions such as diabetes mellitus can affect the presentation. The onset and character of the pain are important. A sudden onset of intense, localized, "somatic" pain suggests peritonitis, as is seen with perforation of the bowel. Crescendo-decrescendo "visceral" pain or colic is more characteristic of bowel, cystic duct, or ureteral obstruction. An evolving pain pattern, visceral at first and later somatic, may suggest appendicitis, cholecystitis, or strangulated bowel. Disproportionate pain compared with a lesser physical finding occurs with ischemia. Characteristic radiation patterns are noted with cholecystitis (scapula), pancreatitis (back), and appendicitis (right lower quadrant).

B. Observe the patient before the examination. Visceral pain usually causes restlessness; parietal pain increases with movement. Auscultate the abdomen for bruits, rubs, and bowel sounds. Palpation should begin away from the site of pain. Involuntary guarding or rebound tenderness, especially with light percussion, implies peritonitis. Deeper palpation can be used to search for organomegaly or masses. Perform rectal and pelvic examinations. Examine the hernial orifices in the groin and, as indicated, examine the external genitalia.

C. A patient who is hemodynamically unstable with possible intraabdominal hemorrhage may require immediate laparotomy. The patient who is acutely ill with hypotension, high fever, leukocytosis, and a suggestive physical examination (involuntary guarding, rigidity, increasing severe tenderness) should also undergo immediate surgical evaluation. Suspected bowel ischemia with acidosis, fever, and evidence of hypovolemia also should be evaluated surgically, as should the patient with evidence of perforation by plain radiography, contrast study, or paracentesis. Resuscitation is critical both before and during further evaluation, including possible ventilatory support IV access and fluids, nasogastric suction, oxygen, and urinary output monitoring; frequent checks of vital signs and preliminary laboratory tests also should be done. Ideally, important medical causes of acute pain can be ruled out before surgery with urinalysis, electrocardiography, and abdominal films.

D. The patient who is more stable should be observed closely. Medical causes of acute abdominal pain can be ruled out, although the list can be extensive. The more common causes are acute pneumonitis, especially lower lobe; pyelonephritis; and mesenteric adenitis. Collagen vascular disease can cause perforation. Multiple metabolic disorders, including diabetic ketoacidosis, Addisonian crisis, uremia, and acute intermittent porphyria, can lead to abdominal pain. A history of chronic liver disease with ascites may suggest spontaneous bacterial peritonitis.

E. Certain patients may present with a discrepancy between severity of disease and physical findings. These include patients who are elderly, malnourished, obese, immunosuppressed, or taking steroids; early postoperative patients; those with mental status changes; and patients with paraplegia.

F. Laboratory evaluation should include hemoglobin/hematocrit, white blood cell count, differential, electrolytes, blood gases, amylase, liver tests, coagulation times, and urinalysis. A serum pregnancy test is mandatory in any woman of childbearing age. Supine and upright abdominal films may suggest obstruction, ischemia, perforation, renal calculi, or intraabdominal abscess. Also a chest x-ray study is helpful in identifying potential thoracic causes of referred pain. Angiography is useful for suspected hemorrhage or ischemia. Contrast studies are

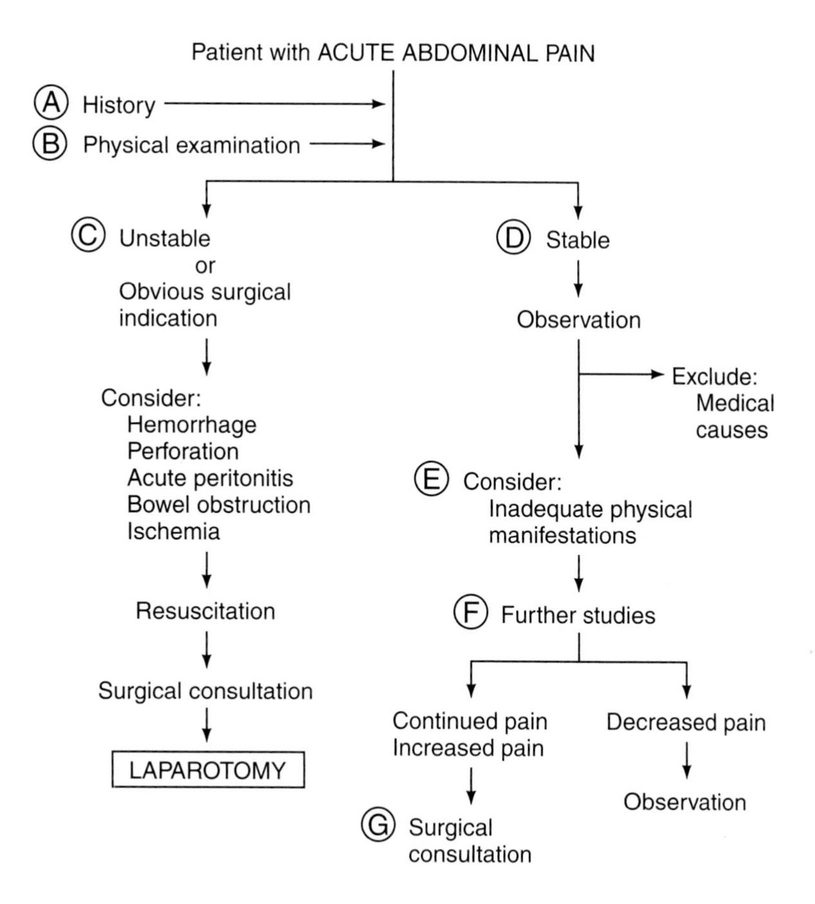

useful for suspected perforation. Ultrasonography and CT imaging can demonstrate pancreatitis, cholecystitis, abscess, retroperitoneal mass, or dilated biliary tree. CT scan has a high diagnostic yield for many causes of abdominal pain. For example, in the diagnosis of appendicitis, it is reported to have a sensitivity and specificity of 98% and 97%, respectively. Ultrasonography may be an initial modality of testing for a suspected hepatobiliary origin of pain and is shown to have similar diagnostic accuracy.

G. Close observation may disclose an evolutionary pattern to the abdominal pain syndrome. If acute pain persists >6 hours, obtain a surgical consultation if this has not already been requested.

References

Flasar MH, Goldberg E. Acute abdominal pain. Med Clin North Am 2006;90(2):481–503.

Glasgow RE, Mulvihill SJ. Abdominal pain. In Sleisenger and Fordtran's Gastrointestinal and Liver Disease: Pathophysiology, Diagnosis and Management, 7th ed. Philadelphia: WB Saunders; 2002:71–82.

Gupta H, Dupuy D. Advances in imaging of the acute abdomen. Surg Clin North Am 1997;77(6):1245–1263.

Raman SS, Lu DS, Kadell BM, et al. Accuracy of nonfocused helical CT for the diagnosis of acute appendicitis: a 5 year review. Am J Roentgenol 2002;178(6);1319–1325.

CHRONIC ABDOMINAL PAIN

Bipin Saud, MD, and Juan Diego Baltodano, MD

Chronic abdominal pain is a common and challenging symptom that is commonly evaluated by primary care providers, gastroenterologists, and surgeons. The vast majority of these patients have a functional disorder. Chronic intractable or undiagnosed abdominal pain is defined by the presence of abdominal pain for at least 6 months without a specific diagnosis after an adequate evaluation. Differentiating functional GI disorders from organic pathology is essential for clinical management. In the United States, it is estimated that the prevalence of chronic functional abdominal pain is 2%, and it occurs primarily in women.

A. A careful, detailed history and physical examination are mandatory to direct further evaluation. Determining the pattern of pain, type of pain, and overall time course of the illness often leads to a systematic and reasonable evaluation. Also, specific details about the pain, such as location, characteristics, alleviating or aggravating factors, and chronology of events, often help to narrow a broad differential diagnosis. Associated symptoms, such as fever, chills, nausea, vomiting, jaundice, weight gain or loss, diarrhea, constipation, melena, hematochezia, change in the color of urine or stool, or change in the diameter of stool should be included in the history. In women, a menstrual history should be obtained.

B. Biliary tract disease leads to intermittent acute pain that is usually localized to the right upper quadrant or the epigastric area that lasts for 15 minutes or a few hours. The pain may radiate to the back or scapula and is often associated with restlessness, sweating, or vomiting. Episodes are typically separated by weeks to months. A history of recurrent pancreatitis or excessive alcohol intake should raise the possibility of chronic pancreatitis. Upper GI symptoms can be related to ulcer or nonulcer dyspepsia. Postprandial abdominal pain may be related to underlying chronic intestinal ischemia, gastroparesis, intermittent intestinal obstruction, pancreatitis, or peptic ulcer disease. Features that suggest organic illness include unstable weight loss, fever, dehydration, electrolyte abnormalities, symptoms or signs of GI blood loss, anemia, and signs of malnutrition and abnormal physical findings.

Routine laboratory testing is mandatory to evaluate for any underlying disease process. CBC, basal metabolic panel (BMP), liver function tests, amylase, and urinalysis (including porphobilinogen in cases of suspected acute intermittent porphyria) are needed. Stool analysis for leucocytes, ova, and parasites should be obtained as clinically indicated. Diagnostic imaging studies such as abdominal x-ray films, abdominal ultrasonography, CT scan of the abdomen, upper GI series with small bowel follow-through, or MRI may be indicated. Endoscopic studies, including upper, lower, capsule endoscopy and endoscopic retrograde cholangiopancreatography (ERCP), are also performed according to each clinical setting.

C. Chronic pain originating from the abdominal wall may be confused with visceral pain, often leading to extensive evaluation. Chronic abdominal wall pain may be related to nerve entrapment, radicular pain radiating from T7 to T12 lesions, or referred pain from abdominal or thoracic lesions. Radicular pain across the abdomen may also be worse with movement and may be caused by irritation of the spinal nerve root from disc and vertebral body disease, a meningeal tumor, tabes dorsalis secondary to syphilis or diabetes, or postherpetic neuralgia. Treatment with a local anesthetic agent is effective for most patients with chronic abdominal wall and radicular pain, which can further confirm the diagnosis.

D. Pelvic pain can be from either GI or gynecologic causes. Common gynecologic sources of pelvic pain include ovarian and uterine tumors, chronic pelvic inflammatory disease, and endometriosis.

(Continued on page 170)

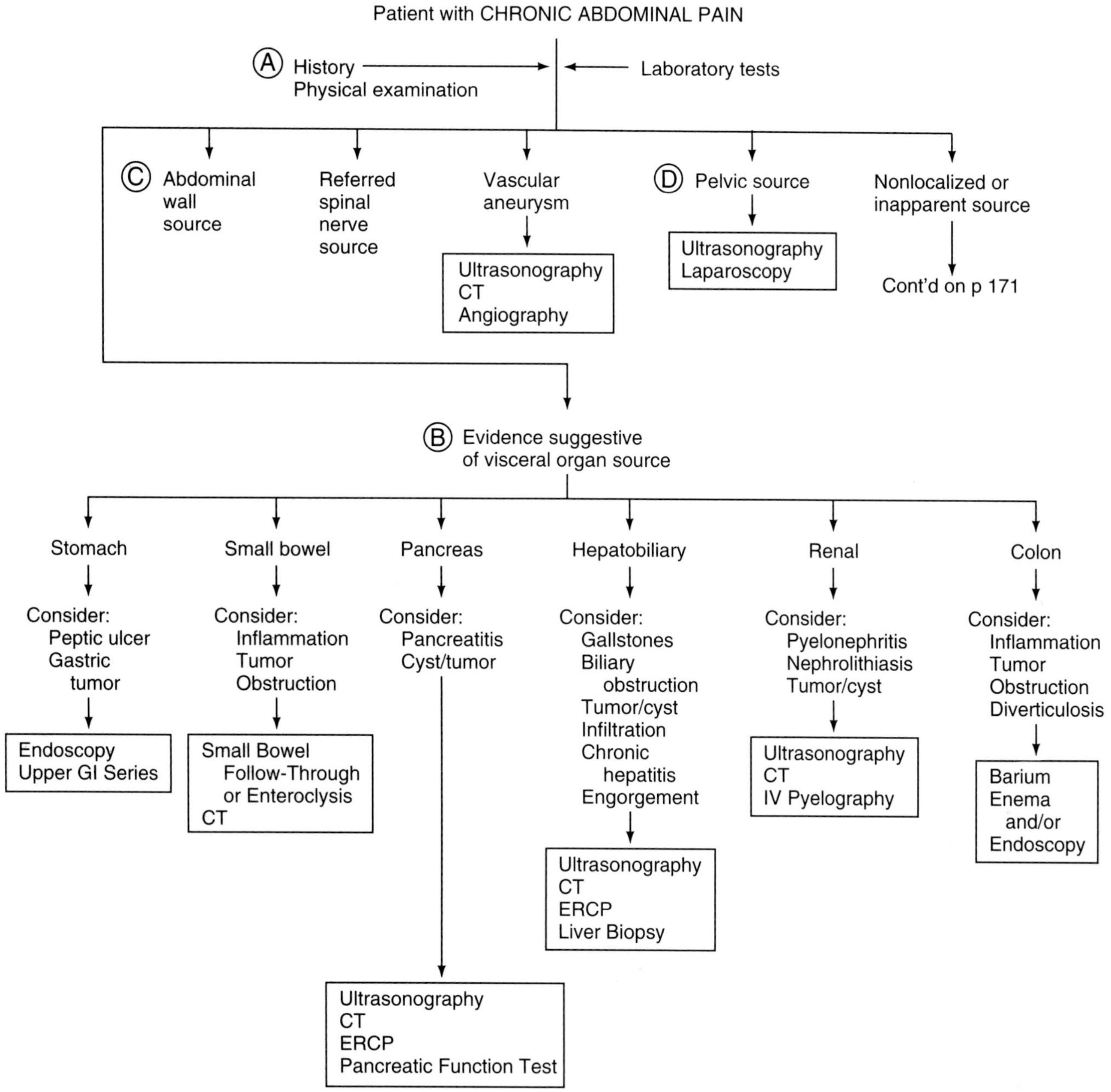

Patient with CHRONIC ABDOMINAL PAIN

(A) History
Physical examination

Laboratory tests

(C) Abdominal wall source

Referred spinal nerve source

Vascular aneurysm
→ Ultrasonography
CT
Angiography

(D) Pelvic source
→ Ultrasonography
Laparoscopy

Nonlocalized or inapparent source
→ Cont'd on p 171

(B) Evidence suggestive of visceral organ source

Stomach
→ Consider:
Peptic ulcer
Gastric tumor
→ Endoscopy
Upper GI Series

Small bowel
→ Consider:
Inflammation
Tumor
Obstruction
→ Small Bowel Follow-Through or Enteroclysis
CT

Pancreas
→ Consider:
Pancreatitis
Cyst/tumor
→ Ultrasonography
CT
ERCP
Pancreatic Function Test

Hepatobiliary
→ Consider:
Gallstones
Biliary obstruction
Tumor/cyst
Infiltration
Chronic hepatitis
Engorgement
→ Ultrasonography
CT
ERCP
Liver Biopsy

Renal
→ Consider:
Pyelonephritis
Nephrolithiasis
Tumor/cyst
→ Ultrasonography
CT
IV Pyelography

Colon
→ Consider:
Inflammation
Tumor
Obstruction
Diverticulosis
→ Barium Enema and/or Endoscopy

E. Metabolic disorders may rarely be associated with abdominal pain. These include acute intermittent porphyria, adrenal insufficiency, hypercalcemia, or hyperthyroidism, and hypothyroidism. Other rare causes include familial Mediterranean fever, hereditary angioedema, diabetic neuropathy, and carcinoid syndrome.

F. Features suggesting irritable bowel syndrome (IBS) are pain for at least 12 weeks (not necessarily consecutive) associated with bowel habit changes, no alarming features, and the absence of nocturnal symptoms. Pain relief with defecation, mucus in the stool, and sensation of incomplete evacuation are typical. Abdominal pain in IBS is usually a crampy sensation of variable intensity and periodic exacerbations. Functional abdominal pain syndrome (FAPS) follows specific diagnostic characteristics. The Rome II criteria for functional abdominal pain include at least 6 months of the following symptoms:
- Continuous or nearly continuous abdominal pain
- None or occasional relationship of pain with physiologic events
- Some loss of daily functioning
- Real pain (i.e., the pain is not feigned)
- Insufficient criteria for other functional gastrointestinal disorders that would explain abdominal pain

G. Chronic mesenteric ischemia, also known as intestinal angina, is manifested by recurrent abdominal pain, which usually develops in patients with mesenteric atherosclerotic disease. Patients complain of dull, crampy postprandial epigastric pain within the first hour after eating. The pain subsides in the next couple of hours. Weight loss is seen in about 80% of the patients.

The goals of treatment in patients with chronic abdominal pain are to identify and manage the underlying cause. It is most important to delineate functional abdominal pain from serious disease processes. Management of patients with functional diseases often requires a multidisciplinary approach.

References

Drossman DA. Functional abdominal pain syndrome. Clin Gastroenterol Hepatol 2004;2(5):353–365.

Drossman, DA, Zhiming, L, Andruzzi, E, et al. US householders survey of functional gastrointestinal disorders: prevalence, sociodemography, and health impact. Dig Dis Sci 1993;38:1569.

Feldman M, Friedman LS, Sleisenger MH. Gastrointestinal and Liver Disease Pathophysiology, Diagnosis and Management. 7th ed. Philadelphia: WB Saunders, 2002.

Friedman HH. Problem-Oriented Medical Diagnosis. 6th ed. Boston: Little, Brown and Company, 1998.

Friedman SL, McQuaid KR, Grendell JH. Current Diagnosis and Treatment in Gastroenterology. 2nd ed. New York: McGraw-Hill, 2003.

Hungin AP, Chang L, Locke GR, et al. Irritable bowel syndrome in the United States: prevalence, symptom patterns and impact. Aliment Pharmacol Ther 2005; 21(11):1365–1375.

Williams RE, Black CL, Kim HY, et al. Stability of irritable bowel syndrome using a Rome II-based classification. Aliment Pharmacol Ther 2006; 23(1):197–205.

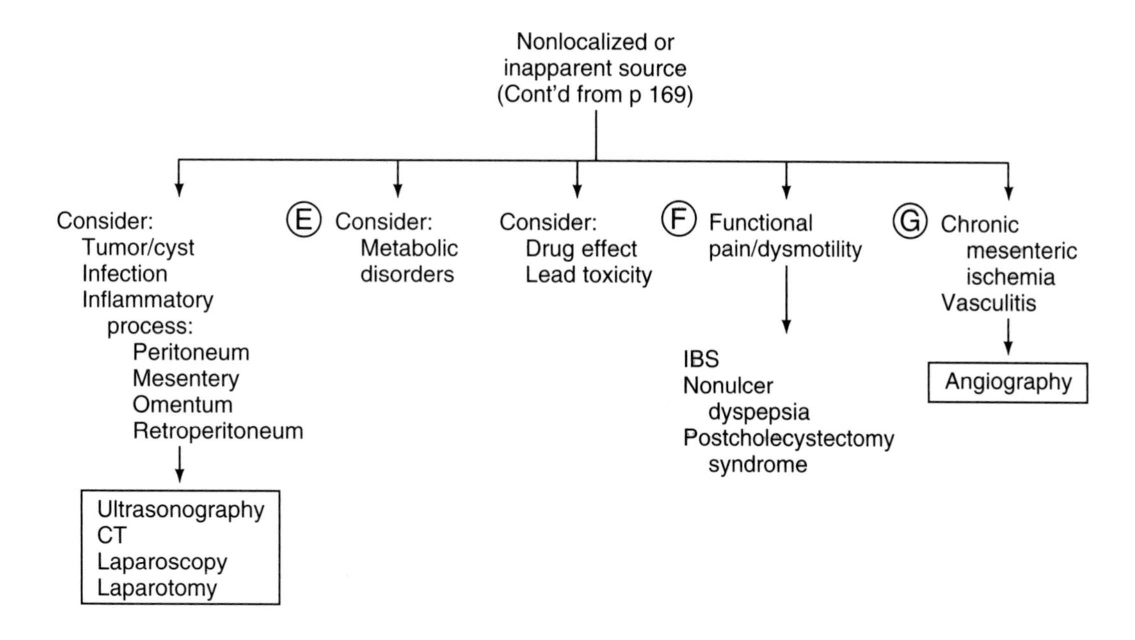

Nonlocalized or inapparent source (Cont'd from p 169)
Consider:
Tumor/cyst
Infection
Inflammatory process:
Peritoneum
Mesentery
Omentum
Retroperitoneum
Ultrasonography
CT
Laparoscopy
Laparotomy
E
Consider:
Metabolic disorders
Consider:
Drug effect
Lead toxicity
F
Functional pain/dysmotility
IBS
Nonulcer dyspepsia
Postcholecystectomy syndrome
G
Chronic mesenteric ischemia
Vasculitis
Angiography

NAUSEA AND VOMITING

Bipin Saud, MD, and Juan Diego Baltodano, MD

Nausea and vomiting are common and distressing symptoms that may result from various underlying causes. Nausea is subjective and is commonly described as a sensation that precedes vomiting. Vomiting is a physical event that results in the rapid, forceful ejection of intestinal contents in retrograde fashion from the stomach via the mouth. Nausea and vomiting should be differentiated from other symptoms such as regurgitation, rumination, and bulimia. Regurgitation is a passive act by which food is brought back into the mouth without the abdominal and diaphragmatic muscular activity that characterizes vomiting. Acid regurgitation, for instance, is an important symptom of gastroesophageal reflux. However, rumination is defined as chewing and swallowing of regurgitated food that has come back into the mouth through a voluntary increase in abdominal pressure within minutes of eating or during eating. Rumination is commonly described among children with mental retardation and those with psychiatric illnesses, but now it is clear that it can occur in adults in the absence of either of these entities.

A. The differential diagnosis of nausea and vomiting is extensive. Therefore, a careful and orderly approach to the evaluation and treatment of patients with nausea and vomiting is needed for cost-effectiveness and to come to a correct diagnosis. When the patient is first seen, the acuteness of the problem should be determined. If there is concern for mechanical obstruction, peritonitis, or perforation, the patient will need to be hospitalized. The patient may require treatment for dehydration and electrolyte abnormalities. Could this be a self-limited viral gastroenteritis? A detailed history may give a clue to an offending medication.

Timing and description of vomiting may also give a clue to the diagnosis. Vomiting in the morning is typically related to pregnancy, uremia, alcohol ingestion, or increased intracranial pressure. The quality of vomiting may also be helpful. A feculent odor to the vomitus is a feature of intestinal obstruction suggestive of bacterial degradation of stagnant intestinal contents.

Associated symptoms such as abdominal pain, fever, diarrhea, or vertigo or a history of similar illness among family and friends may suggest the correct diagnosis. Abdominal pain preceding vomiting usually is suggestive of an obstructive process. Weight loss may indicate a malignant process, although a benign process such as gastric outlet obstruction from peptic ulcer disease may also cause weight loss. The presence of CNS symptoms such as headache, vertigo, neck stiffness, and focal neurologic deficits suggests a central nervous cause of nausea and vomiting. A history of intermittent episodes of vomiting associated with a history of migraine suggests cyclic vomiting syndrome. Postoperative nausea and vomiting (PONV) may complicate 11%–73% of surgical procedures. PONV is more common in women and younger patients and is more likely to occur after general anesthesia.

B. Orthostatic blood pressures should be obtained to evaluate for significant hypotension. A decrease in blood pressure without any change in pulse rate suggests the presence of autonomic neuropathy. General examination may detect jaundice, lymphadenopathy, and occult blood in stool and features that may suggest thyrotoxicosis or Addison's disease. Nausea and vomiting may result in malnutrition and various deficiency states. Examination of the abdomen is important. One should look for masses, abdominal distention, visible peristalsis, and abdominal or inguinal hernias. Assessing for specific areas of abdominal tenderness is also important. Presence of a succussion splash helps identify gastric outlet obstruction or gastroparesis. Extremities should be examined for changes suggesting scleroderma or peripheral neuropathy. Fingernails should be inspected for findings suggestive of self-induced vomiting. Loss of dental enamel may indicate either recurrent vomiting as in bulimia or the consequence of gastroesophageal reflux disease. Neurologic examination is also important, although it is often omitted. Examination of cranial nerves, funduscopic examination, and observation of the patient's gait should be done. In addition, emetic injuries to the esophagus and stomach can also result from vomiting. Vomiting can lead to Mallory-Weiss lacerations and upper GI bleeding. Deeper lacerations in the esophagus can lead to free perforation (Boerhaave's syndrome). Chronic vomiting can lead to dental erosions and caries. Purpura can appear after prolonged vomiting. These are pinhead-sized red macules on the face and upper neck ("mask phenomenon"). These eruptions are probably related to suddenly increased intrathoracic pressure. Nausea and vomiting may occur in congestive heart failure from passive congestion of the liver and gut.

C. Basic laboratory tests include a CBC, ESR, electrolytes, and standard chemistry profiles. In women of childbearing age, a pregnancy test must be done. Screening for thyroid function should be done. Metabolic causes of nausea and vomiting include uremia, diabetic ketoacidosis, hyperparathyroidism, and

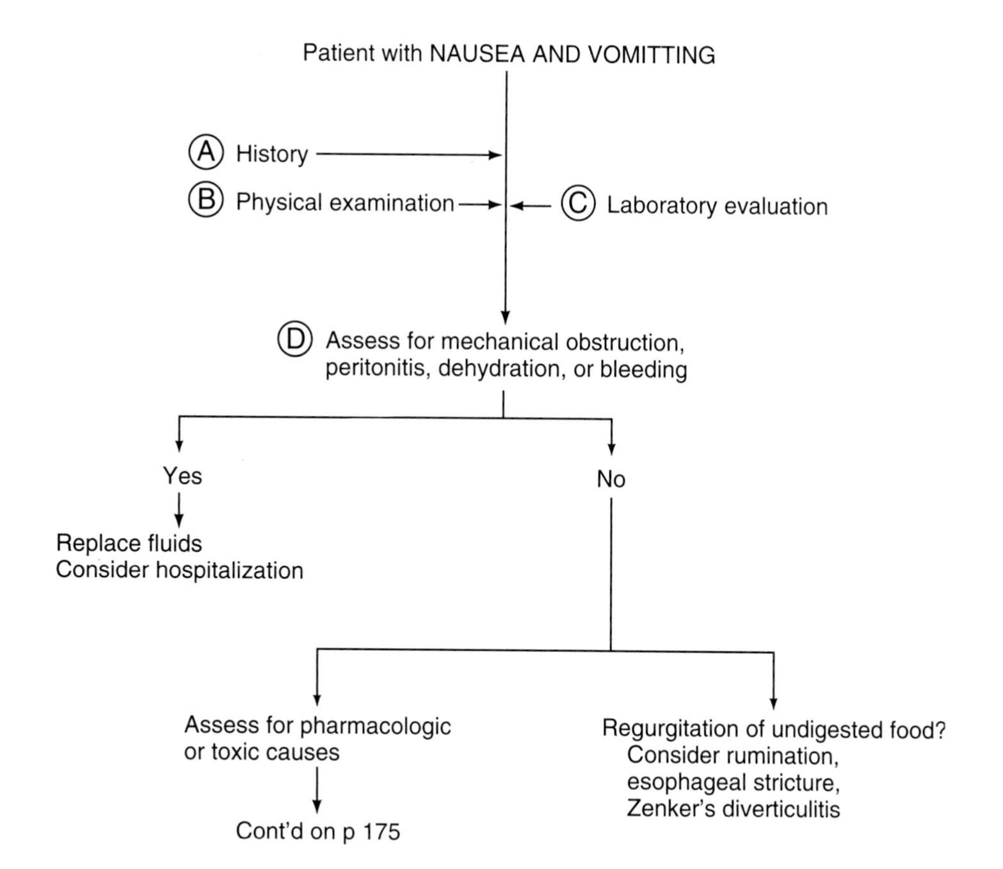

hypoparathyroidism. Serum drug levels may indicate toxicity in patients taking digoxin, theophylline, salicylates, and many other drugs. Hyponatremia on initial blood tests may be a result of Addison's disease. Metabolic derangements can also result from vomiting. Hypokalemia results from loss of potassium in the vomitus and most importantly from renal wasting from secondary hyperaldosteronism. Alkalosis also develops from loss of hydrogen ions in the vomitus, shift of extracellular hydrogen ions into cells caused by cellular potassium deficiency, and secondary hyperaldosteronism. If the clinical presentation is suggestive of mechanical obstruction, upright and supine abdominal x-rays should be obtained.

D. Recent studies suggest that CT scanning may be the technique of choice for the detection and localization of intestinal obstruction. In addition, it may also identify abdominal masses and pancreatic, hepatobiliary, or retroperitoneal pathology. Small bowel follow-through (SBFT) is accurate in the presence of high-grade obstruction but may fail to detect low-grade obstruction and smaller mucosal lesions.

(Continued on page 174)

E. All medications (both prescription and over the counter), dietary supplements, potential toxin ingestions, and environmental toxic exposures should be considered as possible etiologies.

F. Any condition associated with increased intracranial pressure can produce vomiting, with or without associated nausea, by activation of the brainstem structures mediating vomiting. Pregnancy is the most common endocrinologic cause of emesis, occurring in approximately 70% of women during the first trimester.

G. Focal lesions involving the brainstem and posterior fossa may cause and present as nausea and vomiting, as may seizure disorders and migraine. Cyclic vomiting, also referred to as "abdominal migraine," is a rare syndrome. It is characterized by discrete episodes of nausea and vomiting with asymptomatic periods in between and is often associated with migraine headaches and motion sickness. Mean age of onset is 5 years, and it demonstrates a female predominance. Cyclic vomiting has recently been reported among adults and is postulated to result from disordered pituitary prostaglandin release.

H. Electrogastrography (EGG) is performed by placing electrodes over the abdominal skin and recording the frequency and regularity of gastric myoelectrical activity in the fasting state and after a test meal. Gastric dysrhythmias have been observed in patients with idiopathic and diabetic gastroparesis, nausea of pregnancy, and motion sickness. Gastric dysrhythmias have been recorded on occasion in those with unexplained nausea and vomiting in the absence of altered gastric emptying. MRI of the brain should be considered also in those with chronic unexplained nausea and vomiting. Once common organic causes and GI dysmotility have been excluded, consider psychogenic vomiting as a possibility.

Treatment of vomiting should begin with restoration of normal fluid and electrolyte balance. If possible, underlying causes should be treated. When the specific cause of vomiting cannot be determined, antiemetic agents should be used to suppress the symptoms. Scopolamine is used as a transdermal patch principally for prophylaxis and treatment of motion sickness. However, other anticholinergic side effects are not uncommon. Antihistamine drugs with histamine 1 (H_1) receptor antagonists have central antiemetic properties. H_1 receptor antagonists (meclizine or promethazine) are useful in treatment of motion sickness and vestibular disturbances. Neuroleptic agents (e.g., prochlorperazine, chlorpromazine, and haloperidol) are effective in treating nausea and vomiting induced by medications, radiation, or gastroenteritis. Prokinetic agents that are useful in the treatment of nausea and vomiting include dopamine 2 (D_2) receptor antagonists, selective 5-HT_3 receptor antagonists, and motilin receptor agonists. Metoclopramide, a D_2 receptor antagonist, is useful in treating chemotherapy-induced emesis, gastroparesis, or pseudoobstruction. Domperidone is another selective dopamine antagonist with fewer side effects because it does not cross the blood-brain barrier. Selective 5-HT_3 receptor antagonists such as ondansetron and granisetron are effective in controlling chemotherapy-induced emesis refractory to conventional therapy. Erythromycin has been shown to accelerate gastric emptying in patients with diabetic gastroparesis. It acts on motilin receptors on GI smooth-muscle membranes; this effect is unrelated to antibiotic properties. Corticosteroids, especially dexamethasone, have been used in combination with other agents such as metoclopramide and ondansetron in the treatment of chemotherapy-related nausea and vomiting, acting perhaps by reducing prostaglandin formation. Benzodiazepines such as lorazepam and diazepam have also been shown to be effective in the treatment of chemotherapy-related nausea and vomiting. Gastric pacing can be considered in patients with intractable nausea and vomiting related to gastroparesis.

References

AGA Medical Position Statement. Nausea and vomiting. Gastroenterology 2001;120:261–262.

AGA Technical Review. Nausea and vomiting. Gastroenterology 2001;120:263–286.

Hasler WL, Chey WD. Nausea and vomiting. Gastroenterology 2003;125:1860–1867.

Lee M. Nausea and vomiting. In Feldman M, Friedman LS, Sleisenger MH. Sleisenger and Fordtran's Gastrointestinal and Liver Disease: Pathophysiology, Diagnosis and Management. 7th ed., Philadelphia: Saunders, 2002:119–129.

Quigley EM. Gastric and small intestinal motility in health and disease. Gastrenterol Clin North Am1996;25:113.

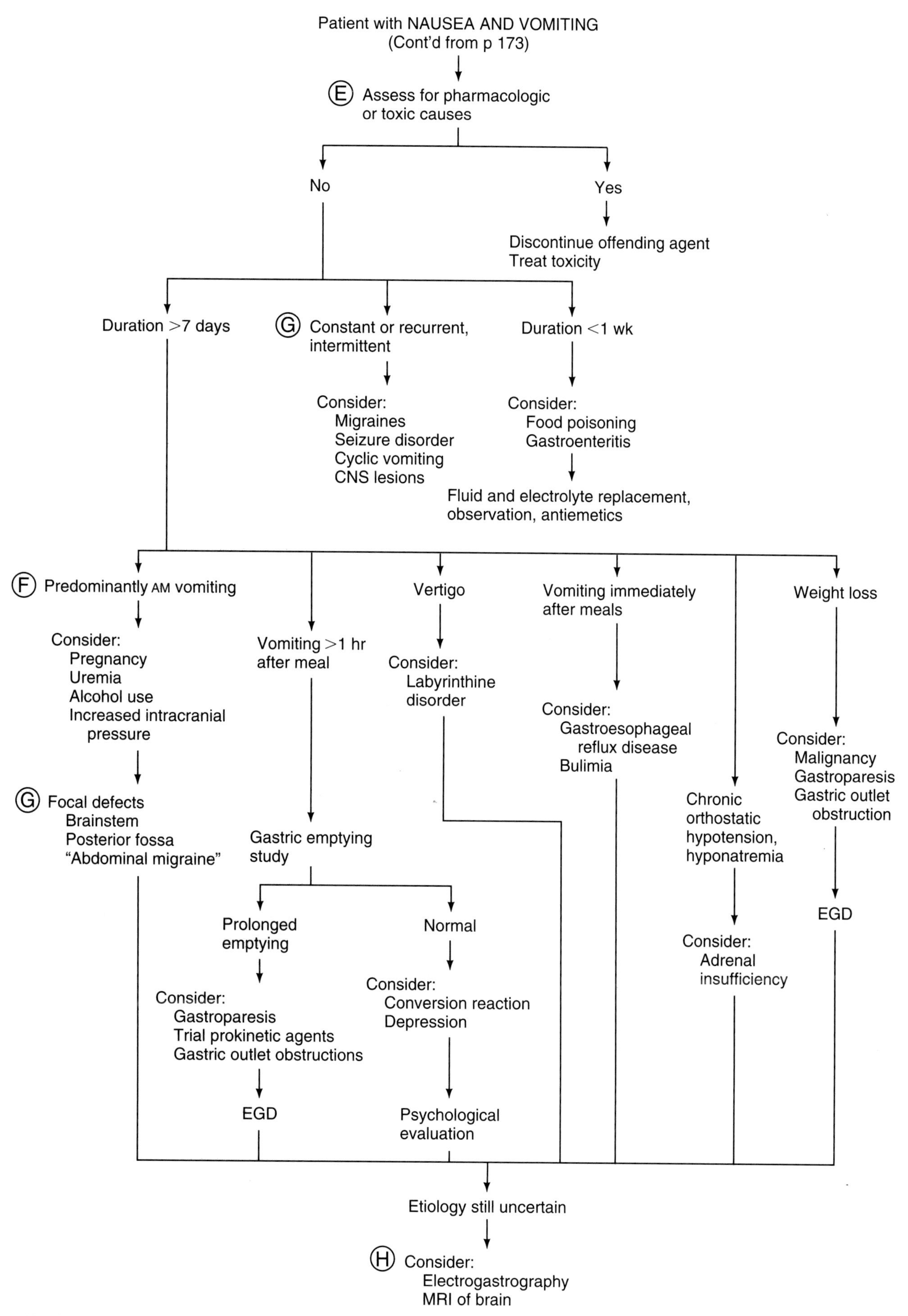

Patient with NAUSEA AND VOMITING
(Cont'd from p 173)
E Assess for pharmacologic or toxic causes
No
Yes
Discontinue offending agent
Treat toxicity
Duration >7 days
G Constant or recurrent, intermittent
Duration <1 wk
Consider:
Migraines
Seizure disorder
Cyclic vomiting
CNS lesions
Consider:
Food poisoning
Gastroenteritis
Fluid and electrolyte replacement, observation, antiemetics
F Predominantly AM vomiting
Consider:
Pregnancy
Uremia
Alcohol use
Increased intracranial pressure
G Focal defects
Brainstem
Posterior fossa
"Abdominal migraine"
Vomiting >1 hr after meal
Gastric emptying study
Prolonged emptying
Consider:
Gastroparesis
Trial prokinetic agents
Gastric outlet obstructions
EGD
Normal
Consider:
Conversion reaction
Depression
Psychological evaluation
Vertigo
Consider:
Labyrinthine disorder
Vomiting immediately after meals
Consider:
Gastroesophageal reflux disease
Bulimia
Chronic orthostatic hypotension, hyponatremia
Consider:
Adrenal insufficiency
Weight loss
Consider:
Malignancy
Gastroparesis
Gastric outlet obstruction
EGD
Etiology still uncertain
H Consider:
Electrogastrography
MRI of brain

*EGD, Esophagogastroduodenoscopy.

ANOREXIA

M. Angelo Trujillo, MD

A. Anorexia (loss of appetite) often is clinically difficult to differentiate from weight loss without an effect of appetite. However, the diagnostic considerations and workup usually are the same for both clinical problems. Perform a careful history and physical examination, including medication history, social history, and psychological screening examination. The causes of anorexia and weight loss may be divided into five major groups: (1) medical conditions, (2) psychological conditions, (3) social factors, (4) age-related factors, and (5) anorexia nervosa and related eating disorders.

B. A medication and treatment profile on patients with anorexia is of utmost importance because it can identify an easily treated cause. The medications listed are commonly associated with anorexia, especially in elderly patients. Therapeutic measures such as radiotherapy (RT) to the mouth or neck region can alter taste and smell and depress appetite.

C. Perform a head CT or MRI scan in patients who have anorexia with suspected CNS disease. Symptoms of visual disturbance, headaches, or signs of increased intracranial pressure (e.g., papilledema or cranial nerve involvement) should alert one to a potential CNS cause. Consider CNS tumors, especially hypothalamic tumors.

D. Several GI disorders can cause anorexia and/or weight loss. Malabsorption syndromes can mimic eating disorders (e.g., parasitic diseases, inflammatory bowel disease, celiac sprue, pancreatic insufficiency). Laboratory findings that can help differentiate organic disease from eating disorders are leukocytosis, steatorrhea, fever, hematochezia, and histologic or radiographic findings typical of certain GI disease states. Malignancy involving the GI tract can cause weight loss by several mechanisms: oral cavity pain or swallowing difficulty, esophageal obstruction or motility problems, gastric outlet obstruction, bowel obstruction, biliary disease, pancreatitis, mesenteric ischemia, and abdominal pain. Distant metastases of GI malignancies also can produce anorexia or weight loss by several mechanisms.

E. Social and cultural factors play an important role in the attitudes and behaviors of eating and body image. These factors are important components in the complex etiology of eating disorders. Other factors, such as difficulty with food acquisition and social isolation, can be important in some patients, especially the elderly.

F. Dementia and depression may cause significant weight loss. These are more commonly seen in the elderly and are important considerations because these disorders are potentially treatable. All cases of depression should be treated and reversible causes for dementia should be sought. Alcoholism is a common cause of anorexia and weight loss. Obtain a careful alcohol and drug abuse history in all cases.

G. Normal physiologic changes in the elderly may cause anorexia and weight loss. Hypogeusia (diminished sense of taste) and decreased olfactory function may result in food being less desirable. Visual and hearing problems may interfere with the usual mealtime socialization and may cause social isolation. Visual disorders and other physical disabilities may interfere with food preparation.

H. Anorexia nervosa and bulimia nervosa are eating disorders that affect 1%–4% of women and are rarely found in men. These disorders usually are diagnosed in the second or third decades, but reports of diagnosis in older persons are increasing. Anorexia nervosa and bulimia nervosa result from complex interactions of physiologic, psychological, and sociocultural dysfunction. Diagnostic criteria for these eating disorders used by most authors are those found in the *DSM-IV* of the American Psychiatric Association. Patient history reveals intense fear of fatness, disturbed perception of body image, and an obsessional desire to lose weight. Patients with bulimia nervosa classically have binge eating commonly associated with self-induced vomiting, abuse of cathartics or diuretics, and fear of loss of control over eating. Treatment of these disorders is complex and should follow a team approach, with a primary care physician managing medical care and coordinating treatment by psychiatric/psychological and nutritional consultants. Many medical complications may result from eating disorders; treatment of these should have priority.

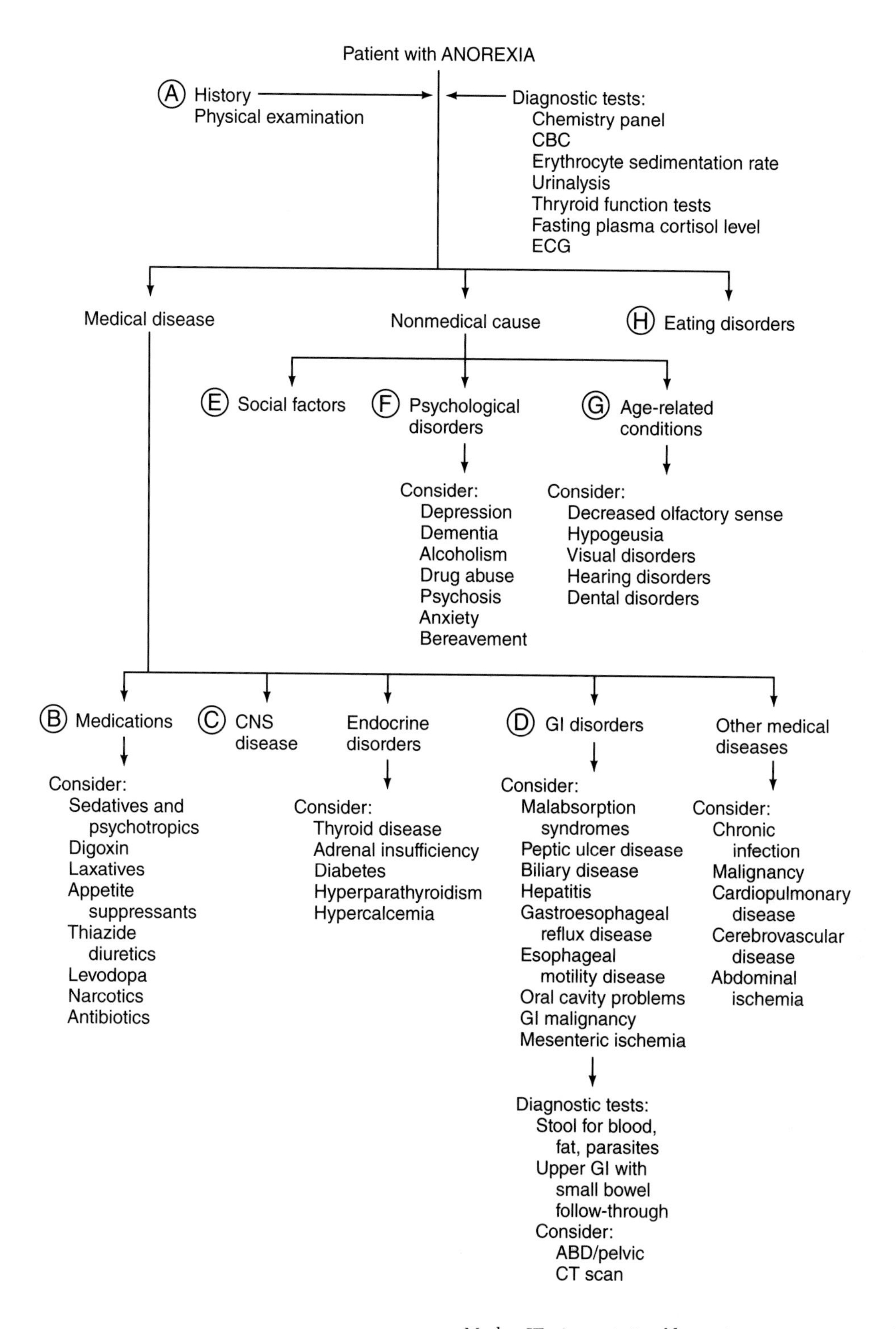

References

Comerci GD. Medical complications of anorexia nervosa and bulimia nervosa. Med Clin North Am 1990;74:1293.

Denke MA. Anorexia nervosa, bulimia nervosa, and obesity. In Sleisenger MH, Foldman M, Freidman LS, eds. Gastrointestinal and Liver Disease, 7th ed, Philadelphia: WB Saunders, 2002:310.

Morley JE. Anorexia in older patients: its meaning and management Geriatrics 1990;45:59.

Olsen-Noll EG, Bosworth MF. Anorexia and weight loss in the elderly. Postgrad Med 1989;15:140.

Rabinovitz M, Pitlik SD, Leifen M, et al. Unintentional weight loss. A retrospective analysis of 154 cases. Arch Intern Med 1986;46:186.

DYSPHAGIA

Philip E. Jaffe, MD

A. The term *dysphagia* is used to describe a sense of food sticking in the throat or difficulty swallowing. It can result from (1) abnormalities in preparing or delivering the food bolus to the esophagus (transfer or oropharyngeal dysphagia), (2) structural abnormalities of the esophagus (e.g., benign strictures, malignancy-related obstruction), (3) compression by extrinsic structures (e.g., the left atrium, aortic aneurysm, lymphadenopathy, tumors), or (4) motility disturbances of the esophagus (achalasia or diffuse esophageal spasm). Obtaining a detailed history is the first and perhaps most important step in evaluating dysphagia. Complaints isolated to solid food usually suggest esophageal obstruction, whereas liquid dysphagia is more often seen with motility disorders. Similarly, difficulty initiating a swallow or difficulty associated with nasal regurgitation in the setting of a recent cerbrovascular accident (CVA), Parkinson's disease, or amyotrophic lateral sclerosis strongly suggests a problem with oropharyngeal neuromuscular coordination. Long-standing intermittent solid food dysphagia in an otherwise healthy individual is commonly seen with benign rings, whereas new onset of progressive solid food dysphagia associated with weight loss is more often seen with malignancy or tight inflammatory strictures. Recently it has become recognized that young adults who present with food impactions may have a distinct condition (allergic eosinophilic esophagitis) that requires a high level of clinical suspicion to diagnose and treat appropriately. In patients with a history or temporal medical history to suggest an oropharyngeal or motility disorder, the evaluation may begin with a barium esophagram or modified barium swallow. Because of the relative insensitivity of barium studies in detecting esophageal mucosal disease, esophagogastroduodenoscopy (EGD) should be part of the evaluation of any patient with the complaint of dysphagia.

B. When endoscopy is performed and a specific etiology for dysphagia is determined, diagnosis-specific treatment is undertaken. Strictures may be dilated with rubber or polyethylene bougies and balloon catheters. Active esophagitis and peptic strictures are treated with antisecretory agents, including H_2-receptor antagonists and proton pump inhibitors. Occasionally severe reflux disease can cause dysphagia without anatomic obstruction. Options for treating obstructing esophageal cancers include laser photocoagulation, radiation therapy, chemotherapy, alcohol injection, and stenting. Their application depends on the extent and location of the tumor and the condition of the patient.

C. If the EGD results are normal, a motility disturbance or subtle esophageal ring should be suspected. Again, history is usually helpful, but esophageal manometry and barium esophagography with ingestion of a barium-soaked marshmallow, cookie, or pill can establish the etiology and exclude such treatable conditions as achalasia.

D. Abnormalities in the preparation and passage of the food bolus from the tongue to the pharynx and then into the esophagus (transfer dysphagia) are most commonly seen with acute CVAs or progressive neurologic disorders (see section A). The dysfunction may slowly improve over several weeks following a CVA, and temporary nasogastric feeding or placement of a gastrostomy tube may be needed. In patients with progressive neurologic disorders and oropharyngeal dysphagia, referral to a speech pathologist for specific directions on the optimal food consistency and neck position to facilitate swallowing can be useful. However, many patients will ultimately require gastrostomy tube placement for enteral feeding.

E. Abnormalities in esophageal peristalsis and lower esophageal sphincter (LES) pressure and coordination with peristalsis are known as motility disorders. Measurement of the esophageal intraluminal pressures via manometric probes may define (1) achalasia—aperistalsis of the esophageal body and incomplete LES relaxation; (2) diffuse esophageal spasm—intermittent, simultaneous contractions; (3) nutcracker esophagus—high-amplitude esophageal contractions; and (4) nonspecific motility disorder—nontransmitted, triple-peaked, or simultaneous contractions that do not meet criteria for the other defined motility disturbances. The frequent association of chest pain with liquid dysphagia in patients with motility disturbances may be the most dominant and disturbing symptom. Treatment of achalasia with forceful pneumatic balloon dilation is effective in 60%–95% of patients but is complicated by esophageal perforation in 2%–5% of cases. Botulinum toxin injection into the LES may provide a relatively short-lived but less risky alternative. Other measures, including serial traditional bougienage, nitrates, and calcium channel blockers, may provide some temporary but generally less effective relief. Surgery (Heller myotomy) provides relief in >90% of patients when performed by an experienced surgeon. The treatment of symptoms related to other motility disorders is more difficult because the effect of nitrates and calcium channel blockers is generally less consistent. Low-dose tricyclic antidepressants may provide effective symptom relief for these patients.

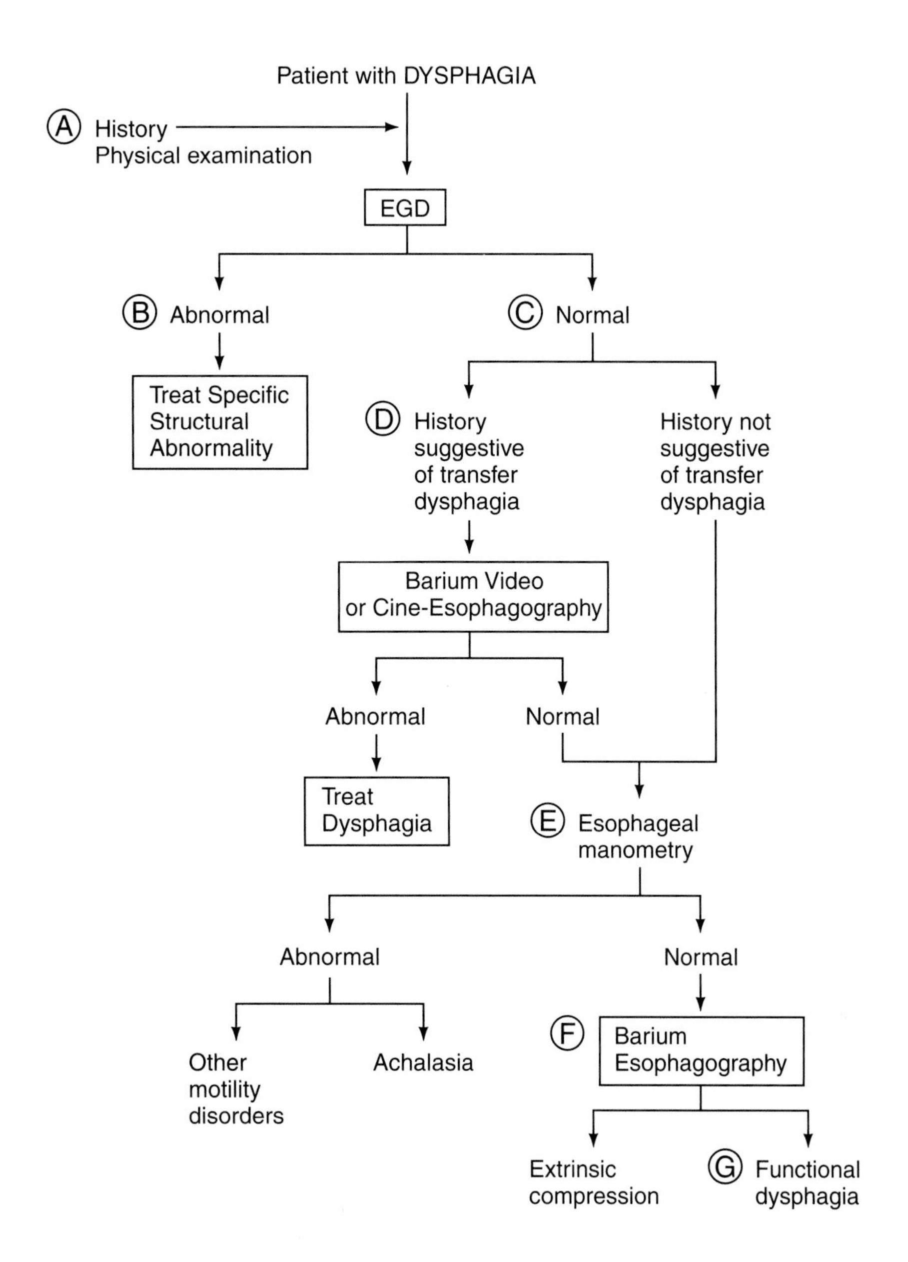

F. If esophagagoscopy and manometry are normal and symptoms persist, consider extraesophageal extrinsic compression by masses or adjacent structures. Barium esophagography may be more useful than endoscopy in this scenario. Mediastinal tumors, left atrial or thoracic aortic enlargement, and osteophytes from cervical degenerative disease are the most common causes.

G. In a substantial number of patients the evaluation yields no specific diagnosis. It is important to confirm the precise nature of symptoms to be certain the other symptoms are not being confused with true dysphagia. This would include the sense of a constant "lump in the throat" ("globus") or postinflammatory sensitivity that could create symptoms interpreted as dysphagia. In the remaining patients, the symptoms may be related to emotional or psychiatric disorders or may be part of a more complex functional gastrointestinal disturbance (global visceral sensitivity).

References

Castell D, Donner M. Evaluation of dysphagia: a careful history is crucial. Dysphagia 1987;2:65.

Gelfand M, Botoman V. Esophageal motility disorders: a clinical overview. Am J Gastroenterology 1987;82:181.

Remedios M, Campbell C, Jones D, Kerlin P. Eosinophilic esophagitis in adults: clinical, endoscopic, histologic findings, and response to treatment with fluticasone propionate. Gastrointest Endosc 2006;63:3.

Rothstein R. A systematic approach to the patient with dysphagia. Hosp Pract (Off Ed) 1997;32:169.

Scolapio J, Gostout C, Schroeder K, et al. Dysphagia without endoscopically evident disease: to dilate or not? Am J Gastroenterol 2001;96:327.

Spechler S. American Gastroenterological Association medical position statement on treatment of patients with dysphagia caused by benign disorders of the distal esophagus. Gastroenterology 1999;117:229.

Trate D, Parkman H, Fisher R. Dysphagia: evaluation, diagnosis, and treatment. Prim Care 1996;23:417.

Varadarajulu S, Eloubeidi MA, Pate RS, et al. The yield and the predictors of esophageal pathology when upper endoscopy is used for the initial evaluation of dysphagia. Gastrointest Endosc 2005;61:804.

HEARTBURN

Richard E. Sampliner, MD

A. Heartburn is the leading symptom of gastroesophageal reflux disease (GERD). It is a substernal sensation of burning that radiates orad and usually reflects the presence of gastric content in the esophagus.

B. Proton pump inhibitor (PPI) therapy is the most effective kind of therapy to relieve symptoms of GERD. At the same time PPI therapy is effective in healing the erosive esophagitis that occurs in a minority of patients who present with heartburn.

C. Step-down treatment is a way to define the lowest level of therapy that will provide symptom relief for a patient. The dose of PPI maybe reduced to every other day, or an H_2-receptor antagonist may be initiated.

D. The alarm symptoms and signs of GERD include dysphagia (difficulty swallowing), weight loss, and anemia. These findings warrant immediate endoscopy to look for complications that need prompt attention, such as esophageal stricture, esophageal ulcer, and cancer.

E. Most patients with GERD have satisfactory symptom control with PPI therapy; a subgroup require twice-daily dosing.

F. Maintenance PPI therapy is whatever dose of PPI that controls the patient's symptoms. It is often necessary to maintain a PPI indefinitely in order to control the symptoms and mucosal disease of the patient with GERD. It is important to recognize that the contemporary indication for laparoscopic fundoplication is not the failure of medical therapy but rather the symptomatic response of the patient to a PPI. Patients who are maintained on a PPI with relief but who still have residual regurgitation indicating volume reflux are appropriate candidates for laparoscopic fundoplication.

G. Initiate 24-hour pH monitoring for patients who fail PPI twice-daily therapy. The goal is to see if there is still abnormal distal esophagus acid exposure. The majority of patients will in fact have a normal 24-hour pH study. However, if the duration of low pH in the distal esophagus is still elevated, an increased dosing of the PPI is appropriate.

H. Upper endoscopy is a consideration in any patient with chronic heartburn. Even if the patient's symptoms are controlled with a PPI, the duration of heartburn should be counted from the onset of reflux symptoms through the course of PPI therapy. Patients most likely to have Barrett's esophagus, according to our current understanding, include older white males with chronic reflux. Unfortunately, we now recognize that a significant group of patients with Barrett's esophagus lack reflux symptoms.

References

Chiba N, De Gara CJ, Wilkinson JM, Hunt RH. Speed of healing and symptom relief in grade II to IV gastroesophageal reflux disease: a meta-analysis. Gastroenterology 1997;112:1798–1810.

DeVault KR, Castell DO. Updated guidelines for the diagnosis and treatment of gastroesophageal reflux disease. Am J Gastroenterol. 2005; 190:100–200.

Klinkenberg-Knol EC, Nelis F, Dent J, et al. Long-term omeprazole treatment in resistant gastroesophageal reflux disease: efficacy, safety, and influence on gastric mucosa. Gastroenterology 2000;118(4): 661–669.

Lundell L, Miettinen P, Myrvoid HE, et al. Continued (5-year) followup of a randomized clinical study comparing antireflux surgery and omeprazole in gastroesophageal reflux disease. J Am Coll Surg 2001;192:172–179.

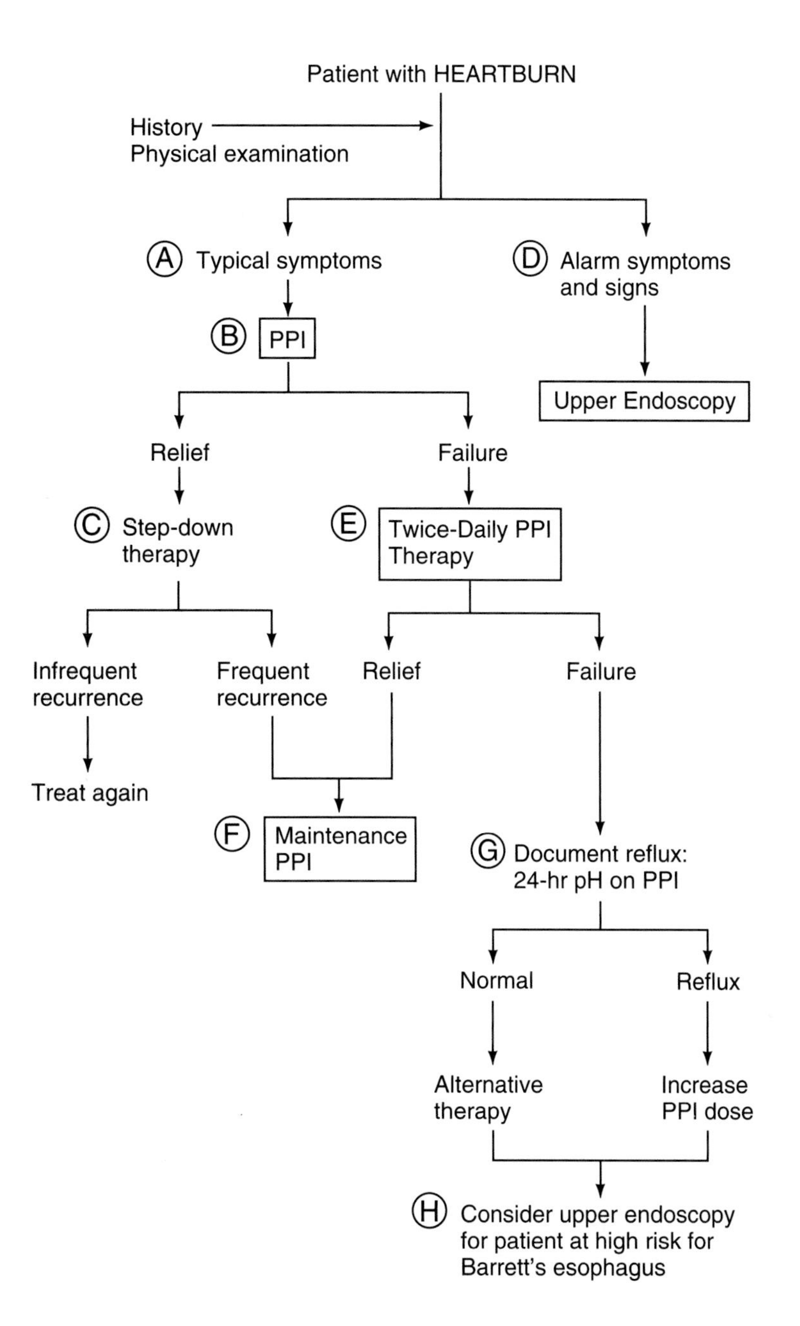
Patient with HEARTBURN
History
Physical examination
A Typical symptoms
D Alarm symptoms and signs
B PPI
Upper Endoscopy
Relief
Failure
C Step-down therapy
E Twice-Daily PPI Therapy
Infrequent recurrence
Frequent recurrence
Relief
Failure
Treat again
F Maintenance PPI
G Document reflux: 24-hr pH on PPI
Normal
Reflux
Alternative therapy
Increase PPI dose
H Consider upper endoscopy for patient at high risk for Barrett's esophagus

NONCARDIAC CHEST PAIN

M. Brian Fennerty, MD

A. Chest pain causes anxiety because of the possibility of cardiac disease. Coronary disease should be excluded before investigating esophageal causes of chest pain. Although microvascular angina is possible with normal coronary arteries, it is not common. More than 600,000 patients a year undergo cardiac catheterization, and one third have normal coronary arteries. Thus, >150,000 patients per year may require evaluation for noncardiac chest pain. Esophageal disorders may cause cardiac-type chest pain in up to 50% of these patients. Associated symptoms of dysphagia, odynophagia, or heartburn are suggestive of an esophageal source but are often absent.

B. Endoscopy is often used initially to exclude structural or mucosal abnormalities such as erosive esophagitis, esophageal strictures/tumors, achalasia, hiatal hernia, and gastric ulcers. Although the diagnostic yield is low, this can be an important test for excluding complicated esophageal disease.

C. Of patients with normal coronary arteries and cardiac chest pain, 35%–50% have gastroesophageal reflux disease (GERD). This may or may not be manifested by erosive esophagitis. Therefore, a normal endoscopic result does not exclude reflux, and reflux may cause cardiac-type chest pain without symptoms of dysphagia or heartburn. In addition, acid perfusion of the esophagus not only lowers the threshold for myocardial ischemia but may induce this condition. The most sensitive test for documenting GERD is ambulatory pH monitoring, which allows correlation of chest pain events with reflux events. Another commonly used "diagnostic" test is a 2- to 4-week therapeutic trial with a proton pump inhibitor (omeprazole or lansoprazole) at a high dosage. Resolution of chest pain implies that it was caused by acid (e.g., reflux); appropriate therapy can then be prescribed, although the accuracy of this test has recently been questioned. An etiologic association can be assumed if cardiac-type chest pain is temporally related to reflux. Unfortunately, pH monitoring is not widely available.

D. Motility disorders of the esophagus account for cardiac-type chest pain in 5%–38% of patients evaluated in noncardiac chest pain series. Manometry measures the pressure and function of the lower esophageal sphincter and the motility of the esophageal body. Most motility abnormalities are intermittent and may be missed during manometry. In addition, the motility abnormality rarely is accompanied by chest pain during the study. High-pressure peristaltic contractions (nutcracker esophagus) are the most common motility disorder diagnosed in patients with chest pain (up to 30%), followed by nonspecific motility disorders (20%–30%), diffuse esophageal spasm (5%–10%), and achalasia (2%–3%). Unless chest pain occurs with the observed motility disturbance, causation cannot be assumed.

E. If motility testing is nonspecific or nondiagnostic, provocative testing may be done. Provocative testing is based on the hypothesis that the esophagus is hypersensitive to normal or physiologic stimuli and that chest pain is simply an altered or heightened perception of these stimuli. Most patients with noncardiac chest pain have personality traits similar to those of patients with irritable bowel syndrome (i.e., they are anxious, depressed, hypochondriacal, and neurotic), and one third meet diagnostic criteria for panic disorder. Provocative tests include perfusing the distal esophagus with acid (Bernstein test), intravenous infusion of a cholinergic agent (Tensilar), or inflation of a balloon in the esophagus (balloon distention). Reproduction of cardiac-type pain is considered diagnostic of an esophageal source of the pain.

References

Browning TH. Diagnosis of chest pain of esophageal origin: a guideline of the Patient Care Committee of the American Gastrointestinal Organization. Dig Dis Sci 1990;35:289.

Cannon RO, Cattau LE, Yokshe PN, et al. Coronary flow reserve, esophageal motility, and chest pain in patients with angiographically normal coronary arteries. Am J Med 1990;88:217.

Just RJ, Castell DO. Chest pain of undetermined origin. Gastrointest Endosc Clin N Am 1994;4:731.

Katz PO, Dalton CB, Richter JE, et al. Esophageal testing of patients with noncardiac chest pain or dysphagia: results of three years' experience with 1161 patients. Ann Intern Med 1987;106:593.

Lieberman D. Noncardiac chest pain: there's often an esophageal cause. Postgrad Med 1989;86:207.

Numans ME, Lau J, de Wit NJ, et al. Short-term treatment with proton-pump inhibitors as a test for gastroesophageal reflux disease: a meta-analysis of diagnostic test characteristics. Ann Intern Med 2004;140:518–527.

Richter JE, Bradley LA, Castell DO. Esophageal chest pain: current controversies in pathogenesis, diagnosis and therapy. Ann Intern Med 1989;100:66.

Voskuil JH, Cramer MJ, Breumelhof R, et al. Prevalence of esophageal disorders in patients with chest pain newly referred to the cardiologist. Chest 1996;109:1210.

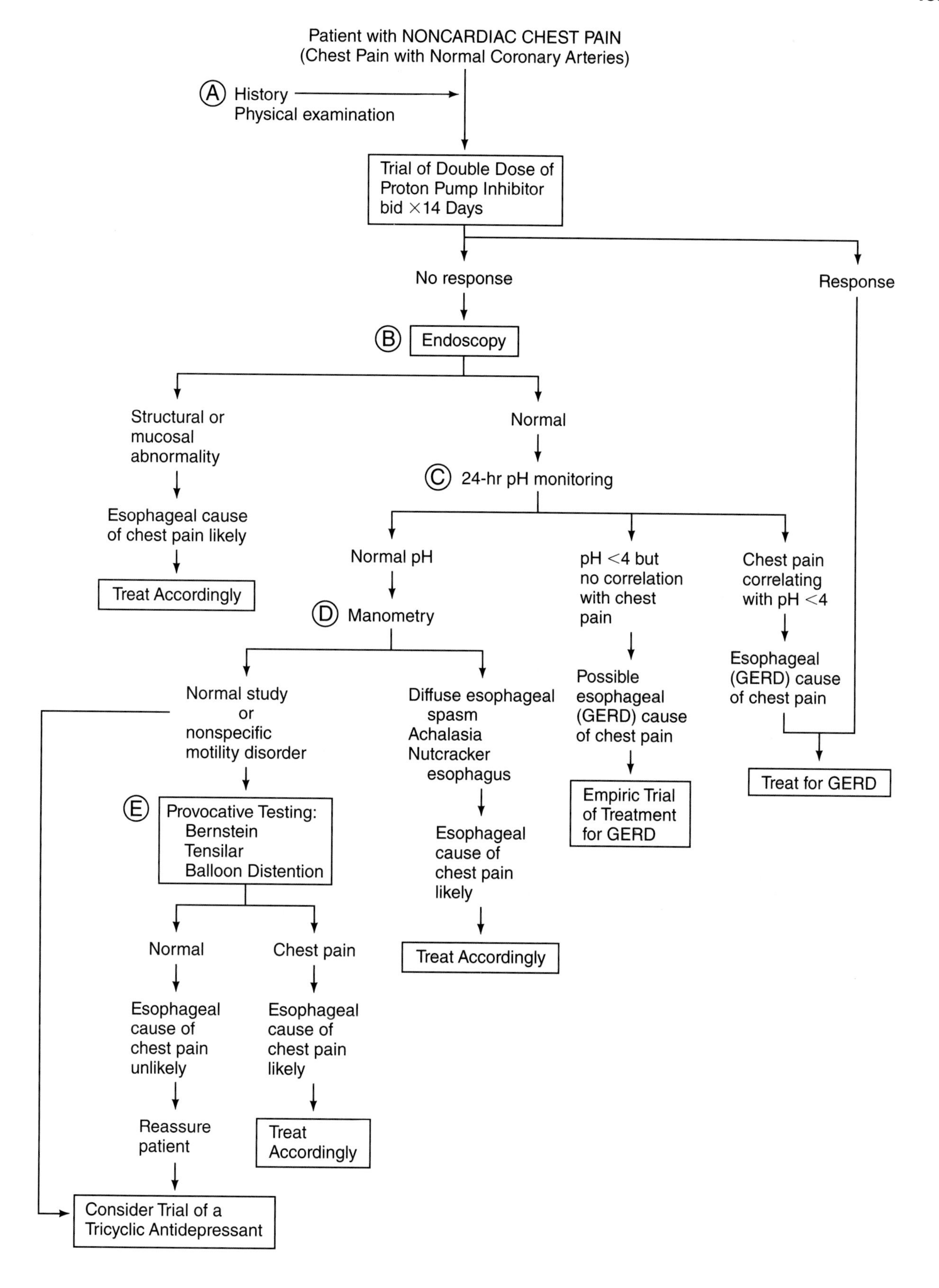

Patient with NONCARDIAC CHEST PAIN
(Chest Pain with Normal Coronary Arteries)
A
History
Physical examination
Trial of Double Dose of Proton Pump Inhibitor bid ×14 Days
No response
Response
B
Endoscopy
Structural or mucosal abnormality
Esophageal cause of chest pain likely
Treat Accordingly
Normal
C
24-hr pH monitoring
Normal pH
D
Manometry
pH <4 but no correlation with chest pain
Possible esophageal (GERD) cause of chest pain
Empiric Trial of Treatment for GERD
Chest pain correlating with pH <4
Esophageal (GERD) cause of chest pain
Treat for GERD
Normal study or nonspecific motility disorder
E
Provocative Testing: Bernstein Tensilar Balloon Distention
Diffuse esophageal spasm Achalasia Nutcracker esophagus
Esophageal cause of chest pain likely
Treat Accordingly
Normal
Esophageal cause of chest pain unlikely
Reassure patient
Chest pain
Esophageal cause of chest pain likely
Treat Accordingly
Consider Trial of a Tricyclic Antidepressant

BELCHING

Gregory L. Eastwood, MD

A. *Belching, burping*, and *eructation* have roughly the same meaning and refer to the passage of gas from the stomach or esophagus through the mouth. In some patients, belching is the only symptom. In others, belching may be accompanied by abdominal discomfort, chest pain, or the passage of excess flatus. All people swallow air in variable amounts, and all people belch from time to time.

B. Most patients who complain of belching swallow excess amounts of air. In fact, they may unwittingly take air into the esophagus before each belch that then is eructated. This practice may be associated with psychological stress or is thought by some patients to relieve other abdominal symptoms. Some patients may improve simply by being made aware of the cause of belching and given reassurance that they are otherwise well. Avoidance of gum chewing and carbonated beverages also is helpful.

C. Occasionally, belching is a sign of organic disease. If the gastric outlet is obstructed partially by peptic disease or carcinoma, swallowed air cannot pass into the bowel and eructation may develop, sometimes accompanied by abdominal pain and vomiting. For unexplained reasons, patients who have symptomatic gallstones may complain of belching. Finally, belching of feculent-smelling gas may indicate prolonged gastric stasis or a gastrocolic fistula that has developed from a carcinoma of the stomach or transverse colon.

D. Upper GI x-ray series or upper GI endoscopy is used to evaluate the stomach for partial gastric outlet obstruction and in rare cases may indicate a gastrocolic fistula complicating a gastric carcinoma. In general, because gastric outlet obstruction or a carcinoma that is large enough to erode into the colon is likely to be diagnosed by an upper GI x-ray series, that study is the appropriate first step in the diagnostic evaluation of belching. However, in some patients with peptic disease who have a small ulcer or have erosions and gastritis, the upper GI x-ray series may be nondiagnostic. In these patients, an upper GI endoscopy may be necessary to confirm the diagnosis.

E. The diagnosis of gallstones and gallbladder disease usually is made by ultrasonography of the upper abdomen.

F. Perform a barium enema if the patient belches foul-smelling gas and if the question of a gastrocolic fistula remains after a nondiagnostic upper GI x-ray series or endoscopy.

G. Testing gut motor function may help diagnose a motility disorder, neuropathy, or systemic disease, such as scleroderma.

References

American Gastroenterological Association website. Gas in the Digestive Tract. www.gastro.org.

Azpiroz F. Intestinal gas dynamics: mechanisms and clinical relevance. Gut 2005;54:893.

Hasler WL. Approach to the patient with gas and bloating. In Yamada T, Alpers DH, Kaplowitz N, et al, eds. Textbook of Gastroenterology, 4th ed. Philadelphia: Lippincott Williams & Wilkins, 2003:802.

Rao SS. Belching, bloating, and flatulence. How to help patients who have troublesome abdominal gas. Postgrad Med 1997;101:275.

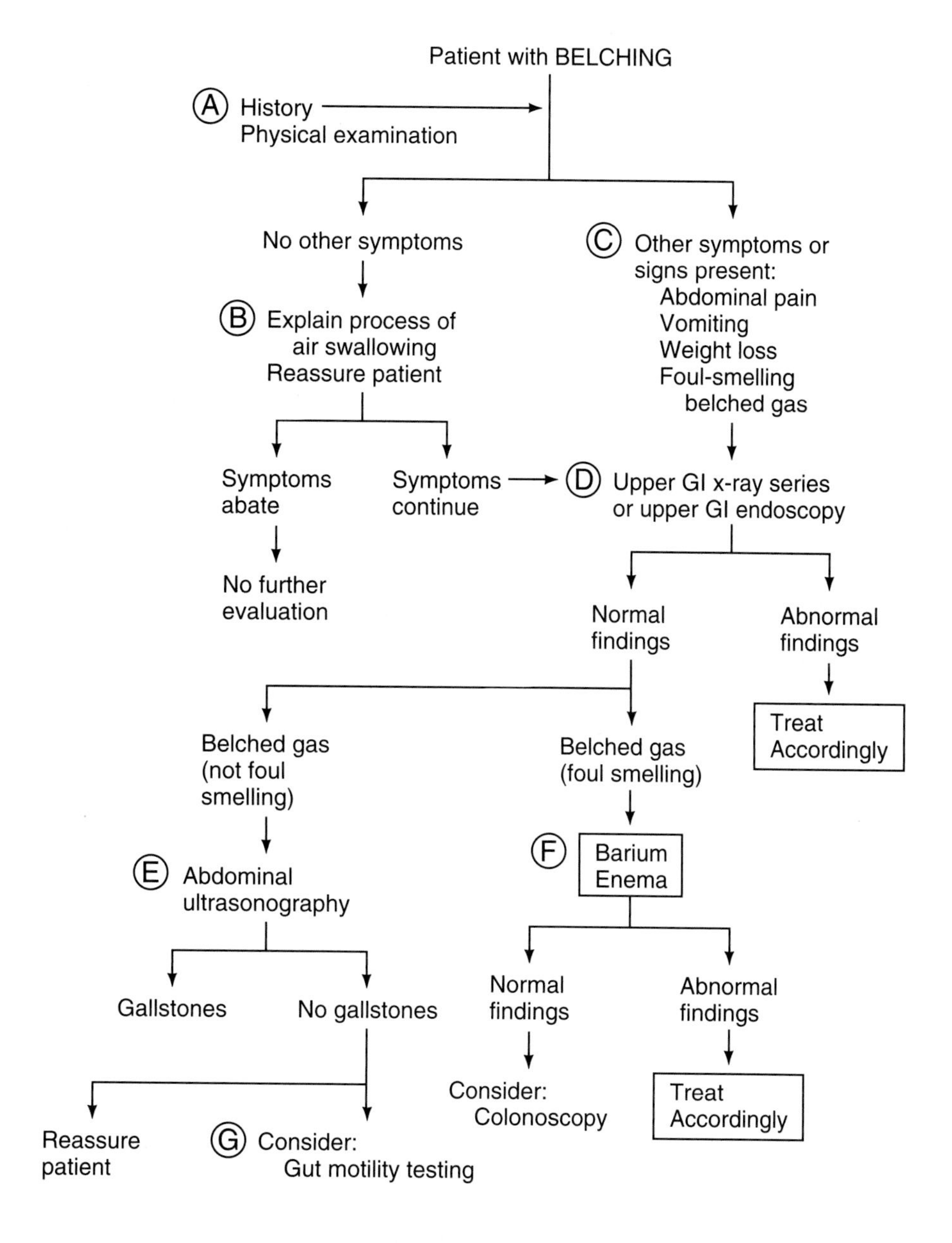
Patient with BELCHING
A History
Physical examination
No other symptoms
C Other symptoms or signs present:
Abdominal pain
Vomiting
Weight loss
Foul-smelling belched gas
B Explain process of air swallowing
Reassure patient
Symptoms abate
Symptoms continue
D Upper GI x-ray series or upper GI endoscopy
No further evaluation
Normal findings
Abnormal findings
Treat Accordingly
Belched gas (not foul smelling)
Belched gas (foul smelling)
F Barium Enema
E Abdominal ultrasonography
Gallstones
No gallstones
Normal findings
Abnormal findings
Consider: Colonoscopy
Treat Accordingly
Reassure patient
G Consider: Gut motility testing

DYSPEPSIA

Bipin Saud, MD, and Juan Diego Baltodano, MD

A. Dyspepsia is defined as chronic or recurrent pain or discomfort centered in the upper abdomen, mainly in or around the midline as opposed to the right or left hypochondrium (Rome II criteria). Discomfort is characterized by or associated with fullness, early satiety, bloating, or nausea. Dyspepsia may or may not be related to eating meals. The annual prevalence of recurrent dyspepsia is approximately 25% over a 3- to 12-month period. If frequent heartburn is included in dyspeptic symptoms, the prevalence exceeds 40%.

The physical examination is usually normal except for mild epigastric tenderness. Examination should assess for GI blood loss, jaundice, abdominal mass or organomegaly, and signs of malabsorption. Screening laboratory tests include CBC and general biochemistries, including liver function tests and amylase. Additional studies may include stool inspection for parasites, abdominal radiography (for obstruction, calcifications), and gastroduodenal motility studies.

Dyspepsia can be caused by a number of disorders. Functional (idiopathic) dyspepsia, also referred to as nonulcer dyspepsia, accounts for up to 60% of cases. Gastroduodenal ulcer disease is found in approximately 15%–25% of patients with dyspepsia but cannot be accurately distinguished from functional dyspepsia based on the symptom pattern. Atypical gastroesophageal reflux disease accounts for 5%–15% of cases. The presence of gastroesophageal reflux disease (GERD) is important to identify because the treatment of this disorder differs from the treatment of other causes of dyspepsia. Gastric or esophageal cancer is present in <2% of cases with dyspepsia. Biliary tract disease is a rare cause of chronic dyspepsia. Association between gallstones and dyspepsia should be made cautiously to avoid unnecessary cholecystectomy because gallstones may silently coexist in patients with dyspepsia.

B. NSAIDs can cause dyspepsia, and their use should be discontinued. Other medications that commonly cause dyspepsia include potassium supplements, iron, antibiotics (especially macrolides, sulfonamides, metronidazole), digitalis, corticosteroids, niacin, gemfibrozil, narcotics, colchicine, quinidine, estrogens, and theophylline.

C. Gastroesophageal malignancy is an uncommon cause of chronic dyspepsia. In addition to age older than 45–55 years, alarm symptoms such as weight loss, persistent vomiting, dysphagia, anemia, hematemesis, palpable abdominal mass, family history of upper GI carcinoma, and previous gastric surgery raise the suspicion of gastric malignancy and should lead to prompt endoscopy. Referral for upper endoscopy is always indicated in older patients presenting with new-onset dyspepsia.

D. It is recommended that young patients with dyspepsia without any alarm features undergo a noninvasive *Helicobacter pylori* test such as *H. pylori* breath or stool test. The rationale for testing for *H. pylori* in patients with dyspepsia is based on peptic ulcer disease as the etiology of a minority of cases of chronic dyspepsia. If *H. pylori* infection is present, then an empiric trial of *H. pylori* eradication treatment is recommended. A 2- to 4-week trial of an antisecretory agent is recommended for patients with negative *H. pylori* results. Endoscopy is recommended for all patients whose symptoms persist or who relapse after empirical therapy.

(Continued on page 188)

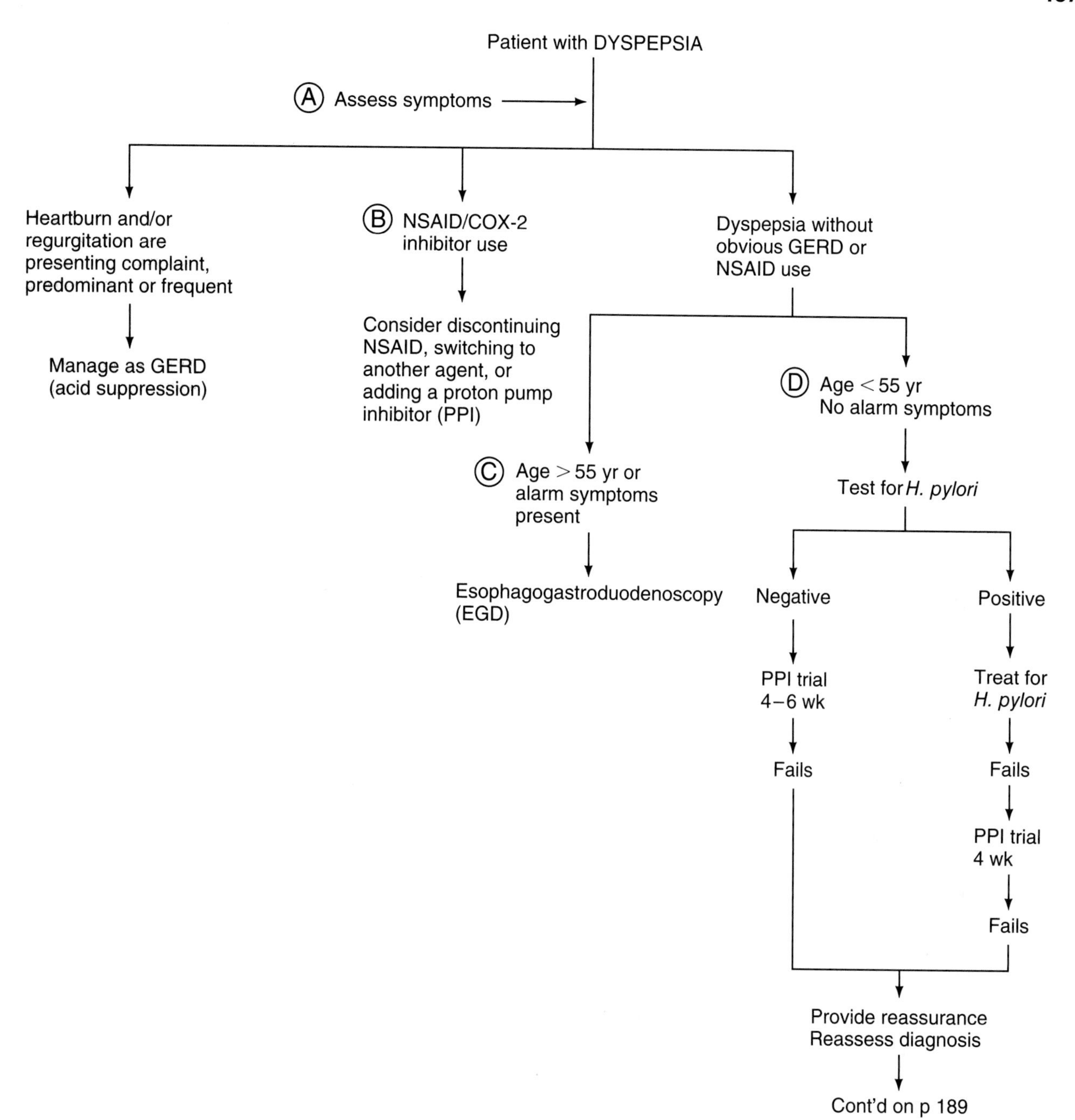
Patient with DYSPEPSIA
A Assess symptoms
Heartburn and/or regurgitation are presenting complaint, predominant or frequent
Manage as GERD (acid suppression)
B NSAID/COX-2 inhibitor use
Consider discontinuing NSAID, switching to another agent, or adding a proton pump inhibitor (PPI)
Dyspepsia without obvious GERD or NSAID use
C Age > 55 yr or alarm symptoms present
Esophagogastroduodenoscopy (EGD)
D Age < 55 yr No alarm symptoms
Test for H. pylori
Negative
Positive
PPI trial 4–6 wk
Treat for H. pylori
Fails
Fails
PPI trial 4 wk
Fails
Provide reassurance Reassess diagnosis
Cont'd on p 189

E. Patients who fail to respond to empiric therapeutic approaches should also undergo endoscopy. The majority of patients will be diagnosed as having functional dyspepsia. These patients may respond to reassurance and if necessary a course of antisecretory or prokinetic therapy. If symptoms persist, other treatments may include behavioral therapy, psychotherapy, or antidepressant therapy.

F. Functional dyspepsia, the most common type of dyspepsia encountered in clinical practice, is defined as follows: at least 12 weeks, which need not be consecutive, within the preceding 12 months of (1) persistent or recurrent dyspepsia (pain or discomfort and centered in the upper abdomen); (2) no evidence of organic disease (including upper GI endoscopic examination) that is likely to explain symptoms; and (3) no evidence that dyspepsia is exclusively relieved by defecation or associated with the onset of a change in stool frequency or stool form (i.e., not irritable bowel syndrome [IBS]).

References

Malfertheiner P, Mégraud F, O'Morain C, et al. Current concepts in the management of *Helicobacter pylori* infection—The Maasstricht 2-2000 Consensus Report. Aliment Pharmacol Ther 2002;16:167.

Ofman JJ, Rabe Neck L. The effectiveness of endoscopy in the management of dyspepsia: a qualitative systematic review. Am J Med 1999;106:335.

Talley NJ, American Gastroenterological Association. American Gastroenterological Association medical position statement: evaluation of dyspepsia. Gastroenterology 2005;129:1753–1755.

Talley NY, Stanghellini V, Heading RC, et al. Functional gastroduodenal disorders. Gut 1999;45(suppl 2):II37–II42.

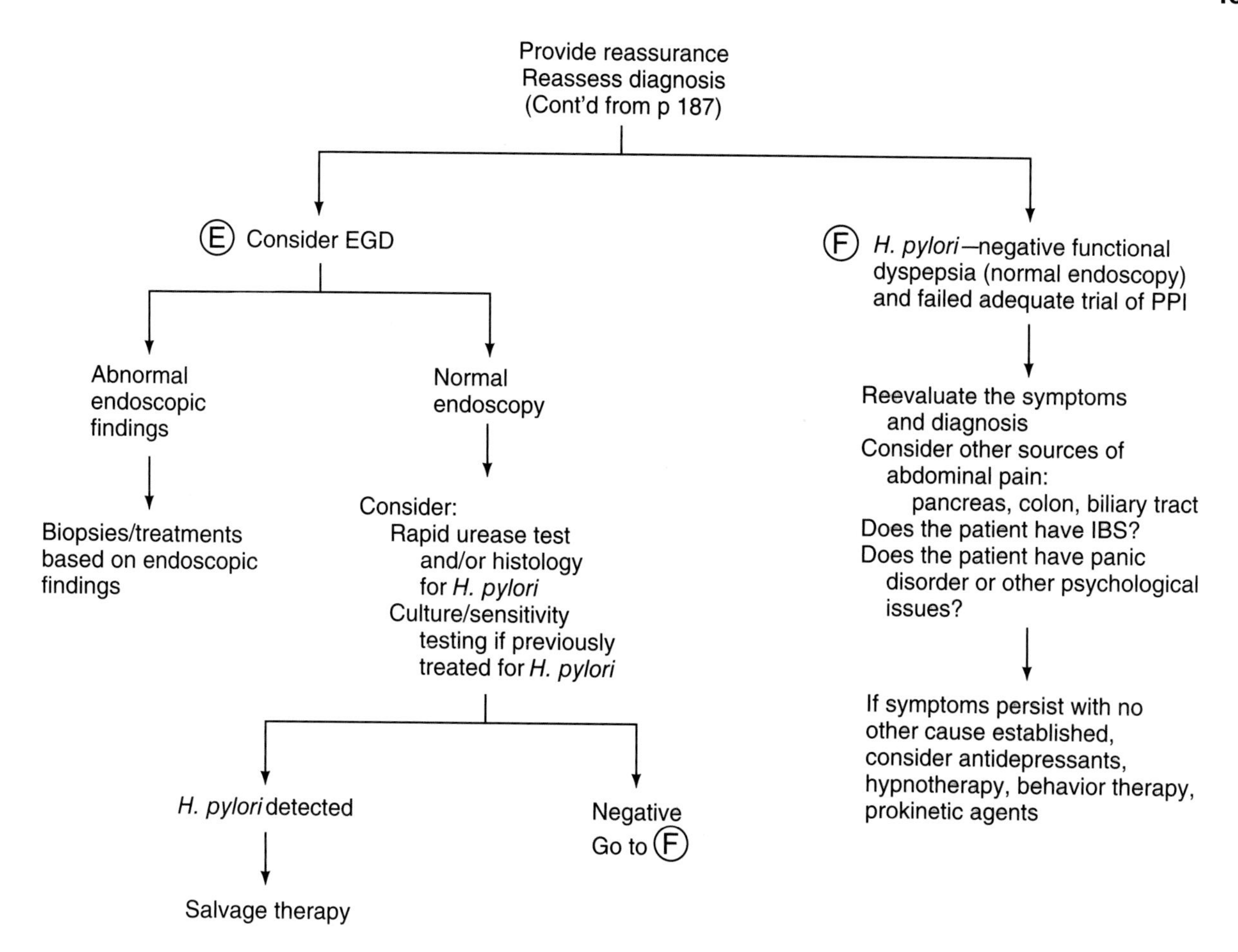
Provide reassurance
Reassess diagnosis
(Cont'd from p 187)
E Consider EGD
Abnormal endoscopic findings
Biopsies/treatments based on endoscopic findings
Normal endoscopy
Consider:
Rapid urease test and/or histology for H. pylori
Culture/sensitivity testing if previously treated for H. pylori
H. pylori detected
Salvage therapy
Negative
Go to F
F H. pylori—negative functional dyspepsia (normal endoscopy) and failed adequate trial of PPI
Reevaluate the symptoms and diagnosis
Consider other sources of abdominal pain:
pancreas, colon, biliary tract
Does the patient have IBS?
Does the patient have panic disorder or other psychological issues?
If symptoms persist with no other cause established, consider antidepressants, hypnotherapy, behavior therapy, prokinetic agents

JAUNDICE

Juan Diego Baltodano, MD, and Bipin Saud, MD

Jaundice is defined as the presence of yellow discoloration of the skin, sclerae, and mucous membranes. This clinical finding results from an elevated serum bilirubin concentration. In general, jaundice is not evident until serum bilirubin concentration exceeds 3 mg/dl. A sequential approach for the diagnosis of jaundice is recommended, which should include a careful history, physical examination, and screening laboratory studies. Once a differential diagnosis is formulated, adequate testing should be directed toward establishing a possible diagnosis.

A. A detailed history must include an assessment of patients' risks factors for intrinsic liver disease, active systemic and abdominal symptoms, medications (including herbs and over-the-counter medications), alcohol consumption, comorbid conditions, prior biliary surgery, and the presence of hereditary liver disease. Physical examination may reveal clues toward a specific condition. For example, high fever or right upper quadrant tenderness suggests cholangitis. Also a palpable gallbladder or a mass may indicate obstructive jaundice from a neoplasm. Intrinsic liver disease is suggested by the presence of ascites; splenomegaly; prominent abdominal veins (consistent with portal hypertension); and signs of chronic liver disease such as spider angiomas, asterixis, and gynecomastia. Initial laboratory studies include serum aspartate and alanine aminotransferase levels (AST, ALT), alkaline phosphatase levels, prothrombin time, albumin levels, and CBC. It is not possible to differentiate intrahepatic from extrahepatic cholestasis on the basis of the serum level of alkaline phosphatase.

B. Initial evaluation of hyperbilirubinemia should determine whether the process is secondary to conjugated (direct) or unconjugated (indirect) bilirubin predominance. In isolated and asymptomatic mild elevation of unconjugated bilirubin, the patient should be evaluated for hemolytic disorders, hereditary disorders of bilirubin metabolism such as Gilbert's or Crigler-Najjar syndrome, and medication-induced disorders (e.g., rifampin).

C. An increase in conjugated bilirubin concentration with abnormal levels of aminotransferases and/or alkaline phosphatase may result from either a hepatocellular cause or the presence of extrahepatic biliary obstruction.

D. Hepatic imaging often complements the findings of the patient's history, physical examination, laboratory studies, and overall clinical presentation. Imaging studies are indicated to confirm the presence or the absence of biliary obstruction. Different accepted modalities to evaluate the biliary system include ultrasonography, CT scan of the abdomen, magnetic resonance cholangiopancreatography (MRCP), endoscopic ultrasonography, endoscopic retrograde cholangiopancreatography (ERCP), and percutaneous transhepatic cholangiography (PTC). Nuclear imaging of the biliary tree that measures hepatic uptake of radiolabeled derivatives of iminodiacetic acid (e.g., HIDA) is not sensitive enough to justify its use in the evaluation of jaundice.

Even if the clinical suspicion for biliary obstruction is thought to be low, evaluating liver parenchyma is as important as excluding that remote possibility of biliary obstruction. In that case, obtaining a CT scan or ultrasound of the abdomen might be an appropriate diagnostic tool. However, if dilated bile ducts are seen, direct imaging modalities such as MRCP, ERCP, or PTC should be obtained. Altogether, the sensitivity and specificity of these tests is 89%–100%.

E. If there is no clinical evidence of biliary obstruction, evaluation for underlying liver disease is mandatory. Obtain the appropriate screening studies, including viral serologies (hepatitis B and C, acute hepatitis A), serum levels of iron, transferrin saturation and ferritin (for hemochromatosis), antimitochondrial antibodies (for primary biliary cirrhosis), antinuclear antibodies, anti–smooth-muscle antibodies and serum electrophoresis (for autoimmune hepatitis), and alpha-1-antitrypsin activity (alpha-1-antitrypsin deficiency). A liver biopsy may be needed to confirm a diagnosis if the previously mentioned serology testing is negative.

F. Once a biliary obstruction is established, therapy is directed toward the relief of the mechanical obstruction. Available endoscopic and radiologic therapies include sphincterotomy, balloon dilation, and stents and drains placement. The optimal strategy depends on the location and the type of obstructing lesion.

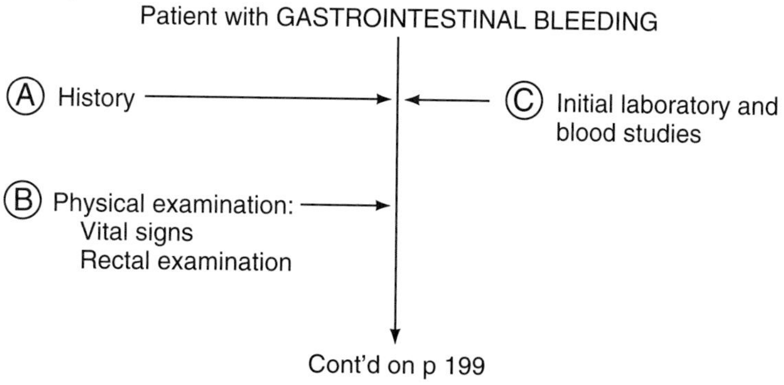

Patient with GASTROINTESTINAL BLEEDING

Ⓐ History

Ⓑ Physical examination:
Vital signs
Rectal examination

Ⓒ Initial laboratory and blood studies

Cont'd on p 199

Table 1 **Diagnostic Considerations in GI Bleeding**

Upper GI Bleeding

Nose, pharynx, or lungs (swallowed)
Esophagogastric mucosal tear (Mallory-Weiss)
Esophageal rupture (Boerhaave's syndrome)
Erosions (esophagitis, gastritis, or duodenitis)
Ulcer (esophagus, stomach, duodenum, or anastomosis)
Dieulafoy's lesion (ruptured mucosal artery)
Angiomas
Varices (esophagus, stomach, or duodenum)
Neoplasm (carcinoma, lymphoma, leiomyoma, leiomyosarcoma, polyps)
Hemobilia
Vascular-enteric fistula (usually aortic aneurysm or graft)

"Middle" GI Bleeding

Presents as either upper or lower GI bleeding
Results from small bowel lesions, such as
 Tumors
 Crohn's disease
 Vascular-enteric fistulas

Lower GI Bleeding

Hemorrhoids
Inflammatory bowel disease (Crohn's disease, ulcerative colitis)
Neoplasm (carcinoma or polyp)
Diverticulosis
Ischemic enteritis or colitis
Angiodysplasia/arteriovenous malformations
Antibiotic-associated colitis
Radiation enteritis or colitis
Amyloidosis
Meckel's diverticulum
Vascular-enteric fistula
NSAID-associated ulcers
Brisk upper GI bleeding

and hematocrit (Hct) are attributable to blood loss, but some patients bleed so rapidly that blood volume has had insufficient time to equilibrate, resulting in normal or only slightly reduced Hgb and Hct. In patients who are actively bleeding, changes in BP and pulse and direct evidence of continued bleeding via nasogastric (NG) tube or per rectum are better indicators of the need to administer electrolyte solutions or replace blood.

Determination of platelet count and clotting factors is important so that abnormalities can be corrected promptly. Extensive blood transfusion dilutes platelets and clotting factors. Also, many patients who bleed while taking therapeutic anticoagulants do so from a clinically significant lesion. Acute GI bleeding may be associated with a modest elevation of WBC count, but usually not more than 15,000/mm^3, so do not attribute leukocytosis to blood loss without considering sources of infection. BUN may increase in upper GI bleeding as a result of absorption of nitrogenous products of blood in the small intestine or as a result of hypovolemia. In patients with marginal liver function, the increased protein load from blood in the gut may induce or aggravate hepatic encephalopathy; gastric lavage and control of bleeding are particularly important in the treatment of these patients.

Table 2 **Prognostic Indicators in GI Bleeding**

Volume of blood loss
Associated medical conditions
Ingestion of mucosal irritants
Age >60 years
Abdominal or pelvic irradiation
Recurrent bleeding
Stigmata of recent hemorrhage in an ulcer

D. For initial management promptly insert a large-bore IV catheter into a peripheral vein; sometimes two IV catheters are needed if bleeding is profuse. If a peripheral vein is not available, use a jugular, subclavian, or femoral vein. A central venous pressure catheter may be useful to evaluate the effects of volume and blood replacement, particularly in the elderly or those with cardiovascular disease. Rapidly infuse normal saline until blood is available. In patients with excess body sodium, such as those with ascites or edema, restoration of intravascular volume takes precedence over concern for sodium overload.

E. Pass an NG tube in every patient with melena or hematemesis. Blood from the esophagus or stomach pools in the stomach, and in >90% of bleeding duodenal ulcers, blood refluxes into the stomach. If the NG aspirate is clear or clears promptly with lavage, the tube may be removed. If there is a large amount of blood or retained material, lavage the stomach with a large-bore tube. Removal of gastric contents facilitates subsequent endoscopy and decompresses the stomach. Because the NG tube is uncomfortable for the patient, predisposes to gastroesophageal reflux and pulmonary aspiration, and may irritate the esophagus or stomach, remove it when it is no longer useful.

F. Upper GI endoscopy or colonoscopy may reveal a specific bleeding site that indicates specific treatment, such as ligation or sclerosis of esophageal varices. Endoscopic treatment of bleeding lesions includes thermal electrocoagulation; laser photocoagulation; and injection of vasoconstrictors, ethanol, or normal saline. The so-called stigmata of recent hemorrhage (SRH) in an ulcer crater—which includes a protruding vessel, an adherent clot, and oozing or spurting of blood—have prognostic and therapeutic implications (Table 2). Patients with SRH are more likely to have uncontrolled or recurrent bleeding and to require therapeutic endoscopy or surgery.

Sigmoidoscopy should be performed early in the evaluation of acute lower GI bleeding. Emergency colonoscopy may be attempted, but its value is limited by stool and blood. If colonoscopy is deemed necessary after the patient is stabilized, the gut can be cleansed with osmotically balanced electrolyte solution by mouth or NG tube.

G. Selective arteriography of the celiac axis, the superior and inferior mesenteric arteries, or their branches may be useful if endoscopy has failed to reveal a diagnosis. Angiodysplastic lesions and vascular tumors can be suspected by their radiographic appearance, and bleeding from other arterial lesions may be identified by a characteristic blush and controlled with autologous clot, gel foam, or vasoconstrictor.

Capsule endoscopy, which uses a wireless camera in a swallowed capsule, creates thousands of pictures and is useful in examining the small intestine beyond the reach of the upper GI endoscope and the colonoscope. Because it requires some bowel preparation and several hours to interpret the pictures, it is more useful in the evaluation of obscure GI bleeding after stabilization of the patient and diagnosis of other small bowel disorders, such as tumors and Crohn's disease.

H. The management of acute GI bleeding requires a team of experienced health professionals. Specific diagnostic studies usually require the skills of an endoscopist or a radiologist. Early surgical consultation may be valuable in managing the patient and the surgeon is better prepared to make a decision regarding operative intervention should the need arise later.

References

American Gastroenterological Association Medical Position Statement: Evaluation and management of occult and obscure gastrointestinal bleeding. Gastroenterology 2000;118:197.

Bounds BC, Friedman LS. Lower gastrointestinal bleeding. Gastroenterol Clin North Am 2003;32:1107.

Comar KM, Sanyal AJ. Portal hypertensive bleeding. Gastroenterol Clin North Am 2003;32:1079.

Eastwood GL. Acute management and identification of risk factors. In Sugawa C, Schuman BM, Lucas CE, eds. Gastrointestinal Bleeding. New York: Igaku-Shoin Medical Publishers, 1992:257.

Elta GH. Approach to the patient with gross gastrointestinal bleeding. In Yamada T, Alpers DH, Kaplowitz N, et al, eds. Textbook of Gastroenterology, 4 ed. Philadelphia: Lippincott Williams & Wilkins, 2003:698.

Huang CS, Lichtenstein DR. Nonvariceal upper gastrointestinal bleeding. Gastroenterol Clin North Am 2003;32:1053.

Kamath PS. Esophageal variceal bleeding: primary prophylaxis. Clin Gastroenterol Hepatol 2005;3:90.

Longstreth GF. Epidemiology of hospitalization for acute upper gastrointestinal hemorrhage: a population-based study. Am J Gastroenterol 1995;90:206.

Longstreth GF. Epidemiology and outcome of patients hospitalized for acute lower gastrointestinal hemorrhage: a population-based study. Am J Gastroenterol 1997;92:419.

Melmed GY, Lo SK. Capsule endoscopy: practical applications. Clin Gastroenterol Hepatol 2005;3:411.

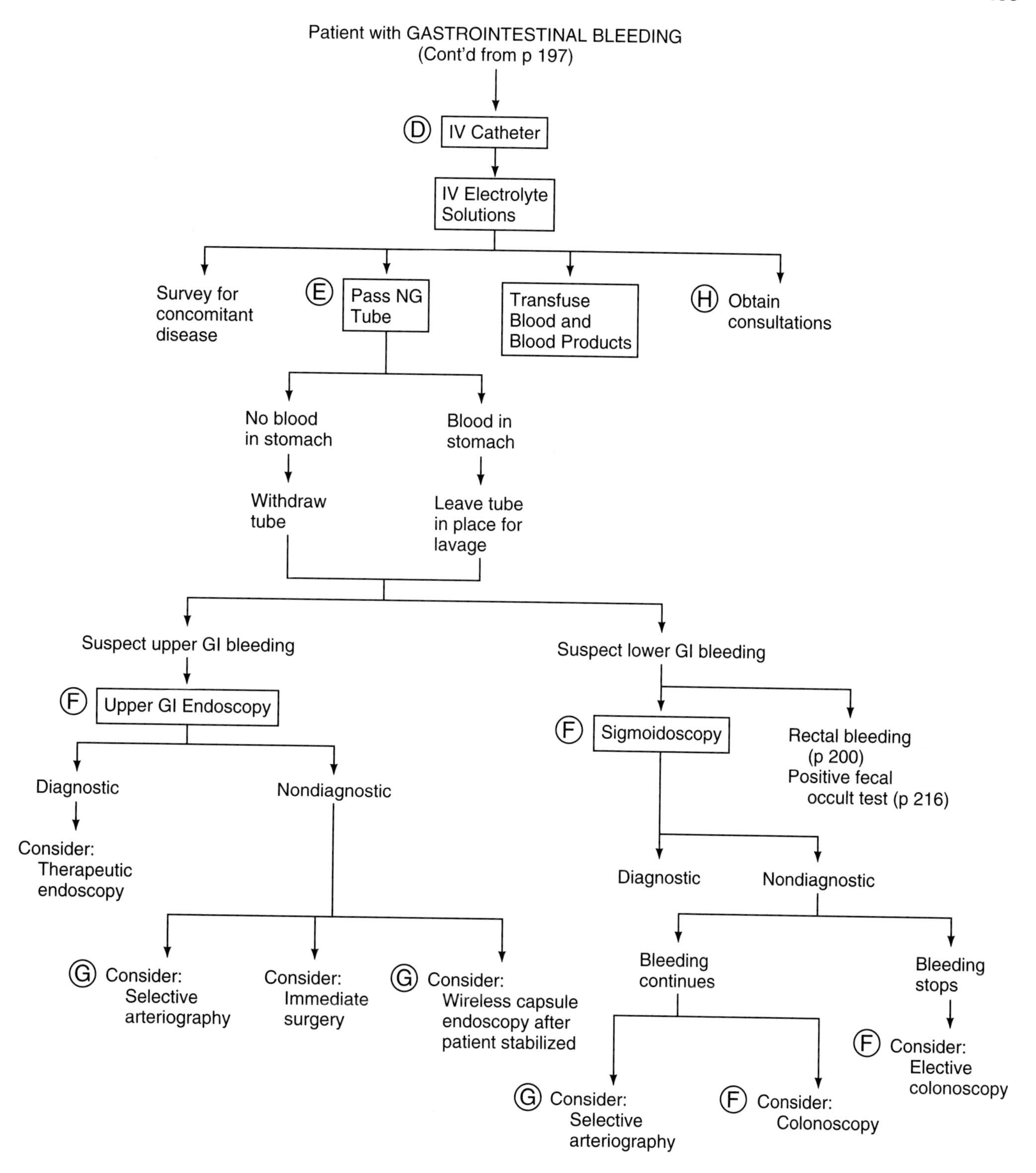

Patient with GASTROINTESTINAL BLEEDING
(Cont'd from p 197)
D
IV Catheter
IV Electrolyte Solutions
Survey for concomitant disease
E
Pass NG Tube
Transfuse Blood and Blood Products
H
Obtain consultations
No blood in stomach
Blood in stomach
Withdraw tube
Leave tube in place for lavage
Suspect upper GI bleeding
Suspect lower GI bleeding
F
Upper GI Endoscopy
F
Sigmoidoscopy
Rectal bleeding (p 200)
Positive fecal occult test (p 216)
Diagnostic
Nondiagnostic
Consider: Therapeutic endoscopy
G
Consider: Selective arteriography
Consider: Immediate surgery
G
Consider: Wireless capsule endoscopy after patient stabilized
Diagnostic
Nondiagnostic
Bleeding continues
Bleeding stops
F
Consider: Elective colonoscopy
G
Consider: Selective arteriography
F
Consider: Colonoscopy

RECTAL BLEEDING

Juan Diego Baltodano, MD, and Bipin Saud, MD

Lower gastrointestinal (LGI) bleeding is anatomically defined as bleeding beyond the ligament of Treitz. Commonly used terms to describe the passage of blood from the lower intestinal tract include rectal bleeding, bright-red blood per rectum, and hematochezia. Rectal bleeding involves a wide clinical spectrum ranging from self-limited trivial bleeding to massive hemorrhage with shock. Unfortunately, these terms do not reflect the acuity, severity, or localization of the bleeding source. Therefore, this broad clinical entity frequently represents a challenge for the clinician. Acute LGI bleed is one of the most common GI indications for hospital admission, and the incidence increases substantially with age. However, because most acute LGI bleeding is self-limited, outcomes are generally favorable.

A. The initial approach to a patient with LGI bleed is based on determining the severity and acuity of bleeding, volume resuscitation, and correction of underlying coagulopathy when necessary. It is also important to exclude an upper GI source of bleeding.

   A thorough history and physical examination is mandatory in the evaluation of patients with LGI bleeding. Epidemiologic factors such as age and associated comorbidities are also important to consider. In patients >65 years, frequent causes include vascular ectasias, diverticular hemorrhage, or ischemic colitis, whereas in younger patients, infectious or inflammatory conditions are more likely.

   Determining the severity of bleeding, duration (acute versus chronic), frequency, and the color of blood passing per rectum is crucial. Commonly, the presence of melena indicates bleeding from an upper GI source, small bowel, or proximal colon, whereas bright-red blood signifies distal colon or rectal origin. It is important to remember that 10% of upper GI bleeds present as hematochezia. Therefore, this should always be considered as a possible source in patients with rectal bleeding, especially in a patient who presents in shock or with orthostatic hypotension.

   Important factors in the patient history include constipation or diarrhea (hemorrhoids, colitis), diverticulosis, prior radiation therapy (radiation enteritis), recent polypectomy (postpolypectomy), abdominal pain (ischemia, inflammatory or infectious), vascular disease, hypotension or recent vascular surgery (ischemia), anorectal disease, and trauma. The use of NSAIDs or anticoagulants also is associated with LGI bleeding, especially diverticular bleeding. Also, family history of colon cancer or polyposis increases the likelihood of colorectal neoplasia. Other uncommon causes include solitary rectal ulcer, vasculitis, endometriosis, intussusception, portal colopathy, and diversion colitis.

   On physical examination, it is mandatory to assess the patient's hemodynamic status, possible amount of blood loss, source of bleeding, and associated comorbidities. The presence of orthostatic tachycardia/hypotension (decrease in systolic blood pressure [SBP] >20 mm Hg or increase in heart rate [HR] >20 bpm) indicates acute blood loss of at least 15%. In more severe cases, these patients may have resting hypotension or shock, which is indicative of 20%–25% of volume depletion. In both clinical settings, aggressive volume resuscitation and close monitoring in an intensive care unit are indicated.

   The presence of mucocutaneous lesions such as telangiectasias (Osler-Weber-Rendu disease), stigmata of chronic liver disease, pigmented lip lesions (Peutz-Jeghers syndrome), abdominal tenderness, palpable masses, and splenomegaly are important to detect. These characteristics can serve as indicators to guide a diagnostic approach and subsequent treatment. A rectal examination serves to identify anorectal lesions and stool color.

B. Performing a nasogastric lavage is a quick and safe method to exclude, for the most part, an upper GI source. Emergent esophagogastroduodenoscopy should be performed if fresh blood is present in gastric lavage or if clinically suspected, especially if the patient has been taking NSAIDs.

C. The utility of anoscopy/sigmoidoscopy in the initial management of LGI bleeding is debatable. Experts believe that anoscopy should be part of the initial assessment. Flexible sigmoidoscopy may be diagnostic for distal colorectal pathology such as ulcerative or infectious colitis, hemorrhoids, proctitis, or solitary rectal ulcer, eliminating the need for emergency colonoscopy. With either modality, the presence of more proximal lesions cannot be ruled out. There are three methods for definitive diagnosis and treatment of LGI bleeding: endoscopic, radiologic, and surgical interventions.

   Colonoscopy is advocated for most cases because it provides the opportunity for early diagnosis and treatment when possible. However, there is great controversy on the appropriate time to perform colonoscopy. Colonoscopic evaluation can be performed within the first 8–24 hours of presentation. It generally requires bowel preparation, which can be given orally or through a nasogastric tube. Endoscopic hemostasis can be attempted by different methods, such

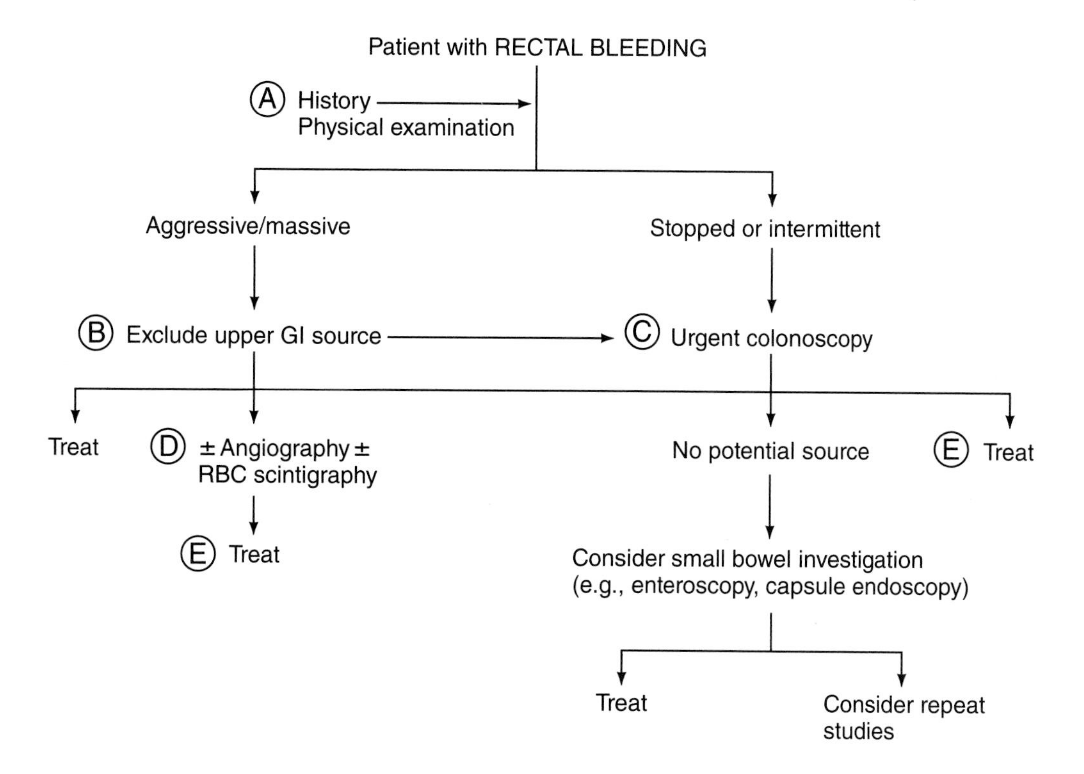

as injection, thermal/electrical coagulation, hemoclips, and band ligation.

D. The use of radionuclide scintigraphy (tagged RBC scan) is controversial because its accuracy in localizing the bleeding site can vary. Among the advantages are its sensitivity to detect active bleeding as low as 0.1–0.5 ml/min and the fact that it is a noninvasive test. The main purposes of obtaining an RBC scan would be to use it as a screening test for possible angiography and/or guide for surgical intervention. Angiography detects bleeding rates of >0.5 ml/min and, in addition to its diagnostic benefit, offers therapeutic possibilities (selective microembolization or injecting pharmacologic vasoconstricting agents), hence reducing the need for surgical intervention. Possible complications include bleeding, formation of a hematoma at the catheter site, arterial dissection, and intestinal ischemia. Currently, angiographic therapy is usually reserved for patients who are poor surgical candidates. Angiography can also be used as a guide for surgical resection if needed.

E. Surgery is indicated when bleeding is continuous and recurrent. In general, in patients requiring large amounts of blood products (>4–6 units over a 24-hour period or >10 units total), a surgical approach is recommended if possible.

F. Finally, if no potential source of bleeding is found, small bowel investigation is required. Small bowel sources represent approximately 2%–15% of causes of LGI bleeding. Patients with small bowel bleeding generally require more diagnostic procedures, blood transfusions, and longer hospital stays when compared with patients with other sources of GI bleeding. Some authors suggest this entity should be considered separately. Endoscopic techniques such as enteroscopy or capsule endoscopy are the appropriate diagnostic modalities in these cases.

References

ASGE Guideline: the role of endoscopy in the patient with lower-GI bleeding. Gastrointestinal Endoscopy 2005;62:656–660.

Green BT, Rockey DC. Lower gastrointestinal bleeding—management. Gastroenterol Clin North Am 2005;34:665–678.

Green BT, Rockey DC, Portwood G, et al. Urgent colonoscopy for evaluation and management of acute lower gastrointestinal hemorrhage: a randomized controlled trial. Am J Gastroenterol 2005;100: 2395–2402.

Rockey DC. Lower gastrointestinal bleeding. Gastroenterology 2006; 130:165–171.

Strate LL. Lower GI bleeding: epidemiology and diagnosis. Gastroenterol Clin North Am 2005;34:643–664.

Strate LL, Syngal S. Timing of colonoscopy: impact on length of hospital stay in patients with acute lower intestinal bleeding. Am J Gastroenterol 2003;98:317–322.

Zuckerman GR, Prakash C. Acute lower intestinal bleeding. Part II: etiology, therapy, and outcomes. Gastrointest Endosc 1999;49:228–238.

ACUTE DIARRHEA

M. Brian Fennerty, MD

A. Diarrhea is one of the most common complaints resulting in visits to a physician. The history and physical examination (including rectal examination) are critical in determining who needs further diagnostic evaluation and in selecting appropriate therapy. Important questions to ask are duration of illness; volume of stool; presence of blood or pus in stool; and symptoms of systemic illness such as fever, anorexia, weight loss, and volume depletion. Most patients should not undergo further evaluation at this time, but they should be treated symptomatically. However, the presence of systemic symptoms dictates that the stool be more closely evaluated for evidence of invasive infection or inflammatory bowel disease (IBD).

B. The simplest test that can be performed in the office to evaluate inflammatory changes of the bowel mucosa is to inspect by microscopy a fecal sample for WBCs/RBCs. The presence of either of these implies infection with invasive organisms and/or IBD.

C. To evaluate infection by an invasive bacterial organism, a stool culture is necessary. Most clinical laboratories routinely test for *Shigella, Salmonella,* and *Campylobacter* spp. If travel or other historical features suggest other pathogens, more specific testing for *Amoeba, Yersinia* spp., or *Clostridium difficile* and others may be necessary. In certain clinical situations, testing for certain types of *Escherichia coli* may be prudent. In patients with HIV disease, testing for unusual pathogens (e.g., cryptosporidia, mycobacteria) may be necessary.

D. In patients who have WBCs/RBCs in the stool and a negative culture, or those without inflammatory cells but continued diarrhea, perform flexible sigmoidoscopy to evaluate for IBD, which may be present even if the mucosa is grossly normal appearing. Therefore, a biopsy is helpful in detecting minimal mucosal changes. In addition, the histologic appearance in the setting of gross inflammatory changes can help differentiate acute infectious self-limited colitis from IBD. Generally, perform a biopsy irrespective of gross findings.

E. In patients with negative cultures and sigmoidoscopy but continued diarrhea, further evaluation may be required.

References

Fedorak R. Antidiarrheal therapy. Dig Dis Sci 1987;32:195.

Harris JC, DuPont HL, Hornick RB. Fecal leukocytes in diarrheal illness. Ann Intern Med 1972;76:697.

Plotkin G. Gastroenteritis: etiology, pathophysiology and clinical manifestations. Medicine 1979;58:95.

Slutsker L, Ries AA, Greene KD, et al. *Escherichia coli* O157:H7 diarrhea in the Unites States: clinical and epidemiologic features. Ann Intern Med 1997;126:505.

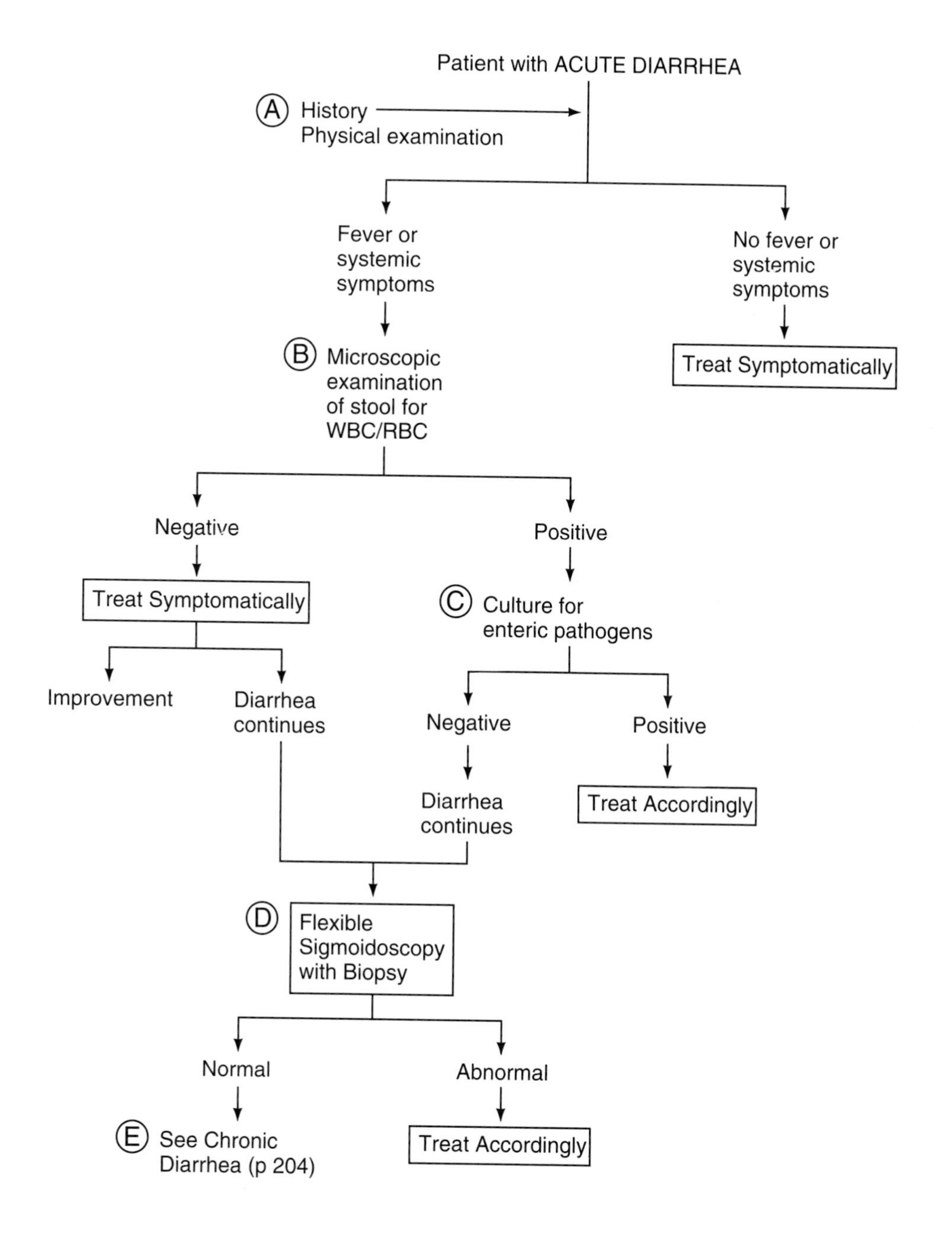
Patient with ACUTE DIARRHEA
(A) History
Physical examination
Fever or systemic symptoms
No fever or systemic symptoms
Treat Symptomatically
(B) Microscopic examination of stool for WBC/RBC
Negative
Positive
Treat Symptomatically
(C) Culture for enteric pathogens
Improvement
Diarrhea continues
Negative
Positive
Diarrhea continues
Treat Accordingly
(D) Flexible Sigmoidoscopy with Biopsy
Normal
Abnormal
(E) See Chronic Diarrhea (p 204)
Treat Accordingly

CHRONIC DIARRHEA

Juan Diego Baltodano, MD, and Bipin Saud, MD

Diarrhea is defined as the passage of stool with liquid consistency and weight >200 g/day. It becomes chronic when symptoms persist for >4 weeks.

The common pathophysiologic mechanism of diarrhea is an incomplete absorption of water from the lumen. This can occur in several ways, such as reduced rate of net water absorption (abnormal electrolyte secretion), intraluminal osmotic water retention (osmotic load), decreased mucosal surface area, and abnormalities in intestinal motility. Several classifications for the clinician guide the evaluation of diarrhea. A practical and widely used approach to facilitate the diagnosis is based on stool characteristics. Chronic diarrhea is then subdivided into watery, inflammatory, or fatty in nature.

A. A detailed medical history is essential for the evaluation of chronic diarrhea. It is important to differentiate functional from organic disorders. A functional etiology may be suggested in the absence of significant unintentional weight loss, nocturnal symptoms, or persistence of symptoms for >1 year. Onset of symptoms, specific patterns, duration, and aggravating/alleviating factors should always be investigated. It is also essential to inquire about a previous history of radiation therapy, prior abdominal surgery, and antibiotic or other medication use because these are common causes of iatrogenic diarrhea. Medication use has been described as the causative factor in up to 4% of patients with chronic diarrhea. The clinician should elicit a history of specific stool characteristics such as the presence of blood, mucus, oil droplets, or undigested food particles. Other coexisting symptoms, including abdominal pain, cramps, fever, excessive flatulence, and bloating, should be further investigated. Other systemic illnesses such as AIDS, diabetes, and thyroid and collagen vascular diseases may play a contributory role in patients with chronic diarrhea. Dietary habits and the presence of food additives (sorbitol, mannitol, and fructose) should also be discussed. Recent travel, sexual history, occupation, source of drinking water, and alcohol or illicit drug abuse are other pertinent pieces of information in the history.

B. On physical examination, prompt determination of the severity of symptoms is mandatory and is initially more important than obtaining a specific diagnosis. A good place to start is to evaluate the patient's intravascular volume status. If detected, dehydration and electrolyte imbalances should be addressed and corrected immediately. A careful abdominal examination should be performed, noting absence or presence of abdominal sounds, bruits, fluid, organomegaly, or palpable masses. A rectal examination may reveal pelvic or sphincter dysfunction. The physical examination can also help in identifying systemic causes of diarrhea such as right-sided heart murmurs, enlarged hard liver and flushing (carcinoid), arthritis (inflammatory bowel disease, Whipple's, and other enteric infections), dermatitis herpetiformis (celiac sprue), and pyoderma gangrenosum or erythema nodosum (inflammatory bowel disease [IBD]).

C. Routine laboratory studies should be obtained as part of the initial evaluation. These include a CBC, electrolytes, thyroid function tests, and a screen for celiac disease. Other studies are also complementary to initial testing. Stool analysis is crucial in the evaluation of chronic diarrhea. These samples can be obtained in a random sample or a timed collection.
   - 24- to 48-hour collection samples are preferred so that stool volume, weight, and different components can be accurately measured.
   - Fecal leukocytes and lactoferrin (iron-binding glycoprotein) are important diagnostic tools for detecting inflammatory diarrhea. This can be secondary to an infectious cause, IBD, or microscopic colitis.
   - Fecal occult blood testing is nonspecific. The utility of this test for detecting inflammatory and neoplastic pathology in chronic diarrhea has not been established. Conditions such as celiac sprue, small bowel lymphoma, and refractory sprue have been associated with positive guaiac results.
   - Stool fat is used to determine the presence of steatorrhea, which is defined as a loss of fat in stool >7 g or 9% of fat intake in 24 hours. A minimal consumption of 70–100 g of fat per day is mandatory for quantitative studies. Fat excretion >14 g per day is strongly suggestive of fat malabsorption. A qualitative Sudan III stain test can predict 90% of patients with clinically significant steatorrhea.
   - Stool osmotic gap is used to differentiate an osmotic from a secretory type of diarrhea. This is determined by the electrolyte concentration in the stool water, using the following formula: $290 - 2(Na + K)$. If the osmotic gap is small (<50), unabsorbed electrolytes retain water in the lumen, which is characteristic of secretory diarrhea. However, if the osmotic gap is large (>125), the nonelectrolyte content in the lumen is accounted for by the retained water, being more consistent with an osmotic diarrhea.

(Continued on page 206)

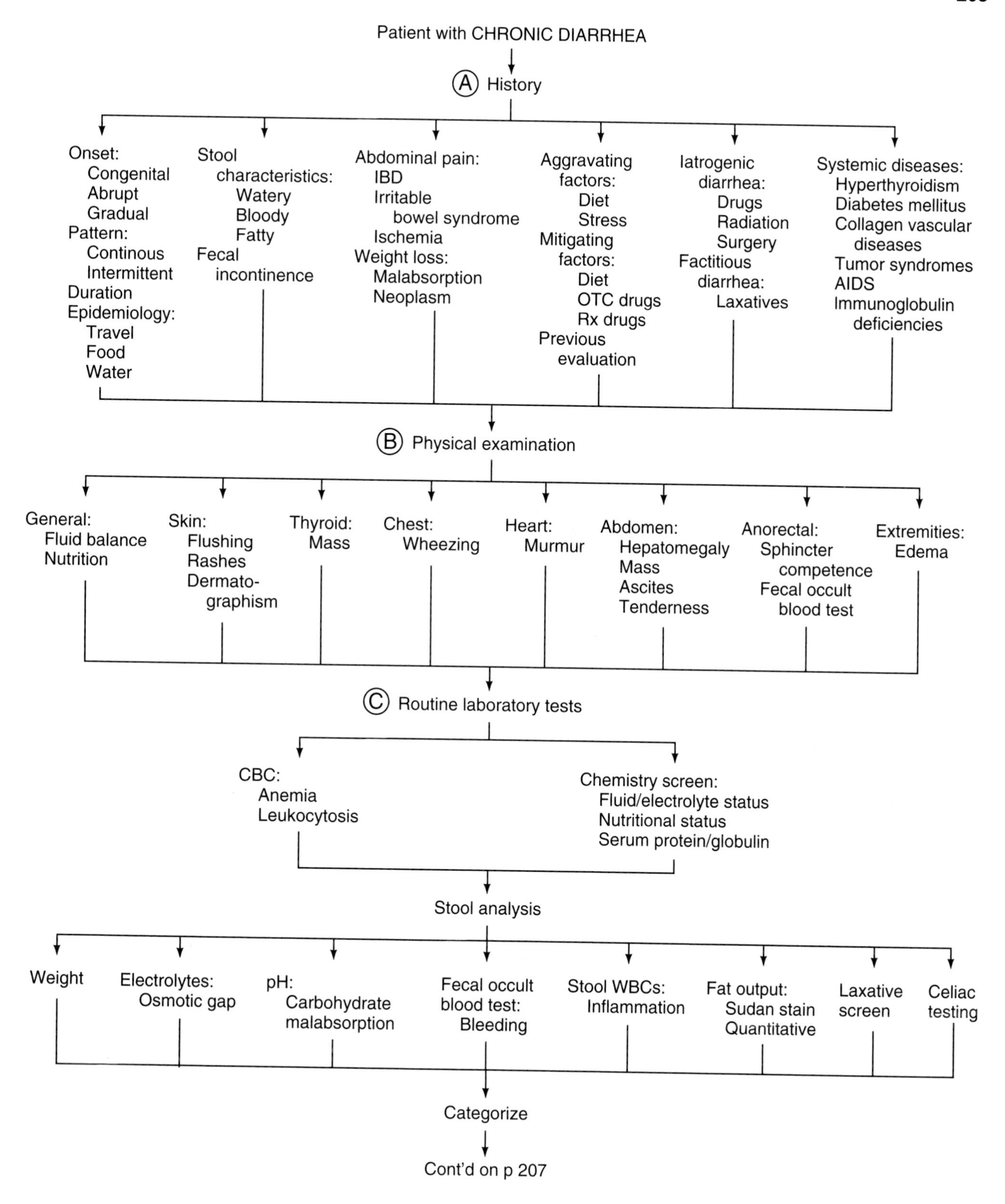

Patient with CHRONIC DIARRHEA
(A) History
Onset:
Congenital
Abrupt
Gradual
Pattern:
Continous
Intermittent
Duration
Epidemiology:
Travel
Food
Water
Stool characteristics:
Watery
Bloody
Fatty
Fecal incontinence
Abdominal pain:
IBD
Irritable bowel syndrome
Ischemia
Weight loss:
Malabsorption
Neoplasm
Aggravating factors:
Diet
Stress
Mitigating factors:
Diet
OTC drugs
Rx drugs
Previous evaluation
Iatrogenic diarrhea:
Drugs
Radiation
Surgery
Factitious diarrhea:
Laxatives
Systemic diseases:
Hyperthyroidism
Diabetes mellitus
Collagen vascular diseases
Tumor syndromes
AIDS
Immunoglobulin deficiencies
(B) Physical examination
General:
Fluid balance
Nutrition
Skin:
Flushing
Rashes
Dermato-graphism
Thyroid:
Mass
Chest:
Wheezing
Heart:
Murmur
Abdomen:
Hepatomegaly
Mass
Ascites
Tenderness
Anorectal:
Sphincter competence
Fecal occult blood test
Extremities:
Edema
(C) Routine laboratory tests
CBC:
Anemia
Leukocytosis
Chemistry screen:
Fluid/electrolyte status
Nutritional status
Serum protein/globulin
Stool analysis
Weight
Electrolytes:
Osmotic gap
pH:
Carbohydrate malabsorption
Fecal occult blood test:
Bleeding
Stool WBCs:
Inflammation
Fat output:
Sudan stain
Quantitative
Laxative screen
Celiac testing
Categorize
Cont'd on p 207

- The measurement of stool osmolality has no use in calculating the osmotic gap. Osmolality values <290 mOsm/kg generally indicate contamination of the stool with water or hypotonic urine.
- Stool pH <5.3 indicates carbohydrate malabsorption. When proper carbohydrate absorption fails to take place in the small intestine, excessive bacterial fermentation occurs in the colon, creating a more acidic environment and reducing stool pH.
- Chemical and chromatographic methods can be used to confirm the surreptitious ingestion of laxatives. In these cases, watery stool can either have a secretory or osmotic component. Fecal concentration of substances such as phosphate, sulfate, magnesium phenolphthalein, and reducing substances can be measured.
- Carbohydrate and protein content can also be tested in stool. However, these are not routinely recommended unless the results would directly alter the management of the patient. These include alpha-1-antitrypsin to look for protein-losing enteropathy and D-xylose absorption test to evaluate specific mucosal defects rather than pancreatic digestive defects.
- Serologic testing for celiac disease is recommended on a routine basis in patients with chronic diarrhea. Measurements of tissue transglutaminase and immunoglobulin A (IgA) antiendomysial antibodies are part of this evaluation.
- Urine testing is useful when carcinoid or pheochromocytoma is suspected. These include measurements of urine levels of 5-HIAA (5-hydroxyindole acetic acid), vanillylmandelic acid (VMA), and histamine (mast cell disease and foregut carcinoids).
- Serum testing for peptide hormones is indicated when causes such as Zollinger-Ellison syndrome, glucagonoma, neuroendocrine vasoactive intestinal peptide (VIP)-producing tumors, or thyroid medullary carcinoma are suspected.
- Other specific physiologic tests are available once a particular diagnosis is pursued.

D. Watery diarrhea is subdivided into two main categories: secretory and osmotic. In secretory diarrhea, infection should be excluded as an initial step. This can be done by performing stool cultures for bacteria and other organisms, such as *Aeromonas, Plesiomonas,* microsporidia, *Giardia,* coccidian, cryptosporidium, and standard ova and parasites. Subsequently, structural diseases such as short gut syndrome, gastrocolic or enteroenteric fistulas, IBD, and malignancies can be diagnosed with radiologic testing (small bowel series or CT scan of the abdomen) and endoscopic studies with biopsy when possible esophagogastroduodenoscopy [EGD]), colonoscopy, or capsule endoscopy). Serologic and other specific testing should be ordered for each suspected diagnosis.

E. Osmotic diarrhea has a more limited diagnosis. It is usually secondary to the ingestion of exogenous magnesium, consumption of poorly absorbed carbohydrates, or carbohydrate malabsorption. Magnesium directly measured in the stool >44 mmol/L is suggestive of laxative abuse.

F. The underlying abnormality present in inflammatory diarrhea is disruption and inflammation of the mucosa. This can be secondary to inflammatory bowel disease, infections, medications (NSAIDs, chemotherapy), pseudomembranous colitis, ischemia, radiation enterocolitis, and neoplasia. Sigmoidoscopy or colonoscopy with biopsy may be indicated to evaluate for structural changes, depending on the clinical circumstances.

G. Fatty diarrhea (or steatorrhea) can be secondary to a maldigestive or a malabsorptive process. Within this category, the three most common related conditions are celiac sprue, pancreatic insufficiency, and bacterial overgrowth. Once this is established, endoscopic studies with small bowel biopsies are necessary to exclude structural disease. If the latter has been excluded, imaging studies of the pancreas are mandatory to evaluate for pancreatic causes. There is no optimal test to assess pancreatic function. Therefore, a therapeutic trial of pancreatic enzyme supplementation with an objective measurement of a response may be the "optimal" physiologic testing.

References

American Gastroenterological Association medical position statement: guidelines for the evaluation and management of chronic diarrhea. Gastroenterology 1999;116:1461–1486.

Headstrom PD, Surawcicz CM. Chronic diarrhea. Clin Gastroenterol Hepatol 2005;3:734–737.

Schiller LR. Chronic diarrhea. Gastroenterology 2004;127:287–293.

Schiller LR, Sellin JH. Diarrhea. In Feldman M, Friedman LS, Sleisenger MH, eds. Sleisenger and Fordtran's Gastrointestinal and Liver Disease: Pathophysiology, Diagnosis and Management, 7th ed. Philadelphia: Saunders, 2002:131–153.

Thomas PD, Forbes A, Green J, et al. Guidelines for the investigation of chronic diarrhoea, 2nd ed. Gut 2003;52 Suppl 5:v1–15.

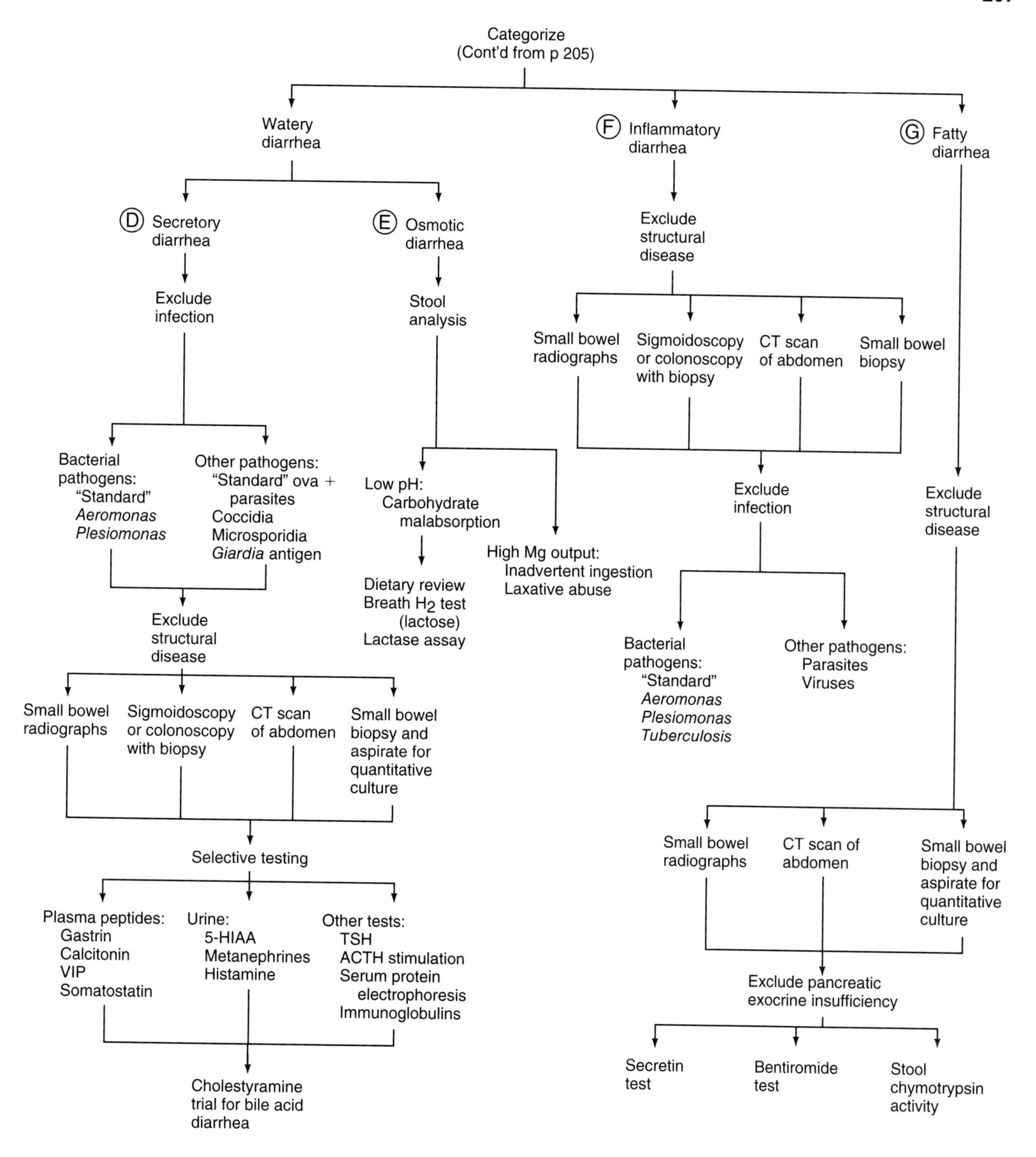

Initial efforts should be directed to classification of chronic diarrhea based on history, physical examination, basic laboratory test results, and stool analysis. Further evaluation is made for secretory diarrhea (D), osmotic diarrhea (E), inflammatory diarrhea (F), and fatty diarrhea (G). It is not necessary to perform every test in a given pathway once a diagnosis is reached. *TSH,* Thyroid-stimulating hormone; *ACTH,* adrenocorticotropic hormone. Modified from American Gastroenterological Association medical position statement: guidelines for the evaluation and management of chronic diarrhea. Gastroenterology 1999;116:1461–1486.

CONSTIPATION

Philip E. Jaffe, MD

A. In Western societies, adults average three bowel movements per week. There is significant variation depending on sex, age, diet, culture, and geographic location. History should be directed at defining the characteristics, frequency, and severity of complaints. New onset of an altered bowel pattern in an older individual who has not undergone recent colorectal cancer screening should suggest mechanical colonic obstruction until proved otherwise. Whenever possible, colonoscopy should be considered as the initial diagnostic study in this situation, whether or not there are other concerning symptoms such as bleeding, pain, or weight loss. Those with more chronic symptoms and younger patients are more likely to have irritable bowel syndrome (IBS), colorectal motility disorders, Hirschsprung's disease, or medication-related constipation. The latter issue is probably underappreciated, but the use of opiates, calcium channel blockers, "antispasmodics," other anticholinergic drugs, and iron supplements should be considered. Systemic diseases, including diabetes mellitus, progressive systemic sclerosis, Parkinson's disease, and thyroid disease, should be considered. Physical examination should include digital rectal examination to assess for anorectal diseases, including fissures and thrombosed hemorrhoids, masses, fecal impaction, and possibly sphincteric abnormalities. If not performed recently, hemoglobin, serum electrolytes, calcium, magnesia, and thyroid-stimulating hormone levels should be obtained. Simple dietary measures such as the addition of fluid and fiber and elimination of potentially offending agents are usually recommended initially; however, persistent symptoms should warrant the exclusion of significant colorectal pathology.

B. In patients 50 years of age and older, colonoscopy can be justified based on current colorectal cancer screening recommendations. In younger patients with a family history of colorectal cancer or unexplained iron-deficiency anemia, colonoscopy should also be considered. Otherwise, barium enema and flexible sigmoidoscopy should be adequate to evaluate for structural colorectal lesions. Barium enema may also be useful in children and adolescents, in whom Hirschsprung's disease is more common. Although important to exclude obstructing processes in the appropriate setting, these studies do not commonly define the source of the problem.

C. The finding of an obstructing colorectal mass, usually adenocarcinoma, generally requires surgical resection. In selected cases where there is obstruction in the setting of widely metastatic disease, palliation with laser photocoagulation or colonic stent placement may be effective alternatives. Stents may also be placed when there is near-complete colonic obstruction to allow for colonic decompression and better colonic preparation prior to elective surgery.

D. Anorectal disorders, including fissures, thrombosed hemorrhoids, and perirectal abscesses, may contribute to constipation by causing fecal avoidance because of pain. Conservative measures including stool bulking agents, softeners, sitz baths, and local nitrates or calcium channel blockers are preferred unless symptoms persist or an abscess develops, requiring surgery.

(Continued on page 210)

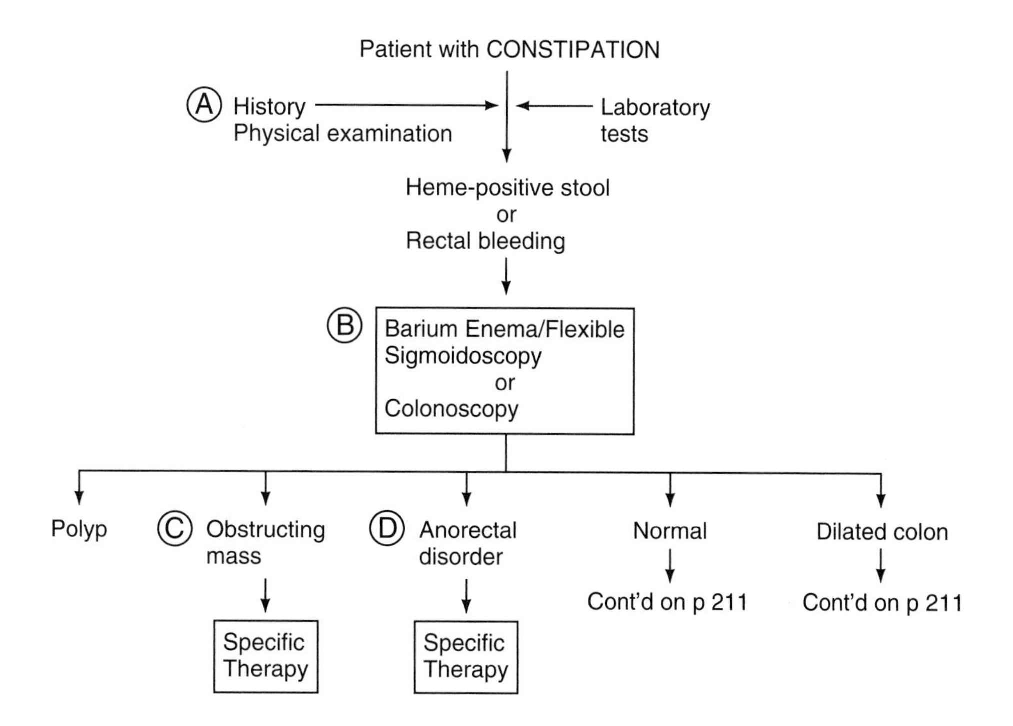
Patient with CONSTIPATION
A
History
Physical examination
Laboratory
tests
Heme-positive stool
or
Rectal bleeding
B
Barium Enema/Flexible
Sigmoidoscopy
or
Colonoscopy
Polyp
C
Obstructing
mass
D
Anorectal
disorder
Normal
Dilated colon
Specific
Therapy
Specific
Therapy
Cont'd on p 211
Cont'd on p 211

E. In patients with complaints of constipation and studies that exclude obstructing lesions, a radiopaque marker colonic transit study confirms the presence of a motility problem and may help define the cause. Commercially available capsules contain 24 tiny radiopaque pellets that can be seen on standard radiographs. A simplified study involves obtaining x-ray films on day 3 following ingestion and 2 days later if markers are seen in the colon on the first study. Often patients misinterpret symptoms of hard stool consistency or problems with fecal evacuation as constipation, and transit studies may provide objective data to support or refute their perception. The finding that all markers are passed by the time of the first radiograph usually suggests that the problem is one of perception rather than delay in fecal transit. When most markers persist in the rectum and rectosigmoid region, the possibility of functional anorectal motility disturbance should be further investigated. Those found to have persistence of radiopaque markers throughout the colon are more likely to have slow transit constipation or a diffuse colonic motility disturbance, which may respond to saline laxatives, prokinetic agents, and fiber supplementation.

F. A large number of patients complaining of constipation will be found to have normal colonic transit as measured by radiopaque marker studies. In some the feeling of constipation may reflect their expectations relative to cultural norms; most probably have a variant of IBS. Empirical treatment generally begins with taking bulking agents, eating a high-fiber diet, and increasing fluid intake. Some patients may require osmotic agents, saline laxatives, and prokinetics agents such as tegaserod. Stimulant cathartics may also be used periodically, although there is anecdotal (and unproven) concern regarding the development of colonic hypomotility when used frequently.

G. The finding of colonic dilation on barium enema suggests the possibility of neurologic impairment of the colon (e.g., Hirschsprung's disease), an anorectal motility disorder, or colonic pseudoobstruction. Rectal biopsy in children is useful in diagnosing Hirschsprung's disease. The finding of melenosis coli on colonoscopy is diagnostic of chronic use of anthraquinone-containing laxatives (e.g., cascara or senna).

H. Anorectal motility studies using catheters that measure anal sphincter pressures and studies measuring the expulsion of water-filled balloons of varying size can be helpful in assessing anorectal physiology. In addition, measurement of nerve conduction velocity of the puborectalis muscle can help to determine the appropriateness of muscular and neurogenic response. Together these studies can define the presence or absence of pelvic relaxation disorders and a number of other motility disturbances that may contribute to constipation. Specific treatment depends on the specific disorder that is discovered but usually involves some combination of bulking agents, prokinetic drugs, and biofeedback therapy aimed at retraining and restoring normal anorectal activity.

I. When specific anatomic definition of the anorectal abnormality is required, defecography is performed by the transrectal instillation of thickened barium pastes or other viscous radiopaque materials. Lateral fluoroscopic views of the distal colon, including the rectosigmoid junction, are obtained during active defecation to determine whether there is normal puborectalis activity leading to straightening of the anorectal angle. This study can help to define abnormalities in perineal descent, rectoceles, and rectal prolapse. Those with chronic colonic dilation, normal anatomic studies and colonic biopsies, and anorectal motility studies are said to have chronic idiopathic colonic pseudoobstruction. Although treatable by ileostomy, this is frequently a highly morbid procedure in these patients.

References

Brandt L, Prather C, Quigley E, et al. An evidence-based approach to the management of chronic constipation in North America. Am J Gastroenterol 2005;100:S1.

Diamant N, Kamm M, Wald A, Whitehead W. AGA technical review on anorectal testing techniques. Gastroenterology 1999;116:735.

Higgins P, Johanson J. Epidemiology of constipation in North America: a systematic review. Am J Gastroenterol 2004;99:750.

Muller-Lissner S, Kamm M, Scarpignato C, Wald A. Myths and misconceptions about chronic constipation. Am J Gastroenterol 2005; 100:232.

Rao S, Ozturk R, Laine L. Clinical utility of diagnostic tests for constipation in adults: a systematic review. Am J Gastroenterol 2005; 100:1605.

Stewart W, Liberman J, Sandler R, et al. Epidemiology of constipation (EPOC) study in the United States: relation of clinical subtypes to sociodemographic features. Am J Gastroenterol 1999;94:3530.

Wald A. Is chronic use of stimulant laxatives harmful to the colon? J Clin Gastroenterol 2003;36:386.

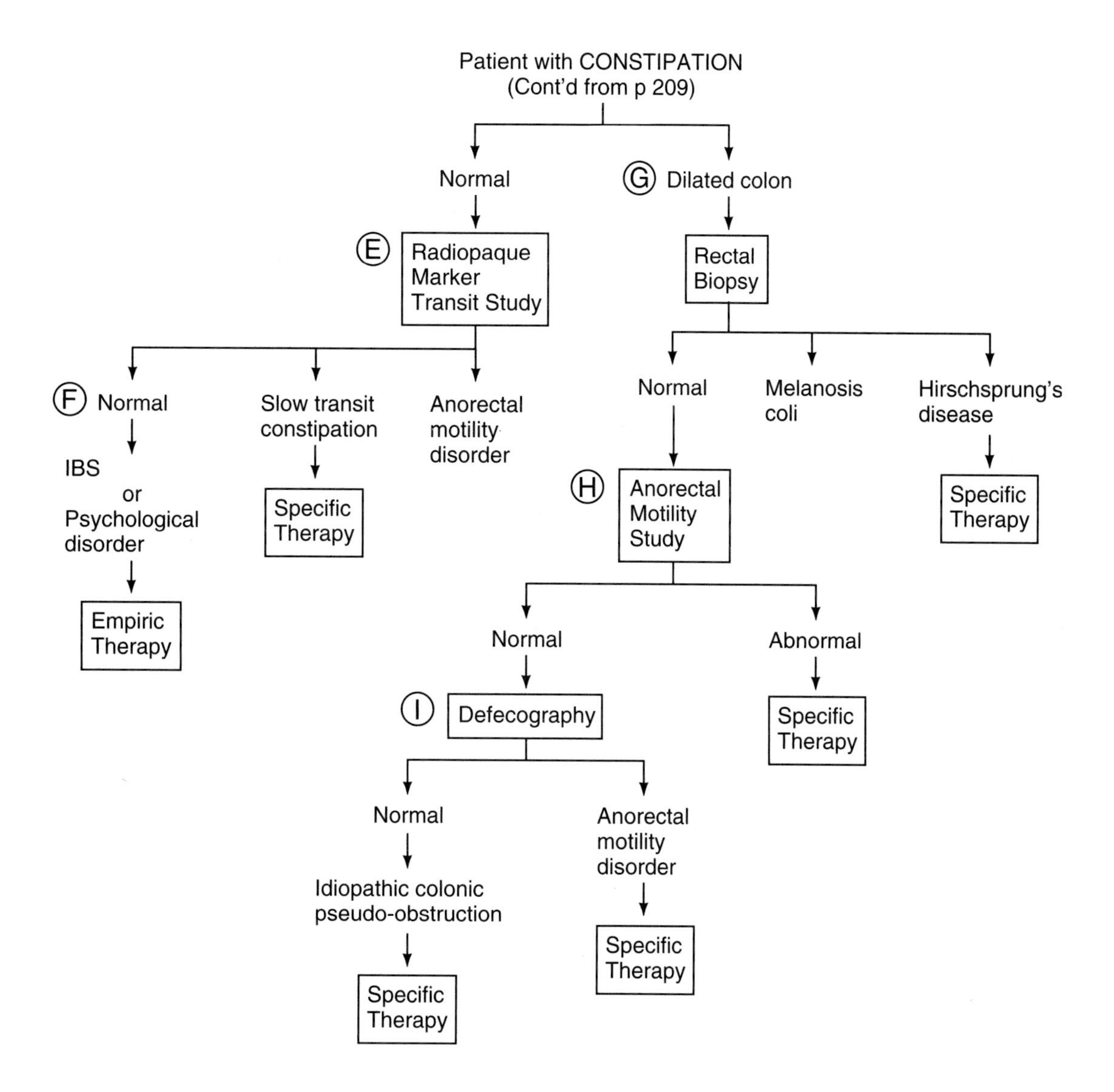
Patient with CONSTIPATION
(Cont'd from p 209)
Normal
G Dilated colon
E Radiopaque Marker Transit Study
Rectal Biopsy
F Normal
Slow transit constipation
Anorectal motility disorder
Normal
Melanosis coli
Hirschsprung's disease
IBS or Psychological disorder
Specific Therapy
H Anorectal Motility Study
Specific Therapy
Empiric Therapy
Normal
Abnormal
I Defecography
Specific Therapy
Normal
Anorectal motility disorder
Idiopathic colonic pseudo-obstruction
Specific Therapy
Specific Therapy

IRRITABLE BOWEL SYNDROME

M. Brian Fennerty, MD

Irritable bowel syndrome (IBS) is a common disease that affects 10%–15% of the population and is thought to be a gut motor-sensory disorder, the basis of which is physiologic but the manifestations of which are affected by various environmental (e.g., foods) and host (e.g., stress, comorbid illness, prior psychological/physiologic trauma) factors. Although there are many functional gut diseases, IBS primarily is a disease of colonic dysfunction. Subclassification of IBS may be helpful in disease management strategies because the various subtypes are associated with different treatment choices and pathophysiologic mechanisms. The subtypes are based on stool consistency alone and include IBS with constipation (IBS-C), IBS with diarrhea (IBS-D), IBS mixed type (IBS-M), and IBS unsubtyped (IBS-U). Patients with IBS-M have both hard and loose stools over periods of hours or days, whereas IBS patients with alternating bowel habits change subtype over periods of weeks and months.

A unifying biochemical cause of IBS is not established, but in many patients the pathophysiology appears to involve serotonergic signaling of colonic motor and sensory function. There is no laboratory test that can be used to diagnose IBS. Instead the diagnosis is based on the characteristic symptoms (Table 1), although it may be necessary to exclude other conditions that can mimic or produce IBS-like symptoms (e.g., colitis, lactose intolerance, sprue) through focused laboratory testing. However, routine laboratory tests are not indicated or necessary to make the diagnosis of IBS. It is important to assess for "alarm flag" symptoms (weight loss, GI bleeding, anemia, or nocturnal symptoms) because these symptoms may indicate underlying serious diseases and should prompt further diagnostic evaluation.

A. Apply the diagnostic criteria for IBS (see Table 1).

B. Assign the patient to an IBS subtype. Avoid routine diagnostic testing (e.g., CBC, chemistry panel, stool studies, endoscopy) unless symptom directed. Serologic screening for sprue may be helpful in some patients, and those with alarm symptoms or those older than age 50 may need more advanced testing with colonoscopy, etc.

C. Reassure the patient that he or she has a common, benign, and treatable chronic disease that rarely progresses.

D. Avoid aggravating factors such as specific foods, dairy products, opiates, and NSAIDs. The predominant symptom or subtype will indicate empirical therapies to be tried. Empirical therapeutic trials include increased fiber (IBS-C), antidiarrheals (IBS-D), and antispasmodics.

E. In those not responding to empirical therapy, directed therapy with serotonin agents (alosetron [IBS-D] or tegaserod [IBS-C]) or prostaglandins (lubiprostone [IBS-C]) may be effective.

Table 1: **Rome III Diagnostic Criteria for Irritable Bowel Syndrome**

Irritable Bowel Syndrome
At least 3 months, with onset at least 6 months previously of recurrent abdominal pain or discomfort associated with 2 or more of the following: • Improvement with defecation; *and/or* • Onset associated with a change in frequency of stool; *and/or* • Onset associated with a change in form (appearance) of stool

References

Camilleri M, Dubois D, Coulie B, et al. Prevalence and socioeconomic impact of upper gastrointestinal disorders in the United States: results of the US Upper Gastrointestinal. Clin Gastroenterol Hepatol 2005; 3(6):543–542.

Drossman DA. The functional gastrointestinal disorders and the Rome III process. Gastroenterology 2006;130:1377–1390.

Drossman DA, Camilleri M, Mayer EA, Whitehead WE. AGA technical review on irritable bowel syndrome. Gastroenterology 2002;123: 2108–2131.

Drossman DA, Morris CB, Hu Y, et al. A prospective assessment of bowel habit in irritable bowel syndrome in women: defining an alternator. Gastroenterology 2005;128:580–589.

Longstreth GF, Thompson WG, Chey WD, et al. Functional bowel disorders. Gastroenterology 2006;130:1480–1491.

Patient with ABDOMINAL DISCOMFORT WITH ALTERED BOWEL MOTILITY

- (A) Rome diagnostic criteria for IBS (Table 1)
  - Positive
    - Physical examination
    - (B) IBS subtype
    - (C) Directed diagnostic testing, if necessary
      - (D) Constipation
        - Osmotic Laxative, Fiber
        - (E) Lubiprostone, tegaserod
      - (D) Diarrhea
        - Loperamide Diphenoxylate
        - (E) Alosetron
  - Negative
    - Consider other functional GI disorders
    - See Chronic Diarrhea (p 204) and Constipation (p 208)

ANORECTAL PAIN

M. Angelo Trujilo, MD

A. Anorectal pain has several potential causes, including local and nonlocal disease processes. A careful history and physical examination, including neurologic, anoscopic, and pelvic examinations, are important in the search for a cause, which may range from an easily treated condition to a life-threatening one. Important considerations in the history are associated symptoms and reported signs (e.g., fever, rectal bleeding, vaginal discharge, hematuria, neurologic dysfunction). Also note rapid onset of symptoms, sexual practices, and any history of inflammatory bowel disease.

B. Careful inspection, along with digital and anoscopic examinations, reveals most local causes of anorectal pain, but further evaluation with proctosigmoidoscopy may be necessary. This also provides a means for obtaining biopsy specimens for culture and histology. Rectal bleeding, mucus discharge, diarrhea, and anorectal pain suggest proctitis from infection or other inflammatory causes.

C. A pelvic examination and consideration of pelvic ultrasonography or CT scan are important in the diagnosis of conditions that may cause referred pain to the anus and rectum. Most of these conditions have a common pathway of irritation of the pudendal nerves that supply sensory innervation to the anus and rectum. Cervical and vaginal cultures and urinalysis with culture are necessary when considering pelvic inflammatory disease, prostatitis, or nephrolithiasis. Consider CT-pyelography if the clinical picture is otherwise consistent with nephrolithiasis.

D. The diagnosis of proctalgia fugax rests on the history and the exclusion of other pelvic or anorectal abnormality. It is a benign condition of unknown cause characterized by paroxysmal anorectal pain of varying severity and sudden onset. Coccygodynia consists of throbbing or aching pain in the coccygeal region. Organic causes include fracture of the coccyx and traumatic arthritis of the sacrococcygeal joint. A functional coccygodynia also exists. Coccygeal tenderness associated with spasm of surrounding muscles is a common finding on physical examination. Tension myalgia of the pelvic floor describes a syndrome of chronic vague discomfort in the rectum, pelvis, or lower back in patients without any other definable cause of pain. Pain typically is constant. Some authorities believe that the pain may be related to poor posture, generalized deconditioning, and possible psychological disorders. Chronic idiopathic anal pain has features that overlap with the other chronic pain syndromes.

E. There are several neurologic causes of anorectal pain. Associated neurologic signs and symptoms, pain characteristics, onset of pain, and spinal pathology are important factors in considering a neurologic cause for rectal pain. After a careful neurologic examination the procedures listed will be helpful in diagnosis of a specific neurologic disorder. Formal neurology consultation is recommended.

F. Pain may originate in sacral spinal cord segments or sacral nerve roots. Neoplasm, abscess, or inflammatory processes of the conus medullaris may present with pain. Associated loss of bowel or bladder function often occurs.

G. Entrapment of the sacral nerve roots of the cauda equina may occur secondary to inflammatory reactions in the cerebrospinal fluid or they may be compressed by tumor, abscess, or lumbosacral disc herniation.

H. The sacral plexus is located against the posterior pelvic wall. The plexus may be compressed by tumor or enlarged lymph nodes. Consider CT or MRI of the sacral spine and pelvis.

I. Spinal subarachnoid hemorrhage is a rare cause of rectal pain. This is most commonly the result of vascular malformation rupture, but it may also be associated with trauma, anticoagulant therapy, blood dyscrasias, or tumor. Ependymoma is the most common tumor associated with spinal subarachnoid hemorrhage. In patients with sudden onset of rectal pain associated with back pain, headache, stiff neck, and fever, consider spinal subarachnoid hemorrhage.

References

Harper MB, Pope JB. Office procedures: flexible sigmoidoscopy. Prim Care 1997;24:341.

Hull T. Examination and diseases of the anorectum. In Feldman M, Friedman LS, Sleisenger MH, eds. Gastrointestinal and Liver Disease, 7th ed. Philadelphia: WB Saunders, 2002:2277.

Lieberman DA. Common anorectal disorders. Ann Intern Med 1984;101:837.

Peery WH. Proctalgia fugax: a clinical enigma. South Med J 1988;81:621.

Rappaport B, Emsellem HA, Shesser R, Millstein E. An unusual case of proctalgia. Ann Emerg Med 1990;19:201.

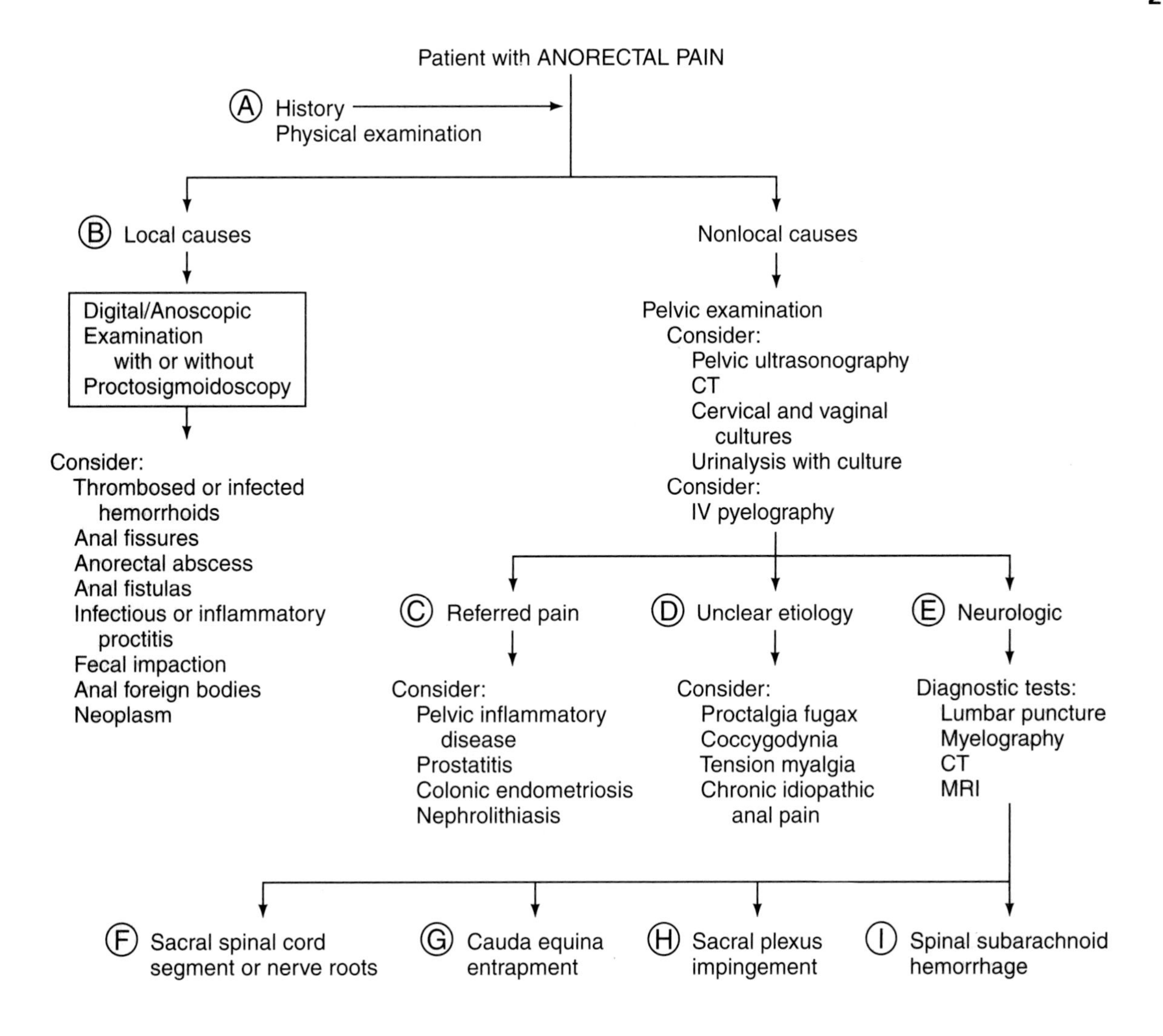
Patient with ANORECTAL PAIN
(A) History
Physical examination
(B) Local causes
Nonlocal causes
Digital/Anoscopic Examination with or without Proctosigmoidoscopy
Consider:
Thrombosed or infected hemorrhoids
Anal fissures
Anorectal abscess
Anal fistulas
Infectious or inflammatory proctitis
Fecal impaction
Anal foreign bodies
Neoplasm
Pelvic examination
Consider:
Pelvic ultrasonography
CT
Cervical and vaginal cultures
Urinalysis with culture
Consider:
IV pyelography
(C) Referred pain
(D) Unclear etiology
(E) Neurologic
Consider:
Pelvic inflammatory disease
Prostatitis
Colonic endometriosis
Nephrolithiasis
Consider:
Proctalgia fugax
Coccygodynia
Tension myalgia
Chronic idiopathic anal pain
Diagnostic tests:
Lumbar puncture
Myelography
CT
MRI
(F) Sacral spinal cord segment or nerve roots
(G) Cauda equina entrapment
(H) Sacral plexus impingement
(I) Spinal subarachnoid hemorrhage

POSITIVE FECAL OCCULT BLOOD TEST (FOBT)

M. Brian Fennerty, MD

Colon cancer will affect 6% of us during our lifetimes. Each year in the United States, there are >140,000 new cases and 50,000 deaths from colorectal carcinoma. Accumulating evidence suggests that screening patients for colorectal neoplasia may either prevent colorectal cancer by detecting colon polyps that may evolve into carcinoma or allow detection of colorectal cancer at a pre-symptomatic earlier stage, making curative therapy more likely. At present this screening strategy consists of (1) testing stool for the presence of blood, most commonly using guaiac-impregnated cards, flushable reagent pads, or immunochemical tests, and (2) directly observing the distal colon by endoscopic or radiographic examinations.

A. The clinical use of a positive fecal occult blood test (FOBT) obtained at the time of digital rectal examination has not been adequately validated. Despite the absence of data regarding accuracy in detecting neoplastic disease, this is a widely accepted and practiced clinical test. It has been estimated that false-positive rates up to 25% occur with FOBT on digital rectal examination. Until the specificity of FOBT by digital rectal examination is clarified, it is recommended that patients undergo FOBT only on spontaneously evacuated stools.

B. Patients should be sent home with FOBT cards, educated about diet and medicine, and asked to provide stool samples. Any one of six samples testing positive should be further evaluated. The test is positive in 4%–6% of asymptomatic patients tested, but only 5%–10% of these have colorectal cancer and 20%–30% have colon polyps; therefore, 60%–70% are false-positive results. In addition, 30%–50% of patients with proven colon cancer have a false-negative test result. Therefore, a positive test leads to further evaluation in many patients without disease, and a negative test result does not exclude disease.

C. For evaluating a patient with a positive FOBT result, two strategies are available: (1) flexible sigmoidoscopy and air-contrast barium enema or (2) colonoscopy, either endoscopic or CT colography. With the first strategy, any positive finding (e.g., polyp or cancer) necessitates colonoscopy. In addition, the first strategy alone misses 10% of cancers and 20% of large polyps. Therefore, colonoscopy is the preferred means of evaluation when available. It also may provide the most cost-effective strategy under certain conditions.

D. If symptoms dictate or if there is iron deficiency, a normal colonoscopy indicates that a further search for GI blood loss from the upper gut is indicated. Esophagogastroduodenoscopy (EGD) should be performed to evaluate the presence of upper GI structural lesions (ulcer, inflammation, tumors, arteriovenous malformations [AVMs]).

E. Although small bowel tumors, or Crohn's disease of the small bowel, usually do not present with heme-positive stools, a negative endoscopic examination of colon and upper GI tract should prompt evaluation of the small bowel, preferably by capsule endoscopy. However, neither of these tests detects small mucosal lesions such as AVM or small tumors.

F. If stools remain positive for fecal occult blood, consider invasive studies such as angiography or small bowel enteroscopy or capsule, which are now widely available. These may permit visualization of small vascular lesions or tumors undetectable by other means.

G. If a colon cancer or large cherry-red polyp is found, this may be presumed to be the cause of bleeding and may be treated endoscopically or surgically. Similarly the presence of mucosal inflammation (i.e., colitis) is also presumably the source. However, the presence of AVMs or diverticula is not sufficient to exclude either proximal source.

References

Barry MJ, Mulley AG, Richter JM. Effect of workup strategy on the cost-effectiveness of fecal occult blood screening for colorectal cancer. Gastroenterology 1987;93:301.

Fleisher ED, Goldberg SB, Browning TH, et al. Detection surveillance of colorectal cancer. JAMA 1989;261:580.

Guittet L, Bouvier V, Mariotte N, et al. Comparison of a guaiac based and an immunochemical faecal occult blood test in screening for colorectal cancer in a general average risk population. Gut 2007;56:210–214. Epub 2006 Aug 4.

Kim DH, Pickhardt PJ, Taylor AJ, et al. CT colonography versus colonoscopy for the detection of advanced neoplasia. N Engl J Med 2007;357:1403–1412.

Knight KK, Fielding JE, Battista R. Occult blood screening colorectal cancer. JAMA 1989;261:587.

Levin B, Bond JH. Colorectal cancer screening: recommendations of the U.S. Preventive Task Force. Gastroenterology 1996;111:1381.

Read TE, Read JD, Butterly LF. Importance of adenomas 5 mm or less in diameter that are detected by sigmoidoscopy. N Engl J Med 1997;336:8.

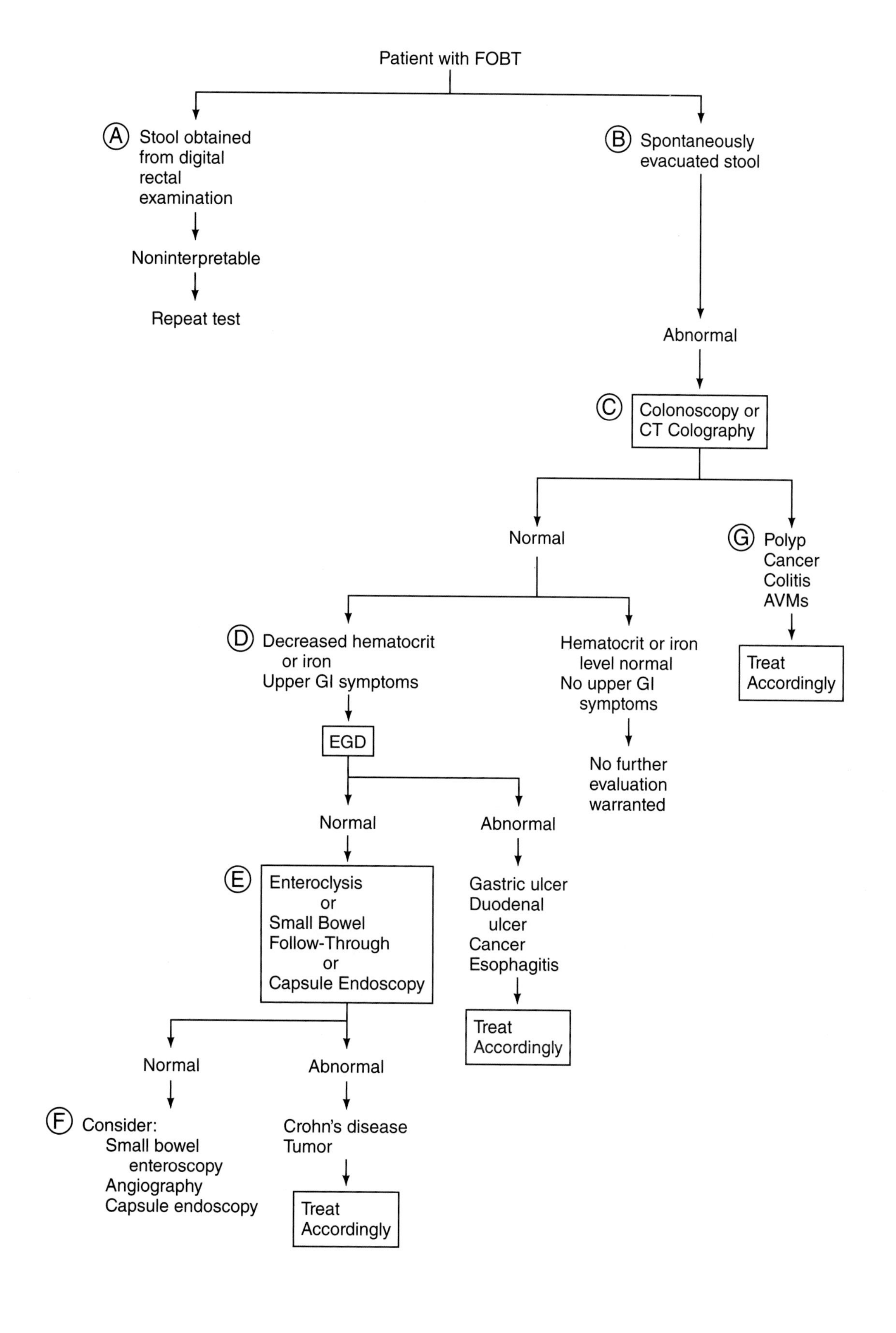
Patient with FOBT
A Stool obtained from digital rectal examination
Noninterpretable
Repeat test
B Spontaneously evacuated stool
Abnormal
C Colonoscopy or CT Colography
Normal
G Polyp
Cancer
Colitis
AVMs
Treat Accordingly
D Decreased hematocrit or iron
Upper GI symptoms
EGD
Hematocrit or iron level normal
No upper GI symptoms
No further evaluation warranted
Normal
Abnormal
E Enteroclysis or Small Bowel Follow-Through or Capsule Endoscopy
Gastric ulcer
Duodenal ulcer
Cancer
Esophagitis
Treat Accordingly
Normal
Abnormal
F Consider:
Small bowel enteroscopy
Angiography
Capsule endoscopy
Crohn's disease
Tumor
Treat Accordingly

FLATULENCE

Gregory L. Eastwood, MD

A. Flatulence is the passage of excess intestinal gas per rectum or the feeling that excessive gas is in the abdomen. Many patients complain of bloating, meaning that the abdomen becomes uncomfortably distended, usually after eating. Often, bloating is attributed to excessive intestinal gas. However, the perception that the passage of flatus or the amount of intestinal gas is excessive may be inaccurate because it may not actually be due to an abnormal amount of intestinal gas. Patients who complain of excessive flatus or of abdominal pain from gas sometimes have disorders of gut motility and a heightened pain response to intestinal gas, rather than excess intestinal gas. Some patients who complain of abdominal pain and bloating do have demonstrable disorders, such as peptic disease, gallbladder disease, Crohn's disease, or recurrent bowel obstruction. If, in addition to complaints of gaseousness, the patient has loss of weight, localized abdominal pain, vomiting, or blood in the stool, the suspicion of an organic GI disorder is increased.

B. Bacterial action on dietary substrates produces gas. Some patients can identify certain foods that aggravate the symptoms. A common offender is lactose, which causes excess intestinal gas production, cramps, and diarrhea in lactase-deficient individuals. Elimination of milk and milk products, legumes, cabbage, and similar foods may be effective in alleviating symptoms.

C. Perform sigmoidoscopy and a barium enema or colonoscopy to look for anorectal disease and colonic disorders. Reflux into the terminal ileum may identify Crohn's disease.

D. Upper GI and small bowel x-ray series may identify Crohn's disease of the small intestine, recurrent small bowel obstruction, or other disorders of the upper GI tract. Ultrasonography of the abdomen and pelvis may identify gallstones or an extraintestinal mass.

E. Testing gut motor function may help diagnose a motility disorder, neuropathy, or systemic disease such as scleroderma. Hydrogen breath testing can suggest carbohydrate malabsorption or small bowel bacterial overgrowth.

F. High-fiber bulking agents or so-called antispasmodics, such as dicyclomine, may be useful in patients who have no demonstrable treatable disorder or in whom a specific food has not been implicated. However, bulking agents, because they contain nondigestible substrates, may cause increased flatus. In some patients, stress reduction therapy may be helpful.

References

American Gastroenterological Association website. Gas in the digestive tract. www.gastro.org.

Azpiroz F. Intestinal gas dynamics: mechanisms and clinical relevance. Gut 2005;54:893.

Hasler WL. Approach to the patient with gas and bloating. In Yamada T, Alpers DH, Kaplowitz N, et al, eds. Textbook of Gastroenterology, 4th ed. Philadelphia: Lippincott Williams & Wilkins, 2003:802.

Rao SS. Belching, bloating, and flatulence. How to help patients who have troublesome abdominal gas. Postgrad Med 1997;101:275.

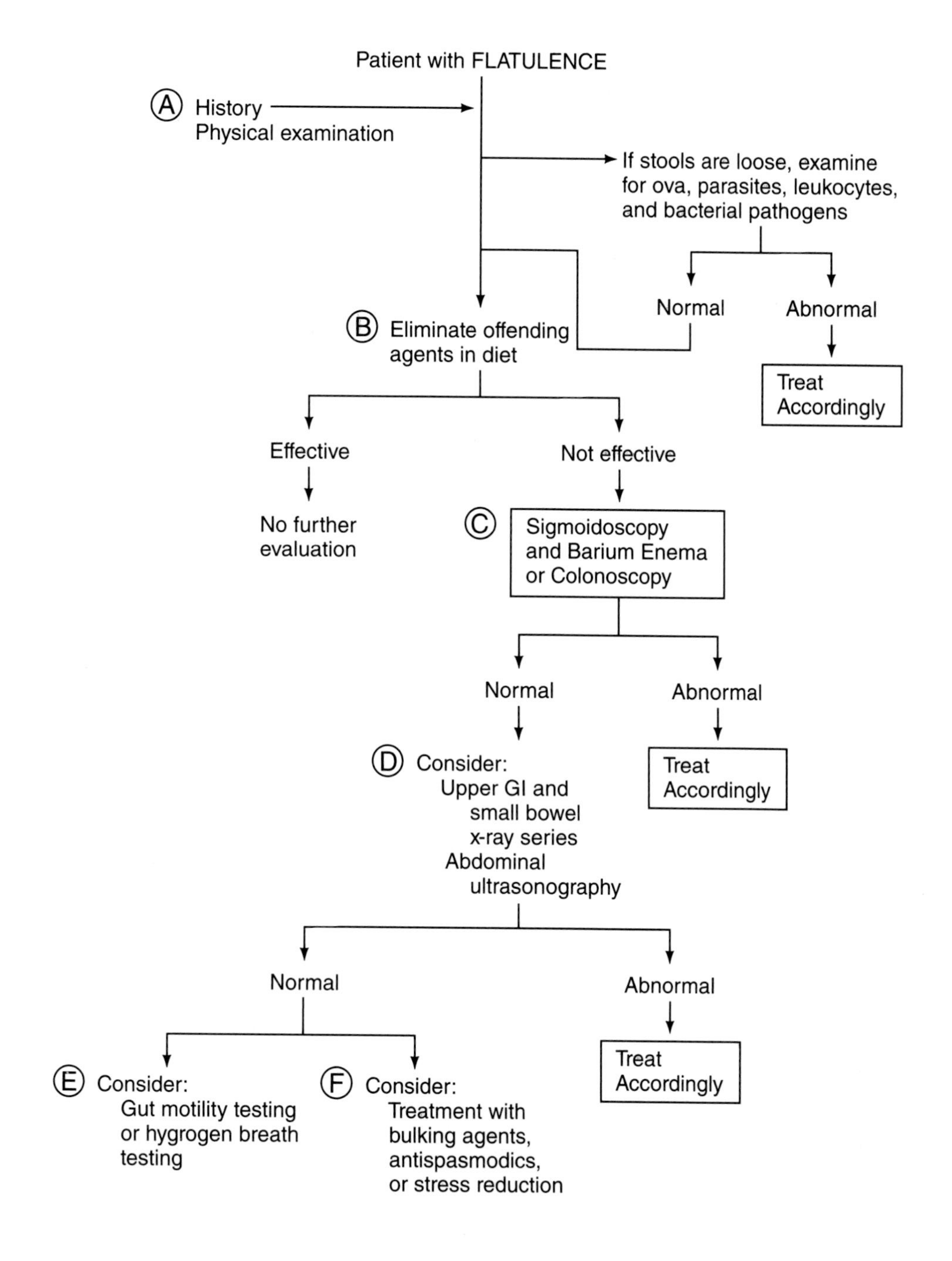
Patient with FLATULENCE
A
History
Physical examination
If stools are loose, examine for ova, parasites, leukocytes, and bacterial pathogens
Normal
Abnormal
Treat Accordingly
B
Eliminate offending agents in diet
Effective
No further evaluation
Not effective
C
Sigmoidoscopy and Barium Enema or Colonoscopy
Normal
Abnormal
Treat Accordingly
D
Consider:
Upper GI and small bowel x-ray series
Abdominal ultrasonography
Normal
Abnormal
Treat Accordingly
E
Consider:
Gut motility testing or hygrogen breath testing
F
Consider:
Treatment with bulking agents, antispasmodics, or stress reduction

FECAL INCONTINENCE

Philip E. Jaffe, MD

A. A history of rectal surgery, trauma, or infections may provide clues to the cause of fecal incontinence. A temporal relation with systemic conditions, including progressive neuromuscular disease, cerebrovascular disease, and diabetes mellitus, can often suggest the etiology. A history of previous anal sphincteric injury during childbirth is an important clue as well. The common anorectal disorders, including fistula, fissures, viral infection, tumors, postinflammatory strictures, distal rectal ulcers, and severe hemorrhoidal disease, may contribute to incontinence through several mechanisms. In addition, any condition that can lead to severe diarrhea can also lead to fecal incontinence by overwhelming the ability of the anus to control the large volume. For this reason all causes of diarrhea, including infectious, malabsorptive, inflammatory, and neoplastic, need to be considered. Paradoxically, fecal impaction is another potential cause and needs to be excluded. A careful history to determine the consistency of the material passed and the circumstances during which this occurs is very helpful. Physical examination should focus on inspection of the perineum and digital rectal examination.

B. Flexible sigmoidoscopy should be performed to exclude distal colonic masses, proctitis, and other common rectal processes. When sigmoidoscopy is normal or if diarrhea without anorectal disease is suspected, colonoscopy should be performed to exclude more proximal colon disease. Additional studies, including small bowel x-ray and biopsy, stool cultures and studies for parasitic infection, and timed quantified stool collections, may all be part of the evaluation.

C. Anorectal manometry with a balloon-tipped catheter is performed to determine anal sphincter resting and squeeze pressures, the threshold for rectal sensation to distention, and the appropriateness of anal sphincter pressure response to rectal distention and defecatory effort. Rectal compliance may also be calculated. Higher-than-normal sensory thresholds are common in diabetic persons with incontinence and may respond to the addition of bulking agents, opioid antidiarrheal drugs, and biofeedback training. In cases in which traumatic disruption of the anal sphincter is considered (usually during childbirth or by previous surgery), anorectal endoscopic ultrasound may be useful in defining areas of muscular injury and directing surgical repair.

D. When available, defecography can demonstrate anatomic defects, including rectal prolapse, that may not be detected during examination or on endoscopic evaluation.

E. Disease of the rectum, including ulcerative proctitis, ischemia, and radiation proctitis, can lead to decreased rectal compliance and incontinence. Infusion of saline into the rectum while intraluminal pressures are measured can define this problem. As in all anorectal conditions that lead to fecal incontinence, proximal fecal diversion (usually by colostomy) may be necessary if other pharmacologic, dietary, behavioral, and local surgical measures fail.

References

Fernandez-Fraga X, Azpiroz F, Malagelada J. Significance of pelvic floor muscles in anal incontinence. Gastroenterology 2002;123:1441.

Madoff R, Parker S, Varma M, Lowry A. Faecal incontinence in adults. Lancet 2004;364:621.

Norton C, Chelvanayagam S, Wilson-Barnett J, et al. Randomized controlled trial of biofeedback for fecal incontinence. Gastroenterology 2003;125:1320.

Rao S. Diagnosis and management of fecal incontinence. Am J Gastroenterol 2004;99:1585.

Sagar P, Pemberton J. Anorectal and pelvic floor function. Relevance of continence, incontinence, and constipation. Gastroenterol Clin North Am 1996;25:163.

Sager P, Pemberton J. The assessment and treatment of anorectal incontinence. Adv Surg 1996;30:1.

Whitehead W. Functional anorectal disease. Semin Gastroenterol 1996; 4:230.

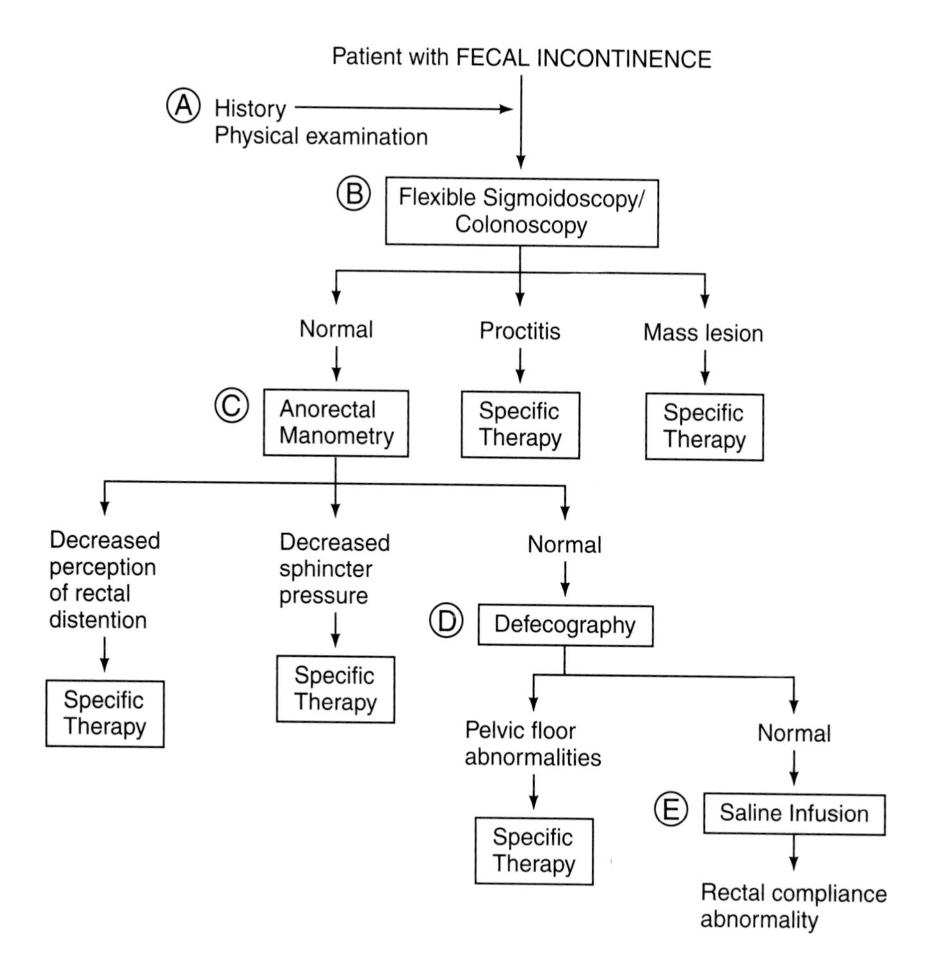

Patient with FECAL INCONTINENCE
A
History
Physical examination
B
Flexible Sigmoidoscopy/ Colonoscopy
Normal
Proctitis
Mass lesion
C
Anorectal Manometry
Specific Therapy
Specific Therapy
Decreased perception of rectal distention
Decreased sphincter pressure
Normal
Specific Therapy
Specific Therapy
D
Defecography
Pelvic floor abnormalities
Normal
Specific Therapy
E
Saline Infusion
Rectal compliance abnormality

ASYMPTOMATIC ABNORMAL LIVER AMINOTRANSFERASES

Juan Diego Baltodano, MD, and Bipin Saud, MD

Liver aminotransferases include aspartate aminotransferase (AST, formerly SGOT) and alanine aminotransferase (ALT, formerly SGPT). They actively participate in the process of gluconeogenesis as mitochondrial and cytosolic enzymes within the hepatocyte. Other liver biochemical enzymes include alkaline phosphatase (canalicular membrane), gamma glutamyl transpeptidase (hepatocyte and biliary epithelia), and 5′-nucleotidase (sinusoidal and canalicular membrane).

Abnormally increased serum liver enzymes are reported in approximately 0.5%–4% of the asymptomatic population, usually when routine health screening testing is performed. The first step when evaluating a patient with increased liver biochemistries is to assess the degree of abnormality. If those are minimal (usually 2–5 times the upper limit of the reference range), retesting is necessary to avoid excessive and expensive workup.

Of significance is that reference laboratory values are defined as the mean of the distribution ± 2 standard deviations of the normal population. Therefore, there will always be a subset of asymptomatic patients (2.5% above and 2.5% below the reference range) without any demonstrable cause of minimally "abnormal" liver chemistries. However, patients with underlying chronic liver disease may have fluctuating levels of "normal" serum liver biochemistries throughout the course of their disease. Physiologic states can also lead to elevated liver enzymes (e.g., pregnancy induces elevation of alkaline phosphatase).

A. If a significant abnormal pattern is detected, use the diagnostic clues to guide further testing. During the initial evaluation, review patient symptoms; risk factors for liver disease (alcohol abuse, illicit drug use, tattoos, history of blood transfusions, sexual history); associated morbid conditions (diabetes or glucose intolerance, obesity, dyslipidemia); medications (including herbal/alternative and over-the-counter medications); and family history. Perform a thorough physical examination. Look for stigmata of chronic liver disease such as spider angiomas, palmar erythema, gynecomastia, testicular atrophy, and Duputyren's contractures during physical examination.

B. The clinical significance of any liver chemistry test abnormality must be interpreted in the context of each clinical setting. Generally, these abnormalities can be further categorized into three main groups: hepatocellular injury predominance (AST/ALT), associated cholestasis (increased alkaline phosphatase and bilirubin), and/or associated impaired metabolic/synthetic liver function (low albumin, prolonged prothrombin time [PT]). Specific ratios and levels of serum AST to ALT may be useful in differential diagnosis. For example, in most forms of acute liver injury this ratio is ≤1, whereas in alcoholic hepatitis it is typically >2. Elevation of these enzymes >1000 U/L suggests ongoing acute viral, drug, or ischemic insult to the liver.

Epidemiologic factors help guide further evaluation and management. Worldwide, viral hepatitides are the most common causes of abnormal liver transaminases. Hereditary hemochromatosis (HH) is also frequent. Therefore, initial testing for mildly elevated aminotransferases must include serologies for hepatitis A, B, and C viruses as well as fasting iron (Fe) studies (serum ferritin and iron saturation). Nonalcoholic fatty liver disease (NAFLD) unfortunately has no specific serologic test available, and it is increasing in frequency. Risk factors for fatty liver include the presence of obesity, hypertriglyceridemia, glucose intolerance, and diabetes mellitus.

(Continued on page 224)

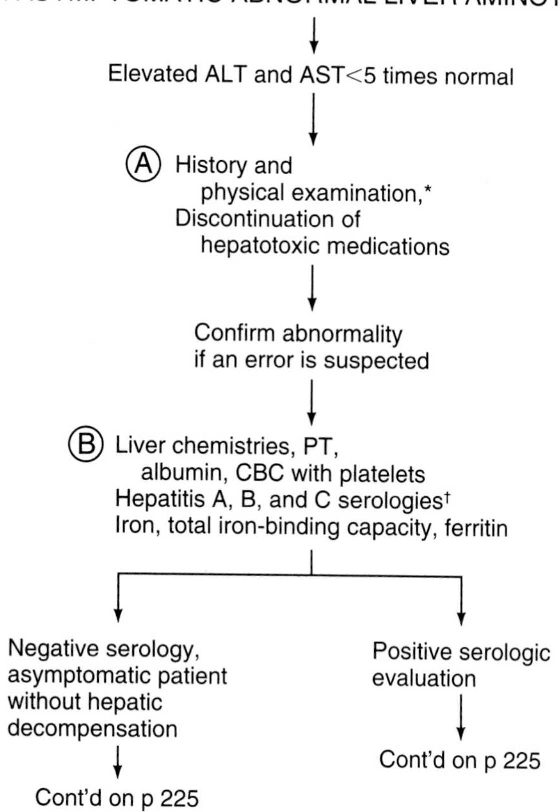

Patient with ASYMPTOMATIC ABNORMAL LIVER AMINOTRANSFERASES
Elevated ALT and AST<5 times normal
(A) History and physical examination,*
Discontinuation of hepatotoxic medications
Confirm abnormality if an error is suspected
(B) Liver chemistries, PT, albumin, CBC with platelets
Hepatitis A, B, and C serologies†
Iron, total iron-binding capacity, ferritin
Negative serology, asymptomatic patient without hepatic decompensation
Cont'd on p 225
Positive serologic evaluation
Cont'd on p 225

C. If hepatitis serologies and iron studies are normal, serum ceruloplasmin and alpha-1-antitrypsin should be measured to screen for Wilson's disease and alpha-1-antitrypsin deficiency disorders, respectively. Chronic autoimmune hepatitis can be another less common cause of liver AST/ALT elevation. It occurs predominantly in women and is often associated with thyroiditis and other autoimmune disorders. Serum serologic markers to screen for autoimmune hepatitis include antinuclear antibody (ANA), anti–smooth-muscle antibody (Ab), and potentially liver kidney microsomal (LKM) antibody. Other hepatotropic viruses (concomitant hepatitis E and D, Epstein-Barr, cytomegalovirus, and herpes) or infiltrating liver disease (sarcoidosis, tuberculosis, amyloidosis, fungal infection, and lymphomas) can be a cause for elevated aminotransferases. Uncommon nonhepatic causes for abnormal transaminases include thyroid disease, muscle disorders, celiac disease, hemolysis, and strenuous exercise.

When the alkaline phosphatase is also found to be abnormally elevated, hepatobiliary or nonhepatic origin should be differentiated. Serum assays of 5′-nucleotidase or gamma glutamyl transferase are generally used to confirm or exclude a liver-specific origin. Once confirmed, liver imaging studies are recommended to complete inital evaluation. Radiologic tests available include utrasonography (US), CT, radionuclide scans, and MRI. For biliary obstruction or parenchymal disease, US or CT are included as a part of the inital evaluation. If a primary or metastasic liver malignancy is suspected, a triple-phase CT of the liver is recommended. For the detection of intrahepatic vascular lesions, a nuclear scan or MRI of the liver is necessary. Finally, magnetic resonance cholangiopancreatography (MRCP) is an effective noninvasive imaging technique to evaluate biliary ductal anatomy.

D. Liver biopsy provides important prognostic and diagnostic information in patients with liver disease. However, it should be performed only if the expected results exceed the low risks of the procedure. In patients with chronically elevated (>6 months) liver enzymes or with impaired hepatic function, liver biopsy should be considered. Recent studies have shown that the most likely diagnosis is steatosis and steatohepatitis when biopsy is performed for abnormal liver chemistries with unremarkable serologies.

References

Daniel S, Ben-Menachem T, Vasudevan G, et al. Prospective evaluation of unexplained chronic liver transaminase abnormalities in asymptomatic and symptomatic patients. Am J Gastroenterol 1999;94(10):3010–3014.

Feldman M, Friedman LS, Sleisenger MH. Biochemical liver test. In Davern TJ, Scharrschmidt BF, eds. Gastrointestinal and Liver Disease: Pathophysiology, Diagnosis, Management. Vol. 2. Philadelphia: Saunders, 2002:1227–1239.

Goessling W, Friedman LS. Increased liver chemistry in an asymptomatic patient. Clin Gastroenterol Hepatol 2005;3(9):852–858.

Green RM, Flam S. AGA Technical review on the evaluation of liver chemistry tests. Gastroenterology 2002;123(4):1367–1384.

Neuschwander-Tetri BA, Caldwell SH. Nonalcoholic steatohepatitis: summary of an AASLD Single Topic Conference. Hepatology 2003;37(5):1202–1219.

Pratt DS, Kaplan MM. Evaluation of abnormal liver-enzyme results in asymptomatic patients. N Engl J Med 2000;342(17):1266–1271.

Sampliner RE. The liver disease of asymptomatic patients with elevated aminotransferases. Hepatology 1989;10(4):524–525.

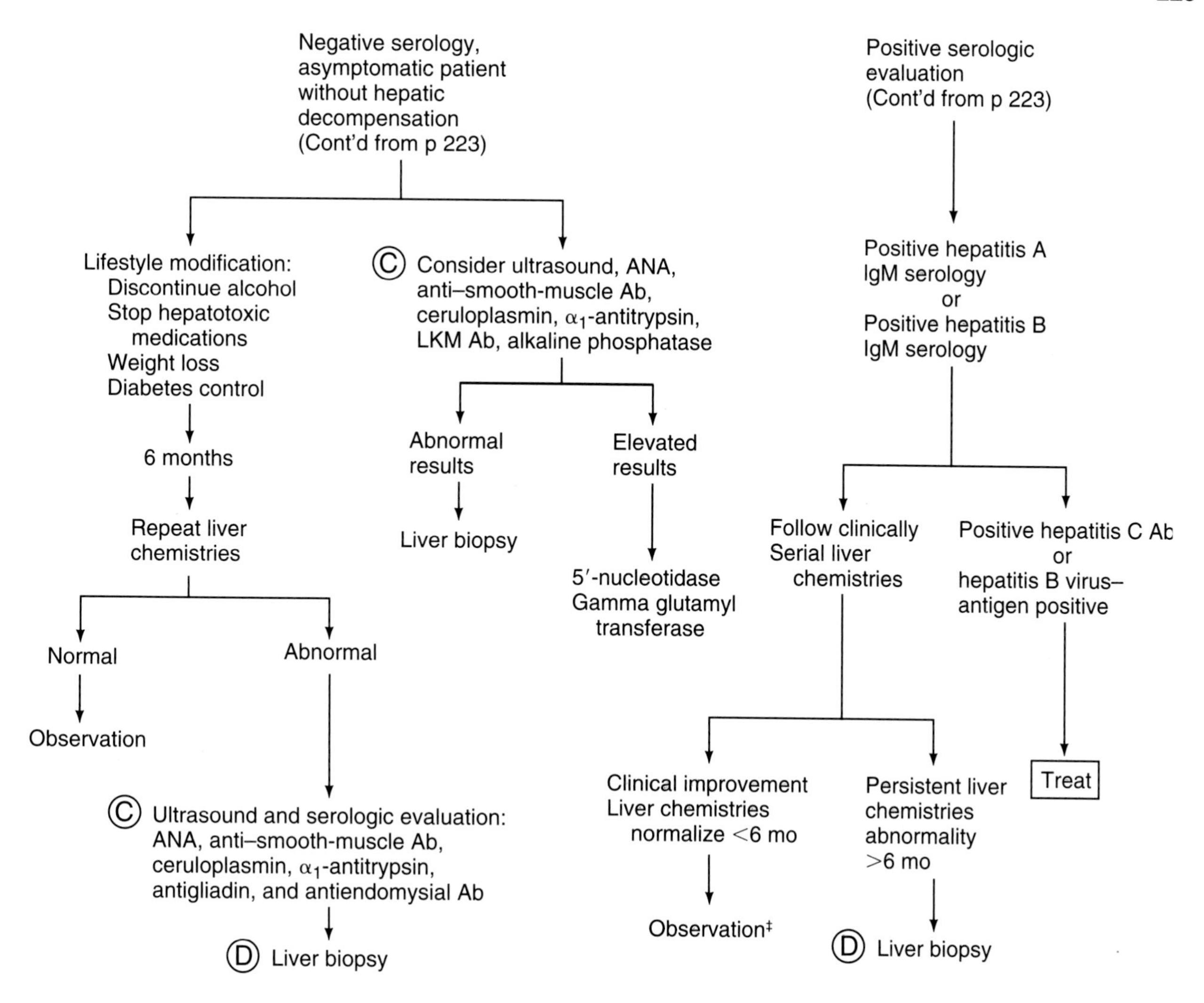

Elective radiologic and serologic evaluations should be dependent on the clinical scenario specific to an individual patient. In addition, depending on the clinical scenario, computerized tomography or abdominal magnetic resonance imaging may be preferable to ultrasonography. Patients with more significant elevations of the ALT or AST, with an abnormal albumin or prothrombin time, or with evidence of chronic liver disease and/or hepatic decompensation should typically have more expeditious evaluations.

* When findings from these indicate that one or more diagnostic considerations are likely, subsequent evaluation should be direct toward establishing these diagnoses.

† HAV–IgM, HBsAg, and Hepatitis B core antibody–IgM fraction (HBcIgM), HCV antibody (consider HCV–RNA).

‡ Liver biopsy may considered in patients with chronic HCV viremia and either normal or abnormal serum ALT levels.

Modified from the American Gastroenterological Association. American Gastroenterological Association medical position statement: Evaluation of liver chemistry tests. Gastroenterology 2002; 123:1364.

ELEVATED SERUM IRON

M. Brian Fennerty, MD

A. Hemochromatosis is an inherited autosomal-recessive disorder characterized by excessive GI absorption of iron and progressive iron deposition in parenchymal organs. The gene frequency in the population is 0.06%. Clinical characteristics include lethargy, weight loss, increased skin pigmentation, loss of libido, abdominal pain, joint pain, diabetes, hepatomegaly, testicular atrophy, and arthropathy. Patients with asymptomatic hemochromatosis with increased serum iron must be differentiated from patients with iron overload secondary to alcoholic liver disease, hemolytic anemias, and medicinal iron. The family history may indicate liver disease.

B. The serum iron is a poor screening test to detect idiopathic hemochromatosis (IHC) because false-positive results occur in those ingesting iron, in alcoholics, and in those with heterozygotes of the hemochromatosis allele. However, calculating the transferrin saturation from the serum iron and the iron-binding capacity proves to have a sensitivity >90% (for saturation >60%). Unfortunately, as many as 24% of people (many heterozygotes) with normal iron stores also have saturation in this range. The serum ferritin reflects total body iron, and an increase in ferritin usually reflects increased body stores. When combined, increased transferrin saturation and elevated ferritin have a sensitivity of 94%.

C. The diagnosis of IHC requires direct documentation of excess iron in the liver. In addition, quantifying the amount of iron and liver damage has important treatment and prognostic implications. Normal hepatic iron concentrations are 300–800 μg/g dry weight. In those with hemochromatosis, the hepatic iron concentration usually is >10,000 μg/g dry weight. Presymptomatic patients with hemochromatosis occassionally may have iron concentrations that overlap with those of persons with alcoholic liver disease. The recent identification of the gene for hereditary hemochromatosis (HFE C282Y and H63D) has resulted in the ability to accurately diagnose the disease through a genetic screening test.

D. To differentiate alcoholic siderosis from hemochromatosis, Bassett et al. compared hepatic iron concentration in predominantly young patients with homozygous hemochromatosis with that in patients with alcoholic liver disease. Hepatic iron index (HII) was calculated by converting micrograms of dry weight to micromoles (1 μg/56 = μmols) and then dividing by the patient's age. This group discovered that all homozygous patients had an HII >2.0, and all patients with alcoholic liver disease and heterozygotes had an HII <2.0. This value appears to be the most discriminating test available to diagnose IHC.

References

Adams PC, Kertesz AE, McLaren CE, et al. Population screening for hemochromatosis: a comparison of unbound iron-binding capacity, transferrin saturation, and C282Y genotyping in 5,211 voluntary blood donors. Hepatology 2000;31:1160–1164.

Bassett ML, Halliday JW, Powell LW. Genetic hemochromatosis. Semin Liver Dis 1984;4:217.

Basset ML, Halliday JW, Powell LW. Value of hepatic iron measurements in early hemochromatosis and determination of the critical iron level associated with fibrosis. Hepatology 1986;6:24.

Bonkovsky HL, Ponka P, Bacon BR, et al. An update on iron metabolism: summary of the Fifth International Conference on Disorders of Iron Metabolism. Hepatology 1996;24:718.

Dadone MM, Kushner JP, Edwards CQ, et al. Hereditary hemochromatosis: analysis of laboratory expression of the disease by gene type in 18 pedigrees. Am J Clin Pathol 1982;78:196.

Edwards CQ, Griffen LM, Goldgar D, et al. Prevalence of hemochromatosis among 11,065 presumably healthy blood donors. N Engl J Med 1988;318:1355.

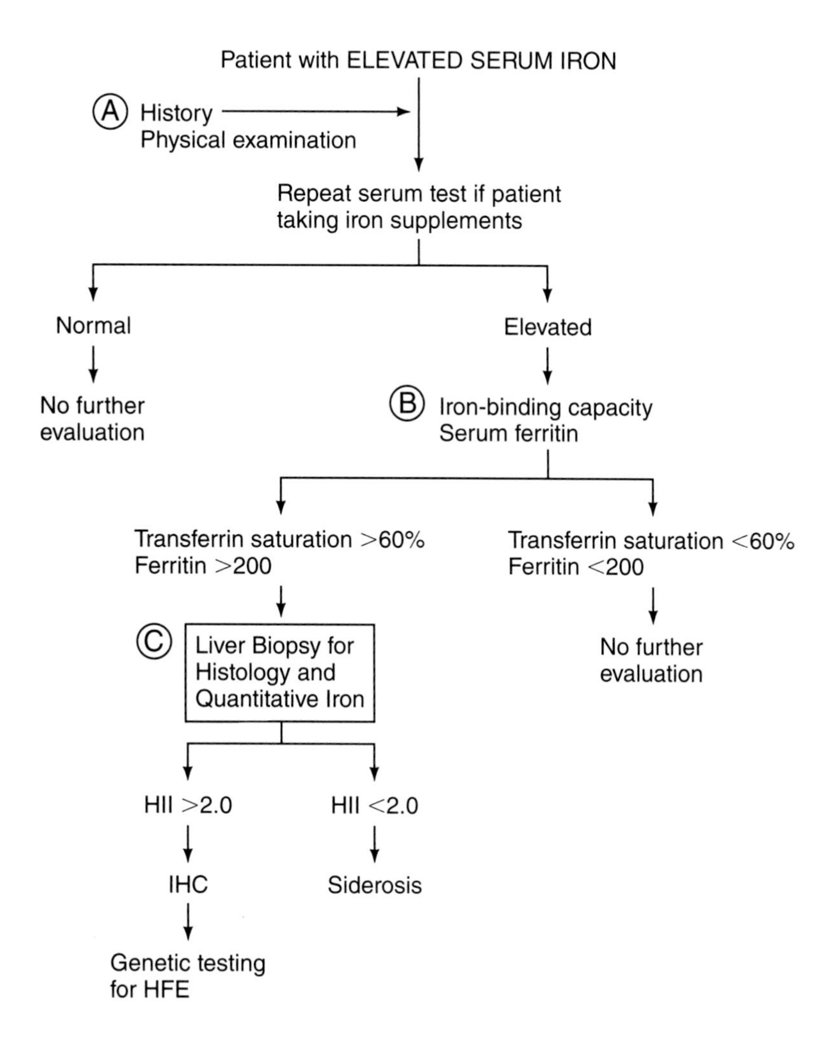

Patient with ELEVATED SERUM IRON
(A) History
Physical examination
Repeat serum test if patient taking iron supplements
Normal
No further evaluation
Elevated
(B) Iron-binding capacity
Serum ferritin
Transferrin saturation >60%
Ferritin >200
Transferrin saturation <60%
Ferritin <200
No further evaluation
(C) Liver Biopsy for Histology and Quantitative Iron
HII >2.0
HII <2.0
IHC
Siderosis
Genetic testing for HFE

ELEVATED SERUM AMYLASE

M. Angelo Trujillo, MD

A. Amylase is an enzyme with a 55,000-dalton molecular weight that hydrolyzes starch. The pancreas and salivary glands contain very high concentrations of amylase. Amylase also is produced by a number of other organs in lower concentrations. Approximately 35%–45% of normal serum amylase is of pancreatic origin. Amylase has a serum half-life of 1–2 hours. Approximately 20% of circulating amylase is excreted in the urine; the remainder is catabolized at an unknown site. Increased serum amylase is most commonly caused by pancreatitis, but hyperamylasemia may be associated with several other nonpancreatic or nonabdominal disorders with similar clinical presentations.

B. In acute pancreatitis serum amylase increases within 24–48 hours of the acute onset of pancreatitis. Levels return to normal within 3–5 days in most cases. A normal serum amylase level occasionally is seen in acute pancreatitis. This may represent early pancreatitis, after a transient rise and fall of amylase, extensive pancreatic necrosis with inability to produce amylase, or cases of acute exacerbation of chronic pancreatitis in which the gland cannot produce amylase. Serum amylase also may be normal when pancreatitis is associated with hypertriglyceridemia. In this case, a urinary amylase measurement usually shows a marked elevation. Cholelithiasis, ethanol, and idiopathic causes are responsible for about 90% of all cases of acute pancreatitis. Commonly used drugs known to cause pancreatitis include ethanol, hydrochlorothiazide, furosemide, sulfonamides, tetracyclines, estrogens, valproate, and azathioprine. A serum amylase level >3 times the upper limit of normal is consistent with pancreatitis. Other abdominal processes usually do not cause amylase levels >2–2.5 times the upper limit of normal, with the exception of salivary gland disease and gut perforation or infarction.

C. In acute pancreatitis with persistent elevated serum amylase levels, complications of acute pancreatitis as listed should be considered. Abdominal CT is useful in identifying pseudocysts, abscesses, ascites, and some tumors: Consider MRI of the pancreas with magnetic resonance cholangiopancreatography (MRCP) or endoscopic ultrasound (EUS), or consider endoscopic retrograde cholangiopancreatography (ERCP) in pancreatitis of biliary origin or idiopathic pancreatitis. This would be of low yield if the CT, MRI, MRCP, and EUS results are negative.

D. In a patient with epigastric pain and elevated serum amylase, rule out causes other than acute pancreatitis. In cases of perforated viscus (esophagus, stomach, small intestine, colon), peritoneal absorption of GI contents results in elevated serum amylase. The patient usually has a more abrupt onset of pain and more peritoneal irritation. Several other nonpancreatic conditions listed also present with more pronounced signs of peritonitis, and most need surgical intervention.

E. The elevation of serum amylase in renal insufficiency usually is modest, seldom >2 times the upper limit of normal. Macroamylasemia is a condition in which the major portion of serum amylase is bound to immunoglobin. A (IgA). These macromolecular aggregates cannot undergo glomerular filtration, so the urine amylase level is low or normal. The amylase/creatinine clearance ratio (ACR) is calculated as follows:

$$\text{ACR} = \frac{\text{A (urine)} \times \text{CR (serum)}}{\text{A (serum)} \times \text{CR (urine)}} \times 100$$

where A = amylase concentration and CR = creatinine concentration. In macroamylasemia, the ACR is abnormally low (usually <0.2%).

F. After the common causes have been considered, more obscure causes should be sought. Isoamylase or lipase measurements may be helpful. Elevated serum amylase secondary to lung disease or certain tumors is commonly of the salivary or s-isoenzyme. Alcoholic patients may have an elevated serum amylase of salivary origin.

References

Jensen DM, Rayse VL, Newell J, et al. Use of amylase isoenzyme in laboratory evaluation of hyperamylasemia. Dig Dis Sci 1987;32:561.

Magno EP, Chari S. Acute Pancreatitis. In: Feldman M, Friedman LS, She is enger MH, eds. Gastrointestinal and Liver Disease. 7th ed. Philadelphia: WB Saunders, 2002:913.

Rabsztyn A, Green PH, Berti I, et al. Macroamylasemia in patients with celiac disease. AM J Gastroenterol 2001;96:1096–1100.

Ranson JH. Diagnostic standards for acute pancreatitis. World J Surg 1997; 21:136.

Salt WB, Schenker S. Amylase—its significance: a review of the literature. Medicine 1976;55:269.

Tietz NW, Huang WY, Rauh DF, Shuey DF. Laboratory tests in the differential diagnosis of hyperamylasemia. Clin Chem 1986;32:301.

Toskes PP. Biochemical tests in pancreatic disease. Curr Opin Gastro 1991;7:709.

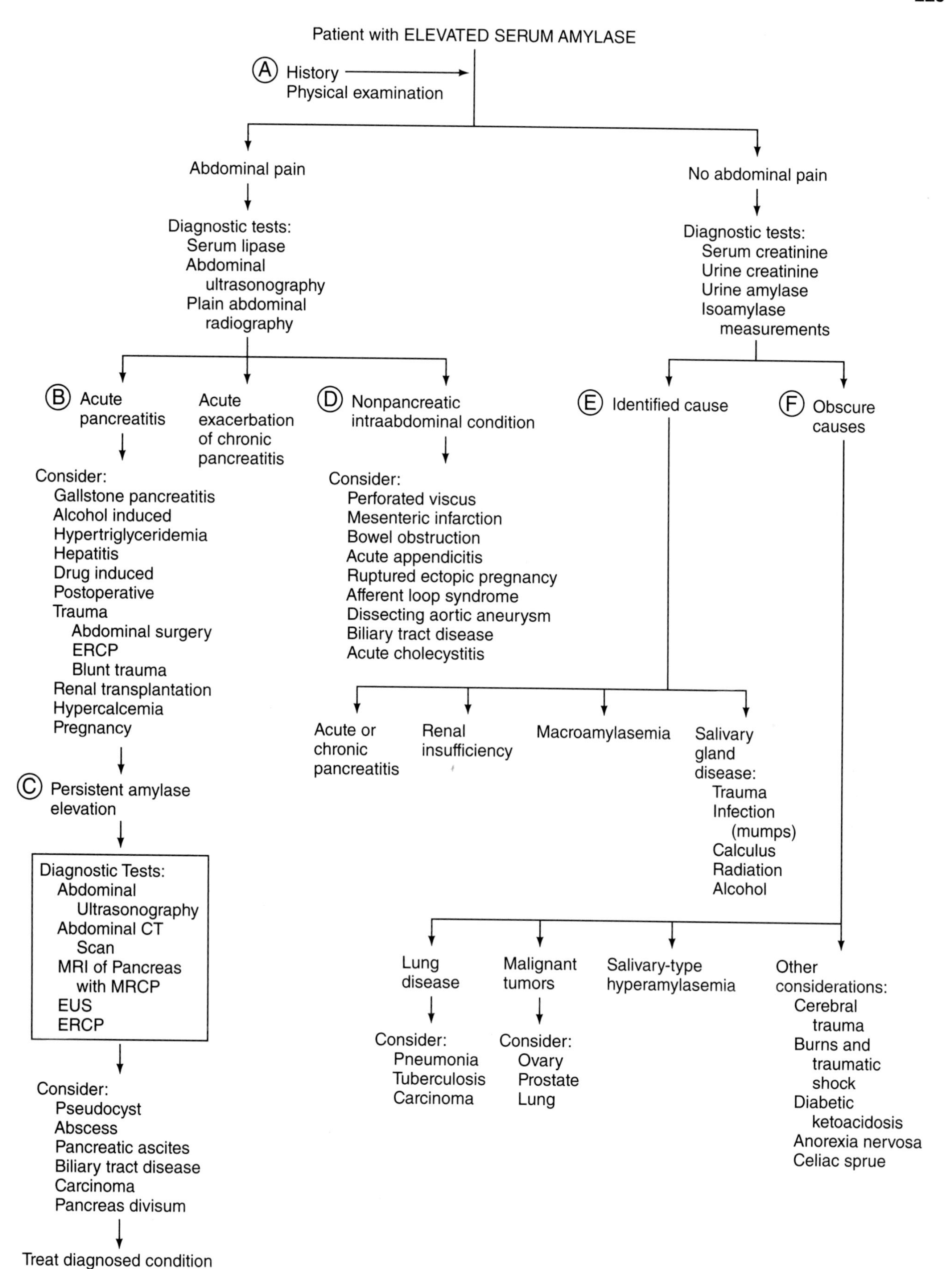
Patient with ELEVATED SERUM AMYLASE
(A) History
Physical examination
Abdominal pain
Diagnostic tests:
Serum lipase
Abdominal ultrasonography
Plain abdominal radiography
(B) Acute pancreatitis
Consider:
Gallstone pancreatitis
Alcohol induced
Hypertriglyceridemia
Hepatitis
Drug induced
Postoperative
Trauma
Abdominal surgery
ERCP
Blunt trauma
Renal transplantation
Hypercalcemia
Pregnancy
(C) Persistent amylase elevation
Diagnostic Tests:
Abdominal Ultrasonography
Abdominal CT Scan
MRI of Pancreas with MRCP
EUS
ERCP
Consider:
Pseudocyst
Abscess
Pancreatic ascites
Biliary tract disease
Carcinoma
Pancreas divisum
Treat diagnosed condition
Acute exacerbation of chronic pancreatitis
(D) Nonpancreatic intraabdominal condition
Consider:
Perforated viscus
Mesenteric infarction
Bowel obstruction
Acute appendicitis
Ruptured ectopic pregnancy
Afferent loop syndrome
Dissecting aortic aneurysm
Biliary tract disease
Acute cholecystitis
No abdominal pain
Diagnostic tests:
Serum creatinine
Urine creatinine
Urine amylase
Isoamylase measurements
(E) Identified cause
Acute or chronic pancreatitis
Renal insufficiency
Macroamylasemia
Salivary gland disease:
Trauma
Infection (mumps)
Calculus
Radiation
Alcohol
(F) Obscure causes
Lung disease
Consider:
Pneumonia
Tuberculosis
Carcinoma
Malignant tumors
Consider:
Ovary
Prostate
Lung
Salivary-type hyperamylasemia
Other considerations:
Cerebral trauma
Burns and traumatic shock
Diabetic ketoacidosis
Anorexia nervosa
Celiac sprue

Hematology/Oncology

Ana Maria López, MD, MPH, FACP
Section Editor

ANEMIA

Raymond Taetle, MD

A. The general evaluation of anemia includes an initial evaluation of volume status. If clinical signs of intravascular volume depletion such as orthostatic hypotension are present, RBC and plasma loss may have occurred. Correct intravascular volume before evaluating the patient for anemia.

B. Begin evaluation of the pathophysiology of anemia by assessing effective RBC production. The normal steady-state reticulocyte production is approximately 50,000/mm^3 per day (1% of 5 million), and the maximum production is approximately 400,000/mm^3. Under extreme stress, reticulocytes may be released from the marrow a day early, and even higher levels of apparent production are achieved. These figures may be used to interpret whether RBC production is increased or decreased.

C. Increased RBC production in a patient with anemia is presumptive evidence of increased RBC destruction (hemolysis). The hemolysis may be intravascular or predominantly extravascular. In either case, haptoglobin, the major plasma heme-binding protein, may be depressed. In intravascular hemolysis, free hemoglobin (Hb) may be present in plasma and iron (Fe) may be in renal tubule cells (urinary hemosiderin). Indirect bilirubin and lactate dehydrogenase may also be elevated. The Coombs' test is used to distinguish immune and nonimmune hemolysis. A positive, direct Coombs' test indicates antibody or complement on the RBC cell surface. Only certain IgG isotypes react with macrophage Fc receptors; therefore, a positive Coombs' test may be present without causing increased RBC destruction. Autoimmune antibodies have maximal binding at either 37° C (warm antibodies, usually IgG) or 4° C (cold antibodies, usually IgM).

D. If the spleen is palpable and thus clinically enlarged, hypersplenism cannot be definitively ruled out as a cause of RBC destruction. This can occur secondary to processes that themselves lead to anemia, such as the ineffective erythropoiesis accompanying thalassemia and hemolysis from an abnormal Hb, such as sickle cell/C disease.

E. If hypersplenism is unlikely, hemolysis may be a result of mechanical trauma, congenital enzyme, or Hb defects within the RBC. Microangiopathic hemolytic anemia (MAHA) results from RBC trauma from fibrin strands in small vessels (thrombotic thrombocytopenic purpura, hemolytic uremic syndrome, disseminated intravascular coagulation [DIC]), or more rarely, prosthetic heart valves. Enzymatic defects can be drug dependent, such as G6PD deficiency, or constitutive, such as pyruvate kinase deficiency. Abnormal Hbs (sickle hemoglobin) and membrane defects (hereditary spherocytosis) also cause hemolysis. Acquired causes of hemolysis include the excess complement sensitivity acquired in paroxysmal nocturnal hemoglobinuria (PNH) and infections such as malaria.

(Continued on page 234)

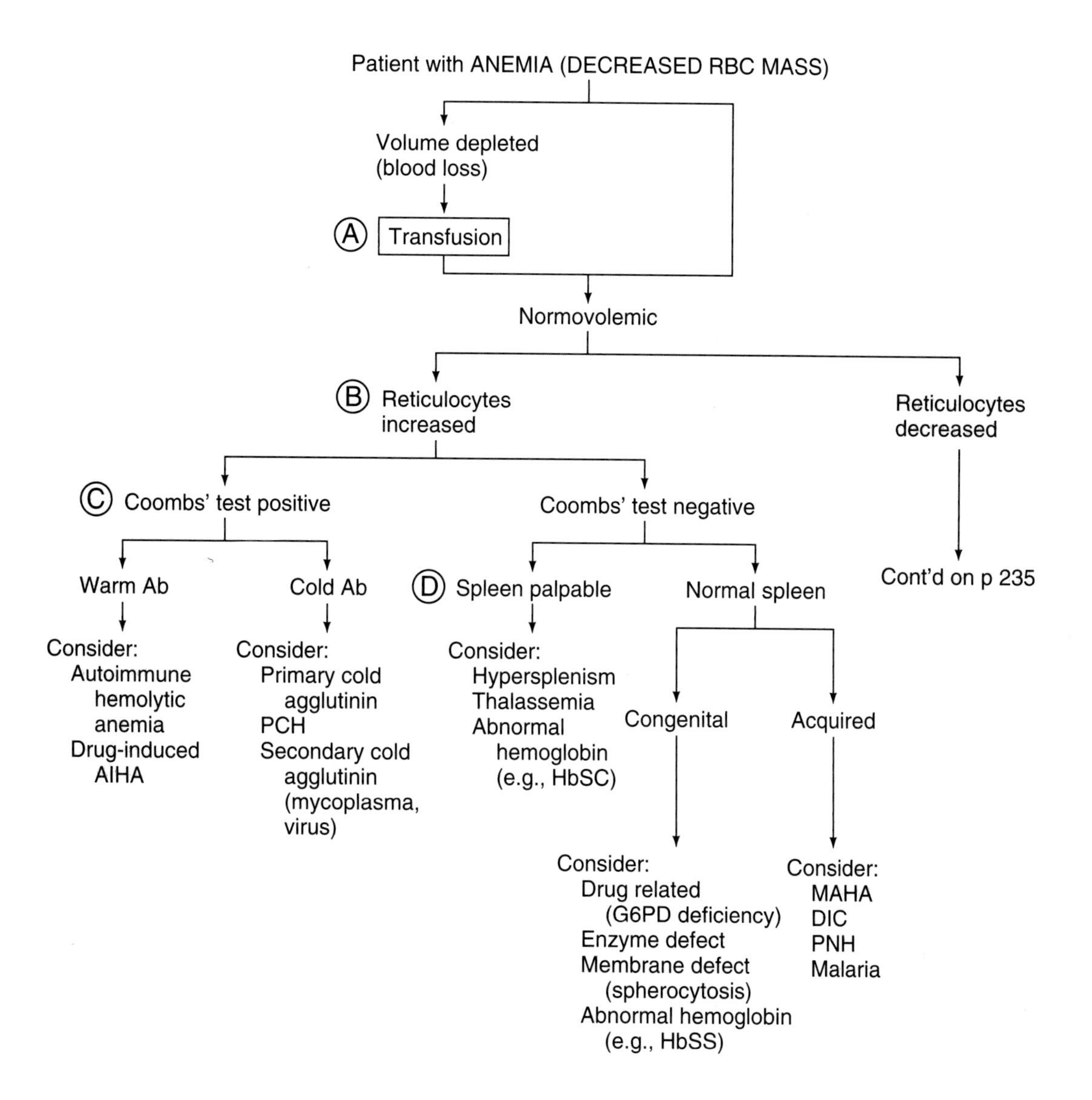
Patient with ANEMIA (DECREASED RBC MASS)
Volume depleted
(blood loss)
Ⓐ
Transfusion
Normovolemic
Ⓑ Reticulocytes
increased
Reticulocytes
decreased
Ⓒ Coombs' test positive
Coombs' test negative
Warm Ab
Cold Ab
Ⓓ Spleen palpable
Normal spleen
Cont'd on p 235
Consider:
Autoimmune
hemolytic
anemia
Drug-induced
AIHA
Consider:
Primary cold
agglutinin
PCH
Secondary cold
agglutinin
(mycoplasma,
virus)
Consider:
Hypersplenism
Thalassemia
Abnormal
hemoglobin
(e.g., HbSC)
Congenital
Acquired
Consider:
Drug related
(G6PD deficiency)
Enzyme defect
Membrane defect
(spherocytosis)
Abnormal hemoglobin
(e.g., HbSS)
Consider:
MAHA
DIC
PNH
Malaria

F. When RBC production is decreased or normal in the face of anemia (normal production with a reduced RBC mass constitutes depressed production), guidance as to the origin of the anemia may be provided by RBC size obtained through automated cell counting. Microcytic anemias generally involve processes in which Hb or heme synthesis is impaired. Thalassemia minor is a common cause of microcytic anemia. Major thalassemias cause more severe anemia and often are accompanied by organomegaly and/or skeletal abnormalities caused by marrow expansion. Anemia of chronic disease is the most common anemia in hospitalized patients; can be mildly microcytic (mean cell volume ≥75); and shows reduced serum Fe, reduced total iron-binding capacity (TIBC), and increased serum ferritin. In contrast, Fe deficiency is the most common outpatient anemia and is characterized by reduced serum Fe, *increased* TIBC, and *reduced* serum ferritin.

G. In normocytic anemias, consider anemia of chronic disease in appropriate clinical settings when the aforementioned laboratory findings are present. If anemia of chronic disease is absent, order a bone marrow aspiration and biopsy to rule out a marrow defect in RBC production resulting from aplasia, processes replacing the marrow (myelophthisic anemia), lymphoproliferative or myeloproliferative disorders, or malnutrition. Protein calorie malnutrition causes anemia in disorders such as anorexia nervosa. Other metabolic disorders also cause severe anemia, including uremia. The primary defect in patients with uremia is a relative lack of the erythroid-stimulating hormone erythropoietin (EPO), which may now be substantially corrected by EPO administration. The Fe status of these patients depends on their transfusion and medication histories.

H. Macrocytic anemias result from either vitamin deficiencies or primary processes involving the marrow. Liver disease also can cause macrocytosis because of excess RBC membrane lipid, but it is not associated with vitamin deficiency. Vitamin B_{12} deficiency may be a result of pernicious anemia or secondary to other causes of B_{12} malabsorption, but it is almost never a result of dietary deficiency. In recent years, many early cases of B_{12} deficiency have been detected by serum B_{12} assays and confirmatory tests (increased serum methylmalonic acid or homocysteine). Folate deficiency usually is a result of dietary deficiency or diet in combination with ethanol ingestion. Some drugs also impair folate absorption (phenytoin) or metabolism (trimethoprim).

I. When folate and B_{12} levels are normal, macrocytic anemias often result from myelodysplasia or unusual congenital dyserythropoietic anemias (types 1, 2, or 3) diagnosed by bone marrow examination.

References

Dallman PR. Biochemical basis for the manifestations of iron deficiency. Ann Rev Nutr 1986;6:13.
Doll DC, Weiss RB. Neoplasia and the erythron. J Clin Oncol 1985;3:429.
Guyatt GH, Oxman AD, Ali M, et al. Tests for determination of iron-deficiency anemia: a meta-analysis. Laboratory diagnosis of iron-deficiency anemia: an overview. J Gen Intern Med 1992;7:145.
Saxena S, Rabinowitz AP, Johnson C, et al. Iron-deficiency anemia: a medically treatable chronic anemia as a model for transfusion overuse. Am J Med 1993;94:120.
Sears DA. Anemia of chronic disease. Med Clin North Am 1992;76:567.
Thompson CE, Damon LE, Ries CA, et al. Thrombotic microangiopathies in the 1980s: clinical features, response to treatment, and the impact of the human immunodeficiency virus epidemic. Blood 1992;80:1890.
Van Wyck DB. Iron management during recombinant human erythropoietin therapy. Am J Kidney Dis 1989;14:9.
Yip R, Dallman PR. The roles of inflammation and iron deficiency as causes of anemia. Am J Clin Nutr 1988;48:1295.

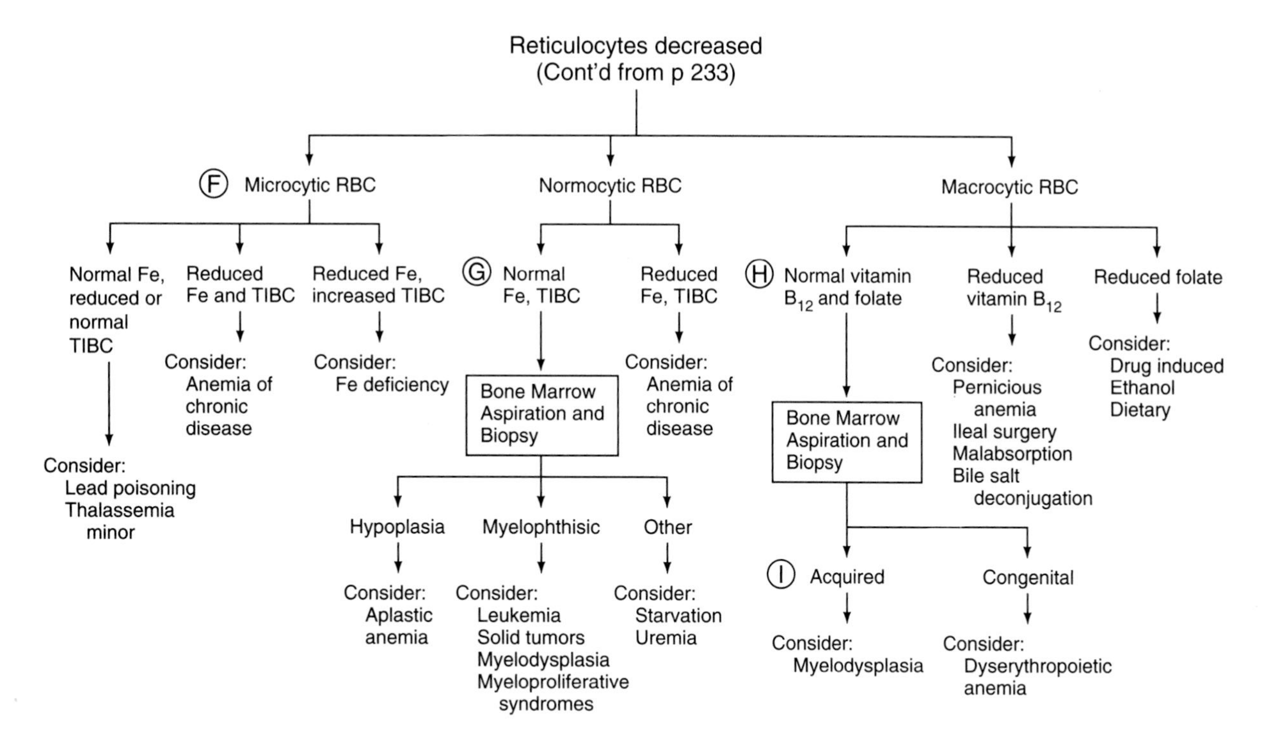

Reticulocytes decreased
(Cont'd from p 233)
F Microcytic RBC
Normocytic RBC
Macrocytic RBC
Normal Fe, reduced or normal TIBC
Consider: Lead poisoning Thalassemia minor
Reduced Fe and TIBC
Consider: Anemia of chronic disease
Reduced Fe, increased TIBC
Consider: Fe deficiency
G Normal Fe, TIBC
Bone Marrow Aspiration and Biopsy
Hypoplasia
Consider: Aplastic anemia
Myelophthisic
Consider: Leukemia Solid tumors Myelodysplasia Myeloproliferative syndromes
Other
Consider: Starvation Uremia
Reduced Fe, TIBC
Consider: Anemia of chronic disease
H Normal vitamin B_{12} and folate
Bone Marrow Aspiration and Biopsy
I Acquired
Consider: Myelodysplasia
Congenital
Consider: Dyserythropoietic anemia
Reduced vitamin B_{12}
Consider: Pernicious anemia Ileal surgery Malabsorption Bile salt deconjugation
Reduced folate
Consider: Drug induced Ethanol Dietary

POLYCYTHEMIA

Nenad Antic, MD

A. Increased plasma hemoglobin (Hb) or hematocrit (Hct) does not necessarily reflect an elevated total body RBC mass. If repeat determinations confirm an increased plasma Hb, RBC mass and plasma volume should be measured using radiolabeled RBC and albumin. This test, however, is performed in only a very small number of centers. The report should contain total RBC mass in percentages (100% being expected normal for the given age, sex, and weight; diagnostic criteria for polycythemia vera [PV] is >25% above the mean) and as total intravascular volume. In the absence of frank volume contraction, a patient with very high Hb (>18.5 g/dl in men and >16.5 g/dl in women) nearly always has an elevated RBC mass and the RBC mass test is not necessary.

B. Increased RBC mass indicates "true" polycythemia. An increase in plasma Hb attributed to a normal or high normal RBC mass and reduced plasma volume is termed *spurious* polycythemia. In the past, many cases of spurious polycythemia resulted from treatment with diuretics for hypertension. Although such patients do not have an expanded RBC mass, the decreased ratio of plasma to RBC in blood results in unfavorable whole blood rheology. Spurious polycythemia therefore may be associated with a high incidence of morbid arterial thrombotic events. Discontinue diuretics and substitute other forms of treatment, or evaluate the patient to delineate other possible causes of the decreased plasma volume.

C. If the RBC mass is elevated, test ABGs for Hb O_2 saturation. When saturation is <90%, hypoxia may cause increased erythropoietin (EPO) production and secondary polycythemia. In some patients, hypoxia occurring only at night is revealed by sleep studies, and it is typically sufficient to elevate EPO levels and cause polycythemia. Nighttime blood gas or oximeter readings may clarify this problem. Regardless of the cause, elevation of Hb levels to above normal generally is considered to result in unfavorable rheology and O_2 delivery. Provide supplemental O_2 if indicated to lower the EPO stimulus. Right-to-left cardiac shunts can also cause decreased blood O_2 content and polycythemia but usually present in childhood.

D. When plasma EPO levels are increased in the absence of hypoxia, consider localized hypoxia within the kidney or impaired O_2 delivery. Renal cysts and tumors and hydronephrosis can compress intrarenal vessels and cause local hypoxia, leading to increased renal elaboration of EPO; renal artery stenosis can cause this as well. Ultrasonography or CT of the kidneys usually is diagnostic, but in some patients arteriography is necessary. Certain rare tumors (e.g., hepatomas, cerebellar hemangiomas, pheochromocytoma) can produce ectopic EPO. Rarely, uterine fibromas have also been associated with this finding.

Other less common etiologies of increased EPO production include Bartter's syndrome, EPO receptor hypersensitivity, androgen therapy, and autotransfusions.

Secondary polycythemia can occur with normal EPO levels in chronic hypoxia or decreased oxyhemoglobin desaturation. During the initial response to hypoxia, EPO levels are elevated, but once steady-state erythrocytosis is achieved, the EPO levels required to maintain an elevated Hb level may fall within the normal assay range.

E. Levels of abnormal Hb that result in reduced O_2 unloading in tissues also cause tissue hypoxia and increased EPO production. The most common cause is probably increased carboxyhemoglobin levels from CO in cigarette smoke. Carboxyhemoglobin levels ≥6% can elevate EPO production and increase Hb levels. Unusual congenital Hbs may also release O_2 poorly and cause polycythemia. Both result in a shift in the oxyhemoglobin dissociation curve.

(Continued on page 238)

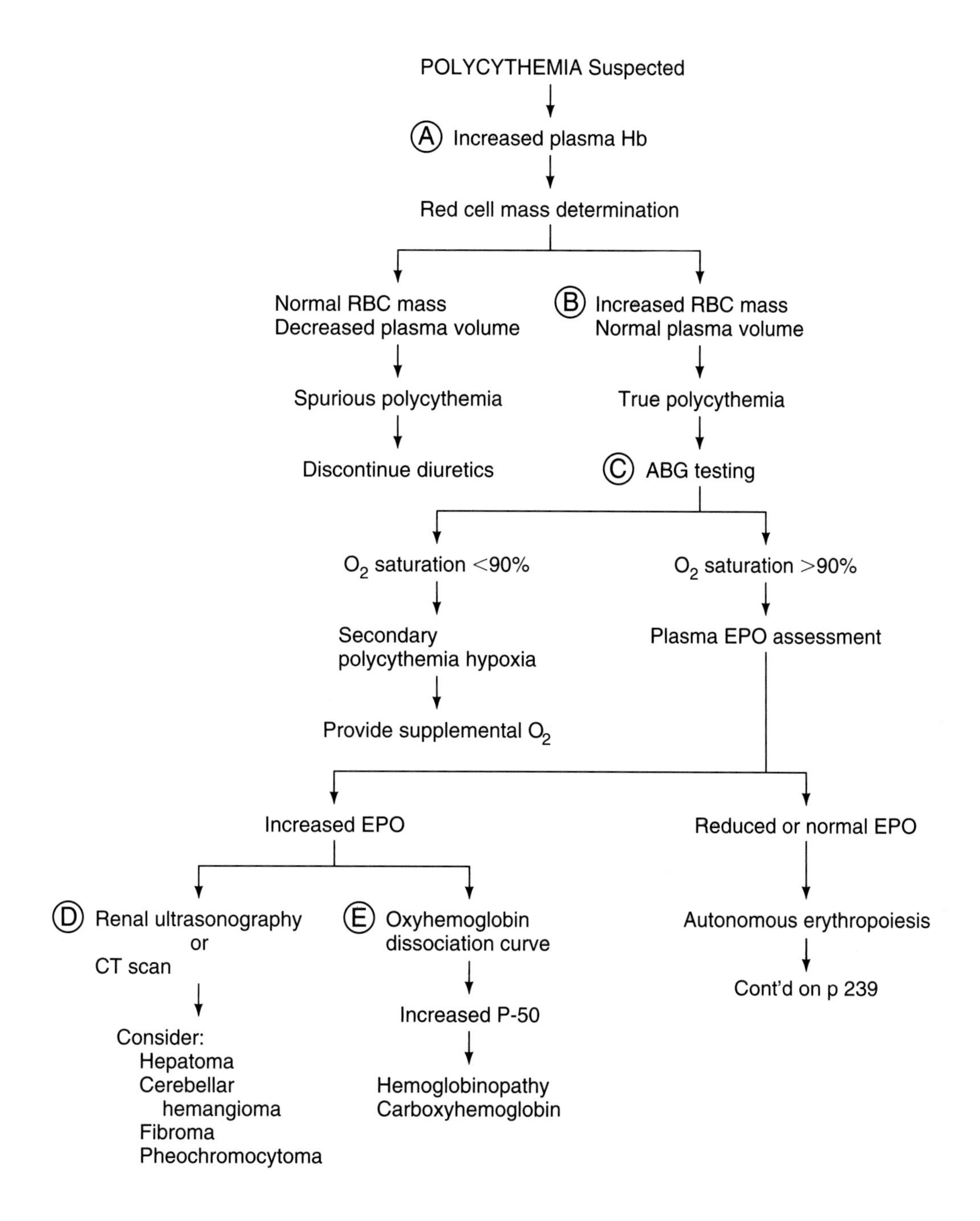
POLYCYTHEMIA Suspected
(A) Increased plasma Hb
Red cell mass determination
Normal RBC mass
Decreased plasma volume
(B) Increased RBC mass
Normal plasma volume
Spurious polycythemia
True polycythemia
Discontinue diuretics
(C) ABG testing
O_2 saturation <90%
O_2 saturation >90%
Secondary
polycythemia hypoxia
Plasma EPO assessment
Provide supplemental O_2
Increased EPO
Reduced or normal EPO
(D) Renal ultrasonography
or
CT scan
(E) Oxyhemoglobin
dissociation curve
Autonomous erythropoiesis
Cont'd on p 239
Increased P-50
Consider:
Hepatoma
Cerebellar
hemangioma
Fibroma
Pheochromocytoma
Hemoglobinopathy
Carboxyhemoglobin

F. Patients with normal plasma EPO levels and increased RBC mass have autonomous erythropoiesis, usually PV. In some cases this diagnosis remains unconfirmed because patients may lack other evidence of PV. Such cases have recently been termed *pure* erythrocytosis and usually are managed by phlebotomy. The Polycythemia Vera Study Group (PVSG) proposed criteria for the diagnosis of PV. In concept, these criteria are clinical findings indicating the presence of a multilineage myeloproliferative disorder. Absence of EPO elevation and normal arterial O_2 saturation are assumed because, in the presence of hypoxia, increased erythropoiesis cannot be definitively confirmed to be autonomous. An increased RBC mass also is required. If these findings are noted in a patient with a palpable spleen (major criterion), the diagnosis of PV is established; two more major criteria are clonal genetic abnormality other than Ph chromosome or bcr/abl fusion gene in marrow cells and endogenous erythroid colony formation in vitro. If a palpable spleen, genetic abnormalty of the bone marrow, and in vitro colony formation are absent, the additional presence of two of the following four minor criteria is required: thrombocytosis >400 million/dl, WBC count >12 million/dl, bone marrow biopsy showing panmyelosis with prominent erythroid and megakaryocytic proliferation, and low serum EPO levels. However, some patients with PV do not meet such criteria. Some present after GI bleeding and may have initially reduced Hb levels. Others lack the full diagnostic criteria but require therapy because of the unfavorable rheologic effects of polycythemia. Presenting symptoms of polycythemia are nonspecific and largely reflect increased blood viscosity. These include headaches, plethora, fatigue, hypertension, pruritus, erythromelalgia, ulceration of fingers and toes, joint pain, epigastric pain, weight loss, paresthesias, visual disturbances, vertigo, tinnitus, and ruddy cyanosis. Some patients have major thrombotic events such as stroke or myocardial infarction or bleeding manifestations. Such patients should not undergo nonemergency surgery until polycythemia has been corrected. For reasons that have not been fully elucidated, polycythemia per se results in a bleeding diathesis. Platelet dysfunction may exacerbate this problem in PV but is often normal at initial presentation.

G. PV is generally managed with phlebotomy to reduce Hb levels to normal. Patients treated with phlebotomy alone show an increased incidence of thrombotic events early in their disease. Management approach to a PV patient should start with a risk stratification.

Patients at low risk are those who are <60 years of age, without a history of thrombosis and cardiovascular risk factors (smoking, obesity) and with a platelet count of <1.5 million per microliter. Patients at high risk are the complete opposite. Intermediate risk is neither high risk nor low risk. Patients at low risk are treated with aspirin in addition to phlebotomy, unless they have a history of a hemorrhagic episode or platelet count >1 million and acquired vonWillebrand syndrome. Patients at high risk also should receive myelosuppressive therapy: interferon-α, hydroxyurea, or busulfan is most commonly used. A relatively new agent with profound effects on platelet production, anegrelide, has been used to control elevated platelet counts in PV and other myeloproliferative disorders, but experience with this agent is limited.

Prognosis of untreated PV is poor; median survival is 6–18 months, with thrombosis being the most common cause of death. Other causes of mortality in PV are transformation to acute leukemia or to "spent phase" (postpolycythemic myeloid metaplasia) and bleeding.

References

Berlin NI. Polycythemia vera. Semin Hematol 1997;34:1–5.

Brodmann S, Passweg JR, Gratwohl A, et al. Myeloproliferative disorders: complications, survival and causes of death. Ann Hematol 2000; 79:312–318.

Kaplan ME, Mack K, Goldberg JD, et al. Long-term management of polycythemia vera with hydroxyurea: a progress report. Semin Hematol 1986;23:167.

Nissenson AR, Nimer SD, Walcott DL. Recombinant human erythropoietin and renal anemia: molecular biology, clinical efficacy, and nervous system effects. Ann Intern Med 1991;114:402.

Prchal JT, Prchal JF. Evolving understanding of the cellular defect in polycythemia vera: implications for its clinical diagnosis and molecular pathophysiology. Blood 1994;83:1.

Spivak JL. Polycythemia vera: myths, mechanisms and management. Blood 2002;100:4272–4290.

Tefferi A. Polycythemia vera: a comprehensive review and clinical recommendations. Mayo Clin Proc 2003;78:174–194.

Wasserman LR. Polycythemia Vera Study Group: a historical perspective. Semin Hematol 1986;23:183.

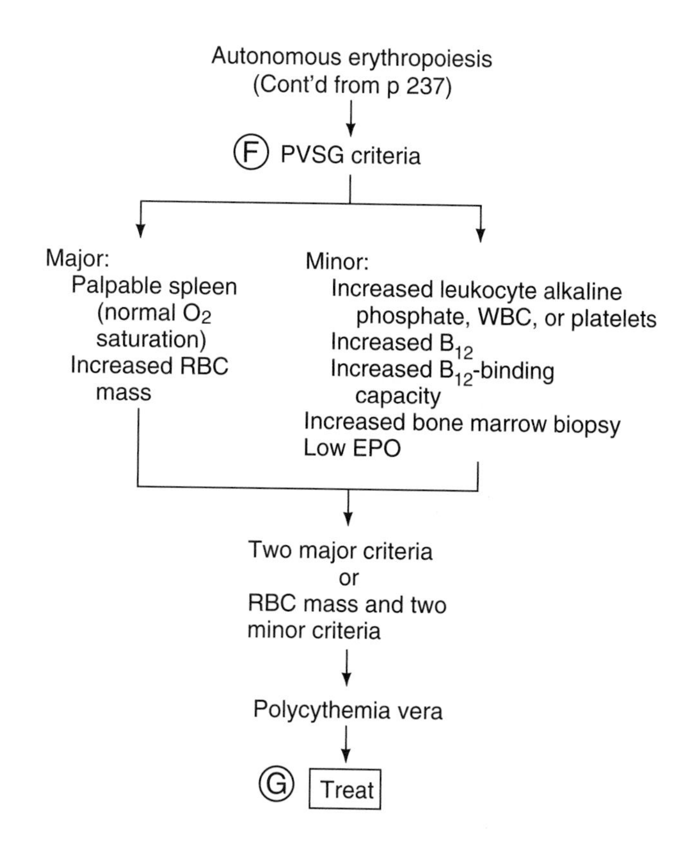

Autonomous erythropoiesis
(Cont'd from p 237)
F PVSG criteria
Major:
Palpable spleen
(normal O_2
saturation)
Increased RBC
mass
Minor:
Increased leukocyte alkaline
phosphate, WBC, or platelets
Increased B_{12}
Increased B_{12}-binding
capacity
Increased bone marrow biopsy
Low EPO
Two major criteria
or
RBC mass and two
minor criteria
Polycythemia vera
G Treat

NEUTROPHILIA

Robert M. Rifkin, MD, FACP

Increases in the number of circulating WBCs may represent either a primary disorder of WBC production or, more commonly, a secondary response to an underlying disease. Leukocytosis is defined by age-adjusted population normal values. Abnormal elevations in mature neutrophil count (neutrophilia) represent the most common cause of leukocytosis and are the subject of this decision matrix.

A. Neutrophilia is best defined as an increase in the absolute blood neutrophil count to a level >2 standard deviations above the mean value for normal adult individuals. From a practical standpoint, this is usually defined as a neutrophil count >10,000/mm^3. Neutrophil counts follow a diurnal variation, with the peak counts occurring late in the afternoon. However, this variation is not enough to produce neutrophilia.

B. Initially, laboratory error should be excluded as a cause of neutrophilia. With the advent of electronic complete blood counting, error has been virtually eliminated. Blood counts that do not make sense in a given clinical context should be repeated. There is no substitute to evaluating the peripheral blood smear. Factitious neutrophilia may result from preanalytic variables such as a blood sample obtained with inadequate anticoagulant.

C. The evaluation of neutrophilia begins with a thorough history and physical examination to search for an underlying disease state. Neutrophilia commonly results from an acute or chronic inflammatory process. A bone marrow examination rarely provides useful information except in those patients in whom a primary marrow dyscrasia is suspected. Bone marrow biopsy with culture may be useful in the detection of chronic infections (fungal or mycobacterial). In patients with very mild neutrophilia, remember that the neutrophil count in 2.5% of the general population must be >2 standard deviations above the mean. The regulation of the neutrophil count is also genetically controlled, and examination of siblings and family members can be helpful in difficult cases.

D. The workup of neutrophilia is greatly simplified when it can be classified as primary or secondary. In normal individuals the neutrophil count varies directly with the serum cortisol level, with both levels peaking in the late afternoon. Neutrophil counts increase slightly after meals, with postural changes, and with stress and emotional stimuli. These physiologic changes are not enough to cause a clinically meaningful increase in the neutrophil count.

E. Primary neutrophilia is that without evidence of an associated disease and may result from a wide variety of bone marrow disorders. These can be idiopathic, familial, or malignant. Benign hematologic disorders, including rebound from agranulocytosis, megaloblastic anemia, or chronic idiopathic leukocytosis, can produce chronic neutrophilia. Malignant hematologic disorders such as chronic myeloid leukemia and myeloproliferative disorders must also be considered as other causes of persistent primary neutrophilia.

F. Secondary neutrophilia may result from a wide variety of stimuli. Both physical and emotional stimuli may cause neutrophilia. These stimuli may include cold, heat, exercise, seizures, pain, labor, surgery, panic, and rage. Localized and systemic bacterial and mycotic infections may result in secondary neutrophilia. Ongoing tissue necrosis with the activation of the complement system is responsible for increases in neutrophil count. Finally, colony-stimulating factors such as filgrastim, sargramostim, and pegylated filgrastim can elicit a striking neutrophilia. Mild chronic neutrophilia most often is the result of smoking. Long-standing chronic inflammation can also produce puzzling cases of secondary chronic neutrophilia. Vasculitis, rheumatoid arthritis, gout, myositis, colitis, dermatitis, periodontal disease, and drug reactions are often associated with chronic neutrophilia. Nonhematologic malignancy can produce chronic neutrophilia; causes commonly include carcinomas of the lung, stomach, breast, kidney, pancreas, and uterus. Neutrophilia in response to drug administration is rare except in the case of the administration of glucocorticoids, epinephrine, and lithium salts. Specific therapy to reduce only the neutrophil counts is not recommended. Instead, treatment of the underlying cause is preferred.

References

Hoffbrand AV, Catovsky D, Tuddenham EGD. Postgraduate Hematology. Oxford: Blackwell, 2005:277.

Hoffman R, Benz EJ, Shattill SJ, et al., eds. Hematology: Basic Principles and Practice, 4th ed. Philadelphia: Elsevier/Churchill Livingstone, 2005:802.

Lichtman MA, Beutler E, Kipps TJ, et al., eds. Williams Hematology, 7th ed. New York: McGraw-Hill, 2006:907.

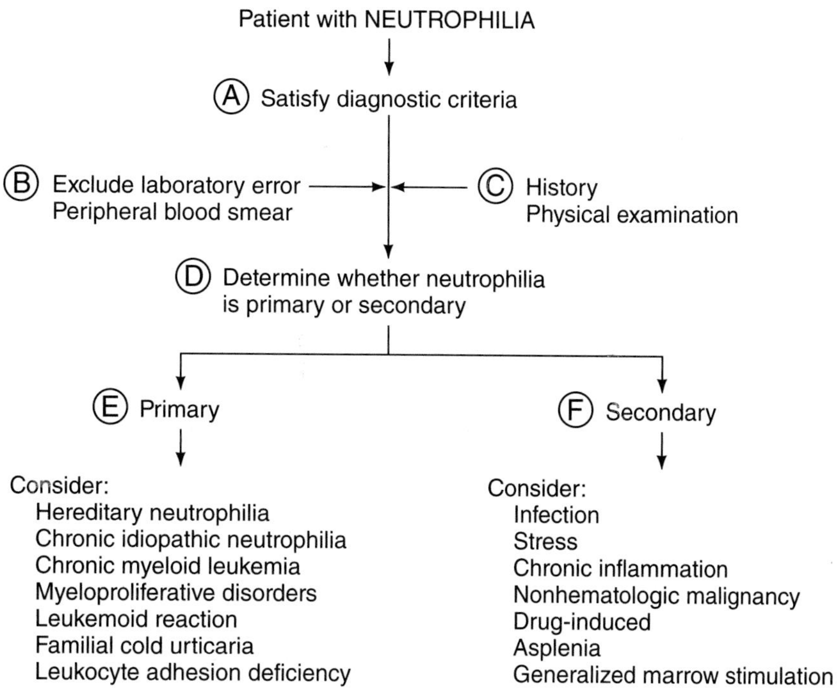

Patient with NEUTROPHILIA

↓

(A) Satisfy diagnostic criteria

(B) Exclude laboratory error
Peripheral blood smear →

← (C) History
Physical examination

↓

(D) Determine whether neutrophilia is primary or secondary

(E) Primary

↓

Consider:
- Hereditary neutrophilia
- Chronic idiopathic neutrophilia
- Chronic myeloid leukemia
- Myeloproliferative disorders
- Leukemoid reaction
- Familial cold urticaria
- Leukocyte adhesion deficiency

(F) Secondary

↓

Consider:
- Infection
- Stress
- Chronic inflammation
- Nonhematologic malignancy
- Drug-induced
- Asplenia
- Generalized marrow stimulation

LEUKOPENIA

William H. Kreisle, MD, and Manuel Modiano, MD

In adults leukopenia is a total WBC count <3700 cells/mm^3. Most cases result from absolute neutropenia (<2500 cells/mm^3); rare cases are secondary to absolute lymphopenia (<1000 cells/mm^3).

A. Initial evaluation should include a thorough history and physical examination. Give special attention to the use of drugs and the presence of adenopathy, splenomegaly, ecchymoses, petechiae, and signs of infection. CBC, differential, and platelet counts are essential to determine absolute neutrophil and lymphocyte counts and to rule out any accompanying anemia or thrombocytopenia. The blood smear provides important information concerning RBC and WBC morphology. The results of these tests often lead to specific diagnoses.

B. Patients with neutropenia usually have signs and symptoms of infection that often are life threatening. Fever in the absence of localizing signs of infection is common. After obtaining cultures, start broad-spectrum antibiotics immediately.

C. Isolated neutropenia and pancytopenia can occur with many commonly used noncytotoxic drugs (e.g., quinidine, penicillins, sulfonamides, phenothiazines, diuretics), alkylating agents, antimetabolites, and other neoplastic agents. If physical examination and laboratory test results are negative for a neoplastic or hematologic disorder, stop the drug and observe the patient by taking frequent blood counts. Order a bone marrow biopsy and aspirate if the neutropenia fails to resolve in 5–7 days or if blood counts continue to decline.

D. Disorders leading to splenomegaly with splenic sequestration can cause neutropenia, but there usually is associated thrombocytopenia. Differential diagnosis includes cirrhosis, sarcoidosis, glycogen storage diseases, and other uncommon conditions.

E. If the bone marrow result is unremarkable and there is no evidence of splenomegaly or an autoimmune disorder, consider rare chronic neutropenic states. Observe the patient with serial blood counts to document the neutropenic pattern.

F. Most cases of neutropenia are associated with anemia and/or thrombocytopenia. Unless a drug is strongly suspected as the cause, order a bone marrow biopsy and aspirate to rule out a primary hematologic disorder that requires prompt treatment.

G. If the only bone marrow abnormality is the absence of mature granulocytes, this suggests maturation arrest or autoimmune destruction. Perform a workup for an autoimmune disorder. If available, an antineutrophil antibody assay may be helpful.

H. Infections that can cause neutropenia with anemia and/or thrombocytopenia include viruses (Epstein-Barr, cytomegalovirus, virus HIV, hepatitis, measles); bacteria (severe gram-negative and gram-positive organisms); *Mycobacterium,* typhoid fever, malaria; and fungi. Bone marrow should be cultured as part of an extensive workup for infection.

I. Lymphopenia without associated neutropenia is uncommon. Most cases are secondary to drugs (e.g., steroids), radiation injury, or renal failure. Some viral infections, particularly HIV, can also cause absolute lymphopenia.

References

Dale DC. Neutropenia and neutrophilia. In Williams WJ, ed. Hematology, 4th ed. New York: McGraw-Hill, 2001:823.

Logue GL, Schimm DS. Autoimmune granulocytopenia. Annu Rev Med 1980;31:191.

Murphy MF, Metcalf P, Waters AH, et al. Incidence and mechanism of neutropenia and thrombocytopenia in patients with human immunodeficiency virus infection. Br J Haematol 1987;66:337.

Vincent PC. Drug-induced aplastic anemia and agranulocytosis. Incidence and mechanisms. Drugs 1986;31:52.

Watts RG. Neutropenia. In Greer JP, Foerster J, Lukens JN, et al. Wintrobe's Clinical Hematology, 11th ed. Philadelphia: Lippincott Williams & Wilkins, 2003:1777.

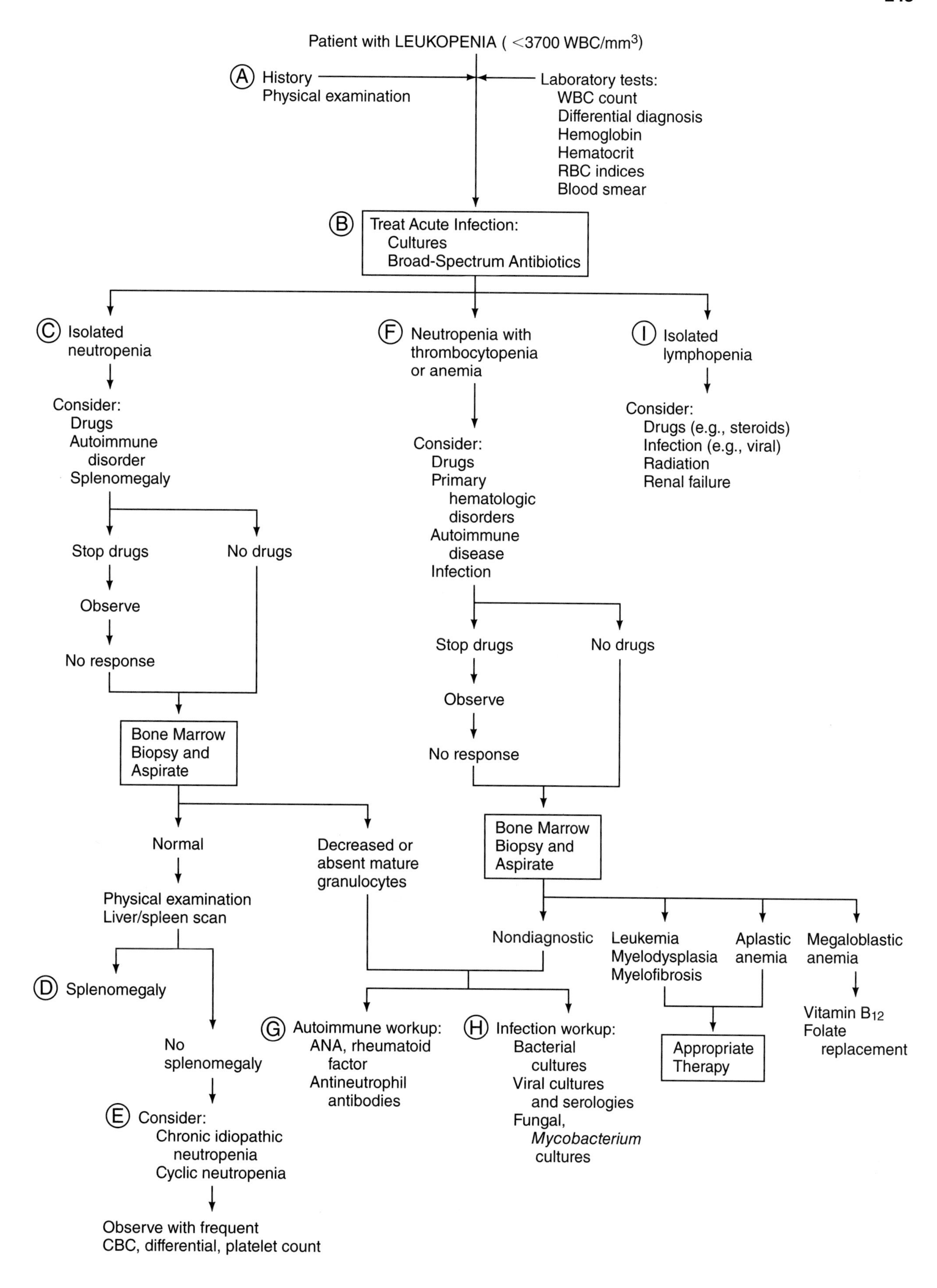

Patient with LEUKOPENIA (<3700 WBC/mm3)
A History
Physical examination
Laboratory tests:
WBC count
Differential diagnosis
Hemoglobin
Hematocrit
RBC indices
Blood smear
B Treat Acute Infection:
Cultures
Broad-Spectrum Antibiotics
C Isolated neutropenia
Consider:
Drugs
Autoimmune disorder
Splenomegaly
Stop drugs
No drugs
Observe
No response
Bone Marrow Biopsy and Aspirate
Normal
Decreased or absent mature granulocytes
Physical examination
Liver/spleen scan
D Splenomegaly
No splenomegaly
E Consider:
Chronic idiopathic neutropenia
Cyclic neutropenia
Observe with frequent
CBC, differential, platelet count
F Neutropenia with thrombocytopenia or anemia
Consider:
Drugs
Primary hematologic disorders
Autoimmune disease
Infection
Stop drugs
No drugs
Observe
No response
Bone Marrow Biopsy and Aspirate
Nondiagnostic
Leukemia
Myelodysplasia
Myelofibrosis
Aplastic anemia
Megaloblastic anemia
Appropriate Therapy
Vitamin B12
Folate replacement
G Autoimmune workup:
ANA, rheumatoid factor
Antineutrophil antibodies
H Infection workup:
Bacterial cultures
Viral cultures and serologies
Fungal, Mycobacterium cultures
I Isolated lymphopenia
Consider:
Drugs (e.g., steroids)
Infection (e.g., viral)
Radiation
Renal failure

DEEP VENOUS THROMBOSIS

Guillermo Gonzalez-Osete, MD, and Manuel Modiano, MD

Deep venous thrombosis (DVT) is caused by intravascular deposits of predominantly fibrin, RBCs, platelets, and WBC components, accumulating in a vein and producing obstruction to venous outflow and/or vessel wall inflammation. The clinical manifestations depend on the severity of these inflammatory processes. Often the initial sign is a pulmonary embolism (PE).

A. Detailed history taking should look for previous episodes and for inherited disorders of protein C and S deficiency, antithrombin (AT) III deficiency, or an abnormal factor V (factor V_{LEIDEN}). With such deficiencies there is a strong family history of recurrent DVT or PE that presents at an early age; >80% of patients with protein C deficiency have had an episode of DVT or PE by age 40. Patients with ATIII deficiency have a similar presentation and also may have a history of failure to be anticoagulated with heparin. Other hypercoagulable causes are the *MTHFR* (5,10-methylenetetrahydrofolate reductase) gene mutation, prothrombin gene mutation, and activated protein C resistance. Some are acquired, such as the anticardiolipin antibodies. It is important to obtain a complete drug and medication history, including use of estrogen or oral contraceptives. A history of frequent abortions with a prolonged partial thromboplastin time (PTT) should make one suspect a lupus anticoagulant (i.e., anticardiolipin antibodies). This also is present in some collagen vascular diseases such as systemic lupus erythematosus. Surgery that requires >30 minutes and certain surgical procedures (orthopedics, those involving trauma to lower limbs [e.g., knee surgery, urologic, gynecologic]) are associated with increased incidence of DVT. Other risk factors are trauma, pregnancy, puerperium, congestive heart failure (CHF), myocardial infarction, cerebrovascular accidents, extremity paralysis, malignancy (especially of the prostate, breast, or pancreas), obesity, varicose veins, immobilization, use of estrogens, smoking, and age. All of these may increase the risk of DVT by stasis and/or increased activation of coagulation.

B. Pain is present in approximately 50% of patients with DVT. Swelling and tenderness to compression also are found in 75% of patients. The clinical diagnosis of DVT is not accurate. Thrombosis does not always produce complete obstruction or inflammation. In 30% of patients who have pain and swelling, there is proven DVT. The classic Homan sign (discomfort in the calf muscles on forced dorsiflexion of the foot) is not sensitive. It is noted in 33% of patients with positive venography and 50% with negative venography. Unilateral swelling associated with discoloration is an important sign that should alert one to the diagnosis.

C. The differential diagnosis includes ruptured Baker's cyst, muscle tear, cramp, hematoma, arthritis, bone disease, varicose veins, and postphlebitic syndrome. If no cause is apparent, consider noninvasive screening.

D. When the history and physical examination suggest DVT, ancillary tests such as noninvasive impedance plethysmography (IPG) and duplex ultrasound or invasive tests such as ^{125}I and contrast venography will corroborate the diagnosis. Laboratory tests should include platelet count, prothrombin time (PT), PTT, and D-dimer. The D-dimer test has emerged as a good screening tool; a positive result supports further workup to rule out DVT and pulmonary embolism in the appropriate clinical setting, and a negative result does not exclude it.

E. Noninvasive diagnostic tests available are IPG and duplex ultrasonography (D-US). IPG is good for detecting proximal vein thrombosis and/or recurrent DVT but is insensitive for detecting nonobstructive proximal thrombosis and calf vein thrombosis. Its sensitivity is 83%–93%; its specificity is 83%–90%. It must be repeated serially to increase its sensitivity. False-positive results may occur with CHF, postoperative leg swelling, excessive leg tension, or external compression. D-US (sensitivity, 95%; specificity, 98%) is the ideal method of screening patients with suspected DVT. It is good for detecting proximal but not calf vein thrombosis. Calf vein thrombosis usually requires no treatment other than bed rest and elevation of the extremity. In 20%–30% of cases, however, the thrombus may extend into the popliteal vein, and full anticoagulation is required because of the increased incidence of PE. Extension into the popliteal system often is missed on initial noninvasive tests but may be seen if the examination is repeated after 3–5 days.

F. ^{125}I with fibrinogen detects fibrin accretion to a thrombus and will be positive with active ongoing clotting. It detects calf vein thrombosis in 90% of cases and proximal vein thrombosis in 60%–80%. Fibrinogen carries with it the risks inherent with the use of any blood product, including allergic reactions and transmittal of infections. It is contraindicated in iodine allergy, pregnancy, and lactation. The combined approach of ^{125}I and IPG was positive in 81 of 86 patients with positive venograms; both tests were negative in 104 of 114 patients who had negative venograms. This is a useful approach if DVT is suspected clinically and ^{125}I is inconclusive. Venography is the gold standard but is invasive, is not

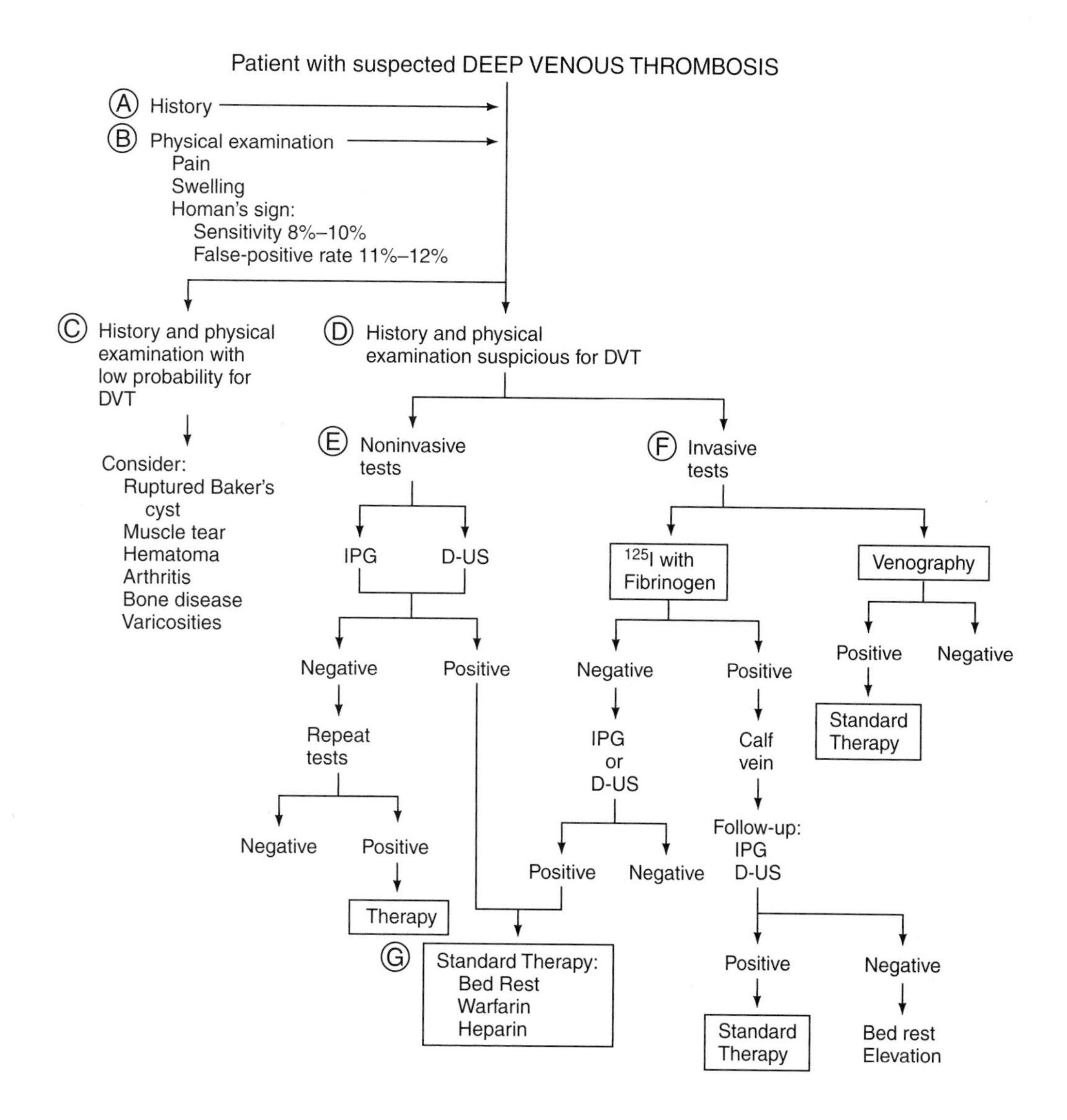

always available, and may not visualize the deep venous system. It may itself cause a DVT.

G. If the diagnosis is confirmed, begin treatment. Standard treatment includes IV heparin, SC heparin, low molecular weight heparins, oral anticoagulants, bed rest, and extremity elevation. Patients with protein C deficiency may have skin necrosis and increased sensitivity to warfarin. Start therapy with IV heparin bolus, 5000 U, followed by continuous infusion of heparin, approximately 1000 U/h or 800–10,000 U SC heparin every 6–8 hours. Monitor activated PTT at 6 hours and thereafter until stabilized at 1.5–2 times control values. Obtain a baseline platelet count and monitor every 3 days while the patient is taking heparin. Watch for heparin-associated thrombocytopenia and heparin-associated thrombosis. Alternatively, Lovenox twice daily at a dosage of 1 mg/kg SC every 12 hours or at dosage of 1.5 mg/kg once a day could be used instead of heparin. Begin warfarin sodium on the first day by instituting the estimated daily maintenance dosage (5–10 mg). Maintain INR at 2.0–3.0. It usually takes 72–96 hours for the INR to reach this range, and heparin should be continued until the INR is at this level. Treatment should last at least 12 weeks.

References

Hommes DW, Bura A, Mazzolai L, et al. Subcutaneous heparin compared with continuous intravenous heparin administration in the initial treatment of deep vein thrombosis: a meta-analysis. Ann Intern Med 1992;116:279.

Hull R, Raskob G, Pineo G, et al. A comparison of subcutaneous low-molecular-weight heparin with warfarin sodium for prophylaxis against deep-vein thrombosis after hip or knee implantation. N Engl J Med 1993;329:1370.

Hull RD, Raskob GE, Rosenbloom D, et al. Heparin for 5 days as compared with 10 days in the initial treatment of proximal venous thrombosis. N Engl J Med 1990;322:1260.

Hyers T, Hull RD, Weg J. Antithrombotic therapy for venous thromboembolic disease. Chest 1989;95:37s.

Lensing AWA, Hirsh J, Buller HR. Diagnosis of venous thrombosis. In Colman RW, Hirsh J, Marder VJ, et al, eds. Hemostasis and Thrombosis, 3rd ed. Philadelphia: JB Lippincott, 1994.

Pini M, Pattachini C, Quintavalla R, et al. Subcutaneous vs. intravenous heparin in the treatment of deep venous thrombosis—a randomized clinical trial. Thromb Haemost 1990;64:222.

Salzman EW, Hirsh J. The epidemiology, pathogenesis, and natural history of venous thrombosis. In Colman RW, Hirsh J, Marder VJ, et al, eds. Hemostasis and Thrombosis, 3rd ed. Philadelphia: JB Lippincott, 1994.

White R, McGahan JP, Daschbach M, et al. Diagnosis of deep vein thrombosis using duplex ultrasound. Ann Intern Med 1989;111:297.

COAGULATION ABNORMALITIES

Deborah Fuchs, MD; Ana Maria López, MD, MPH, FACP; and Manuel Modiano, MD

A. Blood coagulation represents conversion of the soluble plasma protein fibrinogen into an insoluble fibrillar polymer, fibrin. It is the result of complex serial reactions involving procoagulant proteins that circulate in plasma as inert precursors until converted sequentially by specific chain reactions to their active forms. Factors are numbered not by the order in which they become activated but by the order in which they were discovered. The prothrombin time (PT) measures the extrinsic and common pathways of coagulation, including factors VII, X, V, II, and I. The partial thromboplastin time (PTT) measures the intrinsic and common pathways of coagulation, including factors XII, XI, IX, VIII, X, V, II, and I. The thrombin time (TT) measures the time it takes to convert fibrinogen to fibrin, the last stage of the common pathway.

B. When confronted with a prolonged PT or PTT, first take a careful history, including previous bleeding or bruising, spontaneously or after surgery or trauma. A family history of bleeding and a complete list of medications being taken (prescription or not) are essential. Confirm that platelets are normal by count. Also inquire about history of clotting because lupus anticoagulants can prolong PT bleeding time. In 1990 an analysis of 862 publications on the bleeding time concluded that the bleeding time is not a useful test, particularly as a preoperative screening test in a patient with negative bleeding history (see Rodgers reference).

C. Patients with a history of bleeding disorders often know the etiologic factors and corrective measures taken in the past. If so, correct the situation as before (if possible, check with the patient's regular physician for dosage and type of factor correction) or refer the patient to a hematologist.

D. When the cause is unknown or when there is no history of bleeding, first confirm the abnormality of the coagulation times, especially if there has been no previous bleeding with trauma or major surgery. Again, a detailed history, including medications, and a full physical examination are essential.

E. When coagulation tests do not correct with mixing studies, it usually is because an inhibitor or anticoagulant is present. A correction denotes a deficiency of one or more coagulation factors. Inhibitors are either antibodies directed to specific factors (e.g., factor VIII or factor IX antibody) or an antiphospholipid antibody (lupuslike antibody) directed to phospholipid. Inhibition can also occur from a drug such as heparin or protamine, but it is usually known when these substances are present.

F. An isolated prolonged PT that corrects with mixing suggests a factor VII deficiency, and this factor can then be measured directly. If no correction occurs on mixing with normal plasma, there is likely an inhibitor present, most likely a lupuslike inhibitor; however, a specific factor antibody could also be present. Specific assays for a lupuslike inhibitor are available.

G. An isolated prolonged PTT that corrects with mixing suggests one or more factor deficiencies (VIII, IX, XI, or XII). An inherited deficiency is often of a single factor, whereas multiple-factor deficiencies are usually acquired (e.g., liver disease). No correction suggests a lupus or specific inhibitor. Factor VIII deficiency (classic hemophilia A) is an X-linked inherited disorder that affects only males clinically; females are carriers. It is the most common severe coagulation disorder. Coordinate treatment with an experienced hematologist, but emergency replacement can be done with fresh frozen plasma (FFP), cryoprecipitate, or factor VIII concentrates. Von Willebrand's disease is the most common and most heterogeneous of heritable defects of coagulation. It arises from a qualitative or quantitative deficiency of the adhesive glycoprotein, von Willebrand factor (vWF), which is required for platelet adhesion. It serves as a carrier protein for factor VIII and stabilizes factor VIII in the plasma. vWF is an autosomal-dominant disorder with its gene located on chromosome 12. Some of the rare types of vWD are actually autosomal recessive. Last, factor IX deficiency (hemophilia B) is an X-linked disorder that is indistinguishable from factor VIII disease clinically, but it is treated with FFP or with factor IX concentrates.

H. A prolonged TT is often caused by small amounts of heparin that many patients receive in the hospital; therefore, a reptilase time (RT) may be done to exclude heparin. Reptilase is a thrombinlike enzyme from a particular snake venom that is not inhibited by heparin. If both the TT and RT are prolonged, the abnormality is from low fibrinogen or the presence of fibrinogen degradation products (FDPs), a paraprotein, or an abnormal fibrinogen molecule, all of which can be measured directly.

I. When both the PT and PTT are prolonged, the same reasoning can be applied as discussed for each individual test, except that multiple factors in multiple pathways may be deficient (inhibitor mix corrects) or may be inhibited (inhibitor mix does not correct). Again, specific factors can be assayed directly and potential causes can be considered as indicated in the decision tree.

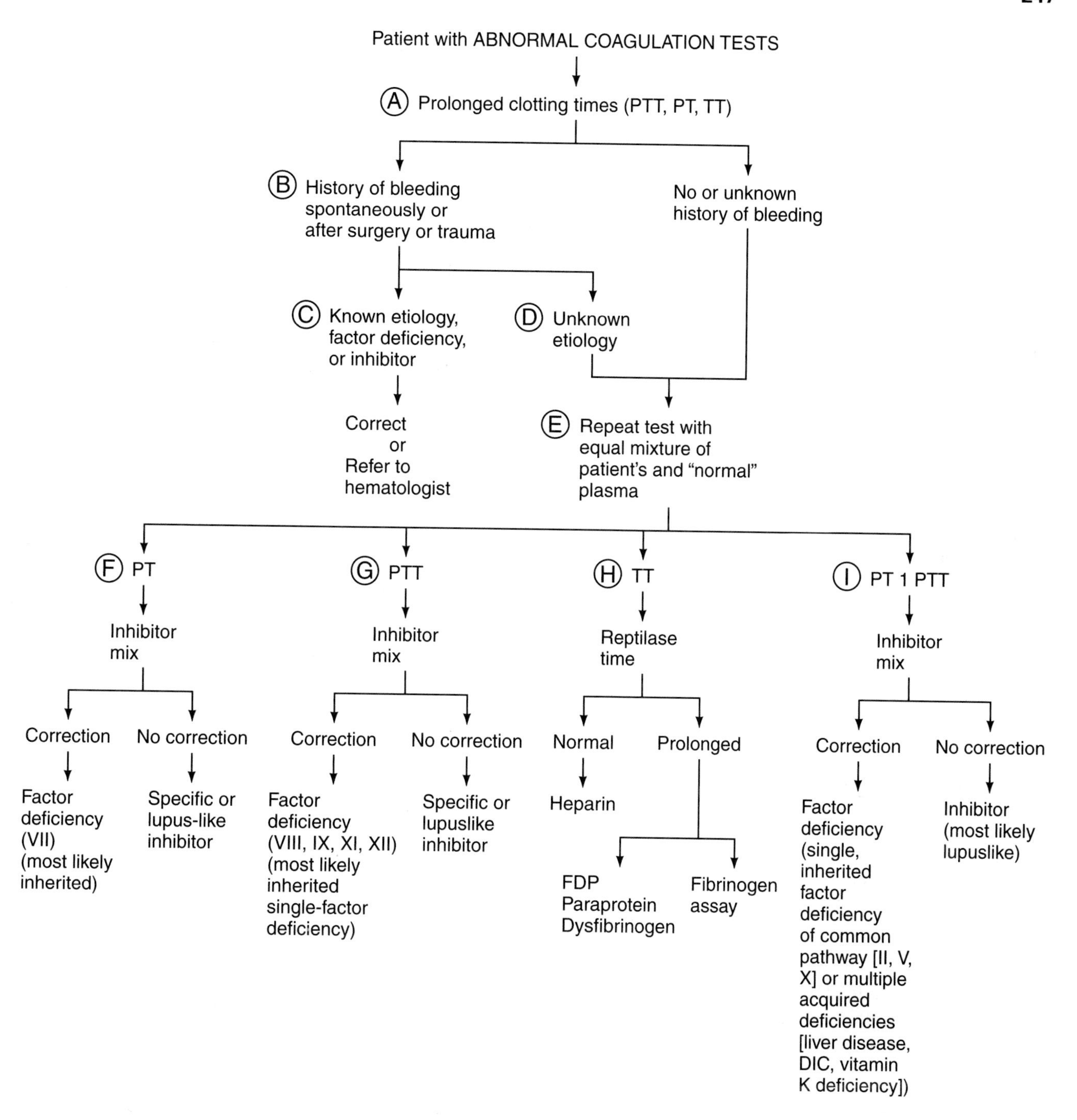

References

Ey FS, Goodnight SH. Bleeding disorders in cancer. Semin Oncol 1990;17:187.

Jandl JH. Disorders of coagulation. In Blood: Textbook of Hematology, 2nd ed. Philadelphia: Lippincott-Raven, 1996.

Levine M, Hirsh J. The diagnosis and treatment of thrombosis in the cancer patient. Semin Oncol 1990;17:160.

Patterson WP. Coagulation and cancer: an overview. Semin Oncol 1990;17:137.

Patterson WP, Caldwell CW, Doll DC. Hyperviscosity syndromes and coagulopathies. Semin Oncol 1990;17:210.

Patterson WP, Ringenberg QS. The pathophysiology of thrombosis in cancer. Semin Oncol 1990;17:140.

Rapaport S. Preoperative hemostatic evaluation: which tests, if any? Blood 1983;61:229.

Rodgers RP. Bleeding time tables. A tabular summary of pertinent literature. Semin Thromb Hemost 1990;16:21–138.

Schaffer AI. The hypercoagulable states. Ann Intern Med 1985;102:814.

TRANSFUSION THERAPY: FRESH FROZEN PLASMA AND CRYOPRECIPITATE

Richard M. Kaufman, MD

Plasma is prepared from whole blood donations by centrifugation or is collected by apheresis. By definition, fresh frozen plasma (FFP) is frozen within 6–8 hours of collection and is stored at –18° C or colder. Each unit of FFP has a volume of approximately 250 ml. FFP contains all of the coagulation factors at normal physiologic levels. The primary use of FFP is to replace coagulation factors in patients with documented coagulopathy (prothrombin time [PT] and/or activated partial thromboplastin time [aPTT] >1.5 times normal) who are bleeding or undergoing an invasive procedure. Dosing is by patient weight (10–20 ml/kg). A discussion of the indications for FFP follows.

A. *Vitamin K Deficiency/Warfarin Reversal:* Vitamin K is required for the γ-carboxylation of coagulation factors II, VII, IX, and X, as well as the anticoagulant proteins C and S. This carboxylation step is critical for the normal activity of these proteins. Warfarin (Coumadin) exerts its anticoagulant effect by rendering patients functionally vitamin K deficient. There are several ways to reverse the effect of warfarin: (1) discontinue warfarin and wait—complete reversal of the coagulopathy will occur within 48 hours; (2) administer vitamin K—reversal occurs in about 12 hours; (3) infuse FFP—a single FFP infusion of 10–20 ml/kg will generally correct hemostasis immediately.
B. *Liver Disease:* The liver produces all coagulation factors except factor VIII. Thus liver disease, regardless of etiology, is often associated with multiple coagulation-factor deficiencies. Several additional features of liver disease may increase the tendency to bleed, including portal hypertension, decreased clearance of activated coagulation complexes, dysfibrinogenemia, and splenomegaly with associated thrombocytopenia. The PT is prolonged to a greater extent than the aPTT; this is due to the short half-life of factor VII (4–6 hours). Because factor VII has such a short half-life, it is rarely possible to infuse a large enough volume of FFP to correct the patient's PT entirely to normal. However, it should be emphasized that a completely normal PT is not required for hemostasis to be achieved.
C. *Isolated Coagulation Factor Deficiency:* FFP carries the same risks of pathogen transmission as other blood products, so FFP is never given in cases where a specific factor concentrate is available (e.g., factor VIII for hemophilia A). Currently FFP is the only product available for inherited or acquired deficiencies of factors II, V, X, and XI.
D. *Dilutional Coagulopathy:* In cases where bleeding patients receive a large volume of RBCs cells and colloid replacement, there may be sufficient dilution of endogenous coagulation factors to impair hemostasis. FFP may be indicated if the patient's PT and/or aPTT are prolonged to >1.5 times the mean of normal.
E. *Other Conditions:* Plasma infusion may be beneficial in DIC for patients with a prolonged PT and aPTT who are bleeding, undergoing an invasive procedure, or both. Plasma exchange with plasma replacement is the mainstay of therapy for thrombotic thrombocytopenic purpura (TTP). Finally, plasma is used to treat C1-esterase deficiency (hereditary angioedema).
F. Cryoprecipitate (CRYO) is prepared by thawing FFP at 4° C and collecting and refreezing the insoluble fraction. Each unit of CRYO has a volume of 10–15 ml and contains an average of 250 mg of fibrinogen. The usual dose is a pool of 10 U. CRYO is indicated for patients who are bleeding and have a fibrinogen level <100 mg/dl (e.g., DIC). In the past, CRYO was used to treat von Willebrand's disease; it is no longer used in this setting because of the availability of factor VIII concentrates that contain high levels of von Willebrand's factor.

References

Brecher, ME, ed. Technical Manual. Bethesda, MD: AABB, 2005.

Fresh-Frozen Plasma, Cryoprecipitate, and Platelets Administration Practice Guidelines Development Task Force of the College of American Pathologists. Practice parameter for the use of fresh-frozen plasma, cryoprecipitate, and platelets. JAMA 1994;271(10): 777–781.

McVay PA, Toy PT. Lack of increased bleeding after liver biopsy in patients with mild hemostatic abnormalities. Am J Clin Pathol 1990;94(6): 747–753.

Segal JB, Dzik WH. Paucity of studies to support that abnormal coagulation test results predict bleeding in the setting of invasive procedures: an evidence-based review. Transfusion 2005;45(9):1413–1425.

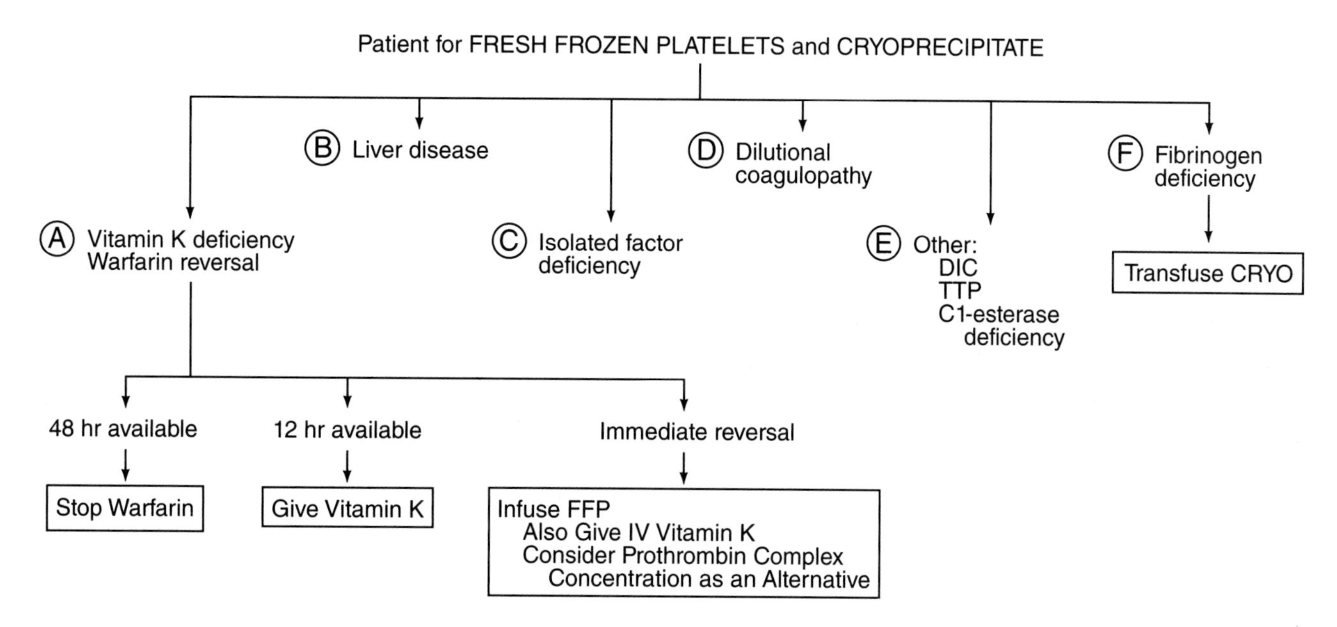

Patient for FRESH FROZEN PLATELETS and CRYOPRECIPITATE
(A) Vitamin K deficiency
Warfarin reversal
(B) Liver disease
(C) Isolated factor deficiency
(D) Dilutional coagulopathy
(E) Other:
DIC
TTP
C1-esterase deficiency
(F) Fibrinogen deficiency
Transfuse CRYO
48 hr available
Stop Warfarin
12 hr available
Give Vitamin K
Immediate reversal
Infuse FFP
Also Give IV Vitamin K
Consider Prothrombin Complex
Concentration as an Alternative

TRANSFUSION THERAPY: PLATELETS

Richard M. Kaufman, MD

Platelets (PLTs) are transfused to prevent or treat bleeding in patients with quantitative or qualitative PLT defects. PLTs are either prepared from a unit of whole blood (random-donor PLT unit, RDP) or are collected by apheresis (single-donor PLT unit, SDP). A pool of four to six RDPs provides about the same total PLT dose as one SDP ($\geq 3 \times 10^{11}$ PLTs).

A. The vast majority of PLT transfusions are given prophylactically to patients who are not bleeding and who have thrombocytopenia. For years, a PLT count of 20,000/μl was used as a standard PLT transfusion trigger. Later, multiple controlled trials demonstrated that prophylactic PLT transfusions can safely be given using a lower trigger (e.g., 10,000/μl), leading to substantial product inventory and cost savings. A PLT transfusion trigger higher than 10,000/μl is often used for patients with comorbidities (fever, coagulation defects, intracranial lesions, high white cell counts, rapid PLT consumption).

B. A published practice guideline has recommended a PLT count of 50,000/μl for most major surgical procedures, with counts near 100,000/μl recommended for neurosurgical or ophthalmologic procedures. PLT counts of 25,000/μl or so are generally adequate for minor procedures, such as central venous line placement.

C. PLT transfusions are indicated to treat bleeding in the setting of thrombocytopenia or a qualitative platelet abnormality. The goal should be to maintain a PLT count >50,000/μl.

D. Bleeding in the setting of pharmacologic inhibitors of PLT function (aspirin, clopidogrel, abciximab, etc.) frequently responds to PLT transfusion. In contrast, uremic bleeding tends to respond less well to PLT transfusion because the infused PLTs rapidly acquire the same defect affecting the patient's own PLTs.

E. The response to PLT transfusion is assessed by observing whether bleeding stops and by measuring a posttransfusion PLT count. The expected PLT increment for an average adult receiving an SDP or a pool of RDPs is 30,000–60,000/μl. Although the posttransfusion increment is the usual value considered in routine practice, a more accurate measure of PLT response is provided by the corrected count increment (CCI):

$$\text{CCI} = \frac{\text{Body surface area (m}^2) \times \text{PLT count increment}/\mu\text{l} \times 10^{11}}{\text{No. of PLTs transfused}}$$

A CCI of ≥7500 indicates an adequate PLT response.

F. Platelet refractoriness may be defined as a poor increment following repeated PLT transfusions. Several nonimmune factors can cause PLT refractoriness, including medications, fever, sepsis, DIC, bleeding, splenomegaly, and graft-versus-host disease. In a subset of cases, PLT refractoriness is immune mediated. A 10-minute to 1-hour posttransfusion PLT count that fails to show an adequate CCI on more than one occasion usually indicates antibody-mediated PLT destruction (alloimmunization). A recipient panel-reactive antibody (PRA) score of ≥20% provides supporting evidence for the role of anti–human leukocyte antigen (HLA) antibodies.

G. PLTs themselves tend to be poor immunogens. For patients who become alloimmunized, the initial antigenic stimulation generally comes from HLA class I molecules expressed on WBCs. Providing leukoreduced blood products is effective at helping to prevent PLT alloimmunization. Once a patient does become alloimmunized to PLTs, a number of strategies may be considered, including administering HLA-matched or cross-matched PLTs. If the specificity of the recipient antibody can be determined, providing antigen-negative PLT units may also be effective.

References

Fresh-Frozen Plasma, Cryoprecipitate, and Platelets Administration Practice Guidelines Development Task Force of the College of American Pathologists. Practice parameter for the use of fresh-frozen plasma, cryoprecipitate, and platelets. JAMA 1994;271(10):777–781.

Heckman KD, Weiner GJ, Davis CS, et al. Randomized study of prophylactic platelet transfusion threshold during induction therapy for adult acute leukemia 10,000/microL versus 20,000/microL. J Clin Oncol 1997;15(3):1143–1149.

Leukocyte reduction and ultraviolet B irradiation of platelets to prevent alloimmunization and refractoriness to platelet transfusions. The Trial to Reduce Alloimmunization to Platelets Study Group. N Engl J Med 1997;337(26):1861–1869.

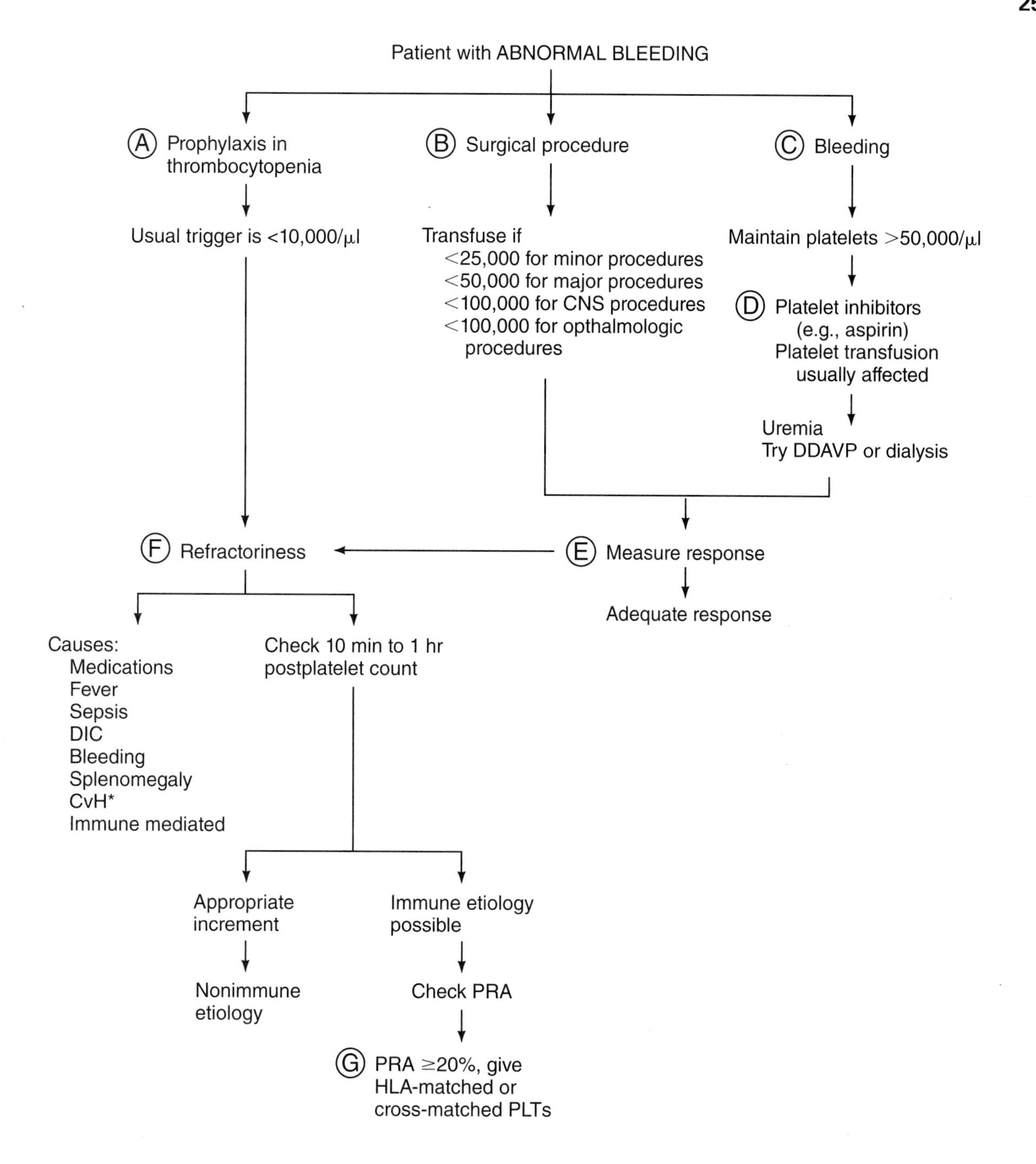

*Common variable hypogammaglobulinemia.

Petz LD, Garratty G, Calhoun L, et al. Selecting donors of platelets for refractory patients on the basis of HLA antibody specificity. Transfusion 2000;40(12):1446–1456.

Rebulla P, Finazzi G, Marangoni F, et al. The threshold for prophylactic platelet transfusions in adults with acute myeloid leukemia. Gruppo Italiano Malattie Ematologiche Maligne dell'Adulto. N Engl J Med 1997;337(26):1870–1875.

Wandt H, Frank M, Ehninger G, et al. Safety and cost effectiveness of a 10 × 10(9)/L trigger for prophylactic platelet transfusions compared with the traditional 20 × 10(9)/L trigger: a prospective comparative trial in 105 patients with acute myeloid leukemia. Blood 1998;91(10):3601–3606.

TRANSFUSION THERAPY: RED BLOOD CELLS

Richard M. Kaufman, MD

RBCs are transfused to increase oxygen-carrying capacity to meet tissue demands. The clinical significance of anemia varies widely, depending on the underlying cause, the time course, and the patient's volume status and clinical condition. Thus RBC transfusion decisions can be complex, and it is inappropriate to rely solely on a hemoglobin (Hgb) trigger. Rather, the risks and benefits of transfusion should be considered on an individual case basis. The patient's clinical status needs to be assessed carefully. Signs and symptoms of anemia (e.g., fatigue, lightheadedness, pallor, tachycardia, dyspnea on exertion) should be sought.

RBC units are derived from whole blood donations, after removal of most of the plasma, which is used for the production of fresh frozen plasma (FFP) and/or platelet concentrates. RBCs may also be collected by apheresis. RBCs are stored at 1°–6° C and have a maximum shelf life of 42 days. A unit of RBCs has a volume of about 250–300 ml and is expected to increase the recipient's Hgb by approximately 1 g/dl or hematocrit by 3%.

A. Because of normal physiologic compensation mechanisms (e.g., increased cardiac output, increased oxygen extraction), anemia may be surprisingly well tolerated, particularly when subacute in onset. For patients with normovolemic anemia caused by a nutritional deficiency, transfusion frequently can be avoided. Instead, the appropriate pharmacologic therapy (i.e., iron, folate, or vitamin B_{12}) should be administered.

B. For patients with severe acute hemorrhage, initial efforts should be focused on preventing hypovolemic shock. Volume resuscitation with crystalloid or colloid solution is of greater immediate importance than restoring oxygen-carrying capacity.

C. A number of RBC transfusion guidelines have been published. In general, it has been suggested that transfusion is almost never indicated with a Hgb level >10 g/dl and is often needed for a Hgb level <6–7 g/dl. Clinical judgment is required for patients with Hgb levels between 6–7 g/dl and 10 g/dl.

D. A particularly valuable study of RBC transfusion was the Transfusion Requirements in Critical Care (TRICC) study, published in 1999. This was a well-designed randomized controlled trial of RBC transfusion in the intensive care setting. Almost 850 patients with anemia who were in the intensive care unit were randomly assigned to either a liberal or a restrictive transfusion strategy. Patients in the liberal group were transfused for a Hgb level <10 g/dl and were maintained with Hgb concentrations of 10–12 g/dl. Patients in the restrictive group were transfused for a Hgb level <7 g/dl and were maintained at hemoglobin levels of 7–9 g/dl. The primary end point, overall 30-day mortality, was similar in the two groups. Mortality during hospitalization was significantly lower in the restrictive group. A reanalysis of the data did reveal a trend (not statistically significant) toward higher mortality among patients in the restrictive group with acute myocardial infarction and unstable angina.

E. Commonly used modifications to RBC products include leukoreduction, irradiation, and washing. Leukoreduction removes >99% of contaminating WBCs and helps prevent febrile nonhemolytic transfusion reactions, human leukocyte antigen (HLA) alloimmunization, and cytomegalovirus (CMV) transmission. Leukoreduction has additionally been proposed to prevent transfusion-associated immunosuppression, but the data are currently unclear. Irradiation is currently the only approved means to prevent transfusion-associated graft-versus-host disease (TA-GVHD). Washing RBCs is done to remove plasma proteins; this is indicated when the recipient has a history of severe allergic reactions that are refractory to antihistamine administration.

References

Consensus Conference. Perioperative red blood cell transfusion. JAMA 1988;260(18):2700–2703.

Hébert PC, Wells G, Blajchman MA, et al. A multicenter, randomized, controlled clinical trial of transfusion requirements in critical care. Transfusion Requirements in Critical Care Investigators, Canadian Critical Care Trials Group. N Engl J Med 1999;340(6):409–417.

Hébert PC, Yetisir E, Martin C, et al. Is a low transfusion threshold safe in critically ill patients with cardiovascular diseases? Crit Care Med 2001;29(2):227–234.

Simon TL, Alverson DC, AuBouchon J, et al. Practice parameter for the use of red blood cell transfusions: developed by the Red Blood Cell Administration Practice Guideline Development Task Force of the College of American Pathologists. Arch Pathol Lab Med 1998;122(2):130–138.

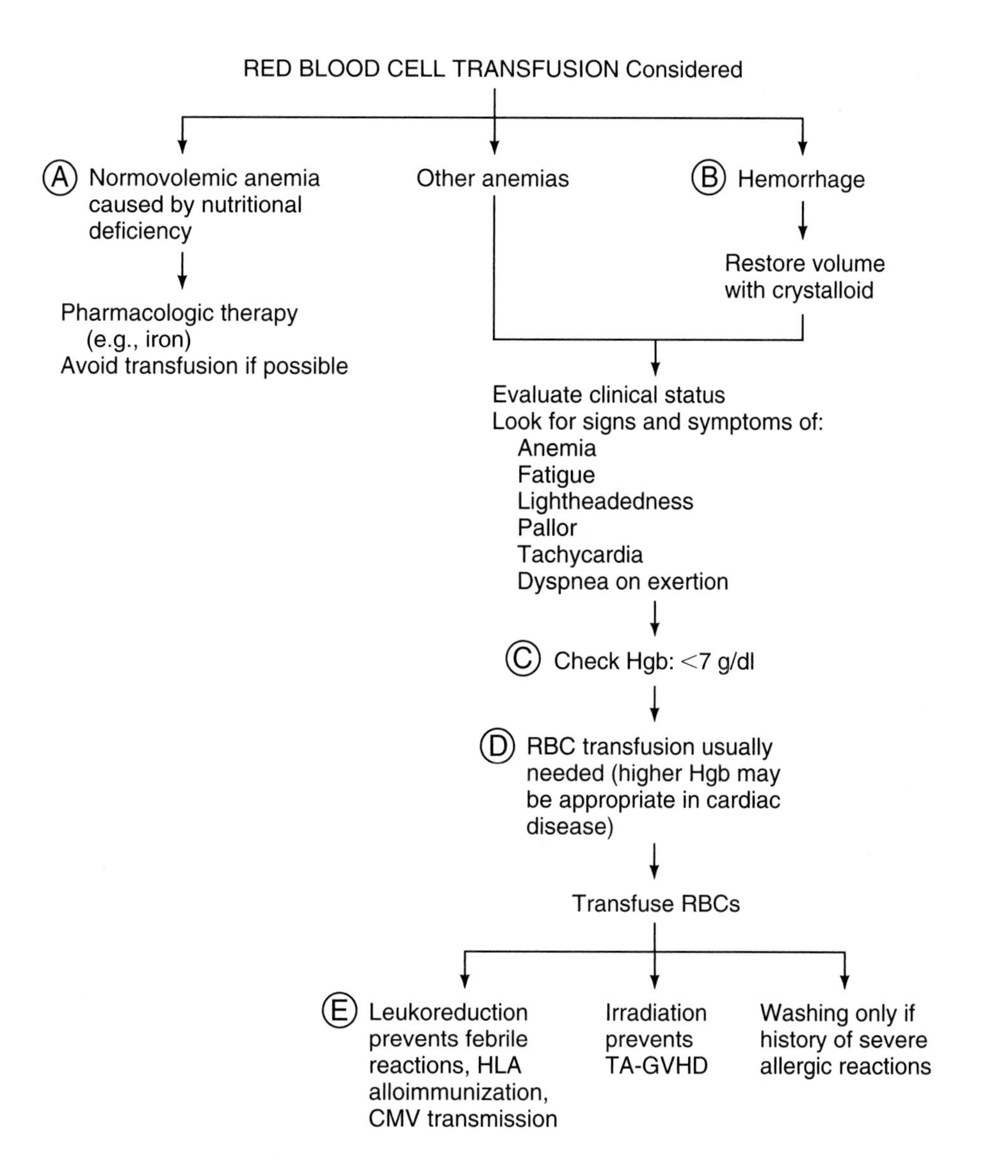
RED BLOOD CELL TRANSFUSION Considered
(A) Normovolemic anemia caused by nutritional deficiency
Pharmacologic therapy (e.g., iron)
Avoid transfusion if possible
Other anemias
(B) Hemorrhage
Restore volume with crystalloid
Evaluate clinical status
Look for signs and symptoms of:
Anemia
Fatigue
Lightheadedness
Pallor
Tachycardia
Dyspnea on exertion
(C) Check Hgb: <7 g/dl
(D) RBC transfusion usually needed (higher Hgb may be appropriate in cardiac disease)
Transfuse RBCs
(E) Leukoreduction prevents febrile reactions, HLA alloimmunization, CMV transmission
Irradiation prevents TA-GVHD
Washing only if history of severe allergic reactions

TRANSFUSION THERAPY: GRANULOCYTES

Richard M. Kaufman, MD

Granulocyte transfusions are sometimes considered for patients with severe neutropenia (absolute neutrophil count [ANC] <500/μl) and a life-threatening bacterial or fungal infection. Cases where granulocyte transfusions are considered are ones in which the patient's own neutrophil counts are expected to recover within a few weeks (e.g., following a chemotherapy-induced nadir). Despite being used for >40 years, the efficacy of granulocyte transfusions remains unclear. Indeed, a multicenter randomized controlled trial of standard antimicrobial therapy, high-dose granulocyte transfusion has recently been proposed to attempt to definitively settle the question of what (if any) role granulocytes have in treating neutropenic sepsis. In the 1970s and early 1980s, seven randomized controlled studies were performed to assess the efficacy of granulocytes. Three trials reported positive results, two trials reported partial positive results, and two trials reported negative results. All these studies were criticized for several reasons, including administration of insufficient granulocyte doses, small patient sample sizes, and excessively high mortality rates observed among the control patients. In the mid-1980s, granulocyte transfusion use fell sharply because the clinical results seen were marginal, there was concern over adverse reactions, and there were marked improvements in antimicrobial agents. Interest in granulocyte transfusions was renewed in the 1990s, when the introduction of recombinant granulocyte colony-stimulating factor (G-CSF) permitted the collection of extremely high doses of granulocytes.

A. Granulocytes are collected by apheresis from healthy donors, either volunteer community apheresis platelet donors, or friends or family members of the patient. To increase the granulocyte yield, donors may be mobilized with a single dose of G-CSF approximately 12 hours before granulocyte collection. G-CSF mobilization permits the harvest of $4–8 \times 10^{10}$ granulocytes. Corticosteroids (e.g., oral dexamethasone) have been shown to increase the granulocyte yield even further. In general, granulocyte mobilization of donors has been reported to be well tolerated, but there are known risks associated with both G-CSF and corticosteroid administration.

B. Granulocyte products are stored at room temperature and must be transfused within 24 hours of collection. Because granulocyte products may contain 40–50 ml of RBCs, they must be ABO compatible with the recipient. All granulocyte products must be irradiated to prevent transfusion-associated graft-versus-host disease. Generally, patients who are negative for cytomegalovirus (CMV) only receive granulocytes from donors who are CMV negative.

C. Adverse reactions to granulocytes are seen in about 10% of granulocyte transfusions. Typical reactions are fever/chills or mild allergic reactions (itching/hives). More rarely, serious reactions are seen, such as anaphylaxis or acute lung injury. Hypoxic reactions have been reported to be associated with the administration of amphotericin, so granulocyte transfusions are typically given several hours apart from doses of amphotericin. Finally, granulocyte products carry the same infectious risks of other blood products. Because granulocytes must be given within 24 hours of collection, infectious disease testing is not available prior to the time of administration. Ordinarily, the granulocyte donor is tested and documented to be negative for all standard infectious disease markers up to 30 days ahead of the granulocyte donation.

References

Hübel K, Carter RA, Liles WC, et al. Granulocyte transfusion therapy for infections in candidates and recipients of HPC transplantation: a comparative analysis of feasibility and outcome for community donors versus related donors. Transfusion 2002;42(11):1414–1421.

Price TH. Granulocyte transfusion therapy: it's time for an answer. Transfusion 2006;46(1):1–5.

Price TH, Bowden RA, Boeckh M, et al. Phase I/II trial of neutrophil transfusions from donors stimulated with G-CSF and dexamethasone for treatment of patients with infections in hematopoietic stem cell transplantation. Blood 2000;95(11):3302–3309.

Strauss RG. Therapeutic granulocyte transfusions in 1993. Blood 1993;81(7):1675–1678.

Vamvakas EC, Pineda AA. Meta-analysis of clinical studies of the efficacy of granulocyte transfusions in the treatment of bacterial sepsis. J Clin Apher 1996;11(1):1–9.

GRANULOCYTE TRANSFUSION Considered

↓

May be considered in patient with ANC
<500/μl and life-threatening infection
unresponsive to conventional therapy

↓

(A) Request blood bank to:
- Mobilize donor
- Collect product

↓

(B) Transfuse within 24 hr

↓

(C) Adverse events may include:
- Fever/chills
- Allergic reactions
- Acute lung injury
- Disease transmission

TRANSFUSION REACTIONS

Richard M. Kaufman, MD

In past decades, three viruses comprised the most important infectious risks of transfusion: hepatitis B virus (HBV), hepatitis C virus (HCV), and HIV. In the United States, improvements in donor screening (e.g., nucleic acid testing) have all but eliminated transfusion transmission of HIV and HCV. The per unit risks are now approximately 1 in 2 million for HIV and HCV and 1 in 200,000 for HBV. With the rates of HIV, HCV, and HBV transmission having dropped so low, other transfusion risks have gained new prominence. The most significant infectious risk of transfusion is now sepsis from a bacterially contaminated platelet unit. Platelets (PLTs) must be stored at room temperature. Bacteria can be cultured from about 1 in 3000 PLT units, and a clinically significant septic reaction is thought to occur in about 1 in 20,000 PLT transfusions. The other most important current risks of transfusion are as follows: (1) transfusion-related acute lung injury (per unit risk of 1/5000) and (2) transfusion of the wrong RBC unit, typically resulting from a patient identification error (per unit risk of 1/12,000 to 1/19,000).

A. In general, any adverse clinical event that occurs during a blood transfusion should be considered a transfusion reaction until proved otherwise. Steps to take when a transfusion reaction is suspected include the following: (1) stop the transfusion and notify the blood bank; (2) reconfirm the identity of the patient and unit immediately; (3) draw a fresh blood sample, and send it plus the remaining blood component to the blood bank. The blood bank will perform a clerical check, examine the recipient's plasma for visible hemolysis, and perform a direct antiglobulin test (DAT) to look for antibody-coated red cells in the recipient.

B. Acute hemolytic transfusion reactions occur when preformed antibodies in the recipient bind to transfused RBCs. The classic example is an ABO-incompatible transfusion (e.g., A donor/O recipient). The antibody-antigen interaction can lead to complement fixation, cytokine effects, renal failure, and DIC. Fever is the most common sign. Other signs and symptoms may include rigors; pain at the infusion site or in the chest, abdomen, or flanks; nausea/vomiting; and shock. In anesthetized patients, red urine may be the only presenting sign. *The transfusion should be stopped immediately.* Blood pressure support and maintaining adequate renal perfusion are primary concerns. Patients should be hydrated with normal saline ± diuretics.

C. Delayed hemolytic transfusion reactions are anamnestic anti-RBC antibody responses that occur 1–2 weeks posttransfusion. Patients are often asymptomatic. Decreased survival of transfused RBCs may be suspected based on a falling hemoglobin/hematocrit level and an increased bilirubin. The DAT is usually positive. Treatment is supportive; the patient's CBC and renal status should be monitored.

D. Febrile nonhemolytic transfusion reactions (FNHTRs) are generally defined as a temperature increase of at least 1° C in the setting of transfusion, for which no other cause can be established. These reactions are typically benign, but other, more serious causes of fever must be excluded (i.e., hemolytic and septic reactions). Proposed mechanisms of FNHTR include (1) recipient antibody interacting with transfused leukocytes and (2) transfusion of cytokines that have accumulated during storage. The use of prestorage leukoreduced blood products has decreased the incidence of FNHTRs. These reactions generally respond well to acetaminophen administration.

E. Allergic transfusion reactions are caused by allergies to donor plasma proteins. Allergic reactions to blood products span the entire spectrum from mild urticarial reactions to full-blown anaphylaxis. For reactions limited to urticaria only (i.e., no bronchospasm or hypotension) it is acceptable to stop the transfusion, treat with antihistamines, and restart the infusion if the symptoms resolve. Epinephrine is the mainstay of treatment for anaphylactic transfusion reactions.

F. Transfusion-related acute lung injury (TRALI) is characterized by acute-onset hypoxemia and the appearance of bilateral infiltrates on chest x-ray within 6 hours of transfusion of a plasma-containing component. The acute respiratory distress syndrome seen is noncardiogenic in nature but may be difficult to distinguish from circulatory overload. Multiple mechanisms for TRALI have been proposed. In at least a subset of cases, TRALI is precipitated by passive transfusion of donor antibodies (usually anti–human leukocyte antigen) that react with recipient cells. Care is supportive. All patients with TRALI require supplemental oxygen, and about 75% need mechanical ventilatory

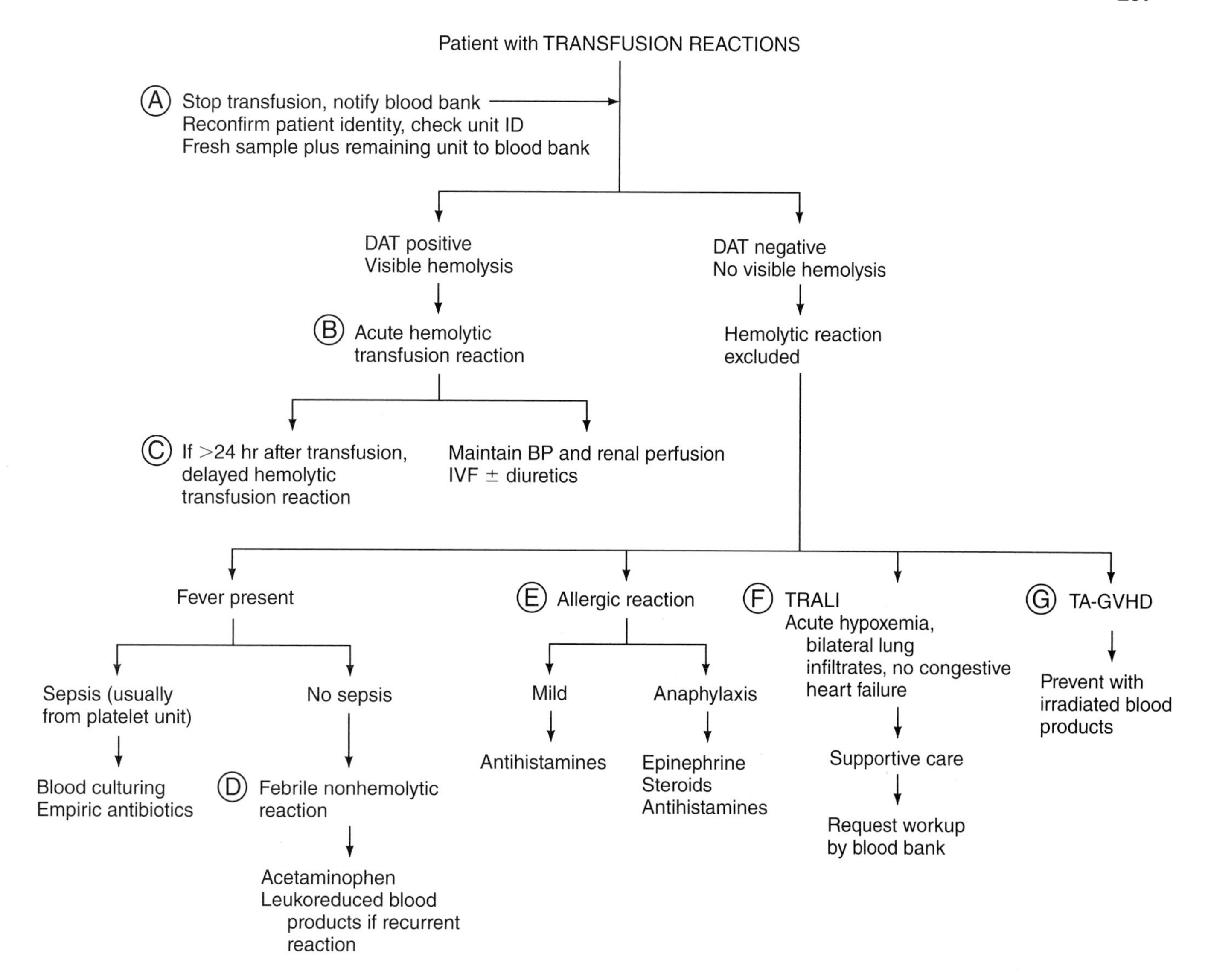

support. Although most patients with TRALI recover spontaneously over 2–4 days, there is a 5%–10% mortality rate.

G. Transfusion-associated graft-versus-host disease (TA-GVHD) is a rare but devastating complication of blood transfusion that primarily affects recipients who are immunocompromised. Viable lymphocytes in the transfused blood component attack host tissues, leading to severe rash, diarrhea, and pancytopenia within 7–10 days of transfusion. TA-GVHD is almost uniformly fatal. There is no treatment, but TA-GVHD can be prevented effectively by providing irradiated blood products.

References

Brecher ME, ed. Technical Manual. Bethesda, MD: AABB, 2005.

Dodd RY, Notari EP 4th, Stramer SL. Current prevalence and incidence of infectious disease markers and estimated window-period risk in the American Red Cross blood donor population. Transfusion 2002; 42(8):975–979.

Hillyer CD, Josephson CD, Blajchman MA, et al. Bacterial contamination of blood components: risks, strategies, and regulation: Joint ASH and AABB educational session in transfusion medicine. Hematology Am Soc Hematol Educ Program 2003:575–589.

Linden JV, Wagner K, Voytovich AE, et al. Transfusion errors in New York State: an analysis of 10 years' experience. Transfusion 2000; 40(10):1207–1213.

Toy P, Popovsky MA, Abraham E, et al. Transfusion-related acute lung injury: definition and review. Crit Care Med 2005;33(4):721–726.

CLASSICAL HODGKIN'S LYMPHOMA

Daniel O. Persky, MD, and Carol S. Portlock, MD

Hodgkin's lymphoma (HL) typically presents with progressive, nontender, rubbery lymphadenopathy in supraclavicular, cervical, axillary, or (rarely) inguinal regions. Most commonly, patients are 15–35 years of age. Mediastinal adenopathy may be detected incidentally or may lead to symptoms of nonproductive cough, shortness of breath, or both.

A. The diagnosis usually is made on excisional lymph node biopsy; extranodal sites may be confirmatory. The pathology should be reviewed by an expert hematopathologist to rule out benign causes or non-Hodgkin's lymphoma.

B. The following baseline studies are performed in all patients to assess clinical stage: (1) CBC, including lymphocyte count; (2) ESR and lactate dehydrogenase (LDH); (3) liver enzymes, including albumin; (4) serum alkaline phosphatase; (5) renal function tests; (6) chest radiograph (Fig. 1); (7) CT scan of the chest, abdomen, and pelvis; and (8) bone marrow biopsy. Bone marrow biopsy may be omitted in stage IA/IIA patients without cytopenias. Positron emission tomography (PET) scanning is now routinely used in HL staging and is becoming a component in treatment assessment. Anthracycline-containing therapy requires a baseline assessment of cardiac function, and bleomycin-containing therapy requires a baseline pulmonary function test.

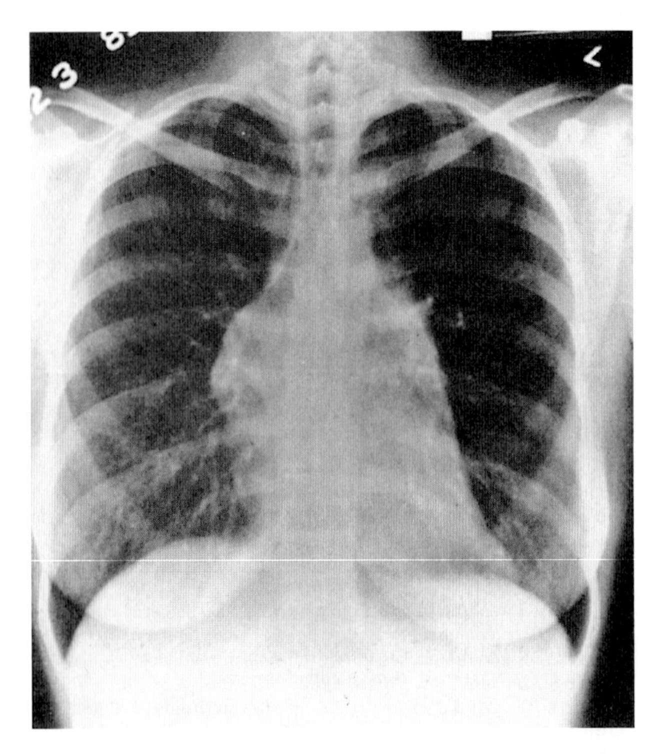

Figure 1. Mediastinal mass >0.3 × the chest diameter.

C. Cotswolds modification of Ann Arbor staging system is used.

D. The risk factors for limited stage (I and II) HL are: (1) bulky disease (designated "X") defined as any mass >10 cm in transverse dimension or mediastinal mass of more than one third of intrathoracic diameter or >35% of thoracic diameter at T5-6; (2) B symptoms (defined as fever higher than 38° C, drenching night sweats, or unexplained weight loss of >10% over 6 months); (3) ESR ≥50 without B symptoms or ≥30 with B symptoms; and (4) more than three involved lymph node sites. Some groups also consider age ≥50 years and extranodal extension as risk factors.

E. Patients without risk factors can be considered for two to four cycles of ABVD (doxorubicin, bleomycin, vinblastine, and dacarbazine) followed by 20–30 Gy of involved field radiation therapy (IFRT). Patients with any risk factors may receive four cycles of ABVD followed by 30–36 Gy of IFRT. Another option in selected patients with limited-stage HL is ABVD alone for four to six cycles.

F. The risk factors for advanced stage HL (IIXB, III, and IV) are enumerated in the International Prognostic Score (IPS) and include the following: (1) albumin <4 g/dl, (2) hemoglobin <10.5 g/dl, (3) male gender, (4) stage IV disease, (5) age ≥45 years, (6) WBC count ≥15,000/mm^3, and (7) lymphocyte count of <600/mm^3 or <8% of WBC.

G. Six cycles of ABVD remains the standard combination chemotherapy for advanced stage HL. Prospective studies comparing ABVD with new regimens, Stanford V and BEACOPP (bleomycin, etoposide, doxorubicin, cyclophosphamide, vincristine, prednisone, and procarbazine), are ongoing. In IPS 0–3 and bulky stage II disease, IFRT is administered after satisfactory ABVD response (30–36 Gy). Another option for patients at the IPS 0–3 advanced stage is the 12-week regimen of Stanford V (vinblastine, doxorubicin, vincristine, bleomycin, mechlorethamine, etoposide, and prednisone) followed by IFRT for initial sites >5 cm. Patients ages ≤60 years with IPS of 4–7 may be considered for escalated BEACOPP followed by IFRT to initial sites >5 cm.

Patients with relapsed or refractory HL should be evaluated for salvage chemotherapy followed by autologous stem cell transplantation.

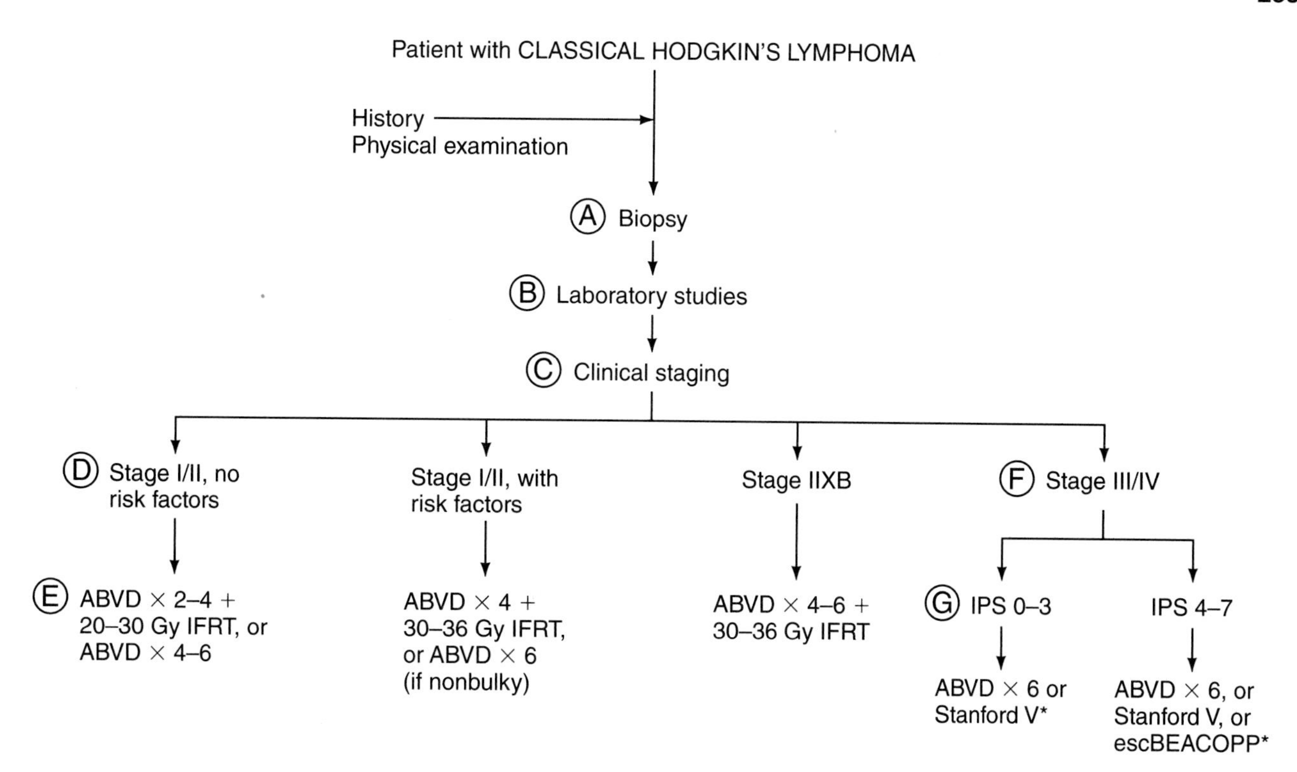

References

Canellos GP, Anderson JR, Propert KJ, et al. Chemotherapy of advanced Hodgkin's disease with MOPP, ABVD, or MOPP alternating with ABVD. N Engl J Med 1992;327:1478.

Connors JM. State-of-the-art therapeutics: Hodgkin's lymphoma. J Clin Oncol 2005;23(26):6400–6408.

Diehl V, Franklin J, Pfreundschuh M, et al. Standard and increased-dose BEACOPP chemotherapy compared with COPP-ABVD for advanced Hodgkin's disease. N Engl J Med 2003;348(24):2386–2395.

Hasenclever D, Diehl V. A prognostic score for advanced Hodgkin's disease. International Prognostic Factors Project on Advanced Hodgkin's Disease. N Engl J Med 1998;339(21):1506–1514.

Horning SJ, Hoppe RT, Breslin S, et al. Stanford V and radiotherapy for locally extensive and advanced Hodgkin's disease: mature results of a prospective clinical trial. J Clin Oncol 2002;20(3):630–637.

Hutchings M, Loft A, Hansen M, et al. FDG-PET after two cycles of chemotherapy predicts treatment failure and progression-free survival in Hodgkin lymphoma. Blood 2006;107(1):52–59.

Lister TA, Crowther D, Sutcliffe SB, et al. Report of a committee convened to discuss the evaluation and staging of patients with Hodgkin's disease: Cotswolds meeting. J Clin Oncol 1989;7(11):1630–1636.

Meyer RM, Gospodarowicz MK, Connors JM, et al. Randomized comparison of ABVD chemotherapy with a strategy that includes radiation therapy in patients with limited-stage Hodgkin's lymphoma: National Cancer Institute of Canada Clinical Trials Group and the Eastern Cooperative Oncology Group. J Clin Oncol 2005;23(21):4634–4642.

CHRONIC MYELOGENOUS LEUKEMIA

Robert M. Rifkin, MD, FACP

Approximately 4300 patients are diagnosed with chronic myelogenous leukemia (CML) each year in the United States, with CML accounting for 14% of all cases of leukemia in adults. CML occurs with an incidence of 1–2 per 100,000 population, and this incidence is constant worldwide. Males are more often affected than females, and the median age at presentation is 45–55 years. One third of the patients are >60 years of age. CML is uncommon in children and adolescents, accounting for <5% of childhood leukemia.

Although CML results from the malignant transformation of a single cell, the causative factors remain unknown. Predisposing factors for CML remain largely unidentified, except that the incidence is significantly higher in survivors of an atomic blast. The molecular-cytogenetic pathology of CML has been extensively described. The molecular events involved in the initiation and transformation of CML have provided the basis for therapies that have changed the natural history of the disease. CML has since become the paradigm for our understanding of leukemogenesis and drug development.

CML is caused by the transforming capability of the protein products resulting from the Philadelphia translocation, t(9;22)(q34;q11), and the cytogenetic-molecular changes acquired during clonal evolution and the progression of the disease. Up to 95% of patients express the Philadelphia chromosome, which results from a reciprocal translocation between the long arms of chromosomes 9 and 22. This process involves the exchange of genetic material from a segment of abl (abelson) gene on chromosome 9q34 with a part of bcr (breakpoint cluster region) on chromosome 22q11, creating a fusion bcr-abl gene on 22q11. Expression of bcr-abl proteins triggers molecular transformations through increased tyrosine kinase activity. Uncontrolled activations of kinases initiate downstream signaling pathways that upregulate transcription of gene complexes, mediating proliferations and transformation of CML progenitor cells. Manifestations of CML result from the unrestrained proliferation of granulocytes.

Classically, the disease pursues a triphasic course. The chronic phase, which usually lasts 3–5 years, features mild constitutional symptoms that vanish with therapy. The disease then transforms to an accelerated phase where drug resistance begins to emerge. Finally, it terminates in blast crisis.

A. CML is characterized by the expansion of myeloid progenitor cells at various stages of maturation, their premature release into the circulation, and their tendency to accumulate in extramedullary sites. In most patients, CML presents in chronic phase. Symptoms at presentation often reflect the increase in cell mass and turnover and may include lethargy, weakness, night sweats, and weight loss. Occasionally there is abdominal discomfort resulting from splenomegaly. In recent series up to 50% of patients display no symptoms and have the diagnosis established through routine blood counts. Presentation in accelerated or blast phase constitutes <10% of patients.

B. Laboratory manifestations of chronic-phase CML are myeloid hyperplasia in the marrow and thrombocytosis, neutrophilic leukocytosis, and basophilia in the peripheral blood. Peripheral blood leukocytosis of >100,000/µl is seen in 70%–90% of patients. Nucleated RBCs are usually seen in the peripheral blood smear and help to comprise the leukoerythroblastic blood picture, which is a nearly universal finding at diagnosis of the disease.

C. The bone marrow is hypercellular, with a myeloid-to-erythroid ratio of between 9:1 and 15:1. Myeloid cells show all stages of maturation, with a preponderance of immature precursors. Marrow fibrosis may be patchy and progress to a diffuse pattern with disease evolution. Metaphase spreads from bone marrow aspiration are the definitive tests for the Philadelphia translocation. Additional karyotypic abnormalities are observed with disease progression. Molecular techniques have now become the mainstay of diagnosis and are utilized in the monitoring of therapy. Patients receiving therapy are usually followed utilizing the polymerase chain reaction (PCR) and fluorescence in situ hybridization (FISH). Both tests provide a higher degree of sensitivity than conventional cytogenetics.

(Continued on page 262)

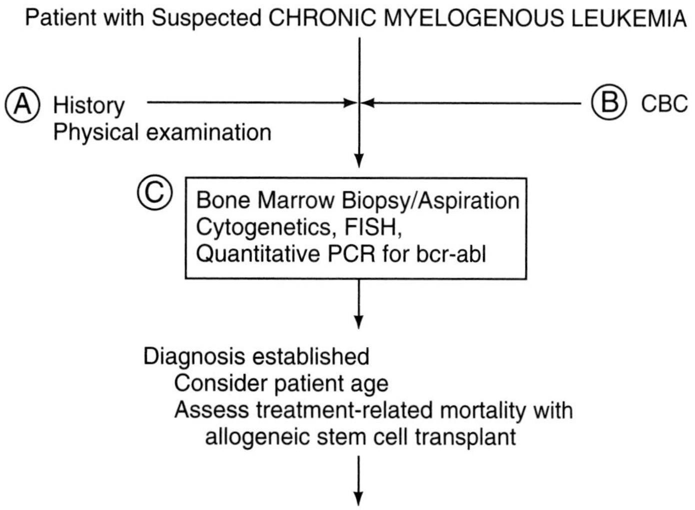

Patient with Suspected CHRONIC MYELOGENOUS LEUKEMIA

(A) History
Physical examination

(B) CBC

(C) Bone Marrow Biopsy/Aspiration
Cytogenetics, FISH,
Quantitative PCR for bcr-abl

Diagnosis established
Consider patient age
Assess treatment-related mortality with allogeneic stem cell transplant

Cont'd on p 263

D. The prognosis for patients with CML has changed dramatically in the past 20 years. Patients diagnosed with chronic-phase CML now have a median survival of 5–7 years and up to 9 years if they have a good prognosis. Therapies such as allogeneic stem cell transplantation, imatinib, and interferon-α have all contributed to this progress utilizing risk-adapted strategies.

E. At the time of diagnosis, most patients with CML are in the chronic phase. The natural history of CML invariably leads to blastic transformation directly or, more frequently, to blastic transformation with an intervening accelerated phase. Median time from diagnosis to transformation is between 36 and 40 months. Blastic transformation may result in death within 3–6 months. Transformation is heralded by loss of response to initial therapy and clinical signs such as unexplained lymphadenopathy, fever, progressive splenomegaly, weight loss, and bone and joint pain. One third of patients have a transformation immunophenotypical of acute lymphoblastic leukemia (ALL) and may respond to ALL therapy. The remaining two thirds transform to acute myeloid or acute undifferentiated leukemia and may respond to acute myelogenous leukemia (AML) regimens.

F. The development of imatinib has revolutionized the therapeutic approach to CML. Imatinib has been confirmed as an active agent in the treatment of chronic and transformed phases of CML. It can readily induce complete hematologic remissions (CHR) within 3 months of the institution of therapy. As the response continues to evolve, major cytogenetic responses (MCGR) may be obtained within 6–9 months. Imatinib is the single most active agent available for the treatment of CML. In a multinational study of 1106 patients, imatinib proved superior to a regimen of cytarabine and interferon with respect to response rates, improved toxicity, and tolerability. Although imatinib is the most effective therapy for CML, allogeneic stem cell transplantation remains the only curative therapy available. Hydroxyurea and busulfan used to be commonly used agents in the treatment of CML, but neither are curative and only rarely result in a cytogenetic response. Thus, therapy with these two agents must be regarded as palliative.

G. In carefully selected patients, allogeneic stem cell transplantation can cure a substantial percentage of patients who have a suitable donor. Allogeneic stem cell transplantation results in long-term survival in 50%–80% of patients. Although relapses can occur following transplantation, this rate is the lowest in younger patients and those who receive transplants during the chronic phase of their disease. Infusion of donor lymphocytes at the time of posttransplant relapse can induce durable and complete molecular remissions. Matched unrelated donor transplants have a high rate of treatment-related morbidity and mortality. However, highly selected younger patients can have 5-year survival rates as high as 70%. Early results of reduced-intensity transplants show rapid engraftment, complete eradication of host hematopoiesis, and minimal procedure-related toxicities.

Given the availability of imatinib and stem cell transplantation, the decision on how best to treat patients with CML remains controversial. Treatment algorithms need to be continuously updated in light of emerging data and the development of a second generation of tyrosine kinase inhibitors that may overcome resistance to imatinib therapy.

References

Druker BJ, Sawyers CL, Kantarjian H, et al. Activity of a specific inhibitor of the BCR-ABL tyrosine kinase in the blast crisis of chronic myeloid leukemia and acute lymphoblastic leukemia with the Philadelphia chromosome. N Engl J Med 2001;344:1038.

Druker BJ, Talpaz M, Resta DJ, et al. Efficacy and safety of a specific inhibitor of the BCR-ABL tyrosine kinase in chronic myeloid leukemia. N Engl J Med 2001;344:1031.

Faderl S, Talpaz M, Estrov Z, et al. The biology of chronic myeloid leukemia. N Engl J Med 1999;341:164.

Jemal A, Murray T, Samuels A, et al. Cancer statistics, 2003. CA Cancer J Clin 2003;53:5.

Kantarjian HM, Talpaz M, O'Brien S, et al. Dose escalation of imatinib mesylate can overcome resistance to standard-dose therapy in patients with chronic myeloid leukemia. Blood 2003;101:473.

Kurzrock R, Kantarjian HM, Druker BJ, et al. Philadelphia chromosome-positive leukemias: from basic mechanism to molecular therapeutics. Ann Intern Med 2003;138:819.

Qazilbash MH, Devetten MP, Abraham J, et al. Utility of a prognostic scoring system for allogeneic stem cell transplantation in patients with chronic myeloid leukemia. Acta Haematol 2003;109:119.

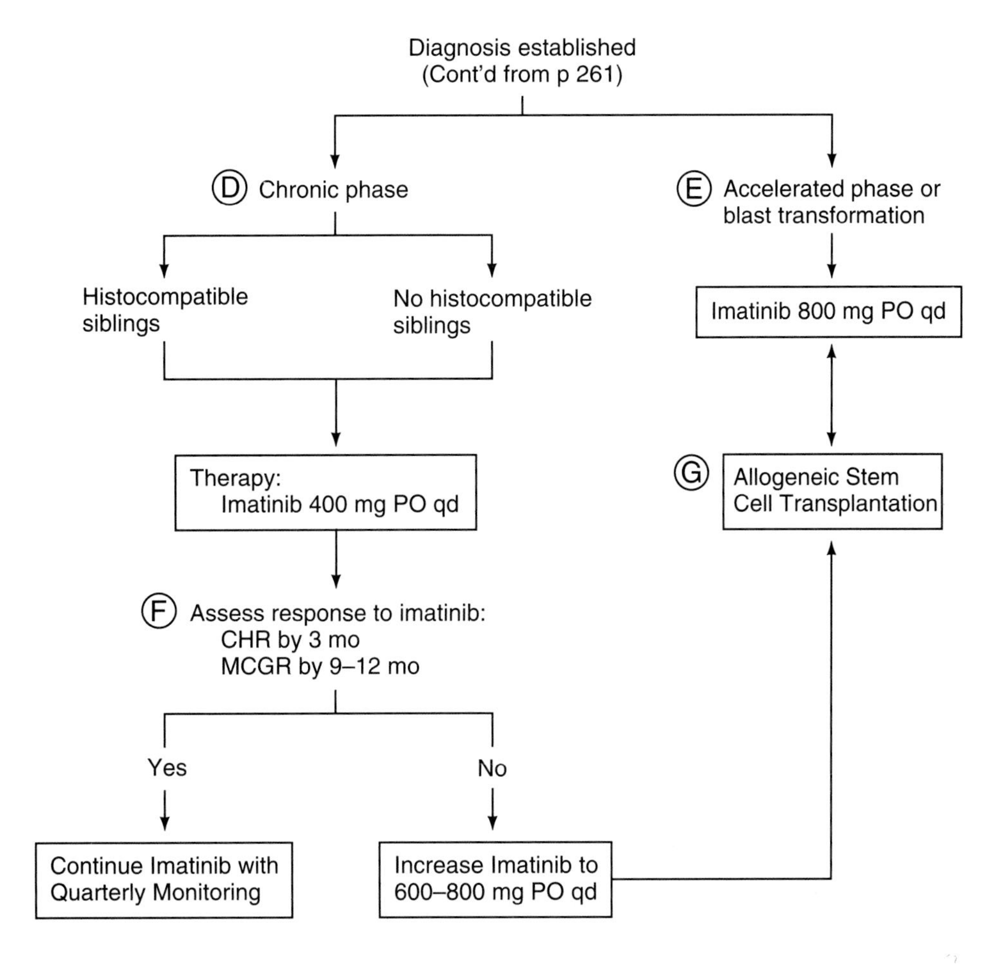
Diagnosis established
(Cont'd from p 261)
D Chronic phase
E Accelerated phase or blast transformation
Histocompatible siblings
No histocompatible siblings
Imatinib 800 mg PO qd
Therapy:
Imatinib 400 mg PO qd
G Allogeneic Stem Cell Transplantation
F Assess response to imatinib:
CHR by 3 mo
MCGR by 9–12 mo
Yes
No
Continue Imatinib with Quarterly Monitoring
Increase Imatinib to 600–800 mg PO qd

ABNORMAL SERUM PROTEIN ELECTROPHORESIS

Sheeba K. Thomas, MD; Michael Wang, MD; and Donna M. Weber, MD

Monoclonal gammopathy is the presence of a monoclonal protein (M protein) in the serum or urine. It consists of one of the immunoglobulins, a heavy chain, and/or a light chain. Biclonal gammopathy is noted in about 2% of cases. Monoclonal gammopathy may be seen in a variety of diseases, both benign and malignant.

A. The focus of the initial workup is to recognize, quantitate, and characterize the abnormal protein present in serum and urine using serum protein electrophoresis (SPEP), immunoelectrophoresis (IEP), urine protein electrophoresis (UPEP), and serum free light chain assay and to determine whether there is evidence of a coexisting disorder that requires treatment. The bone survey and marrow examination are especially helpful in excluding multiple myeloma.

B. Patients with elevated IgG, A, D, or E may have a solitary plasmacytoma of bone, multiple myeloma, amyloidosis, or a monoclonal gammopathy of unknown significance (MGUS). Patients with monoclonal IgM may have MGUS, Waldenstrom's macroglobulinemia, amyloid, or cryoglobulinemia. The listed screening examinations guide the diagnosis. Statistically, most patients with a monoclonal gammopathy have MGUS. Of the 873 cases of monoclonal gammopathy evaluated at the Mayo Clinic as of 1988, 64% had MGUS and 16% had multiple myeloma. Less common diagnoses were amyloidosis (8%), non-Hodgkin's lymphoma (6%), chronic lymphocytic leukemia (2%), solitary or extramedullary plasmacytoma (2%), and Waldenstrom's macroglobulinemia (2%).

C. Solitary plasmacytoma of bone occasionally presents with a monoclonal gammopathy (50%), although half of the patients show no M component in either serum or urine. The diagnosis is based on histologic evidence of a tumor consisting of plasma cells, identical to those seen in multiple myeloma, and confined to a single bone site. Levels of uninvolved immunoglobulins usually are preserved. In addition to standard studies for myeloma, MRI of the thoracic and lumbosacral spine is useful to confirm the diagnosis of multiple myeloma. Radiotherapy of 45 Gy is the treatment of choice. Although >50% of the patients will be alive at 10 years, the disease-free survival is only 15%–45% because most patients develop multiple myeloma. In 60 previously untreated patients with solitary plasmacytoma of bone treated at MD Anderson Cancer Center between 1965 and 2000, median survival from completion of radiotherapy was 11 years. Patients most likely to have a prolonged disease-free survival are those whose M protein completely disappears, as measured by the most sensitive tests, within 1 year of radiotherapy. Accordingly, periodic follow-up with SPEP, IEP, and UPEP is indicated in all patients with an abnormality before treatment.

D. Extramedullary plasmacytoma is a plasma cell tumor that arises outside the bone marrow, most often in the upper respiratory tract, including the nasal cavity and sinuses, nasopharynx, and larynx. Patients generally do not have a detectable M component in either serum or urine, so detection of a monoclonal protein usually indicates multiple myeloma. The diagnosis is based on the finding of a plasma cell tumor in an extramedullary site, the absence of multiple myeloma in the bone marrow, and no lytic lesions in the bone survey. Fewer than 25% of patients have evidence of a monoclonal protein in the serum or urine by electrophoresis or immunofixation. Radiotherapy provides disease-free survival exceeding 10 years in 50%–65% of patients.

E. Because of more frequent screening of blood chemistries and counts, about 20% of patients with multiple myeloma are now recognized by chance without significant symptoms or signs of disease (asymptomatic multiple myeloma). Asymptomatic disease generally is characterized by a serum M protein of <4.5 g/dl and the absence of lytic bone lesions, anemia (hemoglobin >10.5 g/dl), hypercalcemia, renal failure attributable to myeloma, and symptoms of disease. A subset of these patients may have long-term stability of disease. At our center, risk factors for disease progression include IgA subtype and serum M protein >3.0 g/dl. Patients with none of these features may be followed by observation, as are patients with MGUS because they remain stable for many years (low risk to progression), whereas patients with two features have a median time to progression of 18 months (high risk). An abnormal MRI result of the spine appears equally effective in predicting patients at risk for early progression to symptomatic disease (median 18 months). To avoid complications of disease, early chemotherapy may be an option for patients at high risk. Patients with one risk feature (intermediate risk) can be separated into low- or high-risk categories by MRI of the spine.

F. The presence of multiple lytic lesions with >10% plasma cells in the bone marrow, any serum M component, and/or light chains in the urine indicates multiple

(Continued on page 266)

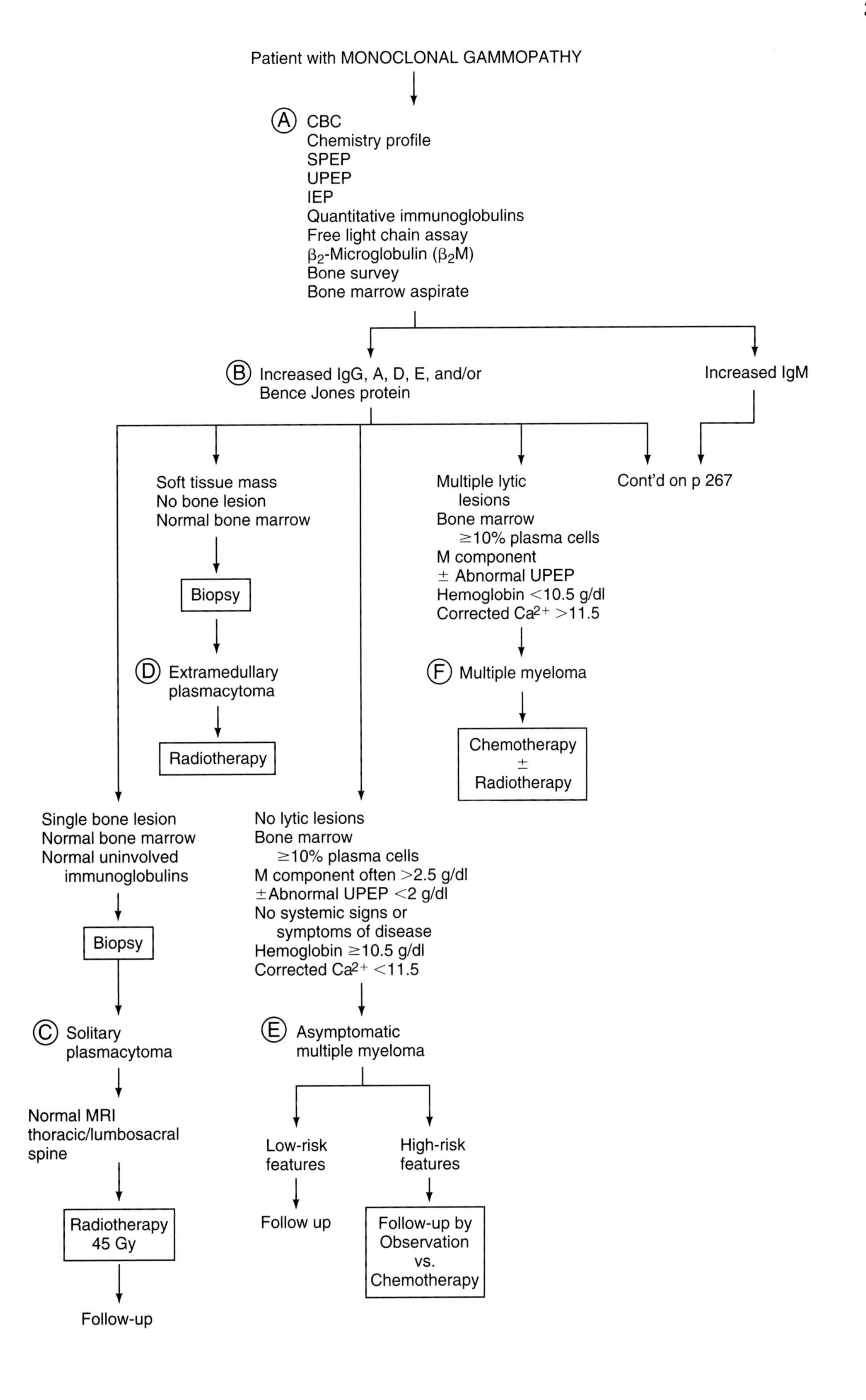
Patient with MONOCLONAL GAMMOPATHY
(A) CBC
Chemistry profile
SPEP
UPEP
IEP
Quantitative immunoglobulins
Free light chain assay
β2-Microglobulin (β2M)
Bone survey
Bone marrow aspirate
(B) Increased IgG, A, D, E, and/or Bence Jones protein
Increased IgM
Soft tissue mass
No bone lesion
Normal bone marrow
Biopsy
(D) Extramedullary plasmacytoma
Radiotherapy
Multiple lytic lesions
Bone marrow ≥10% plasma cells
M component
± Abnormal UPEP
Hemoglobin <10.5 g/dl
Corrected Ca2+ >11.5
(F) Multiple myeloma
Chemotherapy ± Radiotherapy
Cont'd on p 267
Single bone lesion
Normal bone marrow
Normal uninvolved immunoglobulins
Biopsy
(C) Solitary plasmacytoma
Normal MRI thoracic/lumbosacral spine
Radiotherapy 45 Gy
Follow-up
No lytic lesions
Bone marrow ≥10% plasma cells
M component often >2.5 g/dl
±Abnormal UPEP <2 g/dl
No systemic signs or symptoms of disease
Hemoglobin ≥10.5 g/dl
Corrected Ca2+ <11.5
(E) Asymptomatic multiple myeloma
Low-risk features
Follow up
High-risk features
Follow-up by Observation vs. Chemotherapy

myeloma. The most common complications of this disease are bone pain (usually from fractures), hypercalcemia, infection, and renal failure. Chemotherapy with melphalan-based regimens alone results in a median survival of 3 years. However, a study by the Intergroupe Francais du Myelome found that autologous stem cell transplantation improved 5-year overall survival rates from 12% to 52%. Newer thalidomide-, lenalidomide-, and bortezomib-based therapies have improved survival in randomized trials and are expected to affect overall median survival; however, this is not yet reflected in SEER data statistics.

G. MGUS indicates the presence of an M component in patients without multiple myeloma, solitary plasmacytoma of bone, extramedullary plasmacytoma, amyloidosis, macroglobulinemia, or other lymphoproliferative disorders. MGUS is characterized by an M component <3.0 g/dl, generally preserved uninvolved immunoglobulins, normal CBC, low levels of marrow plasmacytosis, no lytic lesions or hypercalcemia, and the absence of renal failure attributable to multiple myeloma. More important, over a long period the M component usually remains stable and no additional abnormalities must develop. The incidence of MGUS increases with age, reaching approximately 7.5% in patients >85 years old. In a large series of 1384 patients with MGUS, the concentration of the M component ranged between unmeasurable and 3.0 g/dl (median 1.2–1.3 g/dl). IEP revealed IgG in 70%, IgA in 12%, IgM in 15%, and biclonal gammopathy in 3% of patients. The light-chain type was kappa in 61% and lambda in 39%. Bone marrow specimens from 160 of these patients revealed a low level of marrow plasmacytosis (0%–10%, median 3%). Multiple myeloma, amyloidosis, macroglobulinemia, or other lymphoproliferative processes developed in 8% of the patients, with an actuarial rate of 10% at 10 years, 21% at 20 years, and 26% at 25 years. Most patients with progressive disease developed multiple myeloma (65%). In a similar study by the same authors, the time from diagnosis of MGUS to development of multiple myeloma ranged from 1 to 32 years (median 10 years), indicating that such patients must be followed indefinitely.

H. The presenting manifestations of primary amyloidosis include weakness, weight loss, ankle edema, dyspnea, parasthesias, lightheadedness, syncope, peripheral neuropathy, carpal tunnel syndrome, congestive heart failure, nephrosis, periorbital purpura, arthralgia, orthostatic hypotension, macroglossia, and diarrhea with malabsorption syndrome. Abdominal fat aspiration at an experienced center, using a 19-gauge needle, has a sensitivity of 70%–80%, and only 13% of patients with amyloidosis will not have evidence of amyloid deposition on either abdominal fat aspiration or bone marrow biopsy. The most effective treatment for primary amyloidosis is high-dose melphalan followed by autologous stem cell transplantation. Other regimens, including melphalan and prednisone, high-dose dexamethasone-based therapies, and thalidomide-based therapies, may also provide some benefit.

I. Patients with an elevated IgM (often <2 g/dl) and peripheral adenopathy often have an underlying B-cell neoplasm. In a series of 213 patients with an IgM MGUS diagnosed at the Mayo Clinic between 1960 and 1994, 14% developed non-Hodgkin's lymphoma, Waldenstrom's macroglobulinemia, primary amyloidosis, or chronic lymphocytic leukemia. The median duration from presentation with MGUS until the diagnosis of the lymphoma was 4 years (range 0.4–22 years). Given the long latency period before development of associated malignancies in some patients, periodic follow-up should continue indefinitely.

J. Waldenstrom's macroglobulinemia is a rare disease (one seventh as common as myeloma) and is the result of an uncontrolled proliferation of lymphoplasmacytoid cells in which a large monoclonal IgM is produced. The presenting signs and symptoms include weakness, fatigue, bleeding (especially oozing from the oronasal area), blurred vision, dyspnea, weight loss, paresthesias, retinal lesions ("sausage" or "boxcar" formation), hepatosplenomegaly, and lymphadenopathy. IgM levels often are >3 g/dl. Initial treatment for symptomatic patients traditionally has been with alkylating agents such as chlorambucil, which produces remission rates of 50%–60%. More recently treatment with nucleoside analogs (cladribine or fludarabine) induced responses of 70%–80% in previously untreated patients. When nucleoside analogs are combined with alkylating agents (e.g., cyclophosphamide) and the monoclonal antibody rituximab, response rates of up to 90% can be seen.

References

Attal M, Harousseau JL, Stoppa AM, et al. A prospective, randomized trial of autologous bone marrow transplantation and chemotherapy in multiple myeloma. Intergroupe Francais du Myelome. N Engl J Med 1996;335(2):91–97.

Gertz MA, Merlini G, Treon SP. Amyloidosis and Waldenstrom's macroglobulinemia. Hematology Am Soc Hematol Educ Program 2004:257–282.

Kyle RA. Monoclonal gammopathy of undetermined significance and solitary plasmacytoma. Hematol Oncol Clin North Am 1997;11:71.

Kyle RA, Therneau TM, Rajkumar SV, et al. A long-term study of prognosis in monoclonal gammopathy of undetermined significance. N Engl J Med 2002;346(8):564–569.

Weber DM. Solitary bone and extramedullary plasmacytoma. Hematology Am Soc Hematol Educ Program 2005:373–376.

Weber DM, Dimopoulos MA, Delasalle K, et al. 2-Chlorodeoxyadenosine alone and in combination for previously untreated Waldenstrom's macroglobulinemia. Semin Oncol 2003;30(2):243–247.

Weber DM, Dimopoulous MA, Moulopoulos LA, et al. Prognostic features of asymptomatic multiple myeloma. Br J Haematol 1997;97:810.

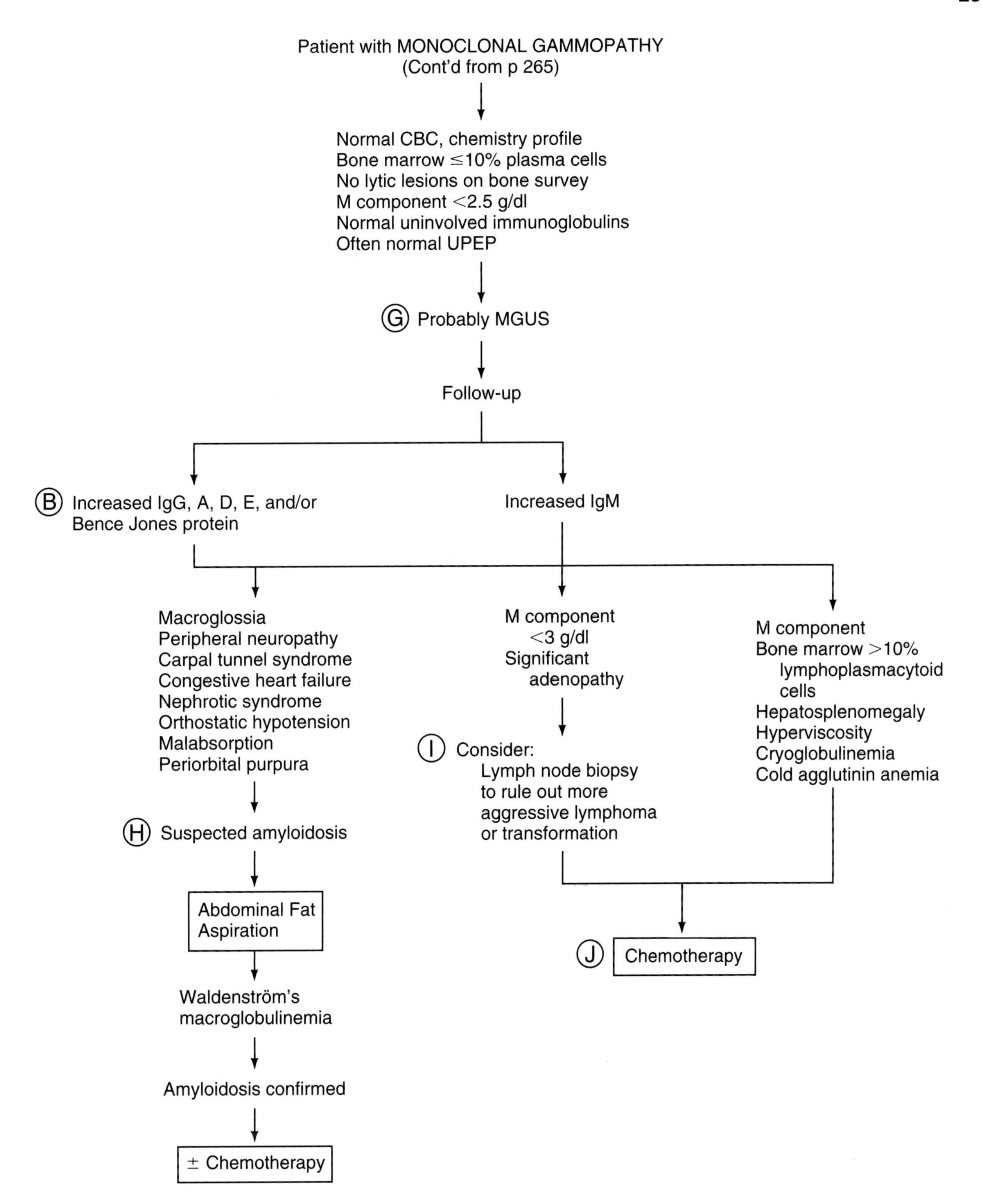

Patient with MONOCLONAL GAMMOPATHY
(Cont'd from p 265)
Normal CBC, chemistry profile
Bone marrow ≤10% plasma cells
No lytic lesions on bone survey
M component <2.5 g/dl
Normal uninvolved immunoglobulins
Often normal UPEP
G Probably MGUS
Follow-up
B Increased IgG, A, D, E, and/or Bence Jones protein
Increased IgM
Macroglossia
Peripheral neuropathy
Carpal tunnel syndrome
Congestive heart failure
Nephrotic syndrome
Orthostatic hypotension
Malabsorption
Periorbital purpura
H Suspected amyloidosis
Abdominal Fat Aspiration
Waldenström's macroglobulinemia
Amyloidosis confirmed
± Chemotherapy
M component <3 g/dl
Significant adenopathy
I Consider:
Lymph node biopsy to rule out more aggressive lymphoma or transformation
M component
Bone marrow >10% lymphoplasmacytoid cells
Hepatosplenomegaly
Hyperviscosity
Cryoglobulinemia
Cold agglutinin anemia
J Chemotherapy

LYMPHADENOPATHY

Guillermo Gonzalez-Osete, MD, and Manuel Modiano, MD

More than 500 lymph nodes in the human body may become enlarged in response to numerous stimuli: (1) infection (bacterial, viral, parasitic, spirochetal, chlamydial, mycobacterial, or fungal), (2) drug reactions (phenytoin, serum sickness), (3) malignancy (head and neck, GI, breast, rectal, lymphoma), and (4) miscellaneous conditions (sarcoidosis, systemic lupus erythematosus).

A. New-onset lymphadenopathy <7 days' duration is unlikely to be malignant.

B. Recurrent or long-term (>7–14 days) lymphadenopathy (unilateral or bilateral) requires a full workup. Most experienced clinicians see the patient again in 2–4 weeks to determine whether the node is increasing before embarking on a full workup. The associated symptoms of fever, weight loss, or night sweats suggest malignancy (lymphoma B symptoms) or infection. Regional symptoms such as chest tightness, dysphagia, shortness of breath, and/or facial swelling suggest mediastinal disease and require a CT scan of the chest. Complaints of fullness in the abdomen, early satiety, and pain radiating to the shoulders or back necessitate abdominal CT to rule out pancreatic, renal, or other intraperitoneal lesions. Unilateral leg swelling (after deep vein thrombosis is ruled out) may require pelvic CT to rule out regional lymphadenopathy causing extrinsic compression.

C. Serologic studies and blood cultures help differentiate among infections, collagen vascular disease, and malignancy. Among the most common infectious causes are infectious mononucleosis, toxoplasmosis, syphilis, Epstein-Barr virus, HIV, and cytomegalovirus. If the history is suspicious and the patient is or was living in an endemic area, these causes must be ruled out.

D. Lymph node enlargement in the head and neck area requires a careful ear, neck, and throat (ENT) evaluation, including biopsy of suspicious lesions; if ENT findings are normal, the patient may need to undergo a triple endoscopy procedure with evaluation of nasal, bronchial, and esophageal passages. Consider fine needle biopsy of the lymph node only if endoscopic findings are normal.

E. The supraclavicular area often is affected by breast cancer, lymphomas (Hodgkin's and non-Hodgkin's), and metastases from the lung and GI tract (esophagus, stomach, pancreas). Supraclavicular nodes are easily biopsied and are highly diagnostic.

F. Enlarged axillary lymph nodes often are a sign of breast or lung cancer. They also are often affected by lymphoma and may be biopsied to obtain a diagnosis if the primary source cannot be found.

G. When inguinal nodes are enlarged, physical examination should focus on the anorectal region, perineum, vulva, penis, and scrotum. Perform sigmoidoscopy to rule out rectal or anal carcinoma; evaluate the genitourinary system by urinalysis. Pelvic CT may provide useful information. If CT findings are normal, proceed with biopsy. Tumor markers carcinoembryonic antigen (CEA), prostate-specific antigen (PSA), and the murine monoclonal antibody OC125 also may provide guidance toward a diagnosis.

H. For a patient with generalized lymphadenopathy but no other signs or symptoms and no other organ involvement, consider biopsy of the most accessible region (not necessarily the largest). The diagnostic yield is better with supraclavicular, axillary, or inguinal nodes (in descending order). A key feature of these biopsies is the need for adequate amounts of tissue with the specimen sectioned to allow for light microscopy, fresh frozen tissue for markers, and a portion in glutaraldehyde for electron microscopy. Patients with nondiagnostic biopsies require close follow-up, especially those with atypical hyperplasia, because many may develop lymphoproliferative disorders. Also, consider angioimmunoblastic lymphadenopathy in patients with "hyperplasia." This can be done by an experienced immunopathologist.

Newer technology, such as positron emission tomography (PET) scans, could be considered as a means of identifying the most appropriate node to biopsy. To assist in the selection of which node to biopsy, one can choose the node that is most active metabolically. This likely would have a better chance of identifying the appropriate node than by random selection, especially in cases in which no known diagnosis is present, other attempts have failed, or review of the literature failed to provide any supporting studies.

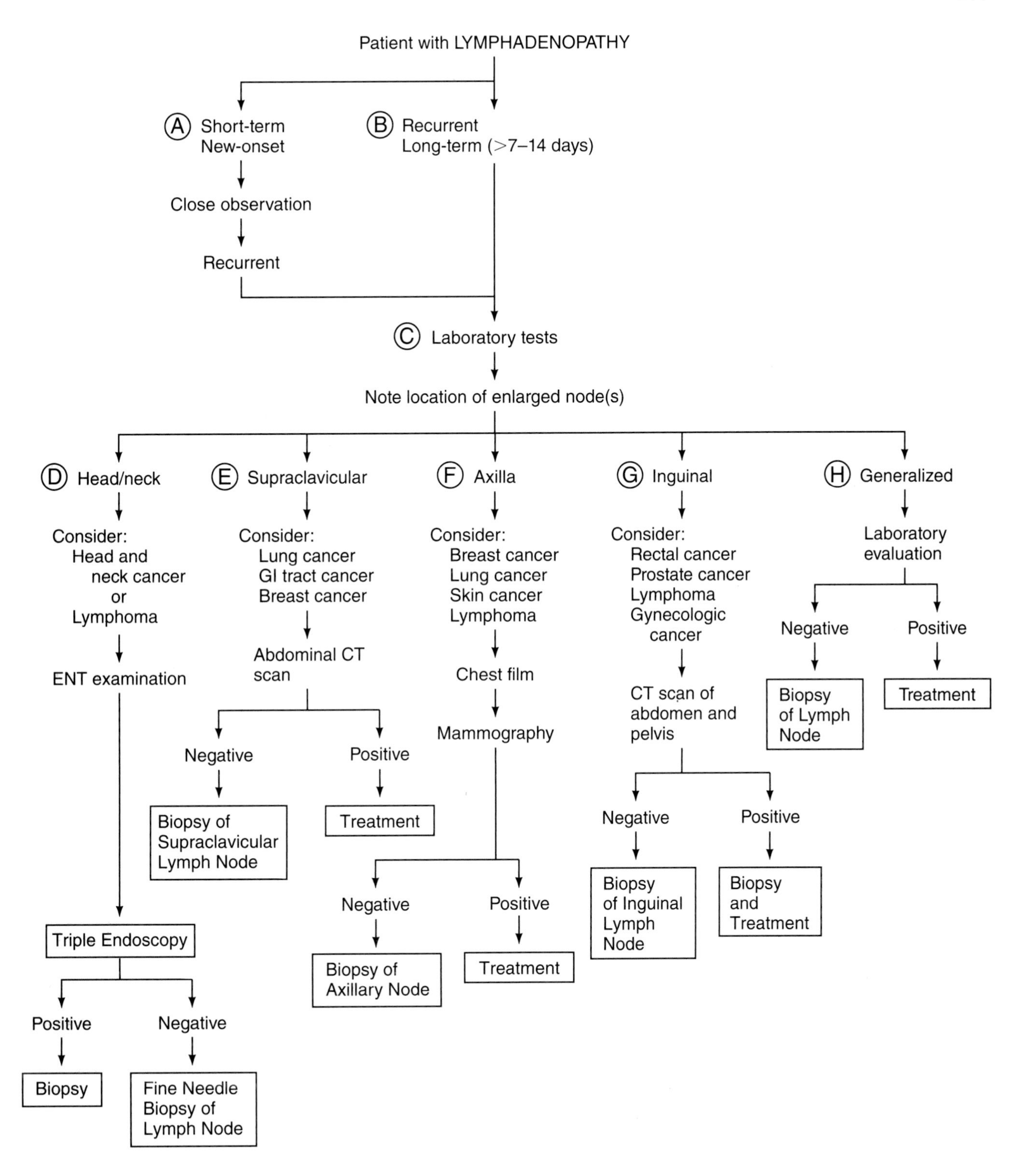

References

Copeland EM, McBride C. Axillary metastases from unknown primary sites. Ann Surg 1973;178:25.

Faller DV. Diseases of lymph nodes and spleen. In Bennett JC, Plum F, eds. Cecil Textbook of Medicine. Philadelphia: WB Saunders, 1996:968.

Moore RD, Weisberger AS, Bowerfind ES. An evaluation of lymphadenopathy in systemic disease. Arch Intern Med 1957;99:751.

Saltzsein S. The fate of patients with nondiagnostic lymph node biopsies. CA Cancer J Clin 1966;16:115.

Schroeder K, Franssila KO. Atypical hyperplasia of lymph nodes: a follow-up study. Cancer 1979;44:1155.

Sinclair S, Beckman E, Eliman L. Biopsy of enlarged superficial lymph nodes. JAMA 1974;228:602.

Zuelzer W, Kaplan J. The child with lymphadenopathy. Semin Hematol 1975;12:323.

CARCINOMA OF UNKNOWN PRIMARY SITE (CUPS)

Daruka Mahadevan, MD, PhD

Carcinoma of unknown primary site (CUPS) is defined as the presence of documented metastatic cancer without an established primary tumor. It is a heterogeneous group of carcinomas; hence, there are no common genetic and phenotypic alterations. In general, CUPS follow an aggressive pathologic and clinical course with no obvious risk factors. Immunohistochemistry (IHC) and pathologic studies are used to characterize CUPS (Table 1).

A. The goal of the diagnostic workup is to identify either the primary site or clinical situations where potentially curative or effective therapy is available. The optimal evaluation required to identify an occult primary carcinoma includes complete history and physical examination, laboratory studies, critical pathologic review, and appropriate imaging studies (Table 2). The incidence of CUPS is 7–12 cases per 100,000 in the United States, accounting for 2.3%–4.2% of cancer in both sexes. Median age of occurrence is ~60 years, and CUPS is the seventh to eighth most frequent cancer and the fourth most common cause of mortality in the world. As a group, median survival for CUPS from diagnosis is approximately 10–12 months.

B. A routine chest x-ray (CXR) is part of the initial evaluation; however, it may be prudent to perform a high-resolution CT scan of the chest, abdomen, and pelvis for staging. CT scans appear to detect 30%–35% of primary sites. The FDG-PET (2-[^{18}F] fluoro-2-deoxy-D-glucose-positron emission tomography) scan is a useful modality, particularly for squamous cell tumors originating in the head and neck areas.

Table 1. **CUPS Histologic Types, Frequency, and Likely Pathobiologic Features**

Histologic Types	Frequency(%)	Pathobiologic Features
Adenocarcinoma (well to moderately differentiated)	50	c-MYC, Ras, Erb-B2, 3p deletion
Adenocarcinoma (poorly differentiated)	30	Chromosomal instability (aneuploidy: 70%), Erb-B2 (11%)
Squamous cell carcinoma	15	PTH-like factor
Neuroendocrine tumors	1	t(11;22)
Lymphoma	1	t(8;14)
Embryonal/germ cell tumors	2	Isochromosome 1(12)p or 12p deletion
Melanomas and sarcomas	1	t(3;13), t(11;22)

Table 2. **Diagnostic Studies Used to Evaluate Patients with CUPS**

Diagnostic Evaluation	Type of Investigations
History	Abdominal pain, persistent cough, bleeding (GI/GU/RS), tobacco/alcohol use, FH
Physical examination	Breast, testicular, pelvic, vulvar, rectal (prostate, blood), lymph node regions, skin
Biopsy and pathology (IHC)	Fine needle aspiration/core; cytokeratin 7 and 20; histology specific markers (ER/PR, PSA)
Staging and radiology	CXR, CT scan of abdomen/pelvis, MRI mammography, FDG-PET
Endoscopy	Upper GI (ERCP), lower GI, laryngoscopy, bronchoscopy, endoscopic ultrasound
Laboratory studies	CBC with differential and platelets, metabolic panel (Ca^{2+}, LDH, β_2M), urine analysis, stool analysis
Serum markers	Histology-specific markers (PSA, CA15.3, CEA, CA27.29, CA125,CA19.9, β-hCG, αFP, Tgb)
Special tests	Electron microscopy

Endoscopic evaluations should be directed toward specific symptoms and signs. Patients with upper respiratory symptoms should be considered for fiberoptic bronchoscopy, laryngoscopy (direct and indirect), or both; patients with GI symptoms should be considered for upper and lower GI endoscopy with random biopsies.

C. An adequate sample of tumor tissue is essential because pathologic examination is the single most important step in determining the primary site. IHC utilizing antibodies to cytokeratins (7 and 20) may guide in identifying certain tumor types (Table 3). Other histology specific markers may also be of diagnostic value in difficult cases (Table 4).

Table 3. **Antibodies to Cytokeratins 7 and 20 May Help in Identifying Certain Tumor Types**

7+/20+	7+/20−
Stomach, biliary, pancreas, ovary (mucinous)	Biliary, pancreas, lung, ovary (nonmucinous), endometrium
7−/20−	7−/20+
Prostate, kidney, liver	Colon, stomach, ovary (mucinous)

(Continued on page 272)

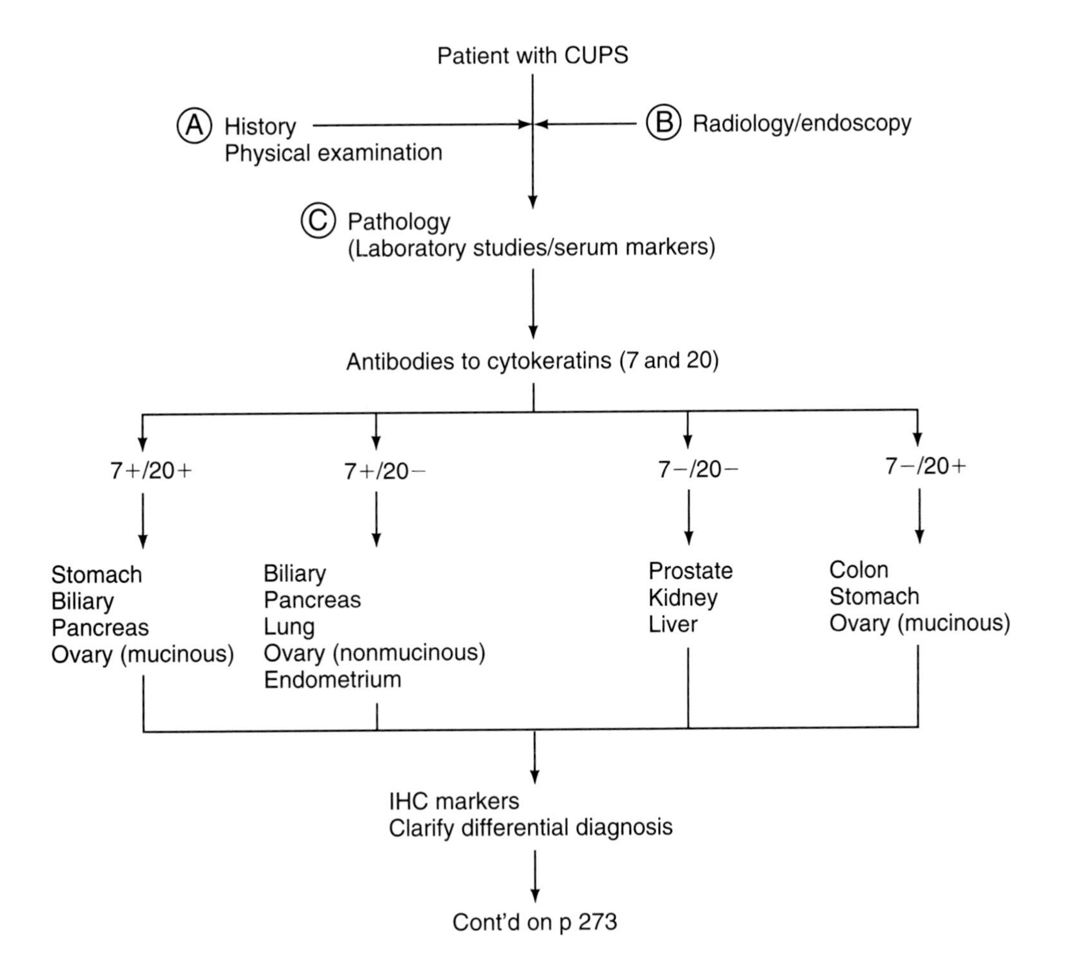

Patient with CUPS
A History
Physical examination
B Radiology/endoscopy
C Pathology
(Laboratory studies/serum markers)
Antibodies to cytokeratins (7 and 20)
7+/20+
7+/20−
7−/20−
7−/20+
Stomach
Biliary
Pancreas
Ovary (mucinous)
Biliary
Pancreas
Lung
Ovary (nonmucinous)
Endometrium
Prostate
Kidney
Liver
Colon
Stomach
Ovary (mucinous)
IHC markers
Clarify differential diagnosis
Cont'd on p 273

Table 4. **Histology-Specific Markers May Be of Diagnostic Value**

Tumor Type	IHC Marker
Carcinoma	Cytokeratins, EMA
Breast	Cytokeratins, EMA, ER/PR, Her2/Neu
Germ cell	Cytokeratins, EMA, βhCG, αFP
Lymphoma	CLA, EMA (±)
Lung	Thyroid transcription factor
Melanoma	S-100, HMB-45, Vimentin, NSE
Neuroendocrine	Chromogranin, synaptophysin, cytokeratin, EMA, NSE
Prostate	PSA, PAP, cytokeratin, EMA
Sarcoma	Vimentin, desmin, CD117, factor VIII
Thyroid	Thyroglobulin, cytokeratin, calcitonin

Serum markers (prostate: prostate-specific antigen [PSA]; breast: CA15.3, CA 27.29, carcinoembryonic antigen [CEA]; lung and colon: CEA; pancreas: CA19.9; ovarian: CA125; germ cell: βhCG, αFP, liver: αFP; thyroid: thyroglobulin) may be useful adjuncts to pathology and imaging studies (see Table 2). The most common epithelial primaries identified by pathology and radiology are lung and pancreatic cancer. Despite extensive workup, <20% will have a primary site identified. However, postmortem studies report about 70% of cases to be undiagnosed.

D. A number of predictive and prognostic factors are characterized as significant in distinguishing favorable from unfavorable groups of CUPS (Table 5). They are certain histopathologic subsets (poorly differentiated carcinoma, squamous cell carcinoma, neuroendocrine carcinoma), number of metastatic lesions (2), female sex, performance status, weight loss, and serum markers (alkaline phosphatase, lactate dehydrogenase, [LDH], CEA).
E. Disease-specific therapy is indicated for the favorable CUPS with a potential for a good treatment outcome (Table 6).
F. However, for unfavorable CUPS, treatment is based on type 3 level of evidence. Chemotherapy regimens include platinum, taxol, or gemcitabine- or irinotecan-based combinations. The availability of gene expression profiling and tissue microarrays may help identify targets for which approved therapies exists (e.g., Avastin, Erbitux, or Herceptin) and may be used alone or in combination with chemotherapy. In general, patients with CUPS should be considered for palliative treatment options suitable for individual clinical use or investigational use on an appropriate clinical trial.

Table 5. **Predictive and Prognostic Factors Characterize Favorable from Unfavorable Groups of CUPS**

Favorable	Unfavorable
Poorly differentiated carcinoma with midline structures (mediastinum, retroperitoneum; men <50 years); extragonadal germ cell sy ndrome	Adenocarcinoma metastatic to the liver or other organs
Papillary adenocarcinoma of the peritoneal cavity (women)	Nonpapillary malignant ascites (adenocarcinoma)
Adenocarcinoma involving only the axillary lymph nodes (women)	Multiple brain metastases (adenocarcinoma or squamous carcinoma)
Squamous cell carcinoma involving cervical lymph nodes	Multiple lung/pleural metastases (adenocarcinoma)
Isolated inguinal adenopathy (squamous carcinoma)	Multiple metastatic bone disease (adenocarcinoma)
Poorly differentiated neuroendocrine carcinoma	—
Blastic bone metastasis with elevated PSA	—
Single small potentially resectable tumor	—

Table 6. **Treatment Modalities for Favorable CUPS That Lead to a Good Survival Outcome**

Favorable CUPS	Treatments
Extragonadal germ cell syndrome	Platinum-based combination therapy for germ cell tumors (50% RR; 15%–25% CR)
Papillary adenocarcinoma of the peritoneal cavity	Surgical debulking followed by platinum-based combination therapy for stage III ovarian cancer (OS similar to stage III ovarian)
Adenocarcinoma involving only the axillary lymph nodes	Breast cancer chemotherapy followed by XRT and adjuvant hormonal therapy if ER/PR+ (5 year OS 75%)
Squamous cell carcinoma involving cervical lymph nodes	N1-Neck dissection followed by XRT N2/3- concurrent chemo-XRT (5-year OS 30%–50%)
Isolated inguinal adenopathy (squamous carcinoma)	Lymph node dissection ± XRT (50% long-term survival)
Poorly differentiated neuroendocrine carcinoma	Platinum or Carbo/Taxol or clinical trial (RR 50%–70%; CR 25%)
Blastic bone metastasis with elevated PSA	Initial treatment: endocrine therapy
Single small potentially resectable tumor	Resection ± XRT

CR, Complete response; OS, overall survival; RR, response rate; XRT, external radiation therapy.

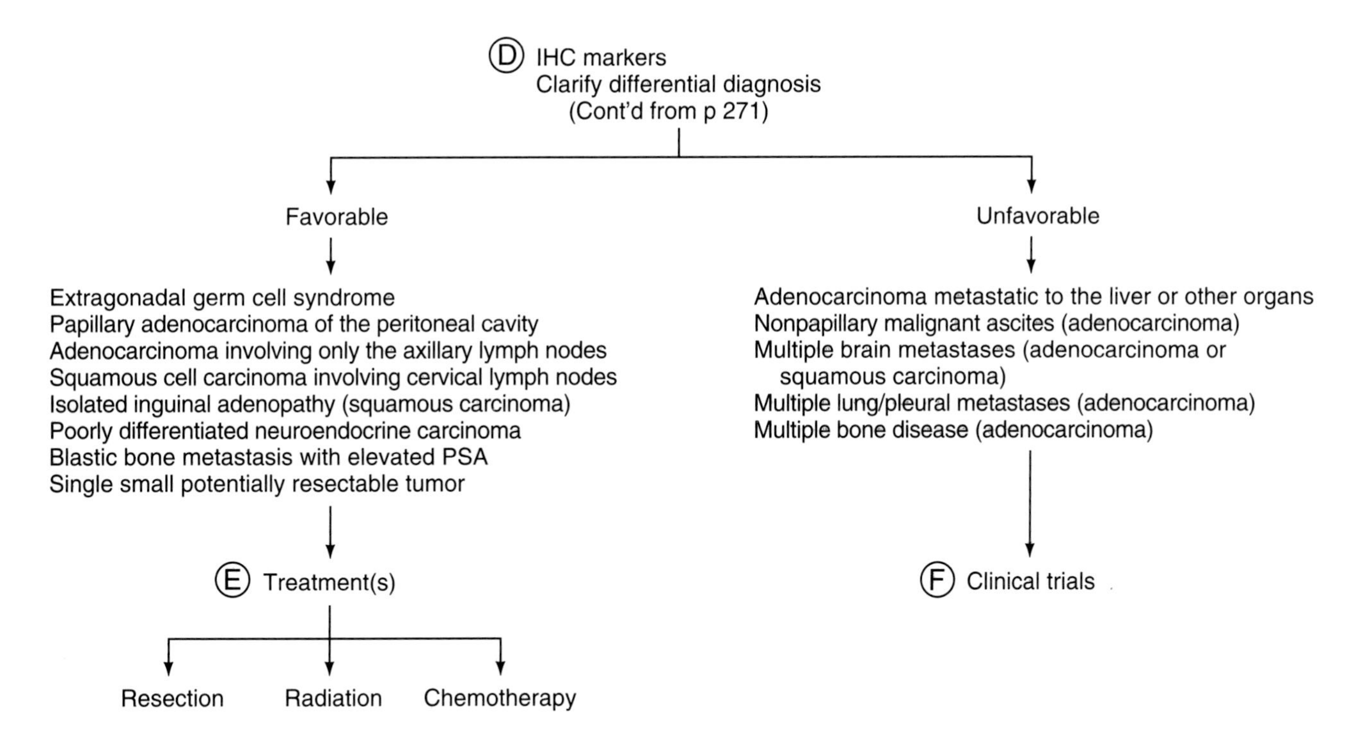

References

Abbruzzese JL, Abbruzzese MC, Hess KR. Unknown primary carcinoma: natural history and prognostic factors in 657 consecutive patients. J Clin Oncol 1994;12:1272–1280.

Abbruzzese JL, Abbruzzese MC, Lenzi R, et al. Analysis of a diagnostic strategy for patients with suspected tumors of unknown origin. J Clin Oncol 1995;13:2094.

Greco FA, Hainsworth JD. Cancer of unknown primary site. In DeVita TV, Hellman S, Rosenberg SA, eds. Cancer: Principles and Practice of Oncology, 4th ed, Philadelphia: JB Lippincott, 1997: 2423–2443.

Lenzi R, Hess KR, Abbruzzese MC, et al. Poorly differentiated carcinoma and poorly differentiated adenocarcinoma of unknown origin: favorable subsets of patients with unknown primary carcinoma? J Clin Oncol 1997;15:2056.

Muir C. Cancer of unknown primary site. Cancer 1995;75:353–356.

Pavlidis N, Fizazi K. Carcinoma of unknown primary (CUP). Crit Rev Oncol Hematol 2005;54:243–250.

NEUTROPENIA AND FEVER

Ana Maria López, MD, MPH, FACP

Infection during episodes of chemotherapy-induced neutropenia is the most common cause of treatment-related mortality in patients with cancer. Most infections originate in the alimentary tract, sinuses, lungs, and skin. The risk of infection in a patient with neutropenia primarily is dictated by the severity and duration of neutropenia. The lower the absolute granulocyte nadir and the more prolonged the neutropenia, the greater the risk of serious infection. Fever is common in patients with cancer and may have many causes, including infection, the tumor itself, inflammation, transfusion of blood products, and chemotherapeutic and antimicrobial drugs. In patients with neutropenia, however, fever (a single temperature ≥38.3° C orally or ≥38° C over at least 1 hour) usually is secondary to infection, especially if the patient has <500 granulocytes/μl.

A. In addition to identifying localizing symptoms, the medical history should focus on special immunologic circumstances or defects that may predispose the patient to opportunistic infections. For example, patients with Hodgkin's disease are at increased risk for herpes zoster and cryptococcal meningitis; those who have undergone bone marrow transplantation are at risk for severe interstitial pneumonia with cytomegalovirus (CMV) or respiratory syncytial virus (RSV); and those taking high-dose steroids are at increased risk for pneumocystis pneumonia and fungal infections. Steroid use may further hide the signs and symptoms of infection, masking the seriousness of the clinical presentation. For instance, delirium may be the only manifestation of a serious infection in a patient receiving high-dose steroids.

B. A thorough physical examination must include careful auscultation of the lungs and meticulous evaluation of the integument, oral cavity, genitalia, and perianal region. Evaluation of the entire integument should focus especially on sites of vascular access and previous invasive procedures as potential portals for infection. The characteristic signs and symptoms of infections may be absent in patients with neutropenia who are unable to mount an adequate inflammatory response.

C. In addition to routine blood tests, culture blood from two separate sites, culture urine, and order a chest radiograph. Perform other tests such as stool culture, lumbar puncture, abdominal radiography, and bronchoscopy only if clinically indicated. For instance, in patients with diarrhea, culture for bacteria, ova, and parasite and perform a toxic screen for *Clostridium difficile.* Even with a comprehensive evaluation, a specific pathogen is initially identified in only 30%–50% of patients. With profound neutropenia (<100 cells/μl), bacteremias can be documented in only 15%–20% of febrile episodes.

D. Antimicrobial therapy is directed against the pathogens most likely to be responsible for the primary infection. Aerobic gram-negative bacilli, especially *Klebsiella, Escherichia coli,* and *Pseudomonas aeruginosa,* account for 30%–40% of all culture-confirmed infections. The incidence of gram-positive cocci (e.g., *Staphylococcus aureus,* coagulase-negative staphylococci, streptococci, pneumococci, *Corynebacterium* spp.) has risen significantly and now represents 60%–70% of isolates in many hospitals. Monotherapy with carbapenems (imipenem or meropenem), cefepime, or occasionally ceftazidime is acceptable for uncomplicated episodes of fever in patients with neutropenia, particularly in those with fever of unknown origin. Although, alternatively, aminoglycosides may be given in combination with an antipseudomonal penicillin in *all* patients with fever and neutropenia, aminoglycosides may be added to a third- or fourth-generation cephalosporin or carbapenems in patients with documented *P. aeruginosa* infection, pneumonia, or sepsis with mental status changes or hypoxemia with the emergence of vancomycin-resistant gram-positives such as *E. faecium.* Use vancomycin only in (1) patients with catheter-related infection with catheter site inflammation, (2) patients who received quinolone prophylaxis, (3) patients with severe mucositis, or (4) patients known to have been colonized with methicillin-resistant *S. aureus* or penicillin-resistant *S. pneumoniae.*

E. If the patient becomes afebrile within 48 hours, no organism is identified, all sites of infection resolve, and the absolute neutrophil count (ANC) is ≥500/μl, discontinue the antibiotic regimen after 7 days.

F. If a patient remains neutropenic but has been afebrile for >5 days, has stable vital signs, and is without mucositis but has an ANC 100–500/μl, discontinue antibiotics and monitor closely. If the temperature increases again, panculture immediately and resume broad-spectrum antibiotics. Patients with neutropenia at high risk (ANC <100/μl or with mucositis or unstable vital signs) should be continued on antibiotics until ANC is ≥500/μl and the patient is clinically improved.

G. Patients who remain neutropenic and febrile at day 4 but are clinically improved may continue the same initial regimen for a total of 7 days. However, if there is clinical deterioration, modify the antibiotic regimen depending on the clinical picture. For instance, for patients with severe mucositis or catheter site inflammation who have

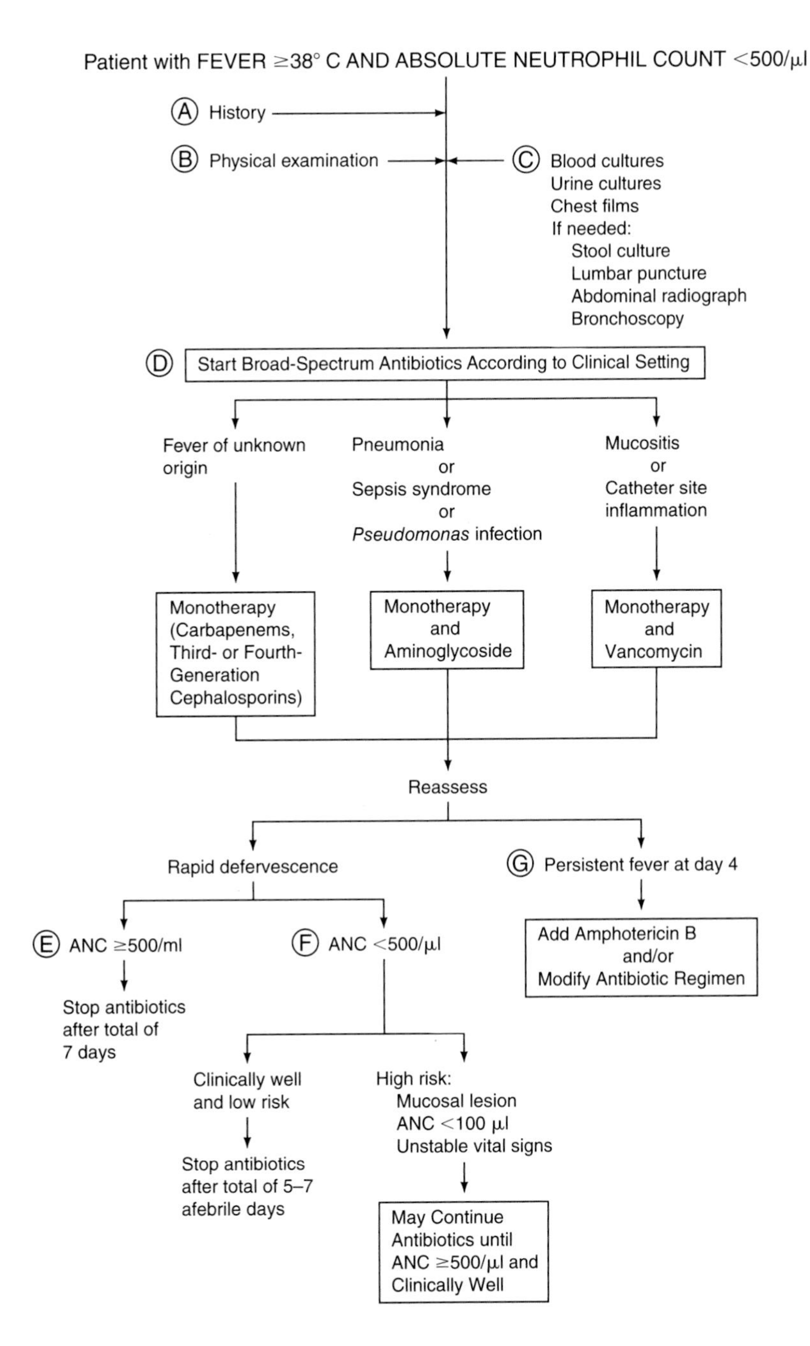

a high likelihood of a gram-positive infection, vancomycin may be added if not previously included. For patients with pneumonia or sepsis syndrome, add aminoglycoside, IV quinolone (e.g., ciprofloxacin), or trimethoprim-sulfamethoxazole (if not previously included) to cover resistant gram-negatives such as *P. aeruginosa* or *Stenotrophomonas maltophilia*, respectively. Add fluconazole if the patient is febrile through day 5 and resolution of neutropenia is not imminent. If the patient received fluconazole prophylaxis before the onset of fever, consider amphotericin B. Even if the patient is clinically improved while receiving antibiotics, perform a thorough examination daily, including the skin, oral cavity, genitalia, perianal area, and sites of venous access as outlined previously. Take seriously any medical complaint, and pursue the cause immediately. For instance, mild discomfort in the maxillary region is often the first sign of a grave fungal infection caused by *Aspergillus* or *Mucor;* tenderness in the perianal area may indicate a superimposed anaerobic infection; and right-sided abdominal discomfort may be the first clue to the diagnosis of typhlitis.

References

Bodey GP. Evolution of antibiotic therapy for infection in neutropenic patients: studies at M.D. Anderson Hospital. Rev Infect Dis 1989;11:1582S.

Hughes WT, Armstrong D, Bodey GP, et al. Guidelines for the use of antimicrobial agents in neutropenic patients with unexplained fever. J Infect Dis 1990;161:381.

Hughes WT, Armstrong D, Bodey GP, et al. 1997 Guidelines for the use of antimicrobial agents in neutropenic patients with unexplained fever. Clin Infect Dis 1997;25:551.

Pizzo PA. Management of fever in patients with cancer and treatment-induced neutropenia. N Engl J Med 1993;328:1323.

PATHOLOGIC FRACTURES

Ana Maria López, MD, MPH, FACP

A. Plain radiography provides most of the information about the underlying lesion and directs future decision making. Technetium-labeled methylene diphosphonate bone scanning is a sensitive indicator of multiple skeletal involvement, except in myeloma, in which little reactive bone is formed. The skeleton is the third most common site of metastasis from adenocarcinoma; skeletal metastases are present in 70% of patients. Diffuse loss of mineral homogeneity throughout the skeleton suggests osteoporosis; osteomalacia; or marrow replacement by leukemia, lymphoma, or myeloma.

B. Of carcinomatous metastases, 90% are solitary, especially those of neuroblastoma and hypernephroma. A solitary bone lesion in a patient >40 years of age is most likely metastasis, whereas it may be a primary bone tumor in a patient <40 years of age.

C. The primary tumor is found in only one third of patients with skeletal metastases; most of those diagnoses have breast or prostate primaries. Undetected primaries are most likely lung or kidney. The recommended diagnostic strategy is history; physical examination; routine laboratory studies; chest radiography; mammography (in women); urinalysis; and ultrasound, CT, or MRI of the kidneys. Additional tests detect primaries in only a few patients.

D. In most cases, tissue diagnosis does not alter surgical therapy, but it may if the lesion is a primary bone tumor or if the metastatic lesion can justifiably be resected, as in hypernephroma, thyroid carcinoma, plasmacytoma, or melanoma. Resection of a solitary hypernephroma metastasis may result in a 30% 5-year survival rate.

E. Patients with metastatic disease have a 2-year average life expectancy; the life expectancy is 6 months for lung metastasis. Restoring the structural integrity of the bone or joint improves function and quality of life. Internal fixation can be supplemented with polymethylmethacrylate (PMMA) cement for immediate stability, and prosthetic replacement can be used even in the young. Treat impending fractures with prophylactic fixation when the lesion is painful, when the lesion is >2.5 cm in diameter, or when the cortex is destroyed >50% across the diameter of the bone on a uniplanar radiograph. Treat shafts of the femur, humerus, tibia, and subtrochanteric femur with intramedullary nail or consider an intercalary metal spacer in selected patients. Use cemented prosthetic replacement for fractures of the femoral neck, distal femoral condyles, proximal tibia, and acetabulum. Percutaneous injection of PMMA into lytic acetabular metastases has been tried in selected patients, although such defects have traditionally been reconstructed using cement-reinforced rods anchored in the surrounding intact ilium. Fractures of the pelvis other than the acetabulum are treated nonsurgically. Radiotherapy follows fracture stabilization.

F. External beam radiotherapy is used to treat other areas that do not require stabilization and fractures or lesions involving the spine, ribs, or nonarticular pelvis. Systemic treatments for metastatic bone disease include chemotherapy, endocrine therapy, and bisphosphonates. Response to bisphosphonates in osteolytic metastases can be assessed by detecting lower bone type I collagen breakdown products, such as N-telopeptide, as measured in serum or urine. Tamoxifen is used in postmenopausal women who have estrogen-positive breast tumors; sometimes tamoxifen is followed by aromatase inhibitors. Men with metastatic prostate cancer are often treated with bilateral orchiectomy and androgen blockade with leuprolide LHRH-A, flutamide, goserelin acetate, or cyproterone acetate. Site-directed radiotherapy using samarium-153, strontium-89, and rhenium-186 has more effectively relieved pain in prostate lesions than in breast lesions. Bisphosphonates treat hypercalcemia, inhibit osteolysis, relieve pain in 50% of patients, and show healing in 25% of patients with breast cancer.

(Continued on page 278)

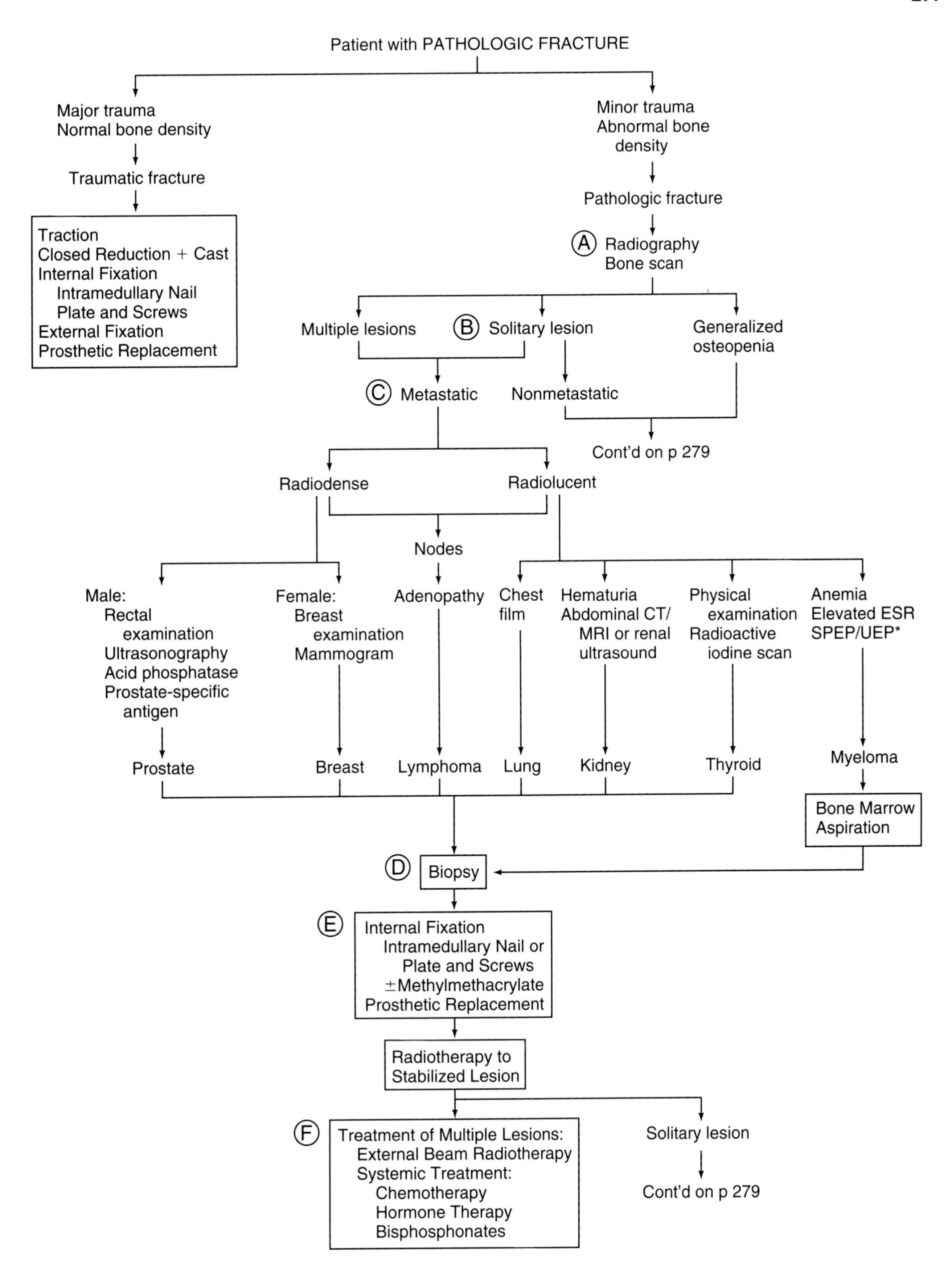

Patient with PATHOLOGIC FRACTURE
Major trauma
Normal bone density
Traumatic fracture
Traction
Closed Reduction + Cast
Internal Fixation
Intramedullary Nail
Plate and Screws
External Fixation
Prosthetic Replacement
Minor trauma
Abnormal bone density
Pathologic fracture
A Radiography
Bone scan
Multiple lesions
B Solitary lesion
Generalized osteopenia
C Metastatic
Nonmetastatic
Cont'd on p 279
Radiodense
Radiolucent
Nodes
Male:
Rectal examination
Ultrasonography
Acid phosphatase
Prostate-specific antigen
Female:
Breast examination
Mammogram
Adenopathy
Chest film
Hematuria
Abdominal CT/ MRI or renal ultrasound
Physical examination
Radioactive iodine scan
Anemia
Elevated ESR
SPEP/UEP*
Prostate
Breast
Lymphoma
Lung
Kidney
Thyroid
Myeloma
Bone Marrow Aspiration
D Biopsy
E Internal Fixation
Intramedullary Nail or
Plate and Screws
±Methylmethacrylate
Prosthetic Replacement
Radiotherapy to Stabilized Lesion
F Treatment of Multiple Lesions:
External Beam Radiotherapy
Systemic Treatment:
Chemotherapy
Hormone Therapy
Bisphosphonates
Solitary lesion
Cont'd on p 279

*SPEP/UEP, Serum protein electrophoresis/urine electrophoresis

G. The differential diagnosis of a fractured solitary bone lesion is listed in the algorithm. Localized osteopenia from failure to use a limb can occur with pain, reflex sympathetic dystrophy, previous cast immobilization, and paralytic conditions. Fractures often are seen in previously irradiated bone and in Paget's disease. The latter is distinguished from prostatic carcinoma by enlargement of the involved bone and coarsened, rather than destroyed, trabeculation.

H. Benign primary bone tumors often have intact cortex, distinct margins, and solid homogeneous periosteal reactions. Malignant tumors show destruction of cortex, indistinct margins, and lamellated or sunburst periosteal reactions.

I. Cast treatment without biopsy is justified for a benign bone tumor having a diagnostic radiographic appearance and self-healing behavior (e.g., unicameral bone cyst, metaphyseal fibrous cortical defect, eosinophilic granuloma, enchondroma, fibrous dysplasia). Biopsy is indicated when the diagnosis is uncertain or when the lesions are unlikely to heal without resection or curettement and grafting (e.g., aneurysmal bone cysts, giant cell tumor, chondromyxoid fibroma, osteoblastoma, chondroblastoma). A cast may be used for healing of the cortex before definitive treatment. Steroid instillation is effective in obliterating unicameral bone cysts if cast immobilization of a fracture is unsuccessful.

J. Before biopsy, order an MRI to determine the extent of marrow and soft-tissue involvement in primary malignant tumors of bone; cortical destruction is better seen on CT. A fracture through a primary bone sarcoma most often necessitates amputation. However, if the cortical fracture is small and displacement is minimal, the patient may still be a candidate for resection and limb salvage, especially if preoperative adjuvant chemotherapy is administered. Treat chondrosarcomas with surgery alone.

K. Both metastatic and metabolic disease may involve the spine, proximal femurs, and ribs. Osteoporosis characteristically results in fractures of the distal radius and femoral neck. Osteomalacia more commonly affects the subtrochanteric femur and successive ribs at the same distance from the spine; 30% of patients with hip fractures have osteomalacia. Osteomalacia, marked by excess of unmineralized osteoid, can be of vitamin D deficiency, poor absorption of calcium or vitamin D enterically, vitamin D–resistant form, or renal osteodystrophy. Osteoporosis can be idiopathic (the type 1 postmenopausal variety is a loss of trabecular more than cortical bone; the type 2 senile variety is an equal loss of both), can result from disuse or immobilization, or can be secondary. The most common causes of secondary osteoporosis in otherwise-healthy males are hypogonadism, steroid use, and alcoholism, and in females are hypercalciuria, malabsorption, hyperparathyroidism, vitamin D deficiency, and too much replacement thyroid hormone. Most of these known causes of osteoporosis in females can be diagnosed by obtaining levels of serum calcium; parathyroid hormone (PTH); 24-hour urine calcium; thyroid-stimulating hormone (TSH); and, if necessary, a 1,25-OH vitamin D_3. For males, a dexamethasone suppression test and a serum testosterone level can be obtained.

Densitometry should be done on men >70 years of age with a fracture or women >50 years of age with a fracture or younger of either gender with risk factors, including weight <127 pounds, small build, menopause before age 45, smoking, alcohol use, steroid use, history of prior fracture, or positive family history. Consider treatment when dual-energy x-ray absorptiometry is <2.0 standard deviations below normal or <1.5 standard deviations below normal if the patient has a fragility fracture or risk factors. Treat the patient with calcium and vitamin D in sufficient doses (currently recommended 1200 mg calcium in two to three divided doses QD and vitamin D at 1000 international units or QD). Calcium carbonate can be used unless the patient has constipation or indigestion, in which case use calcium citrate. Begin bisphosphonates, such as alendronate, risedronate, or ibandronate, 2–6 weeks after fracture and use for as long as 5 years, stopping temporarily if the N-telopeptide decreases to a low level or if another fracture occurs while receiving treatment. PTH can be substituted during fracture healing, or PTH can be used instead when bisphosphonates are ineffective, or if the N-telopeptide is low in low-turnover osteoporosis, or in young females of childbearing age. Hormone replacement with estrogen in postmenopausal women is no longer recommended because of the risk of coronary artery disease, phlebitis, pulmonary embolism, and breast cancer. Raloxifene, a selective estrogen receptor modulator, is effective in reducing spine fractures, but not hip fractures, and reduces the risk of breast cancer and coronary artery disease. Calcitonin, administered as a nasal spray, also has not been shown to protect the hip from future fractures, although it has diminished spine fracture risk and has an analgesic effect on patients with osteoporotic vertebral fractures.

(Continued on page 280)

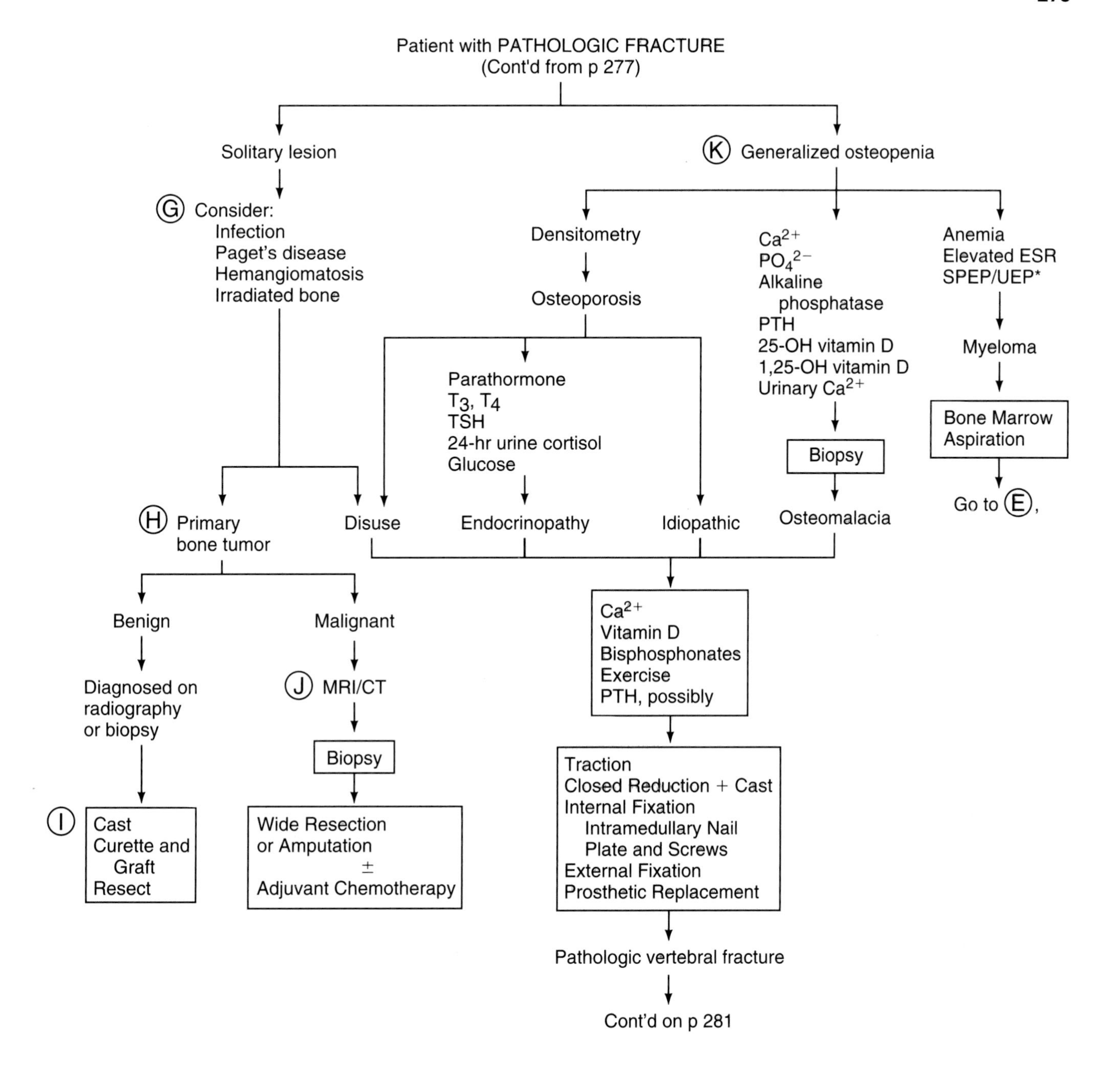

*SPEP/UEP, Serum protein electrophoresis/urine electrophoresis.

L. Most patients with metastatic disease to the spine are treated with radiotherapy alone with 60%–80% improvement, but those who have worsening pain, deformity that may lead to neurologic compromise, or new onset of neurologic deficits are evaluated for structural integrity and possible surgery. CT is best to demonstrate the degree of bone loss or presence of bone fragments in the canal, and MRI is used to determine the extent of involvement of adjacent vertebrae and sagittal deformity. Spinal instability is felt to be present if one of the following is found: bone loss in both the anterior and posterior elements, excessive kyphosis in sagittal alignment, or increased motion when lateral radiographs in flexion and extension are compared. Tumor in the body of the vertebrae with displacement of the posterior cortex into the spinal canal is decompressed with an anterior approach to the spine. Destruction of the pedicles and lamina with compression from the posterior side is decompressed from a posterior approach. The spine is then stabilized with internal fixation anteriorly, posteriorly, or circumferentially, followed by radiotherapy. The vertebral body may need to be replaced with metal, structural bone graft, or a cage containing osteobiologic material. Acute onset of paraparesis is treated with emergency radiotherapy without the need for surgery when the bone is structurally intact and the MRI shows tumor tissue extending into the spinal canal.

M. Osteoporotic vertebral compression fractures are likely to become increasingly common as the population ages and as vitamin D deficiency becomes more common. Of women with hip fractures, 50% have been found to have vitamin D deficiency. Two thirds of acute osteoporotic vertebral fractures are never seen by a physician because the elderly consider the back pain and dysfunction part of the aging process. Most acute pain can be treated with analgesics, decreased activity, or a brace. Occasionally patients have intractable pain, postulated to result from recurrent microfractures related to kyphotic posture, and, very rarely, neurologic deficits requiring surgical treatment.

N. Minimally invasive procedures for the relief of pain in metastasis or osteoporosis of the spine are being studied when the posterior cortex of the vertebrae is intact. When there is no deformity or when the fracture can be reduced posturally, a biomaterial or PMMA in low-viscosity state may be injected percutaneously under pressure into the vertebral body (vertebroplasty). When there is deformity or instability, a percutaneously placed balloon is first inflated to restore vertebral height (kyphoplasty) prior to injecting a higher-viscosity PMMA under lower pressure. Pulmonary embolism and the risk of cement extravasation with consequent neurologic dysfunction are rare but of concern.

References

Bauer HCF. Controversies in the surgical management of skeletal metastases. J Bone Joint Surg Br 2005;87-B:608.

Berman AT, Hermantin FU, Horowitz SM. Metastatic disease of the hip: evaluation and treatment. J Am Acad Orthop Surg 1997;5:79.

Harrington KD. Orthopaedic management of extremity and pelvic lesions. Clin Orthop 1995;312:136.

Houston SJ, Rubens RD. The systemic treatment of bone metastases. Clin Orthop 1995;312:95.

Mankin HJ. Rickets, osteomalacia, and renal osteodystrophy. An update. Orthop Clin North Am 1990;21:81.

O'Connor MI, Ward WG Sr, eds. Metastatic bone disease. Clin Orthop Relat Res 2003(Suppl); 297 pages.

Rao RD, Singrakhia MD. Painful osteoporotic vertebral fracture. Pathogenesis, evaluation, and roles of vertebroplasty and kyphoplasty in its management. J Bone Joint Surg Am 2003;85-A:2010.

Spivak JM, Johnson MG. Percutaneous treatment of vertebral body pathology. J Am Acad Orthop Surg 2005;13:6.

Templeton K. Secondary osteoporosis. J Am Acad Orthop Surg 2005;13:475.

Yazawa Y, Frassica FJ, Chao EY, et al. Metastatic bone disease: a study of the surgical treatment of 166 pathologic humeral and femoral fractures. Clin Orthop 1990;51:213.

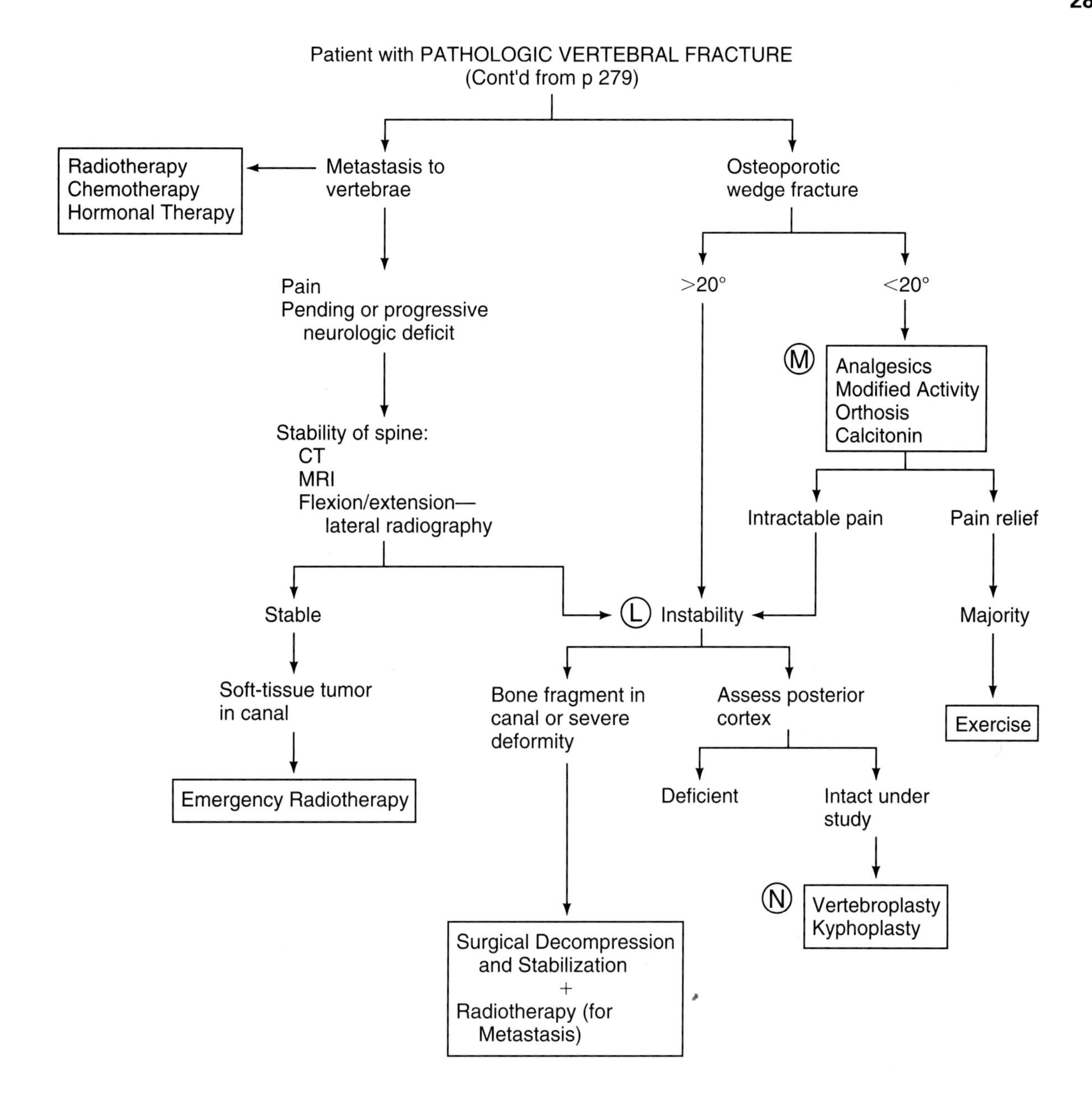

Patient with PATHOLOGIC VERTEBRAL FRACTURE
(Cont'd from p 279)
Radiotherapy
Chemotherapy
Hormonal Therapy
Metastasis to vertebrae
Osteoporotic wedge fracture
Pain
Pending or progressive neurologic deficit
>20°
<20°
M
Analgesics
Modified Activity
Orthosis
Calcitonin
Stability of spine:
CT
MRI
Flexion/extension—lateral radiography
Intractable pain
Pain relief
Stable
L
Instability
Majority
Soft-tissue tumor in canal
Bone fragment in canal or severe deformity
Assess posterior cortex
Exercise
Emergency Radiotherapy
Deficient
Intact under study
N
Vertebroplasty
Kyphoplasty
Surgical Decompression and Stabilization
+
Radiotherapy (for Metastasis)

CLINICAL CONSIDERATIONS FOR STEM CELL TRANSPLANTATION

Philip A. Lowry, MD

Surgery, radiation, and chemotherapy, the traditional pillars of cancer therapy, offer significant improvements in survival and quality of life for patients with malignancies. Although refinements of technique and new agents offer some hope for additional advances, it is likely that further progress in treatment outcome will come from other sources, particularly those that exploit the unique biology of cancer. Recent dramatic successes with agents such as imatinib for the treatment of chronic myelogenous leukemia offer the tantalizing prospect of "magic bullet" treatments that are simple and highly effective, but such breakthroughs are likely to be limited to only a very few diagnoses for the foreseeable future.

One of the first "biological" therapies, bone marrow transplantation, was pioneered almost half a century ago with the initial concept of replacing a diseased organ such as a leukemic marrow with a normal one. Identification of additional sources of cells in peripheral and umbilical cord blood have significantly expanded options in a field now collectively referred to as "stem cell transplantation." In all its forms, stem cell transplantation has the primary and simplistic goal of restoring blood production after aggressive treatment with chemotherapy with or without additional radiation. In *autologous* stem cell transplantation, cells are harvested from the patient in advance and restoration of blood production is the sole goal of the "transplant," which may be better considered a simple rescue from otherwise potentially fatal hematologic toxicities associated with aggressive dosing of chemotherapy required to cure or at least significantly extend survival in diseases such as myeloma and lymphoma.

Allogeneic stem cell transplantation derives cells from another donor for the transplant. Identical twins served as the first successful donors for hematopoietic transplants, but with the characterization of the human leukocyte antigen (HLA) system of transplant antigens, appropriately matched siblings could be identified to serve as donors in successful transplants. Refinements in the molecular characterization of HLA antigens, the development of extensive registries of volunteer adult donors, and rapidly expanding banks of cord blood cells now allow many patients who do not have a suitably matched sibling to identify an adequately matched unrelated donor for transplant.

Even when donor cells are well matched, outside of identical twin transplants there will be "minor" histocompatibility differences between donor and recipient. The risk of rejection has been minimized with modern preparative regimens, but a reverse immunologic reaction of donor cells against normal host tissues is common in allogeneic transplantation—so-called graft versus host disease, or GVHD. In its severe forms, GVHD can be fatal and has been as important as infections in limiting the historical success of allogeneic transplantation, particularly in patients >50 years of age. Better matching of donor and recipient, improved prophylactic pharmacologic regimens for GVHD, and recently the use of less aggressive or "reduced intensity" chemotherapy and radiation regimens preceding the transplant have reduced the impact of GVHD and allowed transplants to be incorporated in the treatment of increasing numbers of patients, including more routine transplant of fit patients up to their early 70s.

It has long been recognized that the immune system plays a key role in surveillance against cancer development and can also be modulated to produce remissions and even cures in a number of cancer diagnoses. In the treatment of malignant disease, allogeneic stem cell transplantation offers an aggressive immune modulation in replacing the patient's immune system with that of the donor. The same minor histocompatibility differences responsible for the problems of GVHD offer the opportunity for a "graft versus tumor" effect, and in many patients it may be this rather than the chemotherapy and radiation per se that ultimately produces a cure.

Allogeneic transplantation is therefore rapidly coming of age, and as it does so it has proved to be a more complex and multifaceted technique than originally appreciated. In nonmalignant diseases, the traditional need to replace a diseased organ with a more functional one remains the primary goal, and patient preparation and stem cell source selection are focused on minimizing technical complications such as GVHD. Allogeneic transplantation has long served to help patients with severe aplastic anemia and life-threatening immunodeficiency disorders. As the technical complications decrease, allogeneic transplantation has and will be increasingly used to treat patients at higher risk and with more chronic blood disorders such as sickle cell anemia and thalassemia.

In the treatment of malignant disease, allogeneic transplantation has been particularly successful in the treatment of chronic myelogenous leukemia where the "graft versus leukemia" effect can be active. It is interesting that the parallel success of imatinib has significantly reduced the number of patients going to transplant, although the latter remains an important option for patients with a poor response or relapsed disease. Allogeneic transplantation for acute nonlymphoblastic leukemia and lymphoproliferative disorders has shown intermediate graft versus leukemia effects but is still an important option for selected patients. For lymphoma and myeloma, many patients may be better served with an autologous transplant, although selected younger patients or patients with more aggressive disease may do better with an allogeneic approach. Results with acute lymphoblastic leukemia have been disappointing, but allogeneic transplant may salvage some patients. The advent of reduced-intensity preparation regimens and better treatments for GVHD are opening up allogeneic transplantation options for the usually older patients with myelodysplasia, and ongoing investigations should define the role in that context.

The future of transplant offers exciting possibilities with in vitro cellular expansion and modulation to optimize posttransplant recovery and augment graft versus leukemia effects yet minimize GVHD. Improving supportive therapy protocols and refinement of pretransplant patient selection and conditioning will increase the success of transplant. Ongoing basic and clinical study should help to characterize the graft versus leukemia effect and better harness its potential in future patient care.

(Continued on page 284)

A. Appropriate identification of potential transplant patients is essential. For nonmalignant blood diseases, transplant for patients at high risk should proceed at the earliest opportunity, ideally before any transfusions are required, especially in patients with aplastic anemia. For patients with malignant disease, disease characteristics at presentation, particularly with respect to cytogenetic changes, will best define candidacy for transplant and its optimal timing. Patients are usually treated with traditional therapy to achieve a remission before transplant, but because pretransplant therapy may affect the rate of complications and success of the transplant itself, coordination with an experienced transplant center at diagnosis is most helpful. Particular attention should be paid in all potential transplant patients to appropriate selection and preparation of transfusions, which should be leukodepleted and irradiated.

B. Transplant candidates must meet minimal criteria for organ function, especially of the lung, heart, and kidney, to ensure tolerance of the rigors of the transplant procedure. They must have no other complicating medical illnesses such as HIV infection that might preclude transplant, and they must be able to give informed consent. Age criteria will vary according to the disease and type of transplant, and performance status will critically modulate the ability of older patients to proceed to transplant. If all other criteria are met, psychosocial, dental, and fertility evaluations should be completed prior to initiating the transplant process.

C. If a patient is suitable for transplant, an appropriate cell source must be determined and steps must be taken for cells to be harvested. This decision initially focuses on determining whether an autologous or allogeneic transplant would be most suitable. The decision to transplant and choice to use an autologous or allogeneic source, and if the latter the best potential donor, should be pursued in collaboration with an experienced transplant center.

D. For patients proceeding with a potential autologous transplantation who have suitably passed previous screening steps, blood and marrow evaluation should ensure the high likelihood of harvesting adequate cells to proceed. Although marrow harvests are still occasionally used, most patients will have cells harvested from the peripheral blood after "mobilization" with growth factors, usually following a chemotherapy treatment. Cells are collected by apheresis and their viability and numbers are assessed for adequacy; then they are cryopreserved until their use for the transplant.

E. For patients requiring an allogeneic transplant, potential suitable donor cells must be matched for HLA-A, B, C, DR, and DQ determinants. Siblings are screened first, but if no appropriately matched sibling donor is available, searches are initiated through adult donor registries and cord blood banks. For sibling or volunteer adult donors, additional physical, psychological, and infectious disease screening must precede consideration for stem cell harvest. Cord blood cells should have been screened for adequate numbers, viability, and lack of infections at the time of banking. ABO compatibility, allosensitization of potential donors by previous pregnancy or blood transfusion, and cytomegalovirus (CMV) infectious status present potential issues with transplant that do not represent absolute contraindications to proceeding but may prioritize choices when several potential donors are available.

F. Following allogeneic transplantation, particular attention must be directed to the prevention, early detection, and, if present, appropriate additional therapy for GVHD.

G. Following all forms of hematopoietic stem transplant, but especially following allogeneic transplantation, the immediate recovery period (3–6 weeks) focuses on pancytopenia with need for transfusion, aggressive treatment of life-threatening infections, and the morbidity of preparative regimen-induced mucositis. Graft rejection or late failure is rare, but blood counts should be closely monitored. Even after count recovery, patients remain at higher risk for infections for prolonged periods, especially following allogeneic transplant. Prolonged pharmacologic prophylaxis, particularly against *Pneumocystis* and viral infections and, in the context of ongoing GVHD therapy, fungal infections, is required. Vaccination against pneumococcus and *Haemophilus influenzae* and revaccination with killed polio and diphtheria/tetanus vaccines is typically given at 1 year posttransplant; because the measles, mumps, rubella (MMR) vaccine is live, there is concern about vaccination-induced infections, so centers vary in their use of it. Intensity and duration of GVHD prophylaxis or treatment will vary from patient to patient. Appropriate follow-up is critical to success and must be conducted at or in collaboration with an experienced transplant center.

H. Posttransplant patients face many other potential long-term issues, including growth alteration in pediatric transplant recipients, increased rates of secondary malignancies, and prolonged physical and psychological morbidities and disabilities. Chronic GVHD may present particular challenges in treatment and morbidity or mortality. Continued involvement of the transplant team with patients experiencing late complications will be critical.

I. If the primary disease relapses after transplant, selected patients may benefit from additional cellular-based therapies. In diseases with a strong potential for graft versus leukemia effects, simple infusion of additional donor cells (donor lymphocyte infusions) sometimes may reinduce remission. Highly selected patients may be candidates for repeated transplant based on disease status and interval from the first transplant.

References

Armitage JO. Bone marrow transplantation. N Engl J Med 1994;330:827.
Blume KG, Forman SJ, Appelbaum FR, eds. Thomas' Hematopoietic Cell Transplantation, 3rd ed. Boston: Blackwell, 2004.

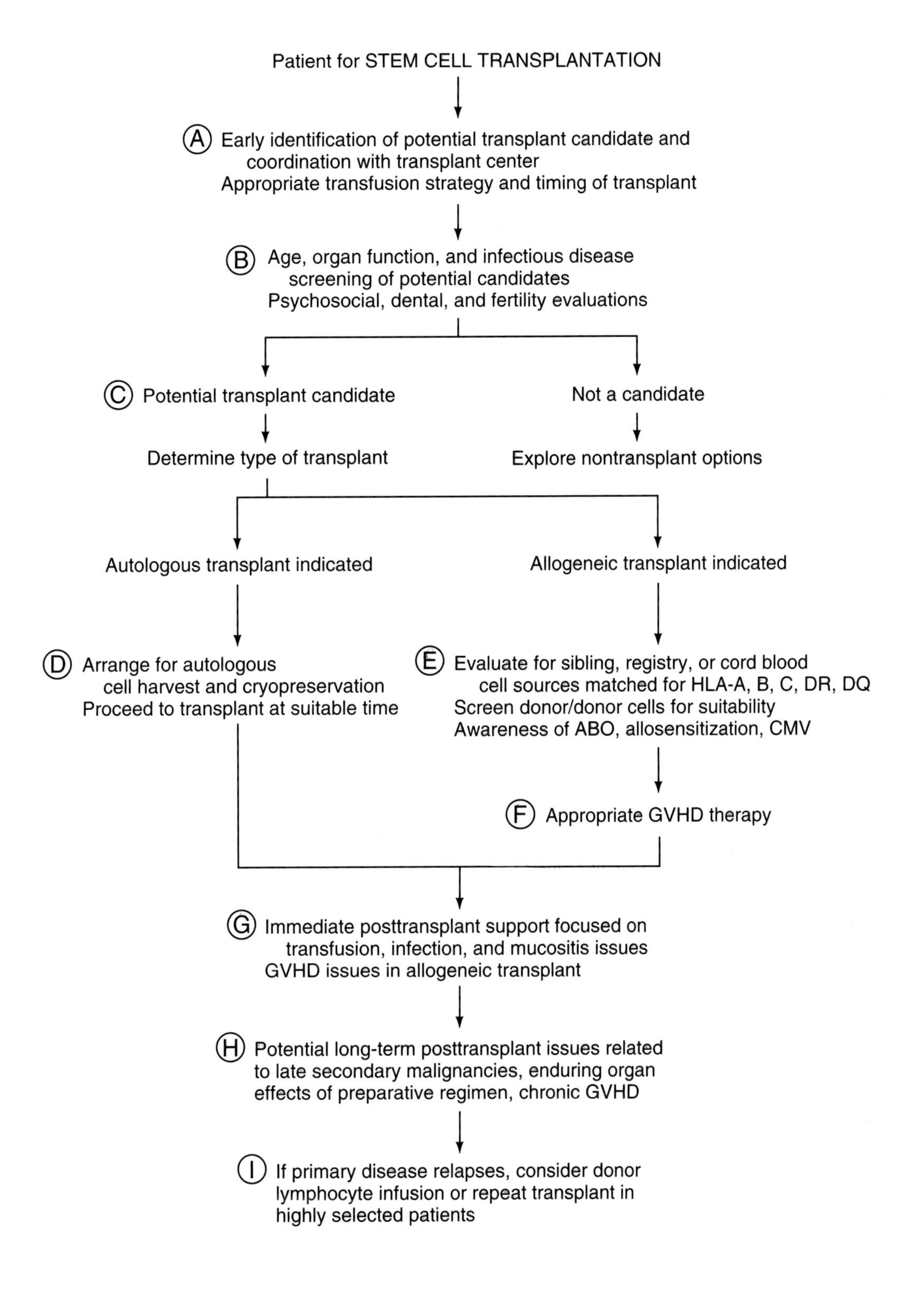
Patient for STEM CELL TRANSPLANTATION
(A) Early identification of potential transplant candidate and coordination with transplant center
Appropriate transfusion strategy and timing of transplant
(B) Age, organ function, and infectious disease screening of potential candidates
Psychosocial, dental, and fertility evaluations
(C) Potential transplant candidate
Not a candidate
Determine type of transplant
Explore nontransplant options
Autologous transplant indicated
Allogeneic transplant indicated
(D) Arrange for autologous cell harvest and cryopreservation
Proceed to transplant at suitable time
(E) Evaluate for sibling, registry, or cord blood cell sources matched for HLA-A, B, C, DR, DQ
Screen donor/donor cells for suitability
Awareness of ABO, allosensitization, CMV
(F) Appropriate GVHD therapy
(G) Immediate posttransplant support focused on transfusion, infection, and mucositis issues
GVHD issues in allogeneic transplant
(H) Potential long-term posttransplant issues related to late secondary malignancies, enduring organ effects of preparative regimen, chronic GVHD
(I) If primary disease relapses, consider donor lymphocyte infusion or repeat transplant in highly selected patients

LATE ISSUES FOR PATIENTS WHO SURVIVE THE INITIAL DIAGNOSIS AND TREATMENT OF CANCER

Philip A. Lowry, MD

Although modern therapy has produced a significant improvement in the rate of control and cure of cancer, the devastation of the disease and its treatment have lasting effects on both patients and family. Successful treatment of patients with cancer requires not only technical expertise in the initial phase of diagnosis and management, but also compassion and commitment in the long term to aid the patient and his or her family in navigating the many complex issues and challenges they will face for years to come.

Following initial cancer therapy, patients and their families will face ongoing needs and issues in five main areas: the potential for relapse of the initial cancer, the physical and physiologic effects of the cancer and its treatment both short and long term, the psychological and emotional sequelae of the disease itself and its treatment, the specific potential for shared genetic risk for cancer development in blood relatives, and the potential for the late development of new cancers, including those that may themselves be a consequence of initial therapy.

Relapse of the primary cancer will be a major concern for patients in the years following initial diagnosis and treatment. A periodic history and physical examination are the key focuses of follow-up and should be coordinated with a cancer specialist, at least during the early phase. In selected malignancies, focused radiologic or laboratory studies will be important, such as mammograms in the follow-up of breast cancer and serial monitoring of prostate-specific antigen (PSA) after treatment for prostate cancer, but for most malignancies repetitive performance of "surveillance" blood and radiologic studies has little additional impact on survival and quality of life while adding significantly to expense. In contrast, prompt and rigorous laboratory and radiologic evaluation of new symptoms or physical findings is key to successful early intervention for possible relapse. For most malignancies, patients should be followed on an interval of every 3 months for 2–3 years after completion of initial successful treatment for cancer. The interval for follow-up can be lengthened thereafter if the patient remains stable. Specific timelines for follow-up and selected ancillary studies that have proved valuable are described for individual cancer diagnoses in the guidelines published by the National Comprehensive Cancer Network (www.nccn.org).

Even when successful, cancer treatment can leave devastating scars and result in significant short- and long-term dysfunction. Radical surgical procedures result in obvious physical effects; radical radiation can produce equally significant scarring in the short term and later endocrine or neurologic dysfunction, accelerated atherosclerosis, or secondary malignancies, as discussed later. Chemotherapy may produce a wide spectrum or early and late organ dysfunction, including immune dysregulation, premature menopause, cardiac dysfunction, pulmonary fibrosis, alterations of renal or hepatic function, neuropathy, or skin pigmentation changes depending on the agents used and dose and duration of therapy. In pediatric populations, intensive cancer therapy may have significant effects on subsequent growth and development.

Interrelated with but sometimes independent of the physical and physiologic effects of cancer therapy, the psychological and emotional consequences are obvious but often persistent well beyond apparently successful initial therapy. Changes in body image, fear of disease relapse, altered interpersonal relationships, disruption of education or career paths, and ongoing alteration of physical capacity may all dramatically and permanently affect cancer survivors. Family members may be equally or even more significantly affected. Although the acute phase of cancer treatment typically includes an extensive framework for psychological and emotional support and therapy, there may be barriers to access to such support following completion of the initial phase of therapy, particularly for patients who find it difficult to return to the setting that reminds them of the trauma of their initial care.

With the characterization of cancer as a disease resulting from alteration of normal genetic programs, it is now possible to explain the clustering of cancers in certain families on the basis of a shared germline mutation placing those families at higher risk. Beyond the many issues described previously that patients must face, they are increasingly aware of and concerned about the potential that they may have transmitted a higher risk for cancer to their children or that they share that risk with other family members. A family cancer syndrome should be particularly suspected when cancer appears in multiple family members or affects particularly young individuals (those <40 years of age). Specific algorithms for genetic counseling, testing, and preemptive intervention have been developed for families with premature or clusters of breast, colon, and ovarian cancer but should be pursued in conjunction with an established genetics clinic.

Cancer survivors are at risk not only for the relapse of their primary malignancy but also of additional and independent malignancies in the years following their diagnosis. The same risk factors that led to the first cancer leave patients at risk for the development of independent cancers of the same organ later, particularly for breast, lung, and head and neck malignancies, with continued tobacco exposure particularly exacerbating that risk in the latter two. Chemotherapy and radiation may also produce secondary malignancies that develop because of the treatment itself. Genetic damage induced by irradiation or by certain classes of chemotherapeutic agents sets into motion a new sequence of cellular degeneration and transformation producing acute leukemia, non-Hodgkin's lymphoma, and virtually the entire spectrum of solid malignancies complicating the late course of cancer treatment. Certain patients, particularly those with Hodgkin's and non-Hodgkin's lymphoma, acute leukemia, retinoblastoma, Wilms' tumor, soft-tissue sarcoma, and testicular malignancies, seem to be at particular risk.

The approach to cancer survivors should be grounded on three important axes: a specific plan for short- and long-term follow-up developed by and usually including the initial oncologic care team to particularly define needed studies and intervals of care; rigorous health maintenance, focusing especially on atherosclerosis risk reduction and general established cancer monitoring such as mammography, colonoscopy, Pap tests, and periodic skin examinations; and access to psychological and emotional counseling and support services. Pediatric cancer survivors should additionally have access to multidisciplinary health care resources that can appropriately respond to and support these patients and their families as they face the unique issues and challenges of changes in subsequent growth and development caused by their treatment.

(Continued on page 288)

A. In the initial discussions of diagnosis and treatment, potential late consequences of treatment choices should be reviewed and evaluated in the context of preexisting medical conditions. Particular attention should be given to reproductive issues, and patients should be offered the possibility of banking sperm or embryos if appropriate and feasible.

B. As primary cancer therapy is completed, a specific follow-up plan designed based on the initial diagnosis and treatment should be developed in collaboration between the oncology and primary care teams. Particular follow-up plans appropriate to specific diagnoses can be reviewed at www.nccn.org. Patients and families should be counseled as to signs or symptoms they should monitor for and report to the care team and issues they may need to anticipate accommodating in their subsequent life and lifestyle choices.

C. Particular design of follow-up must include not only appropriate monitoring for relapse of the primary malignancy but also new cancers in the same organ system and specific secondary malignancies for which the patient may be at risk based on primary therapy. This will include a periodic history and physical examination, with particular attention to a good cancer detection examination in all patients; periodic mammograms and Pap tests in essentially all female patients; and studies in selected patients at higher risk, such as CBC to monitor for secondary myelodysplasia or leukemia, chest x-ray to monitor for lung malignancies in patients following chest irradiation, and the like.

D. Any new signs or symptoms should be promptly and thoroughly evaluated as a possible indication of relapsed or new malignancy. This evaluation should be conducted in conjunction with the oncology care team.

E. Monitoring should include particular attention toward organs at high risk for short- and long-term dysfunction following primary therapy coupled with appropriate risk-reduction strategies. This includes monitoring thyroid-stimulating hormone (TSH) at least annually in patients following radiotherapy to the neck, reproductive counseling and evaluation, and focused cardiovascular monitoring in patients receiving chest irradiation or previous potentially cardiotoxic chemotherapy.

F. Genetic counseling and potential follow-up testing and intervention should be offered to selected patients and their families with a high-risk context and breast, colon, or ovarian malignancies. Families at high risk include those in which multiple malignancies present in one individual or groups of primary relatives, those in which cancer presents at an unusually early age (<40 years old), or those of Ashkenazi Jewish descent in which breast and ovarian cancer occurs. Unusual and extensive clusters of any type of cancer in a single family warrant potential investigation. Approaches are described at www.nccn.org but should be pursued in collaboration with an established genetics clinic.

G. All cancer survivors should resume regular health maintenance procedures as appropriate for age, gender, and general medical history, but this should include particularly vigorous evaluation of and action directed toward cardiovascular risk factors, smoking cessation counseling and intervention, and institution of general positive health habits.

H. Patients and families may need lifelong access to psychosocial counseling and support services.

I. Pediatric cancer survivors and their families may need access to experienced multidisciplinary clinics and resources to focus on the special and profound issues of growth and development alterations induced by their disease and its therapy and the lasting or late-presenting psychosocial consequences of that treatment.

References

Greene MH, Wilson J. Second cancer following lymphatic and hematopoietic cancers in Connecticut, 1935–1982. Natl Cancer Inst Monograph 1985;68:191.

National Comprehensive Cancer Network. www.nccn.org, 2006.

Swinnen LJ. Treatment of organ transplant-related lymphoma. Hematol Oncol Clin North Am 1997;11:963.

Van Leeuwen FE, Travis LB. Second cancers. In DeVita VT, Hellman S, Rosenberg SA, eds. Cancer: Principles and Practice of Oncology, 7th ed. Philadelphia: Lippincott-Raven, 2005.

Witherspoon RP, Fisher LD, Schoch G, et al. Secondary cancers after bone marrow transplantation for leukemia or aplastic anemia. N Engl J Med 1989;321:784.

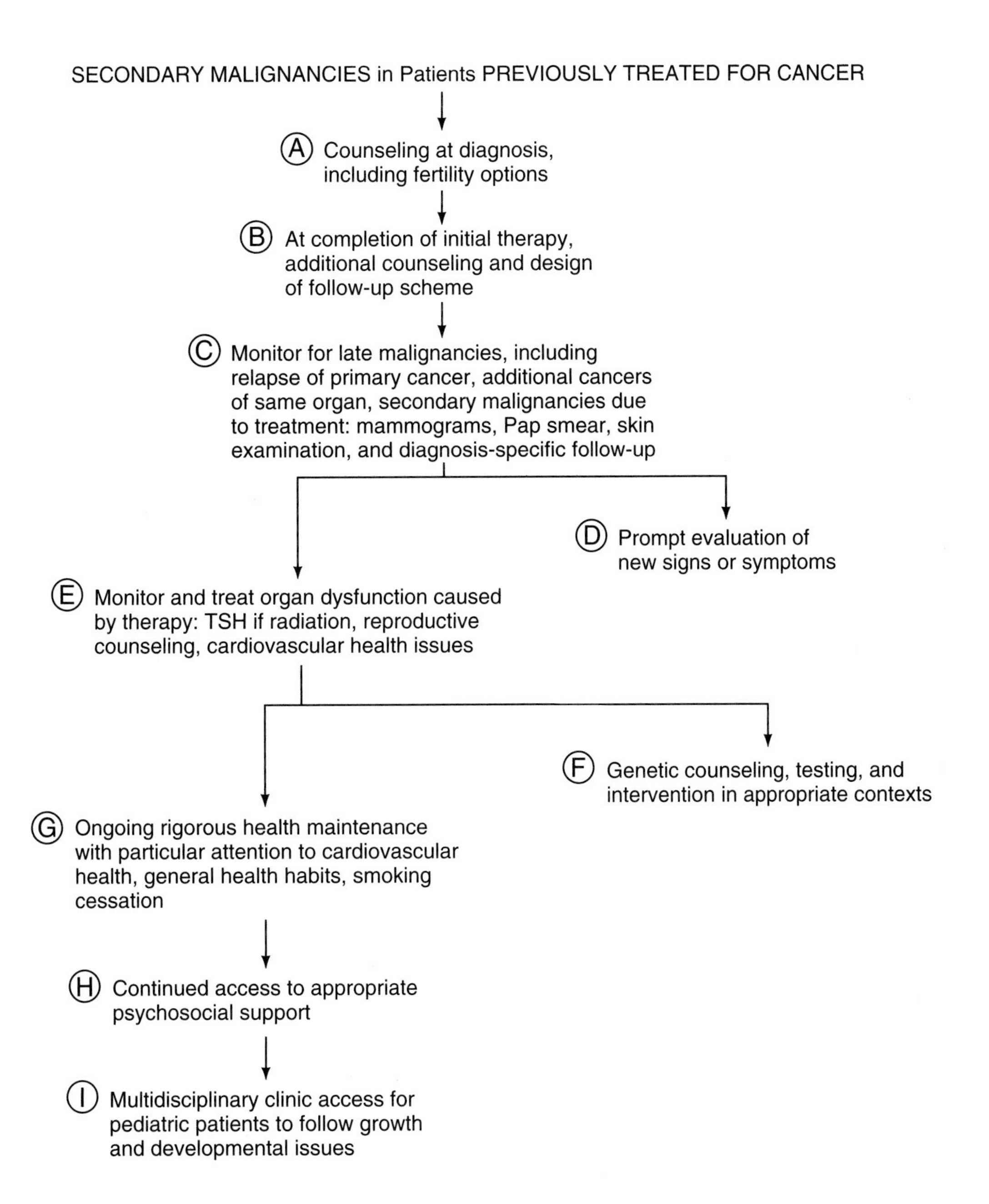
SECONDARY MALIGNANCIES in Patients PREVIOUSLY TREATED FOR CANCER
A Counseling at diagnosis, including fertility options
B At completion of initial therapy, additional counseling and design of follow-up scheme
C Monitor for late malignancies, including relapse of primary cancer, additional cancers of same organ, secondary malignancies due to treatment: mammograms, Pap smear, skin examination, and diagnosis-specific follow-up
D Prompt evaluation of new signs or symptoms
E Monitor and treat organ dysfunction caused by therapy: TSH if radiation, reproductive counseling, cardiovascular health issues
F Genetic counseling, testing, and intervention in appropriate contexts
G Ongoing rigorous health maintenance with particular attention to cardiovascular health, general health habits, smoking cessation
H Continued access to appropriate psychosocial support
I Multidisciplinary clinic access for pediatric patients to follow growth and developmental issues

SUPERIOR VENA CAVAL SYNDROME

Frederick R. Ahmann, MD

A. Obstruction of the superior vena cava (SVC) occurs when this thin-walled vessel is invaded, compressed, or thrombosed. Blockage of the blood flow often leads to development of the easily recognized superior vena caval syndrome (SVCS) with venous distention, facial edema, headache, tachypnea, cyanosis, and plethora. SVCS is commonly characterized as an acute or subacute oncologic emergency. Establishing a diagnosis is essential and can be accomplished safely even if biopsies of tissue exposed to elevated venous pressures and a brief delay in the initiation of therapy are necessary.

B. In a patient with the previously noted signs and symptoms, confirmation that the SVC is obstructed usually is not required because most patients have a mass visible on imaging studies. However, should confirmation be needed, this can be safely accomplished with either contrast or a nuclear venography. Nuclear venography is preferable because of a lower injection volume of contrast, but both are associated with low complication rates.

C. Since the 1950s, bronchogenic carcinomas have been the leading cause of SVCS. In the past decade, with the increased use of intravascular devices, thrombosis associated with such devices now may account for approximately one fourth of cases. For many years histologic confirmation of the diagnosis was thought to be unnecessary because palliative radiotherapy was the only treatment possible. Recent advances in the treatment of lung cancers and lymphoproliferative disorders, in addition to the increasing incidence of benign causes for which radiotherapy is not palliative and is potentially dangerous, mandate accurate pretherapy assessment. Little evidence suggests that diagnostic procedures (including bronchoscopy, lymph node biopsies, mediastinoscopy, and thoracotomies) carry an excessive risk. Therefore, the evaluation of these patients should be similar to that of any patient with a lung mass.

D. Standard palliative therapy for SVCS caused by a malignancy has been radiotherapy. Some debate persists about the optimal dose, schedule, and fields of treatment, but in general, about 50%–70% of treated patients are reported to achieve symptomatic improvement within 2 weeks of initiation of radiotherapy. However, radiotherapy is no longer the sole or even the initial therapy for many patients. In one review, 60% of all cases of SVCS were caused by lung cancer or lymphomas. Thus, a majority of the causes of SVCS are malignancies for which chemotherapy with or without radiotherapy is needed to accomplish the therapeutic objectives of improved quality of life and prolonged survival. SVCS can cause distressing signs and symptoms that should be palliated in a timely fashion. However, because many such patients may have lung cancer or lymphoma together with a definite incidence of benign etiologies, an accurate histologic diagnosis should be pursued in all patients with SVCS unless there are extenuating circumstances. Only with a definite histologic diagnosis can a rational therapeutic choice be made for both relieving SVCS and maximizing survival potential.

References

Ahmann FR. A reassessment of the clinical implications of the superior vena caval syndrome. J Clin Oncol 1984;2:961.

Baker GL, Barnes HJ. Superior vena cava syndrome: etiology, diagnosis and treatment. Am J Crit Care 1992;1:54.

Bigsby R, Greengrass R, Unruh H. Diagnostic algorithm for acute superior vena caval obstruction. J Cardiovasc Surg 1993;34:347.

Perez CA, Presant CA, Van Amburg AL. Management of superior vena cava syndrome. Semin Oncol 1978;5:123.

Rice JW, Rodriguez RM, Light, RW. The superior vena cava syndrome: clinical characteristics and evolving etiology. Medicine 2006;85:37–42.

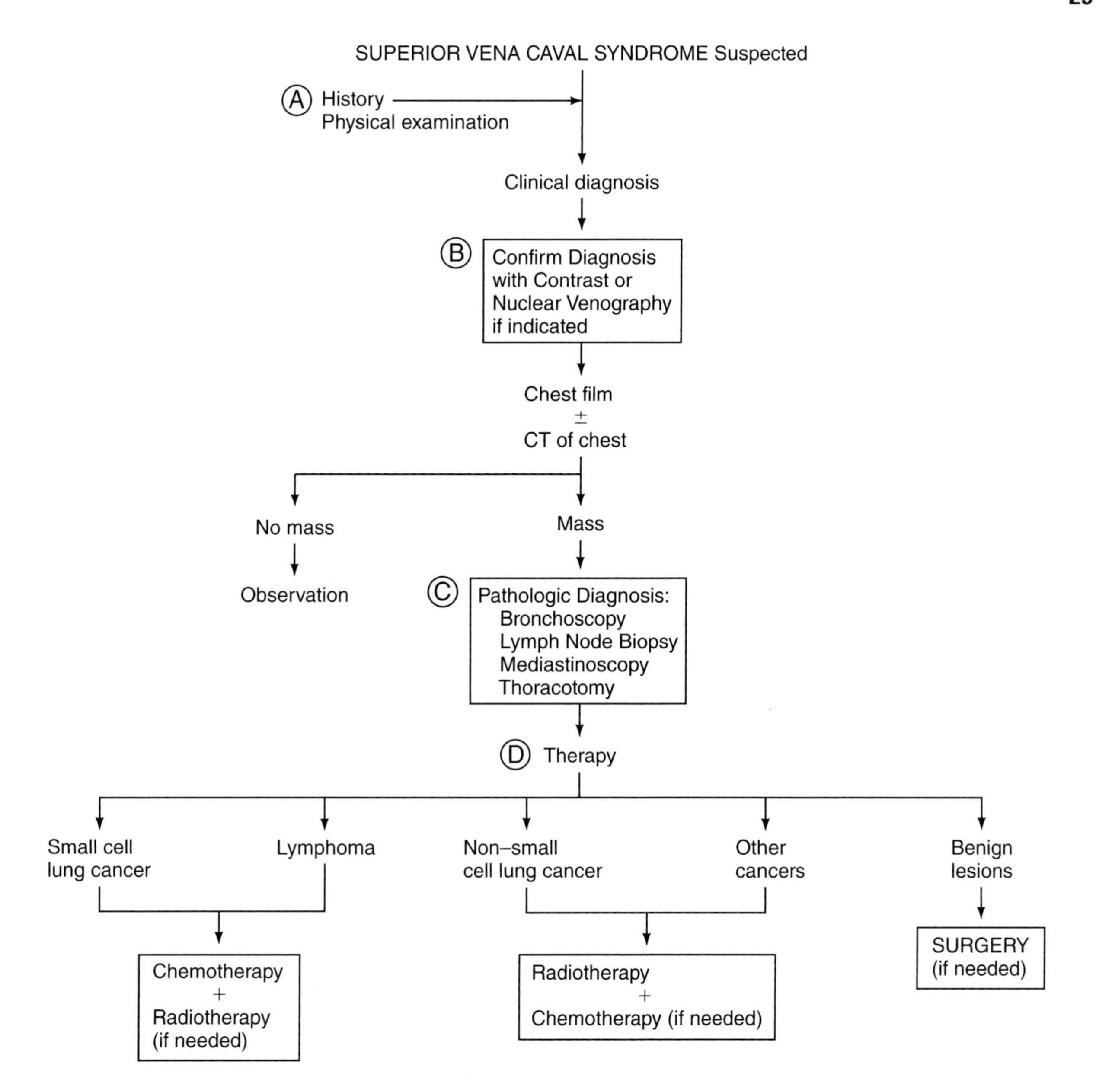
SUPERIOR VENA CAVAL SYNDROME Suspected
A
History
Physical examination
Clinical diagnosis
B
Confirm Diagnosis with Contrast or Nuclear Venography if indicated
Chest film
±
CT of chest
No mass
Observation
Mass
C
Pathologic Diagnosis:
Bronchoscopy
Lymph Node Biopsy
Mediastinoscopy
Thoracotomy
D
Therapy
Small cell lung cancer
Lymphoma
Non–small cell lung cancer
Other cancers
Benign lesions
Chemotherapy + Radiotherapy (if needed)
Radiotherapy + Chemotherapy (if needed)
SURGERY (if needed)

SPINAL CORD COMPRESSION

Guillermo Gonzalez-Osete, MD, and Manuel Modiano, MD

Approximately 5% of systemic cancers involve the spinal cord. Spinal cord compression is a medical emergency in which a delay in treatment often causes irreversible loss of neurologic function.

A. Tumors that most commonly affect the spinal cord are of the lung, breast, prostate, and lymph nodes. Myeloma, melanoma, and genitourinary tract tumors less commonly affect the spinal cord. An important presenting sign is back pain, either of recent onset or old pain that has returned or increased. Pain is present in 97% of all cord compressions, followed in frequency by weakness (76%) and paresthesias (57%) along a bilateral or unilateral dermatomal distribution. Associated bowel and bladder dysfunction is seen in 51% of patients with more advanced disease. A few patients have no history of cancer and pain as the initial presentation.

B. Even when the physical examination does not reveal signs of spinal cord compression, obtain plain radiographs of the painful region to rule out neoplastic involvement. If the plain films are negative, consider nonneoplastic causes (rheumatoid arthritis, aortic aneurysm, spondylosis, herniated disc, spinal tuberculosis, osteoarthritis, osteomyelitis). Proceed with a detailed workup if there is pain with tenderness to percussion over the affected vertebral body, bilateral muscle weakness in the extremities, sensory changes, loss of deep tendon reflexes, or bowel or bladder incontinence.

C. If plain films reveal a lesion in a painful area, follow with MRI or myelography, which have comparable sensitivity and specificity. Myelography is an invasive procedure that requires technical skill and the use of contrast. MRI is not invasive and helps in detecting intramedullary lesions, but patients may have difficulty lying still on the hard table or may have claustrophobia. Also, MRI is not always available. If these studies show a lesion, there is a 90% probability of cord compression.

D. If MRI is negative and clinical findings suggest cord involvement, proceed with myelography. Myelography helps determine the upper and lower extent of the lesion and ascertains whether there is more than one lesion. If a complete block is found on lumbar myelography, cisternal myelography or MRI is required to identify the upper end of the block. If both studies are negative, there is no cord compression.

E. The choice of treatment depends on the type of tumor, the level of the block, the rapidity of onset and duration of symptoms, previous treatment, and the clinical experience available. This medical emergency is treated vigorously with radiation or surgery in addition to steroids. Our current recommendation is to give 10 mg IV dexamethasone immediately, follow with 4 mg every 6 hours daily for at least 72 hours, and then rapidly taper as tolerated. Begin radiotherapy immediately after the diagnosis is established. The earlier a lesion is detected and treated, the better the functional outcome. Response rates are 30%–80%. The total dose of radiation is 3000–4000 Gy delivered over 2–4 weeks.

F. Consider surgery (laminectomy, stabilization) when there is (1) no histologic diagnosis and cord compression is the presenting sign of cancer, (2) history of radiation therapy to the affected area, (3) neurologic progression of disease despite steroids and radiotherapy, (4) instability requiring fixation, or (5) a high cervical lesion. Some more recent articles have reported improved outcomes with surgery followed by radiotherapy. This is a consideration especially in patients who are expected to have longer life expectancy and are in general good physical condition to tolerate such a procedure. After surgery, give radiotherapy to avoid recurrences. Initial response to combined surgery and radiation is 20%–100%, depending on tumor type and timing of treatment. The best prognostic index for eventual recovery of function is pretreatment status: 60% of patients who are ambulatory at diagnosis remain so postoperatively, whereas only 7% of those who are paraplegic at diagnosis are ambulatory after treatment.

G. When plain films are negative and physical examination is not definitive, adjust pain medications and observe. If pain persists or worsens or if the history is highly suspicious, perform MRI and proceed accordingly.

References

Gilbert RW, Kim J-H, Posner JB. Epidural spinal cord compression from metastatic tumor: diagnosis and treatment. Ann Neurol 1978;3:40.

Maranzano E, Latini P, Checcaglini F, et al. Radiation therapy in metastatic spinal cord compression. Cancer 1991;67:1333.

Patchell RA, Tibbs PA, Regine WF, et al. Direct decompressive surgical resection in the treatment of spinal cord compression caused by metastatic cancer: a randomised trial. Lancet 2005;366(9486): 643–638; comment Lancet 2005;366(9486):609–610.

Rodichok L, Harper GR, Ruckdeschel JC, et al. Early diagnosis of spinal epidural metastases. Am J Med 1981;70:1181.

Wasserstrom W, Glass PJ, Posner JB. Diagnosis and treatment of leptomeningeal metastases from solid tumors: experience with 90 patients. Cancer 1982;49:759.

Willson JKV, Masaryk T. Neurologic emergencies in the cancer patient. Semin Oncol 1989;16:490.

Young RF, Post EM, King GA. Treatment of spinal epidural metastases. J Neurosurg 1980;53:741.

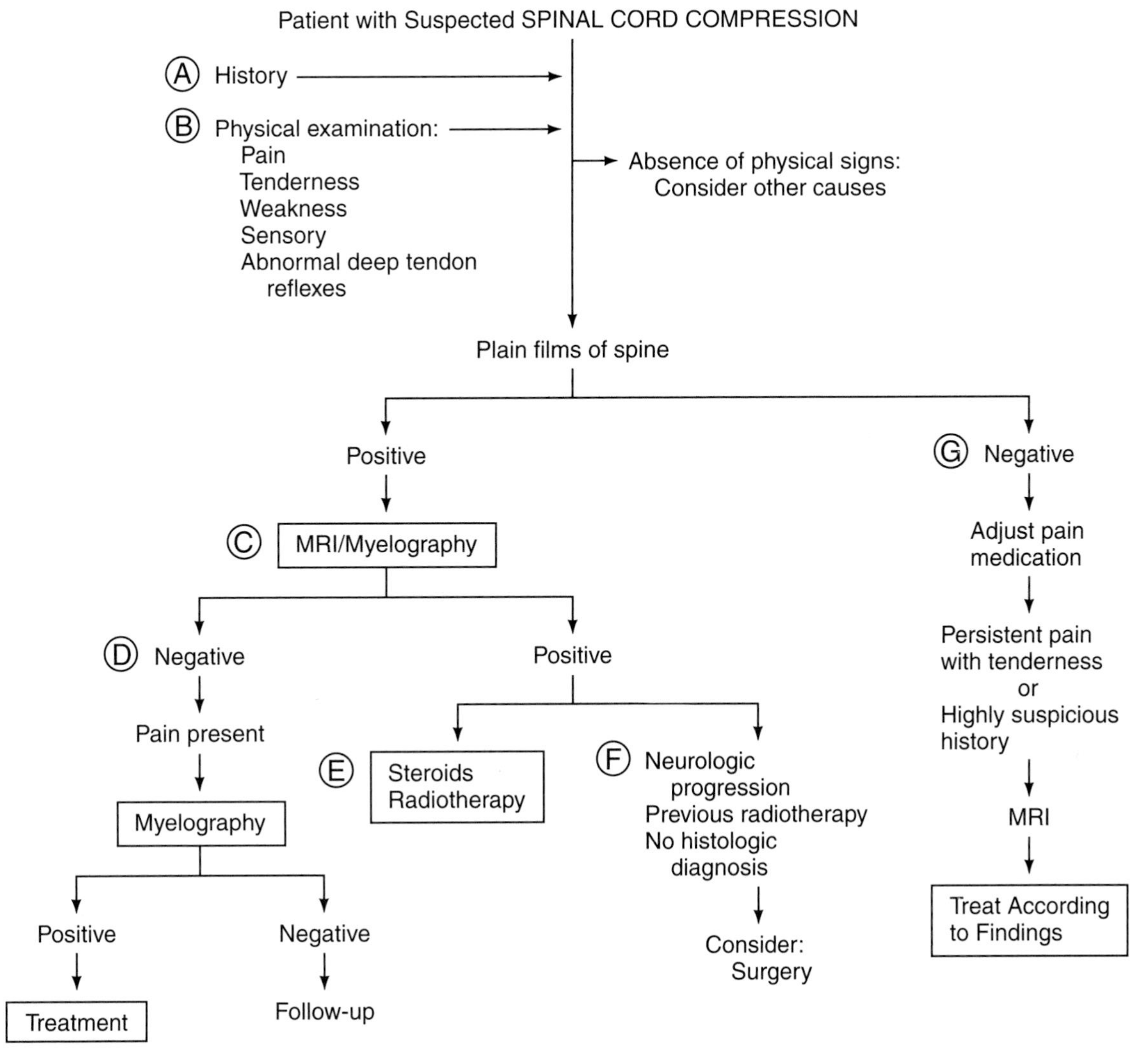

Patient with Suspected SPINAL CORD COMPRESSION

(A) History →

(B) Physical examination: →
Pain
Tenderness
Weakness
Sensory
Abnormal deep tendon reflexes

→ Absence of physical signs: Consider other causes

↓

Plain films of spine

- Positive
  - ↓
  - (C) MRI/Myelography
    - (D) Negative
      - ↓
      - Pain present
      - ↓
      - Myelography
        - Positive → Treatment
        - Negative → Follow-up
    - Positive
      - (E) Steroids Radiotherapy
      - (F) Neurologic progression
        Previous radiotherapy
        No histologic diagnosis
        - ↓
        - Consider: Surgery
- (G) Negative
  - ↓
  - Adjust pain medication
  - ↓
  - Persistent pain with tenderness or Highly suspicious history
  - ↓
  - MRI
  - ↓
  - Treat According to Findings

Infectious Diseases

Michael Klompas, MD, MPH, FRCPC
Section Editor

FOREIGN TRAVEL: IMMUNIZATIONS AND INFECTIONS

Rebeca M. Plank, MD

A. Two questions must be asked in the initial evaluation of a traveler: What is the patient's health status, and where will he or she travel? Variables to consider include countries to be visited, whether travel will be rural or urban, planned activities, and duration of visit. It is important to remember that persons returning to visit their country of origin after living in the United States are also at risk for endemic infections, sometimes more so because they may not feel the need to take special precautions.

B. Infections are acquired through exposure to contaminated food and water, exposure to vectors, such as ticks and mosquitoes, and person-to-person transmission. Travelers should be advised to practice strict hand hygiene and to avoid uncooked food and food from street vendors. They should consume only bottled beverages and use bottled water for ice cubes and for brushing teeth, etc. Fresh water exposure (adventure travel) is a potential source of infections, such as schistosomiasis and leptospirosis. Sexually transmitted diseases, including HIV, are always a risk and travelers should be advised to abstain from sex or to use condoms for all encounters. Travelers should also consider carrying sterile needles and syringes with them in case of medical emergency.

C. One of the first things to be ascertained is that the traveler is up to date with the standard Centers for Disease Control and Prevention (CDC) vaccination schedule for children and adults; this includes pneumococcus, influenza, tetanus, and measle/mumps/rubella (MMR) vaccines because these infections have been acquired overseas. All overseas travelers should be encouraged to be vaccinated against hepatitis A, hepatitis B, polio, and typhoid. Yellow fever occurs only in sub-Saharan Africa and tropical South America, and many countries in these regions require proof of vaccination for entry. A meningitis vaccine is recommended for those traveling to areas in the meningitis belt across central Africa, and Saudi Arabia requires that Hajj and Umrah visitors have a certificate of vaccination. For those who will be traveling to areas where rabies is relatively common but the immune globulin and vaccine would not be immediately available (e.g., trekkers), preexposure vaccination should be considered. Japanese encephalitis vaccine may be indicated in some cases for travelers to Southeast Asia. The cholera vaccine is currently not recommended.

D. Malaria prevention should be a comprehensive endeavor, including remaining in screened areas when possible and using a mosquito net at night, minimizing skin exposure to mosquitos, using insect repellents, and chemoprophylaxis with Malarone (atovaquone-proguanil), doxycycline, or mefloquine. Mefloquine has the advantage of requiring a weekly (rather than daily) dose but has the not uncommon downside of neuropsychiatric side effects. As a result of the emergence of chloroquine resistance, chloroquine prophylaxis is useful only for travelers going to the Caribbean and Central America north of the Panama Canal. Appropriate antimalaria precautions will also protect a traveler from other mosquito and tick-borne illnesses, such as dengue and rickettsial illnesses.

E. Diarrhea is the most common illness in travelers. The importance of adequate hydration in such cases should be emphasized. Increasing resistance to fluoroquinolones limits their usefulness in parts of Asia where azithromycin is recommended. Patients should be given at least a 3-day supply of antibiotics to take with them and instructed to take them in case of moderate to severe diarrhea with fever or pus, mucus, or blood in the stool. If treatment is initiated promptly, even a single dose may reduce the duration of the illness to a few hours. Pepto-Bismol taken every 30 minutes for eight doses has also been shown to decrease stool frequency and shorten illness duration.

(Continued on page 298)

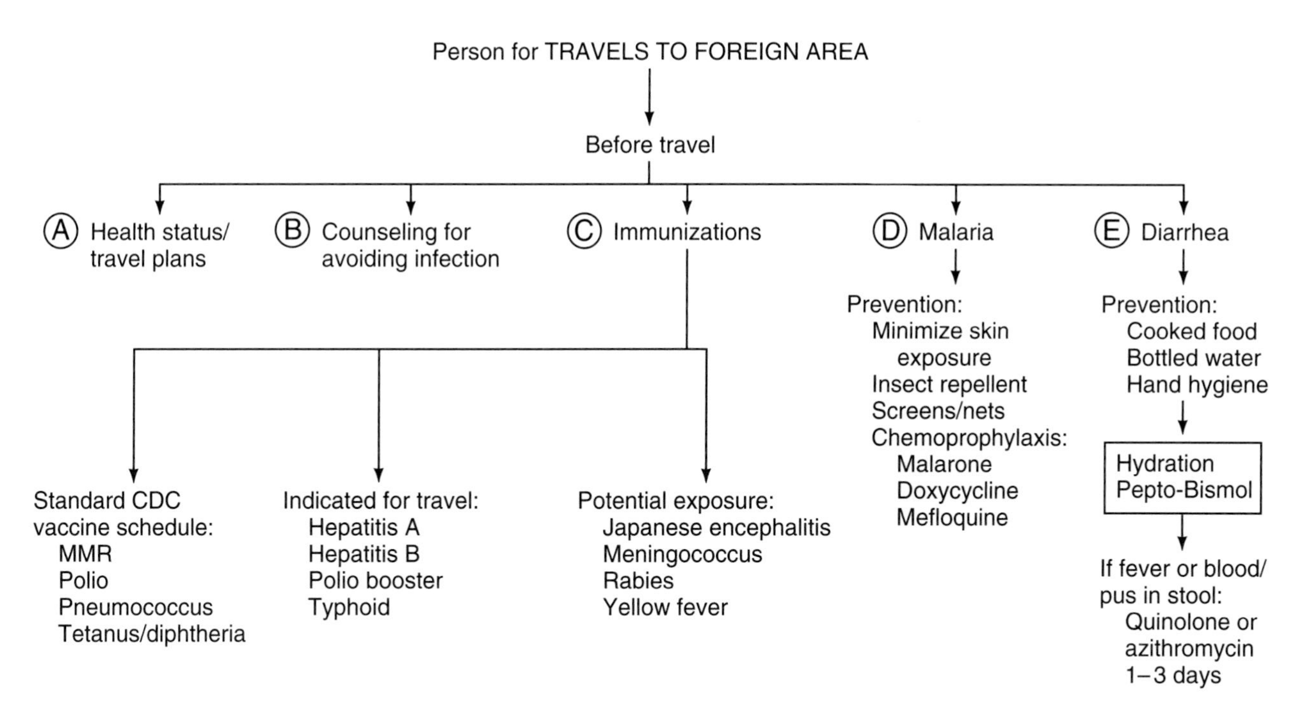
Person for TRAVELS TO FOREIGN AREA
Before travel
(A) Health status/ travel plans
(B) Counseling for avoiding infection
(C) Immunizations
(D) Malaria
(E) Diarrhea
Standard CDC vaccine schedule:
MMR
Polio
Pneumococcus
Tetanus/diphtheria
Indicated for travel:
Hepatitis A
Hepatitis B
Polio booster
Typhoid
Potential exposure:
Japanese encephalitis
Meningococcus
Rabies
Yellow fever
Prevention:
Minimize skin exposure
Insect repellent
Screens/nets
Chemoprophylaxis:
Malarone
Doxycycline
Mefloquine
Prevention:
Cooked food
Bottled water
Hand hygiene
Hydration
Pepto-Bismol
If fever or blood/ pus in stool:
Quinolone or azithromycin 1–3 days

F. If a traveler returns with a nonspecific febrile illness, things that are life threatening, transmissible, or treatable must be excluded immediately. Malaria must be investigated (regardless of prophylaxis history) through thick and thin blood smears. If malaria parasites are seen on smear but no speciation is possible, treatment should be targeted to *Plasmodium falciparum*, which is the most virulent species, and should be assumed to be drug resistant. The incubation period for malaria can be as short as 1 week and as long as several months (even years). Blood cultures for typhoid should be obtained (regardless of vaccination status). Typhoid fever may or may not include GI symptoms. Suspicion for a highly contagious and morbid illness, such as a hemorrhagic fever or the recent severe acute respiratory syndrome (SARS), in patients with compatible symptoms and returning from affected areas should be reported to local health departments immediately.

G. Once investigation is under way for malaria and typhoid, further clinical investigation should be dictated by history (e.g., contact with fresh water, recent unprotected sexual activity) and localizing signs and symptoms (e.g., diarrhea, cough, rash). Dengue is common in travelers and although it causes much discomfort is generally self-limited. Dengue hemorrhagic fever, manifesting with plasma leakage, platelets <100,000 per ml, fever lasting 2–7 days, hemorrhagic tendency, and possibly the development of shock, is generally limited to individuals experiencing repeat dengue infection and treatment is supportive. The CDC maintains a website containing updated information about regional outbreaks that can also help guide workup.

H. If a patient returns with diarrhea, stool should be sent for culture (*Escherichia coli, Salmonella, Shigella, Campylobacter*) and ova and parasite (O&P) three times. Respiratory symptoms may result from viral infections and should be evaluated in much the same way as for nontravelers. Because tuberculosis (TB) is rarely acquired by short-term travelers, it should be more seriously considered in those having been abroad for months or years and an acid-fast bacillus (AFB) smear should be done. Domestic infections should also be considered (e.g., urinary tract infection [UTI], upper respiratory infection [URI]).

I. A partial list of illnesses that can be seen in returning travelers is provided in the algorithm; when in doubt, patients should be referred to a specialized travel clinic and sometimes to an emergency department. See also the useful websites listed in the references.

References

Ryan ET, Kain KC. Health advice and immunizations for travelers. N Engl J Med 2000;342:1716–1725.

Ryan ET, Wilson ME, Kain KC. Illness after international travel. N Engl J Med 2002;347:505–516.

www.cdc.gov/malaria/travel/index.htm.

wwwn.cdc.gov/travel/destinationList.aspx.

wwwn.cdc.gov/travel/notices.aspx.

wwwn.cdc.gov/travel/yellowBookCh4-Diarrhea.aspx.

wwwn.cdc.gov/travel/yellowBookCh9-Immunocompromised.aspx.

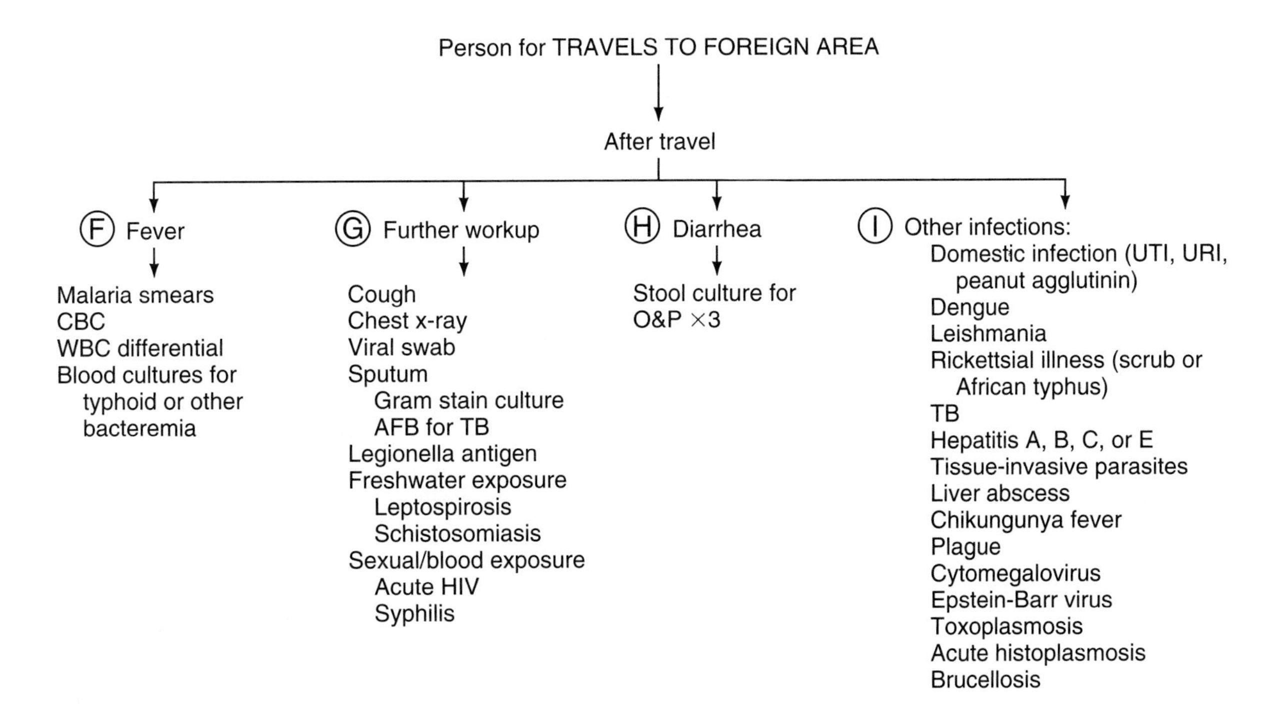

Person for TRAVELS TO FOREIGN AREA
After travel
(F) Fever
Malaria smears
CBC
WBC differential
Blood cultures for typhoid or other bacteremia
(G) Further workup
Cough
Chest x-ray
Viral swab
Sputum
Gram stain culture
AFB for TB
Legionella antigen
Freshwater exposure
Leptospirosis
Schistosomiasis
Sexual/blood exposure
Acute HIV
Syphilis
(H) Diarrhea
Stool culture for O&P ×3
(I) Other infections:
Domestic infection (UTI, URI, peanut agglutinin)
Dengue
Leishmania
Rickettsial illness (scrub or African typhus)
TB
Hepatitis A, B, C, or E
Tissue-invasive parasites
Liver abscess
Chikungunya fever
Plague
Cytomegalovirus
Epstein-Barr virus
Toxoplasmosis
Acute histoplasmosis
Brucellosis

ACUTE AND SUBACUTE MENINGITIS

Alison C. Roxby, MD, MSc

A. Prior to lumbar puncture (LP) brain imaging is recommended to rule out a mass lesion for patients with focal neurologic deficits, abnormal level of consciousness, papilledema, seizure in the past 7 days, or history of CNS disease (mass, stroke, or infection) or for those who are immunocompromised. Brain herniation after LP remains a rare event.

B. If imaging is indicated, blood cultures should be drawn and steroids and antibiotics should be administered before imaging to prevent delay in treatment. Antibiotics should be administered emergently (within 30 minutes) in any patient with suspected bacterial meningitis.

C. If CNS imaging reveals a mass lesion, neurosurgical evaluation may be indicated. Radiologic evidence of temporal lobe abnormalities should be treated empirically as herpes simplex encephalitis pending diagnostic confirmation.

D. Dexamethasone administered at 0.15 mg/kg is recommended in adults with moderate to severe impairment (Glasgow Coma Scale score <12) and suspicion of pneumococcal disease. It should be given just prior to or concomitant with IV antibiotic therapy; it is thought to protect against inflammatory response to bacteria inside the subarachnoid space. Dexamethasone should not be administered after antibiotics have already been given.

E. Antibiotics should be administered empirically and without delay. Antibiotic regimens can be revised once information from the history, physical examination, and the cerebrospinal fluid (CSF) Gram stain is available.

F. In normal adult hosts ≤60 years, the most common organisms are *Streptococcus pneumoniae, Neisseria meningitidis*, and (more rarely) *Haemophilus influenzae*. In patients >60 years, *S. pneumoniae* predominates, but *Listeria monocytogenes* and group B streptococcus are also seen in this age group.

G. In patients who are immunocompromised, including patients with HIV/AIDS, cancer, end-stage renal disease, alcoholism, and diabetes, and in patients taking high-dose steroids, additional organisms should be considered. These include *Cryptococcus neoformans, Mycobacterium tuberculosis, Staphylococcus* species, and aerobic gram-negative bacilli, including *Pseudomonas aeruginosa.*

H. Closed head trauma and basilar skull fractures are linked to infections with *S. pneumoniae* and gram-negative bacilli. Neurosurgical procedures increase risk for meningitis from *Staphylococcus aureus* and *Pseudomonas aeruginosa,* but coagulase-negative *Staphylococcus* species, *Streptococcus*, and aerobic gram-negative bacilli have also been implicated. Upper respiratory flora should be suspected after invasive sinus instrumentation.

I. Intraventricular shunt devices are at high risk of causing infection. The most common organism is *Staphylococcus epidermidis;* other skin flora, including *S. aureus*, diphtheroids, and *Propionibacterium acnes* are also frequent culprits.

(Continued on page 302)

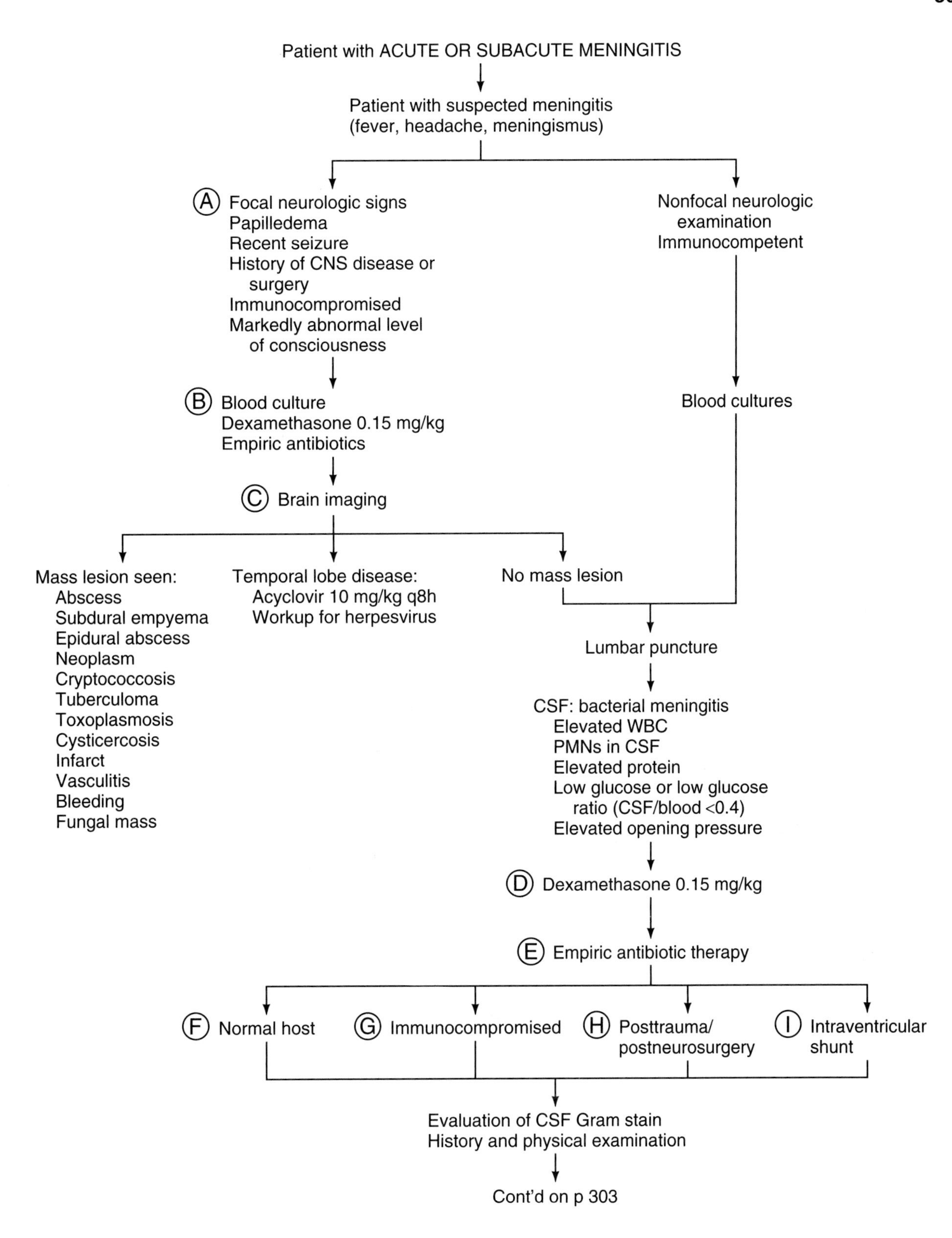
Patient with ACUTE OR SUBACUTE MENINGITIS
Patient with suspected meningitis
(fever, headache, meningismus)
A Focal neurologic signs
Papilledema
Recent seizure
History of CNS disease or surgery
Immunocompromised
Markedly abnormal level of consciousness
Nonfocal neurologic examination
Immunocompetent
B Blood culture
Dexamethasone 0.15 mg/kg
Empiric antibiotics
Blood cultures
C Brain imaging
Mass lesion seen:
Abscess
Subdural empyema
Epidural abscess
Neoplasm
Cryptococcosis
Tuberculoma
Toxoplasmosis
Cysticercosis
Infarct
Vasculitis
Bleeding
Fungal mass
Temporal lobe disease:
Acyclovir 10 mg/kg q8h
Workup for herpesvirus
No mass lesion
Lumbar puncture
CSF: bacterial meningitis
Elevated WBC
PMNs in CSF
Elevated protein
Low glucose or low glucose ratio (CSF/blood <0.4)
Elevated opening pressure
D Dexamethasone 0.15 mg/kg
E Empiric antibiotic therapy
F Normal host
G Immunocompromised
H Posttrauma/ postneurosurgery
I Intraventricular shunt
Evaluation of CSF Gram stain
History and physical examination
Cont'd on p 303

J. The Gram stain should be used to target antimicrobial therapy. If the organism identified is not *S. pneumoniae*, dexamethasone can be discontinued. CSF cultures should be sent to confirm the diagnosis. Blood cultures will also be positive in 50%–75% of patients with bacterial meningitis.

K. If no bacteria are seen on Gram stain, other organisms should be considered. Cryptococcal meningitis should be investigated with India ink stain, cryptococcal antigen testing, and fungal cultures. Only 75% of CSF samples infected with *Cryptococcus* will have positive India ink stains; however, serum and CSF cryptococcal antigen detection has >95% sensitivity. The gold standard remains fungal culture.

L. If *Cryptococcus* is not present, and if CSF glucose levels are normal and CSF is without significant leukocytes, consider a parameningeal focus.

M. Polymorphonuclear leukocytes in the CSF may indicate partially treated bacterial meningitis or a viral meningitis. Empiric antimicrobials should be continued and viral studies, such as enterovirus polymerase chain reaction (PCR), should be done on the CSF sample.

N. In patients with predominantly monocytic white cells in the CSF, a decreased glucose level should prompt consideration for tuberculous meningitis. Partially treated bacterial or fungal meningitis remains a possibility. A monocytic CSF with normal glucose is more indicative of viral infection. PCR sent on CSF can elucidate common viral entities that cause meningitis.

O. Tuberculous meningitis can be an elusive diagnosis. CSF acid-fast bacilli smear is key, as is culture sent from 10 ml of spun CSF sediment. Empiric therapy must be considered in patients with risk factors because culture results can take up to 6 weeks.

References

Attia J, Hatala R, Cook DJ, et al. The rational clinical examination. Does this adult patient have acute meningitis? JAMA 1999;282(2):175–181.

de Gans J, van de Beek D. Dexamethasone in adults with bacterial meningitis. N Engl J Med 2002;347(20):1549–1556.

Hasbun R, Abrahams J, Jekel J, et al. Computed tomography of the head before lumbar puncture in adults with suspected meningitis. N Engl J Med 2001;345(24):1727–1733.

Tunkel AR, Hartman BJ, Kaplan SL, et al. Practice guidelines for the management of bacterial meningitis. Clin Infect Dis 2004;39(9):1267–1284.

Patient with ACUTE OR SUBACUTE BACTERIAL MENINGITIS
(Cont'd from p 301)

- (J) Bacteria on Gram stain
  - → Antimicrobial therapy for bacterial meningitis → Verify culture and adjust antimicrobials accordingly
- (K) No bacteria seen on Gram stain
  - India ink positive for cryptococcus → Treat Cryptococcal Meningitis
  - Cryptococcal antigen positive in CSF → Treat Cryptococcal Meningitis
  - Positive fungal cultures → Treat Cryptococcal Meningitis
  - (L) Negative fungal cultures
    - Increased WBCs in CSF
      - (M) Polymorphonuclear leukocytes → Consider: Partially treated bacterial meningitis; Viral meningitis
      - (N) Mononuclear cells
        - Decreased CSF glucose → Consider: Partially treated bacterial, fungal, or tuberculous meningitis
        - Normal CSF glucose → Consider: Viral meningitis; Partially treated meningitis
    - None or rare WBCs in CSF → Glucose normal, Protein elevated → Consider: Parameningeal focus

(O) Consider empiric treatment for tuberculous meningitis if:
- Hyponatremia
- Exposure to tuberculosis
- History of tuberculosis
- Pulmonary tuberculosis
- Positive AFB smear
- HIV positive

CHRONIC MENINGITIS

Michael Klompas, MD, MPH, FRCPC

A. Chronic meningitis is defined by symptoms and/or signs suggestive of meningeal irritation that have been present for at least 4 weeks. Symptoms usually begin insidiously. Patients typically present with headache, neck stiffness, and mental status changes with or without fever. The differential diagnosis is broad (Table 1) and includes infections, malignancies, inflammatory disorders, and iatrogenesis. The evaluation of chronic meningitis begins with careful history about pattern of headache to exclude recurrent meningitis (classically caused by herpes simplex virus [HSV]) or migraines.

B. Head imaging is essential to evaluate for structural lesions that can cause chronic head pain and meningeal irritation, such as brain abscesses, tumors, hydrocephalus, and cerebral aneurysms with intermittent hemorrhage. The superior detail and resolution achievable with MRI compared with CT can yield additional clues to diagnosis. Lymphoma, toxoplasmosis, cysticercosis, sarcoidosis, and other lesions can have characteristic appearances on high-resolution imaging.

C. The pattern of cerebrospinal fluid (CSF) pleocytosis and chemistry can also guide diagnosis, so a lumbar puncture (LP) should be performed. An eosinophilic pleocytosis is seen with cysticercosis after cyst rupture, coccidiomycosis, *Angiostrongylus,* and schistosomiasis. Neutrophilic pleocytosis is seen with brucellosis, *Nocardia*, actinomycosis, and meningitis with endemic fungi. Lymphocytic pleocytosis is the most common pattern and the least specific—it is seen in lymphomatous meningitis; sarcoidosis; connective tissue disorders; and infections such as neuroborreliosis, syphilis, tuberculosis, and *Cryptococcus.* Low CSF glucose is associated with carcinomatous, tuberculous, and fungal meningitis. Very high CSF protein is usually seen in carcinomatous meningitis.

(Continued on page 306)

Table 1
Etiologies of Chronic Meningitis

Infections	Tuberculosis, brucelllosis, *Nocardia*, actinomycosis, syphilis, Lyme disease, ehrilichiosis, listeriosis Cryptococcus, histoplasmosis, coccidiomycosis, blastomycosis, sporotrichosis Schistosmiasis trypanosomiasis, cysticercosis, toxoplasmosis, *Angiostrongylus* HIV, human T-cell leukemia virus, enterovirus, cytomegallovirus, herpes simplex virus,, varicella zoster virus, Epstein-bar virus
Malignancies	Lymphoma, leukemia, primary brain tumors, metastases of solid malignancies (usually breast, lung, and meleanoma)
Inflammatory disorders	Sarcoidosis, Wegener's granulomatosis, Behçet's disease systemic lupus erythmatosus, granulomatous angiitis
Medications	NSAIDs
Irriants	Indwelling intrathecal devices, intrathecal chemotherapy

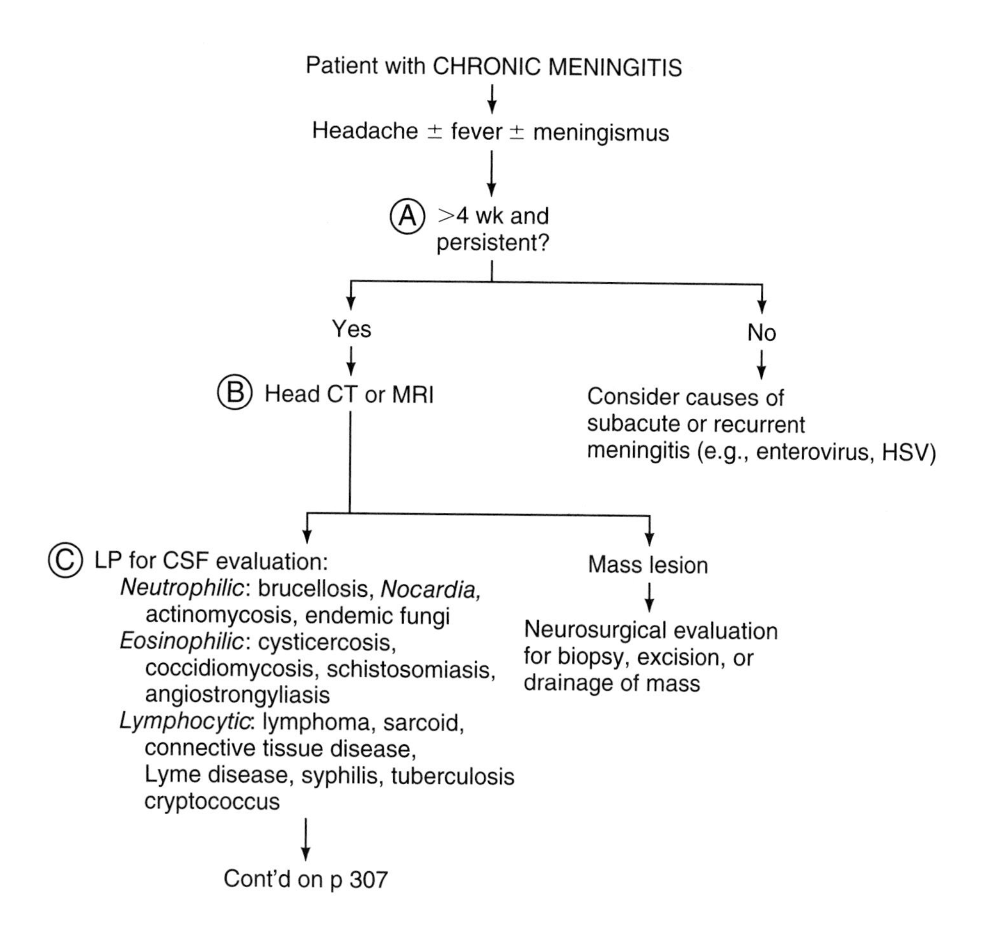

Patient with CHRONIC MENINGITIS
Headache ± fever ± meningismus
(A) >4 wk and persistent?
Yes
No
(B) Head CT or MRI
Consider causes of subacute or recurrent meningitis (e.g., enterovirus, HSV)
(C) LP for CSF evaluation:
Neutrophilic: brucellosis, *Nocardia,* actinomycosis, endemic fungi
Eosinophilic: cysticercosis, coccidiomycosis, schistosomiasis, angiostrongyliasis
Lymphocytic: lymphoma, sarcoid, connective tissue disease, Lyme disease, syphilis, tuberculosis cryptococcus
Mass lesion
Neurosurgical evaluation for biopsy, excision, or drainage of mass
Cont'd on p 307

D. Chronic meningitis is more common among patients who are immunocompromised because of their increased susceptibility to infection. Patients with agammaglobulinemia are susceptible to persistent or recurrent enterovirus meningitis. HIV testing should be routinely performed on all patients with chronic meningitis. Patients with HIV, along with patients who have received a transplant and people receiving chemotherapy, should then be evaluated for tuberculosis, *Cryptococcus neoformans*, neurosyphilis, viral meningitis (HSV, varicella-zoster virus [VZV], cytomegalovirus [CMV], Epstein-Barr virus [EBV]), and other fungal diseases.

E. In patients who are immunocompetent, detailed history and physical examination along with evaluation of the nature of the CSF pleocytosis can guide the differential diagnosis. Travel or residence in areas endemic for tuberculosis (Africa, South America, Caribbean, Asia, Eastern Europe) can be helpful. Likewise, time spent in the southwestern United States or Mexico raises the possibility of coccidiomycosis, residence in the Ohio and Mississippi river valleys or Caribbean suggests evaluation for histoplasmosis, and residence in the southeastern United States can be a clue to blastomycosis. Exposures to farm animals or unpasteurized dairy products suggest brucellosis or listeriosis. Tick bites, gardening, golf, or hiking in Lyme-endemic areas warrant testing for neuroborreliosis.

On examination, cranial neuropathies are suggestive of basilar meningitis associated with tuberculosis, neuroborreliosis, carcinomatous meningitis, or sarcoidosis. Iritis, uveitis, oral and/or genital ulcerations, skin rash, arthritis, and serositis are suggestive of inflammatory disorders such as Behçet's disease, Sjögren's syndrome, systemic lupus erythematosus (SLE), or sarcoidosis.

Blood tests for HIV, syphilis, Lyme disease, cryptococcal antigen, ANA, double-stranded DNA, liver function tests, and blood cultures should supplement the history and physical examination.

CT scanning of the chest can yield further clues to sarcoidosis, Wegener's granulomatosis, tuberculosis, fungal disease, and malignancy. Abnormalities identified outside the brain might be more amenable to biopsy than the meninges or CNS.

F. Once a clinical suspicion has been generated on the basis of history, examination, and preliminary CSF evaluation, it is often necessary to repeat the LP to obtain additional CSF for special studies. A large volume of fluid is necessary to optimize the yield of cytologic and microbiologic studies. At least 5 ml should be sent for cytology and flow cytometry. A minimum of 10 ml is recommended to assess for mycobacteria and fungi via stain and culture. Special CSF studies for suspected infections can include cryptococcal antigen; VDRL; fungal serologies; and polymerase chain reaction (PCR) for mycobacteria, Lyme disease, brucellosis, and herpes family viruses (HSV, VZV, CMV, EBV).

G. If extensive evaluation fails to yield a diagnosis and the patient's symptoms are deteriorating or severe, then consider a brain or meningeal biopsy. These can be particularly helpful in diagnosing elusive malignancy, tuberculosis, and vasculitic disease. The yield of biopsy is greatest if directed to meningeal or parenchymal abnormalities seen on MRI.

H. Consideration should also be given to a trial of empiric therapy. Empiric therapy is usually begun with antituberculous medications. These should be continued for at least 2 weeks before assessing their impact. If antituberculous therapy is not helpful and ongoing investigations fail to yield a diagnosis, then a trial of steroid therapy has been reported to be helpful in up to 50% of cases.

References

Hildebrand J, Aoun M. Chronic meningitis: still a diagnostic challenge. J Neurol 2003;250:653–660.

Sexton DJ. Approach to the patient with chronic meningitis. UpToDate Online 13.3. Available at: www.uptodate.com. Accessed November 22, 2005.

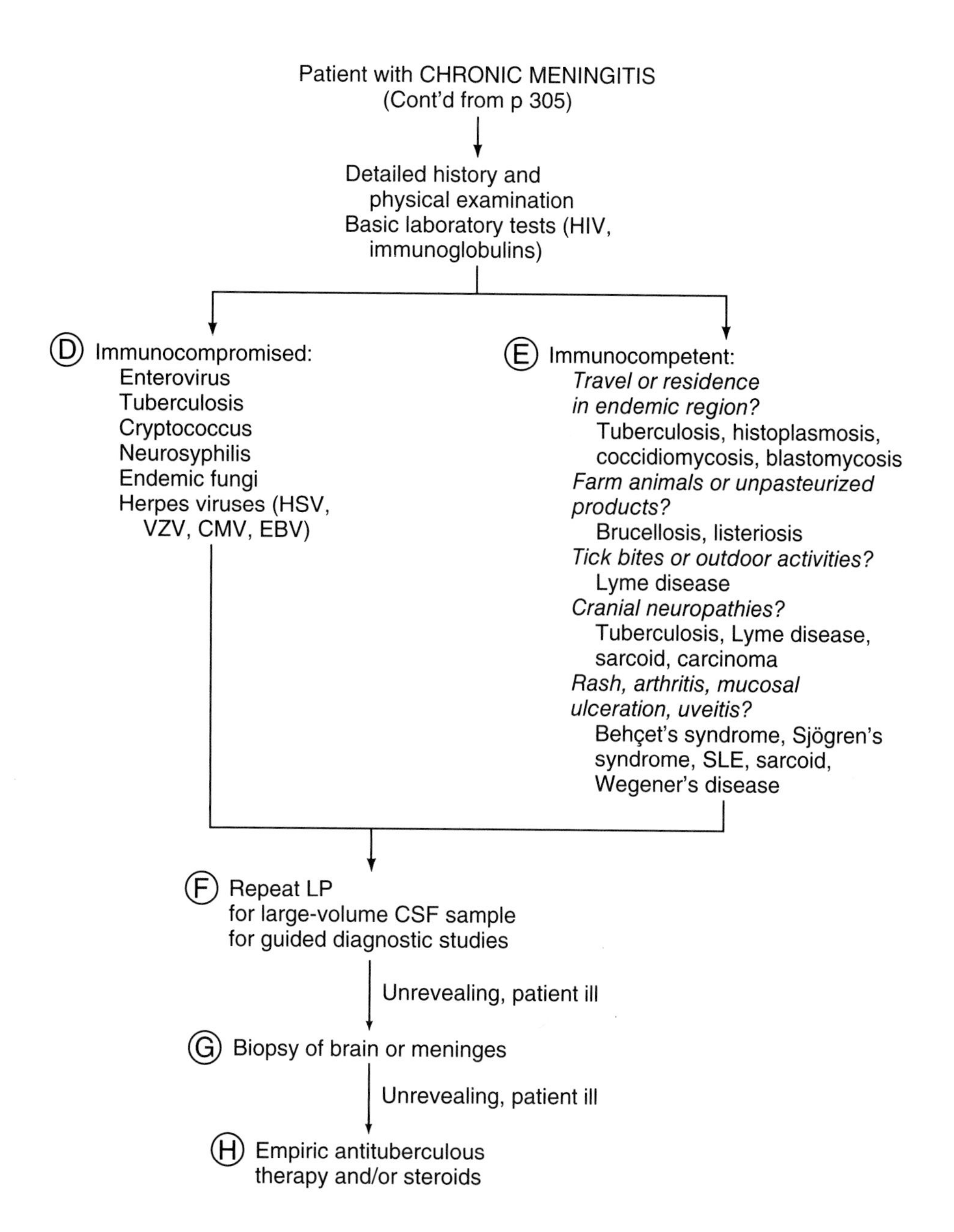
Patient with CHRONIC MENINGITIS
(Cont'd from p 305)
Detailed history and physical examination
Basic laboratory tests (HIV, immunoglobulins)
(D) Immunocompromised:
Enterovirus
Tuberculosis
Cryptococcus
Neurosyphilis
Endemic fungi
Herpes viruses (HSV, VZV, CMV, EBV)
(E) Immunocompetent:
Travel or residence in endemic region?
Tuberculosis, histoplasmosis, coccidiomycosis, blastomycosis
Farm animals or unpasteurized products?
Brucellosis, listeriosis
Tick bites or outdoor activities?
Lyme disease
Cranial neuropathies?
Tuberculosis, Lyme disease, sarcoid, carcinoma
Rash, arthritis, mucosal ulceration, uveitis?
Behçet's syndrome, Sjögren's syndrome, SLE, sarcoid, Wegener's disease
(F) Repeat LP
for large-volume CSF sample
for guided diagnostic studies
Unrevealing, patient ill
(G) Biopsy of brain or meninges
Unrevealing, patient ill
(H) Empiric antituberculous therapy and/or steroids

ASEPTIC MENINGITIS

Rebeca M. Plank, MD

A. If there is clinical suspicion for meningitis, a lumbar puncture (LP) should be performed (prior imaging may be indicated). At a minimum, glucose, protein, cell count, Gram stain, and bacterial cultures should be obtained from the cerebrospinal fluid (CSF). The history and physical examination will dictate what other tests, if any, should be sent (see later). It is prudent to obtain an extra tube of CSF in case further studies become necessary.

B. Aseptic meningitis describes a syndrome of clinical and laboratory findings consistent with meningeal inflammation with negative Gram stain and routine bacterial cultures from the CSF. Glucose, protein, and cell counts can be highly variable and should not be relied on to distinguish between septic and aseptic meningitis; the threshold for initiation of empiric dexamethasone and antibiotics should be low.

Parameningeal bacterial infections (e.g., mastoiditis, epidural abscess) and partially treated bacterial meningitis can have a similar clinical presentation with negative CSF cultures, so these should be excluded.

C. For all patients, risk factors for HIV, herpes simplex virus (HSV), and syphilis should be ascertained. A positive CSF-VDRL is highly specific but insensitive for neurosyphilis; antibody tests specific for *Treponema pallidum* may prove to be more sensitive. Neurosyphilis is classically treated with IV penicillin.

D. HIV itself can cause meningitis, particularly during the seroconversion syndrome of acute HIV and in late-stage disease. It is also a risk factor for opportunistic infections of the CNS, such as *Cryptococcus* (see Central Nervous System Infection in the Patient with HIV). In patients with risk factors for HIV, aseptic meningitis should trigger testing for acute HIV by serum enzyme-linked immunosorbent assay (ELISA) and serum polymerase chain reaction (PCR). CSF PCR for HIV is also available.

E. HSV is a very common cause of aseptic meningitis. It is usually caused by HSV-2. During the primary episode, most patients will also have active or very recent genital lesions. The diagnosis can be confirmed by PCR on CSF.

F. A travel history may reveal risk factors for tuberculosis, coccidiomycosis, and parasites: all possible causes of aseptic meningitis. Special culture media are required to isolate mycobacteria and fungi from the CSF.

Elicit any history of exposure to ticks—which may carry Lyme disease, ehrlichiosis, or Rocky Mountain spotted fever—and to mosquitoes—vectors for viruses such as West Nile, St. Louis, Eastern Equine, and Western and California encephalitides. A history of possible exposure to rodents or their excreta can raise the index of suspicion for lymphocytic choriomeningitis virus and leptospirosis. If one of these is suspected, specific serology and in some cases CSF PCR testing can be obtained.

Enteroviruses (coxsackie A and B and echoviruses) are the most commonly identified cause of aseptic meningitis. The CSF, nasopharynx, and stool can be cultured for enterovirus. CSF PCR for enterovirus is also available.

Other viruses known to cause meningitis include influenza; parainfluenza type 3; mumps; measles; varicella-zoster (primary infection or secondary outbreak); Epstein-Barr; cytomegalovirus; adenoviruses; and human herpes virus types 6, 7, and 8. Serology and in some cases CSF PCR may be useful in making these diagnoses.

Aseptic meningitis has been less frequently associated with a large number of other infectious agents, including *Mycoplasma* spp., *Legionella* spp., Whipple's disease, and *Bartonella henselae* (cat scratch disease).

G. Noninfectious causes of meningitis, such as subarachnoid hemorrhage, carcinomatous meningitis, and rheumatologic causes (e.g., systemic lupus erythematosus, Behçet's disease, vasculitis, and sarcoidosis), should be considered in the appropriate settings. Meningeal inflammation has been reported with the use of NSAIDs, some antibiotics, IV immune globulin, and some cancer therapies.

References

Connolly KJ, Hammer SM. The acute aseptic meningitis syndrome. Infect Dis Clin North Am 1990;4(4):599–622.

de Gans J, van de Beek D, for the European Dexamethasone in Adulthood Bacterial Meningitis Study Investigators. Dexamethasone in adults with bacterial meningitis. N Engl J Med 2002;347(20):1549–1556.

Hasbun R, Abrahams J, Jekel J, et al. Computed tomography of the head before lumbar puncture in adults with suspected meningitis. N Engl J Med 2001;345(24):1727–1733.

Hildebrand J, Aoun M. Chronic meningitis: still a diagnostic challenge. J Neurol 2003;250(6):653–660.

Huang C, Morse D, Slater B, et al. Multiple-year experience in the diagnosis of viral central nervous system infections with a panel of polymerase chain reaction assays for detection of 11 viruses. Clin Infect Dis 2004;39:630–635.

Jolles S, Sewell WAC, Leighton C. Drug-induced aseptic meningitis: diagnosis and management. Drug Saf 2000;22(3):215–226.

Tunkel AR, Scheld WM. Acute meningitis. In Mandell GL, Bennett JE, Dolin R, eds. Principles and Practices of Infectious Diseases, 6th ed. Philadelphia: Elsevier, Churchill, Livingstone; 2005:1083–1126.

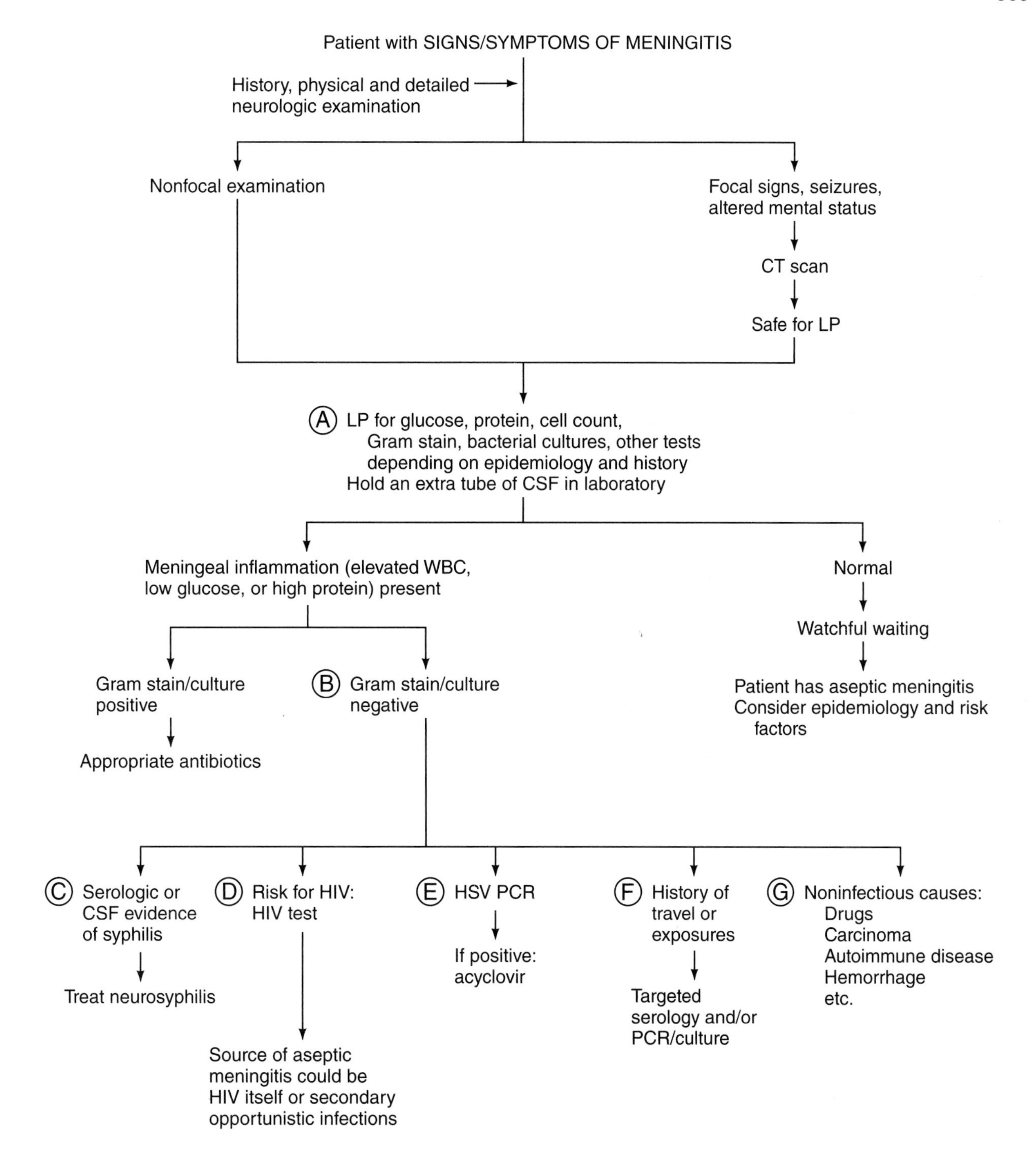

Patient with SIGNS/SYMPTOMS OF MENINGITIS
History, physical and detailed neurologic examination
Nonfocal examination
Focal signs, seizures, altered mental status
CT scan
Safe for LP
(A) LP for glucose, protein, cell count, Gram stain, bacterial cultures, other tests depending on epidemiology and history
Hold an extra tube of CSF in laboratory
Meningeal inflammation (elevated WBC, low glucose, or high protein) present
Normal
Watchful waiting
Patient has aseptic meningitis
Consider epidemiology and risk factors
Gram stain/culture positive
Appropriate antibiotics
(B) Gram stain/culture negative
(C) Serologic or CSF evidence of syphilis
Treat neurosyphilis
(D) Risk for HIV: HIV test
Source of aseptic meningitis could be HIV itself or secondary opportunistic infections
(E) HSV PCR
If positive: acyclovir
(F) History of travel or exposures
Targeted serology and/or PCR/culture
(G) Noninfectious causes:
Drugs
Carcinoma
Autoimmune disease
Hemorrhage
etc.

ENCEPHALITIS

Mohammed Asmal, MD, PhD

Encephalitis should be suspected in patients with acute or subacute presentations of altered levels of consciousness, focal neurologic deficits, seizures, or new psychiatric illness associated with fever and headache. Encephalitis, or meningoencephalitis, is most commonly caused by viral infection but also may be secondary to other infectious agents, malignancy, or autoimmune processes. The differential diagnosis includes isolated meningitis, toxic-metabolic encephalopathy, brain abscess or malignancy, vasculitis, and systemic infection.

A. Define all neurologic deficits, including presence of meningismus and their duration (acute, lasting hours to days, and subacute, present for weeks). Identify a past medical history of HIV or immunosuppression and travel, animal and insect exposure, sick contact, vaccine, and sexual history. List all medications and illicit drugs. In addition to a detailed neurologic examination, assess for papilledema and unusual rashes.

B. Evaluate for decompensated renal or liver failure, drug intoxication, or systemic infection. Although these findings may provide an alternative diagnosis, they do not preclude thorough evaluation for encephalitis. HIV testing should be performed for subacute presentations.

C. Obtain a CT scan of the head if there are focal neurologic abnormalities, papilledema, severely depressed levels of arousal, or seizures or if the patient is immunosuppressed. The CT results will help exclude brain edema and risk of herniation potentially requiring corticosteroids and neurosurgical consultation.

D. Perform lumbar puncture and send cerebrospinal fluid (CSF) for protein, glucose, cell count and differential, Gram stain and bacterial cultures, herpes simplex virus (HSV) types 1 and 2, and varicella-zoster virus polymerase chain reaction (VZV PCR). If the presentation is subacute or there is immunosuppression or HIV, obtain CSF fungal and acid-fast bacillus (AFB) stains and culture, VDRL and PCR for JC virus, human herpes virus (HHV) type 6, cytomegalovirus (CMV), and Epstein-Barr virus (EBV). Depending on the time of the year, exposures, and geographic location, testing is indicated for arboviruses (West Nile, Eastern and Western Equine, and St. Louis encephalitides), enteroviruses, or other pathogens (Table 1). These tests include

Table 1 **Infectious Causes of Encephalitis**

	Pathogen*	Testing
Clinical History		
Lack of Childhood Vaccines	Measles, mumps, polio	Measles, mumps serology
Travel:	Any tropics: Dengue [malaria]	Thick and thin blood smear to rule out malaria, dengue serum ELISA, and serum ELISA for specific arboviruses (acute and convalescent) and CSF PCR if available
1. Africa	1. West Nile [trypanosomiasis]	
2. Asia	2. Japanese encephalitis virus	
3. South America	3. Venezuelan equine encephalitis	
4. Europe	4. Tick-borne encephalitis	
5. North America	5. St. Louis, La Crosse (Midwest), Eastern and Western Equine, West Nile (throughout United States)	
Rodent exposure, transplant	LCMV	Serology
Animal bite, bats, transplant	Rabies	Blood and CSF serology, saliva PCR
Tick bite, woodland exposure	Colorado tick-bite fever [Lyme disease, Rocky Mountain spotted fever]	Serology for CTBF [Lyme ELISA and Western Blot, RMSF serology]
Season:		
1. Summer/fall	1. Enterovirus (coxsackie, echovirus), arbovirus (West Nile, St. Louis, Eastern/Western Equine)	1. CSF, stool and throat PCR and culture for enteroviruses; serum ELISA for arboviruses, and CSF PCR if available
2. Winter/spring	2. Measles, mumps, influenza	2. Serology for mumps and measles, and nasal washings for influenza
Preceding URI	Influenza, adenovirus, mycoplasma	Nasal washings for respiratory virus
Physical Finding		
Vesicular rash	HSV-1/2, varicella	Direct fluorescent antibody, culture
Parotitis, pancreatitis, orchitis	Mumps	Serology
Flaccid paralysis	West Nile	Serology and CSF PCR
Pneumonia	Mycoplasma, respiratory virus, [pneumococcus]	Mycoplasma throat and CSF PCR, Mycoplasma acute/convalescent serology Nasal washings for respiratory virus

*Infections that mimic are in brackets.

(Continued on page 312)

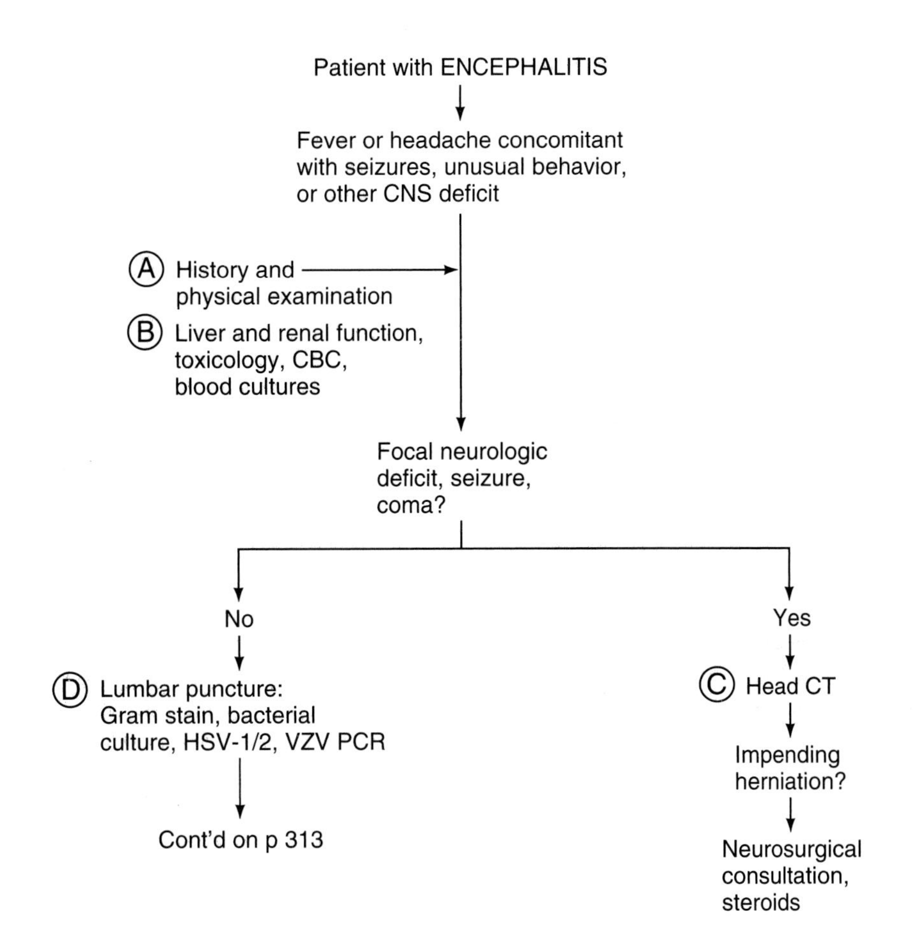
Patient with ENCEPHALITIS
Fever or headache concomitant with seizures, unusual behavior, or other CNS deficit
(A) History and physical examination
(B) Liver and renal function, toxicology, CBC, blood cultures
Focal neurologic deficit, seizure, coma?
No
(D) Lumbar puncture: Gram stain, bacterial culture, HSV-1/2, VZV PCR
Cont'd on p 313
Yes
(C) Head CT
Impending herniation?
Neurosurgical consultation, steroids

virus-specific IgM/IgG enzyme-linked immunosorbent assay (ELISA) of sera, and CSF PCR.

E. Start empiric IV acyclovir 10 mg/kg every 8 hours immediately after the lumbar puncture (adjusted for renal function). If the presentation is acute or includes meningismus, start therapy for bacterial meningitis. Although a low CSF glucose (<50 mg/dl), high CSF protein (>250 mg/dl), or a cell count >1000 with a neutrophilic predominance suggests bacterial meningitis, early viral encephalitis may present with a neutrophilic pleocytosis and early bacterial meningitis may show a lymphocytic predominance. A CSF WBC count of <5 argues against encephalitis, but if suspicion is high, repeat the lumbar puncture in 24–48 hours. If the lumbar puncture, Gram stain, or culture reveal organisms, tailor therapy accordingly. If CSF bacterial culture results are negative at 48 hours, stop antibiotics but continue acyclovir.

F. If no etiology is apparent from initial CSF stains, proceed to MRI of the brain. Leptomeningeal enhancement is a nonspecific finding in meningoencephalitis. Arboviral infection may cause diffuse parenchymal T2 hyperintensity or may center on the brainstem, as may *Listeria* or enteroviruses, whereas HSV often has a predilection for the temporal lobes. White matter–centric T2 hyperintensity often reflects HIV or JC virus infection, in contrast to the focal space-occupying lesions found in toxoplasmosis, abscesses, or malignancy. An EEG is useful in patients with seizures; temporal lobe activity suggests HSV or other herpes viruses. If no diagnosis is made after initial lumbar puncture and imaging, consider repeat lumbar puncture after 48 hours and send for HSV PCR and viral studies not obtained initially. Focal lesions on MRI warrant stereotactic brain biopsy if the patient does not respond to empiric therapy and the diagnosis is uncertain.

G. If CSF PCR is positive for HSV or VZV, continue acyclovir for 14–21 days. If other herpes family viruses are isolated, specific therapy should be initiated with the guidance of an infectious disease specialist. If MRI findings suggest PML or HIV encephalopathy in a patient with HIV, start antiretroviral therapy. For most other causes of viral encephalitis, treatment is supportive, although an experimental protocol has been successful for rabies. If no etiology is evident but the clinical syndrome is highly suggestive of encephalitis, continue acyclovir for presumptive HSV for 14–21 days, unless two separate CSF HSV PCR results 48 hours apart are negative.

H. If an exhaustive infectious evaluation is negative, or if the patient has a past medical history of malignancy, vasculitis, or connective tissue disorder, evaluate for noninfectious etiologies for encephalitis.

References

Centers for Disease Control and Prevention. Information on arboviral encephalitides. Available at: www.cdc.gov/ncidod/dvbid/arbor/arbdet.htm. Accessed June 12, 2009.

Foerster BR, Thurnher MM, Malani PN, et al. Intracranial infections: clinical and imaging characteristics. Acta Radiol 2007;48:875–893.

Mandell G, Bennett J, Dolin R, eds. Principles and Practice of Infectious Diseases, 6th ed. Philadelphia: Elsevier, 2007.

Solomon T, Hart I, Beeching NK. Viral encephalitis: a clinician's guide. Pract Neurol 2007;7:288–305.

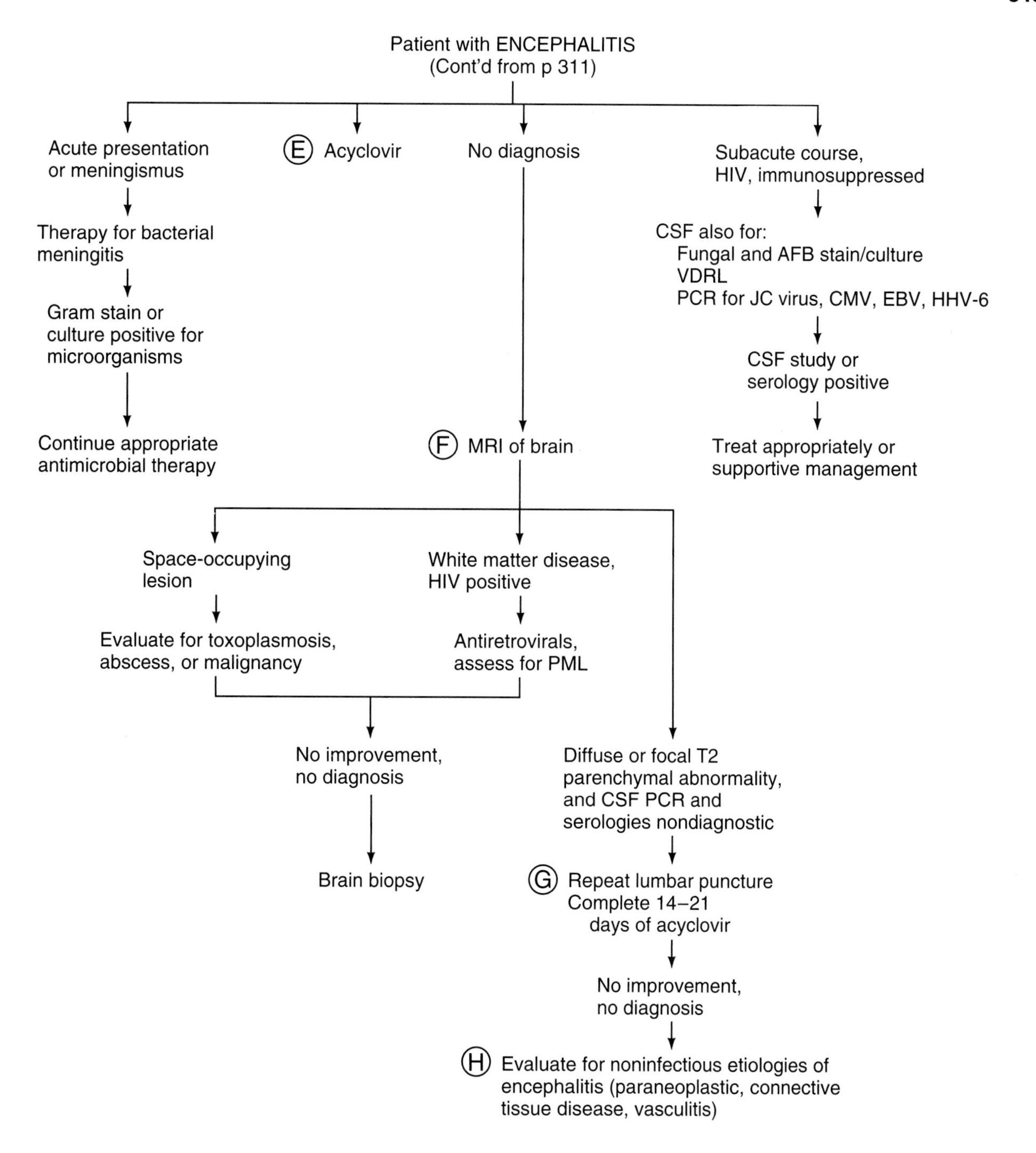
Patient with ENCEPHALITIS
(Cont'd from p 311)
Acute presentation or meningismus
Therapy for bacterial meningitis
Gram stain or culture positive for microorganisms
Continue appropriate antimicrobial therapy
E Acyclovir
No diagnosis
F MRI of brain
Space-occupying lesion
Evaluate for toxoplasmosis, abscess, or malignancy
White matter disease, HIV positive
Antiretrovirals, assess for PML
No improvement, no diagnosis
Brain biopsy
Diffuse or focal T2 parenchymal abnormality, and CSF PCR and serologies nondiagnostic
G Repeat lumbar puncture
Complete 14–21 days of acyclovir
No improvement, no diagnosis
H Evaluate for noninfectious etiologies of encephalitis (paraneoplastic, connective tissue disease, vasculitis)
Subacute course, HIV, immunosuppressed
CSF also for:
Fungal and AFB stain/culture
VDRL
PCR for JC virus, CMV, EBV, HHV-6
CSF study or serology positive
Treat appropriately or supportive management

SEXUALLY TRANSMITTED DISEASES

Bisola Ojikutu, MD, MPH

Sexually transmitted diseases (STDs) are a major cause of morbidity and a significant public health issue both domestically and internationally. Over 15 million cases of STDs are reported annually in the United States alone. These infections can have a devastating impact on the health of individual patients. They also cause adverse social and economic sequelae.

Health care providers play a critical role in diagnosis and treatment of STDs. This chapter will provide a basic overview of some of the more common STDs. HIV infection will be discussed in detail in subsequent chapters.

A. Comprehensive initial evaluation of the patient presenting for treatment or screening for STDs must include the following:
   1. Detailed sexual history (number of sexual partners; date of most recent sexual encounter, including oral and anal sex; record of condom use; use of other forms of contraception; and gender of partners)
   2. Past history of STDs
   3. History of treatment for STDs
   4. Response to treatment
   5. Current complaint (genital lesions, pruritus, abdominal pain, presence of discharge, odor and color of discharge if present, vaginal soreness, dyspareunia, dysuria, fever)
   6. Duration of these complaints
   7. Examination (skin, lymph nodes, mouth and throat, abdomen, external genitalia, speculum examination, evaluation of the rectum and perirectal region

   Questions regarding sexual history should be framed in an open-ended, nonjudgmental fashion. Emphasis should be placed on counseling regarding safer sexual practices.

B. Human papillomavirus (HPV) (particularly types 16, 18, 31, 33, 35, or 45) has been strongly associated with the development of cervical dysplasia and cervical cancer.

C. Partners of patients with suspected or proven chlamydial, gonococcal, or *Trichomonas* infection should be treated to prevent recurrence.

D. All patients who present for STD screening and treatment should be offered HIV testing. Treatment of STDs may reduce the risk of HIV transmission.

E. Male urethritis is most commonly caused by *Neisseria gonorrhoeae*. The most common cause of nongonococcal urethritis is infection with *Chlamydia trachomatis*. Up to 30% of men with urethritis are infected with both pathogens.
   1. Gonococcal urethritis presents asymptomatically in 5% of cases. Evaluation should include urethral smear. More than 4 WBCs per oil immersion field is suggestive but not diagnostic of infection. Urethral smear may also reveal intracellular gram-negative diplococci consistent with gonococcus. Positive leukocyte esterase or >10 WBCs per high-power field on a first-voided urine sample is also suggestive of infection. Diagnosis should be confirmed by culture of urethral discharge. Rapid assays utilizing nucleic acid amplification can be obtained on a urine sample and are also widely used to confirm diagnosis.
   2. Males infected with chlamydial urethritis are often asymptomatic. Both >4 WBCs per oil immersion field and pyuria are suggestive of infection. Diagnosis can be confirmed by rapid nucleic acid amplification on urethral swab or urine. If diagnosis cannot be confirmed, then patients with urethritis should be treated for both gonorrhea and chlamydial infection given the high rate of co-infection. Yearly screening is advocated for sexually active young males. Chlamydia is the most common cause of epididymitis (swollen, red, and tender scrotum) in males <35 years.
   3. Other causes of nongonococcal urethritis are *Mycoplasma genitalium, Ureaplasma urealyticum,* and *Trichomonas vaginalis.*

F. Cervicitis may present with discharge, vaginal pruritus, dyspareunia, and burning. Both *N. gonorrhoeae* and *C. trachomatis* infections are common causes of cervicitis. On speculum examination mucopurulent discharge may be noted on the endocervical canal. The majority of women (>70%) who are infected with *Chlamydia* are asymptomatic. Therefore, the CDC recommends annual screening for all sexually active women regardless of symptoms. Complications of infection include pelvic inflammatory disease/salpingitis, ectopic pregnancy, and infertility. Chlamydia can also cause urethritis in women. Signs of urethritis include urethral discharge, meatal redness, and swelling. Diagnosis of gonococcal cervicitis is by culture, DNA probe, or amplification techniques. Diagnosis of chlamydial cervicitis is accomplished by direct monoclonal antibody staining (DFA), ELISA, DNA probes or amplification techniques (polymerase chain reaction or ligase chain reaction). Use of first-catch urine specimens is a noninvasive means of diagnosing chlamydial and gonococcal infections.

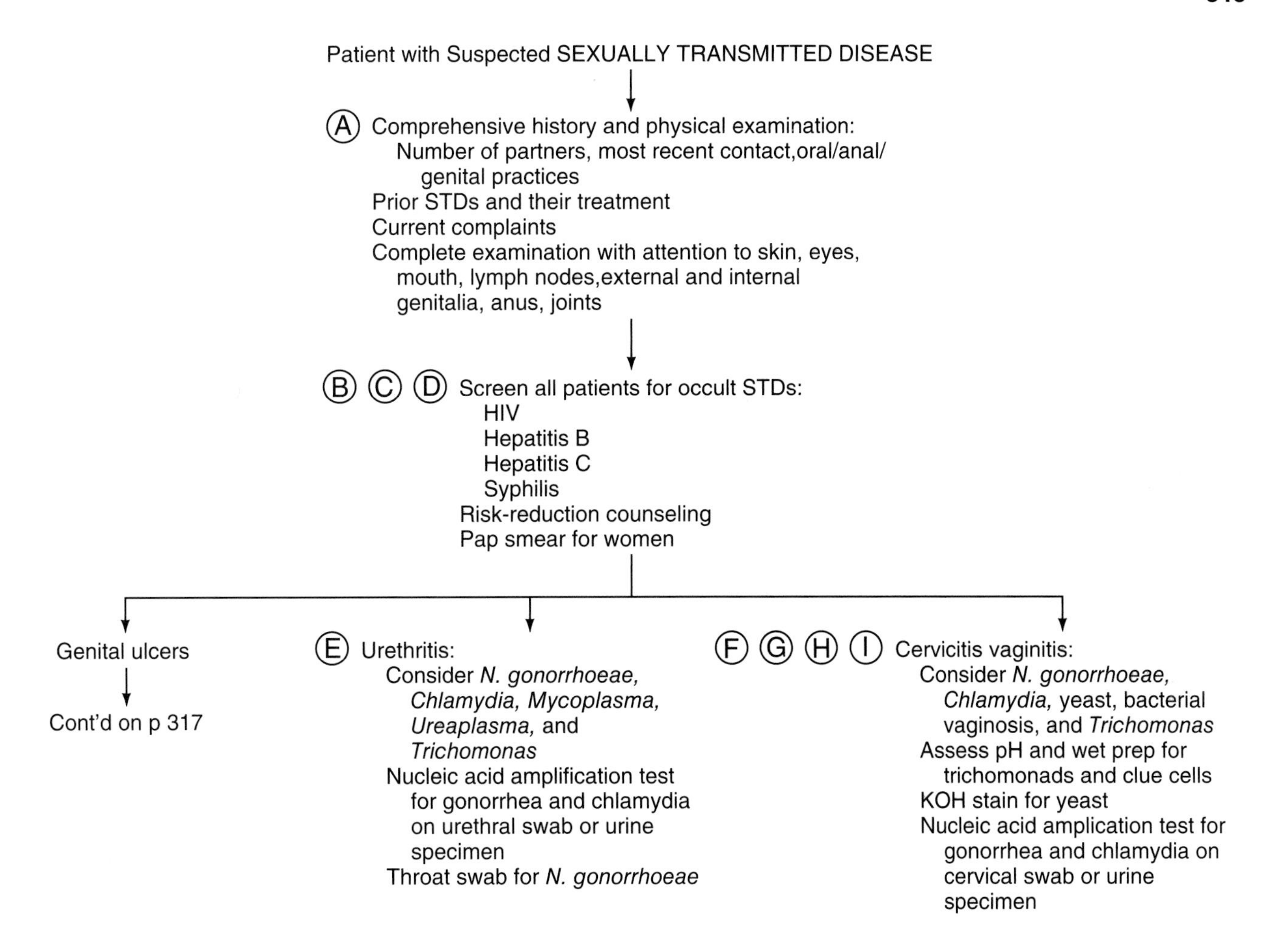

G. Health care providers should be aware that infection with *N. gonorrhoeae* or *C. trachomatis* can cause mucopurulent conjunctivitis and pharyngitis. Sexually active patients with conjunctivitis should be evaluated for these infections. Throat swabs should be performed on all patients who present for STD screening.

H. Bacterial vaginosis is caused by a polymicrobial superficial vaginal infection involving a loss of normal lactobacilli and an overgrowth of anaerobes. This infection is characterized by *clue cells,* which are epithelial cells coated with tiny coccobacillary forms.

I. Vaginal pH is usually >4.5 in cases of *Trichomonas* infection. An abundance of leukocytes and motile, flagellated trichomonads are noted on wet preparation of vaginal secretions.

(Continued on page 316)

J. There are numerous infectious and noninfectious causes of genital ulcers, including (but not limited to) herpes simplex, *Treponema pallidum*, lymphogranuloma venereum (LGV), granuloma inguinale, HIV, *Haemophilus ducreyi*, Behçet's disease, and fixed drug eruptions. The physical examination is insensitive in identifying the underlying cause of genital ulcerations; therefore diagnostic testing is imperative.

K. Genital herpes is most commonly caused by herpes simplex virus (HSV) II, although an increased incidence of genital HSV I has been noted. The characteristic finding of multiple vesicles on an erythematous base may or may not be present on clinical examination. The gold standard for diagnosis is isolation of the virus in tissue culture. A positive Tzanck preparation revealing characteristic giant cells or intranuclear inclusions can also be used. DFA can distinguish between HSV I and HSV II. Serologic tests can be useful if one obtains acute and convalescent serum. A rise in antibody titer may be seen during recurrent infection.

L. The gold standard for the diagnosis of syphilis is darkfield examination (DFE). Samples can be taken from mucocutaneous lesions (except lesions from the oropharynx) or lymph nodes. Three consecutive DFEs are required before a lesion can be considered to be negative. Nontreponemal tests (VDRL and rapid plasma reagent) are used for screening and for monitoring of response to therapy. Specific treponemal tests (e.g., FTA-abs) detect antibody against *T. pallidum* and should be used for confirmation of a positive nontreponemal test. In most patients, the specific treponemal tests remain positive for life. False-negative tests are found in HIV-positive patients, particularly when the patient's CD4 count is <200. PCR testing has also been developed but is available only on a limited basis. Neurosyphilis should be ruled out in patients with late latent syphilis (>1 year from primary infection) by clinical examination. Lumbar puncture should be considered when symptoms or examination are suggestive of neurosyphilis.

M. Syphilitic chancres usually present as solitary, painless lesions with a smooth base and raised borders. However, chancres can sometimes be painful, particularly if secondarily infected. In patients with HIV co-infection, multiple chancres may occur. The external genitalia is most commonly involved. The perianal area, mouth, and anal canal may also be involved in women and in homosexual men.

N. Treatment of primary, secondary, or syphilis of less than a year's duration is benzathine penicillin G 2.4 million U IM × 1 dose. Patients allergic to penicillin should be given doxycycline 100 mg PO bid × 2 weeks. Pregnant patients who are allergic to penicillin should be skin tested, and desensitization to penicillin should be undertaken. Latent syphilis is treated with benzathine penicillin G 2.4 million U IM weekly for 3 weeks. Neurosyphilis is treated with aqueous crystalline penicillin G 24 million U IV daily × 10–14 days followed by penicillin G 2.4 million U IM weekly × 3 weeks. Partner notification and screening is critical. Patients should be offered HIV testing.

O. A single complement fixation titer of >1:64 or a fourfold rise in titer supports the diagnosis of lymphogranuloma venereum. Microimmunofluorescence for the L-type serovar is sensitive and specific. A titer of >1:512 is diagnostic. Definitive diagnosis can be made by aspiration of material from a bubo with growth in cell culture.

P. Granuloma inguinale (caused by *Calymmatobacterium granulomatis*) is a chronic, indolent, ulcerative infection of the skin and lymphatics. Although it is very rare in the United States (<100 cases per year), infection still occurs in tropical regions. Diagnosis is made by the finding of intracellular Donovan bodies (oval rod-shaped organisms) in mononuclear cells.

Q. The genital ulceration caused by *Haemophilis ducreyi* (chancroid) is typically exquisitely painful. Diagnosis is made by culture on special nutrient media. Gram stain may show characteristic "school of fish" gram-negative coccobacilli.

References

Braverman PK. Sexually transmitted diseases in adolescents. Med Clinics North Am 2000;84:869–889.

Emmert D, Kircher J. Sexually transmitted diseases in women. Postgrad Med 2000;107(1):55–65. Available online at www.postgradmed.com/index.php?art=pgm_01_2000?article=815.

Mandell GL, Bennett JE, Dolin R, eds. Principles and Practice of Infectious Diseases, 6th ed. Philadelphia: Churchill Livingstone, 2005.

Workowski KA, Levine WC, Levine WC. U.S. Centers for Disease Control and Prevention guidelines for the treatment of sexually transmitted diseases, an opportunity to unify clinical and public health practice. Ann Intern Med 2002;137:255–262.

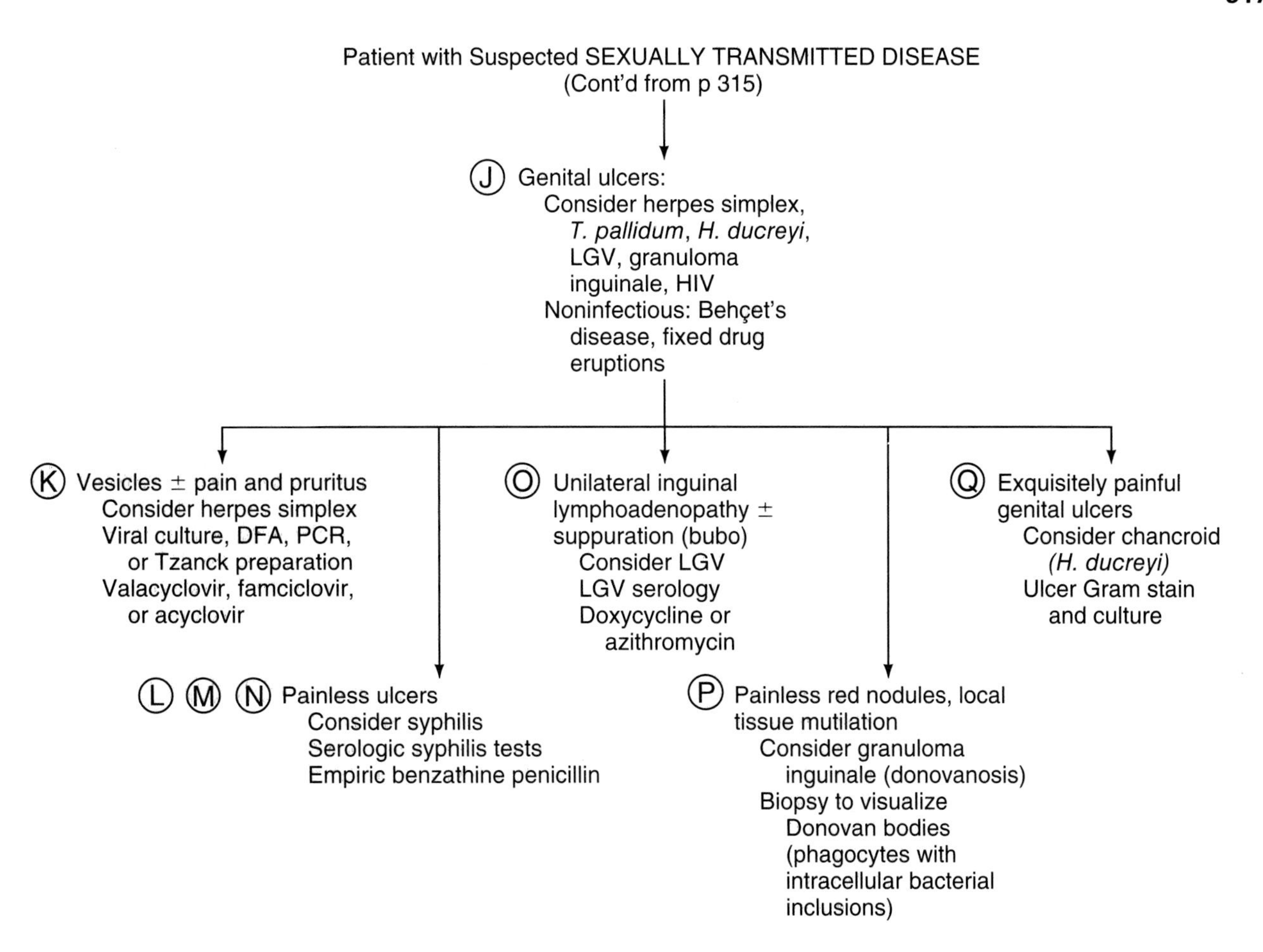
Patient with Suspected SEXUALLY TRANSMITTED DISEASE
(Cont'd from p 315)
(J) Genital ulcers:
Consider herpes simplex, T. pallidum, H. ducreyi, LGV, granuloma inguinale, HIV
Noninfectious: Behçet's disease, fixed drug eruptions
(K) Vesicles ± pain and pruritus
Consider herpes simplex
Viral culture, DFA, PCR, or Tzanck preparation
Valacyclovir, famciclovir, or acyclovir
(L) (M) (N) Painless ulcers
Consider syphilis
Serologic syphilis tests
Empiric benzathine penicillin
(O) Unilateral inguinal lymphoadenopathy ± suppuration (bubo)
Consider LGV
LGV serology
Doxycycline or azithromycin
(P) Painless red nodules, local tissue mutilation
Consider granuloma inguinale (donovanosis)
Biopsy to visualize Donovan bodies (phagocytes with intracellular bacterial inclusions)
(Q) Exquisitely painful genital ulcers
Consider chancroid (H. ducreyi)
Ulcer Gram stain and culture

APPROACH TO THE NEWLY DIAGNOSED HIV-POSITIVE PATIENT

Bisola Ojikutu, MD, MPH

Since the beginning of the AIDS epidemic in the United States approximately 1.6 million patients have been diagnosed with HIV. For over a decade the number of new infections reported annually has remained stable at 40,000 per year. However, the incidence of infection has risen in certain populations, including men who have sex with men, Blacks, Hispanics, and women. Health care practitioners must remain acutely aware of the possibility of new HIV infection and take steps to counsel and test their patients appropriately.

A. Pretest and posttest counseling are critical steps in the evaluation for HIV infection. Pretest counseling should include a description of the blood test, limitations of the test, discussion of high-risk behaviors, risk-reduction counseling, differences between HIV and AIDS, implications of a positive test, and available interventions and treatments. When a test result is obtained, counseling should continue. If the patient's test is positive, then issues such as stigma and disclosure should be discussed. Patients should be advised to inform previous sexual partners of their HIV status. Counseling must also include discussion of adherence to safe sexual practices, use of condoms, avoidance of drugs that disinhibit behavior, and arrangements for follow-up medical care. Patients should also be referred to community resources for supportive counseling.

B. Diagnosis of chronic HIV infection should be made using standard enzyme-linked immunosorbent assay (ELISA) tests. If a patient has HIV infection and is beyond the "window period" (the time after infection has occurred but before evidence of HIV infection is detectable—approximately 6 weeks), then the ELISA test should be obtained. The sensitivity and specificity of this test are estimated to be >98%. If the test is positive, it should be confirmed with a Western Blot, which detects the presence of serologic reactivity to individual viral antigens. The specificity of this test is >99%. Rapid HIV antibody testing has also been approved by the FDA. Confirmatory Western blot testing is still required when rapid-testing kits are used.

C. A detailed history should be obtained. Approximate time and source of infection should be obtained. Particular focus should be placed on risk of co-infection with hepatitis B or C; current sexual activity; substance abuse history; diagnosis and treatment of sexually transmitted diseases (STDs); past medical history of opportunistic infections, including tuberculosis and purified protein derivative (PPD) status; current medications, including herbal supplements; family history of cardiovascular disease and diabetes; most recent Pap smear results (for women); and history of immunizations. Past history of travel to areas endemic for histoplasmosis and coccidiomycosis may also be relevant.

D. An HIV-focused review of systems is critical. Review of systems should include fatigue, weight loss, anorexia, depression, fever, chills, night sweats, adenopathy, skin rash or bruising, headaches, sinus or ear pain, visual changes, oral sores, odynophagia, dysphagia, shortness of breath, dyspnea on exertion, cough, abdominal pain, diarrhea, genital-rectal sores or pain, arthritis, muscle weakness, forgetfulness, and lack of coordination.

E. A complete physical examination for the newly diagnosed HIV positive patient must include a funduscopic examination (risk of cytomegalovirus (CMV) infection in patients with CD4 <50 cells/mm^3), evaluation of the oropharynx for oral candidiasis or oral hairy leukoplakia, skin, lymph nodes, genital and anal region, and neurologic examination.

F. Table 1 provides a list of the basic laboratory studies that should be obtained at the initial visit.

Table 1 Baseline Laboratory Assessment

- CD4 cell count
- Plasma HIV RNA
- CBC with differential
- Chemistry profile, transaminases, BUN/creatinine, rapid plasma reagent or VDRL
- PPD (unless a reliable history of prior tuberculosis or positive skin test can be obtained)
- Serologies for *Toxoplasma gondii*, hepatitis A, B, and C
- Pap smear for women
- G6PD (assessment of risk for hemolysis with receipt of antioxidant drugs like dapsone)—case dependent
- Fasting blood glucose and serum lipids
- Resistance testing should be considered given the risk for acquisition of drug-resistant virus

G6PD, Glucose-6 phosphate dehydrogenase.

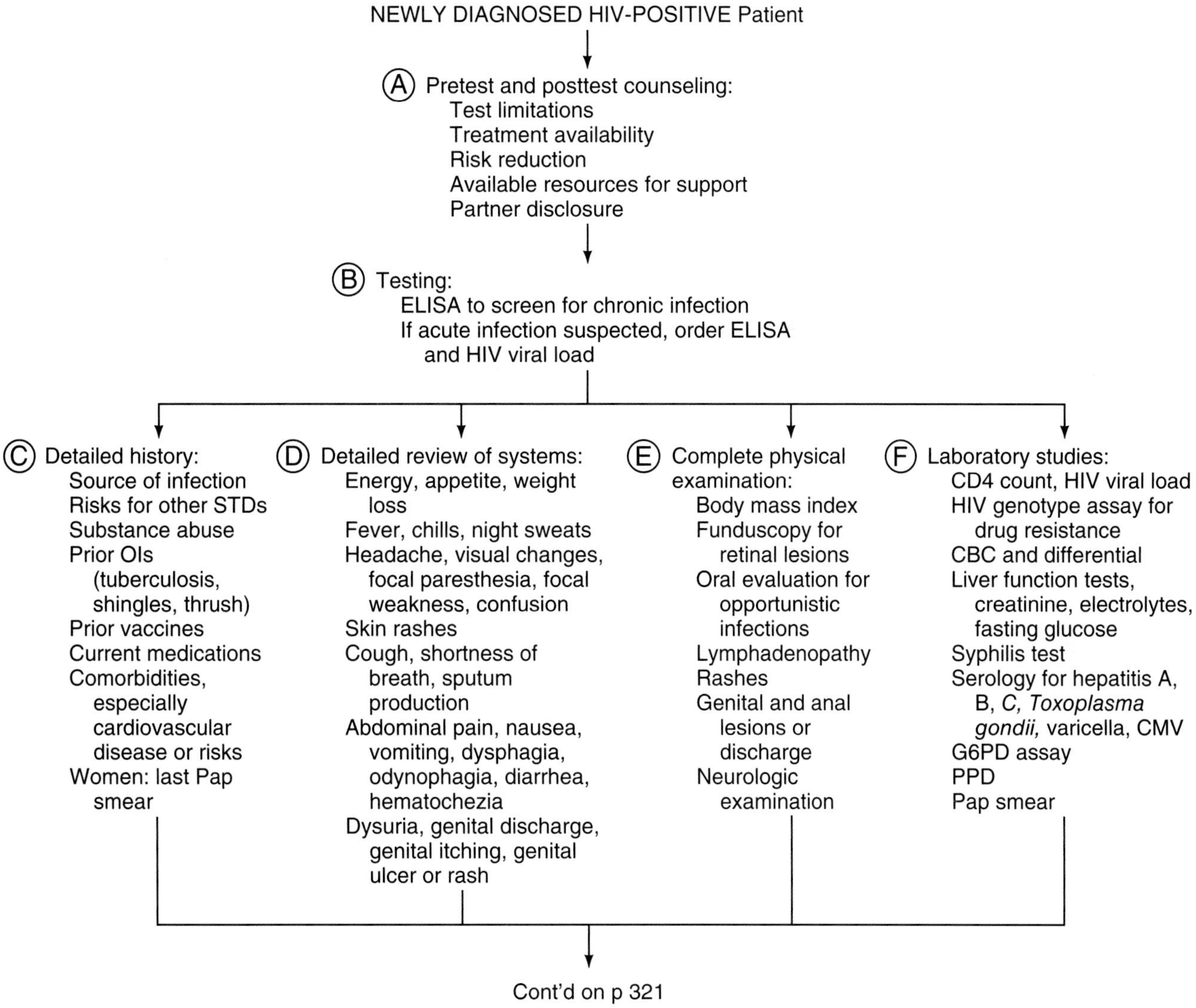

NEWLY DIAGNOSED HIV-POSITIVE Patient

↓

(A) Pretest and posttest counseling:
- Test limitations
- Treatment availability
- Risk reduction
- Available resources for support
- Partner disclosure

↓

(B) Testing:
- ELISA to screen for chronic infection
- If acute infection suspected, order ELISA and HIV viral load

↓

(C) Detailed history:
- Source of infection
- Risks for other STDs
- Substance abuse
- Prior OIs (tuberculosis, shingles, thrush)
- Prior vaccines
- Current medications
- Comorbidities, especially cardiovascular disease or risks
- Women: last Pap smear

(D) Detailed review of systems:
- Energy, appetite, weight loss
- Fever, chills, night sweats
- Headache, visual changes, focal paresthesia, focal weakness, confusion
- Skin rashes
- Cough, shortness of breath, sputum production
- Abdominal pain, nausea, vomiting, dysphagia, odynophagia, diarrhea, hematochezia
- Dysuria, genital discharge, genital itching, genital ulcer or rash

(E) Complete physical examination:
- Body mass index
- Funduscopy for retinal lesions
- Oral evaluation for opportunistic infections
- Lymphadenopathy
- Rashes
- Genital and anal lesions or discharge
- Neurologic examination

(F) Laboratory studies:
- CD4 count, HIV viral load
- HIV genotype assay for drug resistance
- CBC and differential
- Liver function tests, creatinine, electrolytes, fasting glucose
- Syphilis test
- Serology for hepatitis A, B, C, *Toxoplasma gondii,* varicella, CMV
- G6PD assay
- PPD
- Pap smear

↓

Cont'd on p 321

G. The CD4 count correlates well with immune function and is used to gauge the risk for disease progression, development of opportunistic infections (OIs) and the need for OI prophylaxis. Antiretroviral therapy is recommended for all patients with history of an AIDS-defining illness regardless of CD4 count. Therapy is also recommended for asymptomatic patients with CD4 count <200 cells/mm^3. Asymptomatic patients with CD4 counts of 201–350 cells/mm^3 should be offered treatment. For asymptomatic patients with CD4 counts >350 cells/mm^3 and HIV RNA >100,000 copies/ml, most experienced clinicians defer therapy but some clinicians may consider initiating treatment. Therapy should be deferred for patients with CD4 counts >350 cells/mm^3 and plasma HIV RNA <100,000 copies/ml. Patients who are symptom free and have a CD4 count >350 cells/mm^3 and viral load <100,000 copies/ml should be monitored every 3 months for disease progression.

H. Plasma HIV-1 RNA quantification is a factor in determining when to initiate treatment and is critical when assessing response to therapy. The minimal change in viral load considered to be statistically significant is a threefold, or a 0.5 $\log_{10}$ copies/ml, change. The goal of antiretroviral therapy is a viral load below the level of detection (<50 copies/ml using the Amplicor assay). Prior to the initiation of therapy viral load should be measured. Viral load measurement should be repeated at 2–8 weeks following treatment initiation to assess response. There should be a decrease of at least 1.0 $\log_{10}$ copies/ml. Viral load reduction to below the limits of assay detection in a treatment-naive patient should occur within the first 4–6 months of therapy. Once a patient is on standard antiretroviral treatment, viral load testing should be repeated every 3–4 months.

The goal of antiretroviral therapy is to maximally inhibit viral replication and minimize the development of resistant strains of HIV. There are currently four classes of antiretroviral medications: nucleoside/nucleotide reverse transcriptase inhibitors, nonnucleoside reverse transcriptase inhibitors (NNRTIs), protease inhibitors (PI), and entry inhibitors. A summary of preferred initial regimens is found in Table 2.

I. Despite the improving efficacy of antiretroviral therapy, appropriate prophylaxis against opportunistic infection remains a clinical imperative in the care of persons with HIV infection. Prophylaxis against mycobacterium tuberculosis, *Pneumocystis* pneumonia, *Toxoplasma gondii, Mycobacterium avium* complex, and varicella virus are recommended as standard of care (Table 3).

J. Recommended immunizations for HIV positive patients are outlined in Table 4.

Table 2 **Selected Recommended Antiretroviral Therapy Regimens**

Preferred

Efavirenz + (lamivudine or emtricitabine) + (zidovudine or tenofovir)
Lopinavir/ritonavir (coformulation) + (lamivudine or emtricitabine) + zidovudine

Alternative Regimens

Efavirenz + (lamivudine or emtricitabine) + (abacavir or didanosine or stavudine)
Nevirapine + (lamivudine or emtricitabine) + (zidovudine or stavudine or didanosine or abacavir or tenofovir)
- Only administer nevirapine-based regimens to women with CD4 counts <250 cells/mm^3 and men with CD4 counts <400 cells/mm^3

Atazanavir + (lamivudine or emtricitabine) + (zidovudine or stavudine or abacavir or didanosine) or (tenofovir + ritonavir)
Lopinavir/ritonavir + (lamivudine or emtricitabine) + (zidovudine or stavudine or abacavir or tenofovir or didanosine)
Fosamprenavir/ritonavir + (lamivudine or emtricitabine) + (zidovudine or stavudine or abacavir or tenofovir or didanosine)
Fosamprenavir/ritonavir + (lamivudine or emtricitabine) + (zidovudine or stavudine or abacavir or tenofovir or didanosine)
Indinavir/ritonavir + (lamivudine or emtricitabine) + (zidovudine or stavudine or abacavir or tenofovir or didanosine)
Abacavir + zidovudine + lamivudine
- Only when a preferred or alternative NNRTI or PI-based regimen cannot or should not be used

Table 3 **Prophylaxis for Opportunistic Infections**

Organism	Indication	Preferred Prophylactic Regimen
Pneumocystis pneumonia	CD4 count <200 cells/mm^3 or history of oral candidiasis	Trimethoprim-sulfamethoxazole (DS QD, SS QD, DS 3×/wk)
Toxoplasmosis	CD4 count <100 cells/mm^3 and *Toxoplasma gondii* IgG positive	Trimethoprim-sulfamethoxazole 1 DS QD or 1 SS QD
Mycobacterium tuberculosis	Tuberculin skin test > 5 mm induration and active tuberculosis has been excluded	INH 300 mg PO QD × 9–12 mo All persons with HIV exposed to active tuberculosis should receive prophylactic therapy regardless of skin testing results
Mycobacterium avium complex	CD4 <50 cells/mm^3	Azithromycin 1200 mg PO qwk or clarithromycin 500 mg PO bid
Varicella virus	Significant exposure to chicken pox with no history or zoster with no history	Varicella-zoster immune globulin within 96 hr of exposure

NEWLY DIAGNOSED HIV-POSITIVE Patient
(Cont'd from p 319)

↓

(G) Integrate history, physical examination, and laboratory tests to determine:
- Strength of immune system
- Possible presence of active opportunistic infections
- Need for active treatment against opportunistic infections, prohylaxis, and/or antiretroviral therapy (see below)

↓

(H) Antiretroviral treatment:
- Decision to treat based on clinical status, history of opportunistic infections, CD4 counts, and viral load
- Treatment thresholds and recommended agents change frequently
- Refer patient to an HIV specialist or refer to www.aidsinfo.nih.gov for the latest recommendations

↓

Monitoring:
- Repeat CD4 count and viral load 2–8 wk following treatment initiation
- Repeat testing every 3–4 mo

↓

(I) Prophylaxis for opportunistic infections:
- Contingent upon CD4 count and prior infections
- See Table 3 for details

↓

(J) Immunizations:
- Pneumococcal vaccine (often deferred until CD4 count >200 cells/mm^3)
- Hepatitis A (for patients who practice anal intercourse or international travelers) contingent upon CD4 count and prior infections
- Hepatitis B
- Tetanus, diphtheria, and acellular pertussis boosters
- Influenza (yearly)

Table 4 **Immunizations for HIV-Infected Adults**

- Pneumococcal vaccination
- Influenza vaccination (yearly)
- Hepatitis B
- Hepatitis A (particularly MSM patients and those wanting to travel to endemic areas)
- Diphtheria and tetanus boosters (as per protocol in non-HIV infected patients)

With the exception of influenza vaccine, which is given yearly, vaccines should be given early in the course of HIV infection if possible to increase the likelihood of adequate responses

References

Guidelines for the use of antiretroviral agents in HIV-1-infected adults and adolescents, Panel on Clinical Practices for Treatment of HIV Infection convened by the Department of Health and Human Services, October 2006.

Guidelines for preventing opportunistic infections among HIV-infected persons—2002. MMWR 2002;51(RR08):1–46.

Hammer S. Management of newly diagnosed HIV infection. N Engl J Med 2005;353(16):1702–1710.

Mandell GL, Bennett JE, Dolin R, eds. Principles and Practice of Infectious Diseases, ed 6. Philadelphia: Churchill Livingstone, 2005.

RESPIRATORY SYMPTOMS IN HIV-INFECTED PATIENTS

John J. W. Fangman, MD

A. **Risk assessment:** Respiratory complaints are among the most common reasons HIV-positive persons seek medical care and can be the sentinel event that leads to a new diagnosis of HIV. Evaluation of pulmonary symptoms in HIV-positive persons should begin with an assessment of the patient's level of immunosuppression. Although it is widely recognized that the risk of opportunistic pulmonary infections such as *Pneumocystis jiroveci* pneumonia (PCP) is greatest in persons with a CD4 count ≤200 cells/mm^3, the risk is also increased in patients with a CD4/CD8 ratio of ≤14% and in those with a previous history of other opportunistic infections. Clues to advanced immunosuppression in persons whose CD4 count is not immediately available include a history of weight loss, thrush, or marked lymphopenia. Use o at helps to focus the evaluation of HIV-infected persons with respiratory complaints. PCP is rare in persons taking trimethoprim/sulfamethoxazole (TMP/SMX) prophylaxis. Likewise, rates of typical community-acquired bacterial pneumonias as well as unusual causes of pneumonia such as *Nocardia* are less common in those taking TMP/SMX prophylaxis. Use of second-line PCP prophylaxis such as dapsone, atovaquone, and aerosolized pentamidine provide incomplete protection against PCP compared to TMP/SMX and may alter the presentation of opportunistic infections (e.g., upper lobe PCP with aerosolized pentamidine). Unlike TMP/SMX, second-line prophylaxis does not provide protection against other common respiratory pathogens such as *Streptococcus pneumoniae* and *Haemophilus influenzae*.

Given the increased rates of infection with *Mycobacterium tuberculosis* in HIV-infected persons and the important public health challenges co-infection presents, it is important to consider the possibility of active tuberculosis (TB) in persons with HIV who present with respiratory complaints. The pulmonary manifestations of TB are often atypical in persons with HIV, especially those with advanced AIDS. Persons at high risk for TB include those with suggestive radiographic findings (especially cavitary disease), persons with a history of positive purified protein derivative (PPD) tests who did not receive treatment for latent TB infection, individuals from parts of the world where TB is highly endemic, and those at high risk for exposure to TB (history of contact with person with active TB, homelessness, or incarceration). HIV-infected persons suspected of having TB should be placed in respiratory isolation until the diagnosis can be confirmed and effectively treated or an alternative diagnosis ascertained.

B. **Chest radiography:** Although generally not diagnostic, the radiographic pattern of infiltrates can suggest likely etiologies of infection.

Diffuse interstitial infiltrates are common in persons with PCP, as are viral pneumonias (community-acquired such as influenza or more rarely opportunistic infections such as cytomegalovirus), fungal infections (especially endemic fungi), *Toxoplasma gondii,* and TB (especially in persons with advanced AIDS).

Lobar consolidation is more common in community-acquired bacterial pneumonia (*S. pneumoniae* and *H. influenzae*), TB (with higher CD4 counts), and *Legionella pneumophilia*.

Cavitary lesions should prompt consideration of TB; however, bacterial pathogens such as *Staphylococcus aureus*, *Pseudomonas aeruginosa, Rhodococcus equi*, *Nocardia*, and *Mycobacterium avium* complex can also produce cavitary lesions. PCP and fungi (especially *Cryptococcus neoformans*, *Aspergillus*, and *Histoplasma capsulatum*) may also cavitate. Pleural effusions are uncommon in PCP and should prompt consideration of TB or a noninfectious process such as heart failure or lymphoma. A normal chest x-ray (CXR) does not exclude opportunistic pulmonary infections, because both PCP and TB can be seen in up to 10% of persons with a normal CXR.

Although pulmonary infiltrates in persons with HIV are often due to opportunistic infections, such infections are not the only causes of radiographic abnormalities in HIV-infected patients. Noninfectious causes of CXR abnormalities associated with HIV infection include drug reactions (diffuse infiltrates associated with abacavir hypersensitivity), lymphocytic interstitial pneumonitis (diffuse infiltrates seen most commonly in children and older women), Kaposi's sarcoma (peribronchial and nodular lesions), primary pulmonary hypertension (large pulmonary arteries), and malignancies such as non-Hodgkin's lymphoma (NHL) and lung carcinoma (hilar adenopathy or nodular lung lesions).

(Continued on page 324)

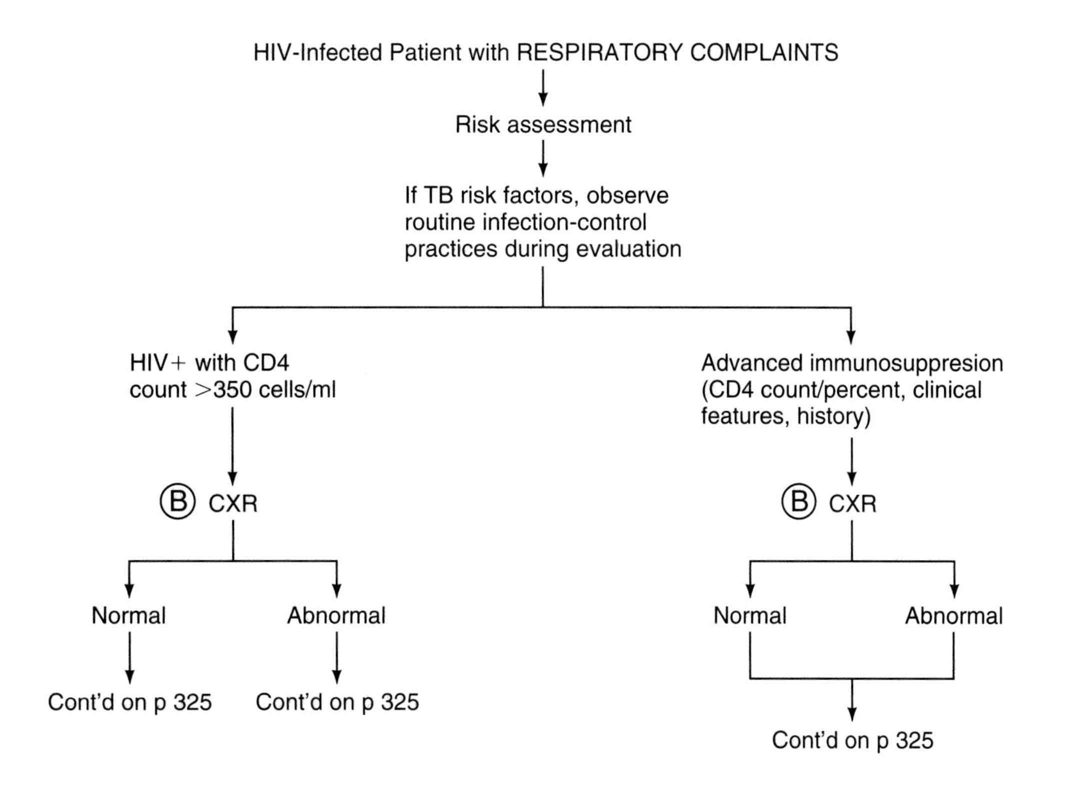
HIV-Infected Patient with RESPIRATORY COMPLAINTS
Risk assessment
If TB risk factors, observe routine infection-control practices during evaluation
HIV+ with CD4 count >350 cells/ml
Advanced immunosuppresion (CD4 count/percent, clinical features, history)
Ⓑ CXR
Ⓑ CXR
Normal
Abnormal
Normal
Abnormal
Cont'd on p 325
Cont'd on p 325
Cont'd on p 325

C. **Clinical clues:** Clinical clues including the duration of symptoms, injection drug use, travel, treatment history, immune status, and physical examination can hint at the etiology of pulmonary infiltrates. Abrupt onset of fever and cough suggests community-acquired pneumonia while subacute evolution of fever and dyspnea (weeks not days) is typical of PCP. Injection drug users are more prone to bacterial pneumonia, TB, and endocarditis. Prior residence or travel to endemic regions should raise suspicion for fungal infections such as histoplasmosis, coccidiomycosis, and blastomycosis as well as parasitic infections such as strongyloidiasis. Antiretroviral therapy history can provide clues both to medication-related toxicity (abacavir hypersensitivity) as well as the development of an immune reconstitution syndrome (new or worsening infiltrates on CXR in patients recently started on antiretrovirals, particularly in conjunction with treatment for active TB). Notably, even patients with preserved CD4 counts suffer greater rates of bacterial pneumonia than uninfected counterparts. Physical examination findings such as weight loss and thrush are signs of advanced immunosuppression and should guide the differential diagnosis accordingly. Funduscopic examination may demonstrate changes associated with a variety of viral, fungal, and mycobacterial pathogens. Regional lymphadenopathy may suggest TB or NHL. Skin lesions are common in cryptococcosis and histoplasmosis, and mucocutaneous lesions are an established risk factor for pulmonary Kaposi's sarcoma.

D. **Microbiologic testing:** Microbiologic testing of respiratory secretions is critical. HIV-infected patients with respiratory complaints and a productive cough should submit sputum for Gram stain and culture, fungal stain and culture, and acid-fast bacillus (AFB) smear and culture. In the proper setting, antigen or molecular testing for respiratory viruses may also be useful in establishing the cause of an HIV-infected person's respiratory complaints. Most patients with PCP have a nonproductive cough and have difficulty producing a deep sputum specimen. HIV-positive patients should have samples collected after induction with hypertonic saline when being evaluated for PCP. Several samples may need to be obtained as the diagnostic yield of a single induced specimen for PCP varies from 50%–90% depending on the prevalence of PCP in the population studied, techniques used to identify the organisms (methenamine silver stain, immunofluorescence, polymerase chain reaction [PCR]), and the expertise of the laboratory performing the test. The evaluation of HIV-infected persons with suspected TB requires three sequential daily samples for AFB smear and culture (samples need not be induced unless the patient is unable to produce a sample). The sensitivity of a single AFB smear may be as low as 30%, but cultures are subsequently positive in 85%–100% of patients.

E. **Assessment of gas exchange:** The evaluation of respiratory complaints in persons with HIV should include an assessment of oxygenation (pulse oximetry or blood gas measurement). PCP commonly produces hypoxemia with exertion, so patients with normal room-air oxygenation saturation should have pulse oximetry assessed during ambulation. Assessment of gas exchange has important therapeutic implications for patients with PCP as well. Because treatment of PCP often results in transient worsening of oxygenation as organisms die, it is important to assess the degree to which gas exchange is impaired. Adjuvant steroids should be considered for those with an alveolar-arterial gradient of ≥35 and/or a Po_2 of ≤70 mm Hg on room air.

F. **Empiric therapy for PCP:** HIV-positive persons with a CD4 count of ≤200 cells/mm^3 who present with fever, progressive dyspnea, and diffuse interstitial infiltrates on CXR are likely suffering from PCP. When such individuals are at low risk for TB, have not been taking PCP prophylaxis, and are not suffering from severe impairment of gas exchange, it is common to begin treatment for PCP while waiting for the results of induced sputum testing. Because of the high pretest probability of PCP, HIV-infected persons with a depressed CD4 count and a normal CXR should be treated empirically if they demonstrate impaired gas exchange. Although nonspecific, elevation of serum lactate dehydrogenase (LDH) can provide additional evidence of PCP in such cases. High-resolution CT of the chest may also be helpful in demonstrating subtle interstitial changes missed with a plain radiograph. In patients at lower risk for PCP or with more severe illness, empiric therapy for PCP may also be considered but further testing should be aggressively pursued so that alternative etiologies for a patient's respiratory complaints can be evaluated.

G. **Additional diagnostic testing:** Steps for further evaluation are dependent upon the patient's degree of immunosuppression and the tempo of the illness. Patients with a CD4 count of ≤50 cells/mm^3 who present with progressive hypoxemia despite appropriate empiric treatment for PCP would likely benefit from early bronchoscopy with bronchoalveolar lavage. By contrast, individuals with preserved CD4 counts and chronic respiratory complaints may benefit first from pulmonary function testing or echocardiography to evaluate noninfectious causes of respiratory difficulties. In patients who remain undiagnosed, bronchoscopy with transbronchial biopsy, video-assisted thoracscopic surgery, and/or open lung biopsy are often needed to make a definitive diagnosis.

Reference

Fangman JW, Sax PE. Human immunodeficiency virus and pulmonary infections. In Fishman AP, Elias JA, Fishman JA, et al. Fishman's Pulmonary Diseases and Disorders, ed 4. New York, McGraw-Hill, 2008, pp. 2241–2264.

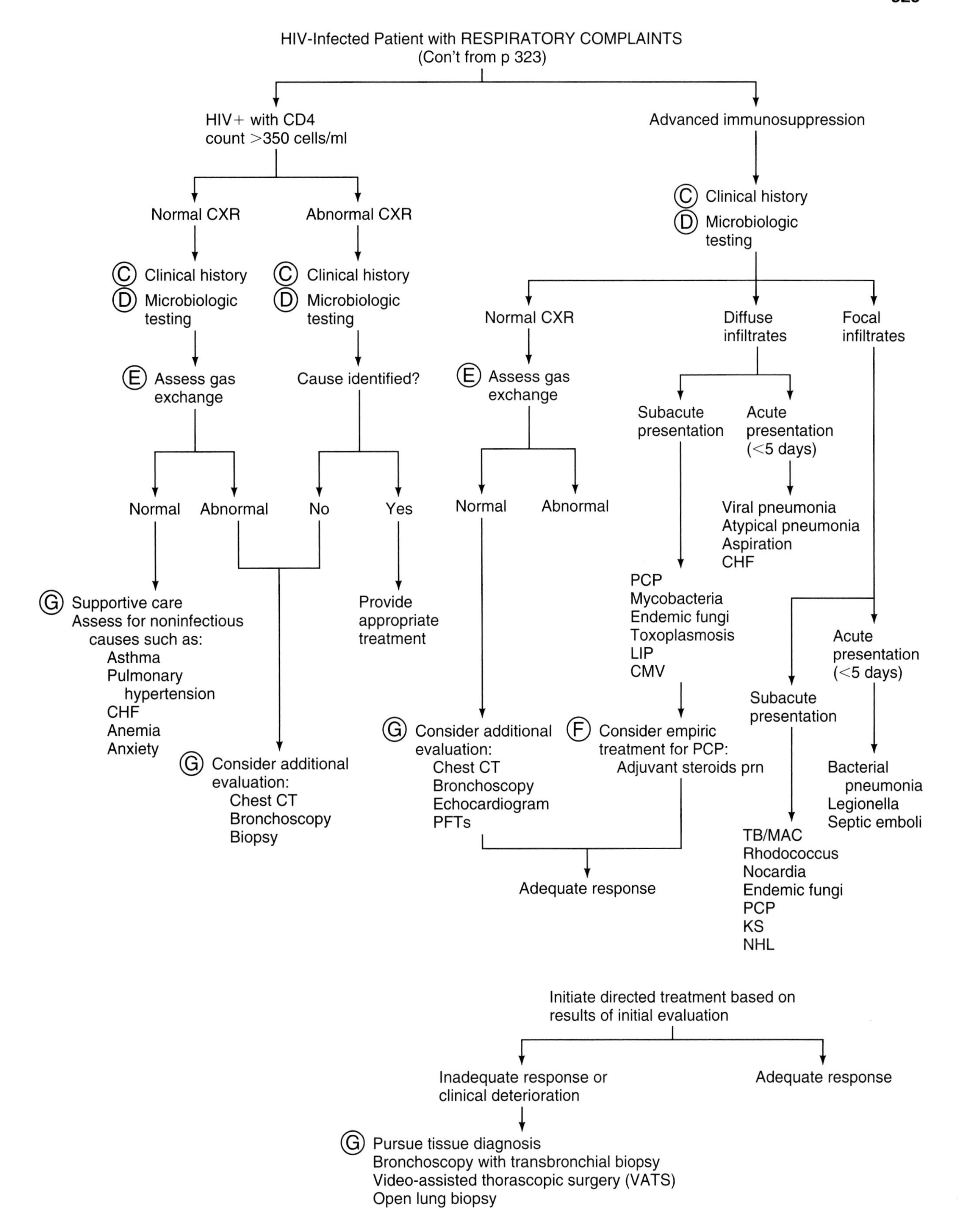
HIV-Infected Patient with RESPIRATORY COMPLAINTS
(Con't from p 323)
HIV+ with CD4 count >350 cells/ml
Advanced immunosuppression
Normal CXR
Abnormal CXR
C Clinical history
D Microbiologic testing
C Clinical history
D Microbiologic testing
E Assess gas exchange
Cause identified?
Normal
Abnormal
No
Yes
G Supportive care
Assess for noninfectious causes such as:
Asthma
Pulmonary hypertension
CHF
Anemia
Anxiety
Provide appropriate treatment
G Consider additional evaluation:
Chest CT
Bronchoscopy
Biopsy
C Clinical history
D Microbiologic testing
Normal CXR
Diffuse infiltrates
Focal infiltrates
E Assess gas exchange
Normal
Abnormal
Subacute presentation
Acute presentation (<5 days)
Viral pneumonia
Atypical pneumonia
Aspiration
CHF
PCP
Mycobacteria
Endemic fungi
Toxoplasmosis
LIP
CMV
G Consider additional evaluation:
Chest CT
Bronchoscopy
Echocardiogram
PFTs
F Consider empiric treatment for PCP:
Adjuvant steroids prn
Adequate response
Subacute presentation
Acute presentation (<5 days)
TB/MAC
Rhodococcus
Nocardia
Endemic fungi
PCP
KS
NHL
Bacterial pneumonia
Legionella
Septic emboli
Initiate directed treatment based on results of initial evaluation
Inadequate response or clinical deterioration
Adequate response
G Pursue tissue diagnosis
Bronchoscopy with transbronchial biopsy
Video-assisted thoracoscopic surgery (VATS)
Open lung biopsy

CENTRAL NERVOUS SYSTEM INFECTION IN THE PATIENT WITH HIV

Rebeca M. Plank, MD

A. A CNS infection may be the initial presentation for patients who are not aware of their HIV status or for individuals with HIV who are not receiving medical care. Initial evaluation should include review of CD4 count and any history of opportunistic infection. If focal findings are present, or if the patient has clinical evidence of increased intracranial pressure such as lethargy, imaging should be performed as soon as possible. Focal lesions may represent surgical emergencies. Prompt initiation of corticosteroids should be considered if there is evidence of significant elevation in intracranial pressure. If no mass effect is detected on imaging, a lumbar puncture (LP) should be performed.

B. If a lesion with mass effect is present, toxoplasmosis or primary CNS lymphoma is at the top of the differential. In those with appropriate risk factors, tuberculosis (TB) should be considered. Gliomas and metastatic malignancy are two noninfectious possibilities.

Patients with CNS toxoplasmosis generally have a positive serum *Toxoplasma* antibody and a CD4 count <100 cells/ml. The lesions are often multiple and ring-enhancing. MRI is more sensitive than CT scan for small lesions. Cerebrospinal fluid (CSF) examination can be consistent with aseptic meningitis, and Giemsa stain of centrifuged CSF samples can occasionally demonstrate organisms. CSF polymerase chain reaction (PCR) for *Toxoplasma gondii* may also be helpful in making the diagnosis.

C. In patients who are clinically stable, have radiographic findings consistent with CNS toxoplasmosis, have a positive *Toxoplasma* serology, and have not been receiving appropriate *Toxoplasma* prophylaxis (e.g., trimethoprim-sulfamethoxazole or atovaquone), it is reasonable to initiate empiric treatment for toxoplasmosis with pyrimethamine and either sulfadiazine (preferred) or clindamycin. Marked improvement or resolution should be seen on follow-up imaging within 10–14 days. If no such improvement is evident, an alternative diagnosis should be sought and brain biopsy may become necessary.

Primary CNS lymphoma can present with solitary or multiple lesions that may or may not enhance. Most patients will have a subacute course and a CD4 count <50 cells/ml. A CSF sample should be sent for cytology and may yield a diagnosis; although these lymphomas are associated with Epstein-Barr virus (EBV), EBV PCR from CSF has had variable sensitivity and specificity and should not be relied on diagnostically.

D. Possible causes of lesions seen on CT or MRI without mass effect include progressive multifocal leukoencephalopathy (PML), HIV encephalopathy, and cytomegalovirus (CMV) encephalitis. PML is caused by reactivation of JC virus in severe immunosuppression; patients usually have CD4 count <200 cells/ml. It presents with progressive neurologic deficits and multifocal areas of demyelination. MRI is more sensitive than CT scan for lesions. It can be diagnosed by CSF PCR for JCV.

CMV encephalitis occurs in the setting of viral reactivation when a patient's CD4 count is <50 cells/ml (sometimes higher). Imaging is highly variable. CMV can present with encephalitis, myelitis, polyradiculitis—manifesting as lower extremity weakness, decreased reflexes, and urinary retention—or as neuropathy that may affect peripheral nerves, including the cranial nerves. CSF examination can be consistent with aseptic meningitis. Diagnosis is made by detecting CMV DNA or CMV antigens in the CSF or by peripheral nerve biopsy.

Primary HIV infection itself can cause a self-limited meningoencephalitis, sometimes accompanied by fever, headache, vomiting, and cranial nerve palsies. HIV encephalopathy occurs in later stages of infection, generally with a CD4 count <200 cells/ml. Patients can present with some combination of cognitive, behavioral, and motor problems. On MRI, the lesions of HIV encephalopathy are usually more symmetric and are less well demarcated than those seen in PML. Elevated protein and a pleocytosis are found in the CSF. The CSF HIV-1 viral load is usually elevated (>1000 copies/ml). Because the signs and symptoms overlap with so many other potential etiologies, HIV encephalopathy should be a diagnosis of exclusion.

(Continued on page 328)

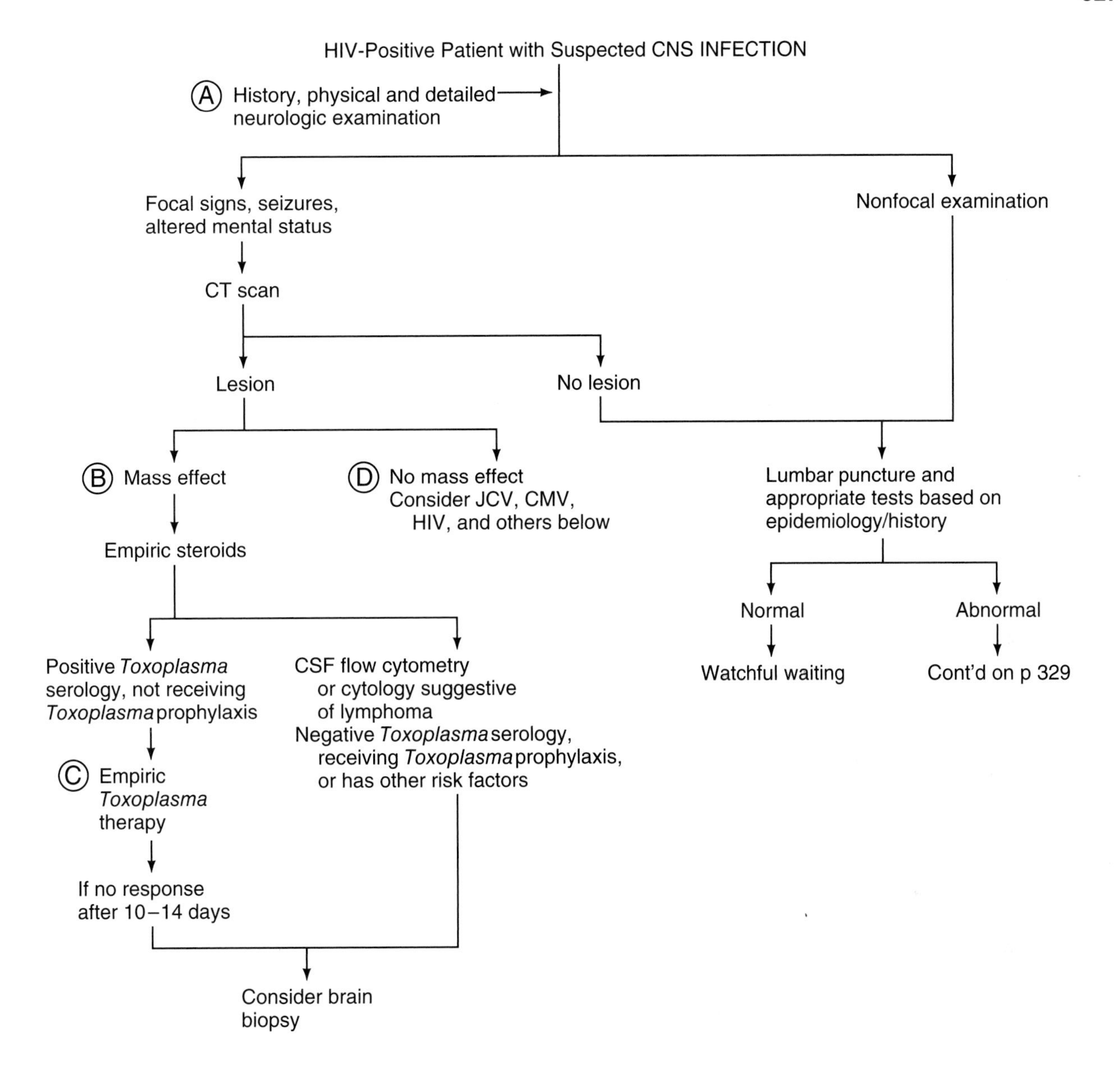
HIV-Positive Patient with Suspected CNS INFECTION
(A) History, physical and detailed neurologic examination
Focal signs, seizures, altered mental status
Nonfocal examination
CT scan
Lesion
No lesion
(B) Mass effect
(D) No mass effect
Consider JCV, CMV, HIV, and others below
Lumbar puncture and appropriate tests based on epidemiology/history
Empiric steroids
Normal
Abnormal
Watchful waiting
Cont'd on p 329
Positive *Toxoplasma* serology, not receiving *Toxoplasma* prophylaxis
CSF flow cytometry or cytology suggestive of lymphoma
Negative *Toxoplasma* serology, receiving *Toxoplasma* prophylaxis, or has other risk factors
(C) Empiric *Toxoplasma* therapy
If no response after 10–14 days
Consider brain biopsy

E. If the previously listed investigations remain unrevealing, then consider other infections. There has been a recent increase in the incidence of syphilis among those also at risk of HIV infection, and neurosyphilis has myriad clinical presentations. In patients with HIV, a CD4 count of ≤350 cells/ml and a serum rapid plasma reagin (RPR) titer of ≥1:32 has been shown to correlate with significantly increased odds of neurosyphilis. Rarely, neurosyphilis may present with a focal lesion (gumma). CSF examination can be consistent with aseptic meningitis. CSF VDRL has a high specificity but low sensitivity; antibody tests specific for *Treponema pallidum* may prove to be more sensitive.

F. Cryptococcal infection of the CNS can present with meningitis and rarely with a local lesion. Patients can present with fever and headache while lacking other signs of meningeal irritation. The CSF is generally found to have low glucose, high protein, and a pleocytosis. Cryptococcal antigen can be detected by agglutination from the CSF, and diagnosis can be confirmed by detection of the organism by India ink stain and culture.

G. Mass lesions may also represent brain abscesses from a variety of organisms, including *Staphylococcus*, *Nocardia*, and *Rhodococcus*, among many others.

H. Cysticercosis should be considered in patients from Central and South America, Asia, and sub-Saharan Africa, particularly if they spent a significant amount of time in rural areas, had contact with pigs, or consumed undercooked pork products.

I. Patients with HIV also remain at risk for bacterial and aseptic meningitis seen in immunocompetent individuals (see Acute and Subacute Meningitis and also Chronic Meningitis).

References

Antinori A, Ammassari A, De Luca A, et al. Diagnosis of AIDS-related focal brain lesions: a decision-making analysis based on clinical and neuroradiologic characteristics combined with polymerase chain reaction assays in CSF. Neurology 1997;48(3):687–694.

Bicanic T, Harrison TS. Cryptococcal meningitis. Br Med Bull 2005;72:99–118.

Griffiths P. Cytomegalovirus infection of the central nervous system. Herpes 2004;11(Suppl 2):95A–104A

Koralnik IJ. Neurologic diseases caused by human immunodeficiency virus-1 and opportunistic infections. In Mandell GL, Bennett JE, Dolin R, eds. Principles and Practices of Infectious Diseases, 6th ed. Philadelphia: Elsevier, Churchill, Livingstone, 2005:1583–1601.

Lynn WA, Lightman S. Syphilis and HIV: a dangerous combination. Lancet Infect Dis 2004;4(7):456–466.

Mamidi A, DeSimone JA, Pomerantz RJ. Central nervous system infections in individuals with HIV-1 infection. J Neurovirol 2002;8(3):158–167.

Marra CM, Maxwell CL, Smith SL, et al. Cerebrospinal fluid abnormalities in patients with syphilis: association with clinical and laboratory features. J Infect Dis 2004;189(3):369–376.

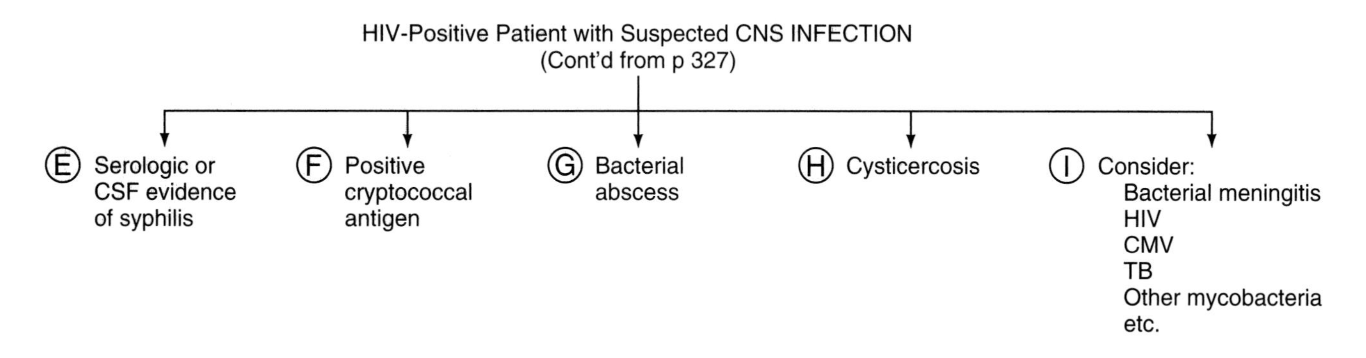
HIV-Positive Patient with Suspected CNS INFECTION
(Cont'd from p 327)
E Serologic or CSF evidence of syphilis
F Positive cryptococcal antigen
G Bacterial abscess
H Cysticercosis
I Consider:
Bacterial meningitis
HIV
CMV
TB
Other mycobacteria
etc.

THE ACUTELY ILL PATIENT WITH HIV

Sarah P. Hammond, MD

A. A careful history and physical examination are crucial to the care of an acutely HIV-positive patient. In particular, the history should focus on localizing features of the illness, recent exposures, prior infections, severity of HIV, and medication history. Attention to localizing symptoms and exposures (including sexual and environmental exposures) help narrow the differential diagnosis and focus the workup. This chapter highlights several common presentations of acute illness in HIV-positive patients: CNS symptoms, respiratory tract symptoms, odynophagia, diarrhea, genitourinary complaints, dermatologic complaints, and systemic febrile illnesses.

B. In addition to focusing on localizing symptoms, the history should focus on the status of the patient's HIV disease. All patients with HIV, regardless of CD4 cell count, are susceptible to community pathogens. However, the CD4 cell count is predictive of their susceptibility to opportunistic pathogens. Patients with a CD4 cell count >200 and a total percentage of CD4 cells of >14% are less susceptible to opportunistic pathogens such as *Pneumocystis jiroveci* pneumonia (PCP). In contrast, patients with CD4 cell counts <50 are susceptible to a large number of opportunistic pathogens, including PCP, toxoplasmosis, *Cryptococcus,* JC virus, cytomegalovirus (CMV), and *Mycobacterium avium* complex (MAC). Thus knowledge of the most recent CD4 count is extremely helpful in directing the workup based on the patient's risk for opportunistic pathogens.

C. The medication history should focus on current antiretroviral and prophylactic medications. Antiretroviral medications have been associated with a number of side effects that mimic acute infectious illnesses. Some of these side effects are specific to the class of antiretroviral medication; whereas others are specific to the particular drug. For example, protease inhibitors commonly cause diarrhea, whereas nucleoside reverse transcriptase inhibitors can infrequently cause lactic acidosis that presents as severe abdominal pain, nausea, and vomiting. In contrast, abacavir and nevirapine cause severe drug-specific side effects. Abacavir infrequently causes a life-threatening hypersensitivity syndromemanifesting as fever, malaise, and rash; nevirapine can cause severe hepatotoxicity.

Prophylactic medications for the prevention of opportunistic infections in patients with HIV sometimes cause severe drug reactions. For example, chronic dapsone use rarely may cause methemoglobinemia (particularly in patients with glucose-6-phosphate dehydrogenase [G6PD] deficiency) that presents with dyspnea and fatigue. Trimethoprim-sulfamethoxazole is a common cause of rash and other symptoms such as nausea and vomiting.

D. *Respiratory System:* The differential diagnosis for an HIV-infected patient with respiratory symptoms regardless of CD4 cell count includes bacterial pneumonia, influenza (if in season), tuberculosis (if exposure history is present), drug toxicity, and other respiratory viruses. In particular, patients with HIV are at increased risk for bacterial pneumonia compared with patients without HIV; the risk is further increased among patients with CD4 counts of <200. Workup of respiratory symptoms should include chest imaging and, if appropriate by history and risk factors, rapid testing for influenza and induced sputum for acid-fast bacillus (AFB). If the CD4 cell count is <200 and the patient is not taking adequate PCP prophylaxis, then PCP should be sought by special stains on induced sputum or bronchoalveolar lavage fluid. Drug toxicity, including abacavir hypersensitivity, dapsone-related methemoglobinemia, and nucleoside reverse transcriptase inhibitor–associated lactic acidosis, can also present as dyspnea and tachypnea and should be considered in patients taking relevant medications. For more details see the chapter Respiratory Symptoms in HIV-Infected Patients (p. 322).

E. *Central Nervous System:* Patients with HIV infection who present with new mental status changes or other neurologic symptoms should be worked up as described in the chapter Central Nervous System Infection in the HIV-Infected Patient (p. 326). Patients with HIV presenting with a new change in vision or eye pain require rapid ophthalmologic evaluation. The differential diagnosis for ophthalmologic symptoms in patients with a low CD4 count includes CMV retinitis, toxoplasmosis, and syphilis, among other diagnoses.

F. *Dysphagia and Odynophagia:* Dysphagia and odynophagia are common problems in the HIV-positive patient. The differential diagnosis, in addition to bacterial pharyngitis and viral upper respiratory tract infection, includes esophageal candidiasis, herpes simplex or CMV esophagitis, and aphthous ulcers. If oral candidiasis is present on examination, then empiric

(Continued on page 332)

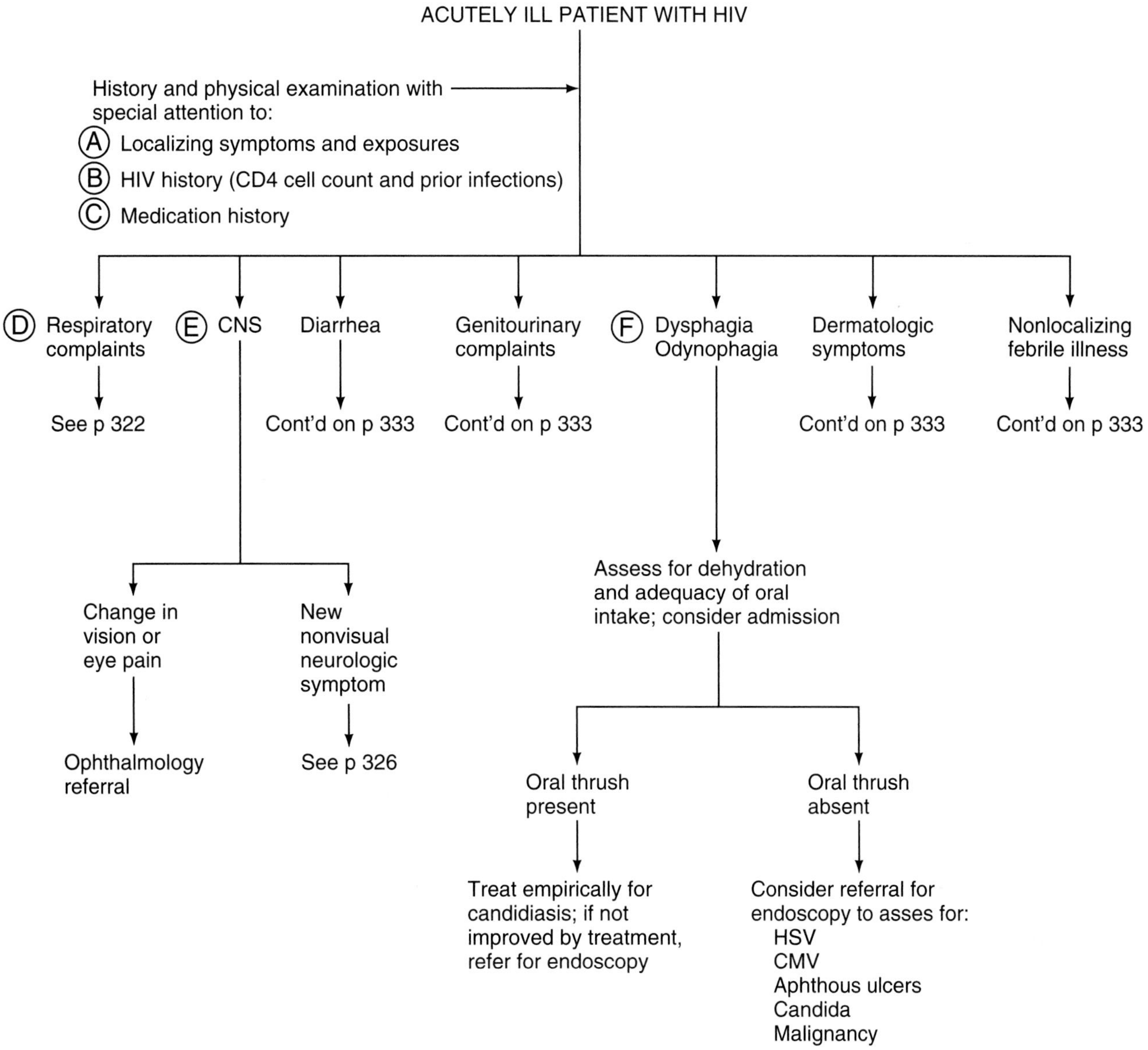

ACUTELY ILL PATIENT WITH HIV

History and physical examination with special attention to:
- (A) Localizing symptoms and exposures
- (B) HIV history (CD4 cell count and prior infections)
- (C) Medication history

(D) Respiratory complaints → See p 322

(E) CNS
- Change in vision or eye pain → Ophthalmology referral
- New nonvisual neurologic symptom → See p 326

Diarrhea → Cont'd on p 333

Genitourinary complaints → Cont'd on p 333

(F) Dysphagia Odynophagia → Assess for dehydration and adequacy of oral intake; consider admission
- Oral thrush present → Treat empirically for candidiasis; if not improved by treatment, refer for endoscopy
- Oral thrush absent → Consider referral for endoscopy to asses for:
  - HSV
  - CMV
  - Aphthous ulcers
  - Candida
  - Malignancy

Dermatologic symptoms → Cont'd on p 333

Nonlocalizing febrile illness → Cont'd on p 333

treatment for esophageal candidiasis is a reasonable approach. However, for cases that limit oral intake or fail to improve with empiric therapy, workup with endoscopic evaluation should be pursued.

G. *Diarrhea.* The differential diagnosis for diarrhea in the HIV-infected patient is broad and includes medication-related diarrhea and infection secondary to bacteria, viruses, or parasites. The risk for bacterial diarrhea in particular is higher among patients with HIV than among patients without HIV. This risk increases with severity of HIV disease. In a large study of HIV-infected patients with diarrhea, *Clostridium difficile* was the most common cause of bacterial diarrhea, followed by *Shigella* and *Campylobacter*. For patients with chronic symptoms, consider medication-related diarrhea and parasitic infection with *Cryptosporidium* and *Giardia.* In patients with CD4 cell counts <50, consider disseminated MAC infection. Workup should include stool culture for *Shigella*, *Salmonella*, *Campylobacter*, *Yersinia*, pathogenic *Escherichia coli*, and *Vibrio;* stool *C. difficile* toxin testing; stool examination for ova and parasites (O&P); and blood isolators for mycobacteria if the CD4 cell count is <50.

H. *Genitourinary Symptoms.* Assessment of genitourinary complaints in HIV-positive patients requires a thorough exposure history, including recent sexual encounters. HIV-positive patients are susceptible to common genitourinary problems such as urinary tract infections; nephrolithiasis; and common sexually transmitted diseases such as syphilis, gonorrhea, chlamydia, and trichomonas. They are also at risk for less common genitourinary diseases such as chancroid, lymphogranuloma venereum (LGV), and adenovirus. Medication side effects such as indinavir-related nephrolithiasis should also be considered. Workup includes a genital examination for ulcers or chancres; urinalysis and urine culture; nucleic acid testing of urine, urethral swab, or cervical swab for chlamydia and gonorrhea; fluorescent antigen testing for herpes simplex virus (HSV) and viral culture of genital ulcers; serum rapid plasma reagin (RPR) test; and, if suggested by history, workup for less common illnesses such as LGV. After a high-risk sexual exposure, chlamydia and gonorrhea are often treated empirically.

I. *Dermatologic Symptoms.* Dermatologic disease is more common in HIV-infected patients than in non–HIV-infected patients. Common dermatologic problems associated with HIV infection include viral infection of the skin and mucous membranes, such as herpes simplex, varicella-zoster, and molluscum contagiosum; systemic bacterial infection with a dermatologic component, such as bacillary angiomatosis (*Bartonella henselae*) and syphilis; superficial bacterial infection of the skin, including ascesses resulting from methicillin-resistant *Staphylococcus aureus* (MRSA); systemic fungal infection (particularly in patients with low CD4 counts), such as cryptococcosis and blastomycosis; parasitic infections, such as scabies; primary dermatologic conditions associated with HIV, such as eosinophilic folliculitis; and hypersensitivity reactions to medications such as trimethoprim-sulfamethoxazole. Workup should be guided by the patient's history (with special attention to medications and exposures), the appearance of the lesion, and the absence or presence of systemic symptoms. Consider admission for patients with systemic or severe symptoms. Promptly refer to dermatology for biopsy in any case in which diagnosis or treatment is not clear.

J. *Systemic febrile illnesses.* Assessment of a febrile patient with HIV infection without localizing symptoms requires a careful history, paying particular attention to exposures, medications, CD4 cell count, and history of previous opportunistic infection. In HIV-positive patients of any CD4 cell count, the differential diagnosis is broad and includes common viral and bacterial infections such as influenza, parvovirus, hepatitis, and MRSA infection; mycobacterial infection with MAC or tuberculosis; endemic mycoses such as histoplasmosis and blastomycosis; medication-related toxicities such as abacavir hypersensitivity and nevirapine-associated hepatitis; and HIV-related malignancies such as HIV-associated lymphoma. In patients with low CD4 cell counts, opportunistic infections are also a major source of fever. Pathogens causing fever in this setting include MAC, PCP, cryptococcus, CMV, and *B. henselae* (bacillary angiomatosis). The workup should include CBC, complete metabolic panel, blood cultures, pathogen-spcifitesting based on exposure (e.g., influenza testing during influenza season and induced sputum to evaluate for tuberculosis), and imaging. In patients with a low CD4 cell count, additional workup should include blood isolators for mycobacteria, serum cryptococcal antigen, and induced sputum for PCP.

References

Bartlett JG, Gallant JE. 2007 Medical Management of HIV Infection. Baltimore: Johns Hopkins Medicine, Health Publishing Business Group, 2007.

Coopman SA, Johnson RA, Platt R, et al. Cutaneous disease and drug reactions in HIV infection. N Engl J Med 1993;328:1670–1674.

Hirschtick RE, Glassroth J, Jordan MC, et al. Bacterial pneumonia in persons infected with the human immunodeficiency virus. N Engl J Med 1995;333:845–851.

Hoffman RM, Currier JS. Management of antiretroviral treatment-related complications. Infect Dis Clin North Am 2007;21:103–132.

Hot A, Schmulewitz L, Viard JP, et al. Fever of unknown origin in HIV/AIDS patients. Infect Dis Clin North Am 2007;21:1013–1032.

Lopez FA, Sanders CV. Fever and rash in HIV-infected patients. UpTo Date 2007.

Sanchez TH, Brooks JT, Sullivan PS, et al. Bacterial diarrhea in persons with HIV infection, United States, 1992–2002. Clin Infect Dis 2005;41:1621–1627.

Wilcox CM, Monkemuller KE. Diagnosis and management of esophageal disease in the acquired immunodeficiency syndrome. South Med J 1998;91:1002–1008.

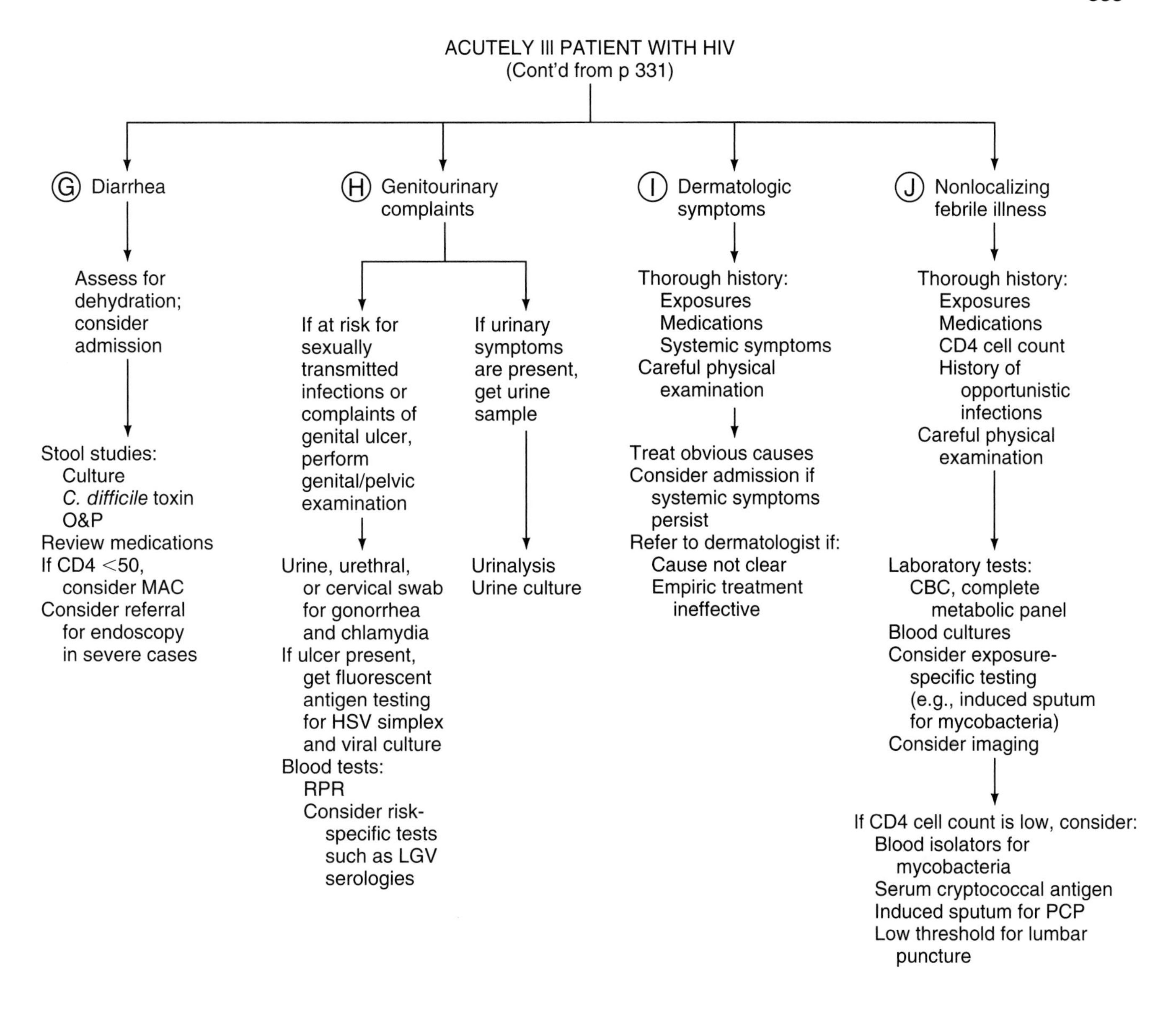
ACUTELY Ill PATIENT WITH HIV
(Cont'd from p 331)
G Diarrhea
Assess for dehydration; consider admission
Stool studies:
Culture
C. difficile toxin
O&P
Review medications
If CD4 <50, consider MAC
Consider referral for endoscopy in severe cases
H Genitourinary complaints
If at risk for sexually transmitted infections or complaints of genital ulcer, perform genital/pelvic examination
If urinary symptoms are present, get urine sample
Urine, urethral, or cervical swab for gonorrhea and chlamydia
If ulcer present, get fluorescent antigen testing for HSV simplex and viral culture
Blood tests:
RPR
Consider risk-specific tests such as LGV serologies
Urinalysis
Urine culture
I Dermatologic symptoms
Thorough history:
Exposures
Medications
Systemic symptoms
Careful physical examination
Treat obvious causes
Consider admission if systemic symptoms persist
Refer to dermatologist if:
Cause not clear
Empiric treatment ineffective
J Nonlocalizing febrile illness
Thorough history:
Exposures
Medications
CD4 cell count
History of opportunistic infections
Careful physical examination
Laboratory tests:
CBC, complete metabolic panel
Blood cultures
Consider exposure-specific testing (e.g., induced sputum for mycobacteria)
Consider imaging
If CD4 cell count is low, consider:
Blood isolators for mycobacteria
Serum cryptococcal antigen
Induced sputum for PCP
Low threshold for lumbar puncture

SEPSIS

Alison C. Roxby, MD, MSc

A. Patients with a life-threatening infection may present with systemic inflammatory response syndrome (SIRS), which can signal severe sepsis and septic shock. It is imperative to recognize this syndrome early and institute prompt and aggressive treatment. The criteria for SIRS are having two or more of the following signs:
   1. Fever (>38° C) or hypothermia (<36° C); tachycardia (heart rate [HR] >90 beats per minute)
   2. Tachypnea with respiratory rate [RR] >20 breaths per minute or $PaCO_2$ <32 mm Hg
   3. Leukocytosis (WBC >12,000 cells/mm^3), leukopenia (WBC <4000 cells/mm^3), or any blood count with >10% bands

   Sepsis is viewed as a continuum with progressive severity. Patients with SIRS and evidence of infection meet criteria for *sepsis;* patients with organ dysfunction have *severe sepsis;* and patients with sepsis and refractory hypotension and perfusion abnormalities despite resuscitation are in *septic shock.* The goal of early therapy is to prevent progression of sepsis to more severe forms.

   Patients who are elderly or immunosuppressed may not manifest the typical vital signs of SIRS; therefore a high index of suspicion should guide management. Elevated arterial lactate levels can indicate impending sepsis in patients whose vital signs do not yet meet criteria.

B. Aggressive resuscitation with fluids is the mainstay of treatment for sepsis-spectrum disease. Patients with sepsis have high volume resuscitation requirements as a result of peripheral vasodilation and have elevated tissue oxygen requirements. Early goal-directed therapy promotes rapid and aggressive treatment of sepsis, similar to the "golden hour" approach to trauma patients. Insert a central venous catheter and use crystalloid fluids to normalize blood pressure, with the goal of keeping central venous pressure (CVP) between 8 and 12 mm Hg and mean arterial pressure (MAP) between 40 and 90 mm Hg. If adequate CVP and MAP goals cannot be met, or if pulmonary edema develops, inotropic agents should be initiated early. ABG measurement can determine the severity of metabolic acidosis. Assess tissue perfusion by checking arterial lactate levels or mixed-venous oxygen saturation. Elevated lactate or low venous O_2 saturation is evidence that tissue perfusion is insufficient and further aggressive measures should continue.

C. Identifying the source of infection is key to effective treatment. Obtaining a history and physical examination is the first step to identifying possible sources. Host factors including immunosuppression, asplenia, recent invasive procedures, and chronic illness are important details. Pneumonia and urinary tract infection remain common causes of sepsis. Intraabdominal disease should always be considered. All patients should have a chest radiograph; urinalysis; standard laboratory tests, including CBC with differential, serum electrolytes, BUN and creatinine; and hepatic panel. Blood cultures should be obtained from two separate venipuncture sites and from any indwelling catheters or lines. Patients with evidence of pneumonia should have sputum Gram stain and culture. Patients with evidence of urinary tract infections should have urine Gram stain in addition to cultures.

D. Empiric parenteral antibiotic therapy should be instituted within 60 minutes of identification of a patient with possible sepsis. The choice of agent depends on the likely source of infection, local antibiotic resistance patterns, and host factors. Initial antimicrobial spectra should include gram-positive and gram-negative bacterial coverage. Additional coverage may be necessary based on host factors such as neutropenia, HIV infection, end-stage renal disease, presence of catheters or hardware, recent surgery, or travel history.

E. Further management of sepsis after initial resuscitation includes intensive monitoring. If respiratory distress is present, positive pressure ventilation may be required. Relative adrenal insufficiency is common in patients with sepsis; cortisol levels should be checked and replacement corticosteroids should be administered in patients who are unstable or in patients with a cosyntropin stimulation response <9 μg/dl. Aggressive glycemic control should be instituted to keep glucose <150 mg/dl. Anemia should be corrected by red cell transfusion. Activated protein C has been proved to increase survival in patients with severe sepsis at high risk of death but can be administered only to patients without risk of bleeding.

F. Patients with evidence of localized infection, such as abscess, should have definitive drainage or surgical evaluation. Any obviously infected hardware should be removed if possible.

G. Antibiotic therapy will need to be revised as culture results or further history are obtained.

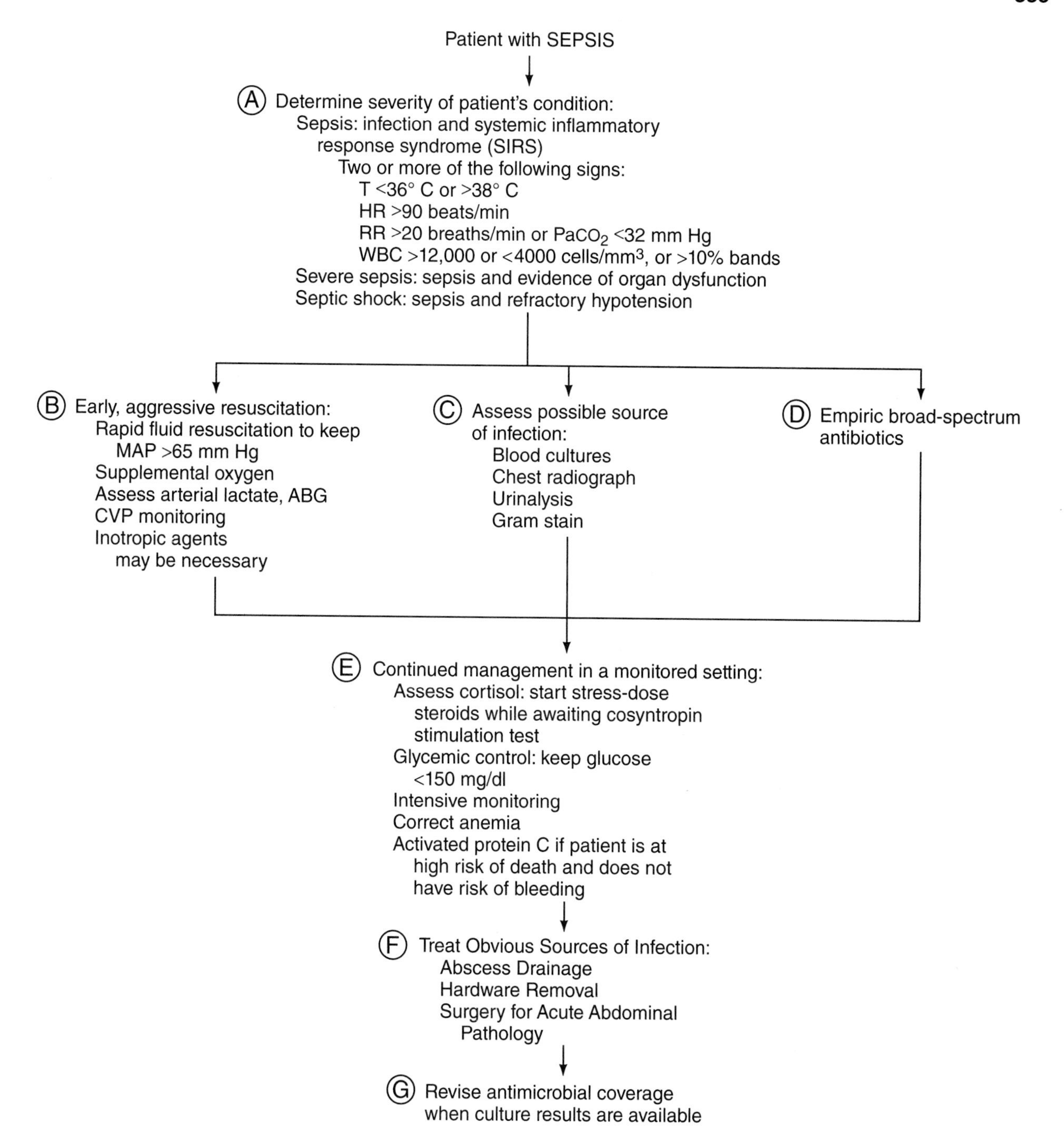

Patient with SEPSIS
(A) Determine severity of patient's condition:
Sepsis: infection and systemic inflammatory response syndrome (SIRS)
Two or more of the following signs:
T <36° C or >38° C
HR >90 beats/min
RR >20 breaths/min or PaCO2 <32 mm Hg
WBC >12,000 or <4000 cells/mm3, or >10% bands
Severe sepsis: sepsis and evidence of organ dysfunction
Septic shock: sepsis and refractory hypotension
(B) Early, aggressive resuscitation:
Rapid fluid resuscitation to keep MAP >65 mm Hg
Supplemental oxygen
Assess arterial lactate, ABG
CVP monitoring
Inotropic agents may be necessary
(C) Assess possible source of infection:
Blood cultures
Chest radiograph
Urinalysis
Gram stain
(D) Empiric broad-spectrum antibiotics
(E) Continued management in a monitored setting:
Assess cortisol: start stress-dose steroids while awaiting cosyntropin stimulation test
Glycemic control: keep glucose <150 mg/dl
Intensive monitoring
Correct anemia
Activated protein C if patient is at high risk of death and does not have risk of bleeding
(F) Treat Obvious Sources of Infection:
Abscess Drainage
Hardware Removal
Surgery for Acute Abdominal Pathology
(G) Revise antimicrobial coverage when culture results are available

References

Bernard GR, Vincent JL, Laterre PF, et al. Efficacy and safety of recombinant human activated protein C for severe sepsis. N Engl J Med 2001;344:699–709.

Dellinger RP, Carlet JM, Masur H, et al. Surviving Sepsis Campaign guidelines for management of severe sepsis and septic shock. Crit Care Med 2004;32:858–873.

LaRosa SP. Sepsis: menu of new approaches replaces one therapy for all. Cleve Clin J Med 2002;69(1):65–73.

Rivers E, Nguyen B, Havstad S, et al. Early goal-directed therapy in the treatment of severe sepsis and septic shock. N Engl J Med 2001;345:1368–1377.

TOXIC SHOCK SYNDROMES

Michael Klompas, MD, MPH, FRCPC

Toxic shock syndromes are rare but life-threatening infectious syndromes characterized by fever, hypotension, and multisystem organ failure. They were first described in 1978 in a case series of young women who became critically ill with fever, rash, and hypotension soon after onset of menstruation. The syndrome was linked to the use of highly absorbent tampons colonized with a toxin-producing strain of *Staphylococcus aureus*. In subsequent years, similar syndromes have been traced to extravaginal infections with *S. aureus*, severe skin and soft-tissue infections with *Streptococcus pyogenes*, and rarely with other bacteria. Approximately one third of cases of toxic shock syndrome are now associated with postpartum and post-surgical wound infections, but cases have been reported of the syndrome arising after infection of virtually any part of the body, including sinusitis, arthritis, osteomyelitis, and respiratory infections.

The syndrome is caused by elaboration of toxins by bacteria colonizing or infecting the body. Both *Staphylococcus* and *Streptococcus* are capable of producing so-called superantigens that can rapidly activate massive numbers of T cells at once. The clinical manifestations of toxic shock syndrome are secondary to cytokine storms precipitated by the activated T cells or directly by the toxins themselves.

Table 1 Toxic Shock Syndrome Clinical Case Definition

- Temperature 38.9° C (102° F)
- Diffuse macular erythroderma
- Desquamation—1–2 weeks after onset of illness, particularly palms and soles
- Systolic blood pressure 90 mm Hg
- Multisystem involvement—three or more of the following:
  1. GI: vomiting or diarrhea at onset of illness
  2. Muscular: severe myalgia or creatine phosphokinase level at least twice the upper limit of normal for laboratory
  3. Mucous membrane: vaginal, oropharyngeal, or conjunctival hyperemia
  4. Renal: BUN or creatinine at least twice the upper limit of normal for laboratory or urinary sediment with pyuria (≥5 leukocytes per high-power field)
     in the absence of urinary tract infection
  5. Hepatic: total bilirubin, ALT, AST at least twice the upper limit of normal
  6. Hematologic: platelets $<100{,}000/mm^3$
  7. CNS: disorientation or alterations in consciousness without focal neurologic signs when fever and hypotension are absent
- Negative results on the following tests, if obtained:
  1. Blood, throat, or cerebrospinal fluid cultures (blood culture may be positive for *Staphylococcus aureusrom*)
  2. Rise in titer to Rocky Mountain spotted fever, leptospirosis, or measles

A. In patients with fever and hypotension an infectious syndrome should be highly suspected and assiduously sought. The presence of a diffuse erythroderma resembling a total body sunburn in a patient who has rapidly become very ill is highly suggestive of a toxic shock syndrome, particularly that caused by *S. aureus*. Evidence of other organ dysfunction, including confusion, profuse diarrhea, severe myalgias, elevated liver enzymes, and thrombocytopenia, confirms the diagnosis. The rash classically desquamates but only 1–3 weeks after presentation; hence, this feature is not helpful for initial diagnosis. The formal case definition for staphylococcal toxic shock syndrome (STSS) is given in Table 1. A thorough examination for a locus of infection should follow, including close assessment of any site of recent surgical intervention and a full gynecologic examination to look for retained tampons or contraceptive sponges. Sites of recent surgery should be opened for irrigation and drainage even if the wound does not appear infected because local inflammatory responses can be blunted in STSS. Any foreign material such as nasopharyngeal packing or tampons should be removed. Blood cultures should be drawn, although bacteremia is rarely found in STSS.

B. Purpura and/or petechiae can be found in toxic shock syndrome, but their presence should prompt a search for other severe disease, including meningococcal or pneumococcal meningitis, bacterial sepsis, Rocky Mountain spotted fever (RMSF), dengue, leptospirosis, and DIC. Both meningococcal and pneumococcal meningitis have been associated with adrenal hemorrhage and necrosis leading to hypotension with purpura and/or petechiae. The presence of meningismus helps to make the diagnosis. RMSF is a bacterial infection caused by *Rickettsia rickettsiae*. It is transmitted by tick bites and is most commonly seen in the southeastern United States. The rash usually first appears on the palms and soles and is accompanied by fever with severe headache. Dengue hemorrhagic fever is a viral illness acquired from mosquito bites predominantly in tropical countries. It is characterized by fever, severe diffuse bone pain, hypotension, and a petechial rash, particularly in parts of the body exposed to pressure (e.g., the skin beneath a blood pressure cuff). Leptospirosis is a severe acute febrile illness caused by the spirochete *Leptospira*. It is classically acquired by contact with animals or their excretions, particularly from rabbits and rats. Patients complain of fever, chills, headache, myalgias, eye

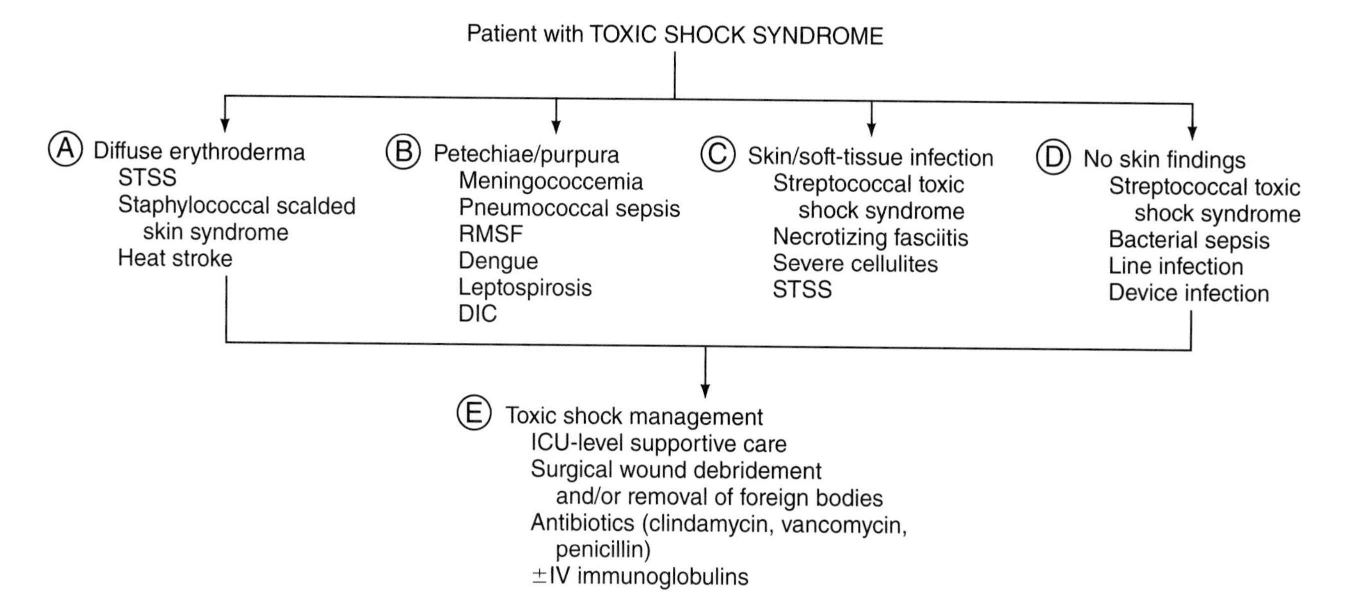

discomfort, and rash. Conjunctival injection, pharyngitis, pulmonary infiltrates, hepatitis, renal dysfunction, and diffuse macular or maculopapular rash can be found on evaluation. DIC is a serious consumptive coagulopathy and hemolytic process that can be precipitated by sepsis, obstetric catastrophe, surgery, pancreatitis, or toxin exposure. It is suggested by laboratory findings of elevated creatinine, prolonged prothrombin time (PT) and partial thromboplastin time (PTT), low fibrinogen, anemia, thrombocytopenia, and the presence of schistocytes on peripheral blood smear.

C. Skin or soft-tissue infection in the presence of fever and hypotension is suggestive of toxic shock syndrome caused by *S. pyogenes* (group A beta-hemolytic *Streptococcusrom*). There is a predilection for these infections to arise from recent surgical wounds. Pulmonary infections, including pneumonia and empyema with *S. pyogenes,* are also well-described precipitants. Severe pain at the site of infection, particularly pain out of proportion to examination findings, is a classic clue to an evolving streptococcal toxic shock syndrome with associated necrotizing fasciitis. The soft-tissue infection is often rapidly progressive. In contrast to STTS, diffuse body rash is rarely seen, whereas blood cultures are frequently positive.

D. Patients presenting with fever and hypotension in the absence of rash should be evaluated for bacterial sepsis. Particular attention should be directed to any indwelling venous access devices or recently implanted hardware that can act as common loci for infection. If present in an unstable patient, every effort should be made to remove these devices as soon as possible.

E. Treatment of toxic shock syndromes consists of supportive care, antibiotic therapy, rapid surgical debridement, and possibly IV immunoglobulins. Patients with toxic shock syndrome often develop capillary leak syndromes leading to refractory, sustained hypotension. Aggressive fluid repletion and ICU-level management are essential. Initial antibiotic therapy should include clindamycin and vancomycin. Clindamycin is recommended because it impairs bacterial toxin production. It has also been shown to be more active than penicillin-derived products against *S. pyogenes* in patients with extremely high bacterial burden. Vancomycin should be included in empiric regimens because of the increasing prevalence of methicillin resistance among community and hospital *S. aureus* isolates. Penicillin can be included if there is a high suspicion that the patient has streptococcal toxic shock syndrome. Rapid, aggressive surgical debridement is essential to decreasing the patient's overall burden of infection. IV immunoglobulins have been shown to be beneficial in streptococcal toxic shock syndrome. If *S. aureus* is isolated from a patient and shown to be methicillin susceptible, then nafcillin should be substituted for vancomycin because it has superior antistaphylococcal activity.

References

Cosgrove SE, Zaleznik DF. Staphylococcal toxic shock syndrome. UpToDate Online 13.3. Available at: www.uptodate.com. Accessed November 16, 2005.

Issa N, Thompson R. Staphylococcal toxic shock syndrome. Postgrad Med 2001;110:55–56, 59–62.

Mandel GL, Douglas RG, Bennett JE, Dolan R, eds. Principles and Practice of Infectious Diseases, 6th ed. New York: Elsevier, 2005.

Stevens DL. Streptococcal toxic shock syndrome. UpToDate Online 13.3. www.uptodate.com. Accessed November 16, 2005.

STAPHYLOCOCCUS AUREUS BACTEREMIA

Caitlin Reed, MD

Staphylococcus aureus is a common and dangerous cause of bacteremia. *S. aureus* bacteremia is increasingly frequent in hospital, health care–associated (e.g., dialysis centers), and community settings. Advances in medical care are implicated in this change in epidemiology. Indwelling vascular catheters, orthopedic hardware, and implanted devices such as pacemakers increase the likelihood of *S. aureus* bacteremia. The increasing incidence of methicillin-resistant *S. aureus* (MRSA) complicates treatment.

A. *S. aureus* is capable of causing extensive destruction of normal tissues such as cardiac valves. *S. aureus* is also particularly prone to metastasize from the original site of infection. Metastatic complications include osteomyelitis, pneumonia, septic arthritis, deep visceral abscesses, and endocarditis. These complications may be occult; however, failure to identify them predisposes to treatment failure. Consequently, a concerted search for endocarditis and metastatic sites of infection is essential. Clinical parameters predictive of complicated bacteremia include positive follow-up blood cultures at 48–96 hours, community acquisition, skin findings suggestive of acute systemic infection, and persistent fever at 72 hours. Even in the absence of any of these risk factors, however, the risk of complication from *S. aureus* bacteremia was 16% in one prospective study. Echocardiography is recommended in most cases to evaluate for endocarditis—the classic stigmata of this condition cannot be relied on to exclude the diagnosis because they are often absent. However, infectious disease consultation is recommended for complicated bacteremia, particularly endocarditis.

B. All vascular catheters must be removed. Although there have been a few reports of success "treating through" infected catheters, the risk of treatment failure is very high. Repeat blood cultures should be drawn in 24–48 hours. Persistently positive blood cultures or signs of clinical failure such as persistent fever or septic shock suggest complicated bacteremia and warrant transesophageal echocardiography to exclude infective endocarditis. Transthoracic echocardiography is useful if positive but can miss one fourth or more of cases of endocarditis. Patients with negative follow-up blood cultures, clinical improvement, and no indwelling devices (valves, hardware, pacemakers, etc.) should be treated for a minimum of 14 days. Because occult infectious foci are common and can have devastating consequences, use caution and err on the side of longer treatment if in doubt about whether there is complicated bacteremia.

C. Strive to identify an eradicable focus of infection because removing foci is vital for successful treatment and decreases mortality. The absence of a known primary focus is associated with an increased probability of endocarditis. Patients with prosthetic devices or hardware should be treated as if that device has been seeded. Obtain appropriate imaging studies to assess for drainable metastatic complications. If identified, it is often uncertain whether these are the cause or the result of the bacteremia. In either case, a prolonged course of at least 4–6 weeks of IV antibiotics is recommended.

D. For deep foci, such as visceral abscess, osteomyelitis, septic arthritis, or infected prosthetic devices, surgical drainage is recommended. Infected prosthetic devices must be removed. Treat with appropriate parenteral antibiotics for 4–6 weeks.

E. Antibiotic selection requires consideration of the possibility of MRSA. Although antistaphylococcal penicillins (e.g., nafcillin) remain the parenteral drug of choice for methicillin-susceptible *S. aureus*, the prevalence of MRSA is increasing rapidly. Initial therapy for known or suspected MRSA bacteremia is vancomycin. Alternatives in cases of vancomycin intolerance or allergy include quinupristin-dalfopristin, daptomycin, and linezolid. The use of aminoglycosides for "synergy" for the first 3–5 days of treatment may decrease the time required for clearance of bacteremia but does not improve the rate of cure or mortality and is not routinely recommended.

F. If treatment fails or relapse occurs, suspect occult endocarditis or metastatic focus of infection. Pursue a careful history and examination to identify areas of possible occult foci, paying particular attention to any prosthetic matter in the body. Transesophageal echocardiography and diagnostic imaging of all suspect areas of the body should be performed. Infected foreign devices should be removed and abscesses should be drained. Antibiotic therapy should be optimized by switching to nafcillin whenever possible or by maximizing the dose of vancomycin. Tight glucose control and minimization of immunosuppressants such as corticosteroids can also be beneficial. Addition of a second antistaphylococcal agent can also be considered. Infectious disease consultation is advised.

NEPHROLOGY

Ajay K. Singh, MBBS, FRCP
Section Editor

CHRONIC KIDNEY DISEASE

Ajay K. Singh, MBBS, FRCP

A. Chronic kidney disease (CKD) is defined as glomerular filtration rate (GFR) <60 ml/min/1.73 m^2 or structural/functional abnormalities of the kidney for ≥3 months; kidney disease <3 months' duration should be evaluated as acute renal failure. The evaluation of the patient with CKD should begin by verifying the duration of kidney damage and identifying potentially reversible causes. Renal ultrasonography should be performed in all patients to rule out obstruction, which is a potentially reversible cause of kidney disease. Important elements of the past medical history that may provide a clue to the cause of kidney disease include type 1 or type 2 diabetes mellitus, hypertension, rheumatologic diseases, malignancy, previous surgery involving the urinary system, viral hepatitis or HIV infection, kidney stones, and recurrent urinary tract infections. Medication history should include over-the-counter and herbal preparations. The review of systems should focus on recent infections; rash; arthralgias or arthritis; and uremic symptoms such as nausea, vomiting, pruritus, sleep difficulties, poor appetite, and abnormal taste. The family history may provide important information such as the possibility of polycystic kidney disease, Fabry's disease, and medullary cystic disease. Laboratory evaluation should include serum electrolytes, BUN, creatinine, urinalysis, urine protein:creatinine, and examination of the urine sediment. More targeted laboratory investigations such as ANAs, serum and urine protein electrophoresis, complement levels, antineutrophil cytoplasmic antibodies, cryoglobulins, and antiglomerular basement membrane antibodies should be undertaken in patients with a suggestive history, laboratory results, or urine sediment. Kidney biopsy can provide definitive diagnosis in patients for whom a diagnosis would alter treatment recommendations or inform prognosis.

B. Potentially reversible causes of CKD include obstructive uropathy, drug-induced interstitial nephritis, Fabry's disease, multiple myeloma, amyloidosis, and certain vasculitides and glomerulonephritides.

C. Serum creatinine should be used to determine the estimated GFR (eGFR) by the following formula: $186 \times \text{creatinine}^{-1.154} \times \text{age}^{-0.203}$ ($\times$ 0.742 if female and $\times$ 1.212 if black). Stage 1 CKD is defined as normal or elevated GFR (≥90 ml/min/1.73 m^2) with kidney damage noted radiographically or on urinalysis (e.g., proteinuria, red cell casts). CKD stages 2–5 are defined as GFR 60–89, 30–59, 15–29, and <15 ml/min/1.73 m^2 (or dialysis), respectively. Medications should be reviewed in patients with reduced eGFR and adjusted accordingly.

D. CKD may progress toward end-stage renal disease. Known risk factors include proteinuria, uncontrolled hypertension, smoking, and obesity. Blood pressure should be treated to below 130/80 mm/Hg. Angiotensin-converting enzyme (ACE) inhibitors or angiotensin receptor blockers should be used, particularly in patients with proteinuria. Diuretics are often required for blood pressure control in patients with CKD. The role of dietary protein intake is controversial. Consultation with a nutritionist is recommended, particularly for patients with stage 3 and higher CKD. Patients with stage 4 CKD should be prepared for the possibility of kidney replacement therapy and referred to a surgeon for evaluation of vascular access for hemodialysis or peritoneal catheter placement for peritoneal dialysis; early referral to a kidney transplant center or specialist is recommended.

E. CKD is a major risk factor for cardiovascular disease. Patients with CKD stages 1–4 should be considered in the highest-risk category for cardiovascular disease risk-reduction strategies. These include treatment of hyperglycemia in patients with diabetes, physical activity, smoking cessation, and use of antiplatelet and lipid-lowering drugs in appropriate patients.

F. Anemia, hyperphosphatemia, and secondary hyperparathyroidism frequently accompany CKD, particularly in its later stages. Hemoglobin and iron indices should be checked regularly in patients with CKD. Recombinant erythropoietin or related analogs should be used to treat anemia; oral and/or IV iron may be necessary for iron deficiency. Treatment of hyperphosphatemia includes dietary modification and the use of oral phosphate binders. Secondary hyperparathyroidism is treated by controlling hyperphosphatemia and replacement of vitamin D with either 25-vitamin D (in deficient patients) or 1,25-vitamin D or its analogs.

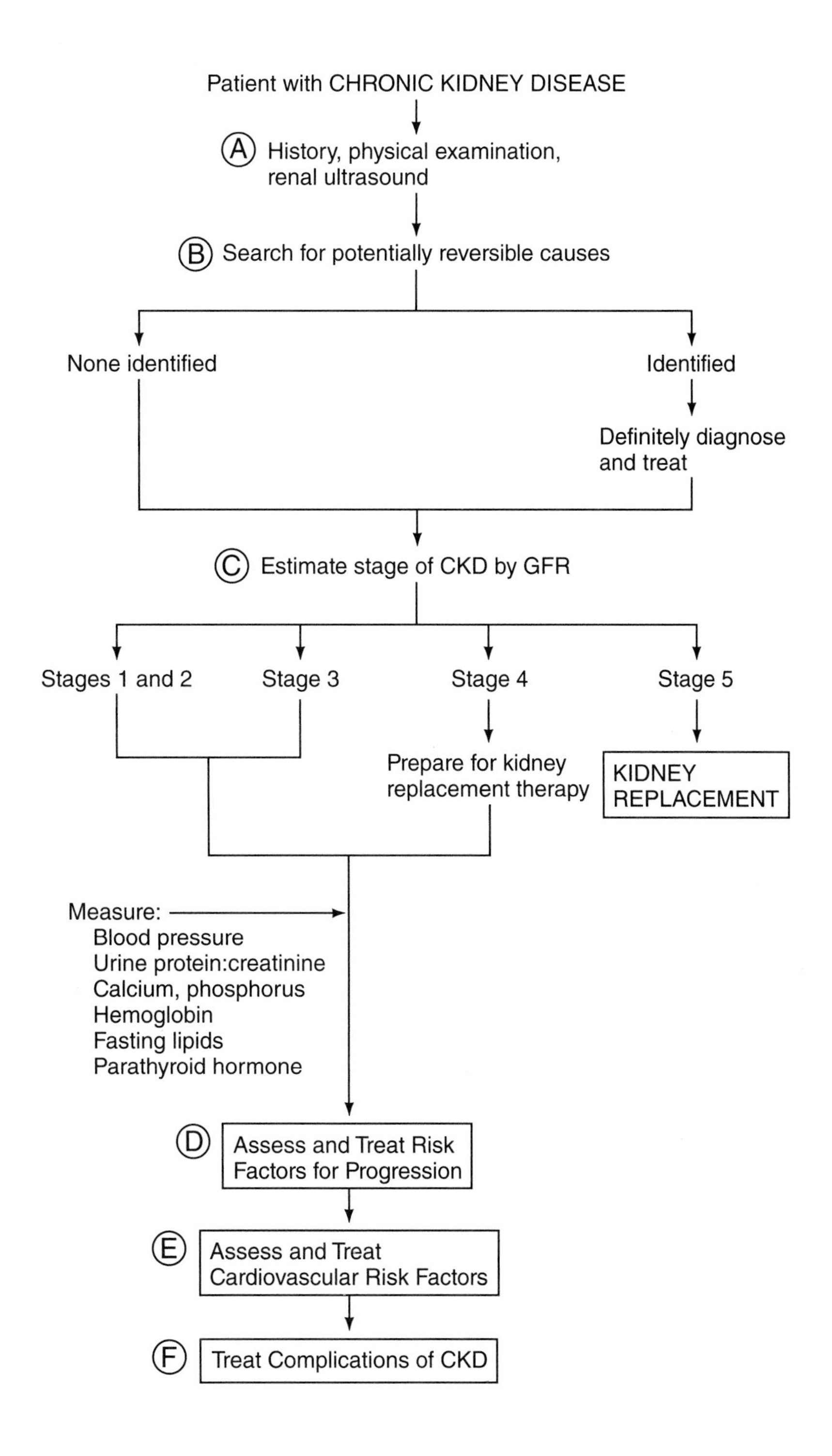

References

Fried LF, Katz R, Sarnak MJ, et al. Kidney function as a predictor of noncardiovascular mortality. J Am Soc Nephrol 2005;16(12):3728–3735.

Jaber BL, Madias NE. Progression of chronic kidney disease: can it be prevented or arrested? Am J Med 2005;118(12):1323–1330.

K/DOQI clinical practice guidelines for chronic kidney disease: evaluation, classification, and stratification. Am J Kidney Dis 2002;39(2 Suppl 1):S1–266.

Levey AS, Bosch JP, Lewis JB, et al. A more accurate method to estimate glomerular filtration rate from serum creatinine: a new prediction equation. Modification of Diet in Renal Disease Study Group. Ann Intern Med 1999;130(6):461–470.

Remuzzi G, Ruggenenti P, Perico N. Chronic renal diseases: renoprotective benefits of renin-angiotensin system inhibition. Ann Intern Med 2002;136(8):604–615.

Sica D, Carl D. Pathologic basis and treatment considerations in chronic kidney disease-related hypertension. Semin Nephrol 2005;25(4):246–251.

ACUTE RENAL FAILURE

Ajay K. Singh, MBBS, FRCP

Acute renal failure (ARF) is defined as a reduction in renal function manifested by an increase in serum creatinine over a period of hours to days. It is often associated with decreased urine output and a failure to excrete nitrogenous waste products and may lead to fluid and electrolyte imbalances. In the absence of a sustained increase, serum creatinine >0.5 mg/dl is a well-established definition of ARF. The causes of ARF may be prerenal (e.g., hypotension, arterial thrombosis), renal parenchymal (e.g., acute tubular necrosis [ATN], glomerulonephritis, tubulointerstitial nephritis), or postrenal (e.g., acute obstruction).

A. The patient with ARF usually presents with abnormal laboratory values, decreased urine output, or both. A thorough history and physical examination are critical in evaluation. Key issues are as follows: (1) ascertaining a history suggestive of bladder outflow obstruction (e.g., secondary to prostatism, such as nocturia, hesitation, and frequency of urination; assessment of any exposures to toxins or nephrotoxic medications, such as exposure to lead or ingestion of NSAIDs; and any systemic symptomatology suggesting an autoimmune etiology, such as arthralgias, arthritis, skin rash); (2) family history of diabetes or kidney disease; and (3) a physical examination focused on assessment of extracellular volume (edema, dry mucous membranes, hypertension, orthostatic hypotension, skin turgor) and detection of systemic process, such as an infection or an autoimmune process.

B. The evaluation of a fresh-voided urine sample for dipstick and microscopy of the urine sediment is essential. The presence of hematuria, proteinuria, or pyuria is important in diagnosis. Careful evaluation of the urinary sediment is key. In a patient with ATN, the presence of tubular cells, amorphous debris representing necrotic cells, and deeply pigmented coarsely granular ("muddy brown") casts are typical. In glomerulonephritis, the presence of red cells, particularly dysmorphic red cells, and red cell casts are characteristic. In acute tubulointerstitial nephritis, the presence of white cells, tubular epithelial cells, and white cell and/or tubular cell casts is typical. Laboratory testing should also include measurement of urine osmolality; sodium, protein, and creatinine in the urine; and serum osmolality, sodium, glucose, anion gap, albumin, total protein, calcium, BUN, and creatinine. In the workup of a patient suspected of having glomerulonephritis, serologic testing, including measurement of complement fractions, and assays for ANA, antineutrophil cytoplasmic antibody (ANCA), and antiglomerular antibody (anti-GBM) should be considered. Early evaluation with a renal ultrasound (US) is essential to exclude urinary obstruction. Severe cases of ATN and some forms of rapid progressive glomerulonephritis (RPGN; e.g., anti-GBM disease) may require a renal biopsy for diagnosis.

C. Prerenal renal failure can result from any condition that leads to decreased renal perfusion, such as intravascular volume depletion (e.g., hemorrhage, GI losses, excessive sweating, third space losses), decreased effective volume (e.g., congestive heart failure), increased renal vascular resistance (e.g., NSAIDs, hepatorenal syndrome), vasoconstrictor drugs (e.g., cyclosporine, radiocontrast), or decreased intraglomerular pressure (e.g., angiotensin-converting enzyme inhibitors). As proximal tubule function is preserved, the urine osmolality (UOsm) is typically >500 mOsm/kg, urine sodium (UNa) is <20 mEq/L, and the fractional excretion of sodium (FeNa) is <1%. In patients receiving diuretics, a fractional excretion of urea of <35% has been found to be more useful. Prerenal azotemia is reversible within 24–72 hours of correction of the hypoperfused state; however, prolonged hypoperfusion may lead to ischemic ATN, which has a more protracted course to recovery (see later). An otherwise bland urine sediment or hematuria with nondysmorphic RBCs calls for evaluation with imaging studies to exclude obstruction.

(Continued on page 356)

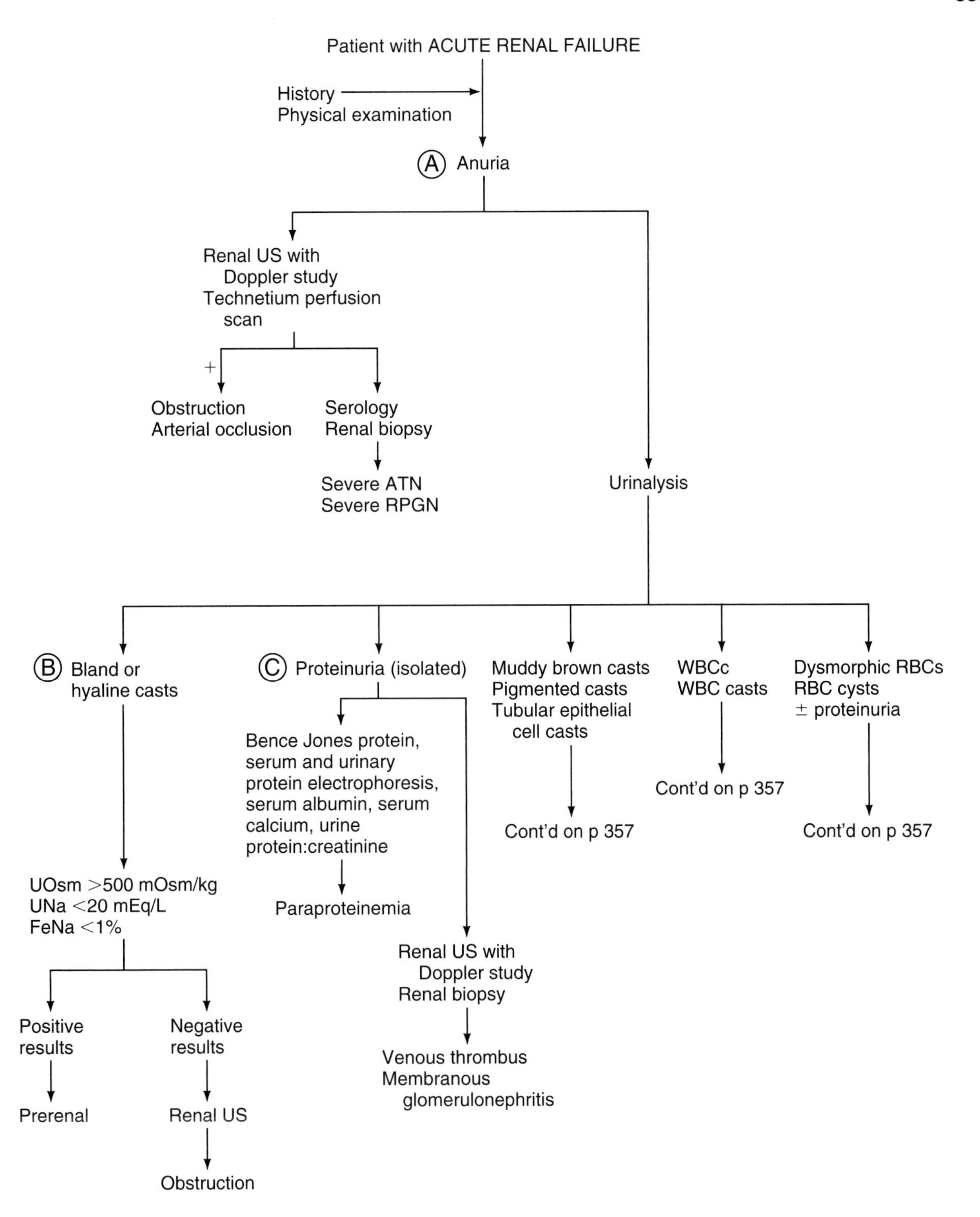

Patient with ACUTE RENAL FAILURE
History
Physical examination
(A) Anuria
Renal US with Doppler study
Technetium perfusion scan
+
Obstruction
Arterial occlusion
Serology
Renal biopsy
Severe ATN
Severe RPGN
Urinalysis
(B) Bland or hyaline casts
UOsm >500 mOsm/kg
UNa <20 mEq/L
FeNa <1%
Positive results
Prerenal
Negative results
Renal US
Obstruction
(C) Proteinuria (isolated)
Bence Jones protein, serum and urinary protein electrophoresis, serum albumin, serum calcium, urine protein:creatinine
Paraproteinemia
Renal US with Doppler study
Renal biopsy
Venous thrombus
Membranous glomerulonephritis
Muddy brown casts
Pigmented casts
Tubular epithelial cell casts
Cont'd on p 357
WBCc
WBC casts
Cont'd on p 357
Dysmorphic RBCs
RBC cysts
± proteinuria
Cont'd on p 357

D. ATN may result from ischemia, exogenous toxins and nephrotoxic drugs (e.g., aminoglycosides, cisplatin, radiocontrast), or endogenous toxins (hemoglobin, myoglobin, uric acid). Urinary oxalate crystals and an osmolar gap point toward ethylene glycol as the etiology, whereas predominance of uric acid crystals should evoke dedicated laboratory studies for gout and other states with high cell turnover such as hematologic malignancies and tumor lysis syndrome. A dipstick positive for hemoglobin in the absence of RBCs in the urine sediment is indicative of myoglobin or hemoglobin in the urine. Serum studies for creatine kinase (CK), haptoglobin, and the clinical context help to make the diagnosis of rhabdomyolysis. A clinically important issue is the differentiation of prerenal azotemia and ischemic ATN that together underlies 75% of cases with acute kidney injury. ATN is characterized by loss of renal tubule epithelial cell function; therefore, urine osmolality is typically <350 mOsm/kg, urine sodium is >40 mEq/L, and FeNa is $>1\%$. In some nonoliguric forms of ATN, such as after radiocontrast or rhabdomyolysis, the FeNa can initially be $<1\%$. Treatment for ATN is supportive; thus far, no therapeutic intervention has been shown to accelerate recovery from ATN, reduce mortality, or improve the length of stay in the hospital. Renal replacement therapy should be provided in a timely fashion when required by volume status or electrolyte imbalances.

E. Dysuria, flank pain, and fever may be associated with an ascending pyelonephritis. Antibiotics are given according to urine and blood culture results. Urinary tract infections in single kidneys (native or transplanted) are particularly prone to decrease renal function. Drug-induced allergic interstitial nephritis (AIN) resulting from a broad variety of medications may be associated with eosinophilia, fever, and skin rash. However, $<10\%$ of patients with AIN present with all three symptoms. Any suspected agent should be discontinued. A renal biopsy is recommended to confirm the diagnosis prior to initiating steroid therapy and to exclude other causes of interstitial nephritis such as the tubulointerstitial nephritis and uveitis (TINU) syndrome or sarcoidosis.

F. Serologic evaluation is usually indicated to diagnose cases of ARF with hematuria, proteinuria, and a sediment that contains dysmorphic RBCs and/or RBC casts. Measurement of a spot urine protein and creatinine is helpful in the differential diagnosis. A urine protein: creatinine ratio >3.5 indicates nephrotic-range proteinuria. If, in addition, the patient has edema and there is a low serum albumin (<3 mg/dl), the patient fits the definition of nephritic syndrome. In this scenario, a renal biopsy can be helpful in establishing the precise diagnosis. In a patient with hypertension and a urine sample that reveals hematuria, proteinuria, and the presence of dysmorphic cells and/or red cell casts, acute nephritis is the most likely diagnosis. A careful clinical evaluation looking for systemic abnormalities and a full serologic evaluation are necessary. Serologic evaluation includes, depending on history and examination, complement levels, ASLO-titer, ANA, ANCA, anti-GBM, hepatitis B and C serologies, cryoglobulins, and syphilis serology. In many instances, a renal biopsy is needed for diagnosis. If signs of systemic vasculitis or pulmonary involvement are present, early intervention with immunosuppressive therapy (IV steroids, cyclophosphamide, plasmapheresis) may be indicated before the results of serologic evaluations are available.

References

Singri N, Ahya SN, Levin ML. Acute renal failure. JAMA 2003;289(6): 747–751.

Thadhani R, Pascual M, Bonventre JV. Acute renal failure. N Engl J Med 1996;334(22):1448–1460.

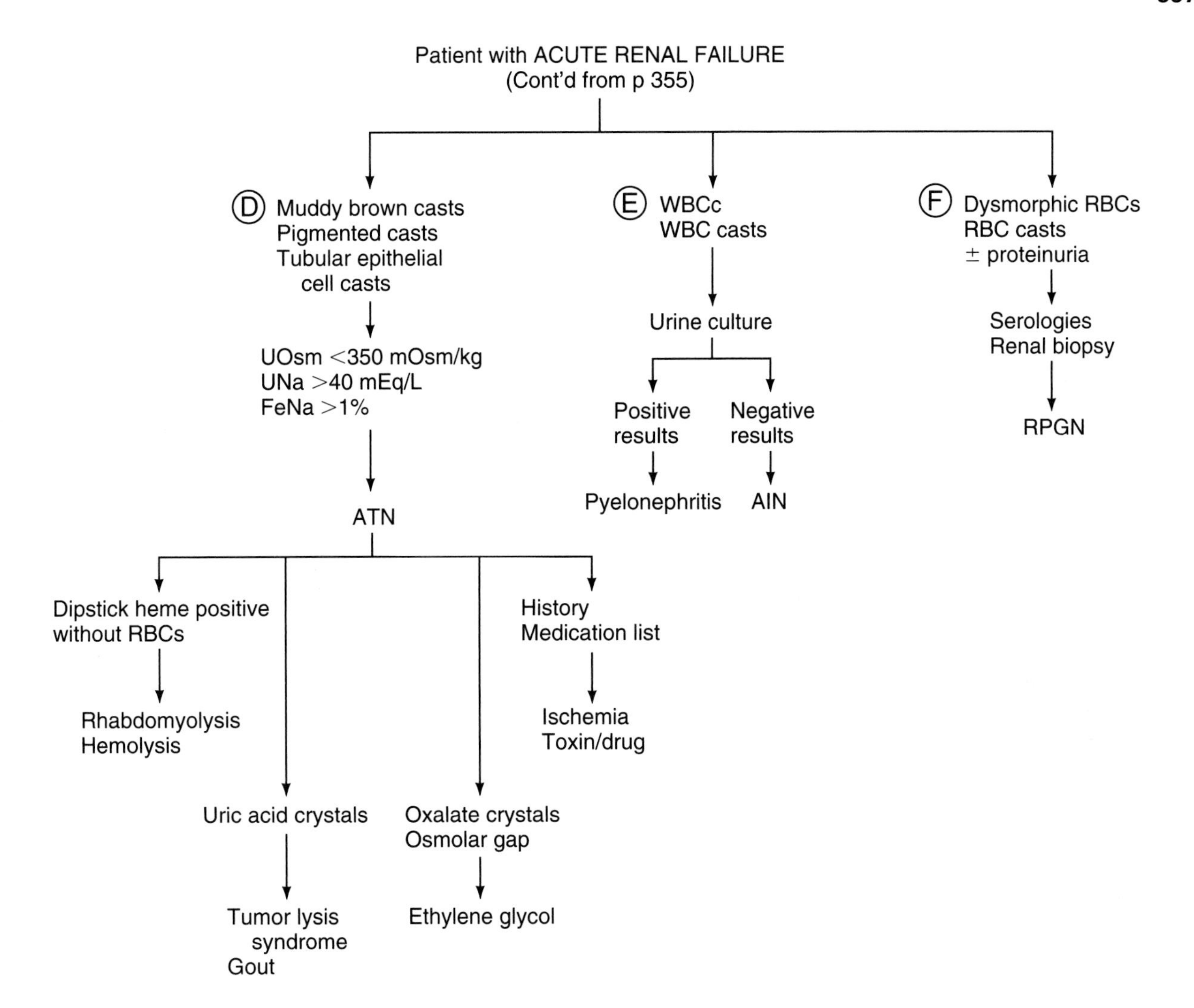

Patient with ACUTE RENAL FAILURE
(Cont'd from p 355)
D Muddy brown casts
Pigmented casts
Tubular epithelial cell casts
UOsm <350 mOsm/kg
UNa >40 mEq/L
FeNa >1%
ATN
Dipstick heme positive without RBCs
Rhabdomyolysis
Hemolysis
Uric acid crystals
Tumor lysis syndrome
Gout
Oxalate crystals
Osmolar gap
Ethylene glycol
History
Medication list
Ischemia
Toxin/drug
E WBCc
WBC casts
Urine culture
Positive results
Negative results
Pyelonephritis
AIN
F Dysmorphic RBCs
RBC casts
± proteinuria
Serologies
Renal biopsy
RPGN

PROTEINURIA

Cynthia Cooper Worobey, MD, and Ajay K. Singh, MBBS, FRCP

A. Proteinuria is the presence of >150 mg/day of protein in the urine. It is often discovered as a positive dipstick test (e.g., Albustix, Multistix) with the degree of proteinuria indicated by a change in color of the reagent, tetrabromophenol blue, ranging from trace (10–30 mg/dl) to 4+ (>1000 mg/dl). Because tetrabromophenol is a pH indicator, the dipstick is buffered to prevent the influence of normal variations in urine pH on color change. False-positive results can occur in very alkaline or concentrated urine; in gross hematuria; in the presence of penicillin, sulfonamides, or tolbutamide; and from contamination with pus, semen, or vaginal secretions. Dipstick protein may be falsely negative with dilute urine or when proteinuria is due to low molecular weight proteins such as light-chain immunoglobulins. Also, dipstick testing is not sufficiently sensitive to detect microalbuminuria (>30 mg/24 hr) and is not appropriate screening for incipient diabetic nephropathy. The sulfosalicylic acid (SSA) turbidity test qualitatively screens for proteinuria. This test should be considered in the workup of patients with suspected paraproteinemia-related renal disease—these patients will be dipstick negative for albumin but will have a positive SSA test because of the presence of Bence Jones protein in the urine. The SSA method requires a few milliliters of freshly voided, centrifuged urine. An equal amount of 3% SSA is added to that specimen. Turbidity will result from protein concentrations as low as 4 mg/dl (0.04 g/L).

B. Functional proteinuria describes a transient increase in urinary protein excretion caused by changes in glomerular hemodynamics, such as can occur with vigorous exercise or fever (Table 1). Postural or orthostatic proteinuria is a type of functional proteinuria typically seen in individuals <30 years of age. Proteinuria is absent after a period of being recumbent, such as after a night's sleep, and develops upon rising. Patients with orthostatic proteinuria are usually <30 years of age, have moderate proteinuria (excrete <2 g/day of protein), and have normal kidney function. Orthostatic proteinuria is relatively common, affecting about 3%–5% of adolescents and young adults. To diagnose orthostatic proteinuria, split urine specimens are obtained for comparison. The first-morning void is discarded. A 16-hour daytime specimen is obtained with the patient performing normal activities and finishing the collection by voiding just before bedtime. An 8-hour overnight specimen is then collected. Functional proteinuria, including orthostatic proteinuria, generally follows a benign course, often with spontaneous resolution.

C. Patients with dipstick-positive urinary protein that persists on repeat testing should undergo a quantitative measurement of protein excretion. The urine protein:creatinine ratio (PCR) in a random urine sample provides an estimate of daily urinary protein excretion. This should be confirmed with a 24-hour urine collection. Urinary creatinine excretion should be included in the 24-hour measurement to determine the adequacy of the specimen. Normal urine creatinine excretion varies by age and sex but is roughly 15–25 mg/kg/day. In the absence of diabetes, isolated urinary protein excretion of <300 mg/day can be followed expectantly.

D. Proteinuria ≥300 mg/day that is persistent should be investigated with a careful history (noting prescription, over-the-counter, and illicit drug use), CBC, and thorough physical examination (Table 2). Renal function tests and a CBC should be obtained. Urinalysis should be performed to detect hematuria or signs of urinary tract infection. Evidence of new renal insufficiency or hematuria without concurrent infection should trigger referral to a nephrologist for further serologic evaluation and possible renal biopsy (see Hematuria chapter). Diabetics should have a funduscopic examination to assess for retinopathy. Renal ultrasound should be obtained to evaluate for signs of chronic obstruction or reflux. Large kidneys can be seen with proteinuria because of HIV, diabetes, and infiltrative processes such as amyloidosis. Any signs or symptoms of hepatitis or HIV infection, connective tissue disease, vasculitis, malignancy, or multiple myeloma should be carefully pursued.

(Continued on page 360)

Table 1 **Common Causes of Functional Proteinuria**

Dehydration
Emotional stress
Fever
Intense physical activity
Most acute illnesses
Orthostatic (postural) disorder

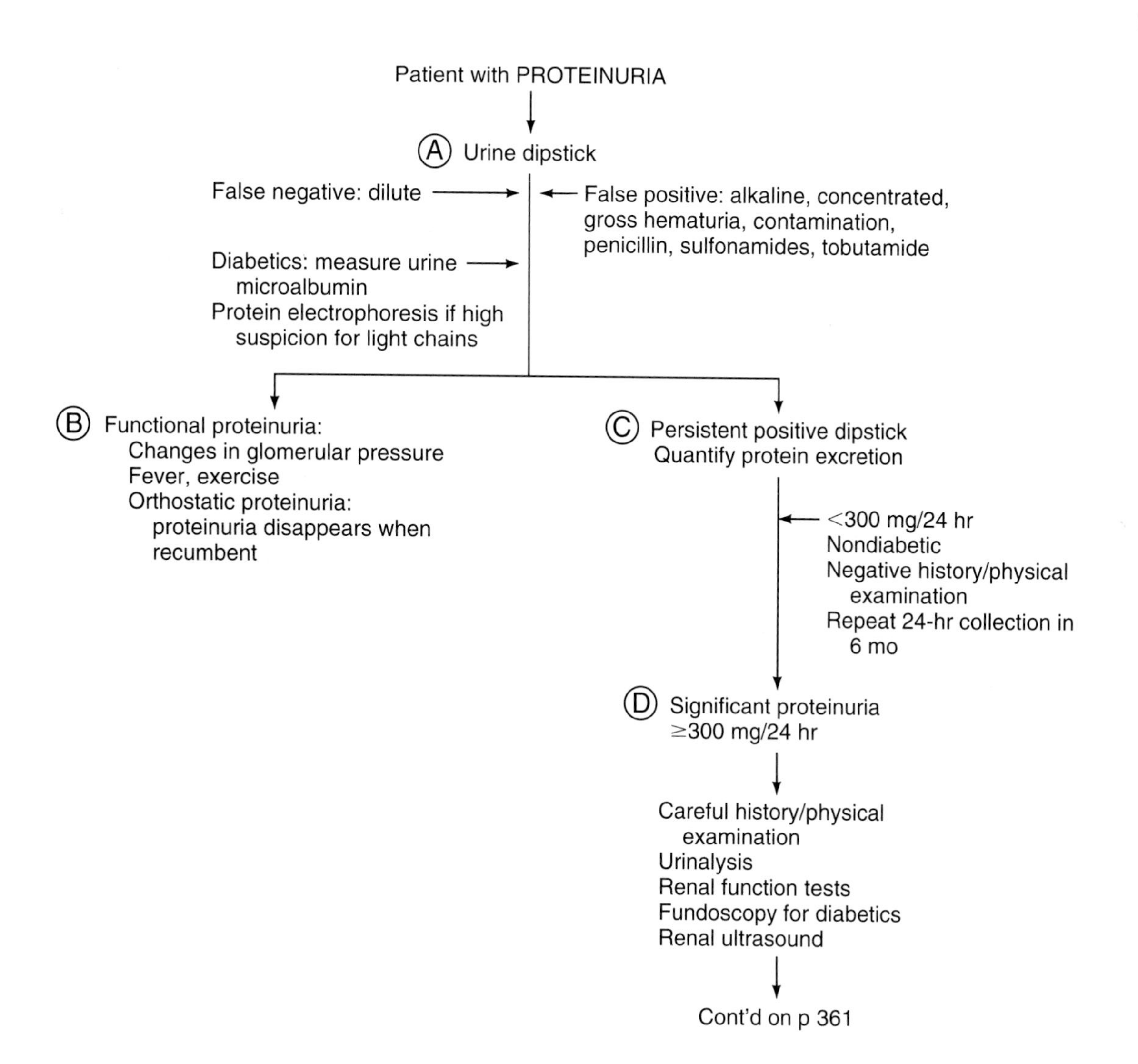
Patient with PROTEINURIA
(A) Urine dipstick
False negative: dilute
False positive: alkaline, concentrated, gross hematuria, contamination, penicillin, sulfonamides, tobutamide
Diabetics: measure urine microalbumin
Protein electrophoresis if high suspicion for light chains
(B) Functional proteinuria:
Changes in glomerular pressure
Fever, exercise
Orthostatic proteinuria: proteinuria disappears when recumbent
(C) Persistent positive dipstick
Quantify protein excretion
<300 mg/24 hr
Nondiabetic
Negative history/physical examination
Repeat 24-hr collection in 6 mo
(D) Significant proteinuria ≥300 mg/24 hr
Careful history/physical examination
Urinalysis
Renal function tests
Fundoscopy for diabetics
Renal ultrasound
Cont'd on p 361

Table 2 **Classification of Proteinuria**

Glomerular
Primary
Minimal-change disease
Idiopathic membranous glomerulonephritis
Focal segmental glomerulonephritis
Membranoproliferative glomerulonephritis
IgA nephropathy
Secondary
Diabetes mellitus
Autoimmune disorders (e.g., lupus nephritis)
Amyloidosis
Preeclampsia
Infection (e.g., HIV, hepatitis B and C, poststreptococcal illness, syphilis, malaria, endocarditis)
Malignancies (e.g., colon and gastric cancers, lung cancer, lymphoma)
Drugs (gold, penicillamine, heroin, NSAIDs)
Tubular
Hypertensive nephrosclerosis
Uric acid nephropathy
Acute allergic interstitial nephritis (e.g., NSAIDs, antibiotics)

E. Nephrotic-range proteinuria (≥3.5 g/day) warrants referral to a nephrologist for further evaluation and possible renal biopsy. The nephrotic syndrome refers to the clinical picture of heavy proteinuria (>3.5 g/day) with edema, hypoalbuminemia (<3.0 g/dl), hyperlipidemia, and lipiduria. The nephrotic syndrome may be a primary process or secondary to a systemic illness. The most common cause of nephrotic syndrome in children is minimal-change disease (accounts for >90% of all cases in children <10 years of age and 50% in children >10 years of age). In adults the most common cause is membranous glomerulopathy in whites and focal segmental glomerulosclerosis in blacks. Important secondary causes of nephrotic syndrome include diabetes mellitus medications including NSAIDs, gold, and penicillamine; infections such as hepatitis B; and autoimmune etiologies such as lupus nephritis. Careful history and evaluation for infection, connective tissue disorder, malignancy, or drug use should uncover most secondary causes. However, serologic evaluation, including for complement, ANA, antistreptolysin assay (ASA titer), hepatitis serologies, and measurement of antineutrophil cytoplasmic antibodies (ANCA), coupled with a renal biopsy, remains the best means of establishing a definite diagnosis for proteinuria. Patients with renal insufficiency, hematuria without infection, or persistent proteinuria without a clear diagnosis should be referred to a nephrologist and considered for renal biopsy.

References

Carroll MF, Temte JL. Proteinuria in adults: a diagnostic approach. Am Fam Physician 2000;62(6):1333–1340.

House AA, Cattran DC. Nephrology: 2. Evaluation of asymptomatic hematuria and proteinuria in adult primary care. CMAJ 2002;166(3):348–353.

Orth SR, Ritz E. Medical progress: the nephrotic syndrome. N Engl J Med 1998;338:1202–1211.

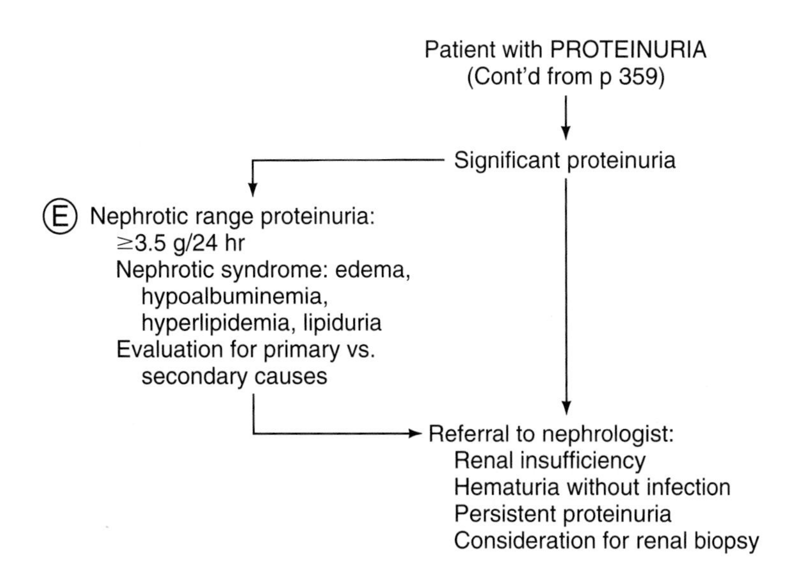
Patient with PROTEINURIA
(Cont'd from p 359)
Significant proteinuria
(E) Nephrotic range proteinuria:
≥3.5 g/24 hr
Nephrotic syndrome: edema, hypoalbuminemia, hyperlipidemia, lipiduria
Evaluation for primary vs. secondary causes
Referral to nephrologist:
Renal insufficiency
Hematuria without infection
Persistent proteinuria
Consideration for renal biopsy

HEMATURIA

Cynthia Cooper Worobey, MD, and Ajay K. Singh, MBBS, FRCP

A. Microscopic hematuria is defined as ≥3 RBCs per high-power microscopic field (hpf) in two of three properly collected centrifuged urine specimens. Urine examined should be from freshly voided, clean-catch, midstream collections. Dipstick testing for heme may be positive in the presence of hemoglobin from as few as 1 RBC/hpf or in the presence of myoglobin or free hemoglobin. Any heme- positive dipstick test should be confirmed by microscopic examination.

B. Renal function tests and a CBC with prothrombin time (PT) and partial thromboplastin time (PTT) should be obtained. If dipstick testing is positive for either bacteruria or pyuria, a urine culture should be sent. If an infection is confirmed, dipstick testing to document resolution of hematuria can be repeated at the completion of antibiotic therapy. If dipstick testing is positive for protein, total urinary protein excretion should be measured. The ratio of the urinary protein concentration to urinary creatinine concentration (PCR) of a random urine sample provides an estimate of daily protein excretion. This should be confirmed with a 24-hour urine collection. A ratio of urinary protein to urinary creatinine >0.3 and/or a 24-hour urinary protein excretion >300 mg suggests the kidney as the source of the microscopic hematuria. The presence of dysmorphic red cells or red cell casts on microscopic examination and/or abnormal renal function further support the diagnosis of a renal parenchymal process.

C. Microscopic analysis of the urine can further distinguish glomerular from nonglomerular bleeding (Table 1). Red cell casts are a specific but insensitive marker of glomerular bleeding. Small, dysmorphic red cells also suggest a glomerular source of microscopic hematuria. Urinary red cells with a uniform biconcave disk shape suggest bleeding from a nonglomerular source.

D. Microscopic hematuria of glomerular origin without proteinuria or renal insufficiency may not require renal biopsy. The most common glomerular causes of isolated microscopic hematuria are immunoglobulin A (IgA) nephropathy, thin basement membrane disease, and hereditary nephritis (Alport's syndrome). If renal function is within the normal range and stable, a renal biopsy may not be necessary for the management of isolated microscopic hematuria of glomerular origin.

E. Microscopic hematuria of glomerular origin with renal insufficiency or proteinuria warrants referral to a nephrologist for evaluation and possible renal biopsy. Serologic tests should be obtained; these include ANA, antineutrophil cytoplasmic antibody (ANCA), antiglomerular basement membrane antibody (anti-GBM), plasma complement (C3 and C4) levels, cryoglobulin, and hepatitis B and C.

F. Once a glomerular source of microscopic hematuria has been ruled out, a rigorous examination of the upper and lower urinary tract for the source of bleeding is warranted. Urothelial cancers are the most common malignancies in patients with isolated microscopic hematuria. Risk factors for cancer that should be borne in mind include age >40 years, a smoking history, occupational exposure to chemical and dyes (e.g., benzene or aromatic amines), history of analgesic abuse, exposure to pelvic radiation, and history of gross hematuria. CT with and without IV contrast should be considered in all patients with nonglomerular hematuria.

Table 1 **Causes of Microscopic Hematuria**

Glomerular

Primary Glomerulonephritis
IgA nephropathy (Berger's disease)
Poststreptococcal
Membranoproliferative glomerulonephritis

Secondary Glomerulonephritis
Immune complex–associated (low C3, C4):
- Lupus nephritis
- Hepatitis C–associated nephritis and cryoglobulinemia
- Essential mixed cryoglobulinemia
- Bacterial endocarditis

Pauci-immune:
- Antiglomerular basement membrane disease
- Antineutrophil cytoplasmic antibody-associated glomerulonephritis
- Polyarteritis

Hereditary Causes
Hereditary nephritis (Alport's syndrome)
Thin GBM nephropathy
Fabry's disease
Nail-patella syndrome

Nonglomerular

Upper Urinary Tract
Renal tumors (renal cell carcinoma, angiomyolipoma, oncocytoma)
Vascular disorders (e.g., arteriovenous malformation, renal vein thrombosis, renal arterial thrombosis with renal infarction)
Polycystic kidney disease
Systemic bleeding disorder or coagulopathy
Infection (acute or chronic pyelonephritis, renal tuberculosis)
Papillary necrosis

Lower Urinary Tract
Tumors (renal pelvis, upper ureter, bladder, urethral)
Stone or foreign body
Trauma
Indwelling catheters
Cystitis
- Infectious
- Drug-induced

Radiation
Prostatitis

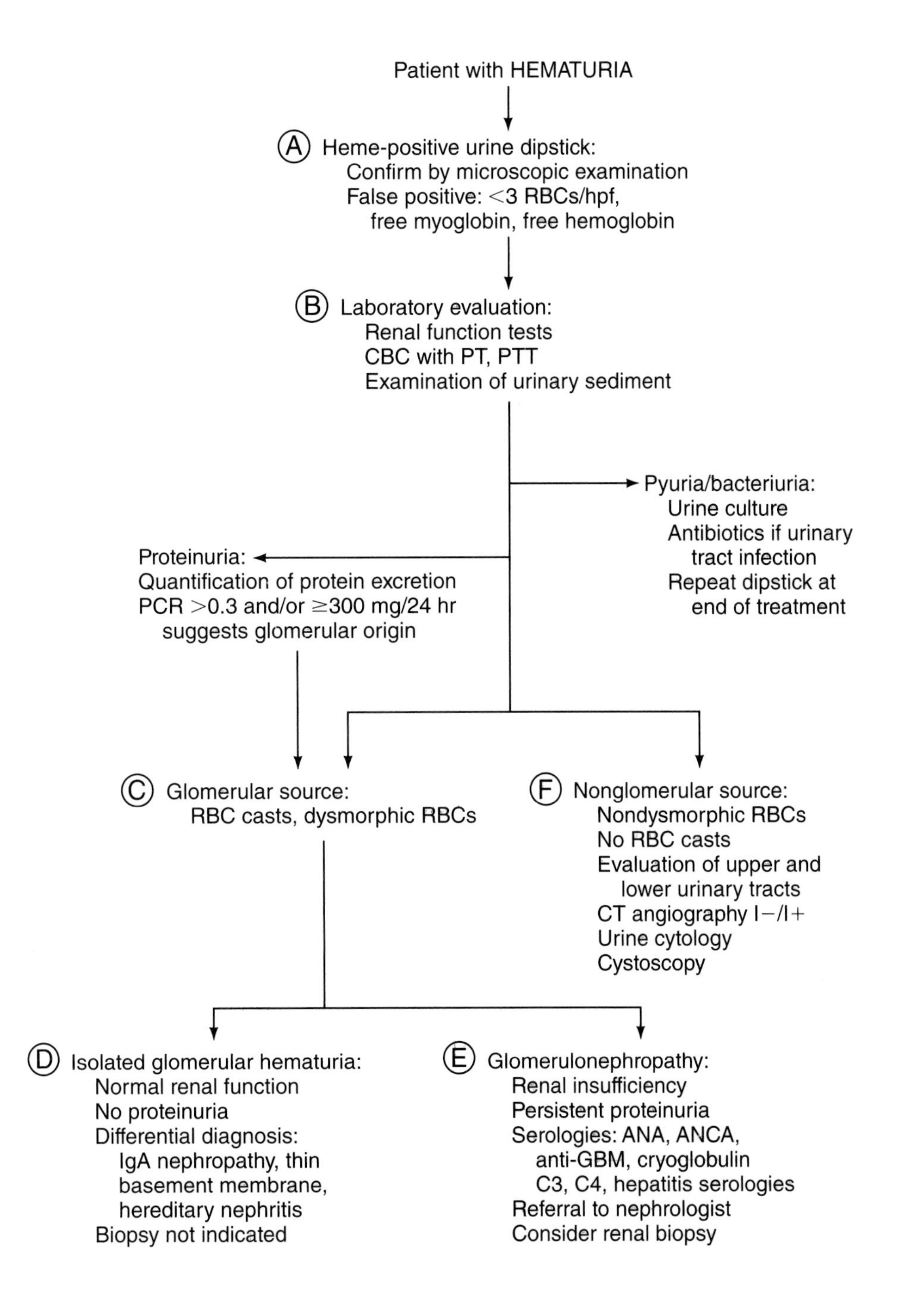

A decision to defer the contrast component of this study (e.g., after demonstration of urolithiasis on noncontrast CT) should be made only after careful risk assessment for concurrent urothelial cancer and with the expectation of close follow-up. If CT is unavailable, excretory urography or ultrasonography are reasonable alternatives to evaluate the upper urinary tract. Cytologic analysis of urine from three serial first-morning specimens should be obtained. Cystoscopic evaluation is recommended for the evaluation of microscopic hematuria in all adults >40 years and for those <40 years with risk factors for urothelial cancer. If the patient is <40 years and has no risk factors, cystoscopy may be deferred. For women with isolated hematuria, urethral and vaginal examinations should be performed to exclude local causes of microscopic hematuria. For uncircumcised men, the foreskin should be retracted to expose the glans penis for examination and urine collection. If phimosis is present, a catheterized urinary specimen may be required.

References

Cohen RA, Brown RS. Microscopic hematuria. N Engl J Med 2003;348: 2330–2238.

Grossfeld GD, Wolf JS Jr, Litwan MS, et al. Asymptomatic microscopic hematuria in adults: summary of the AUA best practice policy recommendations. Am Fam Physician 2001;63(6):1145–1154.

Steele DJR, Michaels PJ. Case 40-2004—a 42-year-old woman with long-standing hematuria. N Engl J Med 2004;351:2851–2859.

Yun EJ, Meng MV, Carroll PR. Evaluation of patient with hematuria. Med Clin North Am 2004;88(2):329–343.

KIDNEY STONES

Ajay K. Singh, MBBS, FRCP

Kidney stone disease is a common cause of morbidity in the Western world. It affects 10%–20% of the population and leads to hospitalization in 1 in 1000 individuals each year. More than 80% of kidney stones occur in white males. White males have a lifetime risk of stone formation approximating 20%. In contrast, the lifetime risk in white females is much lower—approximately 5%–10%. There is also clear racial preponderance of stone disease among whites. Blacks have an incidence rate of stone disease that is 25% that of whites. The peak age of onset for kidney stone formation is 20–30 years. However, there is a high recurrence rate—as high as 50% in 5 years among white males.

Of the four types of kidney stones (Table 1), the most common are calcium-containing stones, which may be calcium oxalate, calcium phosphate, or mixed calcium oxalate/calcium phosphate stones. Magnesium ammonium phosphate stones, also known as struvite stones, are observed mostly in association with an underlying urease-splitting bacterial infection of the urinary tract (e.g., *Proteus* spp). These stones often recur and are usually seen in patients with an associated anatomic abnormality. Approximately 5%–10% of kidney stones are pure uric acid stones. These stones are usually observed in the context of hyperuricemia among patients with a gouty diathesis or a hematologic malignancy. Uric acid stones have a high recurrence rate. Cystine stones are rare. These stones are observed in patients with cystinuria, which results from an autosomal defect in the transport of cystine, ornithine, lysine, and arginine in the kidney and intestine.

The underlying risk factors for stone formation are incompletely understood. The most important risk factors are the supersaturation of urine either by calcium oxalate and/or by uric acid and the pH of the urine (Table 2). The absence or

Table 1 **Frequency of Different Stone Types**

Type	%
Calcium	70–80
Calcium oxalate	70
Calcium phosphate	<5
Mixed calcium oxalate/phosphate	<5
Magnesium ammonium phosphate (struvite)	10–20
Uric acid	5–10
Cystine	<1

Table 2 **Risk Factors for Kidney Stone Formation**

- Supersaturation of urine with solute (examples: hypercalciuria, hyperoxaluria)
- Inadequate inhibition of stone formation (examples: hypocitraturia, reduced levels of urinary osteopontin)
- Anatomic abnormalities (examples: pyelocalyceal diverticula, ureteropelvic junction obstruction, horseshoe kidney)
- Diet (examples: high protein intake, excessive dietary sodium, low urine volume implicated in stone-belt area such as southeastern United States and Middle East)
- Changes in urinary pH (examples: urinary tract infection from urease-splitting organism promotes alkaline urine)
- Certain medication use (examples: acetazolamide by increasing urine pH and urine excretion of calcium; triamterene by crystallizing in urine and forming nidus for stone formation)

reduced level of urinary inhibitors of stone formation, such as citrate, also favors stone formation. The presence of a urinary infection from a urease-splitting organism is a key factor in struvite stone formation. The most common stones are calcium oxalate stones (most often calcium oxalate monohydrate and dihydrate). Less than 5% of calcium-containing stones are composed of pure calcium phosphate (apatite or brushite, $CaHPO_4 \bullet 2H_2O$). The major cause of calcium stone formation is excessive urinary excretion of calcium (hypercalciuria). Hypercalciuria may occur with or without hypercalcemia (Table 3). Hypercalcemia enhances the renal filtered load of calcium and thus results in hypercalciuria. The most common etiology of hypercalcemia is primary hyperparathyroidism. Excessive parathyroid hormone (PTH) secretion causes hypercalcemia by stimulating increased resorption of bone and stimulating increased renal synthesis of dihydroxycholecalciferol (activated vitamin D), which, in turn, stimulates intestinal absorption of calcium. Increased resorption of calcium by the intestine, through a PTH and vitamin D–independent pathway, has also been suggested, but the mechanism remains obscure. Hypercalciuria without hypercalcemia is observed in 60% of calcium stone formers. The primary abnormality appears to be impairment in renal tubular resorption of calcium. Other less common etiologies for calcium-stone formation include hyperuricosuria, which occurs in about 10% of patients; hyperoxaluria; hypocitraturia; and medullary sponge kidney.

Table 3 **Diagnostic Workup of a Patient with a Kidney Stone**

1. Identify the number, size, and location of stones
   a. Radiopaque stones can be seen by a plain abdominal x-ray
   b. Radiolucent stones can be detected by CT
2. Analyze stone's chemical composition
   a. Strain urine (use a coffee filter for straining urine)
   b. Send stone to an experienced laboratory for stone analysis
3. Perform a metabolic workup
   a. Urinalysis and urine culture
   b. Blood chemistries
   c. 24-hour urine collection for volume, pH, calcium, phosphorus, sodium, uric acid, oxalate, citrate, cystine, and creatinine; collect at least two specimens to avoid variability

(Continued on page 366)

A. The clinical presentation varies depending on the location, size, and number of the stones. The majority of kidney stones occur in the upper tracts. The most common presentation is renal colic—the sudden onset of severe pain due to the presence of an obstructive renal or ureteral stone. Renal colic is typically spasmodic in character, lasting several minutes, typically localized to the flank, and often radiating down to the groin. Nausea and vomiting frequently accompany renal colic. Renal colic often occurs in the middle of the night or early morning while the patient is sedentary, and its severity has been described as akin to or worse than childbirth. The severity of pain is a common cause of patients coming to the emergency department. Larger stones may present with painless obstruction or back pain. Stones that reach the ureterovesical junction often present with renal colic accompanied by urgency and frequency. Stones located in the calyces may be completely asymptomatic. The general appearance of a patient with renal colic is of someone writhing in excruciating pain, acting restless, and pacing about the room. The presence of fever usually heralds an accompanying urinary tract infection. Otherwise the physical examination may be completely negative.

B. The laboratory evaluation should be comprised of a CBC; blood chemistries, including measurement of BUN and creatinine; and a urinalysis (Table 3). The presence of a urinary tract infection, particularly with pyelonephritis, will be associated with a leukocytosis. An elevated BUN and creatinine level suggest dehydration and/or the presence of an obstructing stone in a patient with a single kidney or a bilateral obstructing stones. The urine usually demonstrates hematuria and pyuria. Assessment of urine pH is critical because an acid urine with a radiolucent stone will suggest a uric acid stone, whereas very alkaline urine (pH >8.0) suggests an infection with a urease-splitting organism (e.g., *Proteus*, *Pseudomonas*, and *Klebsiella* spp.). The initial radiologic workup should include a KUB (kidney, ureter, and bladder) radiograph and an ultrasound or a noncontrast CT scan.

C. The management of kidney stones can be divided into the management of the acute stone episode and, if the stone is nonobstructing, management of the prevalent stone medically and/or surgically, with an additional focus on prevention of further stones. Management of the acute stone episode rests on optimal pain control using parenteral narcotic agents, hydration, and urologic consultation for potential removal of an obstructing stone. Medical management of a nonobstructing stone requires increasing fluid intake to cause a urine output of >2 L/day, modification in diet, treatment targeted at changing urinary pH, and strategies to prevent further stones from forming. Surgical management depends on the size, location, and number of stones. Surgical options include extracorporeal shock wave lithotripsy (ESWL) and percutaneous or transurethral lithotripsy. General rules are that cystine stones, calcium oxalate monohydrate stones, are generally poorly broken up by ESWL and percutaneous or transurethral lithotripsy for removal are favored. However, other calcium oxalate stones, struvite and uric acid stones, are generally amenable to ESWL and either percutaneous or transurethral routes for removal depending on the size and location of the stones.

References

Asplin JR. Evaluation of the kidney stone patient. Semin Nephrol 2008;28(2):99–110.

Miller NL, Lingeman JE. Management of kidney stones. BMJ 2007;334(7591):468–472.

Reynolds TM. ACP Best Practice No 181: Chemical pathology clinical investigation and management of nephrolithiasis. J Clin Pathol 2005;58(2):134–140.

Sakhaee K. Recent advances in the pathophysiology of nephrolithiasis. Kidney Int 2009;75(6):585–595. Epub 2008 Dec 10.

Unwin RJ, Capasso G, Robertson WG, Choong S. A guide to renal stone disease. Practitioner 2005;249(1666):18, 20, 24 passim.

Worcester EM, Coe FL. Nephrolithiasis. Prim Care 2008;35(2):369–391, vii.

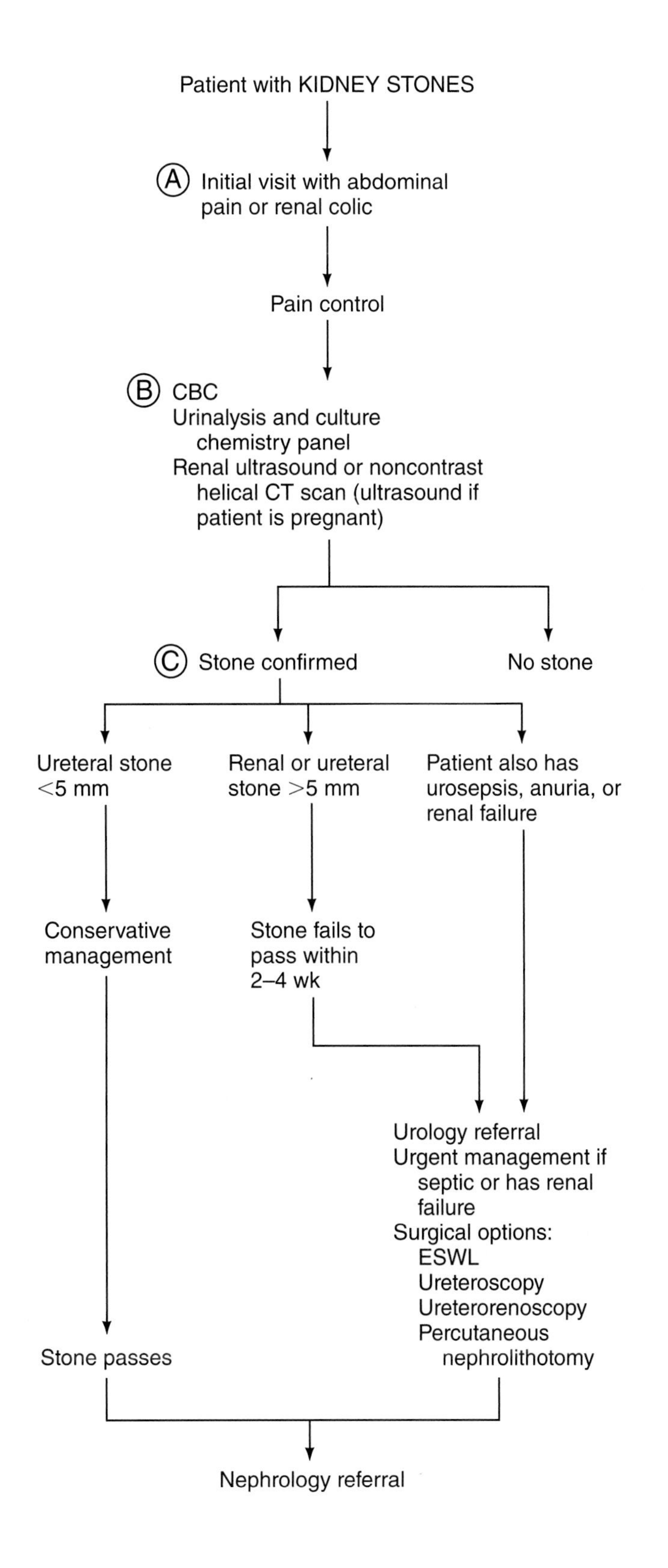
Patient with KIDNEY STONES
(A) Initial visit with abdominal pain or renal colic
Pain control
(B) CBC
Urinalysis and culture chemistry panel
Renal ultrasound or noncontrast helical CT scan (ultrasound if patient is pregnant)
(C) Stone confirmed
No stone
Ureteral stone <5 mm
Renal or ureteral stone >5 mm
Patient also has urosepsis, anuria, or renal failure
Conservative management
Stone fails to pass within 2–4 wk
Urology referral
Urgent management if septic or has renal failure
Surgical options:
ESWL
Ureteroscopy
Ureterorenoscopy
Percutaneous nephrolithotomy
Stone passes
Nephrology referral

RENAL CYSTS AND MASSES

Ana R. Stankovic, MD, and Ajay K. Singh, MBBS, FRCP

A. Hematuria, palpable abdominal mass, and flank pain are the most common clinical manifestations in a patient with a detectable renal lesion. The widespread use of ultrasound (US) and CT scanning has led to an increased detection of renal lesions. The chance of finding an incidental renal mass on CT scan is 33% for patients >50 years of age. With symptoms of hematuria, palpable abdominal mass, or flank pain, the evaluation should begin with an US and/or CT scan. The test sensitivity of a renal US to detect parenchymal masses is 79%. The renal US does not detect masses <5 mm in diameter. Therefore, a renal CT scan with contrast medium should be performed when visualization is inadequate on the US; the mass is small (<1 cm in diameter); or US examination shows evidence of calcifications, septa, or multiple cysts.

B. Most renal lesions are initially discovered on US. US criteria for the classification of simple renal cyst include: (1) spherical or ovoid shape; (2) absence of internal echoes; (3) presence of a thin, smooth wall that is separate from the surrounding parenchyma; and (4) enhancement of the posterior wall, indicating US transmission through the water-filled cyst. If all of these criteria are satisfied and the patient is asymptomatic, no further evaluation of the cyst is necessary because the likelihood of a malignancy is very small. Simple renal cysts are the most common renal masses, occurring in 50% of patients >50 years of age. Symptomatic patients with the same US findings should undergo CT scanning with contrast. The "gold standard" for evaluating renal masses requires CT images <5 mm in thickness before and after contrast is given. The criteria for diagnosing a benign cyst on CT scan include: (1) a homogeneous attenuation value near that of water, (2) no enhancement with IV contrast material, (3) no measurable thickness of the cyst wall, and (4) smooth interface with renal parenchyma. MRI is typically used to evaluate patients with indeterminate lesions. MRI does not detect calcifications. The suspicion for malignancy should be raised if the benign criteria are not met, calcification is present within a cyst, or repeat studies show an enlarging lesion. CT scan has a sensitivity of 94% for detection of renal parenchymal masses, but MRI is statistically superior to CT scan in the correct characterization of benign lesions. If a cyst meets the criteria for being benign, periodic reevaluation is the standard of care. If the lesion is not consistent with a simple cyst, surgical exploration is recommended.

C. Acquired renal cystic disease occurs in as many as 90% of patients who receive dialysis for 5–10 years. The cysts develop as a consequence of chronic renal insufficiency and may be clinically apparent long before dialysis is instituted.

(Continued on page 370)

Key Ultrasonographic Features of the Kidney in Health and Disease

Normal Kidney

- Each kidney measures 10–12 cm in length.
- The renal parenchyma is usually isoechoic compared to the liver or spleen.
- The renal sinuses are hyperechoic.

Hyperechoic Parenchyma Suggests "Medical Disease of the Kidneys"

- Differential diagnosis includes acute or chronic glomerular nephritis, interstitial nephritis, acute rejection, and infiltrative diseases of the kidney (lymphoma, amyloid, etc). Lymphoma most commonly shows rounded hypoechoic masses.

Renal Masses

- 90% of cysts are cortical.
- Cysts become more prevalent with increasing age (in the elderly 1–5 cysts in each kidney are common).
- Simple cysts are smooth, walled structures with distinct anterior and posterior walls and no internal echoes. Posterior acoustic enhancement is often seen.
- Suspect malignant cysts if they are septated or nodular or have thick irregular walls. Thick septations also warrants suspicion of malignancy.
- Solid renal masses: 85% of renal masses are renal cell cancers.
- Renal tumors may be hyperechoic or hypoechoic.
- Approximately 10% of renal tumors are amorphous in appearance and have evidence of calcification.
- Lymphoma should be suspected if there are multiple hypoechoic masses; it is rarely observed as diffuse hypoechoic enlargement.
- Leukemia can be observed either as multiple hypoechoic masses or as diffuse hypoechoic enlargement.
- Metastatic disease is characterized by gross, diffuse, disorganized distortion.
- Angiomyolipomas are benign tumors that are well circumscribed and very echogenic.
  - 80% are idiopathic.
  - More common (×4) in women than in men.
  - In association with tuberose sclerosis, are bilateral and multiple.

Renal Stones

- All types of stones produce acoustic shadow if >2 mm in size.

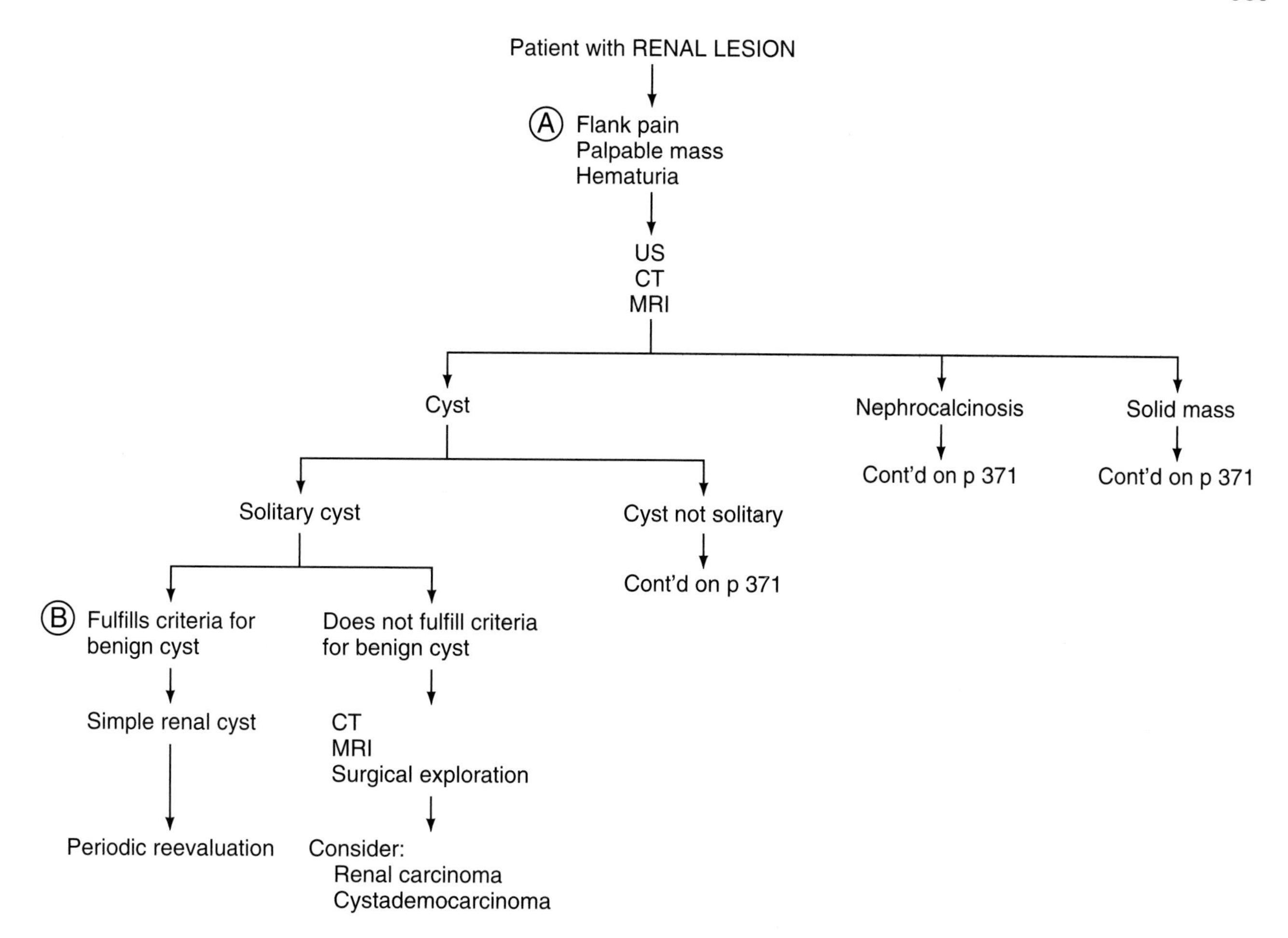
Patient with RENAL LESION
A
Flank pain
Palpable mass
Hematuria
US
CT
MRI
Cyst
Nephrocalcinosis
Solid mass
Cont'd on p 371
Cont'd on p 371
Solitary cyst
Cyst not solitary
Cont'd on p 371
B
Fulfills criteria for benign cyst
Does not fulfill criteria for benign cyst
Simple renal cyst
CT
MRI
Surgical exploration
Periodic reevaluation
Consider:
Renal carcinoma
Cystademocarcinoma

Malignancy and metastases can develop in a small percentage of cases. Screening of all dialysis patients by renal US is recommended after 3 years of dialysis at 1- to 2-year intervals. Major clinical manifestations of acquired cystic disease include flank pain and hematuria in association with rupture of hemorrhagic cysts into the urinary tract or into the perinephric region. Cysts often resolve after successful renal transplantation.

D. Autosomal-dominant polycystic kidney disease (ADPKD) is the most common renal hereditary disease and affects 1 in 400–1000 live births. ADPKD is usually recognized in adults between the third and fourth decades of life. Adult polycystic kidney disease (PKD) causes renal insufficiency in 50% individuals by age 70 years and accounts for 10% of dialysis patients in the United States. ADPKD is caused by defective *PKD1* gene on chromosome 16p in 85% of cases. A positive diagnosis requires (1) at least two cysts (unilateral or bilateral) in patients <30 years of age, (2) at least two cysts in each kidney in patients aged 30–59 years, or (3) four or more cysts in each kidney in patients >60 years. These age-specific data have been developed in reference to *PKD1* patients. Pathology of ADPKD is characterized by massive enlargement of the kidneys secondary to cyst growth and development. The liver also contains cysts in about 40% of patients with ADPKD. Arterial aneurysms of the circle of Willis are found in about 10% of patients. Diagnosis by US is straightforward in advanced disease but may be less reliable in the early stages. CT scan and MRI are more informative, and genetic testing may be required when greater certainty is needed for ADPKD diagnosis.

E. Medullary cystic kidney disease is a rare autosomal-dominant cystic disease characterized by normal- to small-sized kidneys. When cysts are found, they are located at the corticomedullary junction and in the medulla. Diagnosis relies on clinical features with a thorough family history. CT scan is the most sensitive test for cyst detection. The first signs are inability to concentrate the urine and salt wasting, leading to polyuria and polydipsia. Medullary cystic disease progresses inevitably to end-stage renal disease (ESRD) by the age of 20–40 years. Transplantation is the treatment of choice.

F. Medullary sponge kidney usually is not diagnosed before the fourth or fifth decade of life, when patients have secondary calcifications with passage of urinary stones or frequent urinary tract infections. This is a benign disorder with incidence of 1 in 5000 in the general population. The diagnosis is made by IV urography, which shows irregular enlargement of the medullary and interpapillary collecting ducts bilaterally. There is no specific therapy for medullary sponge kidney disease. The patients should be advised to excrete >2 L of urine per day and may benefit from a thiazide diuretic for hypercalciuria, allopurinol for hyperuricosuria, or potassium citrate for hypocitraturia.

G. Renal cell cancer occurs at a rate of 7.5 cases per 100,000 population annually. It accounts for >80% of renal malignancies in adults and occurs more often in men than in women. Risk factors for renal cell carcinoma are smoking, chemicals such as cadmium and nitroso hydrocarbons, acquired cystic disease in ESRD, and Hippel-Lindau disease. Patients may present with hematuria, abdominal mass, flank pain, fever, weight loss, or vericocoele, but many patients are asymptomatic until the disease is advanced. Laboratory findings include anemia or erythrocytosis, hepatic dysfunction, and hypercalcemia. CT scan with radiographic contrast is currently the most widely available, sensitive, and accurate nonoperative method available for making a presumptive diagnosis of renal cancer and its staging. Nuclear MRI is used over CT scanning (1) when detecting tumors in regional lymph nodes and extension into the renal veins and inferior vena cava, (2) in patients with radiographic contrast allergy, and (3) when CT results are equivocal. For patients without distant metastases the treatment of choice is radical nephrectomy. The average survival of patients with metastases is only 6–9 months. Postoperative adjuvant radiation, hormonal therapy, and chemotherapy are not proven to prolong survival.

References

Bosniak MA. The small (less than or equal to 3.0 cm) renal parenchymal tumor: detection, diagnosis, and controversies. Radiology 1991; 179(2):307–317.

Curry NS, Bissada NK. Radiologic evaluation of small and indeterminate renal masses. Urol Clin North Am 1997;24:493–505.

Grantham JJ. Cystic diseases of the kidney. In Stein's Internal Medicine, 5th ed. Philadelphia: Mosby, 1998.

McKinney TD. Renal cell carcinoma. In Stein's Internal Medicine, 5th ed. Philadelphia: Mosby, 1998.

Rizk D, Chapman AB. Cystic and inherited kidney diseases. Am J Kidney Dis 2003;42(6):1305–1317.

Rose BD, Bennett WM, Kruskal JB. Simple renal cysts and evaluation of renal masses in adults. UpToDate 2005. www.uptodate.com.

Watnick S, Morrison G. Approach to renal disease. In Current Medical Diagnosis & Treatment, 44th ed. New York: McGraw-Hill, 2005.

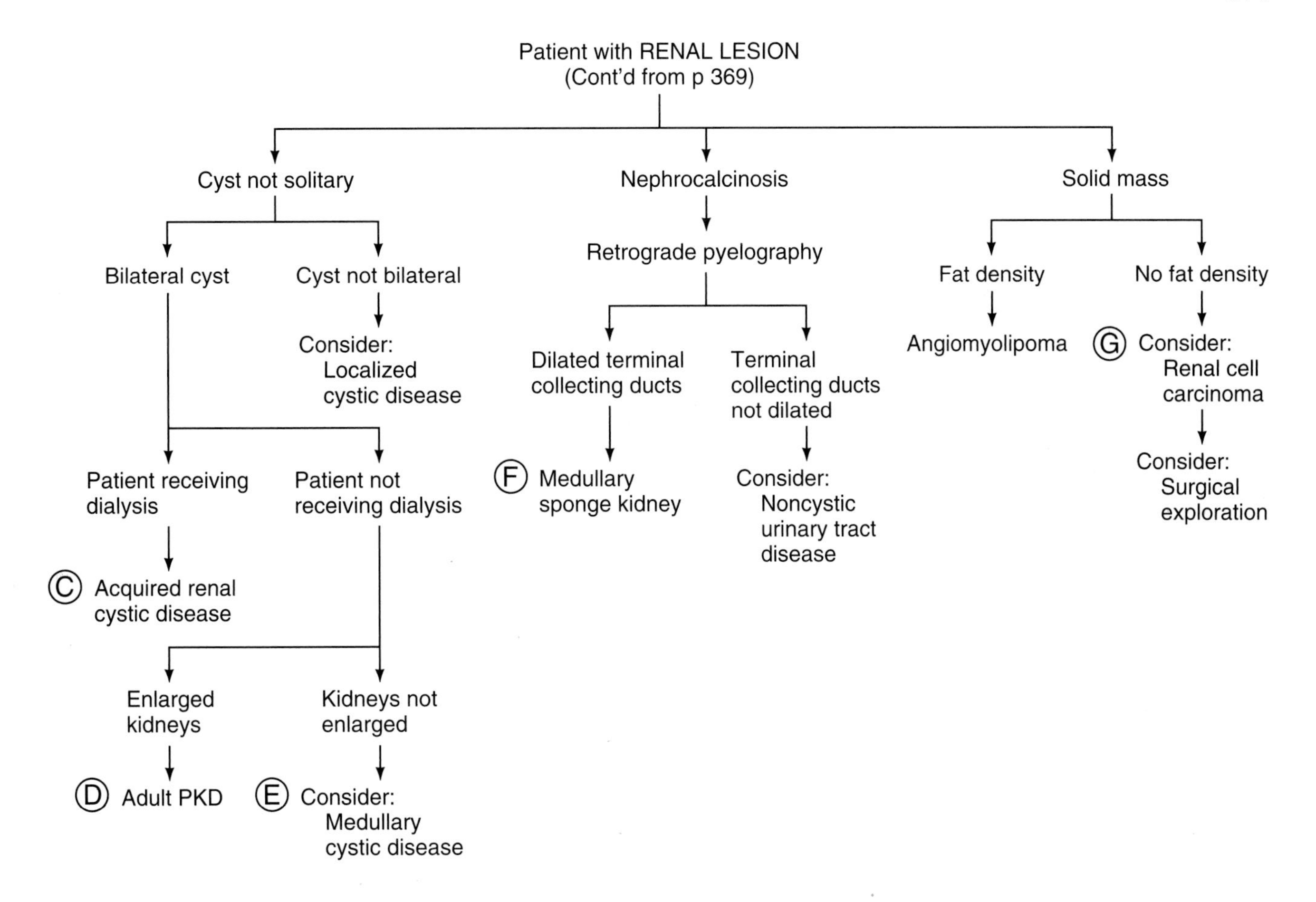
Patient with RENAL LESION
(Cont'd from p 369)
Cyst not solitary
Nephrocalcinosis
Solid mass
Bilateral cyst
Cyst not bilateral
Consider: Localized cystic disease
Retrograde pyelography
Fat density
No fat density
Dilated terminal collecting ducts
Terminal collecting ducts not dilated
Angiomyolipoma
G Consider: Renal cell carcinoma
Consider: Surgical exploration
Patient receiving dialysis
Patient not receiving dialysis
F Medullary sponge kidney
Consider: Noncystic urinary tract disease
C Acquired renal cystic disease
Enlarged kidneys
Kidneys not enlarged
D Adult PKD
E Consider: Medullary cystic disease

METABOLIC ACIDOSIS

Ajay K. Singh, MBBS, FRCP

A. Metabolic acidosis is characterized by a primary decrease in the serum bicarbonate concentration, which is a result of depletion of bicarbonate or by endogenous consumption of bicarbonate to buffer exogenous or endogenous generation of acid. Metabolic acidosis can be subdivided into elevated anion gap (AG) or normal AG acidosis (Table 1). Renal tubular acidosis (RTA) is a classical cause for a normal AG metabolic acidosis (Table 2). In proximal RTA the primary defect is impaired reabsorption of bicarbonate by the proximal tubule. It frequently is associated with defective phosphate, glucose, urate, and amino acid resorption. With distal RTA, the primary defect is an inability to maximally acidify the urine. Type III RTA is a combination of type I and type II RTA. Type IV RTA is characterized by impaired urinary acidification because of hypoaldosteronism. An elevated AG acidosis may occur commonly as a complication of a systemic illness. The AG is equal to the difference between the plasma concentrations of the measured plasma cation (i.e., Na^+) and the measured anions (i.e., chloride [Cl^-], HCO_3^-). AG calculation = $(Na^+) - ([Cl^-] + [HCO_3^-])$. The normal AG is 8−16 mEq/L, with an average value of 12. Causes of a high AG, lactic acidosis, ketoacidosis, renal failure, and ingestions are salicylate, methanol or formaldehyde (formate), ethylene glycol (glycolate, oxalate), paraldehyde (organic anions), sulfur (SO_4^-), phenformin/metformin, and pyroglutamic acidemia (5-oxoprolinemia). The mnemonic MUDPILES is popular: M—methanol; U—uremia; D—diabetic ketoacidosis (DKA), AKA; P—paraldehyde, phenformin; I—iron, isoniazid; L—lactic (i.e., CO, cyanide); E—ethylene glycol; and S—salicylates.

Table 1 **Causes of Metabolic Acidosis**

Normal Anion Gap
GI
Diarrhea
Ureteroileostomy
Renal
Renal tubular acidosis
Aldosterone deficiency (hyporeninemic hypoaldosteronism)
Drugs
Ammonium chloride
Lysine or arginine hydrochloride
Elevated Anion Gap
Diabetic ketoacidosis
Alcoholic ketoacidosis
Starvation ketoacidosis
Lactic acidosis
Toxic ingestion
Methanol
Ethylene glycol
Salicylates
Paraldehyde
Renal failure

Table 2 **Key Features of Renal Tubular Acidosis**

RTA Type	Urine pH	Serum Potassium
Type I RTA (distal)	>5.5	Normal limits or decreased
Type II RTA (proximal)	<5.5	Decreased
Type IV RTA (hyporeninemic hypoaldosteronism)	<5.5	Increased

B. The clinical features of metabolic acidosis are nonspecific. The most common manifestation is hyperventilation because the respiratory center in the brainstem is stimulated to compensate for the acidosis. At its most severe, patients report air hunger. Severe metabolic acidosis may also be associated with hemodynamic instability—a problem most frequently encountered in the intensive care unit. Other manifestations of metabolic acidosis reflect the underlying cause or trigger (e.g., diarrhea, DKA, drug ingestion). The diagnostic approach pivots on the measurement of serum electrolytes, BUN, creatinine, and an ABG level. A low serum HCO_3^- and a pH <7.40 on ABG analysis confirm metabolic acidosis. The AG should be calculated to help with the differential diagnosis of the metabolic acidosis and to diagnose mixed disorders. A high-AG acidosis is present if the AG is >10–12 mEq/L, and a non-AG acidosis is present if the AG is <10−12 mEq/L. If the AG is elevated, the osmolar gap should be calculated by subtracting the calculated serum osmolality from the measured serum osmolality. (Ethylene glycol and methanol poisoning increase the AG and the osmolar gap.) In the case of an increased AG, the ratio of AG and HCO_3^- should be calculated (Δ:Δ). A Δ:Δ <1 suggests mixed normal-AG and high-AG acidosis; an Δ:Δ >2 suggests coexisting metabolic alkalosis. Increases in AG may be observed in nonacidotic states, such as metabolic alkalosis and respiratory alkalosis; however, increases in AG beyond 3–5 mEq/L are unusual. Assessment of the urinary anion gap (UAG) can also be helpful in diagnosis. The urine anion gap (UAG) = $(U_{Na} + U_K) - U_{Cl}$. The UAG is normally positive (range: 30–50). A negative UAG suggests renal excretion of unmeasured cation (e.g., NH_4^+; an extrarenal acidosis). A positive UAG suggests minimal renal

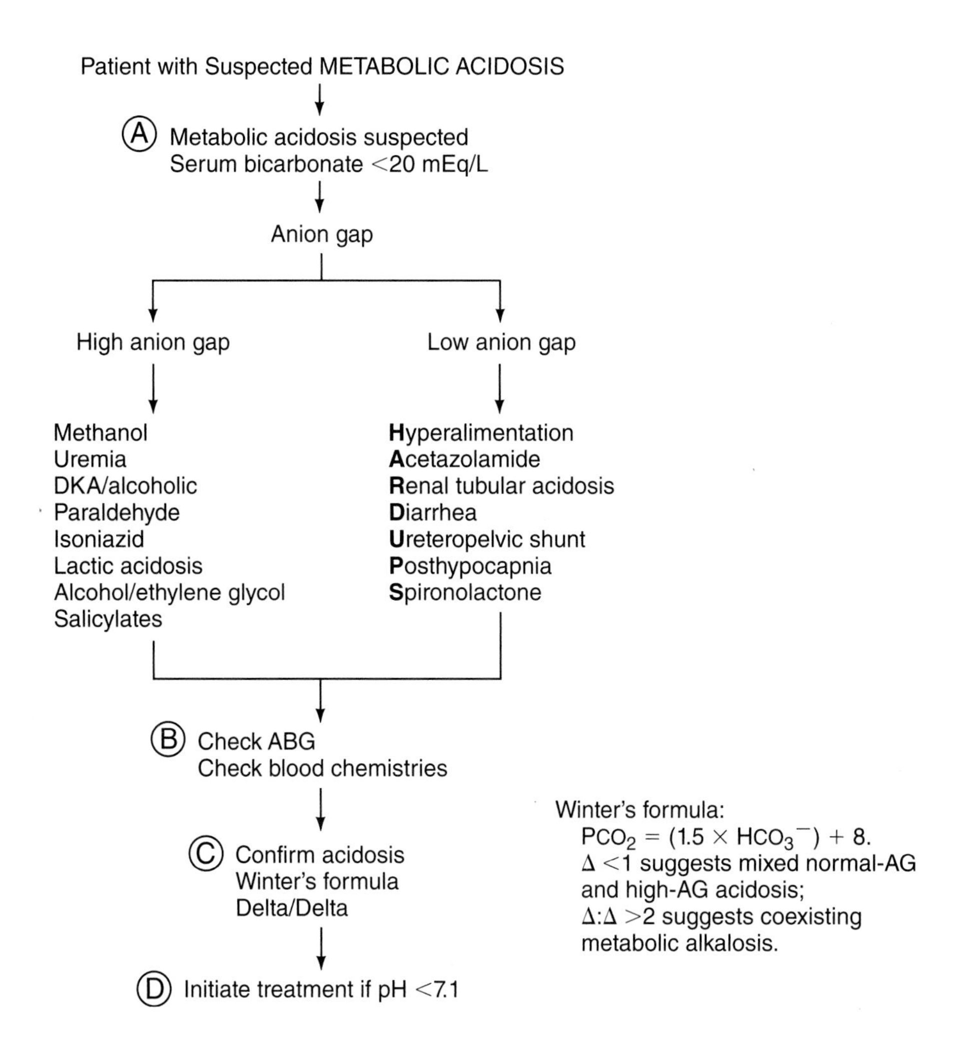

excretion of unmeasured cation (e.g., NH_4^+). Causes include proximal RTA type II, distal RTA or type I, or type IV RTA. Other tests can be performed, including a screen for toxins (e.g., ethylene glycol, salicylate) and tests for metabolic disorders (e.g., ketoacidosis, lactic acidosis) that are known to elevate the AG.

C. Lactic acidosis can be classified as type A, which occurs as a consequence of tissue hypoxia from tissue hypoperfusion or reduced arterial oxygen content. The second category is type B, which does not reflect tissue hypoxia. The most common category is type B1—from sepsis, hepatic failure, renal failure, diabetes mellitus, cancer, malaria, or cholera. The second category is type B2 from drugs or toxins (e.g., acetaminophen, ethanol, salicylates, and ethylene glycol). The third category is type B3, reflecting strenuous muscular exercise, grand mal seizures, and D-lactic acidosis. The clinical presentation of lactic acidosis reflects the underlying etiology (e.g., sepsis or drug ingestion).

D. Treatment of metabolic acidosis depends on the underlying cause and the severity of manifestations. A general rule is that treatment should be initiated if the pH is <7.1, especially when associated with hemodynamic instability. In patients with chronic metabolic acidosis, such as a patient with RTA, oral repletion with sodium bicarbonate is usually sufficient. The HCO_3^- deficit can be calculated by using the following equation: HCO_3^- deficit = deficit/L (desired serum HCO_3^- − measured HCO_3^-) × 0.5 × body weight (volume of distribution for HCO_3^-). Sodium bicarbonate can be administered intravenously.

References

Ayers P, Warrington L. Diagnosis and treatment of simple acid-base disorders. Nutr Clin Pract 2008;23(2):122–127.

Kraut JA, Madias NE. Serum anion gap: its uses and limitations in clinical medicine. Clin J Am Soc Nephrol 2007;2(1):162–174. Epub 2006 Dec 6.

Kwon KT, Tsai VW. Metabolic emergencies. Emerg Med Clin North Am 2007;25(4):1041–1060, vi.

Madias NE. Lactic acidosis. Kidney Int 1986;29(3):752–774.

Morris CG, Low J. Metabolic acidosis in the critically ill: part 2. causes and treatment. Anaesthesia 2008;63(4):396–411.

Rodríguez Soriano J. Renal tubular acidosis: the clinical entity. J Am Soc Nephrol 2002;13(8):2160–2170.

METABOLIC ALKALOSIS

Ajay K. Singh, MBBS, FRCP

A. Metabolic alkalosis is characterized by a primary increase in the serum bicarbonate concentration. This occurs because of a loss of H^+ from the body or a gain in HCO_3^-. In its pure form, it manifests as alkalemia (pH >7.40). As a compensatory mechanism, metabolic alkalosis leads to alveolar hypoventilation with an increase in arterial carbon dioxide tension ($PaCO_2$), which diminishes the change in pH that would otherwise occur. Metabolic alkalosis is the most common acid-base disturbance observed in hospitalized patients, accounting for approximately 50% of all acid-base disorders. Common causes of a metabolic alkalosis are shown in Table 1. Urinary chloride concentration provides a useful paradigm for classification of patients because it represents a convenient measure of extracellular volume. Clinical manifestations are summarized in Table 2.

B. Pathophysiology of metabolic alkalosis should be considered in two phases—initiation and maintenance. Metabolic alkalosis is induced by virtue of a loss of acid, gain of alkali, or the effects of a contracted extracellular fluid compartment (increasing the bicarbonate concentration). Whenever a hydrogen ion is excreted, a bicarbonate ion is gained into the extracellular space. Examples of loss of acid include vomiting, nasogastric (NG) suction, and aldosterone-mediated secretion of hydrogen ions in the collecting duct (e.g., in primary hyperaldosteronism). Gain of alkali may be observed in patients administered alkali in excess of the kidney's excretory capacity. Contraction alkalosis is most frequently observed in patients treated zealously with diuretics or in patients with chloride-rich diarrhea. The maintenance of metabolic alkalosis is influenced by renal hypoperfusion (e.g., in patients who are volume depleted) that results in secondary hyperaldosteronism and thus distal nephron secretion of hydrogen ions. Other important factors include chloride depletion from either GI or renal loss of chloride. Chloride depletion enhances bicarbonate reabsorption through stimulation of the renin-angiotensin-aldosterone system and by inhibition of bicarbonate secretion by the chloride/bicarbonate exchanger.

C. Diagnostic approach to metabolic alkalosis:
   1. Establish the presence of metabolic alkalosis and assess whether the secondary (compensatory) physiologic response is appropriate.
   2. Identify the underlying cause that precipitated alkalosis.
   3. Assess the factors responsible for maintaining alkalosis, such as extracellular volume depletion. The treatment of a metabolic alkalosis depends on identifying and repairing the underlying cause (e.g., repairing the volume, discontinuing NG suction, or stopping diuretic therapy).

D. The treatment of metabolic alkalosis comprises general therapy based on the severity of the alkalosis and more specific therapy based on the underlying initiating cause of the metabolic alkalosis.

   General therapy: Treatment of asymptomatic patients with a mild to moderate alkalosis (pH 7.45–7.6) should involve volume repletion; if necessary, the use of acetazolamide (250–500 mg bid or tid) to cause an alkaline urine rich in bicarbonate may be sufficient. For patients with more severe metabolic alkalosis (pH >7.60) or those who are symptomatic, hydrochloric acid infusion may be necessary. This is usually administered as a 0.1–0.2 M HCl solution into a large vein.

   Specific therapy: This should be determined by whether the patient has a "chloride-responsive" or "chloride-resistant" alkalosis. Chloride-responsive alkalosis in the setting of volume depletion is best treated with IV infusion of isotonic sodium chloride solution. However, chloride-responsive alkalosis in edematous states such as congestive heart failure usually necessitates more

Table 1 **Causes of Metabolic Alkalosis**

Chloride-Sensitive Alkalosis (urinary chloride <20 mEq/L)
Vomiting
Nasogastric suction
Diuretic use
Posthypercapnic
Chloride-Resistant Alkalosis (urinary chloride >20 mEq/L)
Diuretic use
Bartter's syndrome
Potassium depletion
Milk-alkali syndrome

Table 2 **Clinical Manifestations of Metabolic Alkalosis**

Neuromuscular
Twitching
Muscle spasm
Positive Chvostek's and/or Trousseau's sign
Confusion
Lethargy
Seizure activity
Coma
Ventilatory Depression
Hypoxemia in patients with preexisting cardiopulmonary disorders

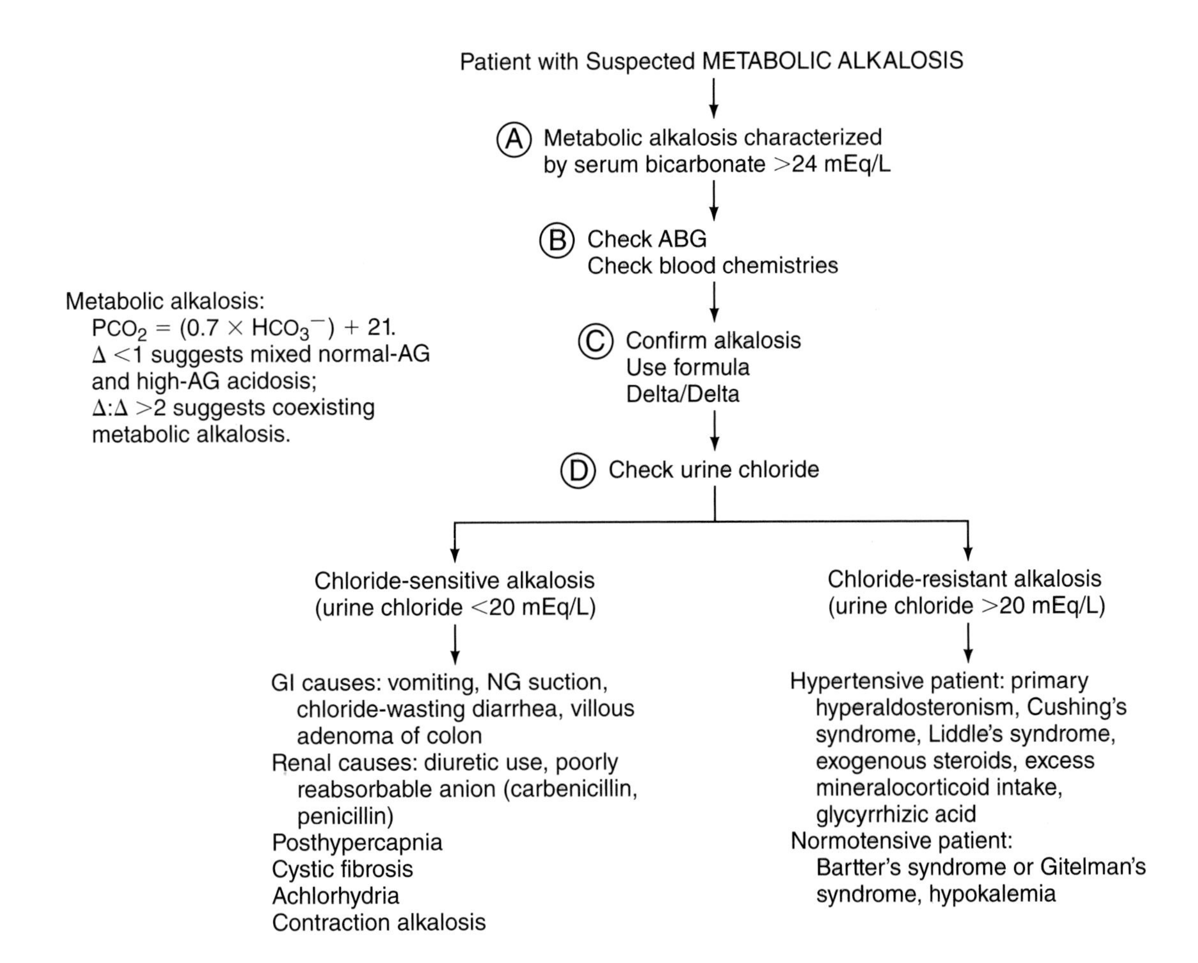

vigorous diuresis (e.g., using a carbonic anhydrase inhibitor [e.g., acetazolamide] or a potassium-sparing diuretic [e.g., spironolactone, amiloride, triamterene]). In patients with a chloride-resistant metabolic alkalosis, if the patient has primary hyperaldosteronism, then surgical resection of the tumor and/or use of an aldosterone antagonist spironolactone should be considered. In glucocorticoid-remediable hyperaldosteronism, metabolic alkalosis and hypertension are responsive to dexamethasone.

In patients with Bartter's syndrome and Gitelman's syndrome, treatment of the metabolic alkalosis necessitates the use of potassium supplementation, potassium-sparing diuretics, NSAIDs, or angiotensin-converting enzyme (ACE) inhibitors. In contrast, metabolic alkalosis in Liddle's syndrome should be treated with amiloride or triamterene but not with spironolactone.

References

Galla JH. Metabolic alkalosis. J Am Soc Nephrol 2000;11(2):369–375.
Khanna A, Kurtzman NA. Metabolic alkalosis. J Nephrol 2006 Mar;19 Suppl 9:S86–S96.
Laski ME, Sabatini S. Metabolic alkalosis, bedside and bench. Semin Nephrol 2006;26(6):404–421.

HYPONATREMIA

Ajay K. Singh, MBBS, FRCP

Hyponatremia is defined as a plasma sodium level <135 mEq/L (135 mmol/L) and is the most commonly encountered electrolyte abnormality in hospitalized patients (prevalence of approximately 2.5%). Acute or symptomatic hyponatremia can lead to significant rates of morbidity and mortality.

A. Clinical features depend on the degree of hyponatremia and the rapidity with which they develop. An abrupt (over 24–48 hours) decrease in the sodium concentration may be associated with symptoms that range from mild anorexia, headache, and muscle cramps to significant alteration in mental status, including obtundation, coma, or status epilepticus. The key diagnostic challenge is to clinically predict total body sodium content. Patients who are hypervolemic have increased total body sodium; patients who are euvolemic have normal body sodium; and patients who are hypovolemic have low body sodium. Hypovolemic hyponatremia develops as sodium (and free water) are lost and replaced by inappropriately hypotonic fluids. Sodium can be lost through renal or nonrenal routes. Nonrenal routes include GI losses, excessive sweating, third spacing of fluids (e.g., ascites, peritonitis, pancreatitis, burns), and cerebral salt-wasting syndrome. Euvolemic hyponatremia is characterized by normal total body sodium and a total body excess of free water. This occurs in patients who take in excess fluids. The most common causes are psychogenic polydipsia, administration of hypotonic intravenously, and the syndrome of inappropriate antidiuretic hormone secretion (SIADH). Hypervolemic hyponatremia occurs in patients with excessive total body sodium (e.g., with congestive heart failure).

B. SIADH is characterized by maximally dilute urine in the face of hypoosmolality and hyponatremia. SIADH is the most common cause of normovolemic (euvolemic) hyponatremia and the most common cause of hyponatremia. SIADH is caused by an increase of arginine vasopressin (AVP) secretion resulting in impairment of water excretion. AVP secretion in these patients is caused by a nonphysiologic release of AVP from the posterior pituitary or another ectopic source. The most common causes of SIADH include neuropsychiatric and pulmonary disease, malignant tumors, major surgery (postoperative pain), and pharmacologic agents. Hyponatremia of SIADH can be explained by the inappropriate secretion of AVP. AVP or antidiuretic hormone (ADH) increases water resorption through the renal tubules in order to conserve water. A pathologic increase of AVP often leads to excessive retention of water. Renal free water excretion is impaired, whereas the regulation of sodium balance is unaffected. In addition, a high volume of water intake is required for significant development of hyponatremia because a high level of AVP alone is usually insufficient to produce hyponatremia. Malignancies may secrete AVP. Also, tumors may cause SIADH secretion by interfering with the normal osmoregulation of AVP secretion from the neurohypophysis through direct invasion of the vagus nerve, metastatic implants in the hypothalamus, or some other more generalized neuropathic changes. Many drugs may also increase production of AVP either directly or indirectly by acting on the kidneys. Examples include chlorpropamide, clofibrate, carbamazepine-oxcarbazepine, vincristine, nicotine, narcotics, and antipsychotic/antidepressant drugs. The most important diagnostic criterion for SIADH is the excretion of inappropriately concentrated urine (>300 mOsm/kg H_2O) despite hypoosmolality and hyponatremia. The absence of any renal, adrenal, or thyroid abnormalities also is important. Appropriate renal response to hypoosmolality is to excrete the maximum volume of dilute urine (i.e., urine osmolality and specific gravity of <100 mOsm/kg and 1.003, respectively). Patients with primary polydipsia will have an appropriate response to the water loading. An inappropriate renal response often implies AVP action on the kidneys. Patients with SIADH tend to be mildly volume expanded secondary to water retention and have a urine sodium excretion rate equal to intake (urine sodium concentration usually >40 mmol/L). Hypouricemia may be an accompanying finding because of the volume expansion (in contrast to hypovolemic hyponatremia). Evaluate for an underlying malignancy (SIADH may precede diagnosis of malignancy by several months). For treatment of mild hyponatremia, water restriction of 1000 ml/day should be adequate. However, patient compliance may be difficult because of the lengthy periods of water restriction that may be required. Pharmacologic agents that antagonize AVP action and maneuvers that increase solute excretion may allow patients with SIADH secretion to drink more water (e.g., demeclocycline). The recommended demeclocycline dose is between 600 and 1200 mg/day with restoration of serum sodium in 5–14 days without restricting water intake. Patients with cirrhosis require dosage adjustments because of fear of developing toxicity. For severe symptomatic hyponatremia 3% hypertonic saline is recommended.

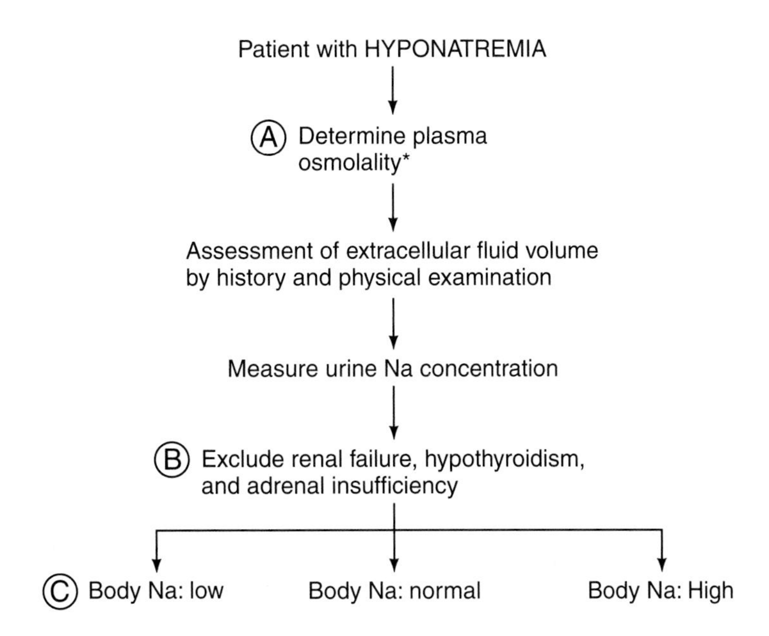

C. The therapeutic strategy for hyponatremia is dictated by the underlying cause of the disorder. It is important to consider the presence or absence of symptoms, the duration of the disorder, and the risk of neurologic complication. It is ideal to raise the plasma sodium concentration by restricting water and increasing water loss. Ultimately, the goal of treatment is to correct the underlying disorder causing hyponatremia, if possible. Symptomatic hyponatremia always requires treatment regardless of severity of the hyponatremia. The issue of how rapid the correction is still of great controversy. For patients who are acute (<48 hours) and severely symptomatic, it is typically recommended to raise the sodium concentration no more than 1–2 mEq/L/hr for the first 3–4 hours with a limit at 15 mEq/L but preferably at 12 mEq/L during the first 24 hours with hypertonic saline. Once symptoms have subsided, the rate of correction can be switched to water restriction. As long as the osmolality of the fluid administered is higher than that of the level of plasma, sodium increases. The quantity of sodium required to increase the plasma sodium concentration by a given amount can be estimated by multiplying the deficit in plasma sodium concentration by the total body water. The treatment of a patient with asymptomatic hyponatremia is less controversial. In patients with chronic hyponatremia, water restriction alone is usually effective. A free water restriction of 1000 ml/day is adequate to achieve negative water balance. In some patients, an even greater restriction of water intake may be necessary because this volume of restriction exceeds total renal and extrarenal water losses. The use of furosemide (40 mg/day) and high salt intake (200 mEq/day), an extension of the treatment of acute symptomatic hyponatremia to the chronic management of euvolemic hyponatremia, has also been reported to be successful.
Patients with hypervolemic hyponatremia, secondary to heart failure or liver cirrhosis, are often asymptomatic. These patients require strict sodium and water restriction and correction of any other electrolyte and metabolic alterations. Patients who have a hypovolemic type of hyponatremia may be treated with isotonic saline in an attempt to replete sodium and remove the hemodynamic stimulus for AVP release.

The most important complication in the treatment of severe hyponatremia is central pontine myelinolysis (osmotic demyelination syndrome). Demyelinating syndrome is most likely to occur in patients whose hyponatremia is more chronic and is rapidly corrected once the adaptive process has set in. Diagnosis can be difficult with small lesions, but more extensive disease is associated with flaccid paralysis, dysarthria, and dysphagia. There is no specific treatment for this disorder, causing a high mortality and morbidity. Because the rate and magnitude of correction seem to play a critical role, it is important to adhere to the suggested rate of correction as stated previously.

References

Adrogué HJ. Consequences of inadequate management of hyponatremia. Am J Nephrol 2005;25(3):240–249. Epub 2005 May 25.

Adrogué HJ, Madias NE. Hyponatremia. N Engl J Med 2000;342(21): 1581–1589.

Upadhyay A, Jaber BL, Madias NE. Incidence and prevalence of hyponatremia. Am J Med 2006;119(7 Suppl 1):S30–S35.

HYPERNATREMIA

Ajay K. Singh, MBBS, FRCP

Hypernatremia is defined as a plasma sodium >145 mmol/L. There is a direct relationship between mortality and increasing plasma sodium. The levels of plasma sodium that are >180 mmol/L carry the highest mortality. Patients who are susceptible are often those who have limited access to water. Commonly, the elderly who are physically incapacitated or very young infants are at an increased risk.

A. Hypernatremia is usually caused by derangement of the cranially mediated neurohormonal control of renal concentrating mechanism (central diabetes insipidus [DI]) or secondary to parenchymal kidney problems (nephrogenic DI) or by losses of free water from other sources. Also needed is the absence of an intact thirst mechanism. In hypernatremia, the hyperosmolar environment causes water to shift from the intracellular compartment to the extracellular compartment and causes overall brain cellular volume reduction. The major symptoms of hypernatremia are neurologic and include altered mental status, weakness, neuromuscular irritability, focal neurologic deficits, and occasionally coma or seizure. The severity of the symptoms depends on the amount of time it takes for the condition to develop. Acute hypernatremia is usually associated with more severe symptoms. These symptoms may include anorexia, restlessness, nausea and vomiting, altered mental status, lethargy or irritability, twitching, ataxia, hyperreflexia, stupor, and/or coma. Hypernatremia that develops over a long period (chronic hypernatremia) gives the adaptive mechanisms (uptake of myoinositol) of the brain a chance to adjust and typically is better tolerated and less symptomatic. Patients are likely to complain of thirst and often have signs of volume depletion.

   DI results in a decrease of arginine vasopressin (AVP) or a decrease in its action on the end organ. DI usually results in the production of abnormally large volumes of dilute urine (>50 ml/kg body weight) with a low osmolality (<300 mmol/kg). Primary DI can be classified into central, nephrogenic, and gestational types. Signs and symptoms are variable depending on the degree and severity of disease. Polyuria, enuresis, and/or nocturia are characteristic. Patients who have intact thirst mechanisms will also be polydipsic. Signs of dehydration and hypernatremia do not develop unless fluid intake becomes restricted. Secondary causes of DI generally develop in patients in whom AVP secretion is inhibited as a response to excessive fluid intake. DI can be classified as central DI (neurohypophyseal DI, neurogenic DI, or pituitary DI), which is caused by a deficient secretion of AVP, which may be congenital, genetic, or acquired. The genetic form is often transmitted by autosomal-dominant transmission but less commonly is transmitted as an X-linked recessive pattern. The common mutation is in the coding region of the AVP-neurophysin II gene that causes an accumulation of the mutant precursor and eventually results in the destruction of the neuron. The acquired form may be the consequence of neurohypophyseal destruction by disease or toxins. Nephrogenic DI can also be classified into genetic, acquired, or congenital. Patients often have normal or increased secretion of AVP, but the kidneys are unresponsive to the secretions. The genetic form is commonly transmitted by an X-linked recessive mutation in the coding region of the V2 receptor gene. Infection, toxins, and other hereditary kidney diseases can disrupt concentrating ability to a point where the AVP becomes ineffective in the acquired form. As opposed to patients with central DI, these patients often present as male infants who cannot express thirst to the caregivers.

   Treatment of uncomplicated central DI comprises replacement of AVP with the synthetic analog DDAVP by either IV or SC route, nasal inhalation, or oral tablet for symptomatic relief. Decrease in urine flow is dose dependent and may vary based on the severity of symptoms. Chlorpropamide can treat patients with central DI who have excessive thirst. Hypoglycemia as a complication may result from decreased caloric intake or exercise. (Chlorpropamide is contraindicated in pregnancy because of uncertain teratogenicity.) Nephrogenic DI cannot be effectively treated with DDAVP as a result of end-organ insensitivity. Thiazide diuretics with amiloride and a low-sodium diet are recommended to reduce the symptoms. Indomethacin can also be effective in some patients.

B. Severe dehydration and hypernatremia may ensue as a result of increased secretion of urine without adequate replacement. Early intervention is often necessary to prevent complications such as convulsions and mental retardation. Gestational DI is often transient but may be severe until weeks after the delivery. The deficiency of AVP during pregnancy largely results from the increased production of an N-terminal aminopeptidase produced by the placenta that metabolizes AVP. These patients often have subclinical deficiency of AVP secretion in the nonpregnant state. The diagnosis of DI relies on documenting an increased 24-hour urine output (>3500 ml/kg in a 70-kg man) and a low urine osmolality (<300 mOsm/kg) with persistent thirst. A key aspect of

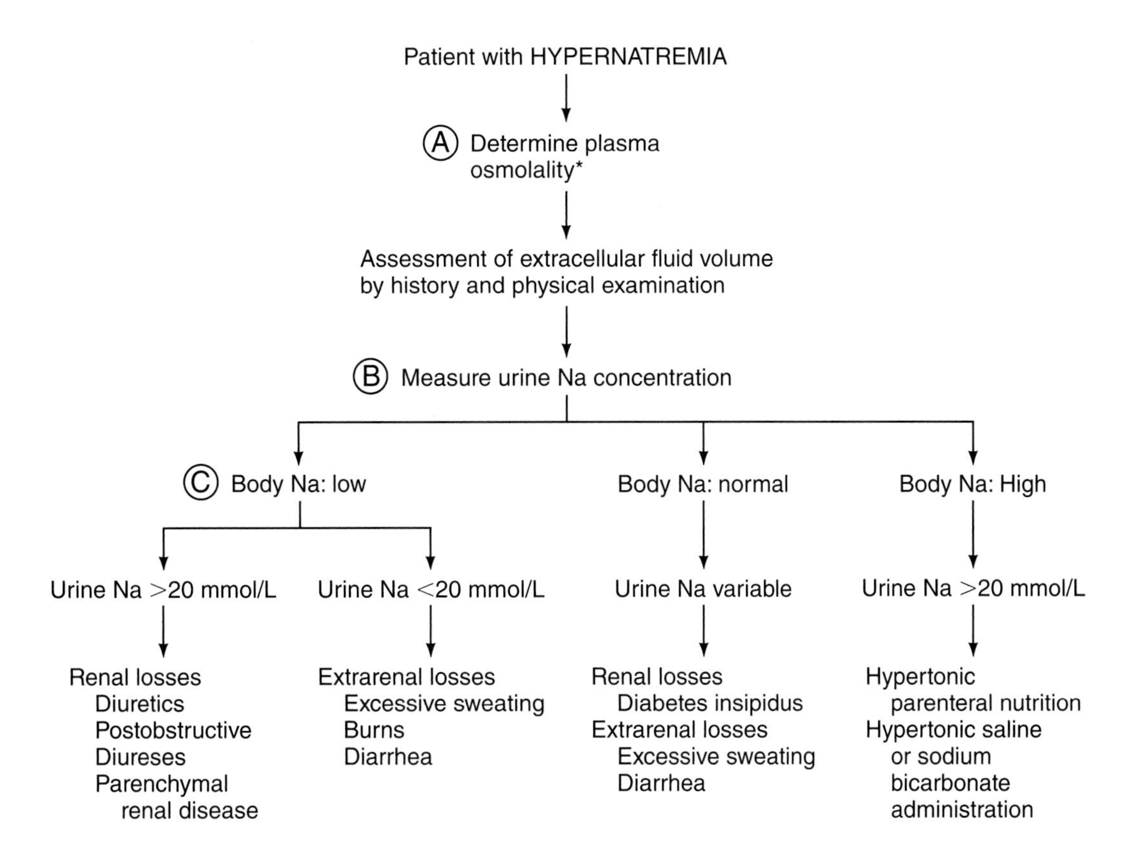

the workup includes a fluid deprivation test, which is often necessary to determine the type of DI. (A positive test characterizes an increase in the urine osmolality >300 mOsm/kg. Nephrogenic DI can be diagnosed by administration of desmopressin [DDAVP] with an increase in the urine osmolality >300 mOsm/kg.) MRI may be useful in visualizing the pituitary and hypothalamus to demonstrate abnormalities.

C. The treatment goals for hypernatremia are to stop ongoing water loss by treating the underlying cause and to correct the water deficit. Water replacement is essential in a patient who is hypovolemic. The amount of fluid deficit can be calculated by the equation:

$$\text{water deficit} = ([\text{plasma Na}^+] - 140)/140 \times \text{total body water}$$

Alternatively, the following formula can be used:

$$\text{water deficit} = [(\text{plasma Na}^+/140) - 1\,] \times \text{total body water}$$

where total body water in a patient with hypernatremia caused by water loss is approximately 50% in men and 40% in women. Water deficit should be corrected over 48–72 hours depending on severity and presentation. When calculating the rate of water replacement, ongoing losses should be taken into account, and the plasma Na^+ concentration should be reduced by 0.5 mmol/L per hour and by no more than 12 mmol/L over the first 24 hours. The fluid should be replaced by an oral route if possible, but if the patient is unconscious, has an altered mental status, or is vomiting, the IV route is preferred with 5% dextrose in water or 0.45% saline solution.

References

Adrogué HJ, Madias NE. Hypernatremia. N Engl J Med 2000;342(20): 1493–1499.

Lin M, Liu SJ, Lim IT. Disorders of water imbalance. Emerg Med Clin North Am 2005;23(3):749–770, ix.

Reynolds RM, Padfield PL, Seckl JR. Disorders of sodium balance. BMJ 2006;332(7543):702–705.

Schrier RW. The sea within us: disorders of body water homeostasis. Curr Opin Investig Drugs 2007;8(4):304–311.

HYPOKALEMIA

Kambiz Zandi-Nejad, MD

Total body potassium (K^+) is estimated to be 3500 mmol. More than 98% of K^+ is intracellular, with the highest contents in skeletal muscle and liver cells. Therefore, a shift of relatively small amounts of K^+ to or from the intracellular pool can have a substantial effect on the extracellular and serum K^+ levels. The daily intake of potassium varies considerably, with an average daily intake of approximately 70–140 mmol in the United States. Despite this variation, the serum K^+ level is tightly maintained between 3.5 and 5.0 mmol/L. This is achieved through homeostatic mechanisms known as *external* and *internal* potassium balance. At steady state, the total daily intake in a healthy person is excreted primarily through the urine (approximately 90%–95%) and stool (approximately 5%–10%); this is known as *external potassium balance.* The rate of potassium excretion by the kidney is related primarily to the flow rate, intraluminal charge, and K^+ concentration in the cortical collecting duct (CCD) segment of the nephron. Kidneys require several hours before they can excrete the added potassium load.

The movement of potassium between intracellular and extracellular fluids is also crucial in maintaining a tight serum K^+ level and is known as *internal potassium balance.* This shift is important because it is the first line of defense when large amounts of potassium enter the circulation over a relatively short period (e.g., following the ingestion of a meal high in potassium). Whereas the main route for potassium entrance and accumulation into the cells is Na-K-ATPase, the main exit mechanism is through potassium channels. The two major stimulants for the movement of potassium into the cells are insulin and agonists of the β_2-adrenergic receptor.

Acid-base disorders can affect the serum K^+ concentration through both *internal* and *external potassium balance*; however, two general rules apply. In chronic acid-base disorders, the effect of external potassium balance is dominant. The effect of acidemia on internal potassium balance is stronger than that of alkalemia for any given change in pH, with this effect being limited primarily to nonorganic acidoses.

A. Hypokalemia is defined as a serum K^+ level <3.5 mmol/L and is one of the most common electrolyte disorders. It can be associated with either a decreased or a normal total body potassium content. It is important to remember that the cause of hypokalemia can be multifactorial, with the involvement of more than one mechanism or etiology. Although the cause of hypokalemia in the majority of cases is obvious from history, physical examination, and/or basic laboratory tests, hypokalemia that is not resolved by the proper initial intervention requires a more rigorous workup to detect and correct the underlying cause; simply replacing potassium will not be sufficient.

B. Look carefully for symptoms and signs such as muscle weakness and ECG changes (e.g., flattened T wave, prominent U waves) suggestive of an impending emergency requiring immediate treatment.

C. Pseudohypokalemia is a condition in which a large number of abnormal leukocytes, seen mainly in patients with myelogenous leukemia, take up plasma potassium when the blood sample is kept at room temperature for a relatively long period.

D. The history should include information about medications (particularly diuretics, laxatives, antibiotics such as certain penicillins and amphotericin B, chemotherapeutic agents such as cisplatin, and β_2-agonists), diet (e.g., potassium intake and supplements such as licorice, which has aldosterone-like effects), associated symptoms (e.g., diarrhea, vomiting, continuous gastric drainage, and profuse sweating), medical history, family history, and high-stress conditions such as head trauma or myocardial infarction. Physical examination should be directed toward vital signs (blood pressure in particular), volume status, and signs of disorders associated with hypokalemia such as hyperaldosteronism and Cushing's syndrome. Initial laboratory tests should include kidney function tests; electrolyte profile, including calcium and magnesium; ABG; CBC; osmolality; and urinary pH, osmolality, creatinine, and electrolyte profile, including Na^+, K^+, and Cl^-. In some cases, urinary Mg^{2+} and Ca^{2+} and plasma renin and aldosterone levels may also be helpful. Of note, low magnesium can enhance renal potassium excretion through a mechanism that is still unclear, and the magnesium level needs to be corrected along with the potassium levels.

E. High levels of either exogenous or endogenous (e.g., following myocardial infarction and alcohol withdrawal) β_2-adrenergic agonists are major causes of K^+ shift into the cells.

F. Kidneys are unable to reduce the potassium excretion to zero, even in the case of no potassium intake. Therefore, in the case of severe reduced intake (e.g., almost no potassium intake with a diet of tea and toast), kidneys will continue to excrete low levels of potassium (usually <10 mmol/L) and hypokalemia will eventually ensue. This is, however, not common, because it requires a virtually potassium-free diet of relatively long duration.

(Continued on page 382)

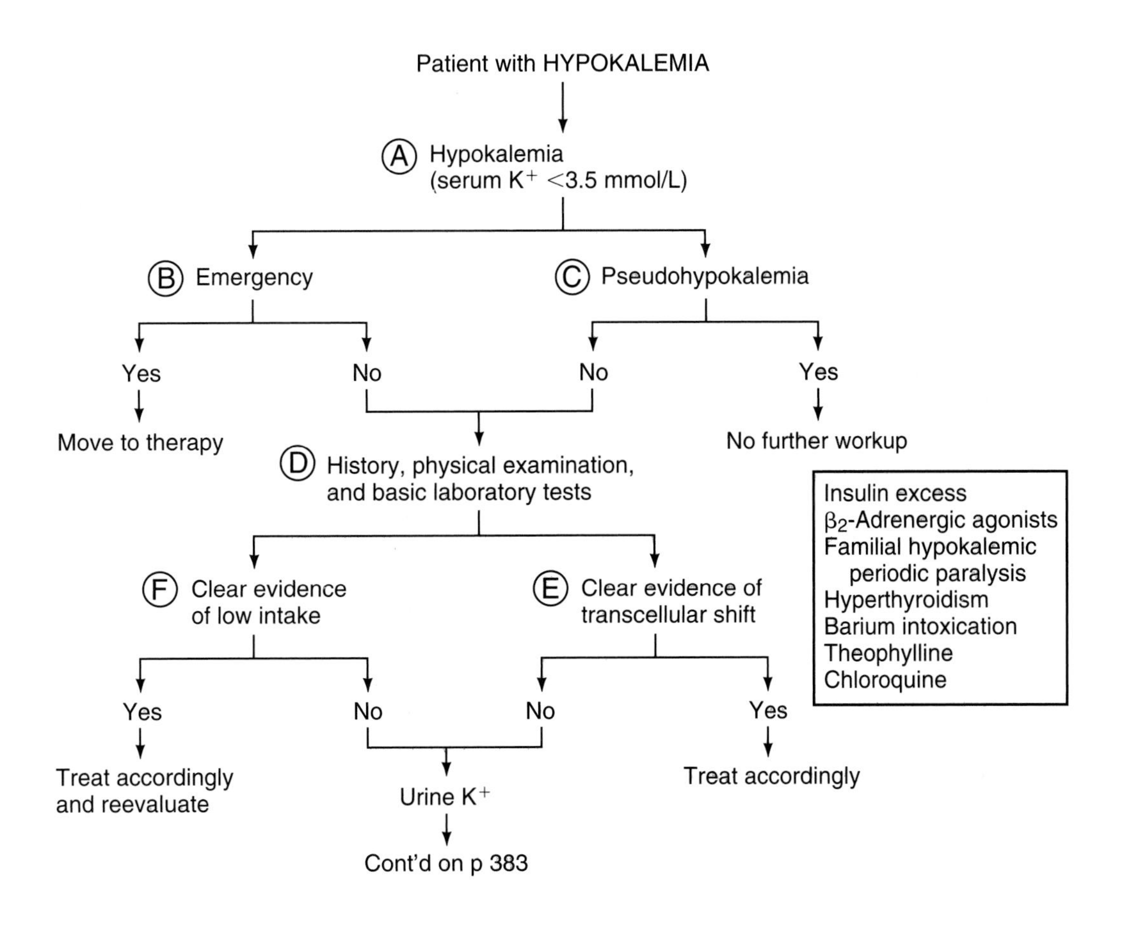
Patient with HYPOKALEMIA
(A) Hypokalemia (serum K+ <3.5 mmol/L)
(B) Emergency
(C) Pseudohypokalemia
Yes
No
No
Yes
Move to therapy
No further workup
(D) History, physical examination, and basic laboratory tests
Insulin excess
β2-Adrenergic agonists
Familial hypokalemic periodic paralysis
Hyperthyroidism
Barium intoxication
Theophylline
Chloroquine
(F) Clear evidence of low intake
(E) Clear evidence of transcellular shift
Yes
No
No
Yes
Treat accordingly and reevaluate
Urine K+
Treat accordingly
Cont'd on p 383

G. The main route of extrarenal potassium loss is the GI tract in the form of diarrhea or GI fistulas. Although gastric fluid contains potassium (6–8 mmol/L), hypokalemia associated with vomiting or continuous gastric drainage mainly results from renal potassium loss in the setting of metabolic alkalosis and volume contraction. Sweat contains approximately 5–10 mmol/L of potassium; therefore, hypokalemia may occur with profuse sweating. In patients with normal kidney function, extrarenal K^+ loss is associated with a urinary K^+ loss of <15 mmol/day.

H. The interpretation of renal excretion of potassium should be based on the serum K^+ level, such that renal potassium excretion should be minimal in the setting of hypokalemia.

I. Transtubular potassium gradient (TTKG) is used to estimate the potassium concentration at the end of CCD. It is useful only if the osmolality of the urine exceeds that of the plasma and if the sodium concentration in urine is at least 25 mEq/L. TTKG can be calculated from the following equation:

$$\frac{\text{Urine } K^+/\text{plasma } K^+}{\text{Urine osmolality/plasma osmolality}}$$

Normal values for TTKG vary and depend on the serum K^+ levels; for hypokalemia, values are <2; for hyperkalemia, values are >6; and for normokalemia, any number is considered normal.

References

Gennary FJ. Hypokalemia. N Engl J Med 1998;339:451–458.
Mount DB, Zandi-Nejad K. Disorders of potassium balance. In Brenner BM, ed. Brenner and Rector's The Kidney, 7th ed. Philadelphia: Elsevier, 2004:997–1040.

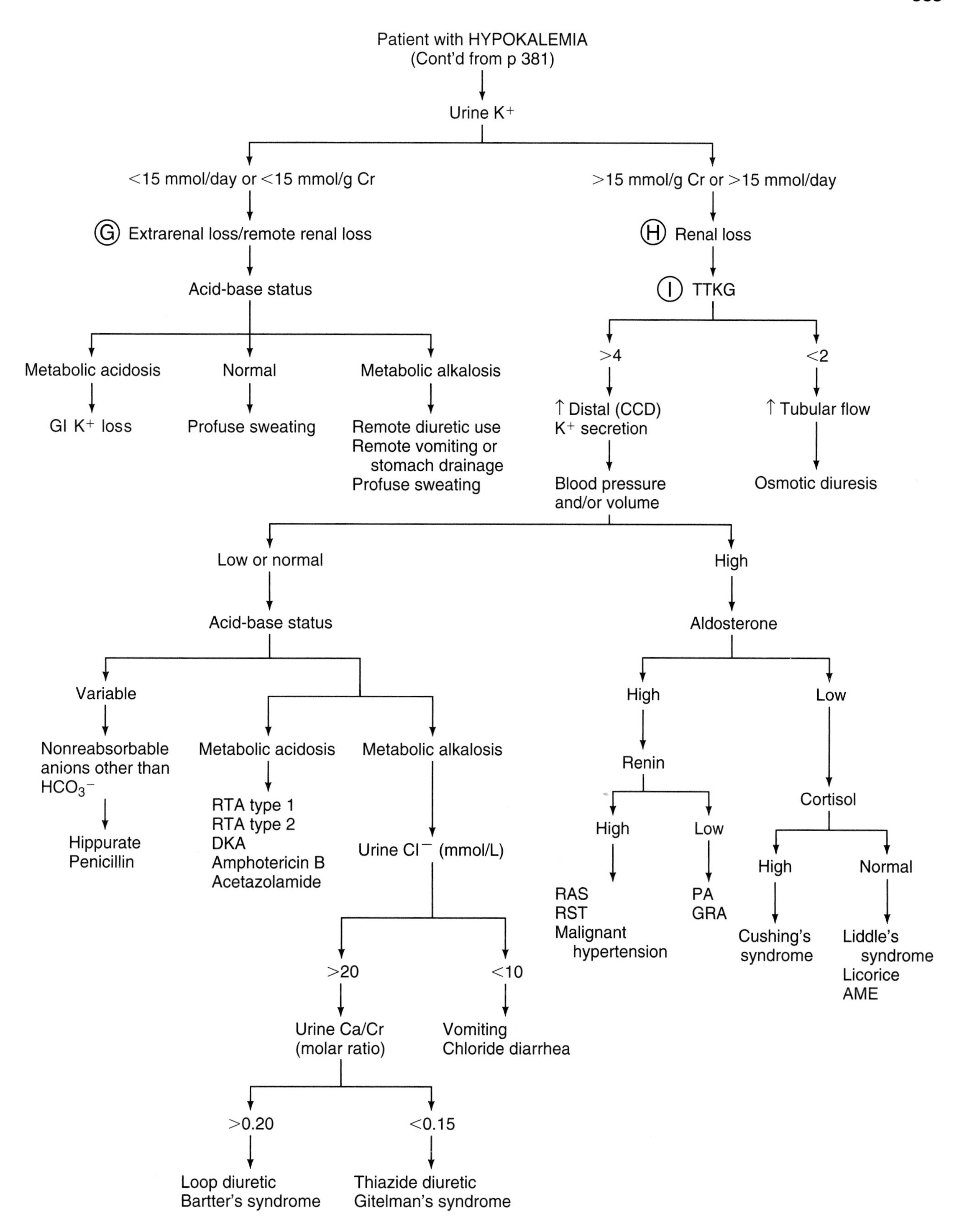

AME, Apparent mineralocorticoid excess; DKA, diabetic ketoacidosis; GRA, glucocorticoid-remediable aldosteronism; PA, primary aldosteronism; RAS, renin-angiotensin system; RST, renin-secreting tumor; RTA, renal tubular acidosis.

HYPERKALEMIA

Kambiz Zandi-Nejad, MD

Please refer to the Hypokalemia chapter for a brief description of potassium homeostasis.

A. Hyperkalemia is defined as serum $K^+ \geq 5.5$ mmol/L. It is a potentially lethal disease requiring immediate attention. The cause of hyperkalemia in a large group of patients is multifactorial, with medications and reduced renal function being the main contributors. It can be associated with either increased or normal total body potassium content and results from external or internal potassium balance disturbances, respectively.

B. Indications for hospitalization of patients with hyperkalemia are not well defined. However, because of the potentially lethal consequences of severe hyperkalemia, it is recommended that all patients with hyperkalemia and ECG changes (including peaked T waves) be admitted and treated emergently. Moreover, given the limitations of ECG changes as a reflection of cardiac toxicity, patients with severe hyperkalemia ($K^+ \geq 6.0$ mmol/L) should also be aggressively managed regardless of the ECG findings. ECG changes of hyperkalemia include peaked symmetric T waves (tenting, most visible in precordial leads), flattened P wave, prolonged PR interval, prolonged QRS duration, and a "sine wave" idioventricular pattern.

C. Pseudohyperkalemia is a factitious increase in serum K^+ level caused by release of K^+ during or after venipuncture. The most common causes are fist clenching or tourniquet use, hemolysis, severe thrombocytosis (usually platelet count >1 million), and severe leukocytosis. Plasma potassium level will be helpful in differentiating pseudohyperkalemia in patients with severe leukocytosis or thrombocytosis.

D. History and physical examination should focus on the risk factors for renal failure, urine output, medications, diet and dietary supplements (e.g., salt substitutes have high potassium content), blood pressure, and volume status. Basic laboratory tests should include kidney function tests; electrolyte profile; blood glucose level; osmolality; ABG; CBC and urinary pH, osmolality, creatinine, and electrolyte profile, including 24-hour urine K^+.

E. Several medications can cause hyperkalemia by altering internal potassium balance favoring potassium exit from cells. Digoxin and similar compounds inhibit Na-K-ATPase and can be associated with hyperkalemia, particularly at supratherapeutic levels. Beta blockers, usually nonselective beta blockers, cause hyperkalemia in part by inhibiting cellular uptake. They can also inhibit renin and aldosterone release. Substances associated with hypertonicity such as hypertonic mannitol or even hypertonic saline can induce hyperkalemia through a "solvent drag" effect, such that potassium will follow the movement of water in response to osmotic gradient. Similarly, hyperglycemia can increase K^+ level; a reduced insulin level can further augment hyperkalemia. Of note, only nonorganic metabolic acidosis is associated with significant hyperkalemia.

F. Increased potassium load may be endogenous or exogenous. The common sources for exogenous potassium are foods rich in potassium, food supplements rich in potassium, massive RBC transfusion, and use of potassium salts of medications (e.g., penicillin K or potassium phosphate). The common sources of *endogenous* potassium are GI bleeding, hematomas, tissue necrosis (e.g., rhabdomyolysis), and tumor lysis syndrome.

G. In the absence of evidence for increased potassium load or transcellular shift, decreased renal potassium excretion is the most common cause of hyperkalemia (occasionally reduced GI excretion of potassium [constipation] in patients with advanced kidney disease can contribute to hyperkalemia).

H. Transtubular potassium gradient (TTKG) is used to estimate the potassium concentration at the end of the cortical collecting duct (CCD). It is useful only if the osmolality of the urine exceeds that of the plasma and if the sodium concentration in urine is at least 25 mEq/L. TTKG can be calculated from the following equation:

$$\frac{\text{Urine } K^+/\text{plasma } K^+}{\text{Urine osmolality/plasma osmolality}}$$

Normal values for TTKG vary and depend on the serum K^+ levels. For hypokalemia values are <2, for hyperkalemia values are >6, and for normokalemia any number is considered normal.

(Continued on page 386)

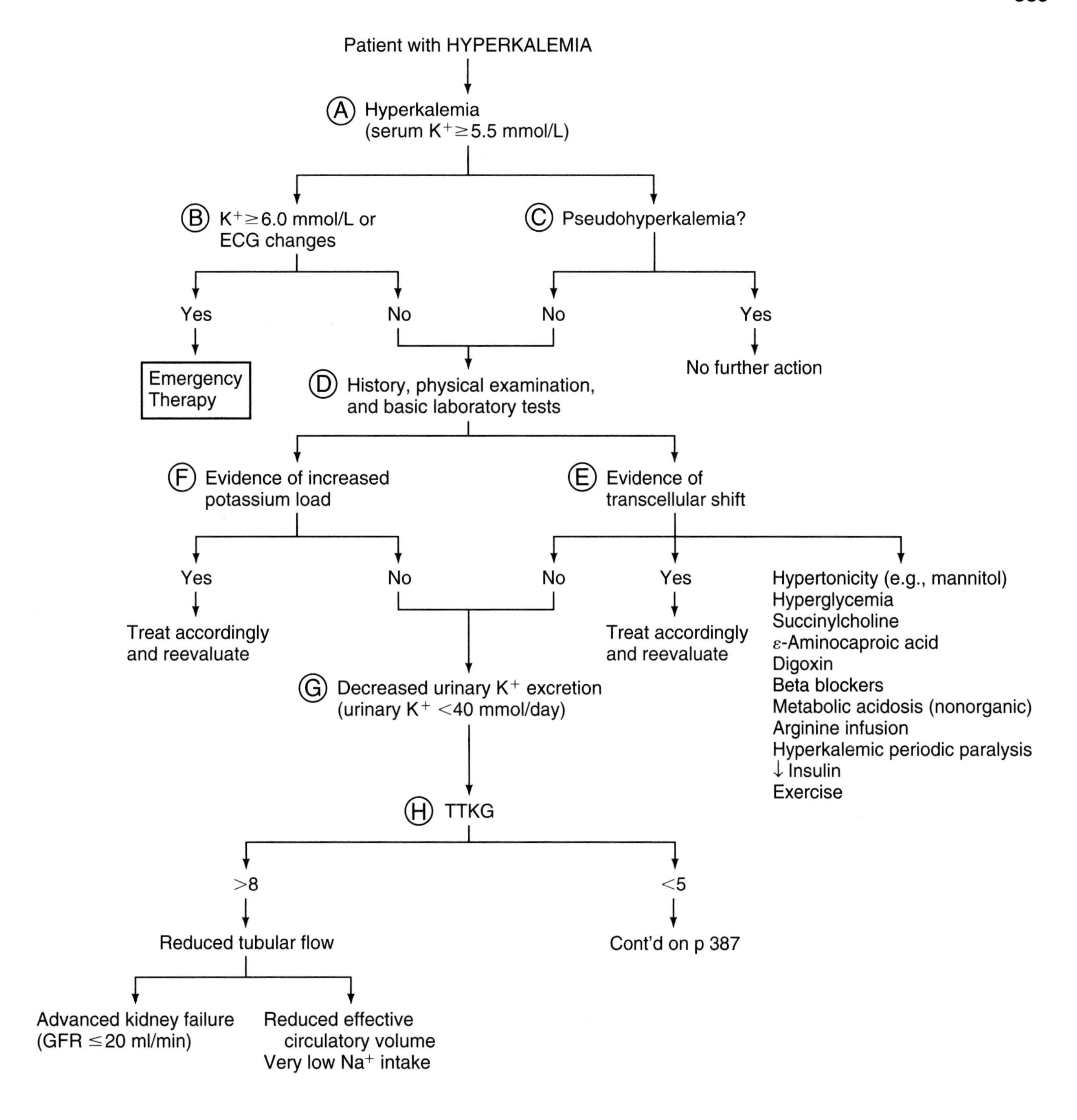
Patient with HYPERKALEMIA
(A) Hyperkalemia (serum $K^+ \geq 5.5$ mmol/L)
(B) $K^+ \geq 6.0$ mmol/L or ECG changes
(C) Pseudohyperkalemia?
Yes
No
No
Yes
Emergency Therapy
No further action
(D) History, physical examination, and basic laboratory tests
(F) Evidence of increased potassium load
(E) Evidence of transcellular shift
Yes
No
No
Yes
Treat accordingly and reevaluate
Treat accordingly and reevaluate
Hypertonicity (e.g., mannitol)
Hyperglycemia
Succinylcholine
ε-Aminocaproic acid
Digoxin
Beta blockers
Metabolic acidosis (nonorganic)
Arginine infusion
Hyperkalemic periodic paralysis
↓ Insulin
Exercise
(G) Decreased urinary K^+ excretion (urinary K^+ <40 mmol/day)
(H) TTKG
>8
<5
Reduced tubular flow
Cont'd on p 387
Advanced kidney failure (GFR ≤20 ml/min)
Reduced effective circulatory volume
Very low Na^+ intake

I. In the absence of advanced kidney failure and low urine flow, a TTKG value <5 is reflective of decreased potassium secretion in CCD, which may result from either aldosterone deficiency or resistance. Whereas an increase in TTKG value to ≥8 in response to 9α-fludrocortisone (a mineralocorticoid) is suggestive of aldosterone deficiency, a lesser or no response is indicative of tubular resistance to aldosterone action.

J. Hyporeninemic hypoaldosteronism is the most common form of hypoaldosteronism in adults. However, several medications are frequent contributors. Among them, potassium-sparing diuretics, NSAIDs, angiotensin-converting enzyme (ACE) inhibitors, angiotensin II receptor blockers (ARBs), heparin and low molecular weight (LMW) heparin, and beta blockers are more common. The usual presentation is in a patient with a mild degree of renal insufficiency and tubulointerstitial involvement. The level of hyperkalemia is usually disproportionate to the degree of renal insufficiency. In many patients, it is associated with mild non–anion gap metabolic acidosis (a condition also known as type IV renal tubular acidosis [RTA]).

References

Mount DB, Zandi-Nejad K. Disorders of potassium balance. In Brenner BM, ed. Brenner and Rector's The Kidney, 7th ed. Philadelphia: Elsevier, 2004:997–1040.

Williams ME. Hyperkalemia. Crit Care Clin 1991;7:155–173.

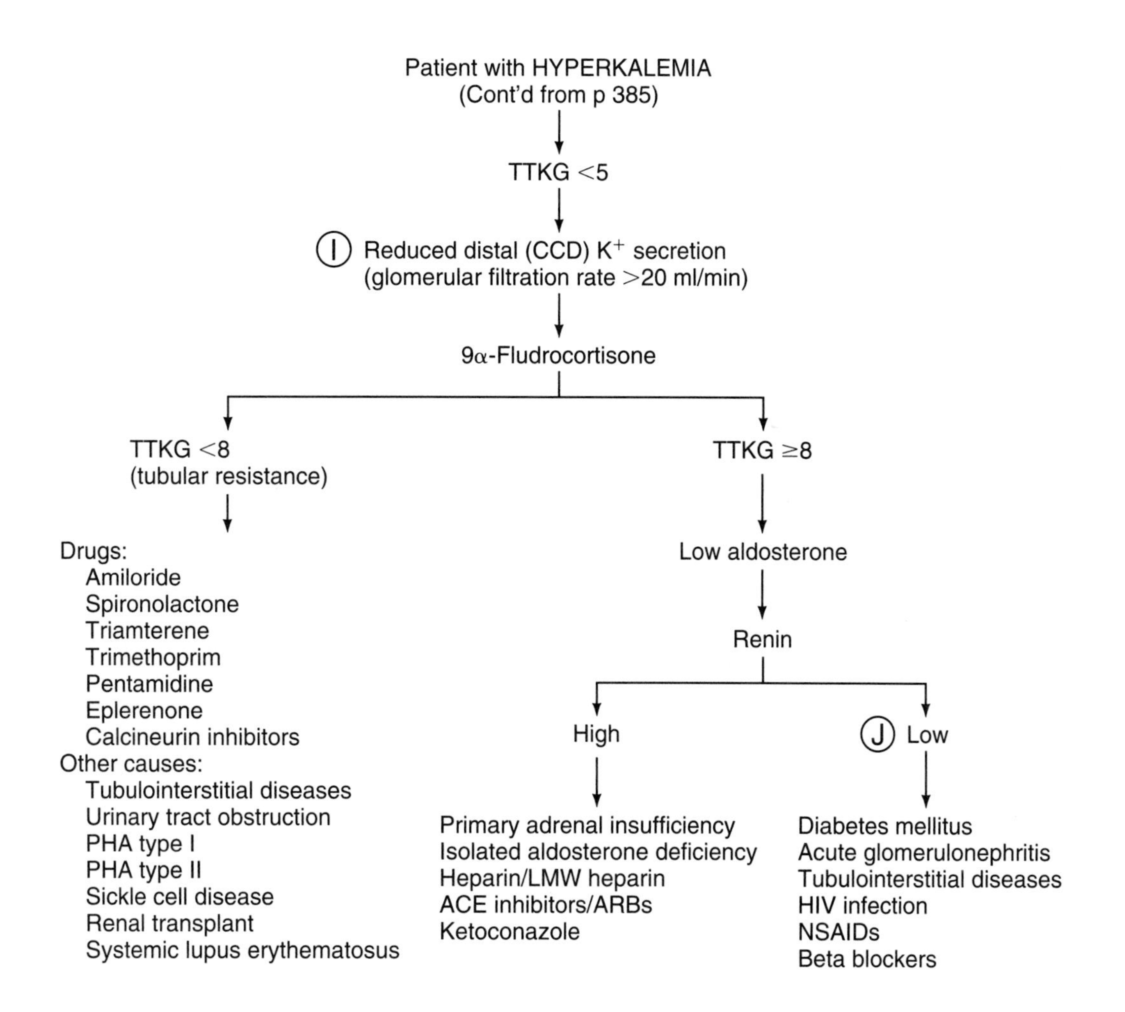

Patient with HYPERKALEMIA
(Cont'd from p 385)
TTKG <5
(I) Reduced distal (CCD) K^+ secretion
(glomerular filtration rate >20 ml/min)
9α-Fludrocortisone
TTKG <8
(tubular resistance)
TTKG ≥8
Drugs:
Amiloride
Spironolactone
Triamterene
Trimethoprim
Pentamidine
Eplerenone
Calcineurin inhibitors
Other causes:
Tubulointerstitial diseases
Urinary tract obstruction
PHA type I
PHA type II
Sickle cell disease
Renal transplant
Systemic lupus erythematosus
Low aldosterone
Renin
High
(J) Low
Primary adrenal insufficiency
Isolated aldosterone deficiency
Heparin/LMW heparin
ACE inhibitors/ARBs
Ketoconazole
Diabetes mellitus
Acute glomerulonephritis
Tubulointerstitial diseases
HIV infection
NSAIDs
Beta blockers

PHA, Pseudohypoaldosteronism.

HYPOMAGNESEMIA

Ajay K. Singh, MBBS, FRCP

Hypomagnesemia is defined as a serum magnesium (Mg^{+2}) level <18 mEq/L (the reference range for serum magnesium level is 1.8–3.0 mEq/L). The prevalence of hypomagnesemia is likely underestimated because of the lack of a good test to predict total body Mg^{+2} status. Approximately 10% of patients in the hospital and up to 60% of the patients in intensive care units are estimated to have hypomagnesemia. Hypomagnesemia is often the result of renal or GI losses and may be related to loop diuretic use, other drug use, alcohol use, and chronic diarrhea. Cutaneous losses are thought to result from excessive sweating on exercise excretion and also may occur in patients with severe burn injury. IV fluid therapy and volume-expanded states may also cause hypomagnesemia resulting from a dilutional effect. Rarely, familial incidence has been reported, primarily in isolated familial hypomagnesemia, familial hypokalemia, and familial hypomagnesemia-hypercalciuria.

A. Patients with hypomagnesemia may be asymptomatic or have a number of clinical manifestations that could reflect other electrolyte abnormalities. Multiple body systems can be involved, including the heart, neuromuscular system, or CNS. Cardiac symptoms include tachyarrhythmias, torsades de pointes, tachycardia, and fibrillation resistant to standard treatment but responsive to Mg^{+2} repletion. ECG changes reflect abnormal cardiac repolarization with bifid T waves, U waves, and prolongation of QT or QU interval. Neuromuscular symptoms are similar to those of hypocalcemia and include tremor, twitching, frank tetany, and positive Trousseau's and Chvostek's signs. CNS symptoms may include generalized, tonic-clonic, or multifocal motor seizures triggered by loud noises and can lead to sudden death. Nystagmus and Wernicke's encephalopathy may also be present. The key element in the diagnosis is to determine whether the hypomagnesemia results from a decreased intake/absorption or increased losses. The workup should be composed of a 24-hour quantitative urinary Mg^{+2} excretion to distinguish increased versus decreased urinary excretion of Mg^{+2}. Increased urinary excretion of magnesium in a patient with hypomagnesemia is invariably a result of renal wasting. However, decreased urinary excretion is usually from renal conservation of magnesium in an attempt to restore Mg^{+2} equilibrium in the face of inadequate Mg^{+2} intake. Renal Mg^{+2} wasting can be seen in patients with defective sodium resorption (diuretic use), use of renal toxins (amphotericin B, cisplatin, aminoglycosides, pentamidine, cyclosporine A), and osmotic diuresis (DM). Extrarenal losses may result from nutrition deficiency (e.g., alcoholism, protein-calorie malnutrition, parenteral nutrition), decreased absorption (e.g., chronic diarrhea, intestinal malabsorption syndromes), and cutaneous losses (e.g., burn patients, marathon runners). Rarely, bone redistribution may occur in patients who have "hungry bone syndrome," in which chronically elevated parathyroid hormone (PTH) is corrected with parathyroidectomy.

B. The treatment of asymptomatic magnesium deficiency is controversial. Patients with hypomagnesemia and associated cardiac disease should receive magnesium supplementation to avoid the risk of developing digoxin cardiotoxicity. The underlying etiology of magnesium losses should be evaluated and treated appropriately. For unknown reasons, patients receiving parenteral nutrition have an increased demand for magnesium. Therefore, magnesium supplementation should be increased to prevent further deficiencies. Symptomatic magnesium deficiency requires repletion to prevent complications such as seizure disorder and ongoing electrolyte imbalance. IV replacement is the route of choice for patients with IV access.

References

Dacey MJ. Hypomagnesemic disorders. Crit Care Clin 2001;17(1): 155–173, viii.

Sedlacek M, Schoolwerth AC, Remillared BD. Electrolyte disturbances in the intensive care unit. Semin Dial 2006;19(6):496–501.

Tong GM, Rude RK. Magnesium deficiency in critical illness. J Intensive Care Med 2005;20(1):3–17.

Topf JM, Murray PT. Hypomagnesemia and hypermagnesemia. Rev Endocr Metab Disord 2003;4(2):195–206.

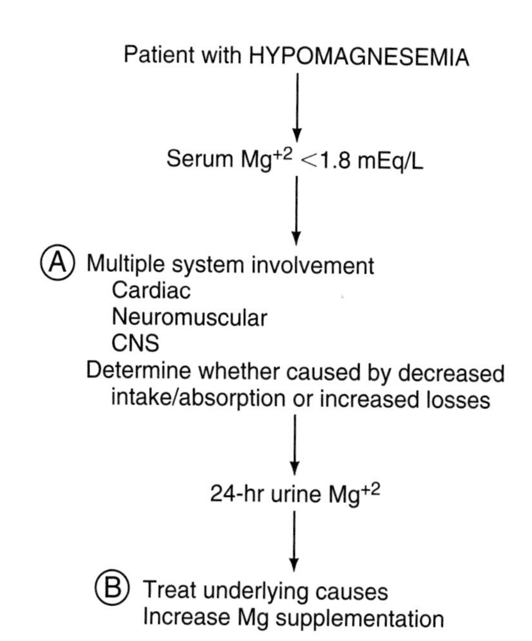
Patient with HYPOMAGNESEMIA
Serum Mg^{+2} <1.8 mEq/L
(A) Multiple system involvement
Cardiac
Neuromuscular
CNS
Determine whether caused by decreased intake/absorption or increased losses
24-hr urine Mg^{+2}
(B) Treat underlying causes
Increase Mg supplementation

HYPERMAGNESEMIA

Ajay K. Singh, MBBS, FRCP

Hypermagnesemia is defined as an increase of serum magnesium (Mg^{+2}) to >1.1 mmol/L (2.2 mEq/L; 2.6 mg/dl). Hypermagnesemia is relatively uncommon but can be seen in patients with acute renal failure (ARF) who are taking magnesium-containing antacids, laxatives, enemas, or infusions. Acute rhabdomyolysis also is associated with hypermagnesemia. Increasing age is an important risk factor for hypermagnesemia in individuals with apparently normal renal function and presumably reflects the decline in glomerular filtration rate that normally accompanies old age. Mg^{+2} is efficiently excreted through the kidneys. Even patients with chronic renal failure can develop an increased fractional excretion of magnesium in the remaining functional nephrons. Generally, the kidneys can maintain Mg^{+2} equilibrium until the creatinine clearance falls below 20 ml/min. Despite declining renal function, patients with end-stage renal disease (ESRD) and ARF rarely develop hypermagnesemia. Exogenous administration is usually necessary to cause significant hypermagnesemia. Even in a patient with normal renal function, exogenous administration may cause toxicity. It is common for patients to have an enhanced absorption of Mg^{+2} as a result of inflammatory disease, obstruction, or perforation of the GI tract. Other causes of hypermagnesemia include lithium therapy, metastatic disease to the bone, milk-alkali syndrome, familial hypocalciuric hypercalcemia, hypothyroidism, pituitary dwarfism, and Addison's disease. The neurologic symptoms often result from the inhibition of acetylcholine release from the neuromuscular end plate by increased extracellular Mg^{+2} levels.

A. Hypermagnesemia can be serious and potentially fatal. Lethargy, drowsiness, hypotension, nausea, vomiting, facial flushing, urinary retention, and ileus may be the initial symptoms observed when the serum Mg^{+2} level exceeds 4–6 mg/dl. If untreated, this condition may progress to flaccid skeletal muscular paralysis and hyporeflexia, bradycardia and bradyarrhythmias, complete heart block, and respiratory depression. Nonspecific ECG changes are often seen and may include prolonged PR intervals and increased QRS duration. Hypotension and cutaneous flushing may be the result of vasodilator effect and inhibition of norepinephrine release from sympathetic postganglionic nerves. Voluntary muscle paralysis and general smooth-muscle paralysis can cause the life-threatening complication of respiratory muscle paralysis and apnea. Coma and cardiac arrest eventually may ensue in patients with severe Mg^{+2} toxicity.

B. The withdrawal of the magnesium infusion is usually sufficient to treat most cases of hypermagnesemia when the patient has normal renal function. Hydration should be initiated with saline diuresis and furosemide. Mg^{+2} can be efficiently cleared through the kidneys in a short amount of time. In patients who have severe complications that may require emergent treatment, administration of Ca^{+2} (1 g for 2–5 minutes of IV calcium chloride or calcium gluconate) may be useful. Patients who have ARF or ESRD may require dialysis against a low magnesium bath. Generally, the expected change in serum Mg^{+2} after 3–4 hours of dialysis with a high-efficiency membrane is approximately one third to one half the difference between the dialysate Mg^{+2} concentration and the predialysis serum ultrafilterable Mg^{+2} level (estimated at 80% of total serum Mg^{+2}). Peritoneal dialysis can also be used to effectively remove Mg^{+2} in patients who cannot tolerate hemodialysis.

References

Moe SM. Disorders involving calcium, phosphorus, and magnesium. Prim Care 2008;35(2):215–237, v-vi.

Topf JM, Murray PT. Hypomagnesemia and hypermagnesemia. Rev Endocr Metab Disord 2003;4(2):195–206.

Sanders GT, Huijgen HJ, Sanders R. Magnesium in disease: a review with special emphasis on the serum ionized magnesium. Clin Chem Lab Med 1999;37(11–12):1011–1033.

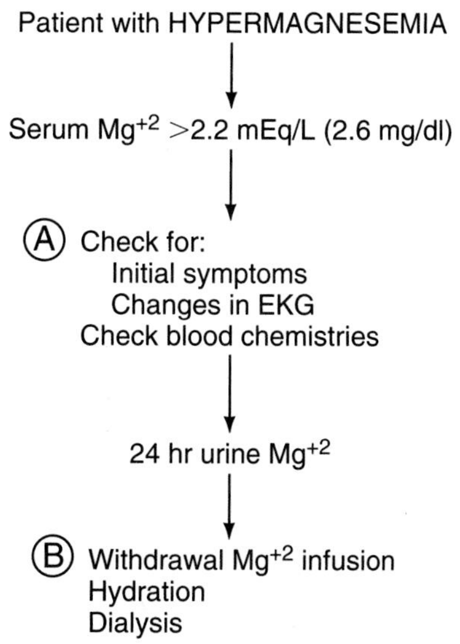

Patient with HYPERMAGNESEMIA

↓

Serum Mg^{+2} >2.2 mEq/L (2.6 mg/dl)

↓

(A) Check for:
- Initial symptoms
- Changes in EKG

Check blood chemistries

↓

24 hr urine Mg^{+2}

↓

(B) Withdrawal Mg^{+2} infusion
Hydration
Dialysis

HYPOPHOSPHATEMIA

Lamioko Shika Pappoe, MD, and Ajay K. Singh, MBBS, FRCP

Phosphorus is a critical component of many cellular compounds (e.g., phospholipids of the cell membrane, nucleic acid, adenosine triphospate [ATP], 2,3-diphosphoglycerate [2,3-DPG]) and plays a key role in an array of metabolic processes. Consequently it is under tight regulatory control. Serum levels of phosphate depend on dietary intake, intestinal absorption, bone turnover, cellular shifts, and renal tubular handling. Homeostasis is maintained primarily by parathyroid hormone (PTH) and vitamin D. The total body phosphorus in a 70-kg adult is estimated to be 700 g: 85% is in the skeleton, 15% is in the soft tissue, and 0.1% is in the extracellular fluid.

A. Hypophosphatemia is defined as a plasma phosphate level <2.5 mg/dl. Causes of hypophosphatemia are shown in Table 1. Hypophosphatemia can occur when there are increased losses, decreased intake, or cellular shifts of phosphate. In order to delineate among the causes, it is important to obtain a thorough history, physical examination, and laboratory evaluation. Hypophosphatemia secondary to decreased input occurs when there is decreased oral intake or intestinal absorption. Hypophosphatemia resulting from poor intake is uncommon, because phosphorus is plentiful in the diet. It can occur, however, when an individual has been chronically and severely malnourished. Malabsorption of phosphorus is often secondary to inflammatory states, surgery, or diarrhea. The most common cause of hypophosphatemia is chronic alcoholism. Over 50% of the hospitalized alcoholics become hypophosphatemic when they are unable to eat for a period of days or develop an alcohol withdrawal state. Increased renal clearance of phosphorus occurs in primary hyperparathyroidism, vitamin D deficiency, vitamin D–resistant and vitamin D–dependent rickets, hyperglycemic states, and oncogenic osteomalacia. There are acquired and hereditary conditions that lead to increased losses of phosphate. Intracellular shifts of phosphorus by insulin infusion can cause an abrupt fall in serum phosphorus, but this is usually transient and usually does not result in a profound deficiency. Finally, cellular shifts can cause hypophosphatemia. This is most often seen with the administration of glucose or total parenteral nutrition (TPN) in malnourished patients. A rise in insulin causes phosphate to move to the intracellular compartment. Additionally, the increased anabolism leads to the formation of high-energy phosphate bonds, further depleting phosphate levels. A similar mechanism is involved in hypophosphatemia resulting from insulin administration in treatment of diabetic ketoacidosis (DKA) or hyperglycemic hyperosmolar nonketotic coma (HONK).

B. The clinical manifestations of hypophosphatemia depend on the severity and duration of low plasma phosphate levels. Patients with moderate hypophosphatemia (1.5–2.5 mg/dl) are generally asymptomatic. Those with severe hypophosphatemia (<1.5 mg/dl) can have metabolic encephalopathy, bone pain, or symptoms secondary to muscle dysfunction (decreased strength, rhabdomyolysis, cardiomyopathy, respiratory failure). Hypophosphatemic patients may also demonstrate hematologic abnormalities (hemolysis secondary to decreased 2,3-DGP and ATP levels, leukocyte dysfunction, thrombocytopenia). When deciding how to manage hypophosphatemia, it is important to keep in mind that serum levels of phosphate do not necessarily reflect total body stores. Hypophosphatemia can occur when total stores are low, normal, or high. Clinically significant hypophosphatemia tends to occur when there is a total-body deficit of phosphorus.

Table 1 **Causes of Hypophosphatemia**

Increased Losses of Phosphate
Acquired
Hyperparathyroidism
Vitamin D deficiency
Renal tubular disease
Extracellular volume expansion
Diuretics (acetazolamide, thiazides)
Osmotic diuresis
Renal transplant
Administration of bicarbonate
Corticosteroids
Hereditary
Fanconi's syndrome
X-chromosome–linked hypophosphatemia
Autosomal-dominant hypophosphatemic rickets
Type 1 distal renal tubular acidosis
Redistribution of Phosphate
Acute respiratory alkalosis
Insulin administration in DKA or HONK
Refeeding of malnourished patients (alcoholics, anorexia)
TPN without phosphate administration
Hungry bone syndrome (after parathyroidectomy or thyroidectomy in the setting of osteopenia)
Increased cellular synthesis
Increased cellular metabolism
Oncogenic hypophosphatemic osteomalacia
Decreased Intake of Phosphate
Vitamin D deficiency
Malabsorption
Alcoholism
Poor nutrition
Antacids containing Mg and Al
Diarrhea/steatorrhea

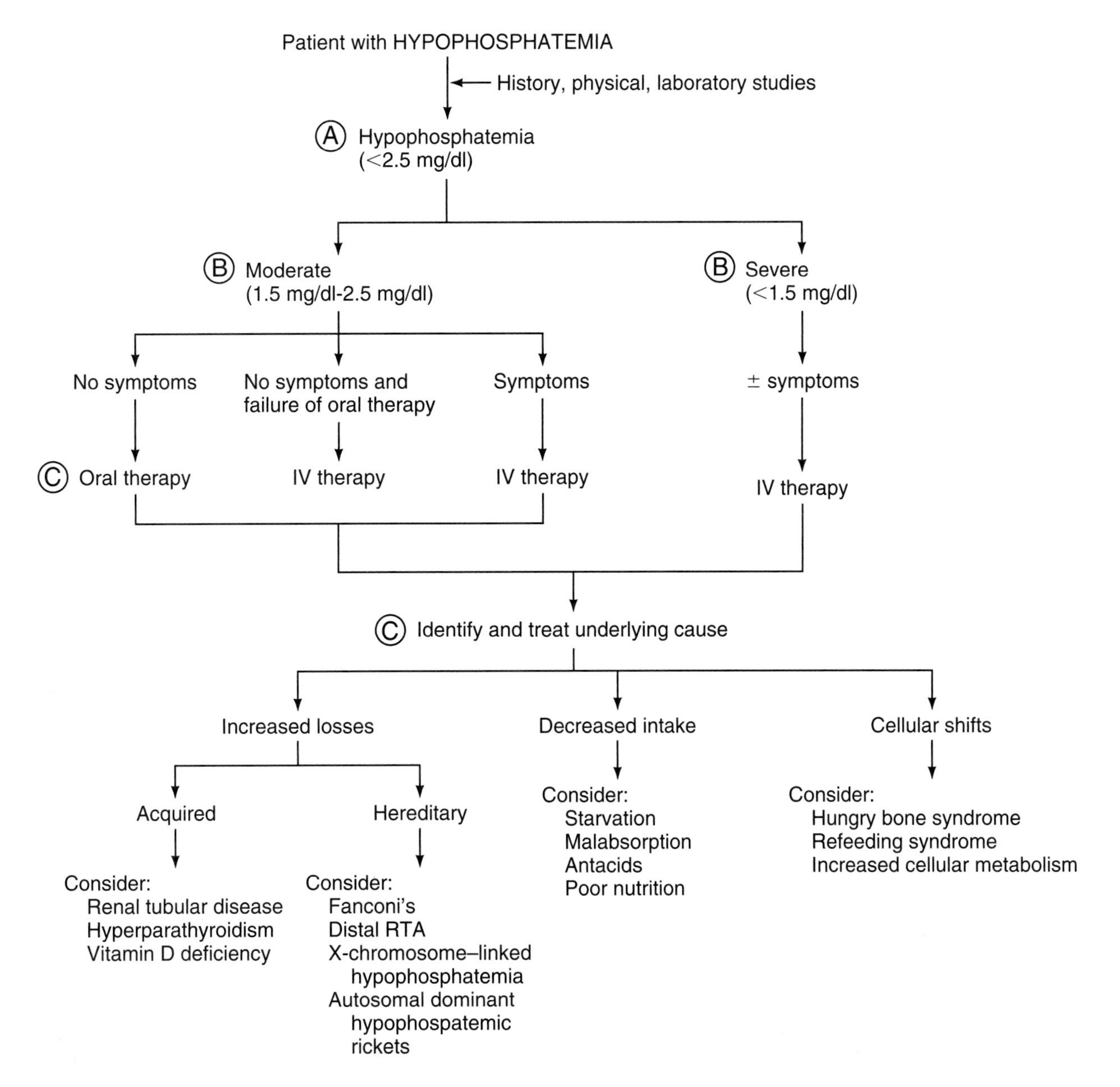

C. Phosphorus can be replaced orally or parenterally. Orally is considered safer. Oral therapies include phosphate-containing salts (sodium phosphate or potassium phosphate) and dairy products (e.g., milk contains 1 mg/ml of phosphorus). Generally, for oral replacement, 60 mmol of phosphate per day in 3–4 divided doses of the preparation of choice, given over 7–10 days is sufficient to correct moderate hypophosphatemia. Parenteral therapy is usually reserved for severe hypophosphatemia or for those who do not tolerate or respond to oral preparations. IV formulations include sodium phosphate and potassium phosphate. A common regimen is 2.5 mg/kg body weight of phosphate over 6 hours in severe hypophosphatemia without overt clinical manifestations, and 5.0 mg/kg body weight over 6 hours in hypophosphatemic emergencies. Phosphate repletion can have side effects. When phosphate-containing salts are used, patients need to be followed closely for hypernatremia, hyperkalemia, hyperphosphatemia, and volume overload. With oral salt supplements patients may have diarrhea. This can be avoided by administering divided doses. During parenteral repletion it is also important to monitor the calcium phosphate product. Overaggressive repletion can lead to metastatic calcium deposition and hypocalcemia.

In addition to correcting plasma levels of phosphorus, the underlying causes of hypophosphatemia need to be identified and treated.

References

Gaasbeek A, Meinders AE. Hypophosphatemia: an update on its etiology and treatment. Am J Med 2005;118(10):1094–1101.

Knochel JP. Disorders of phosphorous metabolism. In Fauci AS et al, eds. Harrison's Principles of Internal Medicine, 14th ed. New York: McGraw-Hill, 1998:2259–2262.

Marinella, MA. Refeeding syndrome and hypophosphatemia. J Intensive Care Med 2005;20(3):155–159.

Paterson CR, Naismith KI, Young JA. Severe unexplained hypophosphatemia. Clin Chem 1992;38(1):104–107.

Subramanian R, Khardori R. Severe hypophosphatemia: pathophysiologic implications, clinical presentations, and treatment. Medicine (Baltimore) 2000;79(1):1–8.

CHOOSING A CHRONIC DIALYSIS MODALITY

J. Kevin Tucker, MD

Patients with chronic kidney disease (CKD) should be informed of the possibility of progression of disease early in the course of their kidney disease. Specific preparation and education about dialysis and transplantation modalities, however, is usually reserved until the patient has reached stage 4 kidney disease (i.e., a glomerular filtration rate [GFR] of 15–29 ml/min).

A. When the patient reaches stage 4 CKD, he or she should be presented with the range of renal replacement options: preemptive transplantation if feasible; hemodialysis (HD), both in-center and home; and peritoneal dialysis (PD). The education of the patient regarding these options may occur in any of a number of settings. The physician may provide education in the course of a routine clinic visit. Alternatively, the physician may refer the patient to a dialysis nurse educator who may spend time with the patient and family members discussing renal replacement options either in an individual session or as a part of a dialysis "options" class. PD is underused in the United States relative to HD. However, when patients are educated about both HD and PD and given a choice as to which modality to use, the percentage of patients choosing PD increases. Although studies comparing HD versus PD in terms of hard outcomes such as mortality continue to generate controversy, there is consensus that patients who choose PD tend to be more satisfied with their treatment and have a higher self-reported quality of life.

B. Because renal transplantation is the best option for long-term renal replacement, patients with stage 4 CKD should be evaluated for their suitability for renal transplantation (see Selection of Patients for Transplantation). The major source of morbidity and mortality in recipients of renal transplants is cardiovascular disease; therefore, particular attention should be paid to screening and/or prevention of cardiovascular disease. If there are no medical contraindications to renal transplantation and there is a suitable living donor, the patient may be a candidate for preemptive renal transplantation.

C. The patient with CKD being considered for PD should be evaluated for medical suitability for this dialysis modality. The key issues include the following:
   (1) Abdominal surgery: The major technical consideration that may affect the decision to choose this modality is a history of major abdominal surgery. The presence of intraabdominal adhesions may adversely affect solute and fluid transport across the peritoneal membrane, making PD technically difficult. However, newer laparoscopic surgical techniques for placement of PD catheters allow for visualization of the peritoneal space and simultaneous lysis of adhesions when they are identified.
   (2) Body habitus: Obesity is not itself a contraindication to PD; however, it does merit special consideration. The patient who is morbidly obese may require placement of a presternal peritoneal catheter (a catheter that has an extension allowing it to exit at the sternum) to reduce the risk of exit site infection. The patient who is obese should also be counseled about the risk of weight gain, development of or progression to more difficult to control diabetes mellitus, and hyperlipidemia associated with PD.
   (3) Diabetes mellitus: Glycemic control often becomes more difficult when a patient with diabetes starts receiving PD. Control of blood sugars usually requires a more intense insulin regimen using subcutaneous and/or intraperitoneal insulin and may require comanagement with the primary care provider or diabetologist. Poor glycemic control in the patient with diabetes is also a risk factor for impaired ultrafiltration because of the diminished osmotic gradient between the blood compartment and the peritoneal compartment.

   Because PD is a home-based, self-directed form of renal replacement, the patient who chooses this form of therapy must be able to learn the technique. Formal education is not a requisite; patients who are illiterate have been successfully taught to perform PD. However, patients with cognitive impairment may not be able to master the technique. These patients may still be managed at home on PD if there is adequate social support at home, such as a spouse or family member who is trained to assist the patient in performing dialysis.

D. The evaluation of the patient with CKD for HD should include examination of the extremities for venous access sites. The arteriovenous (AV) fistula is the preferred dialysis access, and it may require 3–6 months for maturation. The nondominant arm is typically used for the first dialysis access. In elderly patients, diabetic patients with small vessel disease, and patients who have no accessible veins, an AV graft may be necessary. If neither an AV fistula or graft is feasible, a tunneled

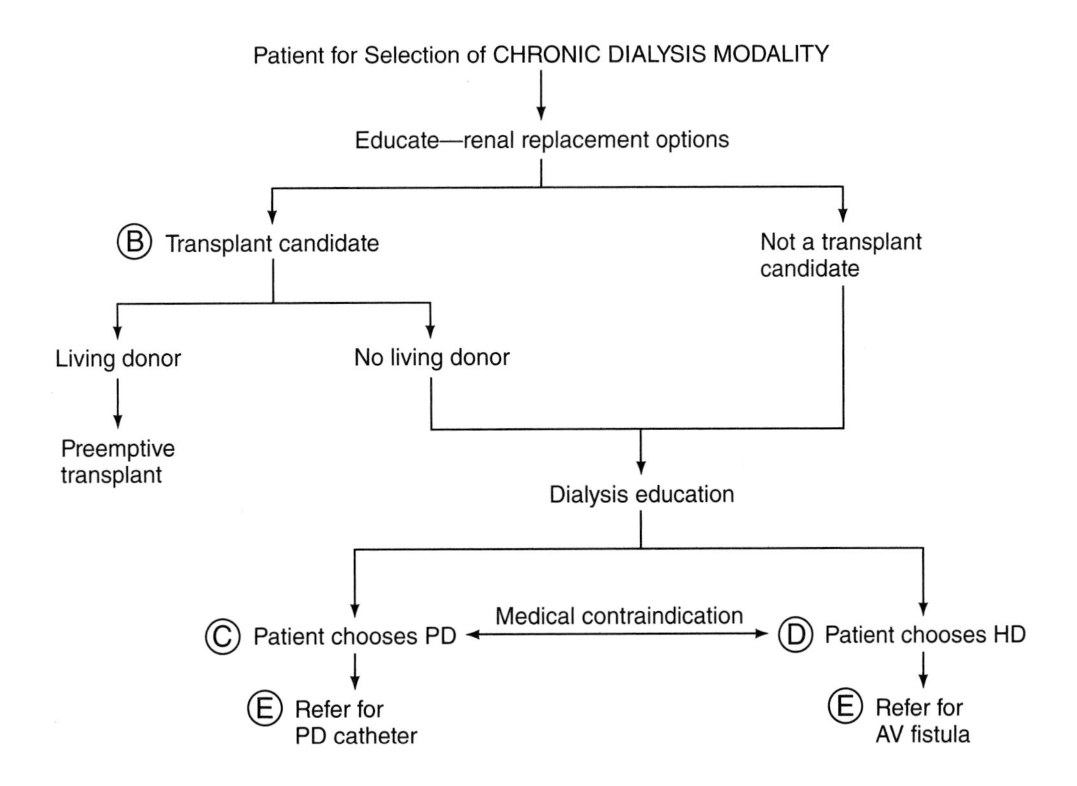

catheter inserted into a central vein (internal jugular or subclavian vein) may be the only recourse. An AV fistula is preferred because of the substantially lower complication rate compared to either an AV graft or a tunneled catheter. These complications include thrombosis, infection, and mechanical failure. The patient should be instructed to avoid venipuncture and blood pressure measurements in that arm to preserve veins for access creation. The cardiovascular system should also be assessed for signs of heart failure. The patient who is volume overloaded and who also has significantly impaired left ventricular function may have difficulty in reaching his or her dry weight because of HD-associated hypotension.

Patients undergoing HD have several options regarding the setting of the treatments. The most common scenario is a patient undergoing treatment in a freestanding outpatient dialysis unit. However, a hospital-based unit or HD at home are other potential possibilities.

E. When the patient with CKD has been educated on renal replacement options and has reached a decision on a preferred modality, the patient should be referred to a surgeon with expertise in either vascular access for HD or PD catheter placement. The native AV fistula will require 3–6 months for maturation; thus, the patient should be referred at a minimum of 6 months before the anticipated need to start HD. A PD catheter usually requires 2–3 weeks to heal. The patient who chooses PD should be seen preoperatively by the surgeon at least 2 months prior to initiation of dialysis.

References

Mange KC, Marshall MJ, Feldman HI. Effect of the use or nonuse of long-term dialysis on the subsequent survival of renal transplants from living donors. N Engl J Med 2001;344:726–731.

Manns BJ, Taub K, Vanderstraeten C, et al. The impact of education on chronic kidney disease patients' plans to initiate dialysis with self-care dialysis: a randomized trial. Kidney Int 2005;68:1777–1783.

Mehrotra R, Marsh D, Vonesh E, et al. Patient education and access of ESRD patients to renal replacement therapies beyond in-center hemodialysis. Kidney Int 2005;68:378–390.

Rubin H, Fink N, Plantinga L, et al. Patient ratings of dialysis care with peritoneal dialysis vs hemodialysis. JAMA 2004;291:697–703.

SELECTION OF PATIENTS FOR TRANSPLANTATION

Colm C. Magee, MD

The evaluation of the patient with chronic kidney disease (CKD) for transplantation should begin *before* initiation of dialysis. This allows preemptive transplantation if a living donor is available. Even if living donation is not feasible, early completion of the evaluation means that the patient can be listed for a deceased donor transplant as soon as dialysis is started. The initial evaluation must be thorough. The general purpose of the initial evaluation is, first, to ensure that there are no medical, surgical, immunologic, or psychosocial contraindications to transplant; second, to extensively educate the patient as to the risks and benefits of transplantation; and third, to determine which type of kidney transplant(s) is best for the patient.

A. A comprehensive history is essential, but one should focus on the following: cause of end-stage renal disease (ESRD), previous transplant history, comorbid illnesses, social supports, and functional status. Certain conditions—such as primary focal glomerulosclerosis or nondiarrheal hemolytic uremic syndrome—can recur in the transplanted kidney, and very careful assessment is required of the risks versus benefits of transplantation in such cases. A comprehensive examination is also required but with focus on overall general health (will this patient tolerate the stresses of transplant surgery and immunosuppression?), signs of decompensated heart or lung disease, and signs of peripheral vascular disease.

B. Standard tests in all patients include ABO blood typing and human leukocyte antigen (HLA) tissue typing; CBC; chemistry panel; calcium; glucose; parathyroid hormone (PTH); chest x-ray (CXR); ECG; urinalysis; urine culture; and tests for exposure to HIV, hepatitis B, hepatitis C, cytomegalovirus, Epstein-Barr virus, and syphilis. Most patients require some form of noninvasive testing for coronary artery disease. Those >50 years should be screened for bowel neoplasia by stool occult blood or colonoscopy. Women should be screened for breast and cervical cancer according to standard guidelines. Many centers check prostate-specific antigen (PSA) in males >50 years.

C. Contraindications to renal transplantation include any major morbidity that would be worsened by transplant or would lead to very short posttransplant survival, severe organ failure (e.g., liver or heart failure), recent cancer, severe obesity, significant infection (e.g., active tuberculosis), and severe psychiatric illness or predicted noncompliance. Depending on the cancer, a recurrence-free period of 2–5 years is usually required before transplant is deemed safe.

D. A current positive T-cell crossmatch (indicating the presence of noxious antibodies against class I HLA antigens of the donor) or incompatibility of the ABO blood group system between potential donor and recipient are both immunologic contraindications because of the very high risk of severe antibody-mediated rejection. In living donation, this problem can sometimes be circumvented by exchange programs or by neutralizing the noxious antibodies of the recipient.

E. The kidney donor options must be carefully discussed with the patient. The best functioning transplants are those derived from living donors; however, many patients do not have suitable living donors and must remain on the waiting list for many years. Certain patients—typically those >60 years or people >50 years with diabetes—should be listed also for expanded criteria donor (ECD) kidneys. By definition, these kidneys have poorer survival than "regular" deceased donor kidneys. However, they are still associated with a survival benefit as opposed to continuing dialysis.

F. Because patients often wait many years on the list, the transplant center should review their overall medical status and suitability for transplant every 1–2 years. This is especially important in people with diabetes, who have such high incidence of cardiovascular disease.

References

Kasiske BL, Cangro CB, Hariharan S, et al. The evaluation of renal transplantation candidates: clinical practice guidelines. Am J Transplant 2001;1(Suppl 2):3–95.

Magee C. Transplantation across previously incompatible immunological barriers. Transplant Int 2006;19(2):87–97.

Merion RM, Ashby VB, Wolfe RA, et al. Deceased-donor characteristics and the survival benefit of kidney transplantation. JAMA 2005;294(21):2726–2733.

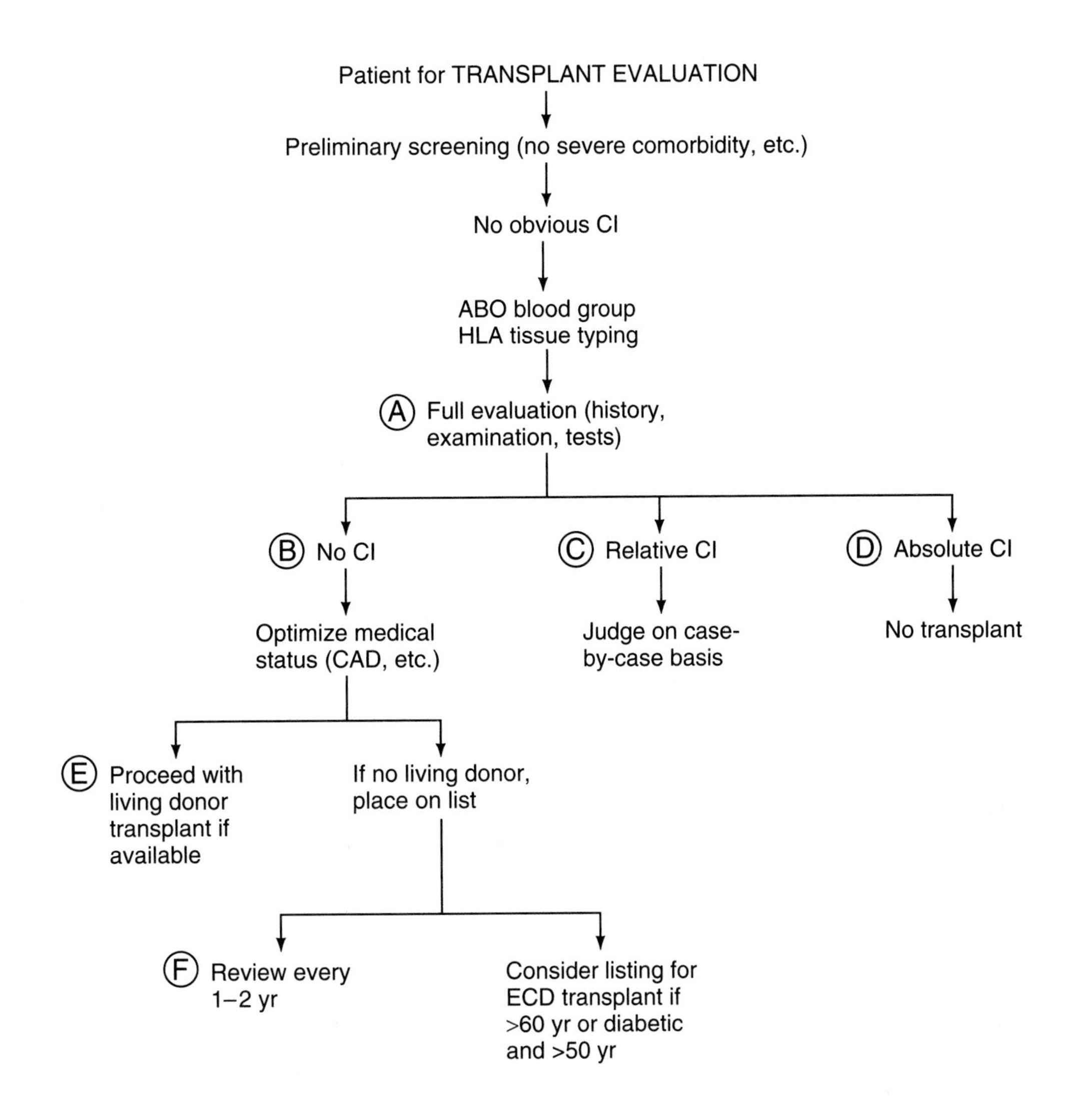

CAD, Coronary artery disease; CI, contraindication.

FEVER IN THE TRANSPLANT RECIPIENT

Colm C. Magee, MD

Fever in the transplant recipient is usually a sign of infection; hence, this review will focus on posttransplant infections. When infections have been rigorously excluded, it may be appropriate to investigate for other causes of fever such as allograft rejection, drug reactions, or neoplasia. Transplant recipients presenting with fever or signs of infection must be investigated urgently. Often, a "tissue diagnosis" (e.g., bronchoscopy with lavage and biopsy) is useful and should be obtained quickly. Empiric antimicrobial therapy is usually required before results are finalized.

A. It is useful to assess fever and infections according to the time period after kidney transplant. In the first month or so, infections are broadly similar to those that affect any hospitalized surgical patient. Thus, bacterial infections (of wounds, urinary tract, or lungs) predominate. Note that patients frequently have indwelling foreign material such as bladder catheters, urinary stents, and central lines; these devices can become infected. Prevention of early infection involves meticulous surgical technique. Treatment typically involves antibiotics and/or removal of infected foreign material. Of note, fever and mild allergic reactions to Thymoglobulin or OKT3 are not uncommon. These can be prevented and treated with acetaminophen + antihistamines + steroids. Other less common nonmicrobial causes of fever include severe allograft rejection and deep venous thrombosis.

B. From about the second to the sixth posttransplant month, the recipient is at relatively high risk of opportunistic infection because the recent cumulative dose of immunosuppression is high. However, "standard" infections of the lungs, urinary tract, and so on, may still occur (see earlier). Opportunistic infections may be viral (e.g., cytomegalovirus [CMV]), bacterial (e.g., pneumocystosis, nocardiosis), or fungal. Probably the most common are CMV infection and pneumocystosis. Symptomatic CMV infection is most common in CMV-positive donor–CMV-negative recipient pairings but can occur when the donor or recipient or both were harboring CMV before transplant. Common features of CMV infection include fever, malaise, leucopenia, and hepatitis; signs of pneumonitis, colitis, or retinitis may also be present. Demonstration of CMV in whole blood (by specialized tests) and in infected tissue (by immunochemistry) confirms the diagnosis. Treatment involves IV ganciclovir or PO valganciclovir and reduction in immunosuppression. *Pneumocystic carinii* pneumonia (PCP) usually presents with fever, malaise, shortness of breath, cough, hypoxia, and infiltrates on chest x-ray (CXR). Demonstration of the organism in induced sputum or lavaged/biopsied lung tissue confirms the diagnosis. Treatment involves high-dose sulfamethoxazole-trimethoprim (SMX-TMP co-trimoxazole) and reduction in immunosuppression. Other opportunistic infections are similarly treated with specific antimicrobial drugs and reduction in immunosuppression.

C. After the first 6 months, the immunosuppressive load is lower and opportunistic infections become less common (although the risk is still somewhat increased). Thus, patients who present years after transplant with fever will often have infective causes similar to the general population. An important exception is the patient who receives late supplemental immunosuppression (e.g., Thymoglobulin for late acute rejection)—they are again at high risk of opportunistic infections.

   Avoiding excess immunosuppression is vital to minimize infection. Many centers prescribe (1) antiviral drugs such as valganciclovir for 3–4 months to prevent CMV infection (if the donor or recipient were CMV positive) and (2) SMX-TMP for 6–12 months to prevent PCP, urinary tract, and other bacterial infections.

D. When allografts fail and the recipients resume dialysis, immunosuppression is usually weaned to zero. Occasionally, this can lead to severe rejection of the failed allograft. Typical features are fever, allograft pain, and tenderness. Pyelonephritis must be excluded. The fever usually responds to steroids, but allograft nephrectomy is sometimes required.

References

Fishman JA, Rubin RH. Infection in organ-transplant recipients. N Engl J Med 1998;338(24):1741–1751.

Preiksaitis JK, Brennan DC, Fishman J, et al. Canadian Society of Transplantation consensus workshop on cytomegalovirus management in solid organ transplantation final report. Am J Transplant 2005;5(2): 218–227.

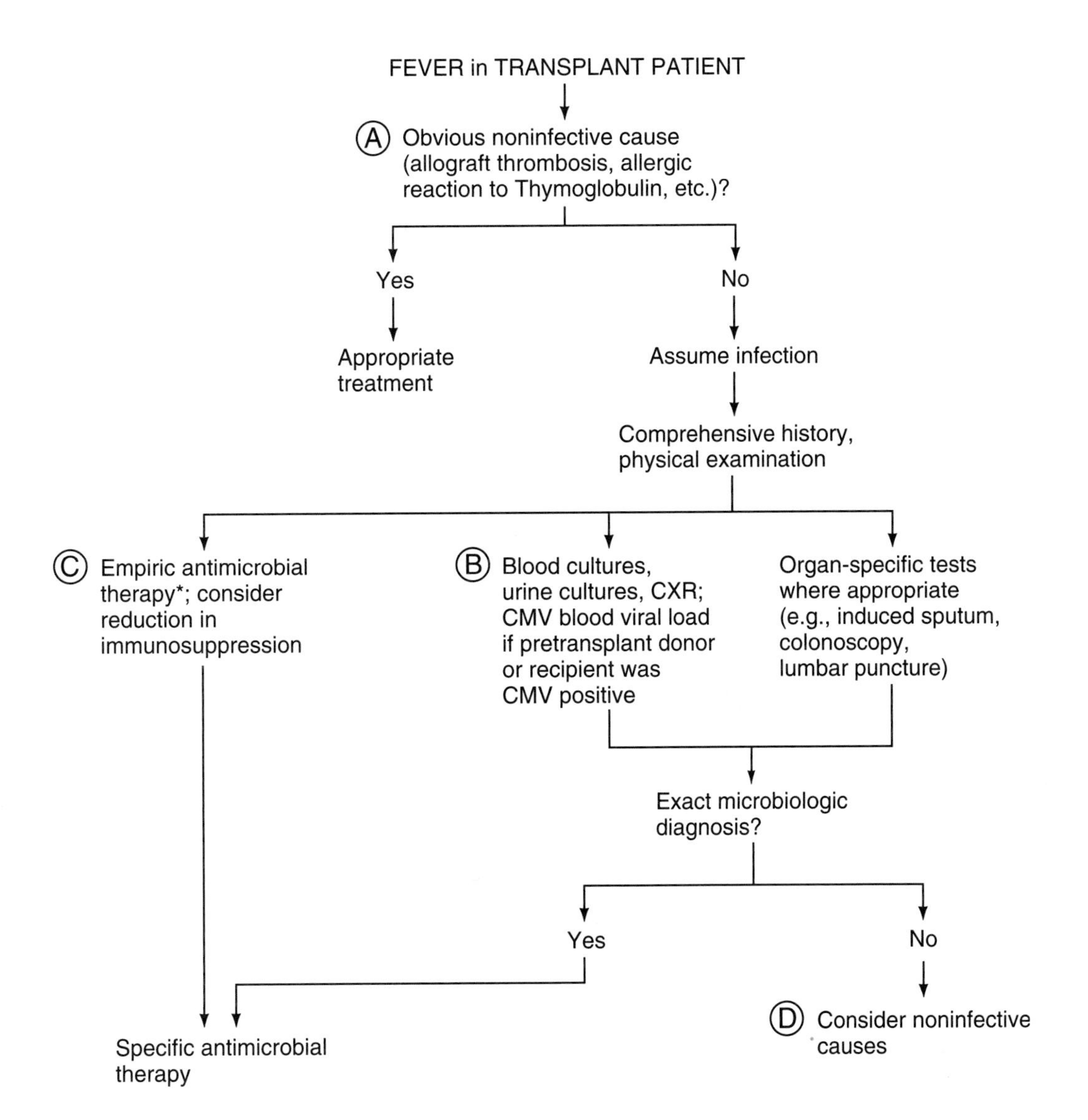

*Empiric therapy will depend on symptoms, signs, and time posttransplant.

NEUROLOGY

Bradford C. Dickerson, MD
Section Editor

ACUTE HEADACHE

Santosh Kesari, MD

Acute headache is a chief complaint in as many as 5% of patients visiting emergency departments and a common problem in outpatient medicine; fortunately, however, most patients with acute headache have benign conditions. The diagnosis of acute headache can be challenging and should proceed in an orderly fashion. Crucial elements include a thorough history, supplemented by general medical and neurologic examinations and laboratory testing and neuroimaging in selected patients. An important first step is to distinguish a primary from secondary headache. Several red flags suggest the possibility of secondary headache: sudden onset, worsening pattern, history of cancer or HIV, fever, focal neurologic symptoms, older age, or pregnancy.

A. Patients with sudden onset of severe headache ("thunderclap") and no history of head trauma require a full neurologic evaluation and a head CT scan to exclude a subarachnoid hemorrhage. Imaging can be negative in up to 15% of those with subarachnoid hemorrhage, so a lumbar puncture is required, regardless of the presence or absence of nuchal rigidity.

B. Every patient with a recent history of head trauma who has focal neurologic complaints or findings or has altered mental status should undergo neuroimaging. Those patients with no focal complaints and a normal neurologic examination can be observed and treated symptomatically. However, if their condition deteriorates or if they fail to improve with conservative treatment, imaging is necessary.

C. Sinusitis is an overdiagnosed cause of headache. The diagnosis of sinus headache should be made only in the context of recent upper respiratory illness, purulent nasal discharge, fever, and localized tenderness over the sinus area. Sinus radiography can confirm the diagnosis but is seldom necessary for the initial evaluation and treatment.

D. The most common category of headache in patients presenting to emergency departments is the nonmigrainous vascular headache secondary to systemic infection. These patients typically are febrile and have other signs and symptoms of systemic illness. The neurologic examination is normal, and there is no nuchal rigidity. Treatment should focus on the underlying illness and on symptomatic management of headache pain.

E. In patients with no history of headache, a new headache may represent a first migraine or tension headache. In the initial evaluation of suspected migraine, it is necessary to perform a complete neurologic evaluation, often including neuroimaging. The role of hypertension in headache is not clearly understood, and it is probably overdiagnosed as a cause of headache. When diastolic blood pressure is >120 mm Hg, this may be the source of headache. Patients in pain from any cause may have elevated blood pressure. Therefore, exclude other causes of headache in patients with headache and high blood pressure.

F. In individuals >50 years of age who have headache, exclude temporal arteritis as a cause. The headache may be unilateral or bilateral, and the temporal arteries are often thickened and tender. Accompaniments may include jaw claudication (pain on chewing food), visual symptoms (e.g., transient diplopia or transient blurring of vision), or transient focal neurologic episodes. It is important to make an early diagnosis to prevent the irreversible visual loss that can occur from thrombosis of the ophthalmic artery. The ESR usually is elevated, but a temporal artery biopsy is diagnostic (although relatively insensitive). Treatment consists of high-dose prednisone and should be started as soon as the diagnosis is suspected, even before biopsy is done.

References

Cortelli P, Cevoli S, Nonino F, et al; Multidisciplinary Group for Nontraumatic Headache in the Emergency Department. Evidence-based diagnosis of nontraumatic headache in the emergency department: a consensus statement on four clinical scenarios. Headache 2004;44(6):587–595.

Mathew NT. Serotonin 10 (5-HT10) agonists and other agents in acute migraine (review). Neurol Clin 1997;15:61.

Robbins LD. Management of Headache and Headache Medications. New York: Springer-Verlag, 1994.

Silberstein SD, Lipton RB, Dalessio DJ. Overview, diagnosis and classification of headache. In Silberstein SD, Lipton RB, Dalessio DJ, eds. Wolff's Headache and Other Facial Pain. New York: Oxford University Press, 2001:6–26.

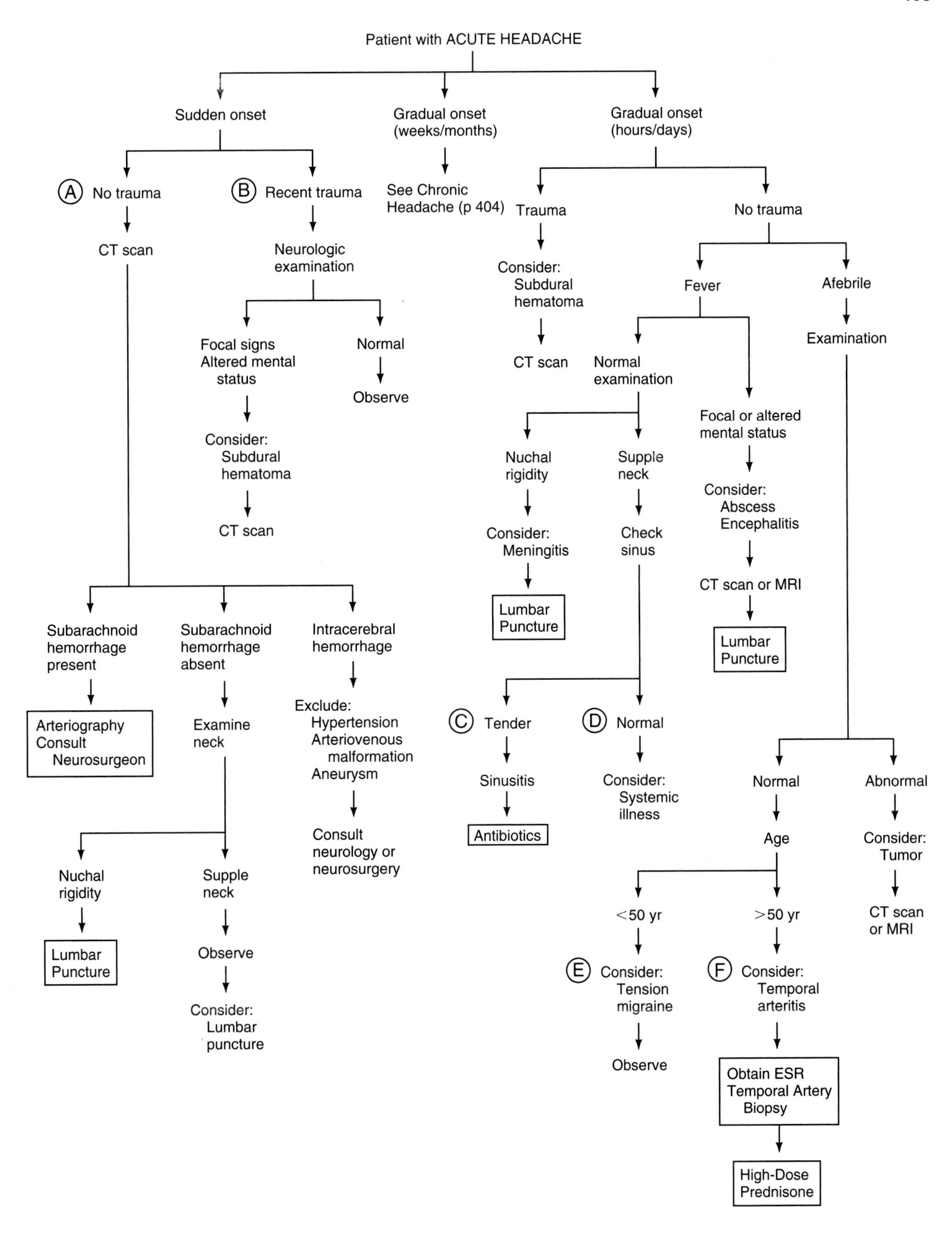

Patient with ACUTE HEADACHE
Sudden onset
Gradual onset (weeks/months)
Gradual onset (hours/days)
Ⓐ No trauma
CT scan
Ⓑ Recent trauma
Neurologic examination
Focal signs Altered mental status
Consider: Subdural hematoma
CT scan
Normal
Observe
See Chronic Headache (p 404)
Trauma
Consider: Subdural hematoma
CT scan
No trauma
Fever
Normal examination
Nuchal rigidity
Consider: Meningitis
Lumbar Puncture
Supple neck
Check sinus
Ⓒ Tender
Sinusitis
Antibiotics
Ⓓ Normal
Consider: Systemic illness
Focal or altered mental status
Consider: Abscess Encephalitis
CT scan or MRI
Lumbar Puncture
Afebrile
Examination
Normal
Age
<50 yr
Ⓔ Consider: Tension migraine
Observe
>50 yr
Ⓕ Consider: Temporal arteritis
Obtain ESR Temporal Artery Biopsy
High-Dose Prednisone
Abnormal
Consider: Tumor
CT scan or MRI
Subarachnoid hemorrhage present
Arteriography Consult Neurosurgeon
Subarachnoid hemorrhage absent
Examine neck
Nuchal rigidity
Lumbar Puncture
Supple neck
Observe
Consider: Lumbar puncture
Intracerebral hemorrhage
Exclude: Hypertension Arteriovenous malformation Aneurysm
Consult neurology or neurosurgery

CHRONIC HEADACHE

Santosh Kesari, MD

Chronic headache is a common complaint (5% of the general population) and, although benign, has a significant negative impact on the quality of life of sufferers and on health care resource utilization. Many patients with chronic headache have comorbid illnesses that require concurrent evaluation and treatment, such as depression, dysthymia, bipolar disorder, anxiety, and fibromyalgia.

A. A careful history is the most important aspect in the evaluation of patients with headache because there are no diagnostic tests for most headache disorders. Important aspects of the history include rapidity of onset, location, the character and temporal pattern of the pain, symptoms of systemic illness, change in pattern of headache, and focal neurologic complaints. The medical context is crucial, including patient age, medical history, and risk factors for other illnesses. Imaging and diagnostic studies maybe necessary to rule out causes of secondary headaches such as brain tumors, meningitis, and sinus disease. Sinus headache commonly causes facial pain, and prognosis is good if recognized and treated properly. Typically, pain is located in the forehead, bridge of nose, or cheeks and is usually of a dull-pressure quality and associated with nasal congestion. Sinus CT may be needed to rule out chronic bacterial sinusitis. A careful search for allergens or irritants should be done. Treatment includes corticosteroid nasal spray, antihistamines, and antibiotics.

B. Migraine headaches are more common in women (3 to 1), with onset before age 50 years and relatively high prevalence (as high as 12.6% in some populations). Classic migraine is a headache preceded by a focal neurologic deficit, usually lasting 15–30 minutes. The most common auras are visual, but sensory, motor, speech, or brainstem symptoms may occur. The headache is usually unilateral; throbbing in quality; and accompanied by nausea and/or vomiting, photophobia, and phonophobia. Migraines may have specific identifiable triggers in some patients, such as physical activity, stress, menstrual cycle, alcohol, and caffeine withdrawal. The headache pain may last hours to a few days.

C. Individuals who have ≤3 migraines per month usually can be treated with abortive and symptomatic medications only. The most effective abortive agents are triptans (selective serotonin agonists); isometheptene, usually in combination with dichloralphenazone; high doses of NSAIDs; or dihydroergotamine. Symptomatic medications include antiemetics, NSAIDs, mild tranquilizers, and narcotic analgesics.

D. Patients with >3 migraines per month are candidates for prophylactic medications, including beta blockers, tricyclic antidepressants, calcium channel blockers, or anticonvulsants (valproic acid, topiramate). Each prophylactic agent should be given in adequate doses and for 3–4 weeks before its effectiveness can be determined.

E. Cluster headaches are severe, unilateral (usually periorbital), sharp, steady (not throbbing) pain episodes that are of relatively short duration (30–120 minutes). Classically, they are nocturnal, often awakening the patient from sleep, but may recur many times throughout a 24-hour period. They are more common in men (14 to 1), may be precipitated by alcohol ingestion, and are usually associated with autonomic symptoms (lacrimation, rhinorrhea, conjunctival injection, nasal congestion, forehead and facial sweating, ptosis, or miosis). The attacks occur in clusters, each cluster lasting 2 weeks to 3 months, with an average of 2 months. Acute headaches can be treated with sumatriptan, ergotamine, and high-flow oxygen. Because of their severity, prophylactic therapy is recommended for all patients and includes verapamil, lithium, valproic acid, or, rarely, prednisone.

(Continued on page 406)

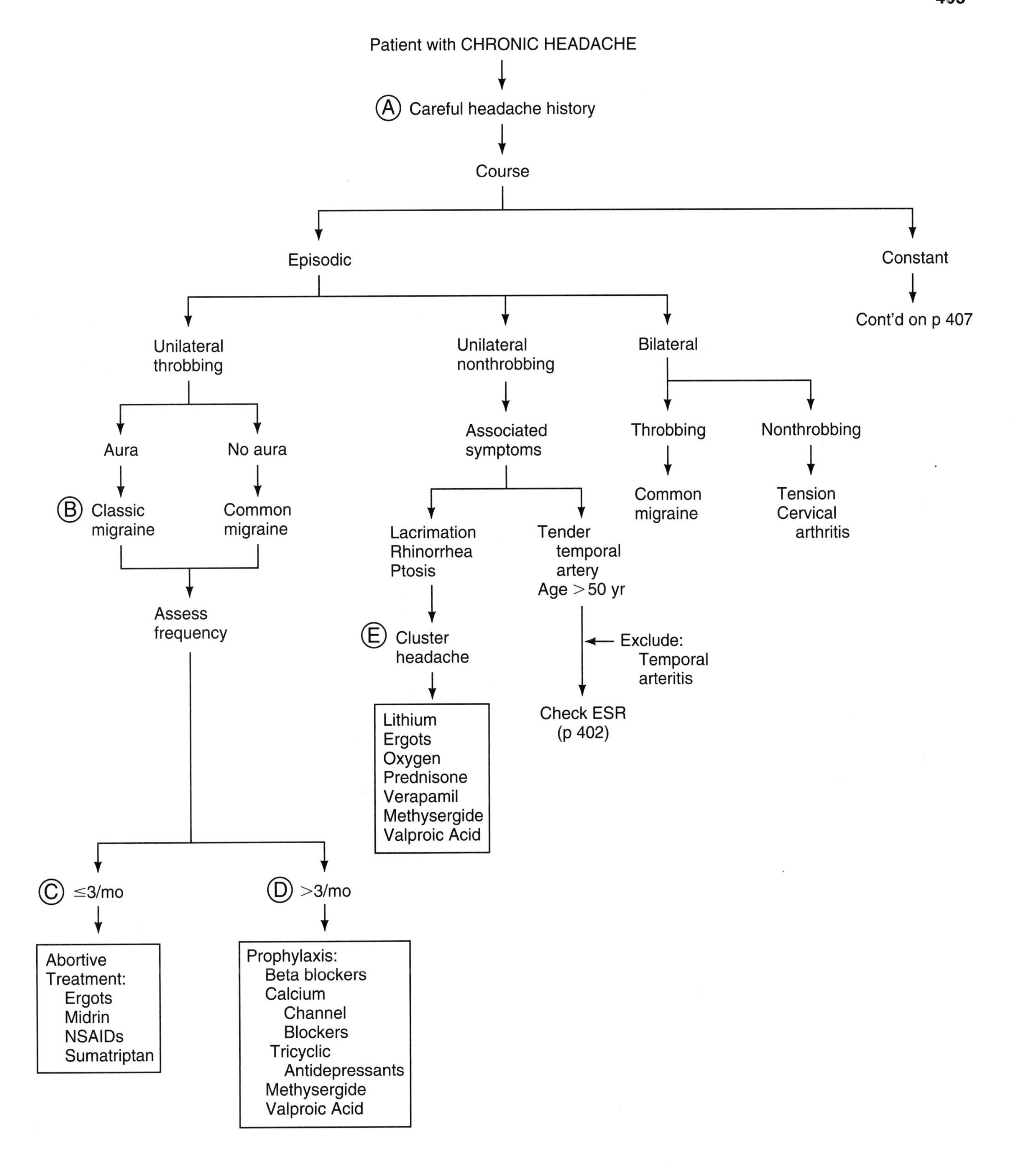

Patient with CHRONIC HEADACHE
(A) Careful headache history
Course
Episodic
Constant
Cont'd on p 407
Unilateral throbbing
Unilateral nonthrobbing
Bilateral
Aura
No aura
(B) Classic migraine
Common migraine
Assess frequency
(C) ≤3/mo
(D) >3/mo
Abortive Treatment:
Ergots
Midrin
NSAIDs
Sumatriptan
Prophylaxis:
Beta blockers
Calcium Channel Blockers
Tricyclic Antidepressants
Methysergide
Valproic Acid
Associated symptoms
Lacrimation
Rhinorrhea
Ptosis
(E) Cluster headache
Lithium
Ergots
Oxygen
Prednisone
Verapamil
Methysergide
Valproic Acid
Tender temporal artery
Age > 50 yr
Exclude: Temporal arteritis
Check ESR (p 402)
Throbbing
Nonthrobbing
Common migraine
Tension
Cervical arthritis

F. Medication-overuse headaches are very common. They arise from use of analgesics (acetaminophen or aspirin), narcotics, ergotamine, or those combined with caffeine and minor tranquilizers. Chronic, daily overuse causes a cycle of treatment and withdrawal that perpetuates and escalates the headache. Some patients require hospitalization during the withdrawal period for symptomatic treatment of the often severe withdrawal headaches and the associated nausea, vomiting, and dehydration. An aggressive prophylactic treatment program may be necessary after withdrawal of analgesics. One of the most common such headaches is caffeine overuse, and slow tapering of caffeine is often extremely effective.

G. Patients with ergotamine dependency have daily or almost-daily headaches alleviated only by ergotamine. When attempts to discontinue the ergotamine are made, a severe and protracted withdrawal headache occurs. Prophylactic medications usually are ineffective while the excessive ergotamine use continues. These patients usually require hospitalization. An effective treatment of the withdrawal headache consists of IV phenothiazines or metoclopramide and IV dihydroergotamine. Once the patient has been withdrawn from the ergotamine, institute an aggressive prophylactic regimen.

H. Tension headache has a lifetime prevalence of 69% in men and 88% in women. The pain level is mild to moderate, intermittent, and usually worse in the late afternoon, and it lasts for several hours. The location is typically bilateral and diffuse, often in a bandlike pattern across the forehead or the back of the head. Pain is described as tightness or pressure and associated with neck muscle tightness and often precipitated by emotional stress. There is rarely nausea, vomiting, photophobia, or phonophobia. Carefully search for aggravating or precipitating factors. Relaxation and biofeedback can reduce the severity and frequency of the headaches. Some patients may require prophylactic medications such as muscle relaxants (tizanidine), tricyclic antidepressants, or beta blockers.

References

Bigal ME, Sheftell FD, Rapoport AM, et al. Chronic daily headache in a tertiary care population: correlation between the International Headache Society diagnostic criteria and proposed revisions of criteria for chronic daily headache. Cephalalgia 2002;22(6):432–438.

Castillo J, Munoz P, Guitera V, et al. Epidemiology of chronic daily headache in the general population. Headache 1999;39(3):190–196.

Curioso EP, Young WB, Shechter AL, et al. Psychiatric comorbidity predicts outcome in chronic daily headache patients. Neurology 1999;52(6):471.

Guitera V, Munoz P, Castillo J, et al. Quality of life in chronic daily headache: a study in a general population. Neurology 2002;58(7):1062–1065.

Ryan CW. Evaluation of patients with chronic headache (review). Am Fam Physician 1996;54:1051.

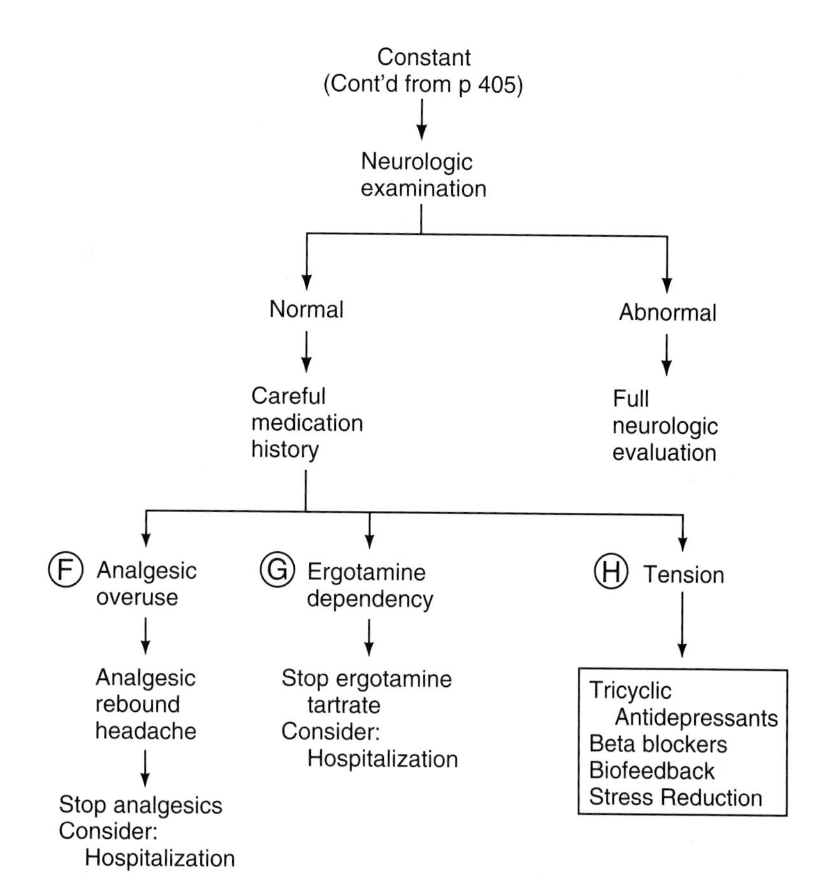
Constant
(Cont'd from p 405)
Neurologic examination
Normal
Abnormal
Careful medication history
Full neurologic evaluation
F Analgesic overuse
G Ergotamine dependency
H Tension
Analgesic rebound headache
Stop analgesics
Consider: Hospitalization
Stop ergotamine tartrate
Consider: Hospitalization
Tricyclic Antidepressants
Beta blockers
Biofeedback
Stress Reduction

TRANSIENT ISCHEMIC ATTACK AND STROKE EVALUATION

Sherry Chou, MD, and MingMing Ning, MD

Transient ischemic attacks (TIAs) are classically defined as brief episodes of focal neurologic deficits, usually lasting <24 hours and affecting cerebral blood flow. They are generally thought not to cause permanent damage to the brain. However, TIAs lasting more than 1 hour are associated with brain tissue damage in up to 50% of all cases. Although the definition remains controversial, TIAs continue to be an important indicator and prognosticator of cerebrovascular and cardiovascular disease. Because the risk of stroke can be as high as 20% within the first 3 months after a TIA and about 5% within 48 hours, early workup to identify the specific etiology and prompt intervention are crucial for stroke prophylaxis.

A. Focal neurologic deficits occur in a number of conditions other than vascular ischemic events. Vascular events have an abrupt onset; the maximal effect is usually seen within minutes. The subacute development of focal neurologic deficits is typically seen in conditions such as subdural hematoma, demyelinating disorders, brain abscesses, mass lesions, and venous sinus thrombosis. Occasionally, these pathologies present with transient deficits, but more commonly persistent abnormalities remain. A focal seizure or migraine may present with transient focal neurologic deficits but is usually accompanied by other symptoms. Involuntary movements, loss of consciousness, incontinence, or confusion suggests a seizure. Visual scintillations or headache may accompany transient episodes in patients with migraine.

B. The primary cause of TIAs is neural tissue ischemia from lack of blood flow. Ischemic etiologies of TIA include large vessel (e.g., carotid or vertebral-basilar stenosis), small vessel (e.g., hypertensive lacunar infarcts), embolic (e.g., cardiac, artery-to-artery, or paradoxical emboli via patent foramen ovale), and other (e.g., trauma-related dissection, vasculitis). The workup to determine the specific pathophysiologic mechanism underlying a TIA is crucial because treatment options differ.

C. The pattern of neurologic deficits indicates the vascular territory involved. Carotid artery ischemia (anterior circulation) can cause blindness (amaurosis fugax) on the ipsilateral (same side) of the affected artery and weakness or sensory loss on the contralateral face, arm, and leg. Aphasia (trouble with speech), including difficulty finding words or understanding others, may be present. In the posterior circulation, ischemia involving the brainstem is common and may cause a constellation of symptoms, including ataxia, dysarthria, diplopia, and facial weakness.

Neurologic evaluation of TIA should include imaging, laboratory, and/or cardiac workup, depending on the clinical suspicion. CT scan of the brain can help to rule out hemorrhage. Carotid duplex ultrasonography, including B-mode and Doppler evaluation of the extracranial carotid system, is a good screening tool to assess the degree of stenosis present and the plaque characteristics. Ultrasonography is also a noninvasive method for follow-up evaluation. If surgery is considered, the patient may need a CT cerebral angiogram or conventional arteriography to provide an accurate assessment of the degree of extracranial stenosis and amount of intracranial vascular disease.

D. Vertebrobasilar TIAs (posterior circulation), which can more easily be missed, may involve a combination of gait or balance problems (ataxia), double vision (diplopia), vertigo, slurred speech (dysarthria), binocular blindness, swallowing difficulty (dysphagia), sleepiness, and varying patterns of limb weakness.

When TIAs involve the vertebrobasilar system, MRI is the imaging method of choice. A CT scan of the region may be less revealing because of bony artifacts in the neck region. Therefore, MRI gives a more detailed view of the cerebellum and brainstem.

For both anterior and posterior circulation TIA workup, laboratory evaluation includes CBC (differential, platelet count), prothrombin and activated partial thromboplastin times, ESR, fasting glucose, electrolytes, liver and kidney function, lipid profile, and urinalysis. Cardiac evaluation includes chest film and ECG. If these are abnormal or if there is clinical evidence of cardiac disease, echocardiography and/or a Holter monitor may identify thrombi or arrhythmias.

E. In patients <45 years old, consider toxic screen, attention to history of trauma to look for carotid/vertebral dissection, transthoracic echo with bubble study to look for patent foramen ovale, or hypercoagulable panel (especially in women taking oral contraceptives to look for venous disease).

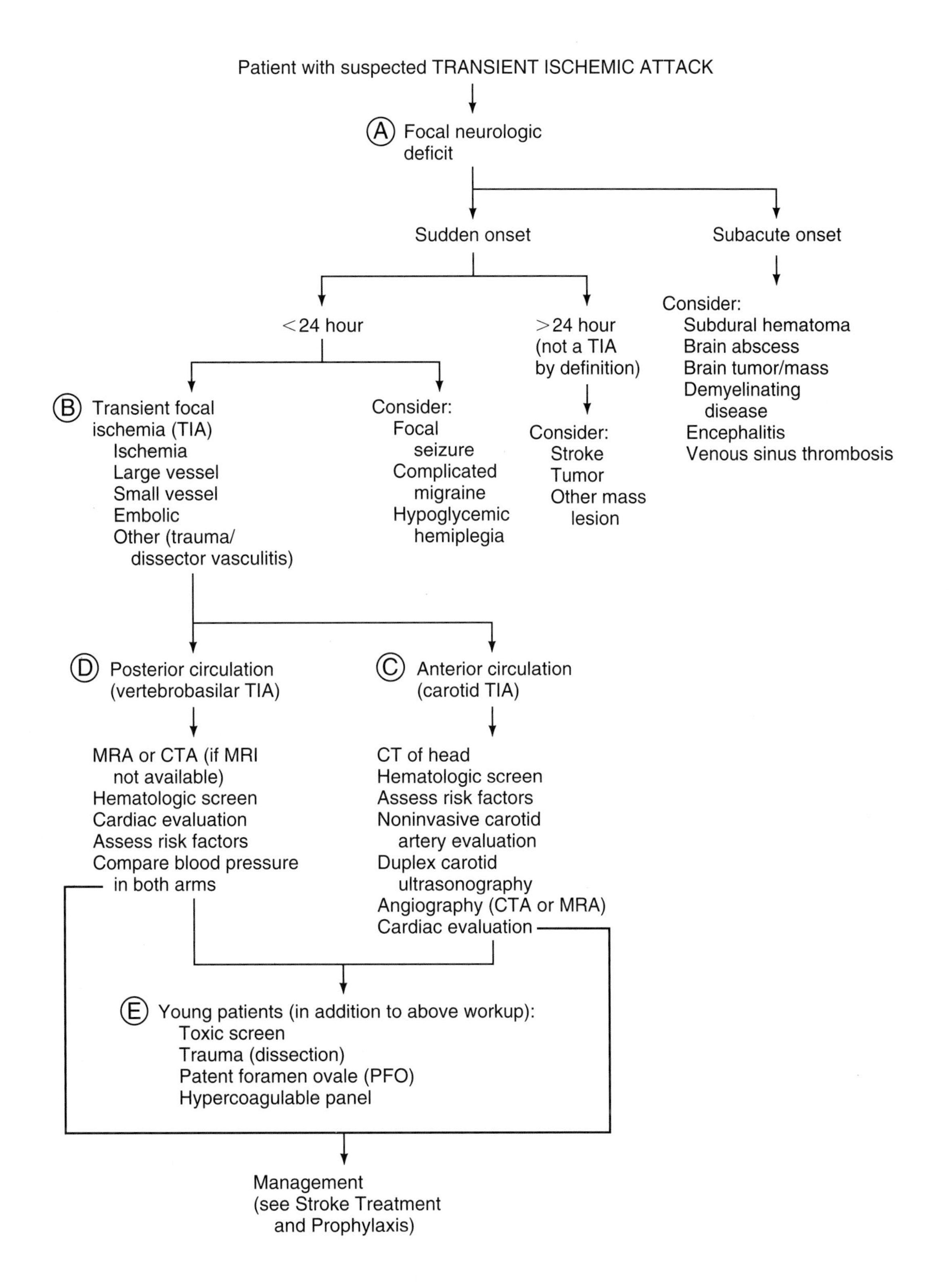

References

Albers GW, Amarenco P, Easton JD, et al. Antithrombotic and thrombolytic therapy for ischemic stroke: the Seventh ACCP Conference on Antithrombotic and Thrombolytic Therapy. Chest 2004;126:483S.

Albers GW, Caplan LR, Easton JD, et al. Transient ischemic attack—proposal for a new definition. N Engl J Med 2002;347:1713.

Caplan LR. TIAs: we need to return to the question, "What is wrong with Mr Jones?" (editorial). Neurology 1988;38:791.

CAPRIE Steering Committee. A randomised, blinded trial of clopidogrel versus aspirin in patients at risk of ischaemic events (CAPRIE). Lancet 1996;348:1329.

Fisher M. Occlusion of the internal carotid artery. AMA Arch Neurol Psychiatry 1951;65:346.

Johnston SC, Gress DR, Browner WS, et al. Short-term prognosis after emergency department diagnosis of TIA. JAMA 2000;284:2901.

Kidwell CS, Alger JR, Di Salle F, et al. Diffusion MRI in patients with transient ischemic attacks. Stroke 1999;30:1174.

TRANSIENT MONOCULAR VISUAL LOSS

Maria K. Houtchens, MD

Transient monocular blindness (TMB) is a medical emergency. The most common etiologies include embolic disease, hemodynamic changes, primary ocular pathology, or primary neurologic disease other than vascular compromise. If the temporary visual loss is caused by vascular ischemia, whether from embolic disease or hemodynamic changes, it is commonly called *amaurosis fugax* (AF).

A. Embolic disease: AF typically is described as impairment of vision that begins in the upper field of vision of one eye and progresses to involve the entire visual field of that eye. It usually lasts seconds to minutes. AF may stop with a hemifield loss, ascend, or rarely progress across the visual field laterally. Repeat episodes of AF tend to follow a stereotypical pattern for each patient.

   Of emboli, 50% are cholesterol plaques, most often originating from the ipsilateral carotid bifurcation or from the distal internal carotid artery. Funduscopy rarely, but diagnostically, reveals a glistening yellow or white object within the retinal vessel (Hollenhorst plaque). Of emboli, 4% may contain fibrin clot and originate from ulcerated vascular plaques or mural cardiac thrombi. Pure calcific emboli are rare and arise exclusively from cardiac valves. An episode of TMB is an indication of increased risk of stroke similar to a hemispheric transient ischemic attack (TIA). Of patients with TMB, 11% later develop strokes; in 41% of those, strokes occur within 1 week of the event.

   In younger patients with history of trauma or neck manipulations who present with TMB, embolic disease or hypoperfusion state from carotid dissection needs to be considered.

B. Temporal arteritis may cause blindness as a result of thrombosis of the central retinal artery as a result of giant cell arteritis. Patients are usually older and complain of visual loss or changes in a setting of headache. They may also have fever, anorexia, and weight loss. Leukocytosis, anemia, and elevated ESR are common. The disease process is self-limited over a period of months. The risk of permanent visual loss from temporal arteritis is approximately 35%, and timely evaluation and treatment with high-dose steroids can prevent further visual loss, although restoration of vision is rare.

   Migraine may present with unilateral visual changes and headache. Homonymous hemianopsia may be misinterpreted by the patient as a monocular loss of vision. Retinal migraine, a rare diagnosis of exclusion that is truly monocular, is presumed to be a vasospastic event. Positive visual phenomena such as scintillating scotoma or "white-outs" may be seen. Most patients with retinal migraines respond well to calcium channel blockers.

   In a young individual, transient unilateral loss of central vision associated with pain on eye movement and headache is seen in acute retrobulbar optic neuritis—either as a clinically isolated syndrome or as a manifestation of a known diagnosis of multiple sclerosis. Symptoms of optic neuritis tend to worsen with increased body temperature (Uhthoff's phenomenon). Inflammation and demyelination of the optic nerve are responsible for visual loss. High-dose IV steroids given once daily for 3–5 days shorten the duration of symptoms but seem to have little effect on the degree of visual recovery based on Optic Neuritis Treatment Trial data.

C. Vascular ocular diseases causing anterior ischemic optic neuropathy (AION), occlusion of the central retinal vein, and malignant arterial hypertension sometimes begin with attacks of TMB. AION involves infarction of the anterior portion of the optic nerve that can be visualized with direct ophthalmoscopy. It has recently been described as a rare complication from use of drugs for erectile dysfunction (the PDEF5 inhibitors). Nonvascular causes of TMB include increased intraorbital pressure and congenital anomalies. Subacute attacks of angle-closure glaucoma can present with transient visual loss and should be considered especially if patients complain of halos around lights. This symptom is a result of corneal edema resulting from rapid elevation of intraorbital pressure. Papilledema from any cause can present with visual obscurations. These disorders can be identified with the aid of a careful ophthalmologic examination showing abnormal ocular findings with a normal retina.

(Continued on page 412)

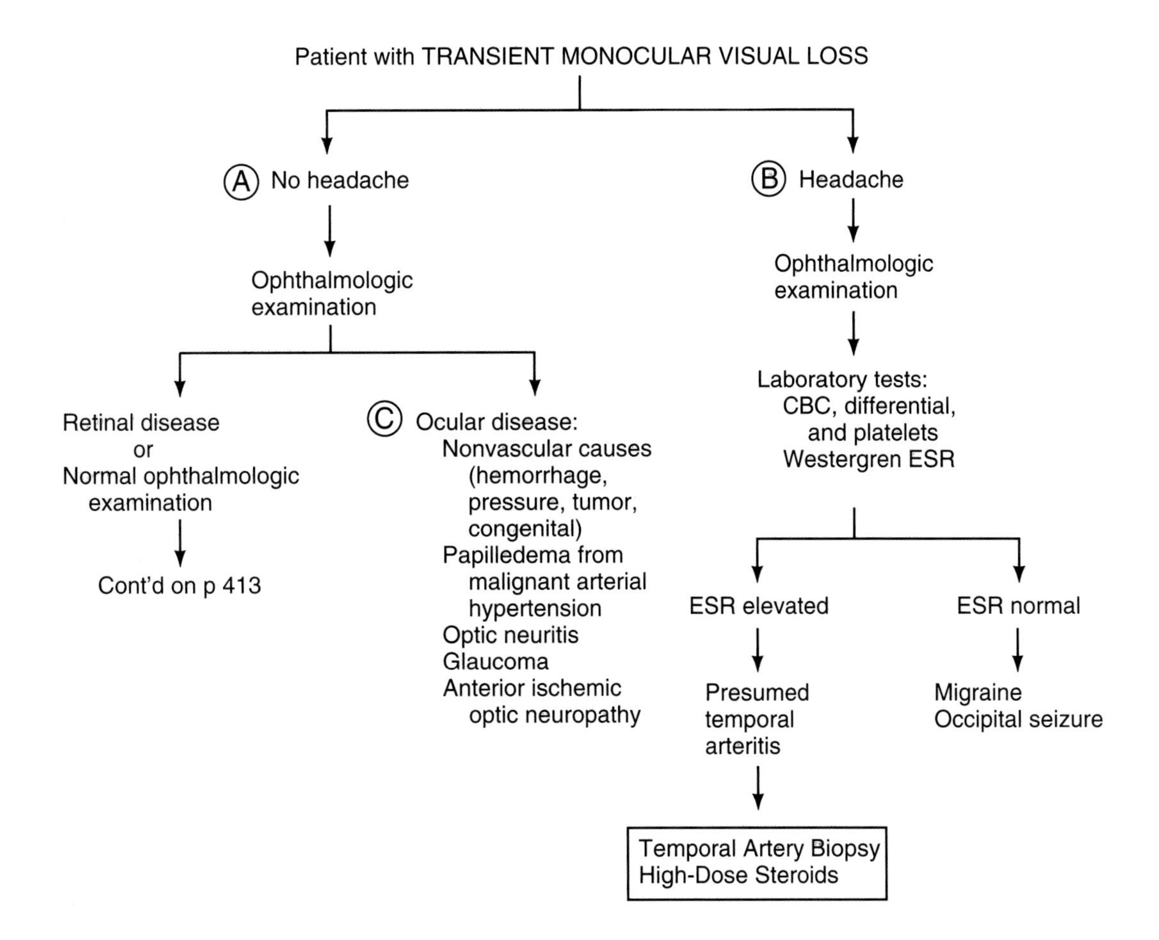

Patient with TRANSIENT MONOCULAR VISUAL LOSS
(A) No headache
Ophthalmologic examination
Retinal disease or Normal ophthalmologic examination
Cont'd on p 413
(C) Ocular disease:
Nonvascular causes (hemorrhage, pressure, tumor, congenital)
Papilledema from malignant arterial hypertension
Optic neuritis
Glaucoma
Anterior ischemic optic neuropathy
(B) Headache
Ophthalmologic examination
Laboratory tests:
CBC, differential, and platelets
Westergren ESR
ESR elevated
Presumed temporal arteritis
Temporal Artery Biopsy
High-Dose Steroids
ESR normal
Migraine
Occipital seizure

D. Laboratory evaluation of patients with a history of transient monocular visual loss includes CBC, differential, and platelet count (e.g., for polycythemia, leukemia, thrombocytosis), ESR (e.g., for evidence of arteritis—giant cell or Takayasu's), fasting blood glucose (diabetes mellitus), prothrombin and partial thromboplastin times (if prolonged, check antiphospholipid antibodies), and lipid profile (hyperlipidemia).
E. Noninvasive vascular studies include duplex (B mode and Doppler) ultrasonography, transcranial Doppler, and ophthalmodynamometry. Identification of the percent stenosis and plaque characteristics helps to inform the need for further, possibly more invasive, evaluation. Ipsilateral carotid artery stenosis ≥70% (severe) in the setting of TMB indicates the need for carotid endarterectomy. Surgical intervention was shown to be superior to medical treatment for symptomatic high-grade stenosis in a multicenter randomized trial. Benefits of surgical versus medical treatment in patients with ipsilateral carotid stenoses of 30%–69% (moderate) who have had an ischemic event (stroke, TIA, TMB) are questionable. Antiplatelet and hydroxymethyl glutaryl coenzyme A HMG-CoA reductase inhibitors (statins) can be used in combination for maximum antiplatelet aggregation effects. Patients with chronic, complete occlusion of the internal carotid artery should be prescribed maximal antiplatelet therapy. Anticoagulants can be used in the setting of symptomatic acute occlusion of carotid artery while a decision about surgical treatment or interventional radiology treatment is made.
F. Transcranial Doppler studies can provide further information about intracranial stenosis in patients in whom cerebral CT angiogram is not performed. MRI scans can reveal "clinically silent" cerebral infarctions or nonvascular lesions. Cardiac evaluation is important in the evaluation of a potential embolic source. Transthoracic or transesophageal echocardiography is performed to assess for potential sources of cardiac emboli, patent foramen ovale, or low cardiac output that occasionally can cause TMB through hypoperfusion mechanism, particularly with concomitant severe ipsilateral carotid disease.

References

Feinberg AW. Recognition and significance of amaurosis fugax. Heart Dis Stroke 1993;2:382.

Laskowitz D, Liu GT, Galetta SL. Acute visual loss and other disorders of the eyes. Neurol Clin 1998;16:323–353.

Liu GT. Disorders of the eyes and eyelids. In Samuels MA, Feske SK, eds. Office Practice of Neurology. Philadelphia: Churchill-Livingstone, 2003:35–68.

Miller NR. Walsh and Hoyt's Clinical Neuro-ophthalmology, 5th ed. Baltimore: Williams & Wilkins, 2004.

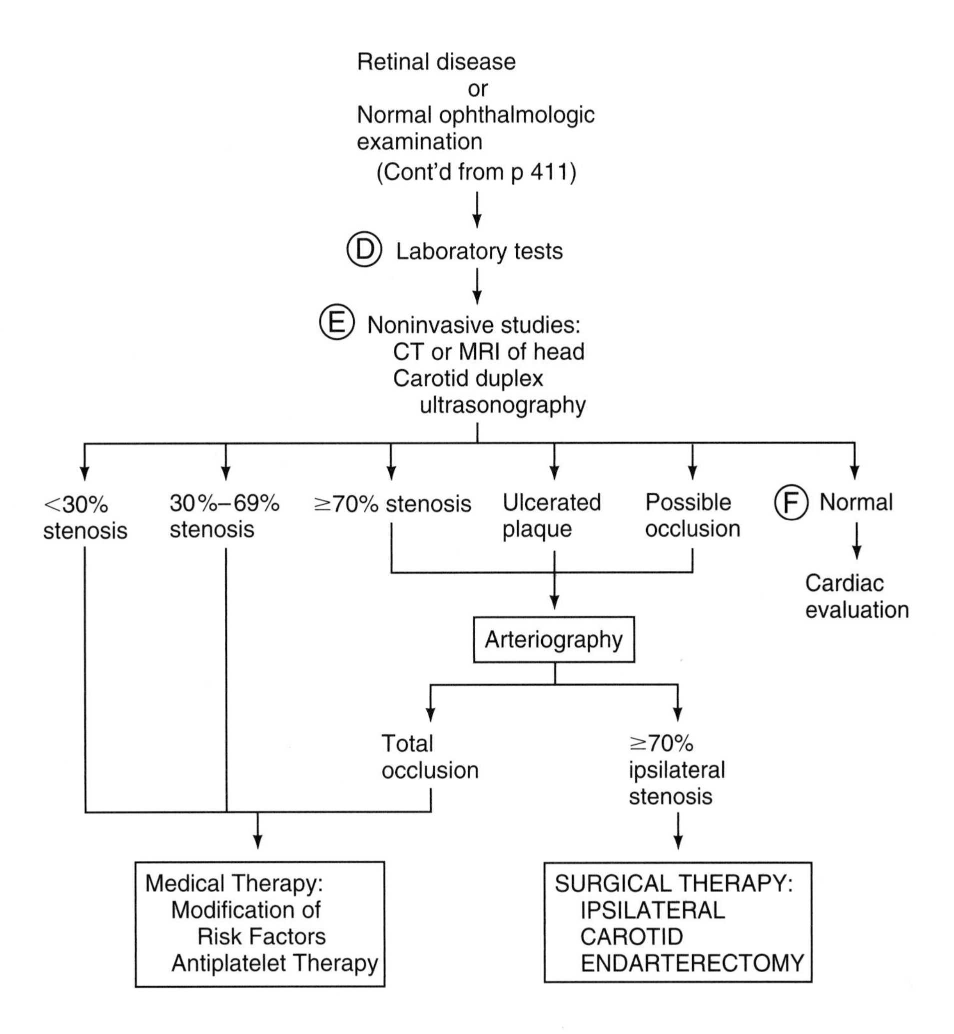
Retinal disease
or
Normal ophthalmologic
examination
(Cont'd from p 411)
D Laboratory tests
E Noninvasive studies:
CT or MRI of head
Carotid duplex
ultrasonography
<30%
stenosis
30%–69%
stenosis
≥70% stenosis
Ulcerated
plaque
Possible
occlusion
F Normal
Cardiac
evaluation
Arteriography
Total
occlusion
≥70%
ipsilateral
stenosis
Medical Therapy:
Modification of
Risk Factors
Antiplatelet Therapy
SURGICAL THERAPY:
IPSILATERAL
CAROTID
ENDARTERECTOMY

ACUTE STROKE

Leigh R. Hochberg, MD

Stroke is the acute onset of a focal neurologic deficit or disturbance in the level of arousal resulting from cerebral ischemia, hemorrhage, or venous occlusion. It is a medical emergency and requires full attention of the practitioner until a diagnosis is made and therapy is initiated.

A. Initial evaluation consists of ensuring the "ABCs" of airway, breathing, and (cardiopulmonary) circulation. Even if ABCs are intact at first assessment, ischemic and hemorrhagic strokes can evolve rapidly and cause depressed consciousness or coma, ultimately requiring assisted ventilation. Vital signs should be noted on initial contact with the patient. Patients with ischemic stroke may benefit from hypertension in the acute setting (ensuring continued perfusion to areas of brain tissue at risk for ischemia), whereas patients with hemorrhagic stroke may require urgent blood pressure reduction. Management of elevated blood pressure should thus be deferred until CT imaging clarifies the presence or absence of intracranial hemorrhage.

B. A focused history obtained from the patient and/or eyewitness is vital; often the history alone will distinguish between stroke types. Particular attention to the time of symptom onset can be critical to subsequent diagnostic and treatment decisions. If someone witnessed the patient become ill, document the onset time. Otherwise, determine the time when the patient was last seen as his or her normal self. Additional questions to ask of witnesses (and the patient, when possible) include: Has anything like this ever happened before? Was there a headache? What was the onset and severity of the headache? Was there a loss of consciousness? Was there a recent head or neck injury? Were there any rhythmic limb, head, or eye movements? It is important to maintain a broad differential, particularly for stroke mimics (e.g., seizure with postictal paralysis, complicated migraine, metabolic/infectious exacerbation of deficits from a prior stroke) while quickly obtaining the history.

C. A focused neurologic examination should then be performed. Completion of the National Institutes of Health Stroke Scale (NIHSS) provides a valuable summary of neurologic function that is easily communicated to other providers and can be used to track clinical improvement or decline over time. Because stroke severity can fluctuate, particularly in the first few hours after onset, repeated examination is warranted. Baseline laboratories (Chem-7, CBC with differential, platelet count, coagulation parameters, cardiac enzymes) should be drawn and sent as soon as stroke is considered in the differential diagnosis.

D. An urgent noncontrast CT scan of the head is indicated for all persons presenting with possible stroke. If an ischemic stroke is suspected, the CT may show only subtle signs of ischemia or may even appear normal. Patients who present with ischemic stroke symptoms of <3 hours' duration and a CT scan without evidence of intracranial hemorrhage should be considered immediately for IV thrombolysis with tissue plasminogen activator (tPA) according to locally developed protocols. In some centers, urgent imaging of the cerebral vasculature (by CT or magnetic resonance angiography) as well as diffusion-weighted MRI can provide further information about stroke size and/or the precise location of cerebrovascular occlusion, but the availability of these tests should not delay thrombolysis.

E. For those patients with acute ischemic stroke for whom IV or intraarterial thrombolysis can be performed, subsequent care will be dictated by locally developed protocols. For those not receiving thrombolysis, oral or rectal administration of aspirin is usually appropriate. Many other IV medications and therapeutic maneuvers (e.g., desmoteplase, hyperoxia, neuroprotective agents, induced hypertension) are currently under study. Acute anticoagulation with heparin is generally limited to patients with critical carotid or basilar artery stenosis, extradural arterial dissection, fluctuating symptoms suggestive of impending thrombosis, or venous occlusion (discussed later). Heparinoid-like compounds are also commonly used during the initiation of warfarin treatment for patients with newly diagnosed atrial fibrillation. Acute anticoagulation is relatively contraindicated following a large stroke (roughly greater than one third of the middle cerebral artery territory) because of an increased risk of hemorrhagic conversion.

F. Patients with a large stroke (ischemic stroke or intraparenchymal hemorrhage) can develop delayed-onset brain edema, which can occur several days following the initial stroke. Repeat CT imaging can help to identify the onset of edema, and judicious use of medications (e.g., mannitol, hypertonic saline) can reduce this edema. Malignant cerebral edema following stroke can cause herniation of the brain across meningeal planes or through narrow bony apertures (e.g., the foramen magnum), resulting in further cerebral injury or death. Hemicraniectomy—the removal of a large portion of the skull over one hemisphere, often accompanied by anterior temporal lobectomy and duraplasty—expands the cranial vault and can be lifesaving by preventing fatal herniation.

G. The subacute management and secondary prevention of ischemic stroke will be influenced by the presenting stroke's "mechanism": cardioembolic (e.g., resulting from left atrial clot formation in a patient with atrial fibrillation), large vessel thromboembolism (stenosis; occlusion; or embolism of a carotid, vertebral, or basilar artery), lacunar/small vessel disease (resulting from prolonged hypertension), or cryptogenic. Evaluation of stroke mechanism (with, as indicated, Holter monitoring, echocardiography, vessel imaging with CT/MR/Doppler ultrasound/angiography, hypercoagulable workup, etc.) can help guide subsequent therapy. Rehabilitation therapy can promote increased functional recovery following stroke. Targeted use of antiplatelet agents, anticoagulants, vascular intervention, blood pressure control, lipid-lowering agents, glucose control, smoking cessation, and other lifestyle modifications (diet, exercise) can reduce the risk of subsequent stroke.

H. If intracranial hemorrhage is present, the location of the hemorrhage and its intracranial compartment (epidural, subdural, subarachnoid, intraparenchymal, intraventricular) should be defined. For those patients with hemorrhage, the presence of a coagulopathy or supratherapeutic prothrombin time (PT) should be excluded by laboratory tests. If the PT/INR is elevated, both vitamin K (administered intravenously but carries small risk of anaphylaxis) and fresh frozen plasma should be provided immediately; this will both help to reduce the risk of the hematoma expanding and will permit neurosurgical intervention if indicated. Protamine may be useful for patients receiving heparinoid-like compounds. Reduction in blood pressure with IV beta blockers (e.g., labetalol) or calcium channel blockers (e.g., nicardipine) may also be needed; nitrates (e.g., nitroprusside, nitroglycerin) should be used only for acute hypertension that is refractory to other agents because nitrates can dilate the cerebral vasculature, resulting in a deleterious increase in intracranial pressure.

I. Intraparenchymal hemorrhage may result from acute or prolonged hypertension, arteriovenous malformations, an underlying malignancy (primary or metastatic), amyloid angiopathy, or supratherapeutic anticoagulation. In addition to blood pressure control and reversal of coagulopathy, imaging (CT, MR, or angiography) can clarify the likely underlying etiology. Neurosurgical consultation is appropriate, although many intraparenchymal hemorrhages may not warrant surgical intervention. Another important cause of intraparenchymal hemorrhage is cerebral venous thrombosis (CVT, sometimes referred to as venous sinus thrombosis). Usually occurring in the setting of dehydration, hypercoagulability, or the postpartum state, venous occlusion typically manifests as a headache of gradual onset, sometimes accompanied by neurologic signs, seizure, or focal hemorrhage. CVT, even in the setting of secondary hemorrhage, should be treated with anticoagulation because the risk of continued venous congestion and hemorrhage continues until the thrombosed venous system becomes sufficiently patent.

J. Subarachnoid hemorrhage (SAH) is usually heralded by the acute onset of the "worst headache of life" accompanied by nausea, vomiting, transient or continuing loss or depression of consciousness, and possible cranial nerve palsy. SAH most commonly results from rupture of a cerebral aneurysm of an artery of the circle of Willis. CT scan will usually reveal diffuse subarachnoid blood; the absence of visible blood on a CT scan, however, does not fully exclude SAH as an etiology. If the CT scan appears normal in the proper clinical context for SAH (acute-onset worst headache of life), a lumbar puncture (LP) should be performed. Four tubes of cerebrospinal fluid should be withdrawn with no more than 1–2 ml each (an extended microbiology panel is not usually indicated), and tubes 1 and 4 should be clearly labeled and sent for cell count. In addition, the person performing the LP should note the presence or absence of xanthochromia (a yellowish tint, indicating blood products). Comparisons of tubes 1 and 4 will permit distinction of a "traumatic tap" (a small vessel punctured by the LP needle, more RBCs in tube 1 than tube 4) versus SAH (no change in RBC count). Immediate neurosurgical consultation is indicated for all patients with SAH. Elevated blood pressure should also be controlled. Definitive management requires surgical or endovascular occlusion of the aneurysm, followed by intensive care management of the delayed neurologic, cardiopulmonary, and other systemic sequelae of SAH.

K. Although not usually categorized under "stroke," epidural and subdural hemorrhages most commonly result from trauma sufficient to cause skull fracture (e.g., being hit by a baseball) and can present as a sudden posttraumatic loss of consciousness that is sometimes followed by immediate recovery and then gradual drowsiness over a period of hours. Subdural hemorrhages result from the tearing of dural bridging veins. These subdural hemorrhages may be nontraumatic (spontaneous, particularly in elderly individuals), in which case they can develop slowly over weeks or months, or they can be secondary to trauma (e.g., following a fall).

Unlike intracerebral and intraventricular hemorrhages, small, acute epidural and subdural hemorrhages can have a subtle appearance on CT, so care must be taken to look for them. Neurosurgical consultation should be sought immediately for epidural and subdural hemorrhages, although small epidural or chronic subdural hemorrhages may not require surgical management. In cases where surgical management is not required, close observation and repeated clinical and radiologic examination of the patient is imperative so that any early hematoma expansion is noted quickly and discussed with the neurosurgeon.

References

Broderick JP, Adams HP Jr, Barsan W, et al. Guidelines for the management of spontaneous intracerebral hemorrhage: a statement for healthcare professionals from a special writing group of the Stroke Council, American Heart Association. Stroke 1999;30(4):905–915.

Coull BM, Williams LS, Goldstein LB, et al. Anticoagulants and antiplatelet agents in acute ischemic stroke. Report of the Joint Stroke Guideline Development Committee of the American Academy of Neurology and the American Stroke Association (a division of the American Heart Association). Neurology 2002;59:13–22.

Hochberg LR, Schwamm LH. Stroke, seizure, and encephalopathy. In Hurford WE, Bigatello LM, Haspel KL, et al, eds. Critical Care Handbook of the Massachusetts General Hospital, 4th ed. Philadelphia: Lippincott, Williams & Wilkins, 2005.

van Gijn J, Rinkel GJ. Subarachnoid haemorrhage: diagnosis, causes and management. Brain 2001;124:249–278.

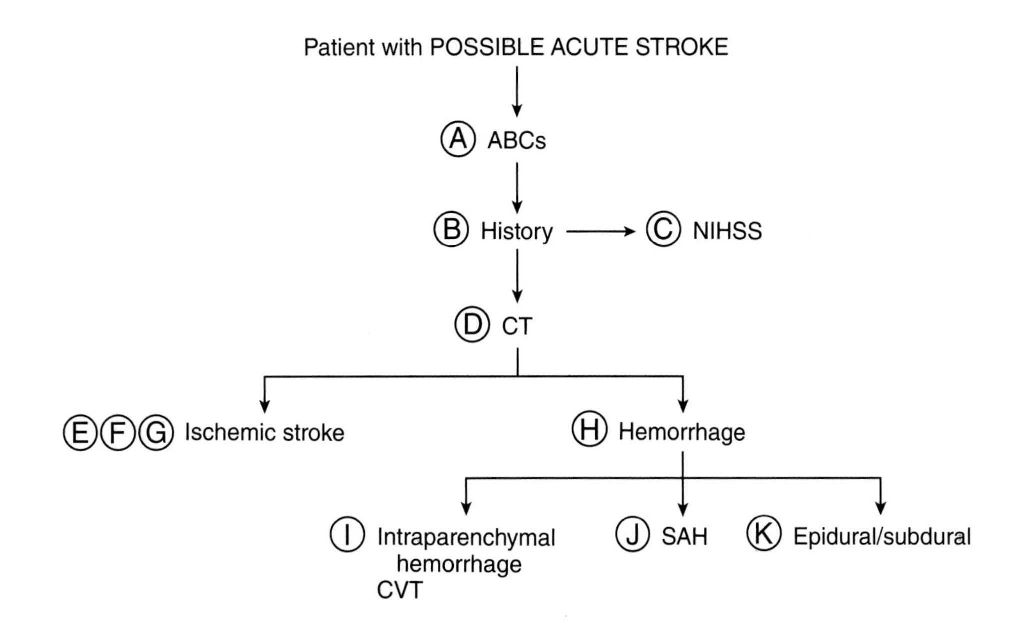
Patient with POSSIBLE ACUTE STROKE
(A) ABCs
(B) History
(C) NIHSS
(D) CT
(E)(F)(G) Ischemic stroke
(H) Hemorrhage
(I) Intraparenchymal hemorrhage CVT
(J) SAH
(K) Epidural/subdural

STROKE TREATMENT AND PROPHYLAXIS

Sherry Chou, MD, and MingMing Ning, MD

A. In patients with stroke or transient ischemic attack (TIA) who are candidates for anticoagulation, it is important to evaluate any evidence of cerebral hemorrhage to triage the possibility of thrombolysis or anticoagulation. The timing of the presentation of stroke is crucial for acute stroke therapy (see Acute Stroke chapter).

B. Beyond the acute phase, management of stroke and TIA centers around secondary prophylaxis. This management includes modification of risk factors such as hypertension, diabetes mellitus, hypercholesterolemia, smoking, and obesity. Myocardial infarction (MI) is one of the most common causes of death in patients with TIA; therefore, a thorough cardiac history and evaluation are indicated.

C. Antiplatelet agents (aspirin, aspirin plus dipyridamole, or clopidogrel) are the treatment of choice for noncardioembolic TIA or stroke of atherothrombotic, lacunar, or cryptogenic etiology. Anticoagulant therapy (warfarin, bridged by low molecular weight heparin or IV heparin) is the mainstay medical therapy for the management of stroke related to atrial fibrillation. Consider anticoagulation also for patients with a thrombus, mechanical prosthetic valve, or carotid/vertebral dissection. However, because of the hemorrhagic risks, anticoagulation is a relative contraindication for embolic stroke from endocarditis. Clinical suspicion of endocarditis would warrant the withholding of anticoagulation therapy.

D. For noncardioembolic stroke, the 2004 American College of Chest Physicians (ACCP) guidelines suggest use of either aspirin-dipyridamole or clopidogrel over aspirin, if there is no added financial strain to the patient. The risk of agranulocytosis makes ticlopidine a second-line antiplatelet agent for those who do not tolerate first-line agents. CBC must be checked every 2 weeks for the first 3 months.

E. Management of carotid artery TIAs involves the determination of the degree of carotid stenosis. If there is an ipsilateral stenosis of ≥70%, carotid endarterectomy along with best medical treatment (antiplatelet agent or anticoagulation) is more beneficial than medical therapy alone. Stent placement or angioplasty are still under investigation but may offer a better risk/benefit profile in selected higher-risk patient populations.

References

Adams HP Jr, Brott TG, Furlan AJ, et al. Guidelines of thrombolytic therapy for acute stroke: a supplement to the guidelines for the management of patients with acute ischemic stroke. A statement for healthcare professionals from a Special Writing Group of the Stroke Council, American Heart Association. Stroke 1996;27:1711.

Hacke W, Albers G, Al-Rawi Y, et al. The Desmoteplase in Acute Ischemic Stroke Trial (DIAS): a phase II MRI-based 9-hour window acute stroke thrombolysis trial with intravenous desmoteplase. Stroke 2005;36:66.

Hacke W, Donnan G, Fieschi C, et al. Association of outcome with early stroke treatment: pooled analysis of ATLANTIS, ECASS, and NINDS rt-PA stroke trials. Lancet 2004;363:768.

Furlan A, Higashida R, Wechsler L, et al. Intra-arterial prourokinase for acute ischemic stroke. The PROACT II study: a randomized controlled trial. Prolyse in Acute Cerebral Thromboembolism. JAMA 1999;282:2003.

Kase CS, Furlan AJ, Wechsler LR, et al. Cerebral hemorrhage after intra-arterial thrombolysis for ischemic stroke: the PROACT II trial. Neurology 2001;57:1603.

Smith WS, Sung G, Starkman S, et al. Safety and efficacy of mechanical embolectomy in acute ischemic stroke: results of the MERCI trial. Stroke 2005;36:1432.

Tissue plasminogen activator for acute ischemic stroke. The National Institute of Neurological Disorders and Stroke rt-PA Stroke Study Group. N Engl J Med 1995;333:1581.

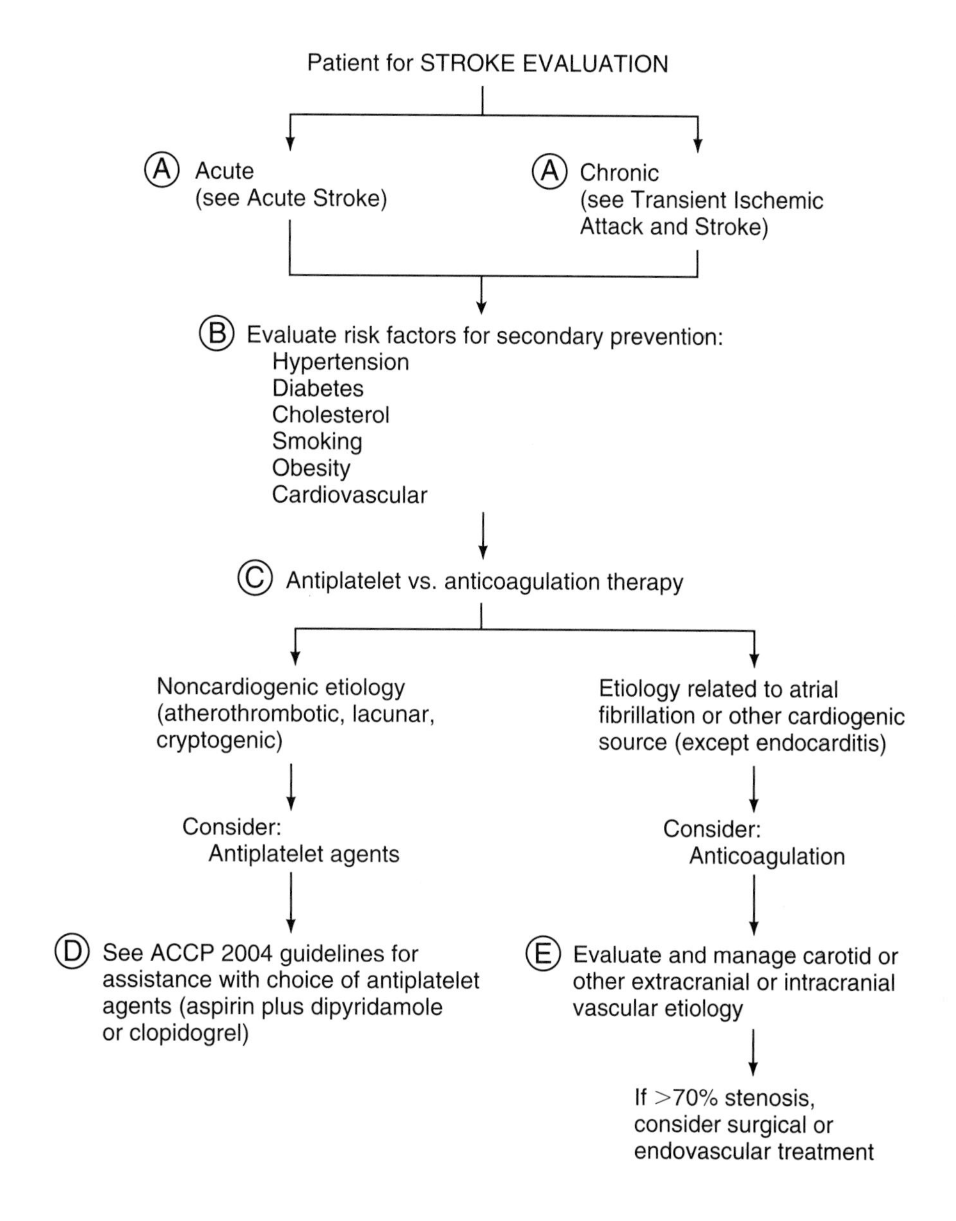
Patient for STROKE EVALUATION
(A) Acute
(see Acute Stroke)
(A) Chronic
(see Transient Ischemic Attack and Stroke)
(B) Evaluate risk factors for secondary prevention:
Hypertension
Diabetes
Cholesterol
Smoking
Obesity
Cardiovascular
(C) Antiplatelet vs. anticoagulation therapy
Noncardiogenic etiology (atherothrombotic, lacunar, cryptogenic)
Etiology related to atrial fibrillation or other cardiogenic source (except endocarditis)
Consider:
Antiplatelet agents
Consider:
Anticoagulation
(D) See ACCP 2004 guidelines for assistance with choice of antiplatelet agents (aspirin plus dipyridamole or clopidogrel)
(E) Evaluate and manage carotid or other extracranial or intracranial vascular etiology
If >70% stenosis, consider surgical or endovascular treatment

MEMORY LOSS

Bradford C. Dickerson, MD

Memory loss, once thought to be a common accompaniment of aging, is now known to be caused by a variety of pathologic insults, many of which are more prevalent in older age. The challenges for clinicians are to take memory complaints by individuals of any age seriously; take a detailed history from the patient and a family member or friend who knows the patient well; generate a differential diagnosis based on the patient's history and risk factors; and pursue the relevant workup, monitoring, and treatment. It is also important to recognize that although a family member or friend may bring memory loss to the attention of the clinician, the patient may deny a problem. Lack of insight into memory impairment is a common occurrence and should be taken very seriously by the clinician.

One approach to the evaluation of the patient with complaints of memory loss involves the answering of the following questions: Is there true memory loss, and is daily function affected? What type of memory loss is present, and are other aspects of cognition or behavior affected? What is the pathophysiology of memory loss ("where is the lesion")?

A. Patients and families may complain of memory loss when in fact impairments in attention, language, or visuospatial function are the source of the problem. A careful, structured history focused on daily activities can often better delineate the problem. Were there particular incidents that prompted the evaluation? Does the patient have difficulty keeping track of appointments, plans, or schedules, or ask questions repeatedly? This may be a symptom of anterograde memory impairment—difficulty learning and retaining new information. Is the patient unable to remember details of recent events, either in personal/family life (e.g., a holiday gathering) or in the news? Such symptoms may indicate a retrograde memory impairment—difficulty retrieving previously learned information. Complaints that "I walk into another room and forget why I was going there" and the like may indicate problems with attention or concentration. Difficulties retrieving the names of friends, family members, or celebrities, or words in conversation may indicate language dysfunction. Incidents in which the patient became lost while driving or disoriented while walking suggest visuospatial dysfunction or problems with spatial memory. Concerns surrounding judgment, decision making, ability to follow the steps of a process, or multitasking may indicate executive dysfunction. In addition to delineating symptom details, a discussion about the impact of symptoms on routine daily life is essential. Has the patient given up activities that were previously performed? Does the patient make mistakes, require additional assistance, or take longer to perform tasks because of memory or cognitive difficulties? In an older person, the presence of cognitive complaints in the setting of impaired routine activities is the hallmark of dementia (see the section Chronic Behavior Change). A detailed history taken from the patient and a reliable informant and emphasis on these areas will usually reveal the nature of the symptoms and suggest how to tailor the approach to examination and testing.

B. Once the history has illuminated the specificity of symptoms, the office examination can be focused on determining the presence and severity of signs. Behavioral observation of the patient with amnesia during the interview will often reveal a normal-appearing (awake, alert, interactive) person who is able to carry on a seemingly routine conversation, although careful attention by the clinician will often detect a relatively limited repertoire of vague statements lacking substantive detail. The clinician should note the patient's awareness of cognitive difficulties and reactions to test performance. Denial of symptoms/signs (anosognosia) can be striking to observe, and usually indicates significant impairment of memory and possibly other cognitive systems. The purpose of a focused mental status examination in the office is to pursue clinical hypotheses generated by the history (see the References for resources describing the mental status examination). Are attention, language, and visuospatial function in fact relatively preserved? What type of memory loss is present? There are multiple memory systems of the brain, and they can be subdivided a number of ways. One useful heuristic is to consider episodic, semantic, procedural, and working memory. Episodic memory involves the ability to learn and retrieve "episodes of life." It is subserved by the medial temporal lobe (including the hippocampus) and other components of the limbic system (including the basal forebrain and mammillothalamic tract), as well as the prefrontal cortex. Dysfunction of episodic memory usually adheres to Ribot's law, which states that recently learned information is more likely to be lost than remotely learned information. In patients with episodic memory loss, there are typically impairments in the learning of new information (which can be tested with word or picture lists in the office) and the retrieval of recently learned information (testable by asking about details of recent experiences in the

(Continued on page 422)

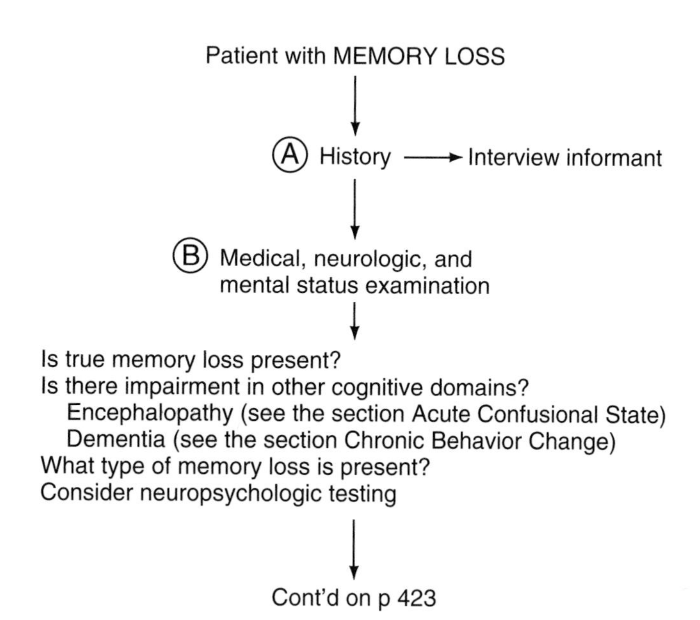
Patient with MEMORY LOSS
A History
Interview informant
B Medical, neurologic, and mental status examination
Is true memory loss present?
Is there impairment in other cognitive domains?
Encephalopathy (see the section Acute Confusional State)
Dementia (see the section Chronic Behavior Change)
What type of memory loss is present?
Consider neuropsychologic testing
Cont'd on p 423

patient's personal life [e.g., a family gathering] and corroborating with an informant), but memory for remote information is often retained (e.g., where the patient went to high school). Episodic memory impairment may be caused by pathologic processes that affect the medial temporal lobe and other limbic system anatomy; these include Alzheimer's disease, Korsakoff's syndrome, hippocampal sclerosis, and posterior cerebral artery or thalamic infarcts. Semantic memory refers to general knowledge about the world, the source of which is usually not remembered. Brain systems underlying semantic memory include the lateral and ventral temporal cortices, as well as the prefrontal cortex. Patients may have difficulty retrieving information about important historical events, recalling the names of presidents, or recognizing and describing the use of common objects (e.g., a wristwatch or scissors). Semantic memory dysfunction may be seen in Alzheimer's disease and other neurodegenerative dementias or with focal lesions of the temporal lobe, such as posterior cerebral artery stroke. Procedural memory involves the learning of skills, such as riding a bicycle or playing an instrument. It is subserved by the supplementary motor cortex, basal ganglia, and cerebellum, and is often spared in patients with episodic or semantic memory dysfunction. Disorders of the basal ganglia, such as Parkinson's disease and Huntington's disease, may cause procedural memory impairment. Working memory involves the ability to keep information in mind and manipulate it (usually to solve a problem). The complex concept of working memory includes aspects of attention, concentration, and executive function, as well as "short-term memory." Problems with working memory usually present with difficulties concentrating or paying attention, which can lead to impairment in learning, judgment, and problem solving. Tests of serial subtraction (7s from 100) or reverse spelling (WORLD) or recitation (months of the year backward) are useful to illuminate working memory deficits. Working memory is subserved primarily by the dorsolateral prefrontal and lateral parietal cortices, as well as the caudate nucleus and other subcortical structures. Since these brain regions are affected in a variety of neurodegenerative diseases, including Alzheimer's disease, Parkinson's disease, and Huntington's disease, working memory deficits can be seen in these conditions. Moreover, they are often seen in multiple sclerosis and other conditions that affect the white-matter tracts that interconnect these regions. The specific nature of memory and cognitive dysfunction can be illuminated further with neuropsychological testing.

C. It is important to define the character and severity of memory loss through the history and examination, which leads to a pathophysiologic differential diagnosis. Additional history regarding medical conditions or risks (e.g., thyroid dysfunction, anemia, cerebrovascular risk factors, toxins or side effects of medications such as anticholinergics) and a systems review (e.g., for depression, sleep disorders, seizures, head injury) can be very useful in narrowing the differential. Systemic conditions may cause impairment in multiple memory systems. Herpes simplex encephalitis is classically associated with chronic amnesia because it affects the medial temporal lobes, but often presents with a febrile acute confusional state. The acuity of onset is also a key historical element. Onset over seconds to minutes may indicate stroke, seizure, or transient global amnesia; onset over days to weeks may indicate inflammatory, toxic/metabolic, or neoplastic processes; onset over months to years often indicates neurodegenerative, neoplastic, nutritional deficiency, or psychiatric etiologies. Transient global amnesia involves the acute onset of isolated memory impairment in the absence of other cognitive or focal neurologic signs and typically affects predominantly episodic memory, usually resolving within 24–72 hours. Patients with a history of seizure disorders, particularly complex partial seizures, may have chronic memory loss. In some cases, this results from mesial temporal sclerosis. Patients with a history of immunosuppression (e.g., after bone marrow transplant) may be susceptible to human herpesvirus-6, which can present with a subacute focal amnesic state. Chronic alcohol use or nutritional deficiency can lead to Korsakoff's syndrome, a chronic amnesia.

D. Next, the clinician should determine whether to pursue neuroimaging, electroencephalography, and laboratory (including lumbar puncture) evaluation. Routine laboratory screening is important (e.g., for thyroid dysfunction or vitamin B_{12} deficiency) and should be tailored by the history and examination. The clinician should strongly consider a neuroimaging study in all cases of memory impairment. Both structural (e.g., MRI) and functional (e.g., positron emission tomography) neuroimaging can be useful.

References

Budson AE, Price BH. Memory dysfunction. N Engl J Med 2005;352 (7):692–699.

Mesulam M-M. Aphasia and other focal cerebral disorders. In Kasper DL, Braunwald E, Fauci AS, et al, eds. Harrison's Principles of Internal Medicine, 16th ed. New York: McGraw-Hill, 2005:145–151.

Petersen RC. Disorders of memory. In Samuels MA, Feske SK, eds. Office Practice of Neurology. Philadelphia: Churchill-Livingstone, 2003:902–912.

Weintraub S. Examining mental state. In Samuels MA, Feske SK, eds. Office Practice of Neurology. Philadelphia: Churchill-Livingstone, 2003:850–858.

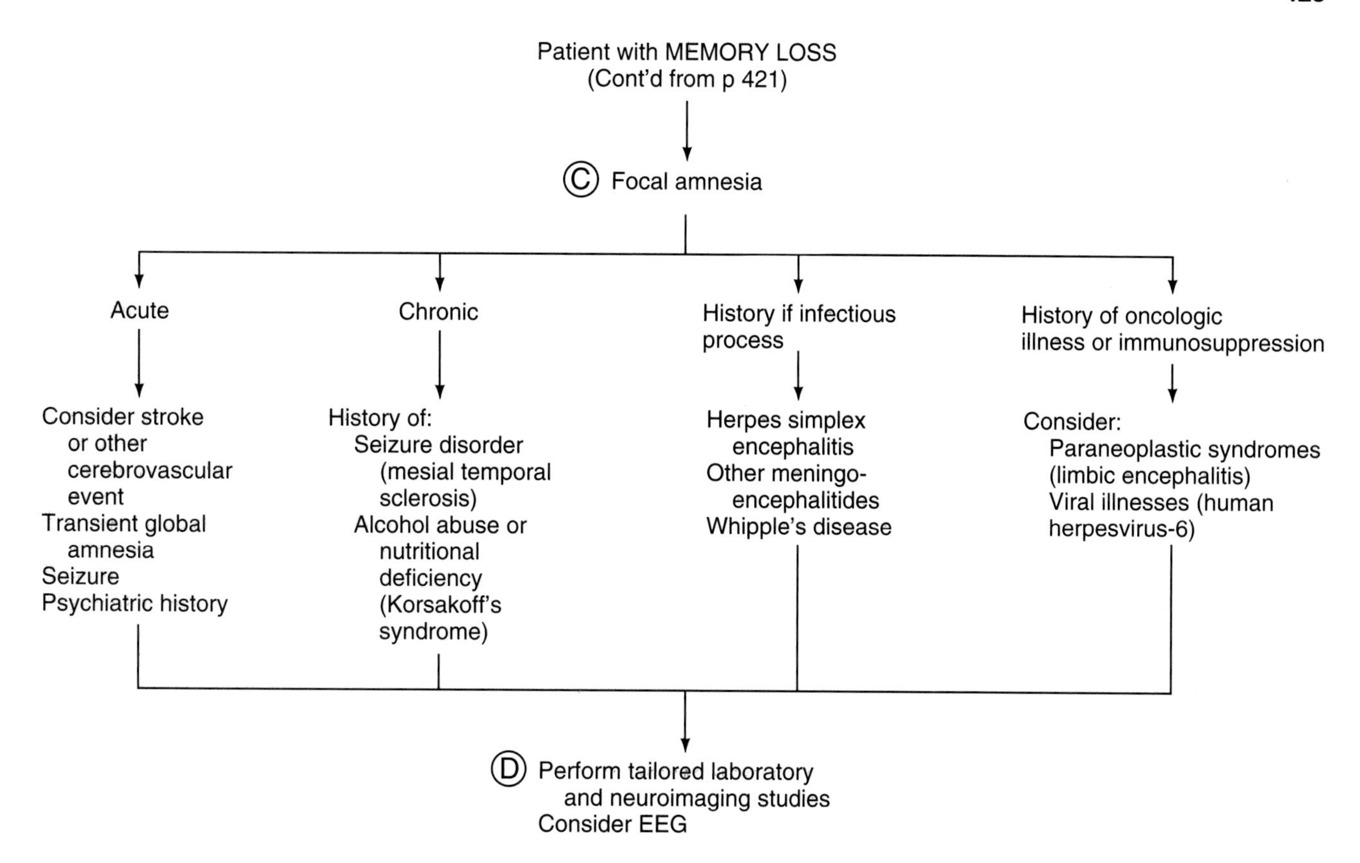
Patient with MEMORY LOSS
(Cont'd from p 421)
Ⓒ Focal amnesia
Acute
Chronic
History if infectious process
History of oncologic illness or immunosuppression
Consider stroke or other cerebrovascular event
Transient global amnesia
Seizure
Psychiatric history
History of:
Seizure disorder (mesial temporal sclerosis)
Alcohol abuse or nutritional deficiency (Korsakoff's syndrome)
Herpes simplex encephalitis
Other meningo-encephalitides
Whipple's disease
Consider:
Paraneoplastic syndromes (limbic encephalitis)
Viral illnesses (human herpesvirus-6)
Ⓓ Perform tailored laboratory and neuroimaging studies
Consider EEG

DIZZINESS

Maria K. Houtchens, MD

Complaints of dizziness from a patient may represent a variety of different sensations. Therefore, a careful history is extremely important to identify, as best as possible, the specific sensations experienced by the patient, which will assist the clinician in narrowing the differential diagnosis of this common symptom.

Specific words are often used by patients to describe vestibular versus nonvestibular dizziness. A feeling of "spinning," motion sickness, or being "drunk," with the sense of imbalance, falling, or tilting to one side is common in vestibular dizziness. The sensation of spinning "inside the head" while the environment remains stable may imply nonvestibular causes. Light-headedness or a "swimming" sensation without specific motion is a common complaint suggestive of low perfusion or glucose states.

A. Nonvestibular dizziness has a variety of etiologies. The light-headedness experienced before a faint is known as a presyncopal event. The mechanism of this symptom is reduced blood flow to the entire brain. Disorders that can cause a decrease in systemic blood pressure include the vasovagal response and orthostatic hypotension. Reduced cardiac output in arrhythmias, cardiomyopathy, or cardiac valvular disease results in cardiogenic presyncope. Hypoglycemia in patients with diabetes who are taking insulin or sulfonylureas may cause shakiness, palpitations, fatigue, and presyncope. Hyperventilation that results in reduced arterial Pco_2 causing cerebral vasoconstriction is a common cause of dizziness in young patients with anxiety or panic disorder. These patients often complain of perioral or bilateral finger numbness and tingling. Nausea and diaphoresis, blurring and dimness of vision, and skin pallor may accompany any of the previously mentioned presyncopal events. A variety of drug reactions can cause dizziness, either through direct ototoxicity (aminoglycosides) or through cerebellar damage (phenytoin, primidone, alcohol). Sedating medications produce a sensation of cloudiness or giddiness that may be interpreted by a patient as dizziness.

B. Acute vertigo involves an intense sense of rotation often exacerbated by head movement. It may result from a peripheral lesion (of the labyrinth or vestibular nerve) or a central lesion (i.e., brainstem or cerebellar vestibular system) and represents unilateral loss of vestibular function. Nausea, vomiting, pallor, and fatigue are often present. Walking is difficult. Spontaneous nystagmus is nearly always present on examination.

C. Central vertigo is suspected in an older patient with a history of hypertension, hypercholesterolemia, and cardiovascular or cerebrovascular disease. Hearing loss is rare, inability to walk is prominent, and nystagmus changes directions of the fast phase when the patient looks away from the lesion. Brainstem or cerebellar infarction or hemorrhage needs to be ruled out with urgent head CT or MRI. Treatment should focus on treatment of the underlying pathophysiology. Antiplatelet or anticoagulation therapy may be indicated. Acute surgical decompression of the brainstem may be necessary to treat a rapidly expanding cerebellar hemorrhage. Recovery from a central insult to vestibular system takes days to weeks. Multiple sclerosis (MS) may present with an attack of central vertigo in a younger patient (5% of MS cases). MRI of the brain may show a multifocal white matter disease on T2 or FLAIR (fluid-attenuated inversion recovery) sequences.

D. Peripheral vertigo is suspected in a patient with history of previous infection involving the ear, prominent hearing loss, systemic symptoms, and severe nausea and vomiting. Vestibular neuronitis accounts for 90% of cases of peripheral vertigo in younger patients. Flu-like illness within 2 weeks of the onset of dizziness is reported by 50% of patients. Steroids and antiviral agents have no proven use in this condition in randomized trials but are often used. Acute suppurative labyrinthitis is a rare bacterial infection of a labyrinth leading to rapid and profound loss of auditory and vestibular function. Diagnosis is suspected in patients with recent history of bacterial otitis media, meningitis, or cholesteatoma with persistent severe ear and mastoid pain, fever, and loss of hearing and vestibular function. An urgent head CT scan with special attention to temporal bone windows and rapid treatment with antibiotics is imperative.

E. Recurrent spontaneous vertigo is caused by sudden temporary and usually reversible impairment of resting neural activity in one labyrinth or its central connections. The typical length of dysfunction is minutes (central vertigo, transient ischemic attacks) to hours (peripheral vertigo).

F. Meniere's disease involves recurrent attacks of peripheral vertigo associated with fluctuating low-frequency hearing loss. The classic symptomatic triad is vertigo, tinnitus, and hearing loss. The pathophysiology is

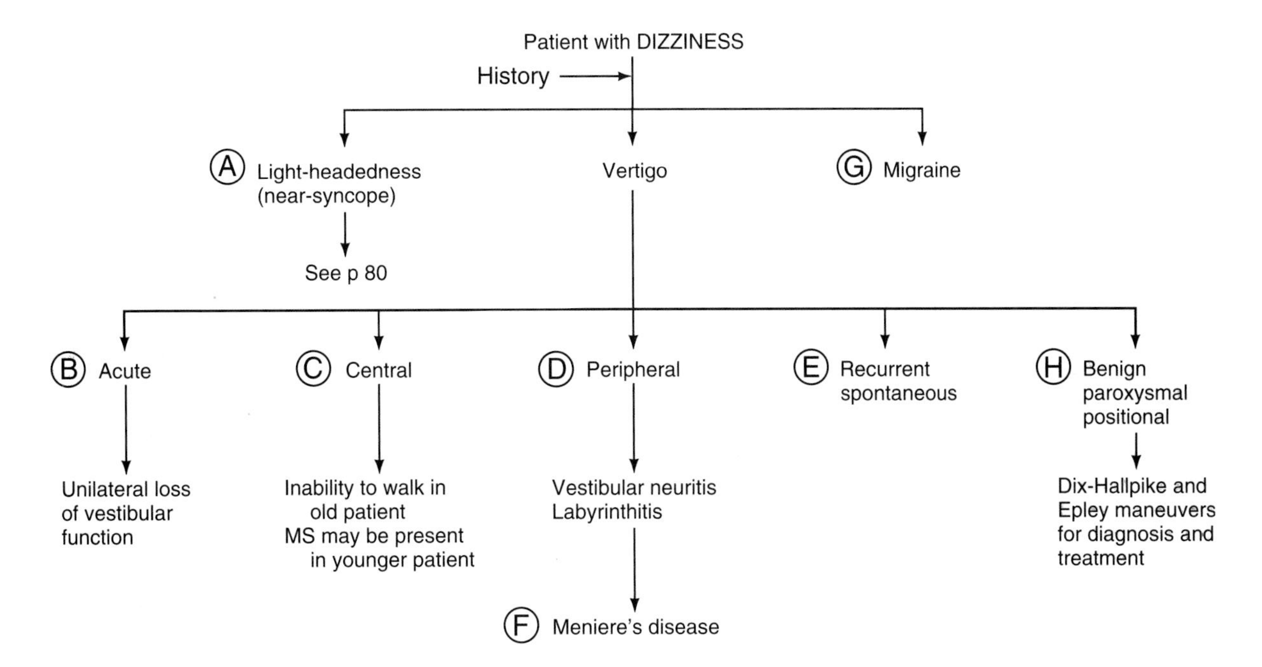

thought to involve distention of the membranous labyrinth in one or both ears that changes in severity. During a period of increased pressure in the labyrinth, patients have a feeling of fullness in the affected ear, an increase in the chronic tinnitus and deafness in that ear, and acute vertigo. The severity of each attack varies greatly; at the onset of severe vertigo, some patients lose consciousness briefly. The duration is typically hours (in rare cases, attacks may last up to a few days). With repeated attacks, deafness increases. In most patients with Meniere's disease, deafness precedes episodic vertigo, but in some, episodes of vertigo precede deafness.

G. Patients with migraine may have attacks of vertigo accompanying headaches (up to 25% of migraine cases). Rarely, it may be the only manifestation of migraines. A trial of migraine prophylactic medication may be diagnostic.

H. Benign paroxysmal positional vertigo is a syndrome involving vertigo precipitated by specific head positions (e.g., looking up, lying on one side). Vertigo usually begins after a brief latent interval (a few seconds) after the head assumes the offending position. A change of position usually relieves symptoms rapidly. Most cases begin suddenly, without apparent cause; others follow head trauma. In older persons the syndrome may be caused by vascular insults in the inner ear. Symptoms commonly subside in a few months but may recur. In 50% of cases, no etiology can be identified. Bedside maneuvers (Dix-Hallpike, Epley) may be used in both the diagnosis and treatment of this disorder. Cases with atypical aspects of history or examination should raise suspicion for positional vertigo caused by posterior fossa lesions, including cerebellar tumors, medulloblastomas, cerebellar atrophy, and Chiari type I malformation.

References

Baloh RW. Clinical practice. Vestibular neuritis. N Engl J Med 2003;348: 1027–1032.

Baloh RW. Dizziness and vertigo. In Samuels MA, Feske SK, eds. Office Practice of Neurology. Philadelphia: Churchill-Livingstone, 2003:78–87.

Froehling DA, Silverstein MD, Mohr DN, et al. Does this dizzy patient have a serious form of vertigo? JAMA 1994;271:585.

SEIZURES

Tracey A. Milligan, MD

A seizure involves temporary abnormal electrical activity in a group of brain neurons resulting in alteration of brain function. Approximately 2%–5% of the population will have at least one nonfebrile seizure during their lifetime. Seizures can be the result of an acute process, a previous intracranial insult, or a developmental lesion, or they may be idiopathic.

A. The differential diagnosis of a seizure-like episode, or spell, includes syncope and postsyncopal convulsive movements, movement disorder or tremor, cerebrovascular events, sleep disorders such as narcolepsy/cataplexy, migraine, and a psychogenic seizure. At times, the diagnosis may require consultation with a neurologist and inpatient video EEG monitoring.

B. There are many types of seizures. Seizures can cause involuntary changes in body movement or function. Seizures typically last 30 seconds to 2 minutes but can last much longer, resulting in status epilepticus (see Status Epilepticus chapter). Seizures can be symptomatic of an acute neurologic, metabolic, or toxic process. Drug or alcohol withdrawal may result in seizures. In pregnancy and the postpartum period a seizure can be a sign of eclampsia. Classification of seizure type has important implications for possible etiologies, diagnostic tests, and treatment recommendations.

C. Seizures that begin focally are classified as focal or partial seizures. Often the patient does not recall the seizure, and a detailed history of the event from a witness can be helpful. Even when the seizure is reported as a convulsion, it may be the result of a secondarily generalized seizure, and a search for a history of auras or signs of a focal onset by history is important. The symptoms of a focal seizure depend on where in the brain the abnormal electrical activity occurs. A focal seizure can be rhythmic focal motor activity that either remains localized or progresses to involve other parts of the body (Jacksonian march). Focal seizures can also be subtle, such as a marching paresthesia of a part of the body, a feeling of déjà vu or fear, a strange epigastric sensation, an unpleasant odor, or visual hallucinations. Focal seizures are typically classified as motor, sensory, autonomic, or psychic. Focal seizures with preservation of consciousness are simple partial seizures. If there is alteration of consciousness, the seizure is classified as a complex partial seizure. During a complex partial seizure, the patient may appear confused or dazed, exhibit automatisms (e.g., lip smacking, hand picking behavior), or not respond to questions. Focal seizures may begin as either simple or complex and may progress very quickly to convulsions (i.e., secondarily generalized seizures, grand mal seizure).

D. A primary generalized seizure can be convulsive or nonconvulsive. Nonconvulsive seizures include petit mal seizures that begin in childhood and consist of brief episodes of eye fluttering and unresponsiveness with a characteristic 3-Hz spike and wave pattern seen on EEG during the seizure. Tonic and atonic seizures result in sudden "drop attacks." Myoclonic seizures consist of brief jerks of muscle contraction and relaxation with epileptiform activity seen on EEG. Primary convulsive seizures are also referred to as grand mal seizures.

E. Important features of the history include possible provocative factors (e.g., alcohol/drug withdrawal, seizure-provoking drugs, or medications), other risk factors for seizure (known history of brain injury, stroke, brain infection, or other cerebral disorder), family history of seizure, and history of previous seizures or transient neurologic events (including febrile seizures). A complete medical and neurologic examination is critical. A history of malignancy; immunocompromise; and/or physical signs of fever, change in mental status, or focal neurologic deficit should prompt urgent evaluation.

F. The initial management of a patient with acute seizure starts with stabilization of airway, breathing, and circulation (ABC). Thiamine and glucose should be provided acutely unless hypoglycemia has otherwise been ruled out. If the patient is febrile, consider brain infection, empiric meningitis/encephalitis treatment, CT, and lumbar puncture. Other testing includes MRI (with gadolinium if there are clinical signs of infection or a history of malignancy), EEG, metabolic profile, human chorionic gonadotropin (hCG) in women of childbearing age, and toxicology screen.

(Continued on page 428)

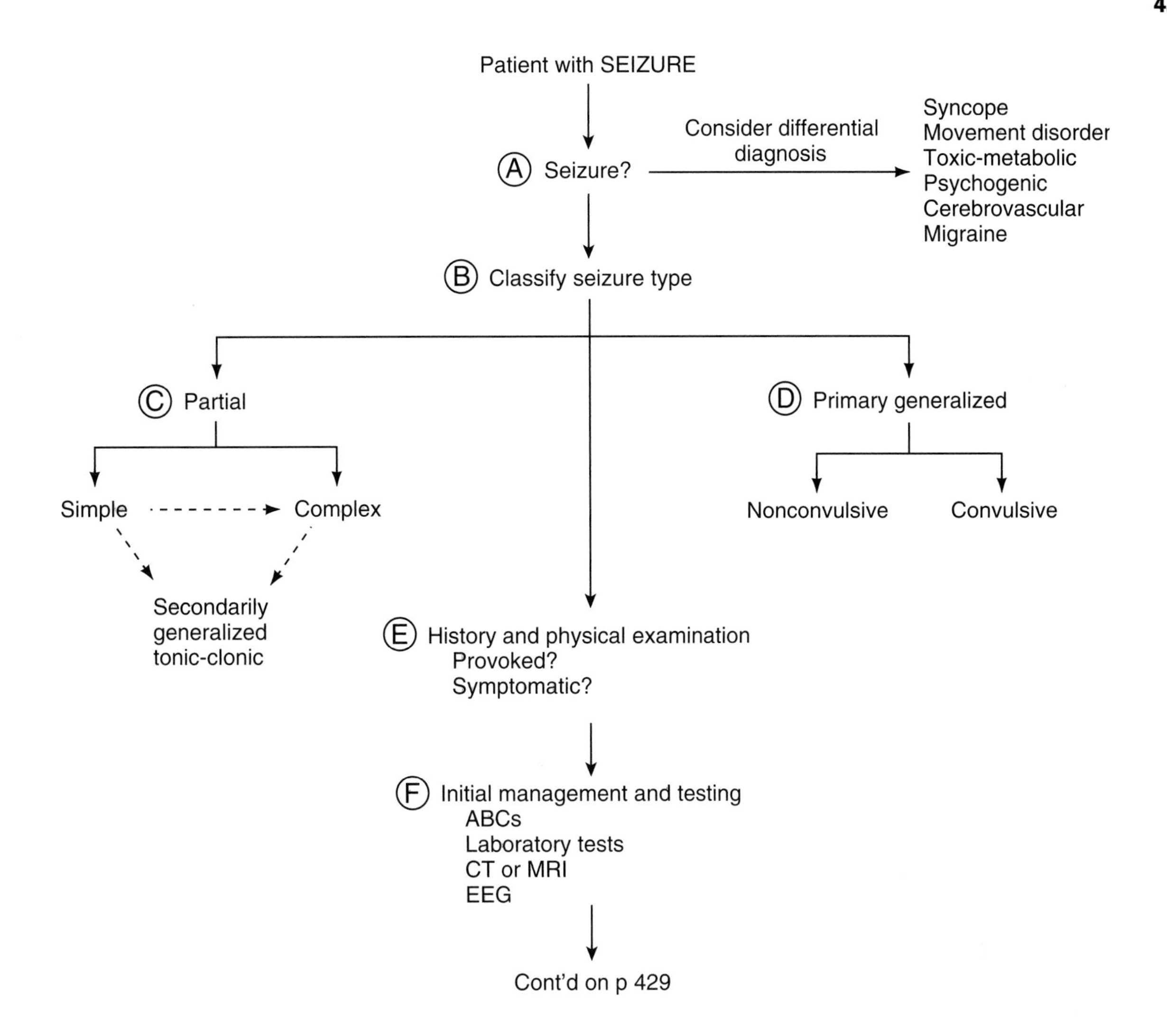
Patient with SEIZURE
(A) Seizure?
Consider differential diagnosis
Syncope
Movement disorder
Toxic-metabolic
Psychogenic
Cerebrovascular
Migraine
(B) Classify seizure type
(C) Partial
Simple
Complex
Secondarily generalized tonic-clonic
(D) Primary generalized
Nonconvulsive
Convulsive
(E) History and physical examination
Provoked?
Symptomatic?
(F) Initial management and testing
ABCs
Laboratory tests
CT or MRI
EEG
Cont'd on p 429

G. Epilepsy is defined as a tendency for recurrent seizures and is diagnosed if there is a history of more than one unprovoked seizure. In most cases antiepileptic medication in indicated. Information regarding driving, safety precautions, medication options, and seizure first aid is available at www.epilepsyfoundation.org and www.epilepsy.com.

H. If there is one uncomplicated, unprovoked seizure, the risk of recurrence is 34% at 3-year follow-up. With a normal MRI and EEG result, it is reasonable to not treat prophylactically depending on physician and patient preference.

I. Structural lesions, preexisting neurologic deficits, focal neurologic examination, and abnormal EEG are associated with an increased risk of recurrence of at least 60%. In many circumstances, antiepileptic prophylaxis is warranted. An acute symptomatic seizure, such as in the setting of stroke or brain infection, may be treated prophylactically, although the exact indications for and duration of treatment are individualized.

J. A variety of antiepileptic medications are currently available. Lorazepam and other benzodiazepines are helpful acutely. Phenobarbital, phenytoin, and valproic acid can be given intravenously. Carbamazepine, gabapentin, lamotrigine, levetiracetam, oxcarbazepine, pregabalin, and zonisamide are all commonly used agents. The specific agent recommended will depend on the seizure type, comorbidities, and patient characteristics and lifestyle.

References

ACEP Clinical Policies Committee; Subcommittee on Seizures (Jagoda AS, Kuffner EK, Huff JS, Sloan EP, Dalsey WC). Clinical policy: critical issues in the evaluation and management of adult patients presenting to the emergency department with seizures. Ann Emerg Med 2004;43:605–625.

French JA, Kanner AM, Bautista J, et al. Efficacy and tolerability of the new antiepileptic drugs I: treatment of new onset epilepsy. Neurology 2004;62:1252–1260.

Hauser WA, Annegers JF, Kurland LT. Incidence of epilepsy and unprovoked seizures in Rochester, Minnesota: 1935–84. Epilepsia 1993;34:453–468.

Hauser W, Rich SS, Annegers JF, et al. Seizure recurrence after a first unprovoked seizure: an extended follow-up. Neurology 1990;40:1163–1170.

Proposal for revised classification of epilepsies and epileptic syndromes. Commission on Classification and Terminology of the International League Against Epilepsy. www.epilepsyfoundation.org and www.epilepsy.com Epilepsia 1989;30:389–399.

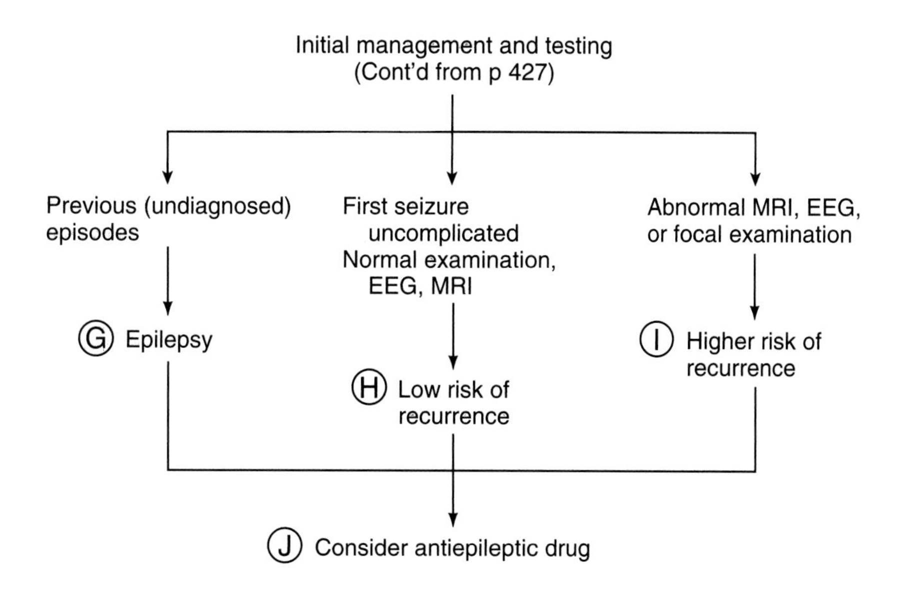
Initial management and testing
(Cont'd from p 427)
Previous (undiagnosed) episodes
First seizure uncomplicated
Normal examination, EEG, MRI
Abnormal MRI, EEG, or focal examination
G Epilepsy
H Low risk of recurrence
I Higher risk of recurrence
J Consider antiepileptic drug

STATUS EPILEPTICUS

Tracey A. Milligan, MD

Status epilepticus is generally defined as 30 minutes of either continuous seizure activity or repetitive seizures without recovery. Convulsive status epilepticus is a medical emergency. Delay in treatment may result in difficult seizure control and poor outcome. Given these risks, aggressive therapy is appropriate for any convulsion lasting >5 minutes. After a convulsion has ended, the patient should be carefully assessed for the possibility of nonconvulsive or subtle ongoing seizures.

A. Types of simple partial status epilepticus include somatomotor (including epilepsy partialis continua), somatosensory, aphasic, visual, oculoclonic, and affective. The electroencephalogram (EEG) shows focal or lateralized discharges. Treatment is with benzodiazepines, phenobarbital, phenytoin, valproate, carbamazepine, and the newer antiepileptic drugs (AEDs).

B. Complex partial status epilepticus (CPSE) consists of complex partial seizures that alternate with a postictal state and may eventually evolve into a continuous epileptic state. It often occurs in patients with known partial epilepsy. Diagnosis may require EEG monitoring. The EEG shows rhythmic activity beginning focally and spreading bilaterally. Treatment is similar to that of simple partial status epilepticus. The use of more aggressive treatment is controversial and should be individualized.

C. Absence status epilepticus is also referred to as petit mal status epilepticus or spike-wave stupor. Clinically, there is a variable degree of responsiveness from slowing of ideation and confusion to lethargy. There is no cycle between levels of responsiveness and unresponsiveness as in CPSE. It is usually seen in children with absence epilepsy but can also be seen in adults, particularly with benzodiazepine withdrawal or use of specific AEDs such as tiagabine. The EEG shows generalized spike-wave discharges. Traditional treatment consists of IV benzodiazepines, valproate, or ethosuximide. The newer broad-spectrum AEDs may also be helpful.

D. True myoclonic status epilepticus is rare and limited to children and adolescents. In adults, myoclonic movements associated with an EEG showing periodic discharges on an attenuated background (burst-suppression pattern) can be seen following an anoxic-ischemic event and portends a bad prognosis. It can also be seen following prolonged convulsive seizures and may indicate a need for more aggressive treatment.

E. Convulsive status epilepticus is the most common and the most dangerous form of status epilepticus. The initial evaluation consists of assessing the airway and assessing and monitoring cardiorespiratory status, providing oxygen and suctioning, obtaining IV access, and sending blood for laboratory tests. Thiamine and glucose are administered unless the patient has a documented normal glucose level. A focused history and neurologic examination are performed, assessing for a known seizure disorder or other illnesses, trauma, focal neurologic signs, and signs of medical illness (e.g., infection, substance abuse).

F. Administer a benzodiazepine as a first-line therapeutic agent. Lorazepam is the preferred agent because of a longer duration of antiseizure action and is given up to 0.1 mg/kg at 1–2 mg/min. Diazepam can also be used at up to 0.25 mg/kg at 2–4 mg/min or midazolam 0.2 mg/kg at 1–4 mg/min.

G. Phenytoin (or fosphenytoin) is administered immediately following lorazepam. It is given at 20 mg/kg (<50 mg/min). The fosphenytoin dose is 20 mg phenytoin equivalents (PE)/kg (<150 mg/min). An additional 10 mg/kg can be administered if seizures continue. Phenytoin is associated with risk of hypotension and bradycardia. These side effects are less frequently seen with fosphenytoin, but the increased cost of fosphenytoin limits its availability. Other agents that may be used instead of phenytoin, or may follow phenytoin infusion if seizures continue, include IV valproate at 20–30 mg/kg (200 mg/min) or phenobarbital 10–20 mg/kg (100 mg/min). Phenobarbital is also associated with a risk of hypotension. Once the patient is stabilized, further diagnostic workup may include CT, lumbar puncture (LP), EEG, and MRI. Immediate EEG assessment is required if there is use of a long-acting paralytic agent, when there is no improvement or return to baseline mental status after controlling overt convulsive movements, or in cases of refractory status epilepticus.

(Continued on page 432)

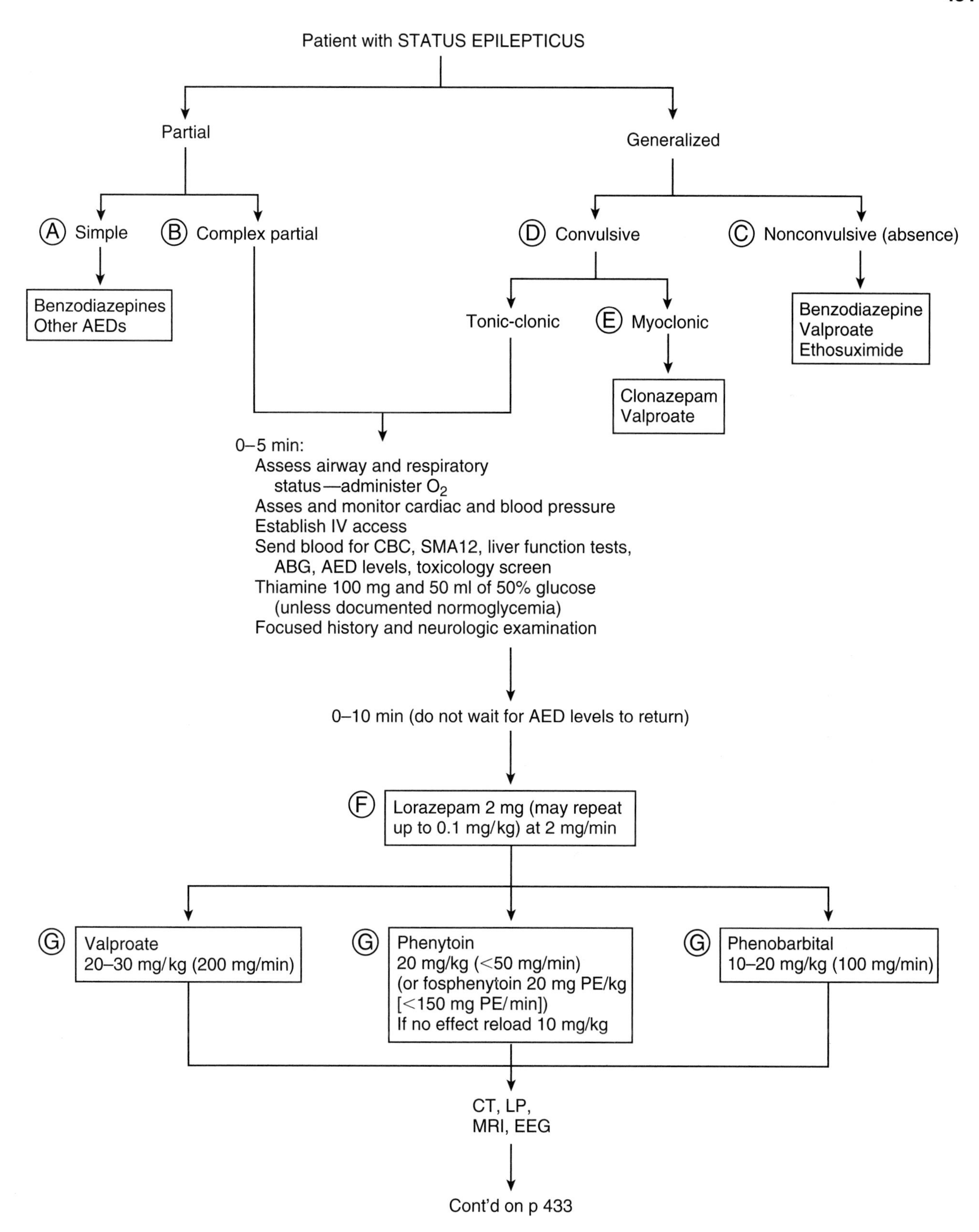
Patient with STATUS EPILEPTICUS
Partial
Generalized
(A) Simple
(B) Complex partial
(D) Convulsive
(C) Nonconvulsive (absence)
Benzodiazepines
Other AEDs
Tonic-clonic
(E) Myoclonic
Benzodiazepine
Valproate
Ethosuximide
Clonazepam
Valproate
0–5 min:
Assess airway and respiratory status—administer O_2
Asses and monitor cardiac and blood pressure
Establish IV access
Send blood for CBC, SMA12, liver function tests, ABG, AED levels, toxicology screen
Thiamine 100 mg and 50 ml of 50% glucose (unless documented normoglycemia)
Focused history and neurologic examination
0–10 min (do not wait for AED levels to return)
(F) Lorazepam 2 mg (may repeat up to 0.1 mg/kg) at 2 mg/min
(G) Valproate
20–30 mg/kg (200 mg/min)
(G) Phenytoin
20 mg/kg (<50 mg/min)
(or fosphenytoin 20 mg PE/kg
[<150 mg PE/min])
If no effect reload 10 mg/kg
(G) Phenobarbital
10–20 mg/kg (100 mg/min)
CT, LP,
MRI, EEG
Cont'd on p 433

H. If seizures persist despite therapy with benzodiazepines and a second AED, status epilepticus is considered refractory and will likely require drug-induced coma with intubation, intensive care unit (ICU) admission, and continuous EEG monitoring. Medication is titrated to induce a burst-suppression pattern on EEG or suppression of epileptiform activity. Medication-induced hypotension is to be expected and can be treated by slowing or stopping the infusion, giving fluid boluses, and using vasopressors as necessary. Historically, pentobarbital has been the agent most widely used. More recently midazolam and propofol have been used with success. These agents are thought to exert their antiseizure action by increased GABAergic activity. Pentobarbital has a higher lipid solubility than phenobarbital, allowing a more rapid passage through the blood-brain barrier, and has a longer half-life than either midazolam or propofol. It is bolused at 5–20 mg/kg and infused at a rate of 0.5–5.0 mg/kg/hr. For breakthrough seizures, another bolus should be administered and the drip should be increased by 0.5 to 3.0 mg/kg/hr. Propofol is increasingly being used as an alternative to pentobarbital and has a rapid onset and the shortest half-life, allowing for the ability to periodically monitor the neurologic examination. It is bolused at 1–3 mg/kg and infused at a rate of 2–10 mg/kg/hr. Higher infusion rates are associated with more adverse reactions. Midazolam has a very rapid onset of action, but tachyphylaxis can often occur. It is bolused at 0.15–0.2 mg/kg and infused at a rate of 0.02 mg/kg/hr.

I. With failure to respond to the previous treatments, status epilepticus is considered severely refractory with a high risk of mortality. Further treatment options include ketamine, lidocaine, thiopental, and isoflurane. Paraldehyde may also be helpful, but availability is limited. Other AEDs via a nasogastric tube, such as topiramate and levetiracetam, can be tried as well.

References

Alldredge BK, Gelb AM, Isaacs SM, et al. A comparison of lorazepam, diazepam, and placebo for the treatment of out-of-hospital status epilepticus. N Engl J Med 2001;345:631–637.

Claassen J, Hirsch LJ, Emerson RG, et al. Treatment of refractory status epilepticus with pentobarbital, propofol, or midazolam: a systematic review. Epilepsia 2002;43:146–153.

Gastaut H. Classification of status epilepticus. Adv Neurol 1983;34:15–35.

Lowenstein DH, Alldredge BK. Status epilepticus. N Engl J Med 1998;338:970–976.

Sinha S, Naritoku DK. Intravenous valproate is well tolerated in unstable patients with status epilepticus. Neurology 2000;55:722–724.

Treatment of convulsive status epilepticus. Recommendations of the Epilepsy Foundation of America's Working Group on Status Epilepticus. JAMA 1993;270:854–859.

Treiman DM, Meyers PD, Walton NY, et al. A comparison of four treatments for generalized convulsive status epilepticus. N Engl J Med 1998;339:792–798.

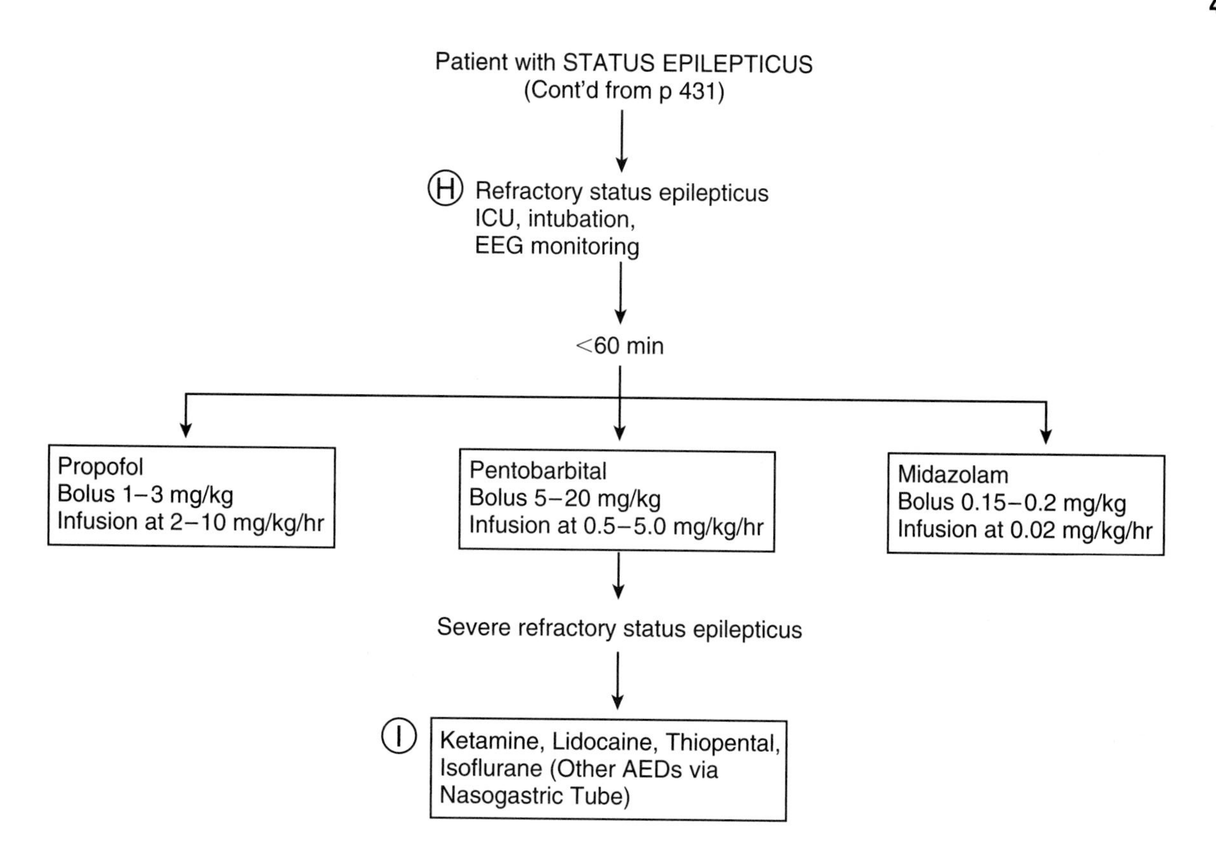

Patient with STATUS EPILEPTICUS
(Cont'd from p 431)
H
Refractory status epilepticus
ICU, intubation,
EEG monitoring
<60 min
Propofol
Bolus 1–3 mg/kg
Infusion at 2–10 mg/kg/hr
Pentobarbital
Bolus 5–20 mg/kg
Infusion at 0.5–5.0 mg/kg/hr
Midazolam
Bolus 0.15–0.2 mg/kg
Infusion at 0.02 mg/kg/hr
Severe refractory status epilepticus
I
Ketamine, Lidocaine, Thiopental,
Isoflurane (Other AEDs via
Nasogastric Tube)

WEAKNESS

Allitia B. DiBernardo, MD

Clinical weakness can be caused by disorders affecting the muscle, the junction of nerve and muscle, the axon, or the motor neuron. A diagnostic approach to the patient who is clinically weak should attempt to resolve weakness into one of these categories. Information from the clinical course and paraclinical testing is rationally applied to narrow the differential diagnosis within each broad category.

A. The degree of diagnostic resolution that can be achieved with the history and physical examination is unmatched by any other mode of investigation. Broadly speaking, the history should provide information about the onset, context, and duration of weakness (acute, subacute, chronic, episodic; outpatient vs. hospitalized vs. critically ill patients), triggers or exacerbating factors (exertion, cold, mechanical pressure), symmetry and distribution (proximal, distal, focal), clinical accompaniments (pain, paresthesias, rash, constitutional symptoms, cramps, fasciculations), comorbidities (diabetes, thyroid disease, vascular risk factors, autoimmune disorders, malignancies), pertinent exposure history (infection, arthropod-borne diseases, medications, and toxins [including alcohol]), and family history. The physical examination should survey the entire central and peripheral nervous systems (a complete neurologic examination) to attempt lesion localization. Lesions anywhere along the course of the anterior horn cell to motor endplate can produce similar clinical signs, making discernment of muscular versus neural pathology in the lower motor neuron distribution difficult. Symmetric proximal weakness and/or muscle tenderness are more typical of muscle than nerve pathology. Myotonia, paramyotonia, or periodic paralysis implicates ion channel defects. Fatigability, atrophy, fasciculations, and loss of reflexes can occur with myopathy, neuromuscular junction (NMJ) disorders, peripheral neuropathy, or anterior horn cell disease. These signs, although not specific to lower motor neurons (LMN), are lumped under the rubric of "LMN signs." Hyperreflexia, increased tone, and slowing of movement are signs characteristic of upper motor neurons (UMN) or their processes in long tracts from the motor cortex to white-matter tracts through the brainstem and into the spinal cord. The physical examination should document whether weakness is associated with UMN signs, LMN signs, or both.

B. When UMN signs of hyperreflexia, bradykinesis, and/or increased tone accompany pure motor weakness, diagnosis depends both on the pattern of weakness and the acuity of onset. UMN weakness evolving over minutes to hours suggests a vascular or demyelinating etiology and should be urgently evaluated by MRI. Unilateral pure motor syndromes can be produced acutely by small lesions in the contralateral primary motor cortex, internal capsule, thalamus, cerebral peduncles, or ipsilateral brainstem and pyramidal tracts. Bilateral isolated weakness can be caused acutely by a lesion of the anterior spinal cord. Pure upper motor syndromes evolving over days to weeks are unusual but could potentially occur in the context of demyelinating lesions from multiple sclerosis (MS) or viral infection or expanding mass lesions, including tumor, hematoma, parasites, or abscess in brain or spinal cord. Weakness resulting from progressive lesions affecting the spinal cord is virtually always accompanied by corresponding sensory level deficits. The presence of constitutional symptoms would support an inflammatory process. Focal pain (headache, neck or back pain) can suggest the region of interest to be evaluated by MRI. White-matter involvement seen on MRI in the brain or spinal cord should prompt cerebrospinal fluid (CSF) evaluation for markers of inflammation and infection. Any mass lesion should be evaluated with neurosurgical consultation, and those that distort normal CNS architecture by exerting "mass effect" should be evaluated urgently. UMN weakness that progresses over months to years suggests degenerative disease. Primary lateral sclerosis is a clinical diagnosis of isolated UMN degeneration affecting the face and limbs, and diagnosis can be aided by electromyography (EMG).

C. Regardless of tempo, CNS pathology more often than not produces mixed modality (motor and sensory) deficits and "neighborhood" signs to aid in localization and diagnosis. UMN-type weakness with accompanying cortical deficits in language, speech, praxis, vision, or sensation (e.g., higher-level sensation, such as stereognosis) generally indicates pathology at the level of the cerebral hemispheres. UMN-type weakness without cortical deficits but with cranial nerve deficits places the lesion in the brainstem. A clinically evident sensorimotor level suggests spinal cord pathology. At any level, in the absence of trauma, an acute evolution of deficits suggests a vascular or demyelinating event that must be emergently evaluated by MRI. The differential diagnosis for mixed-modality subacute and chronic lesions of the hemispheres, brainstem, or spinal cord is too broad to review here. A good first step in narrowing the differential, however, is gadolinium-enhanced MRI of the region of interest. Because

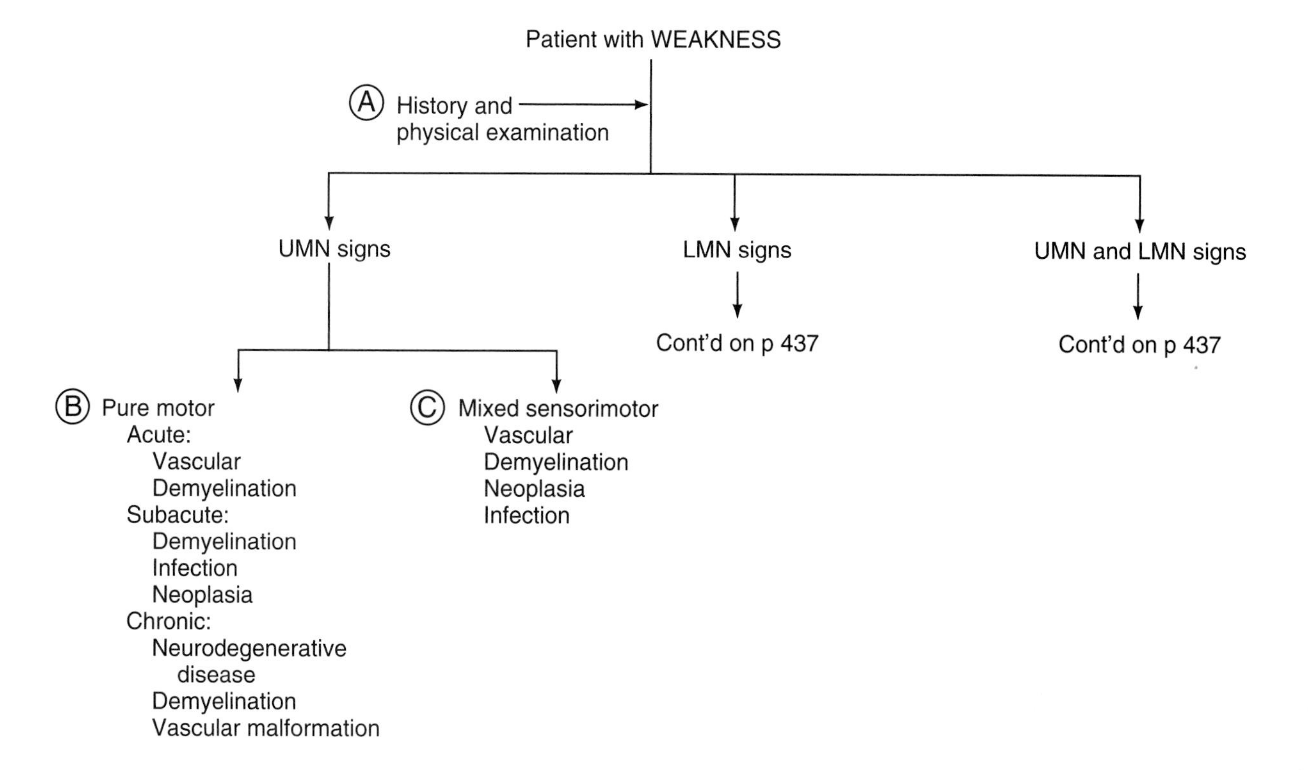

rapid recognition and intervention often are necessary to preserve remaining neurologic function in the setting of spinal cord pathology, special mention will be made of key findings. In hyperacute spinal cord lesions, clear UMN signs may be absent. The presence of a sensory and motor level with decreased sphincter tone, however, is diagnostic of cord injury. Spinal cord lesions are generally divided into compressive (i.e., extramedullary) and intramedullary lesions. Pain tends to be a more prominent feature of compressive cord lesions. Intramedullary lesions, including tumors, demyelination, or syrinx, are often painless. Transverse myelitis is a rapid myelopathy that may be of viral, demyelinating, or vasculitic origin. Insidious myelopathies can result from vitamin deficiencies (B_{12}, E) or HIV infection and should be investigated because deficits can be partially reversed with appropriate treatment.

(Continued on page 436)

D. The presence of LMN signs such as atrophy, fasciculations, or depressed reflexes in the context of weakness should prompt a thorough evaluation of the peripheral nervous system, including assessment of muscle strength and all sensory modalities. Weakness with accompanying sensory deficits can suggest a problem of the root, plexus, or peripheral nerve. The pattern and acuity of sensorimotor deficit are of key diagnostic importance. Symmetric, distal deficits (glove-and-stocking pattern) suggest a generalized length-dependent peripheral neuropathy, which should be further characterized as demyelinating or axonal by electrodiagnostic (EMG/nerve conduction study [NCS]) testing (see the section Peripheral Neuropathy chapter). Unilateral sensorimotor deficits in a dermatome-myotome pattern suggest a lesion of the relevant nerve root, which can be confirmed by MRI and/or EMG. In the context of trauma, root avulsion or neurapraxia are possible. The most common causes of radiculopathy, however, are disc herniation and neural foraminal narrowing. Sensorimotor deficits in a distribution of multiple cervical or sacrolumbar roots suggest either multilevel radiculopathy or plexopathy. Workup of these lesions can be challenging and generally begins with EMG and spinal MRI but can potentially include lumbar puncture (LP) to evaluate for cytomegalovirus, Lyme disease, or malignant cells or MRI of the affected plexus. Finally, sensorimotor deficits in the distribution of a single nerve (mononeuropathy) or multiple nerves (mononeuritis multiplex) should be evaluated first by EMG to guide subsequent workup and treatment.

E. LMN signs in the context of isolated weakness (without sensory loss) can be seen in the setting of motor neuropathy, anterior horn cell disease, NMJ disorders, or myopathy. Evaluation is greatly aided by EMG to assess for myopathic motor units, effects of repetitive stimulation, and exercise on motor unit amplitude and by NCS to rule out demyelination.

F. Disorders of the LMN include acute poliomyelitis, postpolio syndrome, spinal muscular atrophy (SMA), and progressive muscular atrophy (PMA). Although poliomyelitis is rarely seen, degeneration of previously affected anterior horn cells can occur decades after childhood disease as a postpolio syndrome. A family history of LMN disease should raise clinical suspicion for SMA, a heterogenous group of inherited motor neuronopathies that can vary in age of onset, distribution, and inheritance patterns. PMA is a sporadic LMN disease characterized by progressive weakness and atrophy that typically spares facial musculature. Often amyotrophic lateral sclerosis (ALS) presents initially with LMN-only signs and thus must be maintained on the list of differential diagnoses.

G. Of disorders of the NMJ, by far the most common is myasthenia gravis (MG), caused by antibodies that block the acetylcholine (ACh) receptor on the motor endplate. A typical history is one of diurnal variations in fatigue, ptosis, and/or diplopia with symptoms exacerbated by exercise and relieved by rest. Facial musculature is most frequently affected, particularly the eyelid and extraocular muscles. Larger muscles, including neck flexors and extensors, shoulder, and hip girdle muscles, may also be affected. A purely ocular form with low circulating titers of anti-ACh receptor antibodies can occur in older males. Diagnosis can be confirmed by specialized EMG testing, resolution of weakness with administration of edrophonium, and the detection of elevated titers of ACh receptor antibodies. The Eaton-Lambert myasthenic syndrome is a paraneoplastic condition most commonly seen in patients with small cell lung cancer. It can be differentiated from MG by increasing rather than decreasing strength with exercise on both clinical and electrophysiologic testing. Less commonly, acute intoxication with certain drugs can impair neuromuscular transmission, including penicillamine, gentamicin, kanamycin, magnesium salts, quinidine, procainamide, and lidocaine. Botulism poisoning is another relatively rare cause of acute paraparesis from NMJ dysfunction and is characterized by GI upset followed by weakness, ophthalmoplegia, and pupillary abnormalities.

H. Diseases of muscle are generally classed as *dystrophies* or *myopathies.* Disorders of the muscle can be difficult to discern clinically. Diagnosis is often supported by EMG findings and elevated serum creatinine kinase (CK) and confirmed by muscle biopsy.

I. Acquired myopathies fall into three main groups: endocrine, infectious/inflammatory, and drugs and toxins. Dysthyroid states are the most common cause of endocrine myopathies. Hyperthyroidism can produce chronic thyrotoxic myopathy, which may include ophthalmoplegia. Hypothyroid myopathy is associated with increased muscle mass and slowed reflexes. Hyperaldosteronism, acromegaly, Cushing's syndrome, hypophosphatemia, and hyperparathyroidism can also cause myopathic weakness. Inflammatory myopathies include polymyositis (PM), dermatomyositis (DM), and inclusion body myositis (IBM). PM is characterized by proximal weakness, dysphagia, and myalgia, particularly when associated with connective tissue disease. DM is similar but often has a violaceous rash in or around the orbits or scaly papules on the dorsum of the hands. IBM tends to spare the deltoids and affects the wrist and finger flexors. Other infectious/inflammatory causes of myopathy include bacteria and viruses, sarcoidosis, toxoplasmosis, trichinosis, and cysticercosis. Steroids and ethanol are the most significant causes of toxic myopathy. Other drugs to consider include guanethidine, chloroquine, hydroxychloroquine, clofibrate, lovastatin, gemfibrozil, colchicine, zidovudine, doxorubicin, emetine (in ipecac), pentazocine, potassium-lowering diuretics, and heroin. Diagnostic evaluation of acquired myopathy will typically include serum CK, ESR, or C-reactive protein (CRP); screening thyroid function tests (TFTs) and autoimmune antibodies; review of medications and alcohol use; and EMG. Definitive diagnosis usually depends on findings from a muscle biopsy.

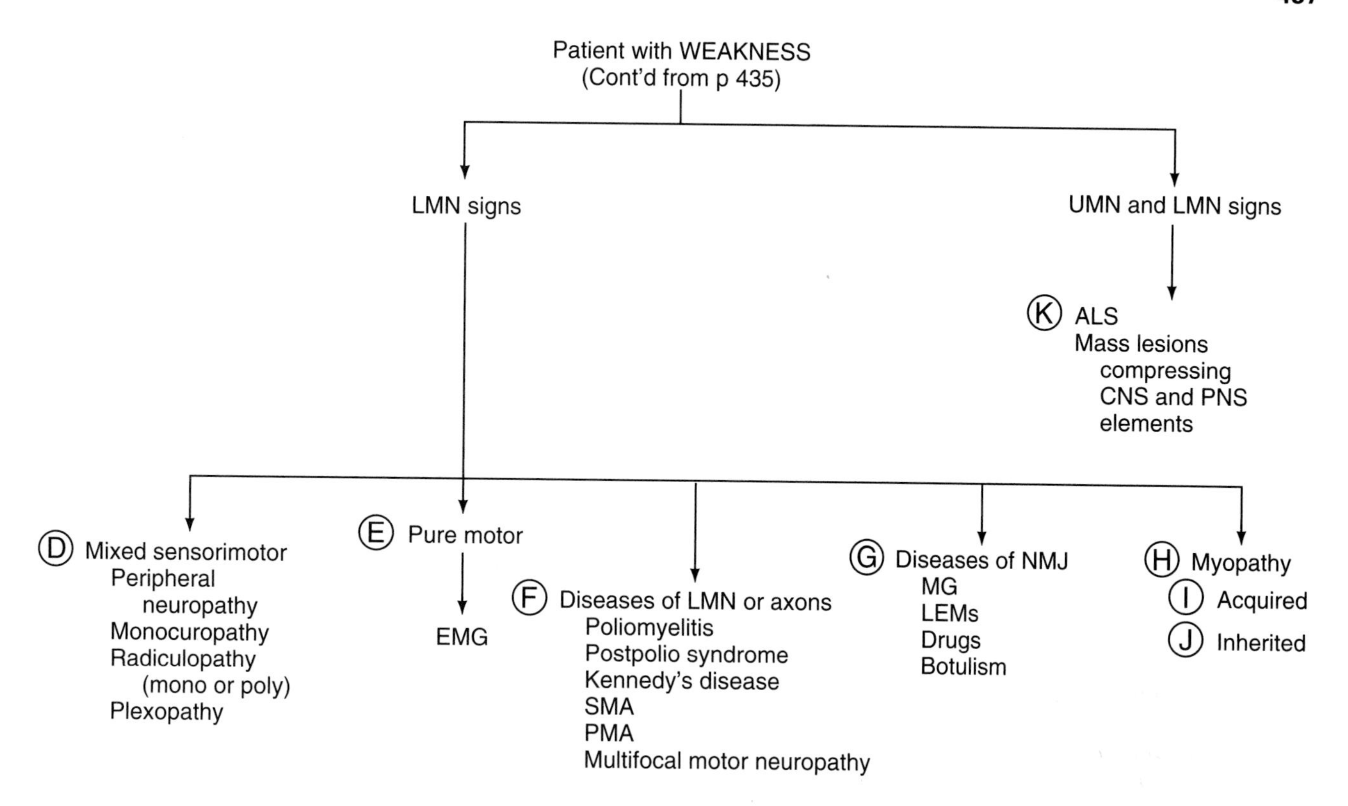

J. Inherited muscle disorders are less commonly encountered in the adult population. Duchenne's and Becker's muscular dystrophy (MD) are X-linked, early-onset diseases characterized by severe proximal weakness, pseudohypertrophy, cardiac involvement, and high CK levels. Myotonic dystrophy is an autosomal-dominant muscle disorder characterized by myotonia, distinctive "hatchet facies," distal weakness, and multisystem involvement. Mitochondrial myopathies are a heterogeneous group of disorders characterized by weakness, fatigability, and multisystem involvement. Diagnosis of inherited myopathies is confirmed by muscle biopsy and in some cases by genetic testing.

K. The presence of both UMN and LMN signs in one or more CNS region (bulbar, cervical, thoracic, and lumbar) is classically seen in ALS, a rapidly progressive degenerative disease of motor neurons that leads to death from respiratory failure within 1–5 years. Because of its grim prognosis and lack of effective treatment, a diagnosis of ALS should be made with EMG support after exclusion of any possible alternative diagnosis, including cervical spine disease and heavy metal poisoning.

References

Ronthal M. Weakness. In Samuels MA, Feske SK, eds. Office Practice of Neurology, 2nd ed. Churchill Livingstone, 2003:8–13.
Ross MA. Acquired motor neuron disorders. Neurol Clin 1997;15:481.
Targoff IN. Diagnosis and treatment of polymyositis and dermatomyositis. Comp Ther 1990;16:16.
Younger DS. Advances in the diagnosis, pathogenesis and treatment of myasthenia gravis. Neurology 1997;48(Suppl 5).

GAIT DISTURBANCES

Marsha Smith, MD

Gait disturbances denote a problem with the initiation and/or maintenance of walking. Many gait disturbances are not primarily of neurologic etiology (e.g., medication effects, illness-related deconditioning). Neurologic systems subserving gait include the frontal cortex and white matter, basal ganglia, diencephalon, midbrain, cerebellum, vestibular system, spinal cord, peripheral nervous system, and muscle. Thus, the initial evaluation of gait disturbances seeks to localize the dysfunction. Some common neurologic etiologies of gait disturbance are reviewed here.

A. A thorough history and physical examination should aim to determine the character and time course of the gait disturbance and associated symptoms and signs, such as rest tremor, bradykinesia, rigidity, numbness, weakness, back pain, urinary incontinence, dementia, and headaches. Alcohol use history, general medical history, and medication use should be reviewed.

B. A spastic gait typically results from upper motor neuron (UMN; cerebral or spinal cord) dysfunction from conditions such as cerebrovascular disease or demyelinating disorders, including multiple sclerosis (MS). In the older population, a common myelopathic etiology of spastic gait is cervical spondylosis. In the younger population, myelopathy may be associated with a demyelinating illness or trauma. This gait is characterized by stiffness in the lower extremities and circumduction of the leg. Scissoring can also be seen and results from increased tone in the adductors. Patients may exhibit exaggerated deep tendon reflexes (DTRs) and may exhibit a unilateral or bilateral Babinski's sign. Neuroimaging of the brain and spinal cord, typically with MRI, is important, as is a laboratory screen (e.g., for vitamin B_{12} deficiency). If a demyelinating illness is suspected, then MRI with and without contrast should be performed.

C. Gait disturbance from sensory dysfunction is typically wide-based with a stamping or slapping character. The examination may reveal reduced deep tendon reflexes, weakness and sensory loss that are greatest distally, and the presence of Romberg's sign (an abnormality in stance that occurs with eye closure). Sensory gait disturbance is usually from disorders affecting the peripheral nervous system or dorsal columns of the spinal cord. This type of gait was classically seen in patients with tabes dorsalis and neurosyphilis. Today it is more commonly seen as a result of large-fiber neuropathy secondary to certain vitamin deficiencies (B_{12}) or diabetic peripheral neuropathy.

D. Neuromuscular disease can also cause an abnormal gait. The distinguishing features are that of high steppage gait to compensate for problems such as foot drop. Patients with illnesses such as myopathy will present with proximal weakness and report difficulty climbing stairs. Weakness of the hip girdle can also lead to a waddling gait, which is a result of excess pelvic rotation. Electromyography would be helpful in either of these scenarios to look for signs of neuropathy or myopathy.

E. Extrapyramidal disorders arise from basal ganglia dysfunction. Associated symptoms and signs include rest tremor, slowness, and rigidity, which could suggest Parkinson's disease. The parkinsonian gait is usually associated with flexed posture, shuffling, decreased arm swing, difficulty initiating, en bloc turning, and festination. Chorea is seen in Huntington's disease. Dystonia, an involuntary contraction of muscles, can also be a cause of gait abnormality.

F. A cerebellar gait disorder can result from an infarct, tumor, alcohol, or demyelination. The lesion is primarily found in the flocculonodular or anterior lobes of the cerebellum. The typical cerebellar gait is ataxic—wide-based and unsteady. Tandem walking may be difficult or impossible. Cerebellar gait disorders are usually, but not always, associated with other cerebellar signs such as intention tremor, dysmetria, rebound, and hypotonia. MRI is the diagnostic test of choice.

G. A frontal gait disturbance is common in older patients and is also known as gait apraxia. Typically no weakness or sensory loss is found. Patients walk with a wide base, short stride, and shuffling steps, and feet appear to be "sticking to the floor," with difficulty initiating gait and en bloc turning. Dementia, bilateral grasp reflexes, and a history of urinary incontinence may be present. Etiologies of frontal gait disorder include normal-pressure hydrocephalus, severe small vessel disease in the basal ganglia or periventricular white matter, or large frontal lobe tumors. MRI is essential to demonstrate ventricular size, the degree of white matter disease, and presence of tumors.

H. Toxins are one of the most common causes of gait difficulty, including excess alcohol intake. Certain prescription or nonprescription drugs and metabolic derangement can also have important effects on balance and gait.

I. Psychogenic gait is a diagnosis of exclusion. *Astasia–abasia* is the term used to denote such bizarre gait; patients may exhibit dramatic fluctuation over time, exaggerated caution, and slowness.

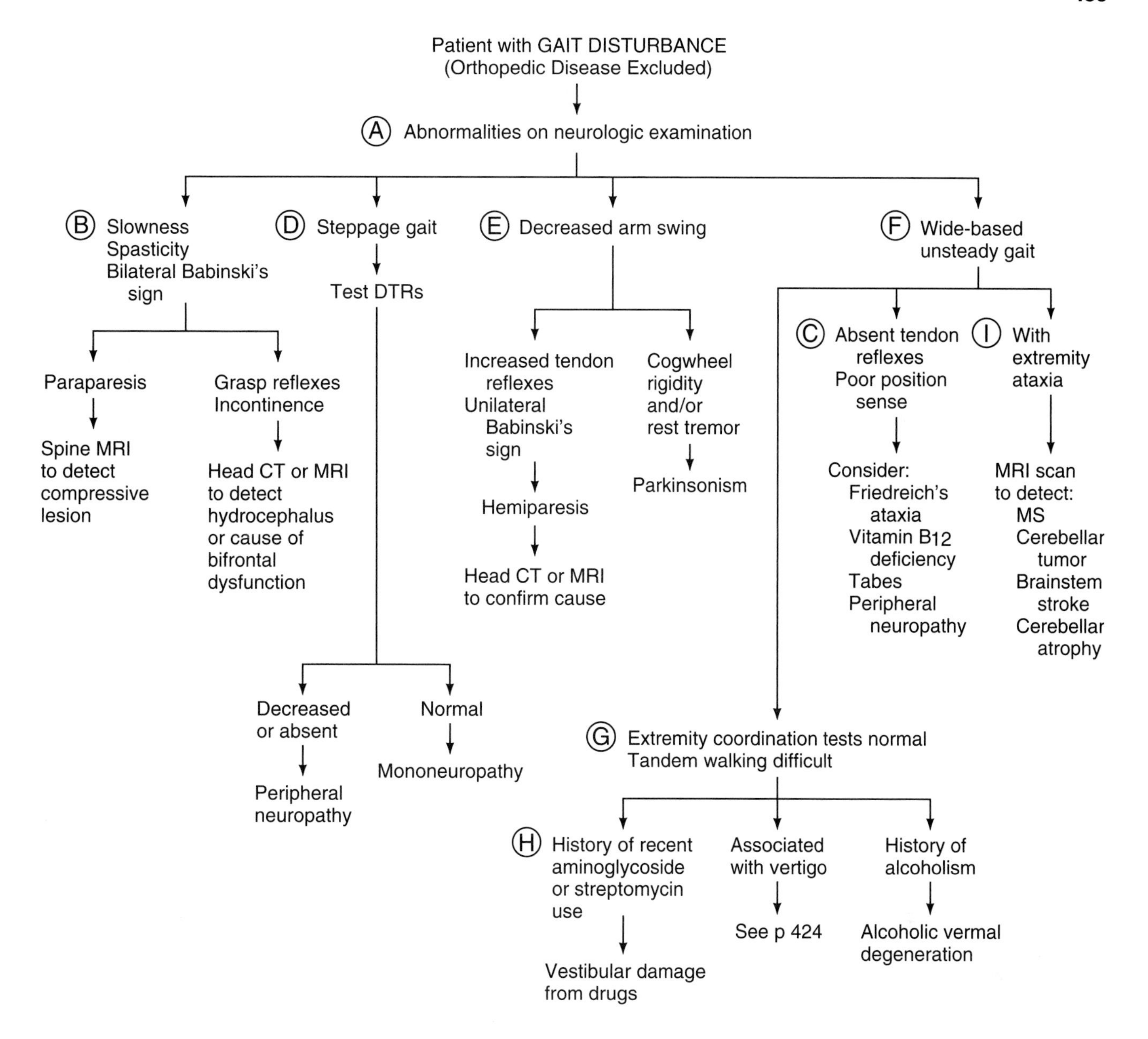

References

Gilman S. Gait disorders. In Rowland LP, ed. Merritt's Textbook of Neurology, 9th ed. Baltimore: Williams & Wilkins, 1995:51–56.

Nutt JG, Horak FB. Gait and balance disorders. In Watts RL, Koller WC, eds. Movement Disorders: Neurologic Principles and Practice. New York: McGraw-Hill, 1997:649–660.

Sudarsky L. Gait impairment and falls. In Samuels MA, Feske SK, eds. Office Practice of Neurology, 2nd ed. Philadelphia: Churchill Livingstone, 2003:25–29.

TREMOR

Yvette M. Bordelon, MD, PhD

Tremor results from involuntary, alternating, rhythmic contractions of agonist and antagonist muscles and is typically classified by the position of the limb in which it is manifest: rest, postural, or action (kinetic). Rate, amplitude, and rhythmicity are also useful descriptors for tremor when considering its potential causes. Although there is overlap in the clinical manifestation of tremor among the various etiologies, it is useful to consider four major categories: parkinsonian, cerebellar, essential, and enhanced physiologic tremor. The categorization of tremor rests primarily on history and neurologic examination.

A. Parkinsonian tremor is characteristically a 3- to 6-Hz rest tremor described as "pill-rolling." Associated hypokinetic features of rigidity, bradykinesia, and gait and postural instability are seen in idiopathic Parkinson's disease (PD). Parkinsonian tremor is less commonly seen in atypical parkinsonian syndromes (also known as Parkinson-plus syndromes), such as multiple-system atrophy and progressive supranuclear palsy. Treatment with levodopa, dopamine agonists, and anticholinergics can alleviate the tremor seen in PD (see also Parkinson's Disease chapter).

B. Cerebellar dysfunction resulting from lesions to the cerebellum or its pathways (by infarcts, mass lesions, demyelination, or degenerative diseases) can result in a large-amplitude, coarse tremor of the limbs (formerly known as rubral tremor) or trunk (known as titubation) that occurs primarily with action or maintenance of a posture. Benzodiazepines and some antiepileptic medications can alleviate this form of tremor.

C. Essential tremor is a common movement disorder that is manifested by an 8- to 12-Hz postural and/or action tremor typically in the upper extremities that is most often familial and alcohol responsive. Clinical trials have shown that propranolol and primidone are the most effective treatments for essential tremor, but other medications can be useful as can deep brain stimulation in medication-refractory cases.

D. Enhanced physiologic tremor is typically a postural tremor of 8–12 Hz, similar to that of essential tremor. It may result from metabolic disorders (hyperthyroidism, hypoglycemia), drugs (caffeine, lithium, amphetamines), or stress (fatigue, anxiety). Treatment is typically not indicated except to address the underlying cause.

References

Louis ED. Essential tremor. Lancet Neurol 2005;4:100–110.

Zesiewicz TA, Elble R, Louis ED, et al; Quality Standards Subcommittee of the American Academy of Neurology. Practice parameter: therapies for essential tremor: report of the Quality Standards Subcommittee of the American Academy of Neurology. Neurology 2005,64:2008–2020.

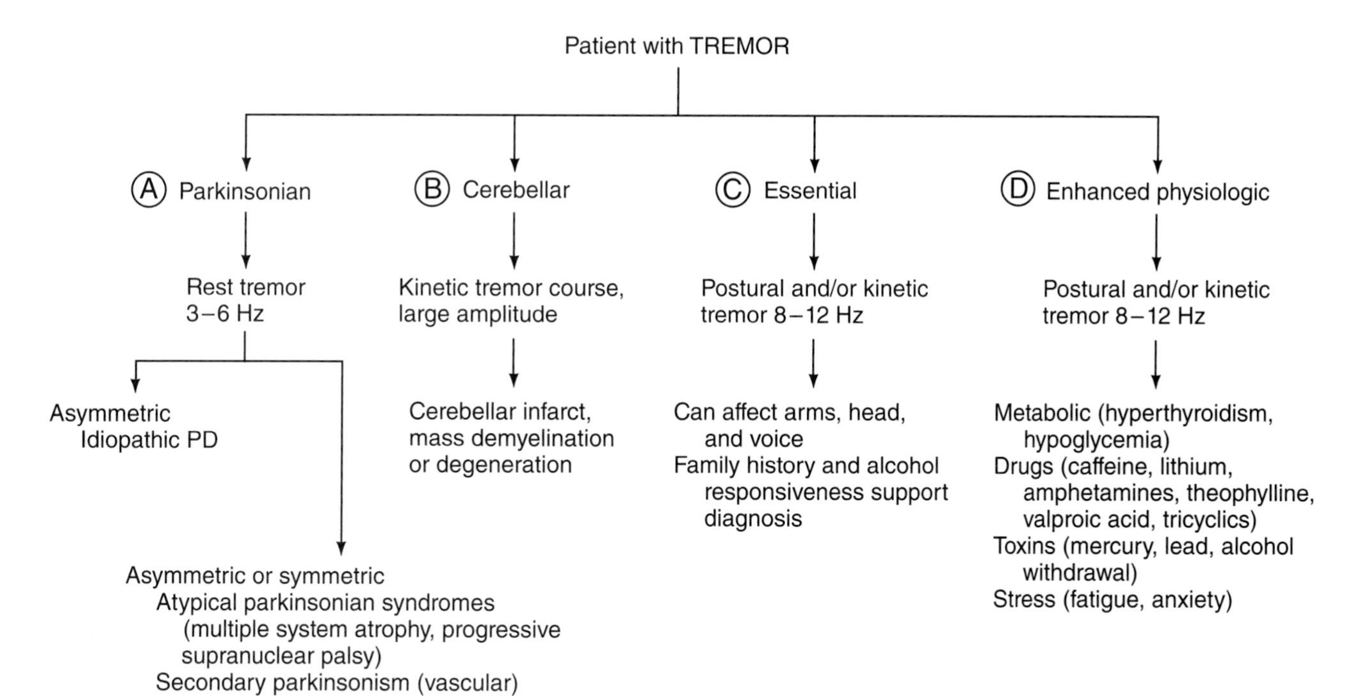

Patient with TREMOR
(A) Parkinsonian
Rest tremor 3–6 Hz
Asymmetric Idiopathic PD
Asymmetric or symmetric
Atypical parkinsonian syndromes (multiple system atrophy, progressive supranuclear palsy)
Secondary parkinsonism (vascular)
(B) Cerebellar
Kinetic tremor course, large amplitude
Cerebellar infarct, mass demyelination or degeneration
(C) Essential
Postural and/or kinetic tremor 8–12 Hz
Can affect arms, head, and voice
Family history and alcohol responsiveness support diagnosis
(D) Enhanced physiologic
Postural and/or kinetic tremor 8–12 Hz
Metabolic (hyperthyroidism, hypoglycemia)
Drugs (caffeine, lithium, amphetamines, theophylline, valproic acid, tricyclics)
Toxins (mercury, lead, alcohol withdrawal)
Stress (fatigue, anxiety)

PARKINSON'S DISEASE

Marsha Smith, MD

Parkinson's disease (PD) was first described by James Parkinson in "An Essay on the Shaking Palsy" in 1817. Clinically, PD is now classically diagnosed as a triad of rest tremor, bradykinesia/akinesia, and cogwheel rigidity. These clinical findings result from degeneration of the dopaminergic neurons in the substantia nigra pars compacta of the midbrain. The histopathologic hallmark of PD is the Lewy body. These neuronal cytoplasmic inclusions are typically found in the midbrain.

A. The diagnosis of PD requires the presence of the following symptoms: resting tremor, cogwheel rigidity, bradykinesia/akinesia, and postural instability. In addition to motor symptoms, patients may also have cognitive impairment (see Chronic Behavior Change chapter). The incidence increases with age, from 0.50 per 100,000 in the 30- to 39-year age range to 119.01 per 100,000 in the 80- to 89-year age range.

B. The decision to treat a patient with suspected idiopathic PD is based on several considerations, including age. The first-line therapy, levodopa/carbidopa is preferred in older patients because of a lesser risk of cognitive side effects in this age group compared with the dopamine agonists. The dopamine agonists are classified as ergot or nonergot alkaloids. The ergot compounds are bromocriptine and pergolide. Nonergot agonists include ropinirole, pramipexole, and apomorphine. Pergolide, ropinirole, and pramipexole are frequently used to treat younger patients with PD. Bromocriptine, one of the oldest dopamine agonists, is now rarely used to treat idiopathic PD. The agonists have a higher incidence of hallucinations and somnolence. As a class, they can also cause nausea and dyspepsia. Recently they have been linked to pathologic behavior such as compulsive gambling. The incidence seems to be dose-dependent, and a higher incidence has been noted in patients being treated with pramipexole. Apomorphine was accepted as treatment for PD in the United States in 2004. Because of its strong emetic effect, apomorphine requires premedication with domperidone, an antiemetic. It is administered subcutaneously, has a rapid onset (about 10 minutes), and can last up to 2 hours. Pergolide, an ergot-derived agonist, has been linked to valvular heart disease and to retroperitoneal and pleuropulmonary fibrosis.

C. Two medications may provide neuroprotective benefits in PD. The DATATOP study suggested that selegiline, a monoamine oxidase inhibitor, may exhibit neuroprotective effects. Similar benefit may be seen with high dosages (1200 mg/day) of coenzyme Q10. Some clinicians add these medications to the treatment regimen with the hope that they may provide neuroprotection.

D. As the disease progresses, higher doses of a levodopa/carbidopa or a dopamine agonist are inevitably required. Patients taking dopamine agonist monotherapy will eventually need levodopa/carbidopa for symptomatic relief. For those patients already taking levodopa/carbidopa, entacapone (a COMT [catechol-*O*-methyltransferase] inhibitor) can be added to lengthen the half-life of the drug. If levodopa/carbidopa begins losing effect ("wearing off") between doses, the dosing interval can be shortened. A controlled-release form of levodopa/carbidopa is often used at nighttime to help reduce symptoms in the morning.

E. Dyskinesias are involuntary movements that can be seen in patients with PD. Their varieties are described in relation to medication dose, usually in relation to peaks and troughs of medication levels. For example, peak-dose dyskinesias usually respond to a decrease in the dose; if the patient is taking a COMT inhibitor, this should be stopped. "Off" dyskinesias can be treated in several ways, including shortening the dosing interval, increasing the dose of levodopa/carbidopa, or adding entacapone.

F. Surgical therapies for PD are another modality of comprehensive therapy for some patients. Deep brain stimulation (DBS) of the subthalamic nucleus is typically reserved for refractory tremor and severe dyskinesia. Extensive evaluation is required prior to the surgery to ensure correct diagnosis and to document the neurologic examination before and after medications. Psychiatric screening is required. Generally, the benefit from DBS is only as good as the patient's best response to medication ("on" time). In most cases, DBS may enable a reduction but not an elimination of dopaminergic therapy.

References

DATATOP. A decade of neuroprotective therapy. Parkinson study group. Deprenyl and Tocopherol Antioxidant Therapy of Parkinsonism. Ann Neurol 1998;44(3 suppl 1):S160–166.

Driver-Dunckley E, Samanta J, Stacy M. Pathological gambling associated with dopamine agonist therapy in PD. Neurology 2003;61(3):422–423.

Lang AE, Widner H. Deep brain stimulation for Parkinson's disease: patient selection and evaluation. Mov Disord 2002;17(Suppl 3): S94–101.

Parkinson Study Group. Effects of coenzyme Q10 in early Parkinson disease: evidence of slowing of the functional decline. Arch Neurol 2002;59(10):1541–1550.

Van Camp G, Flamez A, Cosyns B, et al. Treatment of Parkinson's disease with pergolide and relation to restrictive valvular heart disease. Lancet 2004;363(9416):1179–1183.

Van Den Eden SK, Tanner CM, Bernstein AL, et al. Incidence of Parkinson's disease: variation by age, gender and race/ethnicity. Am J Epidemiol 2003;157:1015–1122.

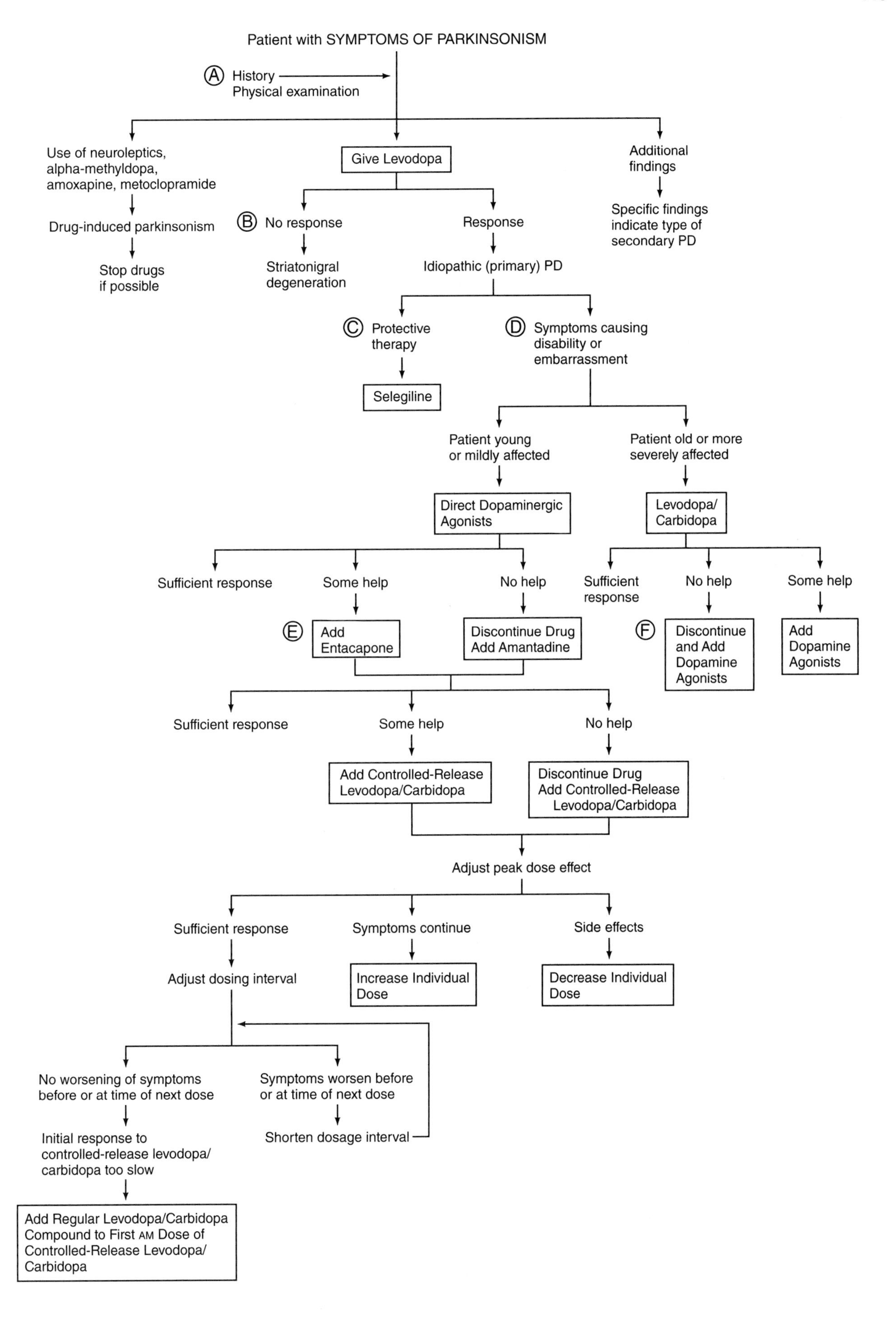
Patient with SYMPTOMS OF PARKINSONISM
(A) History
Physical examination
Use of neuroleptics, alpha-methyldopa, amoxapine, metoclopramide
Drug-induced parkinsonism
Stop drugs if possible
Give Levodopa
(B) No response
Striatonigral degeneration
Response
Idiopathic (primary) PD
Additional findings
Specific findings indicate type of secondary PD
(C) Protective therapy
Selegiline
(D) Symptoms causing disability or embarrassment
Patient young or mildly affected
Direct Dopaminergic Agonists
Patient old or more severely affected
Levodopa/ Carbidopa
Sufficient response
Some help
No help
(E) Add Entacapone
Discontinue Drug Add Amantadine
Sufficient response
No help
Some help
(F) Discontinue and Add Dopamine Agonists
Add Dopamine Agonists
Sufficient response
Some help
No help
Add Controlled-Release Levodopa/Carbidopa
Discontinue Drug Add Controlled-Release Levodopa/Carbidopa
Adjust peak dose effect
Sufficient response
Symptoms continue
Side effects
Adjust dosing interval
Increase Individual Dose
Decrease Individual Dose
No worsening of symptoms before or at time of next dose
Symptoms worsen before or at time of next dose
Initial response to controlled-release levodopa/ carbidopa too slow
Shorten dosage interval
Add Regular Levodopa/Carbidopa Compound to First AM Dose of Controlled-Release Levodopa/ Carbidopa

PERIPHERAL NEUROPATHY

Ronan J. Walsh, MD

Peripheral neuropathies can affect peripheral sensory, motor, and autonomic nerves and on occasion the cranial nerves. Diagnosis is challenging because of the multiplicity of peripheral neuropathies. Thus, it is essential to perform a detailed history and examination to narrow the differential diagnosis.

A. In taking a detailed history, consider the following questions. What systems are involved? Are the symptoms mainly sensory, motor, or a combination of both? Is there an autonomic neuropathy (e.g., orthostatic hypotension, impaired sweating, constipation, diarrhea, impotence, gastroparesis)? Sensory nerve fibers are commonly involved, but this may be a result of large- or small-fiber dysfunction. Patients with a small-fiber neuropathy present with severe neuropathic pain. Complaints of positive phenomena (e.g., burning, prickling, tingling) are useful in differentiating hereditary from acquired forms of peripheral neuropathy. Patients with hereditary motor and sensory neuropathy (HMSN) generally do not have positive symptoms. In addition, patients whose main complaint is severe incoordination and ataxia from loss of proprioception typically have loss of the sensory nerve ganglion, known as ganglionopathy or neuronopathy. What was the temporal nature of the neuropathy in terms of onset and progression? Neuropathies may be acute (evolution over hours to 1 month), subacute (evolution over 1–2 months), or chronic (progression over 2 months) in onset, and the subsequent course can be monophasic, relapsing-remitting, stable, or slowly or rapidly progressive. It is important to inquire into past medical history, medications, illicit drug use, toxic exposures, and family history. Primary systemic disorders (e.g., diabetes mellitus, HIV infection, cancer) can cause peripheral neuropathy and may be the presenting manifestation of the disease. Patients should be asked about their work to see if they are exposed to toxins. Also, risk factors for HIV infection should be explored, particularly in patients with otherwise unexplained peripheral neuropathy. A detailed family history is essential to address whether the neuropathy is hereditary or acquired. Some family members may be only very mildly affected, so a family history is not always apparent to the patient or other family members. Electrophysiologic studies of family members may clarify this.

B. What is the pattern of motor and sensory involvement? Is it symmetric or asymmetric? Is weakness proximal and/or distal? Is the face or trunk affected? Axonal neuropathies manifest in a length-dependent manner, so the distal territories of the longest nerves are the most severely and initially affected. As a result, a symmetric stocking-glove distribution of symptoms and signs is seen. If the arms are more involved than the legs, or the proximal extremities are more affected than distal extremities, this suggests a demyelinating neuropathy or ganglionopathy, which is not length dependent. If there is proximal weakness with no or minimal sensory symptoms, this should raise the concern of a myopathy, neuromuscular junction defect, or spinal muscular atrophy instead of a peripheral neuropathy. Nevertheless, severe proximal weakness can be seen in certain types of peripheral neuropathy. Also, although distal weakness is most often seen in peripheral neuropathies, a few myopathies can present with significant distal weakness (distal muscular dystrophy, myotonic dystrophy, and inclusion body myositis). Additionally, myasthenia gravis can also rarely present with distal weakness. The different sensory modalities (pain, touch, temperature, vibration, and proprioception) should be assessed in all patients. Large-diameter sensory nerves mainly convey deep touch and proprioception, whereas temperature and pain are conveyed by small-diameter nerve fibers. Vibratory perception is carried by both large- and small-diameter nerve fibers. Small-diameter nerve fibers are preferentially affected in some neuropathies (e.g., amyloid neuropathy), whereas other neuropathies have a predilection for larger fibers (e.g., chronic inflammatory demyelinating polyradiculoneuropathy [CIDP]). In amyotrophic lateral sclerosis (ALS), myopathy, or myasthenia gravis, the sensory examination should be normal unless the patient has a concurrent neuropathy. Detailed motor strength testing elucidates the distribution of muscle weakness and atrophy. Muscles should be inspected for evidence of abnormal movements (e.g., fasciculations, myokymia), which are seen in certain neuropathic conditions (e.g., ALS, radiation plexopathy). Muscle tone is usually normal or diminished in a peripheral neuropathy, whereas spastic tone is suggestive of ALS. Ankle jerks are usually lost relatively early on in axonal neuropathies. If upper extremity reflexes are lost or there is a generalized early areflexia, this is suggestive of a demyelinating process or ganglionopathy. Upper motor neuron signs such as pathologically brisk reflexes and extensor plantar responses are not seen in peripheral neuropathies unless there is additional CNS dysfunction, as in ALS. Patients should be asked to walk on their heels and toes because this can unmask subtle distal leg weakness. Asking the patient to stand with feet together and eyes closed assesses the

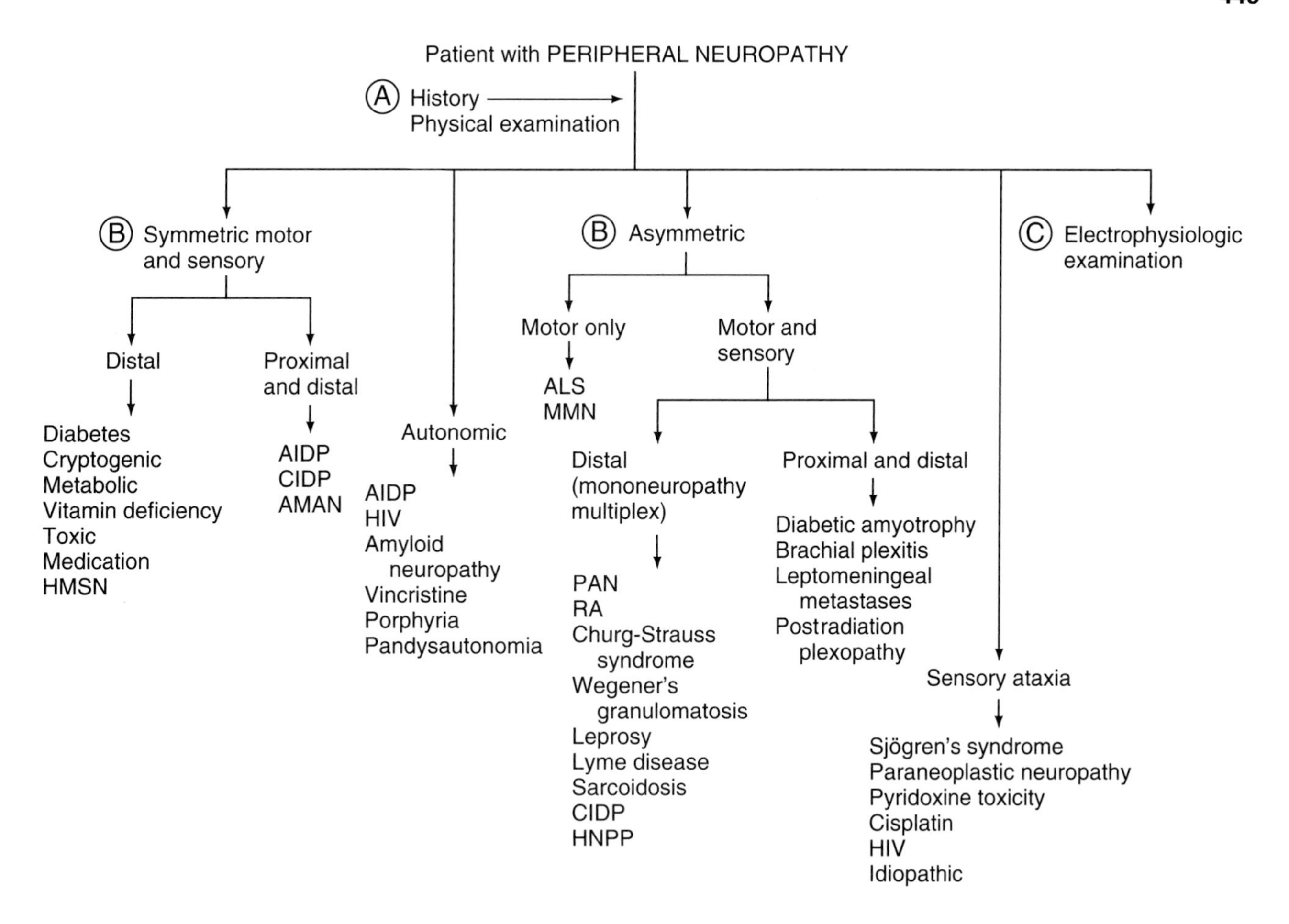

AIDP, Acute idiopathic demyelinating polyneuropathy; AMAN, acute motor axonal neuropathy; HNPP, hereditary neuropathy with liability to pressure palsies; MMN, multifocal motor neuropathy; PAN, polyarteritis nodosa; RA, rheumatoid arthritis.

function of the large-diameter sensory neurons and the posterior columns, which are abnormal in ganglionopathy or a spinocerebellar degeneration (Romberg's sign will be present in these disorders).

C. The electrophysiologic evaluation involves electromyography (EMG) and nerve conduction studies (NCS). These studies are often essential in the evaluation of peripheral neuropathies, can illuminate patterns that are consistent with particular families of disorders, and will often essentially rule out other disorders. A consultation with a neurologist can be valuable in planning the approach to electrodiagnostic testing.

References

Adams RD, Victor M, Ropper AH. Principles of Neurology, 6th ed. New York: McGraw-Hill, 1996.

Amato AA, Zwarts MJ, Dumitru D. Electrodiagnostic Medicine, 2nd ed. Philadelphia: Hanley and Belfus, 2001.

Barohn RJ. Approach to peripheral neuropathy and neuronopathy. Semin Neurol 1998;18:7–18.

Dyck PJ, Thomas PK, eds. Peripheral Neuropathy, 4th ed. Philadelphia: WB Saunders, 2005.

Logigian EL, Herrmann DN. Approach to and classification of peripheral neuropathy. In Samuels MA, Feske SK, eds. Office Practice of Neurology, 2nd ed. Philadelphia: Churchill Livingstone, 2003:569–575.

Wolfe GI, Baker NS, Amato AA, et al. Chronic cryptogenic sensory polyneuropathy: clinical and laboratory characteristics. Arch Neurol 1999;56:540–547.

HYPERKINESIAS

Yvette M. Bordelon, MD, PhD

Disorders of movement are generally classified into two categories: those with too little movement (hypokinesias) and those with excess movement (hyperkinesias). Hypokinetic movement disorders include Parkinson's disease (see Parkinson's Disease chapter) and atypical parkinsonian syndromes. The focus of this chapter is hyperkinesias, which include involuntary movements such as chorea, dystonia, myoclonus, tics, and tremor (see Tremor chapter). Most movement disorders result from impairment of the basal ganglia circuitry. The key to diagnosis of hyperkinesias is history and neurologic examination.

A. Chorea is defined as brief, irregular, nonsustained movements that flow between muscle groups and can be partially suppressible. Other similar types of irregular, flowing movements include athetosis and ballism. Athetosis is slower than chorea and more typically affects distal extremities. Ballism describes large-amplitude choreic movements. The etiologies of chorea encompass primary causes such as inherited disorders (e.g., Huntington's disease, neuroacanthocytosis, Wilson's disease, and ataxia-telangiectasia), secondary causes (e.g., infections, structural lesions, and metabolic abnormalities), and physiologic chorea (seen in infancy). Treatment of chorea is challenging, but symptoms may be controlled with amantadine, neuroleptics, and dopamine-depleting agents such as tetrabenazine and reserpine.

B. Dystonia results from uncontrolled co-contraction of agonist and antagonist muscles causing abnormal postures of the affected body part. It can be classified by location (focal or generalized) or by etiology. Examples of focal dystonia include cervical dystonia (torticollis), blepharospasm, task-specific dystonia (writer's cramp, embouchure dystonia), and spasmodic dysphonia. Generalized dystonia can result from inherited disorders, including DYT-1 dystonia (Oppenheim dystonia) and dopa-responsive dystonia; from perinatal injury; or from heredodegenerative diseases (e.g., Wilson's disease, Huntington's disease). Dystonia may be alleviated by anticholinergics, baclofen, or benzodiazepines. Botulinum toxin injections into affected muscles work well for many types of focal dystonia. Deep brain stimulation of the globus pallidus internus is used to treat medication-refractory dystonia, particularly DYT-1 dystonia. Dopa-responsive dystonia is exquisitely sensitive to low doses of levodopa.

C. Myoclonus is a rapid involuntary movement; it can be positive, as in a muscle contraction, or negative if there is a lapse of muscle tone. Asterixis is a form of negative myoclonus and is seen in patients with metabolic or toxic encephalopathies such as hepatic dysfunction. Myoclonus can be generalized, focal, or segmental. It may result from damage to the cortex, brainstem spinal cord, or peripheral nerves. It is common in some types of seizure disorders (e.g., juvenile myoclonic epilepsy) and is frequently seen after global hypoxic injury. Myoclonus may respond to treatment with benzodiazepines.

D. Tics are also rapid movements of particular body parts but range in severity from being simple motor tics involving one muscle group to complex and repetitive movements of multiple muscle groups. Tics are considered to be involuntary, but they are associated with a premonitory "urge" and can be suppressed briefly. Tics may change in severity, location, and frequency over time. When motor tics appear in combination with vocal tics, a diagnosis of Tourette's syndrome should be considered. Tics are commonly treated with clonidine, neuroleptics, or dopamine depleters when necessary.

Tardive dyskinesia is a term describing a potentially permanent movement disorder that results from the use of dopamine-blocking agents such as neuroleptics and antiemetics (metoclopramide). It is characterized by choreic and/or dystonic movements affecting any part of the body but particularly affecting the mouth and tongue (orobuccal lingual dyskinesias).

References

Agarwal P, Frucht SJ. Myoclonus. Curr Opin Neurol 2003;16:515–521.
Bhidayasiri R, Truong DD. Chorea and related disorders. Postgrad Med J 2004;80:527–534.
Bressman SB. Dystonia genotypes, phenotypes and classification. Adv Neurol 2004;94:101–107.

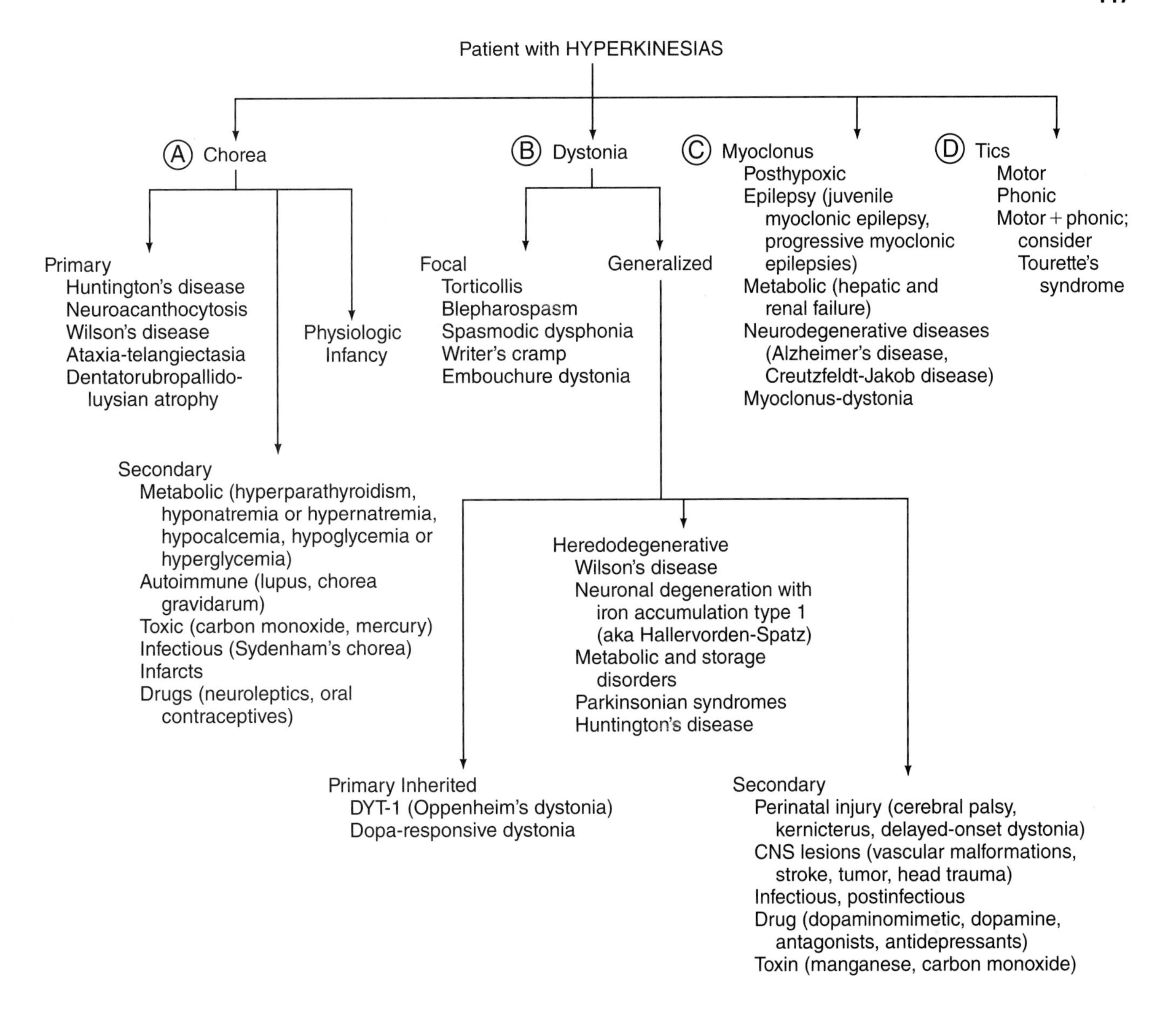
Patient with HYPERKINESIAS
(A) Chorea
Primary
Huntington's disease
Neuroacanthocytosis
Wilson's disease
Ataxia-telangiectasia
Dentatorubropallido-luysian atrophy
Physiologic
Infancy
Secondary
Metabolic (hyperparathyroidism, hyponatremia or hypernatremia, hypocalcemia, hypoglycemia or hyperglycemia)
Autoimmune (lupus, chorea gravidarum)
Toxic (carbon monoxide, mercury)
Infectious (Sydenham's chorea)
Infarcts
Drugs (neuroleptics, oral contraceptives)
(B) Dystonia
Focal
Torticollis
Blepharospasm
Spasmodic dysphonia
Writer's cramp
Embouchure dystonia
Generalized
Heredodegenerative
Wilson's disease
Neuronal degeneration with iron accumulation type 1 (aka Hallervorden-Spatz)
Metabolic and storage disorders
Parkinsonian syndromes
Huntington's disease
Primary Inherited
DYT-1 (Oppenheim's dystonia)
Dopa-responsive dystonia
Secondary
Perinatal injury (cerebral palsy, kernicterus, delayed-onset dystonia)
CNS lesions (vascular malformations, stroke, tumor, head trauma)
Infectious, postinfectious
Drug (dopaminomimetic, dopamine, antagonists, antidepressants)
Toxin (manganese, carbon monoxide)
(C) Myoclonus
Posthypoxic
Epilepsy (juvenile myoclonic epilepsy, progressive myoclonic epilepsies)
Metabolic (hepatic and renal failure)
Neurodegenerative diseases (Alzheimer's disease, Creutzfeldt-Jakob disease)
Myoclonus-dystonia
(D) Tics
Motor
Phonic
Motor + phonic; consider Tourette's syndrome

MUSCLE CRAMPS AND ACHES

Ronan J. Walsh, MD

"True" cramps are sudden, periodic, involuntary, painful contractions of a muscle, or part of a muscle, that last from seconds to several minutes. They are usually relieved by stretching of the muscle. Cramps must be differentiated from *myalgias:* muscle pains that are not associated with muscle contractions. Contractions may also occur without pain. These may be associated with specific activities or occupations, such as "writer's cramp." These contractions are actually *dystonias* that typically affect "overlearned" tasks, such as writing or playing an instrument. Cramps are often confused with *contractures,* seen in certain metabolic myopathies such as phosphorylase deficiency (McArdle's disease). Contractures usually occur with intense exercise and result from depletion of muscle energy stores. There may also be a history of myoglobinuria. Contractures, unlike cramps, are electrically silent on electromyography (EMG). True cramps may occur spontaneously at rest, but more often they are precipitated by a muscle contraction. They are neural in origin, caused by a hyperexcitability of the motor neurons supplying the muscle. In many cases the reason for recurrent cramps remains unclear even after a complete diagnostic evaluation. Treatment with quinine sulfate often is helpful in controlling nocturnal cramps. Frequent daytime cramps may respond to carbamazepine or amitriptyline. After establishing through history that the patient suffers with true cramps, the physician should then explore whether they occur at rest or with exercise.

A. In older patients, children, and pregnant women, leg cramps tend to occur at rest, often at night, after unusual daytime activity, and especially when the feet are cold. The neurologic examination and serum creatine kinase (CK) and aldolase levels are normal. These may require no treatment or be improved by stretching the affected muscle three times a day.

B. Cramps occurring at rest or precipitated by minor exercise may have a specific underlying cause and are listed in the accompanying diagram. These causes should be identified by a thorough history and laboratory examinations, including thyroid-stimulating hormone (TSH), routine chemistry panel (including renal and liver function studies), CK, B_{12}, and folate. These cramps usually lessen or resolve with treatment of the underlying problem.

C. For frequent cramps precipitated during or after exercise, in addition to the laboratory tests listed previously perform a forearm exercise test in which serum lactate, pyruvate, and ammonia are measured at rest and after 1 minute of exercise every minute for 5 minutes. EMG should be performed, looking for evidence of myopathy. Muscle biopsy should be considered. A history of myoglobinuria must be sought.

D. Exercise intolerance, along with cramps or myalgia, characterizes the metabolic myopathies. These disorders commonly result in myoglobinuria after especially strenuous exercise. All but the last two listed are abnormalities of glycogen or glucose metabolism. A "second-wind phenomenon" is a specific feature of myophosphorylase deficiency in which, after the onset of mild exertional cramps, patients rest briefly and then may resume the exercise at the previous or a slightly reduced level. Carnitine palmitoyl transferase deficiency is a disorder of lipid metabolism in which cramps are precipitated by more prolonged strenuous exercise.

E. Cramps, and other entities that may be confused with cramps, occur in a variety of neurologic and neuromuscular disorders. These disorders are accompanied by weakness and/or sensory loss on neurologic examination. Because investigations to evaluate the diagnostic possibilities vary from patient to patient in this situation, such cases are usually best handled by a neurologist. Many of the conditions are treatable.

F. It is important to remember that leg pain and cramps in adults that are precipitated by exercise and promptly relieved by rest often are the result of ischemia from peripheral vascular disease. These patients with "vascular claudication" may have risk factors for cardiovascular disease along with trophic changes and reduced pulses in their legs. Surgical treatment and addressing the cardiovascular risk factors can be successful.

References

Joekes AM. Cramp: a review. J R Soc Med 1982;75:546.

Layzer RB. Muscle pain, cramps, and fatigue. In Engel AG, Franzini-Armstrong C, eds. Myology, 2nd ed, Vol 2. New York: McGraw-Hill, 1994:1754.

McGee SR. Muscle cramps. Arch Intern Med 1990;150:511.

Miller TM, Layzer RB. Muscle cramps. Muscle Nerve 2005 32(4): 431–442.

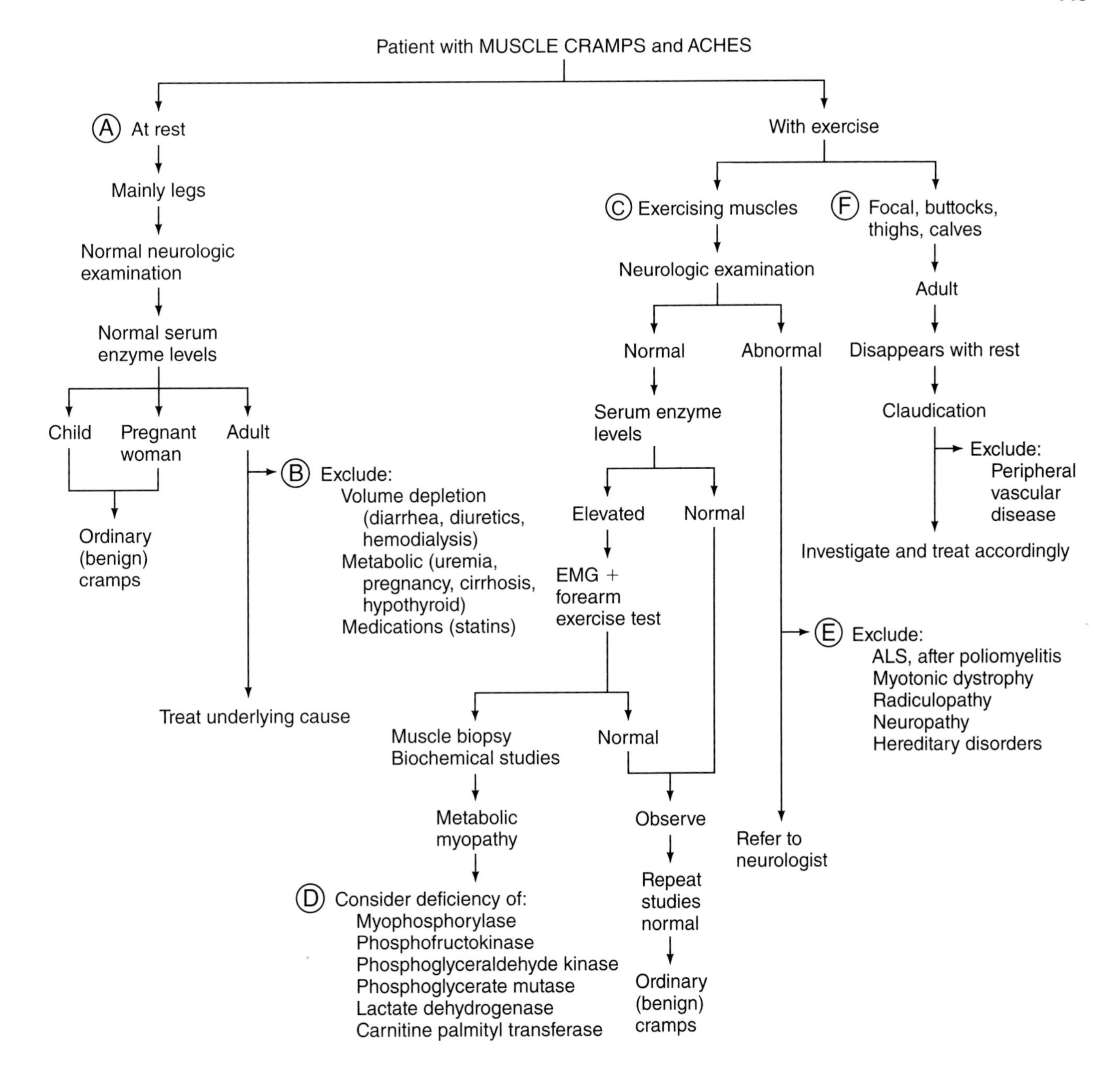
Patient with MUSCLE CRAMPS and ACHES
(A) At rest
Mainly legs
Normal neurologic examination
Normal serum enzyme levels
Child
Pregnant woman
Adult
Ordinary (benign) cramps
(B) Exclude:
Volume depletion (diarrhea, diuretics, hemodialysis)
Metabolic (uremia, pregnancy, cirrhosis, hypothyroid)
Medications (statins)
Treat underlying cause
With exercise
(C) Exercising muscles
Neurologic examination
Normal
Abnormal
Serum enzyme levels
Elevated
Normal
EMG + forearm exercise test
Muscle biopsy
Biochemical studies
Normal
Metabolic myopathy
(D) Consider deficiency of:
Myophosphorylase
Phosphofructokinase
Phosphoglyceraldehyde kinase
Phosphoglycerate mutase
Lactate dehydrogenase
Carnitine palmityl transferase
Observe
Repeat studies normal
Ordinary (benign) cramps
(E) Exclude:
ALS, after poliomyelitis
Myotonic dystrophy
Radiculopathy
Neuropathy
Hereditary disorders
Refer to neurologist
(F) Focal, buttocks, thighs, calves
Adult
Disappears with rest
Claudication
Exclude:
Peripheral vascular disease
Investigate and treat accordingly

ACUTE CONFUSIONAL STATE

Bradford C. Dickerson, MD

Acute confusional states encompass a range of clinical syndromes, variably labeled as encephalopathy or delirium. The dominant clinical sign is inattention. Nearly all other cognitive functions will also appear to be impaired, but this is usually attributable to the attentional deficit. The most common causes of acute confusional states are systemic medical conditions, such as infectious processes, metabolic derangements, toxins, and the effects of medications. Some primary pathologies of the brain can produce acute confusional states, as may primary psychiatric illnesses that impair attention and concentration. A patient presenting with acute confusion should be evaluated emergently and monitored intensively; confusion may herald serious pathologic processes that can lead rapidly to compromised vital function, coma, and death.

A. The critical keys to the diagnosis of most acute confusional states can be found in the history, but most patients will be unable to provide useful information themselves. Thus, it is essential to attempt to obtain as much collateral history as possible, ideally from family members or friends, but additionally from medical personnel or others. In hospitalized patients, chart review may provide important clues to the timing of onset or possible etiologies, such as medications. Next, clinical examination and laboratory testing are crucial, followed in many cases by neuroimaging or other studies. The mental status examination should focus on attentional and arousal systems, and should attempt to provide semiquantitative information for the record that can be used as a comparison against which to judge clinical decline or improvement. Tests that the patient is unable to perform are typically less useful than tests that can be performed, at least in part. The Mini-Mental State Exam is often not particularly useful in this setting. Rather, simple bedside attentional tests may be helpful, such as a continuous performance test in which the patient is asked to remember a single letter (e.g., "A") and to raise a finger when that letter is heard. The examiner then states a series of random letters, approximately one per second, and observes the patient's responses, noting the number of targets (A's) missed and the number of foils (non-A letters) endorsed. Other useful tests include the timed recitation of days of the week or months of the year—first forward and then backward. Observe for easy distractibility (due to externally or internally generated stimuli, possibly suggesting hallucinations) or perseveration. The neurologic examination can be particularly valuable in providing etiologic clues; for example, metabolic derangements may induce signs that accompany confusion, such as asterixis or myoclonus. Focal neurologic signs such as hemiparesis, visual-field defects, asymmetric reflexes, an upgoing toe, or hemineglect suggest the presence of focal brain lesions, which may produce confusional states (e.g., posterior cerebral or right middle cerebral artery infarcts). Laboratory tests and neuroimaging or other studies often provide critical information in this setting.

B. Focal brain lesions of various etiologies may present with acute confusional states. Confusion and agitation may result from focal pathology in right frontal and parietal lobes, unilateral medial temporal lobe lesions in either hemisphere, or midbrain-diencephalic lesions. Ischemic cerebral infarcts of tissue supplied by middle cerebral arteries (usually right), posterior cerebral arteries, or the basilar artery may cause acute confusional states, sometimes with minimal or no accompanying focal neurologic signs. Mass lesions of different types (e.g., tumor, subdural hematoma, intracerebral hemorrhage, abscess) may produce similar clinical features. In many cases involving mass lesions or midbrain-diencephalic pathology, there is an accompanying alteration in arousal.

C. Other primary cerebral processes may present with confusional states. Patients with mild traumatic brain injury may exhibit transient loss of consciousness (i.e., concussion), with or without residual problems with attention, concentration, and memory (post-concussion syndrome). More significant brain injury (e.g., contusion) may produce permanent deficits; the profile of cognitive deficits depends on the areas involved. Severe head injury may result in coma, and evaluation and treatment should proceed according to intensive care protocols (see the section Coma). In older patients, subdural hematoma may result from trivial head trauma. In young patients, migraine may present with confusion with or without headache or other focal neurologic findings.

D. Acute confusion may be the presenting sign of systemic or CNS infection. In febrile confusional states, aggressive workup for infectious etiologies is key, yet infectious etiologies must be kept in mind even when a fever is not obviously present, particularly in older patients or those with immunologic compromise (including patients with an oncologic history). Bacterial and viral agents are more likely to cause acute behavior changes than fungal agents, which tend to produce a

(Continued on page 452)

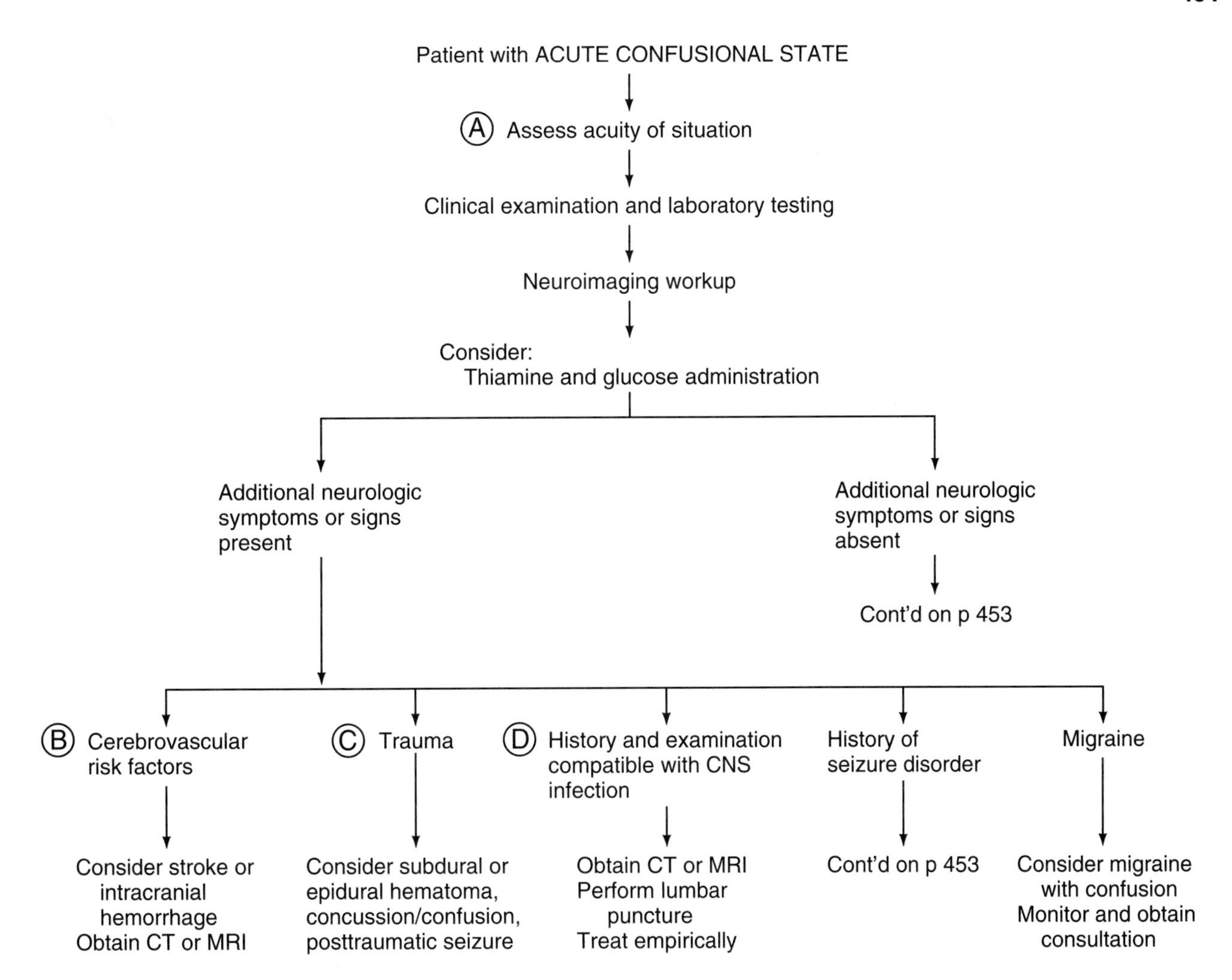
Patient with ACUTE CONFUSIONAL STATE
(A) Assess acuity of situation
Clinical examination and laboratory testing
Neuroimaging workup
Consider:
Thiamine and glucose administration
Additional neurologic symptoms or signs present
Additional neurologic symptoms or signs absent
Cont'd on p 453
(B) Cerebrovascular risk factors
(C) Trauma
(D) History and examination compatible with CNS infection
History of seizure disorder
Migraine
Consider stroke or intracranial hemorrhage
Obtain CT or MRI
Consider subdural or epidural hematoma, concussion/confusion, posttraumatic seizure
Obtain CT or MRI
Perform lumbar puncture
Treat empirically
Cont'd on p 453
Consider migraine with confusion
Monitor and obtain consultation

more indolent course of symptoms. Empiric treatment of herpes simplex encephalitis should be strongly considered in most febrile confusional states until other etiologies can be identified, because significant permanent neurologic impairment may be preventable. Also consider CNS abscesses whether or not focal signs are present. In older patients, common systemic infections such as urinary tract infection may induce significant confusion, which may persist longer that expected after treatment. A low clinical threshold for lumbar puncture must be maintained.

E. Confusional states may be secondary to metabolic derangements resulting from systemic illness. The potential causes are numerous and include thyroid and other endocrine, hepatic, renal, and pulmonary dysfunction. Any condition leading to hypoxia, such as myocardial infarction or cardiac arrhythmia, may lead to a confusional state. Along with a history and neurologic examination, a general medical examination surveying all organ systems is essential in the initial evaluation of a patient with acute confusion. Patients with a history of dementia often develop acutely worsened mental status during periods of intercurrent systemic illness. Treatment of the underlying cause is the primary intervention, but confusion may resolve slowly, particularly in older individuals.

F. Exogenous substances may cause a toxic confusional state. Medications (particularly those with prominent anticholinergic effects) may adversely affect cognitive function. Neuroleptic malignant syndrome must be considered in patients receiving these medications or in patients withdrawn rapidly from levodopa or dopamine agonists. A toxicology screen will reveal drugs of abuse or other agents. Acute confusional syndromes in patients who use alcohol include intoxication, withdrawal, and Wernicke's encephalopathy (classically ophthalmoplegia, ataxia, and encephalopathy, but often presenting without the full triad). The administration of thiamine prior to glucose is essential. Other toxic agents include organic chemical substances (e.g., insecticides), heavy metals, and carbon monoxide.

G. Consider postictal confusion in a patient with a known seizure disorder. Anticonvulsant medication effects—particularly abruptly increased levels due to drug-drug interactions—may cause confusion. Alterations in consciousness may result from absence or complex partial seizures. Although relatively uncommon, nonconvulsive status epilepticus should always be considered in confused patients with or without a seizure history. If the diagnosis is in doubt, treat with benzodiazepines and obtain an urgent EEG, if available.

H. Patients with known psychiatric disorders may present with confusion or inattention. The effects of psychiatric medications must always be considered in this setting.

References

Lipowski ZJ. Delirium: Acute Confusional States, Revised Edition. New York: Oxford University Press, 2005.

Mesulam M-M. Attentional networks, confusional states, and neglect syndromes. In Mesulam M-M, ed. Principles of Behavioral and Cognitive Neurology, 2nd ed. New York: Oxford University Press, 2000:174–256.

Ronthal M. Confusional states and metabolic encephalopathy. In Samuels MA, Feske SK, eds. Office Practice of Neurology. Philadelphia: Churchill-Livingstone, 2003:886–890.

Weintraub S. Examining mental state. In Samuels MA, Feske SK, eds. Office Practice of Neurology. Philadelphia: Churchill-Livingstone, 2003:850–858.

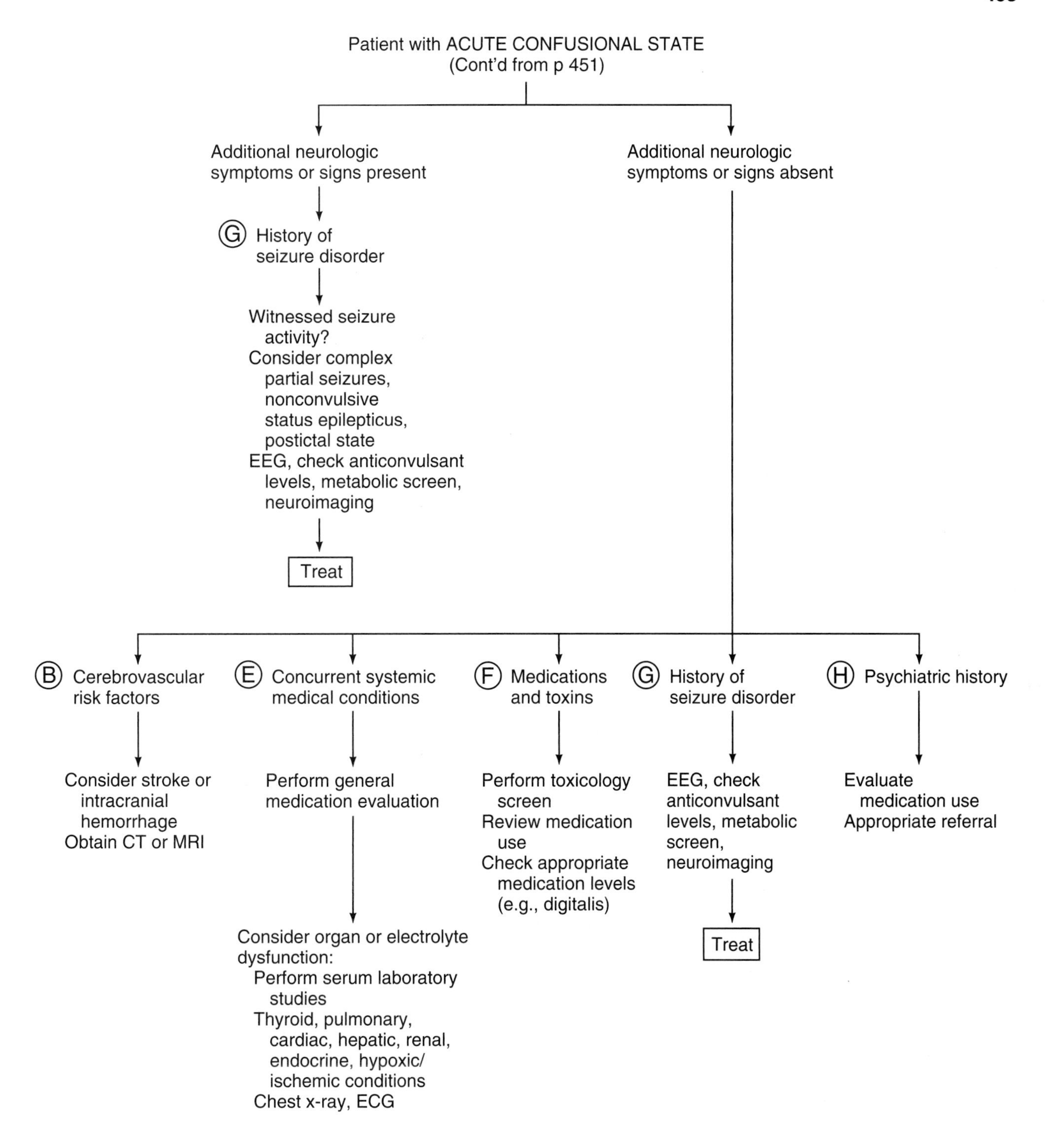
Patient with ACUTE CONFUSIONAL STATE
(Cont'd from p 451)
Additional neurologic symptoms or signs present
G History of seizure disorder
Witnessed seizure activity?
Consider complex partial seizures, nonconvulsive status epilepticus, postictal state
EEG, check anticonvulsant levels, metabolic screen, neuroimaging
Treat
Additional neurologic symptoms or signs absent
B Cerebrovascular risk factors
Consider stroke or intracranial hemorrhage
Obtain CT or MRI
E Concurrent systemic medical conditions
Perform general medication evaluation
Consider organ or electrolyte dysfunction:
Perform serum laboratory studies
Thyroid, pulmonary, cardiac, hepatic, renal, endocrine, hypoxic/ ischemic conditions
Chest x-ray, ECG
F Medications and toxins
Perform toxicology screen
Review medication use
Check appropriate medication levels (e.g., digitalis)
G History of seizure disorder
EEG, check anticonvulsant levels, metabolic screen, neuroimaging
Treat
H Psychiatric history
Evaluate medication use
Appropriate referral

CHRONIC BEHAVIOR CHANGE

Bradford C. Dickerson, MD

Chronic behavior change is a useful descriptor that encompasses dementia, aphasia and other focal cognitive disorders, chronic encephalopathy, and psychiatric disorders. Dementia is a clinical syndrome defined as sustained or progressive decline in cognition or behavior that interferes with routine daily activities. Any domains of mental function may be affected, including memory, language, visuospatial skills, attention, executive function, judgment, and social or emotional behavior. The persistence of the deficit(s) differentiates dementia from acute confusional state or delirium (see the section on acute confusional state). Although many types of dementia are progressive, some (e.g., posttraumatic) are relatively static. Aphasia and other focal cognitive disorders are often chronic but are not considered dementias because they may not encompass multiple domains of cognition or behavior and may not significantly interfere with routine activities outside the specific impairment. They may result from residual static damage following acute brain insults, such as stroke, abscess, or tumor. *Chronic encephalopathy* is a loosely defined term that implies an ongoing medical etiology, such as hepatic or renal encephalopathy. Chronic psychiatric disorders, by definition, involve chronic behavior change and are discussed elsewhere (see the section on behavioral medicine). The list of possible causes of these varieties of chronic behavior change is long, so it is useful to pursue an organized approach to evaluation, with the goal of identifying the most specific diagnosis and treatment. It is critical to remember that, although most forms of dementia or chronic behavior change are irreversible, they are all treatable. Treatment may (rarely) reverse or partly reverse the overall level of impairment, may produce modest improvements in specific aspects of cognition, may alleviate behavioral symptoms, or may improve safety. Comprehensive, multidisciplinary treatment programs for dementia include pharmacologic and nonpharmacologic therapy for cognitive and behavioral symptoms, patient and family support and education, the maximization of safety, and referral to social services and community resources.

A. As is the case for acute behavior change, a detailed history is the essential first step in the evaluation of chronic behavior change. The first office visit is often best devoted primarily to the gathering of information from the patient and a knowledgeable informant (spouse, child, friend). A structured approach to history taking is helpful, focusing first on specific symptoms and reviewing all domains of cognition and behavior (memory, language, visuospatial skills, attention, executive function, mood, personality, social behavior) and general neurologic function (vision, motor behavior, gait). It is critical to determine the degree to which a patient's routine activities have been altered by these symptoms (slowing, increased mistakes, the need for supervision, the relinquishment of activities). A comprehensive review of systems can reveal important relevant history regarding possible etiologies or potential contributors (e.g., transient ischemic attacks, symptoms suggestive of endocrine dysfunction, sleep disturbance, or depression). A medical and family history can be useful to identify additional clinical context and risk profiles (e.g., cerebrovascular risk, family history of Alzheimer's disease [AD]). Social history is key to the establishment of a premorbid baseline, against which current symptoms should be compared. Highly educated patients may perform surprisingly well on mental status testing but have significant impairment in complex social or vocational activities.

B. The evaluation should include medical and neurologic examination and mental status examination. The presence of medical (e.g., cardiac arrhythmia or carotid bruit) or neurologic (e.g., visual field loss, focal weakness, upgoing toe) signs may provide important etiologic clues. The mental status examination should include observations of the patient's behavior during the interview, particularly focused on arousal and attention, affect, motivation, insight, comportment, and spontaneous use of language. Waxing and waning attention, depressed affect, apathy, denial of deficits or anosognosia, disinhibition or lack of concern, dysarthria, word-finding pauses, or circumlocutory or emptiness of speech may be important signs helpful in the characterization and localization of cerebral dysfunction. A detailed yet focused cognitive examination can yield additional useful information and may yield surprising deficits in patients with relatively preserved social skills. If the mental status examination provides information consistent with the history, the clinician may be satisfied with the characterization of symptoms and signs and wish to pursue an etiologic workup. If questions remain regarding the presence, absence, or nature of cognitive dysfunction, referral for neuropsychologic testing is often helpful. Patients' and family members' reports of cognitive-behavioral symptoms should be taken seriously, and if the constraints of office practice do not allow for the detailed testing of cognitive function, additional resources should be brought to bear, including the expertise of colleagues in behavioral neurology, neuropsychiatry, and neuropsychology.

(Continued on page 456)

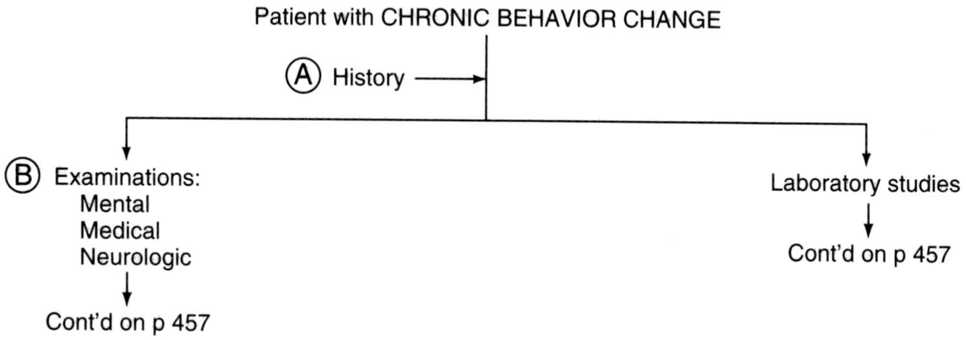

Patient with CHRONIC BEHAVIOR CHANGE

(A) History

(B) Examinations:
- Mental
- Medical
- Neurologic

Cont'd on p 457

Laboratory studies

Cont'd on p 457

C. Laboratory testing, neuroimaging studies, and other tests are essential to consider as part of the workup of patients with chronic behavior change. Just as the cardiologist seeks abnormalities of cardiac structure and function in the evaluation of a patient with chest pain, the neurologist should assess the integrity of brain anatomy (e.g., using MRI) and function (e.g., using positron emission tomography [PET] or single photon emission computed tomography) in the patient with behavioral change. Electroencephalography and lumbar puncture should be considered. Routine screening for thyroid, nutritional, and metabolic abnormalities is important. Depending on local prevalence patterns, syphilis screening should be considered. The medical context may dictate additional laboratory studies.

D. AD classically presents as an insidiously progressive dementia primarily involving memory and executive function, although other forms of the disease may present primarily with visuospatial or language dysfunction. No focal signs are usually found on neurologic examination. Some patients with AD present with affective change, including depression, anxiety, or apathy. Frontotemporal dementia (FTD), much less common than AD and usually presenting at a younger age (50s or 60s), may present with inappropriate or bizarre behavior, personality change, language impairment, or executive dysfunction. This presentation may lead to erroneous primary psychiatric diagnoses. The neuropathologic process of AD usually preferentially affects the medial temporal lobe and temporoparietal cortex, whereas FTD usually involves the frontal and anterior temporal cortex. These changes are often detectable in patients as atrophy of these regions on MRI scans or hypometabolism of these regions on PET. Current treatments follow the rubric outlined previously, with cholinesterase inhibitors and Memantine aimed toward improvements in cognitive function.

E. Cerebrovascular dementia may present with a history of stepwise cognitive decline, often primarily involving executive dysfunction, accompanied in many cases by focal findings on neurologic examination. A clinical context involving cerebrovascular risk factors and neuroimaging evidence of white matter hyperintensities is supportive of this diagnosis. Prophylactic treatment of cerebrovascular risk factors and cholinesterase inhibitors are the current mainstays of therapy.

F. In patients with movement-related symptoms and signs and cognitive changes including slowed thinking and inattention, executive dysfunction, often accompanied by hypophonic or dysarthric speech and apathetic or depressed appearance, the major diagnoses to consider are the dementias associated with one of the extrapyramidal syndromes. These include dementia with Lewy bodies (DLB), Parkinson's disease (PD), progressive supranuclear palsy (PSP), corticobasal ganglionic degeneration (CBD), and Huntington's disease (HD). Characteristic features include fluctuating cognition with pronounced variation in attention and alertness, well-formed visual hallucinations, and parkinsonism in DLB; bradykinesia, rigidity, and tremor in PD; eye movement abnormalities and axial rigidity in PSP; akinetic rigidity (often asymmetric), apraxia or alien limb syndrome, and cortical sensory loss in CBD; and choreoathetosis in HD. Differentiation of these syndromes is often difficult. An empiric trial of levodopa or other prodopaminergic agents may be beneficial. Avoid neuroleptics in patients with DLB, given severe sensitivity reactions. Cholinesterase inhibitors may be beneficial, as are symptomatic therapies for behavioral symptoms, such as depression.

G. Rapidly progressive cognitive decline accompanied in some cases by neurologic signs including dysarthria, gait disturbance, and myoclonus suggests prion dementias, such as Creutzfeldt-Jakob disease. Periodic epileptiform discharges are classically present on electroencephalogram. Treatment is palliative. The triad of dementia, incontinence, and gait disturbance suggests normal-pressure hydrocephalus (NPH). Neuroimaging typically demonstrates ventricular enlargement disproportionate to cerebral atrophy (ex vacuo ventricular enlargement results from cerebral atrophy but is typically proportionate to atrophy). Removal of a large volume of cerebrospinal fluid via lumbar puncture or drain may result in transient improvement of symptoms and suggests potential responsiveness to ventriculoperitoneal shunt procedure.

H. Exogenous substances may result in a toxic confusional state. Drugs (prescription or otherwise) commonly cause cognitive difficulties. If possible, eliminate from the patient's regimen any agents known to do this (particularly anticholinergic agents). Chronic alcohol use leads to executive dysfunction. Korsakoff's syndrome is primarily an amnesic disorder resulting from thiamine deficiency, often related to alcoholism. Other classes of agents capable of inducing cognitive changes include heavy metals (e.g., arsenic, lead, thallium, manganese, mercury), organic agents (e.g., solvents, organophosphate insecticides), and carbon monoxide.

I. Mass lesions, such as frontal lobe tumors or subdural hematomas, may present primarily with chronic behavior change. In patients with a history of cancer, consider metastases, carcinomatous meningitis, and the effects of chemotherapy or radiation therapy. In paraneoplastic disorders, such as limbic encephalitis, cognitive and behavior change may be the presenting symptom prior to the oncologic diagnosis. Primary or secondary seizure disorders may produce chronic behavioral changes unrelated to ictal events.

J. If history and examination are compatible with CNS infection, consider chronic meningoencephalitis. Nonbacterial infectious agents (e.g., cryptococcal, tuberculous infections) may have a relatively indolent

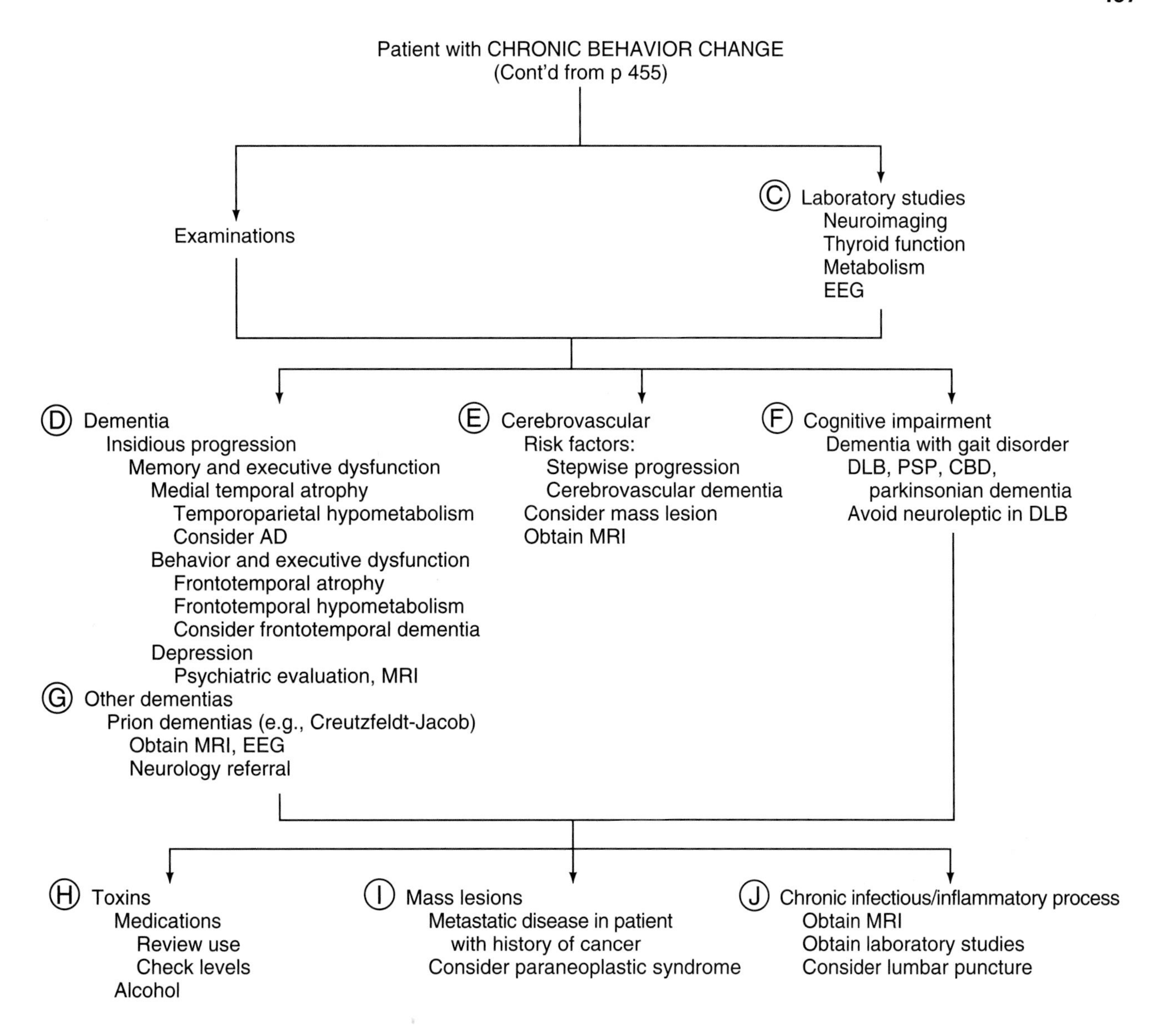

course. Neurosyphilis should be considered, although routine serologic screening is no longer recommended except in endemic regions. Herpes simplex encephalitis classically produces a syndrome of chronic amnesia and behavior change; many patients who succumb to viral encephalitides are left with residual cognitive and behavioral symptoms after acute recovery. Consider HIV dementia in the appropriate setting. Whipple's disease is an amnesic disorder accompanied by a pathognomonic movement disorder of the face (oculomasticatory myorhythmia), caused by the intestinal bacterium *Tropheryma whippelii.*

References

Cummings JL. Alzheimer's disease. N Engl J Med 2004;351:56–67.

Doody RS, Stevens JC, Beck C, et al. Practice parameter: management of dementia (an evidence-based review). Report of the Quality Standards Subcommittee of the American Academy of Neurology. Neurology 2001;56:1154–1166.

Knopman DS, DeKosky ST, Cummings JL, et al. Practice parameter: diagnosis of dementia (an evidence-based review). Report of the Quality Standards Subcommittee of the American Academy of Neurology. Neurology 2001;56:1143–1153.

McKeith IG, Dickson DW, Lowe J, et al. Diagnosis and management of dementia with Lewy bodies. Third report of the DLB consortium. Neurology 2005;65:1–10.

Mendez MF, Cummings JL. Dementia: A Clinical Approach, 3rd ed. Boston: Butterworth-Heinemann, 2003.

DISTURBANCES OF SMELL AND TASTE

Santosh Kesari, MD

Dysfunction of smell or taste usually is not a disease entity in itself; it is usually secondary to another disease process such as sinus disease, medications, toxins, neurodegenerative conditions, tumor, or trauma. Both are insidious symptoms; the patient often does not notice loss of taste, especially when the onset is gradual. Loss of smell, however, may be noticed by the patient as a change in taste sensation. *Anosmia* is the absence of smell sensation; *dysosmia* or *parosmia* is a distorted smell perception, either with or without an odorant stimulus present; and *hyposmia* is a reduced sense of smell. Abnormalities in taste sensation are classified into *ageusia* (absence of taste perception), *hypogeusia* (diminished taste), and *dysgeusia* (distortion of taste resulting in a persistent metallic, bitter, sour, sweet, or salty taste).

A. Diagnostic workup of a patient with smell or taste impairment proves difficult because the complaints are subjective, thus making objective assessment challenging. Evaluation includes a thorough history (gradual or acute onset and other associated findings), physical examination (includes ear, nose, and throat and neurologic examination), and special examination of taste and smell. Head CT with particular attention to the nasal cavities, anterior cranial fossa, and nasal sinuses are important in evaluating for anatomic abnormalities. Further imaging studies, such as MRI, are indicated according to the pathophysiologic process suspected. Biopsy of the olfactory neuroepithelium can be obtained by a needle and is generally a safe procedure. Biopsy utility rests in its ability to demonstrate changes that occur in steroid-dependent anosmia, posttraumatic anosmia, posttrial olfactory dysfunction, and congenital anosmia. Medications affecting the sense of smell and taste are numerous and include opioid analgesics, flunisolide, promethazine, terbinafine, antibiotics, antifungal agents, antiinflammatory drugs, cytotoxic agents, cardiovascular drugs, antiepileptics, psychotropics, nasal decongestants, and antithyroid medications. The true incidence of drug-induced taste and smell disturbances is likely higher because of the infrequency of reporting. Drug-induced smell and taste disturbances can be minimized by avoiding the use of drugs known to induce such disturbances in patients with diseases that make them susceptible to smell and taste disorders. Good nutritional support with zinc supplementation may reduce the possibility of the onset of drug-induced smell and taste disorders. Good oral hygiene coupled with prevention of dry mouth may reduce the incidence of taste disturbances. Once a patient shows signs of such disturbance, an early discontinuation of the offending drug may prevent complete loss or irreversible distortion of smell or taste.

B. Congenital anosmia appears to be caused by absence of olfactory epithelium. The most common congenital disorder is Kallmann's syndrome, in which there is agenesis of the olfactory bulbs in combination with hypogonadism and other developmental abnormalities.

C. Tumors implicated as causes of anosmia are olfactory groove meningiomas, frontal lobe gliomas, and pituitary adenomas with suprasellar extension. Another cause is a large aneurysm of the anterior cerebral or anterior communicating artery. Diseases such as chronic rhinitis and sinusitis or conditions leading to nasal obstruction are common causes of decreased smell. Anosmia caused by these conditions is frequently amenable to treatment; if untreated, it may steadily worsen.

D. Anosmia may occur after even mild head trauma, especially after a blow to the occiput, which causes shearing of the olfactory filaments as they course through the cribriform plate. Although there is no treatment for posttraumatic loss of smell, gradual recovery of smell function occurs in about one third of patients. The olfactory bulbs and their nerves can be damaged during subfrontal craniotomy or as the result of a subarachnoid hemorrhage, meningitis at the base of the skull, or a frontal lobe abscess. Sudden loss of smell, and sometimes also of taste, may occur after an upper respiratory infection. This is more common in older patients and is thought to result from viral damage of the olfactory mucosa. Recovery, if it occurs at all, may take years.

E. Dysosmia is common in elderly persons with or without dementia. In Alzheimer's disease, there may be deficits in central processing of smell, rather than a primary sensory impairment. Uncinate fits, a form of temporal lobe seizures, consist of brief periods of unpleasant or foul odor perception, together with an alteration of consciousness. Gustatory hallucinations may be part of a temporal lobe seizure and manifestations of other temporal-parietal dysfunction. The diagnosis can be confirmed with EEG, and the seizures can be treated with anticonvulsant medication. Olfactory hallucinations also have been described with illnesses such as depression, schizophrenia, Alzheimer's disease, and alcohol withdrawal.

F. A unilateral loss of taste on the anterior two thirds of the tongue can be found in Bell's palsy and results from involvement of the chorda tympani. Loss of taste as a result of head injury is less common than loss of smell. It may

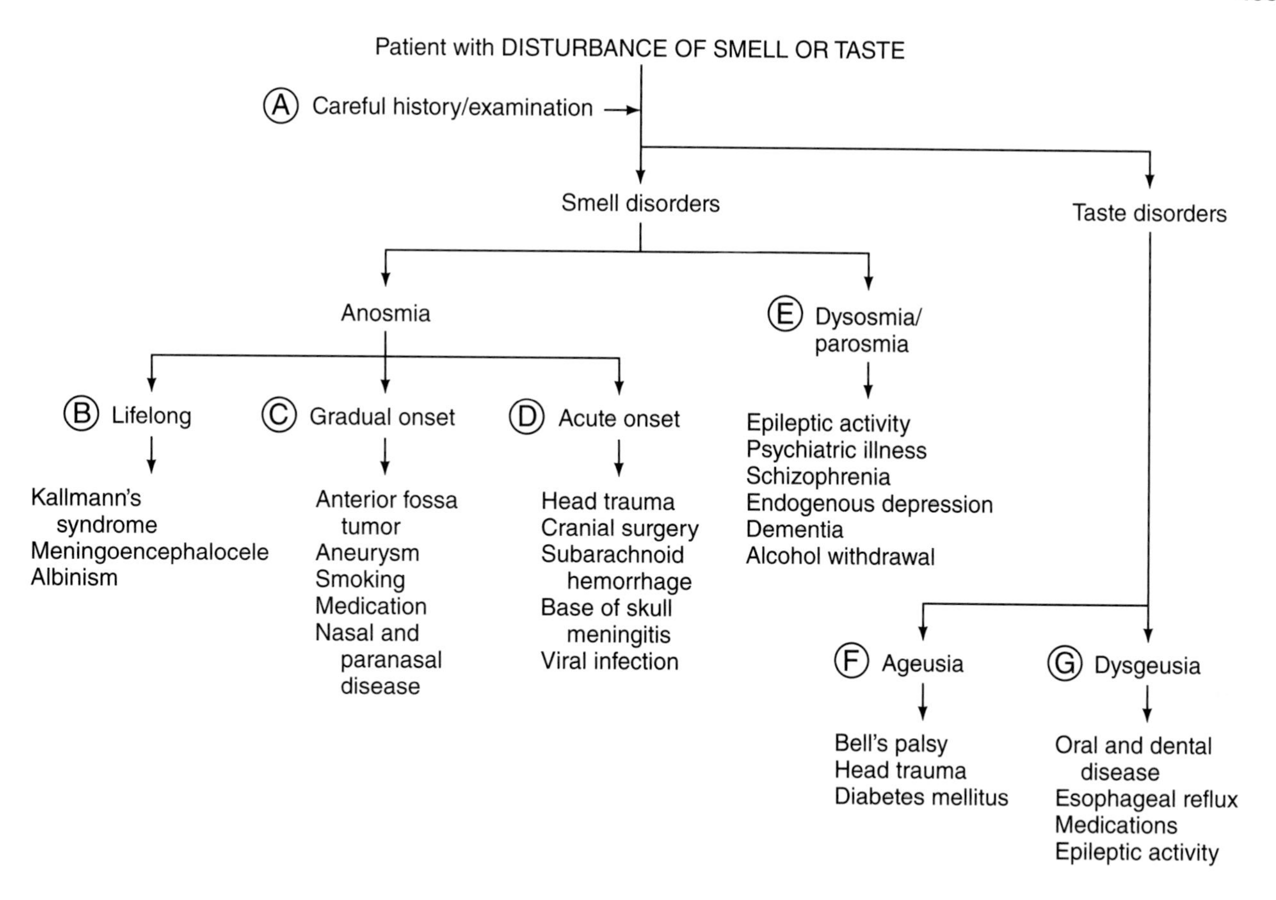

be unilateral or bilateral, presumably caused by damage to the chorda tympani. Patients with diabetes mellitus often have a decreased sensation of sweet, bitter, and sour flavors. This is more common in patients with long-standing diabetes and in those with associated diabetic neuropathy. Cigarette smoking has been demonstrated to cause progressive loss of smell in a dose-related manner, with a gradual restoration of smell perception once patients have stopped smoking. Likewise, chronic alcoholism may lead to dysosmia and dysgeusia.

G. Oral disorders causing taste disturbances include gastroesophageal reflux, oral candidiasis, lichen planus, leukoplakia, carcinoma of the tongue, and other tongue afflictions; xerostomia and sialoadenitis; and palatal clefts and facial hypoplasia. Periodontal disease and other infectious processes may produce abnormal oral secretions, resulting in taste changes. Dental restorations or prostheses can give a metallic taste, whereas dentures may block taste reception.

References

Arcavi L, Shahar A. Drug-related taste disturbances: emphasis on the elderly. Harefuah 2003;142(6):446–450, 485, 484.

Comeau TB, Epstein JB, Migas C. Taste and smell dysfunction in patients receiving chemotherapy: a review of current knowledge. Support Care Cancer 2001;9(8):575–580.

Doty RL, Bromley SM. Effects of drugs on olfaction and taste. Otolaryngol Clin North Am 2004;37:1229–1254.

Frye RE, Schwartz BS, Doty RL. Dose-related effects of cigarette smoking on olfactory function. JAMA 1990;263:1233.

Jafek BW, Gordon ASD, Moran DT, et al. Congenital anosmia. Ear Nose Throat J 1990;69:331.

Jain KK. Drug-Induced Neurologic Disorders, 2nd ed. Göttingen-Bern-Toronto: Hogrefe & Huber, 2001.

Hawkes CH. Disorders of smell and taste. In Samuels MA, Feske SK, eds. Office Practice of Neurology. Philadelphia: Churchill-Livingstone, 2003:102–120.

COMA

David M. Greer, MD

Coma is defined as a "sleeplike unresponsiveness without evidence of awareness of the self or the environment, a state from which patients cannot be aroused." Patients in coma do not show any meaningful responsiveness to their environment but may have variably intact brainstem reflexes. To be considered in coma, the patient may exhibit reflex posturing in response to noxious stimuli but cannot withdraw to pain or otherwise show signs of awareness of external or internal stimuli. The responsibilities of the physician include stabilization of the patient's vital functions and institution of the initial steps in evaluation and management.

Consciousness is predicated on both arousal and awareness and is mediated by the ascending reticular activating system, which originates in the rostral brainstem and then projects into both cerebral hemispheres. Thus, to produce coma, a cerebral process must either affect the rostral brainstem primarily, both cerebral hemispheres concomitantly, or all of the above. Primary brainstem processes include vascular events (e.g., ischemic stroke, hemorrhage), drug intoxication, and compression from a supratentorial or infratentorial mass lesion. Diffuse hemispheric processes include hypoxic-ischemic injuries (e.g., from cardiac arrest), drug intoxication, seizures, infection (e.g., meningoencephalitis), and metabolic disorders (e.g., hypoglycemia, hyponatremia, renal failure, liver failure).

Table 1. **Glasgow Coma Scale**

Function	Score*
Motor response	
Obeys	6
Localizes	5
Withdraws	4
Abnormal flexion	3
Extensor response	2
No response	1
Verbal response	
Oriented	5
Confused conversation	4
Inappropriate words	3
Incomprehensible sounds	2
No response	1
Eye opening	
Spontaneous	4
To command	3
To pain	2
No response	1

*The best score from each of the three areas is summed. Scores can range from 15 (essentially a normal examination) to 3 (no response in any area).

A. The foremost clinical goal in the management of a patient presenting in coma is the ABCs of basic life support. IV access should be obtained promptly, as should nasogastric and urinary catheters. Endotracheal intubation is usually necessary, secondary to poor airway protection or ineffective respiratory efforts. Blood should be sent for CBC, extended chemistries, ammonia level, ABGs, liver function studies, and toxicology screen (including urine). Thiamine (100 mg IV) and glucose (1 amp D_{50} IV) should be administered early. Naloxone (0.4–2.0 mg IV) administration should be considered in cases of suspected narcotic overdose.

B. A rapid medical and neurologic examination should be performed, preferably prior to intubation, because sedating and/or paralytic medications are often administered for intubation. Specific attention should be paid to the cranial nerves and to movements in the extremities to noxious stimulation. The Glasgow Coma Scale (Table 1) provides a quick, systematic way to assess brain dysfunction in patients who are comatose. It most often is used in traumatic coma. The skull should be palpated for hematomas, and one should look for Battle's sign (ecchymosis over the mastoid) or "raccoon eyes" (ecchymosis around the eyes), either of which suggest a basal skull fracture. Other signs include hemotympanum and cerebrospinal fluid (CSF) leakage from the nose or ears. The cervical spine should be immobilized, especially in cases of trauma or if the patient's loss of consciousness was unwitnessed.

C. Neuroimaging should be performed in *all* patients who are comatose to rule out a structural lesion. Initially, CT is preferable to MRI because of its ability to detect acute blood and bone abnormalities, but results can be normal in the early stages of stroke, meningitis, or following cardiac arrest. MRI is superior to CT for the detection of acute cerebral infarction or early signs of encephalitis. CT of the C-spine is performed to evaluate for stability in the acute setting, but MRI may also be required to assess for ligamentous injury.

(Continued on page 462)

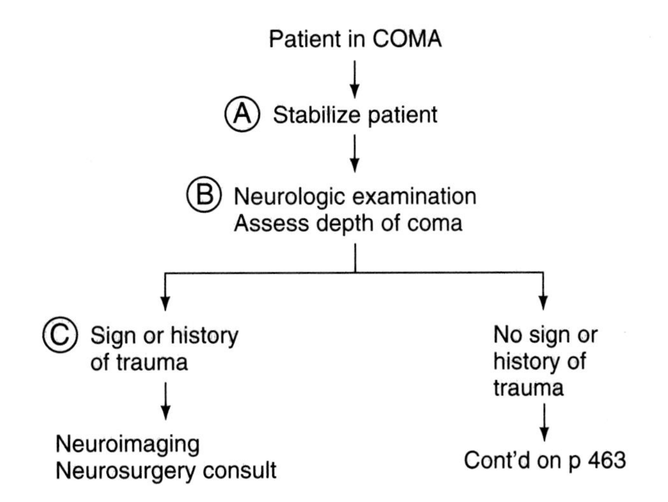
Patient in COMA
(A) Stabilize patient
(B) Neurologic examination
Assess depth of coma
(C) Sign or history of trauma
Neuroimaging
Neurosurgery consult
No sign or history of trauma
Cont'd on p 463

D. A nonfocal examination should raise suspicion of a toxic or metabolic etiology. Dysfunction in virtually any organ system may lead to confusional states and coma. Look for systemic signs of renal or liver insufficiency/failure. Consider drug ingestion or toxin exposure. In most cases, metabolic dysfunction does not cause nonreactive pupils or focal neurologic signs. However, atropine-like substances and glutethimide can abolish pupillary reflexes, and opiate overdose may cause the pupils to be so constricted that a very bright light and a magnifying glass may be needed to detect any reactivity. Toxic-metabolic insults also may result in seizures and lateralizing neurologic signs that may wax and wane or even shift from side to side. Extensor plantar responses also may be seen. However, metabolic causes of coma (especially intoxication) may obscure signs of an underlying focal lesion. Therefore, neuroimaging should still be performed.

E. If a focal lesion is responsible for coma, it is useful to localize the lesion to a supratentorial or infratentorial location. The examination should emphasize the following: eye opening to loud auditory or vigorous physical stimulation, blinking to visual threat, pupillary response to bright light (size, symmetry, reactivity), eye movement abnormalities (including the oculocephalic reflex or "doll's eyes" and the oculovestibular reflex or "cold calorics"), corneal reflex, gag reflex, respiratory pattern (e.g., Cheyne-Stokes, central neurogenic hyperventilation, ataxic and apneustic breathing), extremity movements to noxious stimulation (e.g., symmetric vs. asymmetric responses, decorticate/decerebrate posturing), deep tendon reflexes, and the Babinski reflex. A complete discussion of the abnormalities observed with lesions in different brain areas is beyond the scope of this chapter. The key is to carefully and systematically perform and document the neurologic examination so that clinical stability or progression can be appreciated by the medical team.

F. Signs of meningismus include nuchal rigidity and Kernig's and Brudzinski's signs. Such findings may accompany either a nonfocal or focal examination. Nonfocal examinations may reflect subarachnoid hemorrhage (SAH) or meningoencephalitis. Focal lesions may induce meningismus through direct meningeal irritation (e.g., parenchymal hemorrhage with rupture into the subarachnoid space) or through increased intracranial pressure, which may lead to herniation. After obtaining neuroimaging to rule out a mass lesion, a lumbar puncture should be performed, looking for evidence of blood, xanthochromia, or infection. Approximately 6% of SAHs are diagnosed by lumbar puncture after a falsely negative CT scan. Furthermore, signs of meningismus may be absent in deep coma, so consider performing a lumbar puncture if the history suggests an infectious etiology or if there is no alternative explanation for the patient's state.

G. Prolonged or sustained seizure activity (i.e., status epilepticus) may lead to impaired consciousness and coma. Patients may be in status epilepticus without overt signs of seizures (i.e., nonconvulsive status epilepticus). Seizures also may reflect an underlying process that itself leads to coma. Observe patients carefully for evidence of seizure activity, especially the eyes, which may be deviated to one side or moving rhythmically. Focal seizures suggest a focal lesion, and generalized seizures or myoclonus suggest a toxic–metabolic insult, although these rules are not absolute. Laboratory studies should include anticonvulsant levels as well as metabolic parameters. An EEG may be useful not only to assess seizure activity but also to look for abnormalities compatible with metabolic abnormalities (e.g., rhythmic discharges in hepatic encephalopathy) or focal lesions (i.e., focal slowing).

References

Adams RD, Victor M, Ropper AH. Coma and related disorders of consciousness. In Adams RD, Victor M, Ropper AH, eds. Principles of Neurology, 6th ed. New York: McGraw-Hill, 1997:344.

Brust JCM. Coma. In Rowland LP, ed. Merritt's Textbook of Neurology, 9th ed. Baltimore: Williams & Wilkins, 1995.

Plum F, Posner J. The Diagnosis of Stupor and Coma, 3rd ed. Oxford: Oxford University Press, 1982.

Young GB, Ropper AH, Bolton CF. Coma and Impaired Consciousness. New York: McGraw-Hill, 1998.

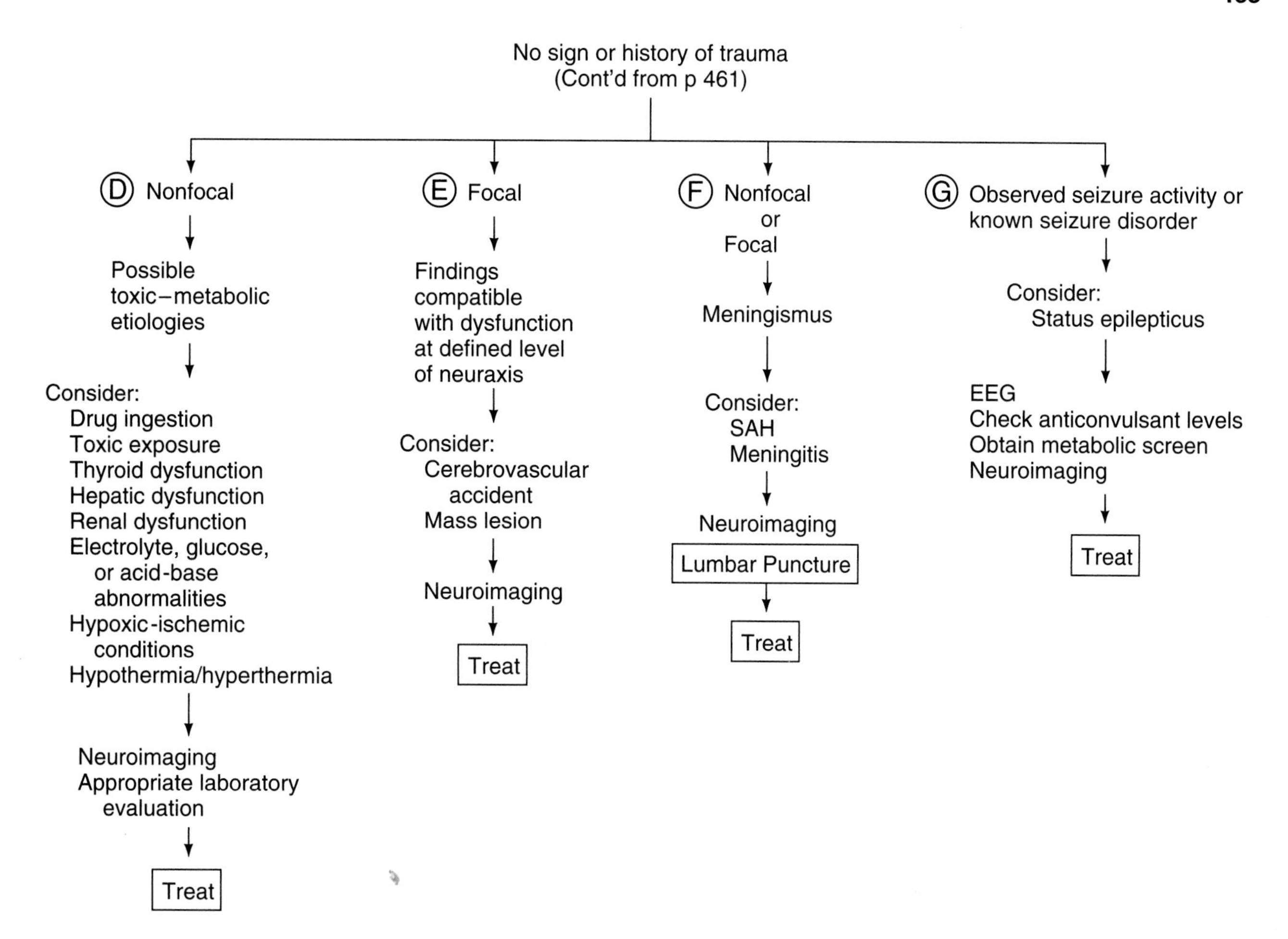
No sign or history of trauma
(Cont'd from p 461)
D Nonfocal
Possible toxic–metabolic etiologies
Consider:
Drug ingestion
Toxic exposure
Thyroid dysfunction
Hepatic dysfunction
Renal dysfunction
Electrolyte, glucose, or acid-base abnormalities
Hypoxic-ischemic conditions
Hypothermia/hyperthermia
Neuroimaging
Appropriate laboratory evaluation
Treat
E Focal
Findings compatible with dysfunction at defined level of neuraxis
Consider:
Cerebrovascular accident
Mass lesion
Neuroimaging
Treat
F Nonfocal or Focal
Meningismus
Consider:
SAH
Meningitis
Neuroimaging
Lumbar Puncture
Treat
G Observed seizure activity or known seizure disorder
Consider:
Status epilepticus
EEG
Check anticonvulsant levels
Obtain metabolic screen
Neuroimaging
Treat

BRAIN DEATH

David M. Greer, MD

Molleret and Goulon introduced the term *brain death* in 1959, when they described 23 patients with "irreversible coma" involving unresponsiveness, loss of brainstem reflexes and spontaneous respiration, and flat EEGs. Advances in mechanical ventilation have enabled survival of systemic organ functioning after devastating neurologic injury, thereby creating the possibility for the person's brain to be "dead" or nonfunctional, while the systemic organs are still viable if supported by external means. In 1981, the President's Commission for the Study of Ethical Problems in Medicine and Biomedical and Behavioral Research issued a report on "Guidelines for the Determination of Death." This included a model statute called the *Uniform Determination of Death Act,* which stated: "An individual who has sustained either (1) irreversible cessation of circulatory and respiratory functions, or (2) irreversible cessation of all functions of the entire brain, including the brain stem, is dead. A determination of death must be made in determination with accepted medical standards." The correct determination of brain death is essential in medical care to ensure that inappropriate measures are not undertaken, to provide finality for families concerned with prognosis, and for possible organ donation. Most states now have statutes or judicial decisions recognizing this concept. However, significant local variations in guidelines exist, and at present individual hospitals are responsible for developing their own guidelines. The following is a description of the necessary requirements for determination of death by brain criteria in adults.

A. The cause of brain dysfunction must be known and must be known to be irreversible. Neuroimaging is often required to establish the cause radiographically and to exclude potentially treatable conditions. There must be no confounding medical conditions that may influence the clinical examination, including severe electrolyte disturbances, acid–base disorders, elevated ammonia level, or endocrine disorders—particularly, profound hypothyroidism or hyperthyroidism or severe cortisol deficiency. Body temperature must be >96.8° F (36.5° C). The systolic blood pressure must be maintained >90 mm Hg. There must be no evidence of drug intoxication, poisoning, or recent use of neuromuscular blocking agents. The barbiturate level must be <10 μg/ml. If significant doses of CNS depressant medications (e.g., narcotics, sedatives, hypnotics, anticholinergics) have been administered recently, the reliability of the clinical examination should be questioned and ancillary testing should be performed. There should be a demonstrated absence of neuromuscular blockade (e.g., with a method of four nerve stimulation) if the patient has received recent or prolonged use of neuromuscular blocking agents. In the presence of confounding variables, brain death may still be determined with the aid of ancillary tests.

B. The three cardinal findings in clinical brain death are coma, absence of brainstem reflexes, and apnea. Coma is defined as the absence of any cerebrally mediated response to noxious stimuli, including pain in all extremities. Brainstem reflexes should include the following:
   - Pupils—no response to bright light (a magnifying glass may be useful if response is questionable). Small or pinpoint pupils should alert the clinician to the possibility of narcotic intoxication but can also be seen with pontine damage.
   - Ocular movement—no oculocephalic reflex ("doll's eyes"—tested only when the integrity of the cervical spine is ensured) and no oculovestibular reflex ("cold calorics"). Testing may be confounded by blood or cerumen in the auditory canal, a disrupted tympanic membrane, or injury to the globes or orbits.
   - Facial motor response—no corneal response, no jaw jerk reflex, no facial grimacing to noxious stimuli. Facial myokymias, resulting from denervation of the facial nerve, are permissible.
   - Pharyngeal and tracheal reflexes—no response to stimulation of the posterior pharynx with pressure, no coughing or significant bradyarrhythmia to bronchial suctioning.
   - Motor response to pain—no purposeful or posturing (extensor or flexor) movements to noxious stimuli (e.g., nail bed pressure). Deep tendon reflexes are permissible because they are spinally mediated.

   Apnea testing requires hemodynamic stability; if the patient is not stable, then ancillary testing should be performed. The patient should have correction of the pH (7.35–7.45) and Pco_2 (35–45) at least 20 minutes prior to testing if possible. The patient should be preoxygenated with 100% Fio_2 for at least 5 minutes prior to testing to an arterial Po_2 of ≥200 mm Hg. (This is to ensure that the patient does not become hypoxic at any time during testing.) Ensure proper functioning of a pulse oximeter. Provide an oxygen source (typically via a catheter to the endotracheal tube to the level of the carina with a continuous flow of oxygen). Disconnect the ventilator, and observe closely for respiratory movements, cyanosis, or hemodynamic instability. If any of

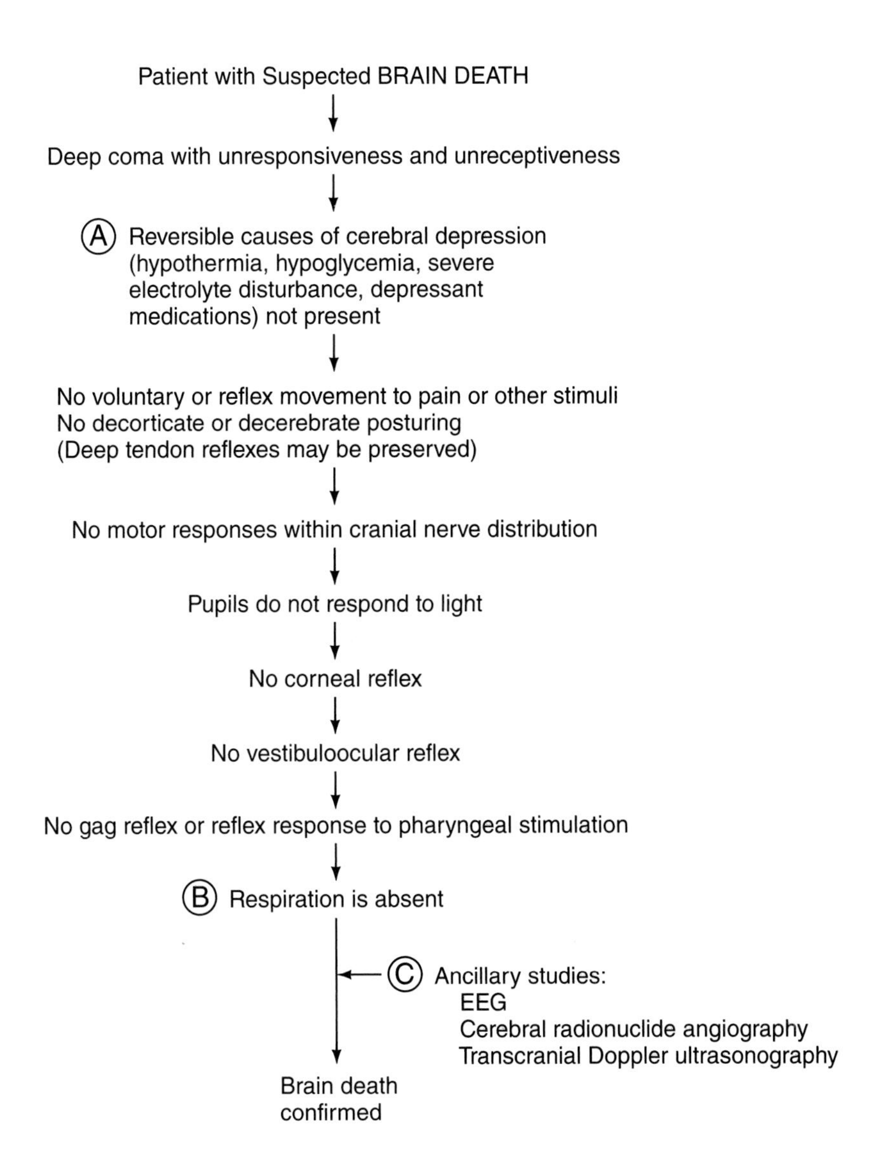

these occur, the test should be aborted. If not, after 8 minutes an ABG measurement is drawn and the patient is reconnected to the ventilator. The apnea test is positive if the pH is ≤7.30 (from a pretest baseline of ≥7.40) or PCO_2 increases from 40 to ≥60 mm Hg, or if there is a 20 mm Hg increase from the pretest baseline. If the test is indeterminate, ancillary testing may be required.

C. Brain death is a clinical diagnosis and does not require ancillary testing, unless the clinical examination cannot be performed or is considered unreliable. Ancillary studies include cerebral angiography, single photon emission computed tomography (SPECT), EEG, or transcranial Doppler ultrasound.

Pitfalls in brain death testing include severe facial trauma; preexisting pupillary abnormalities; sleep apnea or severe pulmonary disease resulting in severe chronic retention of CO_2; or toxic levels of any sedative drugs, including aminoglycosides, tricyclic antidepressants, anticholinergics, antiepileptic drugs, chemotherapeutic agents, or neuromuscular blocking agents.

References

Greer DM. Brain death. In Layon AJ, Gabrielli A, Friedman WA, eds. Textbook of Neurointensive Care. Philadelphia: Saunders, 2004.

Guidelines for the determination of death: report of the medical consultants on the diagnosis of death to the President's Commission for the Study of Ethical Problems in Medicine and Biomedical and Behavioral Research. JAMA 1981;246:2184–2186.

Quality Standards Subcommittee of the American Academy of Neurology. Practice parameters for determining brain death in adults (summary statement). Neurology 1995;45:1012–1014.

Wijdicks EFM. Brain Death. Philadelphia: Lippincott, Williams & Wilkins, 2001.

Wijdicks EFM. The diagnosis of brain death. N Engl J Med 2001; 344:1215–1221.

OCULAR

Sherleen Chen, MD, FACS
Section Editor

DILATED PUPIL

Sherleen Chen, MD, FACS

One must ensure that the dilated pupil is the abnormal pupil by examining the patient in both bright and dim ambient light. If the anisocoria is greater in bright lighting and the larger pupil constricts poorly to penlight examination, then the dilated pupil is the abnormal pupil.

Physiologic anisocoria occurs in approximately 20% of the population. It is characterized by anisocoria that is similar in both bright and dark, normal pupillary constriction to light, and anisocoria that is usually <1 mm in diameter.

A. Acute angle-closure glaucoma is characterized by acute pain with blurred vision and colored halos around lights. On examination, the pupil is unreactive and fixed in a mid-dilated position. The conjunctiva is typically hyperemic, with corneal edema demonstrated by a dulled reflection of light from the corneal surface. The intraocular pressure is acutely elevated.

   This is a medical emergency that requires prompt treatment to prevent permanent visual loss. If a Tono-Pen is available to confirm acutely elevated intraocular pressure, Timoptic 0.5% 1 gtt and/or Diamox 500 mg PO/IV should be given. The patient should be immediately referred to an ophthalmologist for definitive management.

B. In a patient with a dilated pupil, an extraocular motility deficit with or without associated ptosis indicates a third nerve palsy until proved otherwise. The patient may have periorbital pain or headache. Immediate neuroimaging should be obtained, with MRI/MRA of the brain with gadolinium to rule out an aneurysm or mass.

C. Unilateral or asymmetric exposure to adrenergic agents will cause mydriasis associated with a widened palpebral fissure and blanched conjunctiva resulting from vasoconstriction. Common agents include over-the-counter vasoconstrictors for "red eyes" and adrenergic glaucoma medications. Accommodation remains unaffected.

D. Parasympathetic blockade of pupillary constriction typically results in a very large pupil and is associated with loss of accommodation. Common causative agents include atropine, scopolamine patch, and night-blooming flowers.

E. Surgery, prior ocular trauma, or prior inflammation may cause a dilated pupil that may have irregular margins.

F. An Adie's tonic pupil demonstrates cholinergic supersensitivity; the dilated pupil constricts significantly more than the contralateral pupil in response to dilute pilocarpine (0.125%). Additional signs seen without pharmacologic intervention include: (1) The affected pupil constricts slowly in response to light, but constricts quickly with accommodation (looking at a near target. It also remains tonic (redilates slowly) after a prolonged accomodative effort. (2) Segmental palsy of the iris sphincter, seen as an irregularly constricting pupil margin.

References

Bradford CA, ed. Basic Ophthalmology, 8th ed. San Francisco: American Academy of Ophthalmology, 2004.

Kaiser PA, Friedman NJ, Pineda R II. The Massachusetts Eye and Ear Infirmary Illustrated Manual of Ophthalmology, 2nd ed. Philadelphia: Saunders, 2003.

Trobe JD. The Physician's Guide to Eye Care, 3rd ed. San Francisco: American Academy of Ophthalmology, 2006.

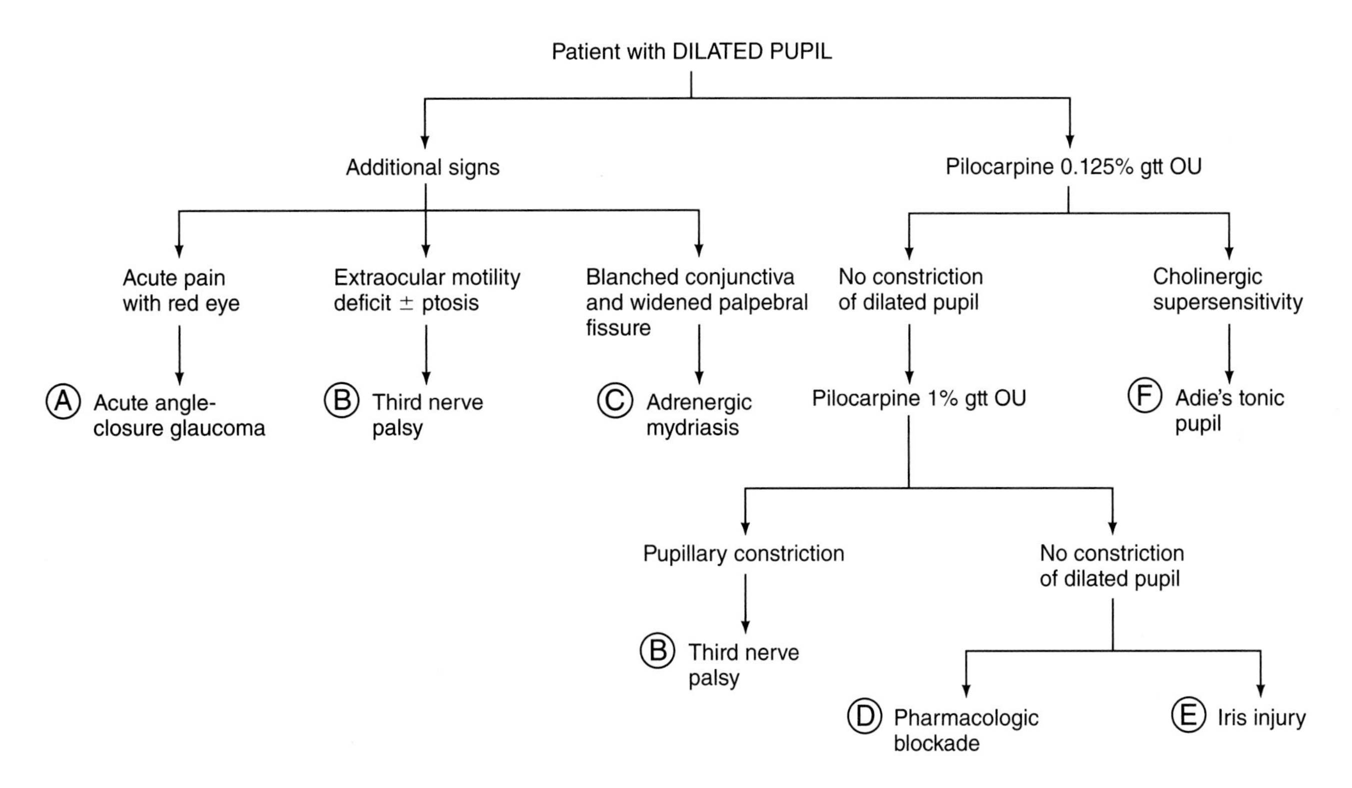
Patient with DILATED PUPIL
Additional signs
Pilocarpine 0.125% gtt OU
Acute pain with red eye
Extraocular motility deficit ± ptosis
Blanched conjunctiva and widened palpebral fissure
No constriction of dilated pupil
Cholinergic supersensitivity
(A) Acute angle-closure glaucoma
(B) Third nerve palsy
(C) Adrenergic mydriasis
Pilocarpine 1% gtt OU
(F) Adie's tonic pupil
Pupillary constriction
No constriction of dilated pupil
(B) Third nerve palsy
(D) Pharmacologic blockade
(E) Iris injury

CORNEAL ABRASION

Sherleen Chen, MD, FACS

Corneal abrasions typically heal rapidly (within 1–2 days) depending on the extent of injury and the patient's age and health. The most important management issues are to exclude more severe injury and to allow healing without infection. Topical anesthetics should never be prescribed for pain control because chronic use is toxic to the corneal epithelium.

A. If the abrasion is associated with a significant mechanism of injury (e.g., high-velocity foreign body), contact with vegetable matter such as a bush or tree, or associated contact lens wear, the patient should be referred to an ophthalmologist for examination because these situations have potential for more serious injury or more virulent or atypical pathogens.

B. On penlight examination, a corneal abrasion may show a normal corneal light reflection or an isolated irregular corneal light reflection in the area of the abrasion. Fluorescein staining and examination under cobalt blue light will outline the area of denuded epithelium as a yellowish-green stain.

C. Patients with recurrent erosion syndrome report a history of recurrent episodes of awakening with symptoms of a corneal abrasion. The examination is often normal because the abrasion has often healed by the time the patient is seen. Patients should use aggressive lubrication with artificial tears QID and erythromycin or another bland ointment QHS for 1 month. An ophthalmology referral should be pursued if the patient is still symptomatic.

D. Multiple linear streaks of fluorescein staining indicate a foreign body embedded in the upper lid until proved otherwise. After everting the upper lid to remove the foreign body, the abrasion is treated as indicated for small abrasions (see section E). The upper lid also should be everted if the patient reports a history of a foreign body in the eye.

E. Small abrasions are treated with ophthalmic ointment tid–qid, such as erythromycin, polymyxin/bacitracin, or bacitracin ointment. Antibiotic ointments with steroids are contraindicated. Patients are seen within 1–2 days to ensure complete resolution of the abrasion without complication.

F. Large abrasions are treated with antibiotic ointments as noted in section E. In addition, pressure patching for 24 hours may decrease pain and aid in healing. A folded eye pad is placed over the closed lid and covered with a second eye pad. Tape is applied diagonally across the forehead to the patient's cheekbone to tightly secure the pad and prevent blinking. An eye patch should never be applied if there is recent history of contact lens wear, potential vegetable matter, or a potential infection. Oral analgesics can be prescribed as needed for 1 day. Topical anesthetics should never be prescribed. Patients should be seen within 24 hours to ensure healing is progressing without infection, or they should be referred to an ophthalmologist.

G. The branching pattern of a corneal dendrite indicates herpetic eye disease. The patient should be referred to an ophthalmologist for further evaluation and management.

H. Immediate ophthalmology referral should be sought for concerning findings such as a corneal opacity, embedded foreign body, a shallow anterior chamber, or an irregular pupil. These signs indicate significant injury or potential infection.

References

Bradford CA, ed. Basic Ophthalmology, 8th ed. San Francisco: American Academy of Ophthalmology, 2004.

Kaiser PA, Friedman NJ, Pineda R II. The Massachusetts Eye and Ear Infirmary Illustrated Manual of Ophthalmology, 2nd ed. Philadelphia: Saunders, 2003.

Trobe JD. The Physician's Guide to Eye Care, 3rd ed. San Francisco: American Academy of Ophthalmology, 2006.

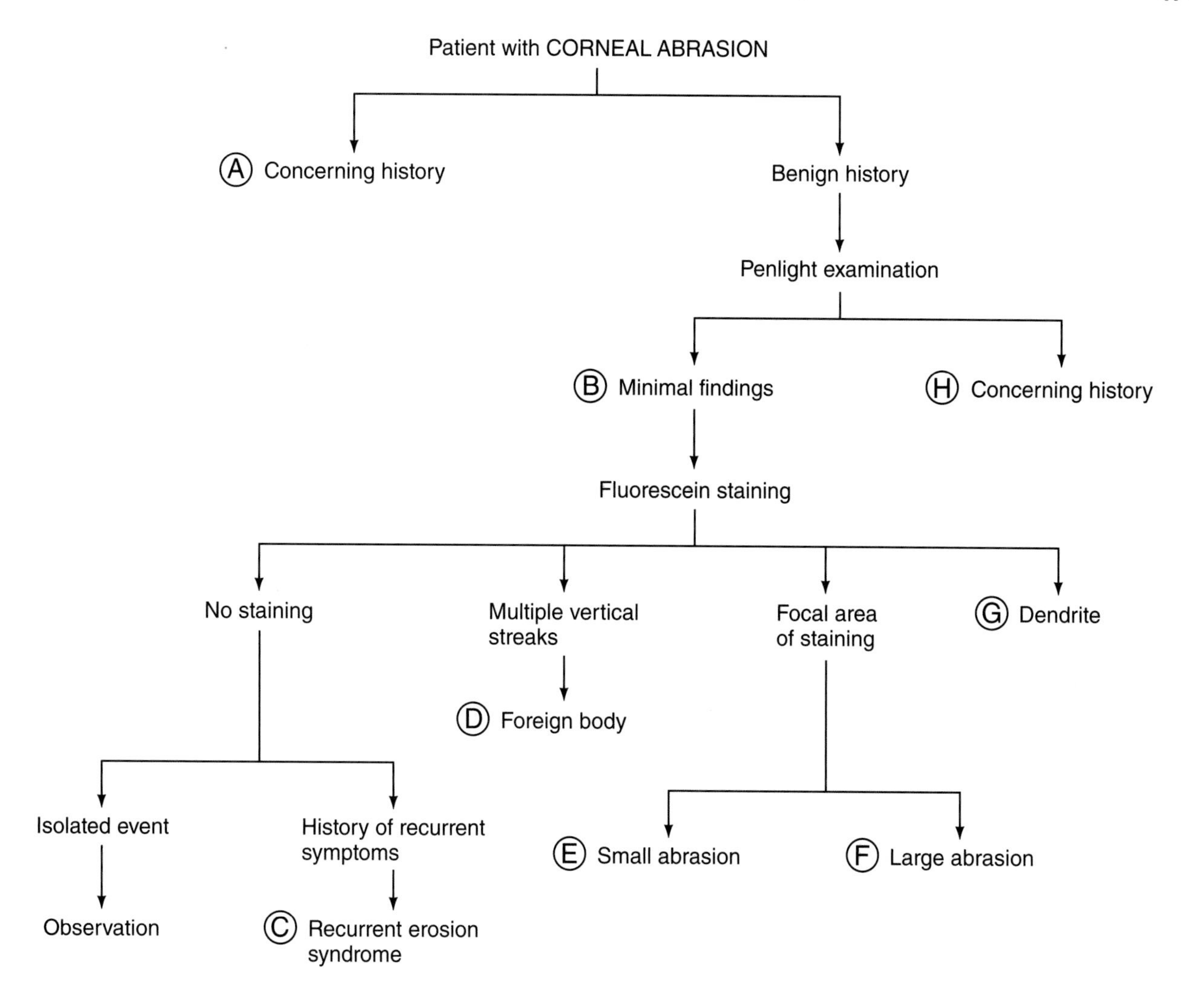
Patient with CORNEAL ABRASION
A Concerning history
Benign history
Penlight examination
B Minimal findings
H Concerning history
Fluorescein staining
No staining
Multiple vertical streaks
Focal area of staining
G Dendrite
D Foreign body
Isolated event
History of recurrent symptoms
E Small abrasion
F Large abrasion
Observation
C Recurrent erosion syndrome

CONJUNCTIVITIS

Sherleen Chen, MD, FACS

A. Chronic conjunctivitis lasting >4 weeks has a large differential, and therefore patients with chronic conjunctivitis should be referred to an ophthalmologist.

B. The acute mucopurulent discharge of bacterial conjunctivitis is typically yellowish-white, thick, and creamy. This is in contrast to the thin, grayish-white, watery, or stringy mucus seen in nonbacterial conjunctivitis.

C. Concerning history includes contact lens wear, recent eye surgery or any history of glaucoma surgery, or any history or symptoms of sexually transmitted disease. These patients should be referred immediately to ophthalmology for further evaluation.

D. If there is no prior or concerning history, the discharge should be cleaned from the eye with frequent flushing using artificial tears and warm compresses to the lids. Antibacterial drops should be given QID for 1 week, with polymyxin-trimethoprim or a fourth-generation fluoroquinolone.

E. Viral conjunctivitis is typically associated with an upper respiratory tract infection (URI) and tender swollen preauricular nodes. Because viral conjunctivitis is extremely contagious when the discharge is present, meticulous hygiene should be maintained with frequent handwashing, avoidance of touching the eyes, and avoidance of sharing towels or linens. Cool compresses and artificial tears can provide symptomatic relief.

F. If conjunctivitis is associated with vesicles of the periocular skin, an ophthalmologist should be consulted to evaluate for more extensive herpetic ocular involvement.

G. Allergic conjunctivitis is typically bilateral, with significant itching and watery discharge. Systemic antihistamines and allergen exposure control are helpful. Cool compresses and artificial tears may be sufficient for mild symptoms. Topical antihistamine/vasoconstrictor drops QID (over the counter) can be used for a few weeks, but chronic use may cause rebound hyperemia and tachyphylaxis. Alternatively, topical antihistamine/vasoconstrictor/mast cell stabilizer drops QD–bid can be prescribed for use as needed.

References

Bradford CA, ed. Basic Ophthalmology, 8th ed. San Francisco: American Academy of Ophthalmology, 2004.

Kaiser PA, Friedman NJ, Pineda R II. The Massachusetts Eye and Ear Infirmary Illustrated Manual of Ophthalmology, 2nd ed. Philadelphia: Saunders, 2003.

Trobe JD. The Physician's Guide to Eye Care, 3rd ed. San Francisco: American Academy of Ophthalmology, 2006.

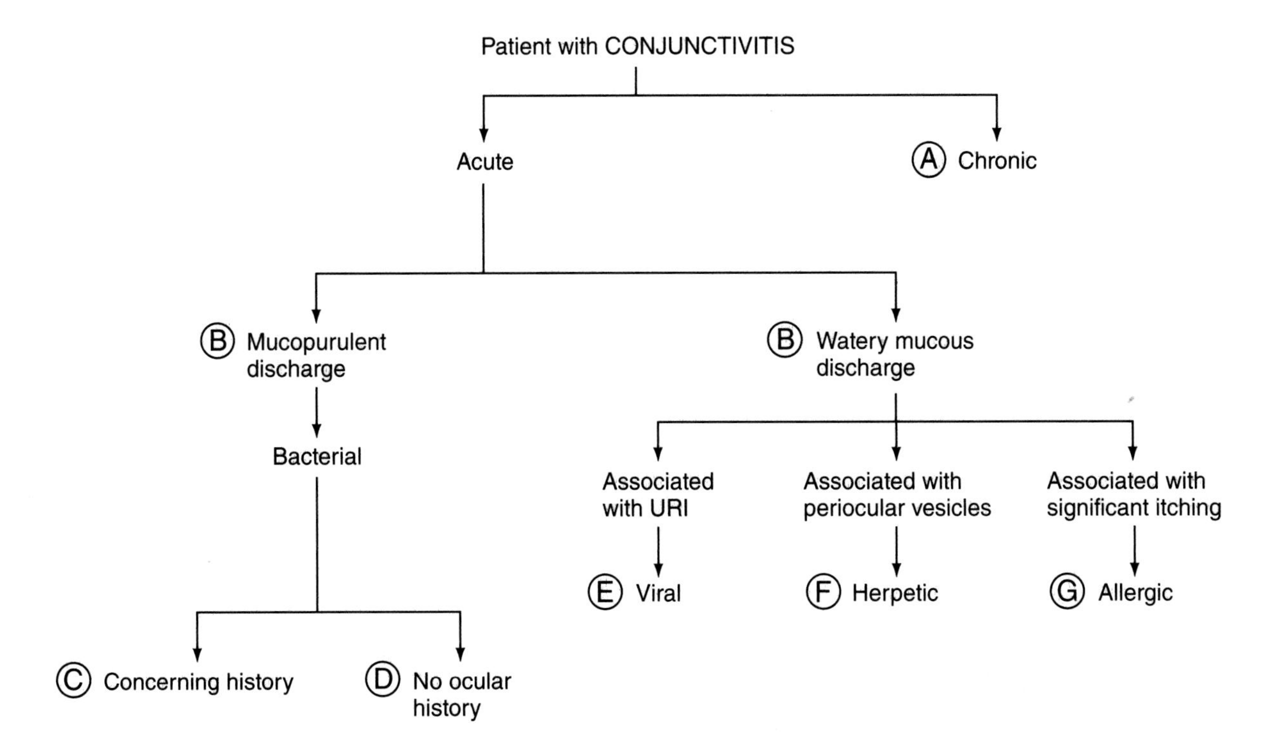

Patient with CONJUNCTIVITIS
Acute
(A) Chronic
(B) Mucopurulent discharge
(B) Watery mucous discharge
Bacterial
Associated with URI
Associated with periocular vesicles
Associated with significant itching
(E) Viral
(F) Herpetic
(G) Allergic
(C) Concerning history
(D) No ocular history

ACUTE VISUAL LOSS

Sherleen Chen, MD, FACS

Patients with acute unilateral visual loss require emergent evaluation. Visual loss occurring over minutes to hours is usually a result of retinal or optic nerve ischemia. Associated symptoms may help to differentiate among the etiologies, a few of which require emergency treatment to prevent permanent or bilateral visual loss.

A. Acute angle-closure glaucoma is characterized by acute periocular pain, which may be severe and associated with nausea and vomiting. Patients experience blurred vision and colored halos around lights. On examination, the pupil is unreactive and fixed in a mid-dilated position. The conjunctiva is typically hyperemic, with corneal edema demonstrated by a dulled reflection of light from the corneal surface. The intraocular pressure is acutely elevated.

   This is a medical emergency that requires prompt treatment to prevent permanent visual loss. If a Tono-Pen is available to confirm acutely elevated intraocular pressure, Timoptic 0.5% 1 gtt and/or Diamox 500 mg PO/IV should be given. The patient should be immediately referred to an ophthalmologist for definitive management.

B. Optic neuritis typically causes eye pain, particularly with extraocular movements. The pupil looks normal, but further evaluation shows a relative afferent pupillary defect (APD). Visual loss usually occurs over days, but it may rarely occur over hours. The eye appears white and quiet. Patients are typically between 18 and 50 years of age. Urgent referral should be made to a neuro-ophthalmologist or neurologist for neuroimaging with MRI of the brain and orbits with gadolinium to assess for demyelinating lesions.

C. Symptoms of giant cell arteritis include jaw claudication, scalp tenderness, headache, malaise, anorexia, and proximal joint or muscle aches. Patients are typically >50 years of age. Confirmatory labs should be ordered, with stat ESR, C-reactive protein (CRP), and CBC with platelets. Immediate methylprednisolone 1–1.5 g IV is given in divided doses to prevent bilateral visual loss. Emergent ophthalmology evaluation should be sought to evaluate for arteritic anterior ischemic optic neuropathy or central retinal artery occlusion. A temporal artery biopsy should be performed within 7 days of starting steroids to confirm the diagnosis.

D. Symptoms of retinal detachment include photopsias (brief monocular flashes of light), floaters (flies or cobwebs that move with eye movement), and a curtain or shadow moving in the field of vision. An urgent ophthalmology referral should be obtained to evaluate for retinal detachment or a vitreous hemorrhage, which is less likely, not urgent, and most commonly seen in patients with a history of diabetic retinopathy.

E. Central retinal artery occlusion causes sudden, profound, painless visual loss. On ophthalmoscopy, the infarcted retina appears whitish and opacified, with a cherry-red spot in the center of the macula. No ocular treatment has been proved to be effective, but an emergent ophthalmology evaluation should be obtained to confirm the diagnosis. Further management involves controlling hypertension and other medical problems and evaluating for carotid or cardiac emboli. In patients >50 years of age, a stat ESR and CRP should be considered to rule out giant cell arteritis as a potential etiology. Patients <50 years of age may need an evaluation for collagen vascular disease; hypercoagulable state; or other rare causes such as syphilis, sickle cell, or Behçet's disease.

F. Ophthalmoscopic examination in central retinal vein occlusion reveals diffuse retinal hemorrhages, dilated retinal veins, and often cotton-wool spots. Blood pressure should be checked, and hypertension and other contributors to cardiovascular disease should be managed. If clinically indicated, a hypercoagulable state should be excluded. An urgent ophthalmology evaluation is obtained to evaluate for elevated intraocular pressure and future potential neovascularization.

G. Patients with nonarteritic anterior ischemic optic neuropathy are typically >50 years of age and experience painless visual loss over hours to days. An emergent ophthalmology referral should be obtained to confirm the diagnosis. Management involves controlling cardiovascular disease.

References

Bradford CA, ed. Basic Ophthalmology, 8th ed. San Francisco: American Academy of Ophthalmology, 2004.

Kaiser PA, Friedman NJ, Pineda R II. The Massachusetts Eye and Ear Infirmary Illustrated Manual of Ophthalmology, 2nd ed. Philadelphia: Saunders, 2003.

Trobe JD. The Physician's Guide to Eye Care, 3rd ed. San Francisco: American Academy of Ophthalmology, 2006.

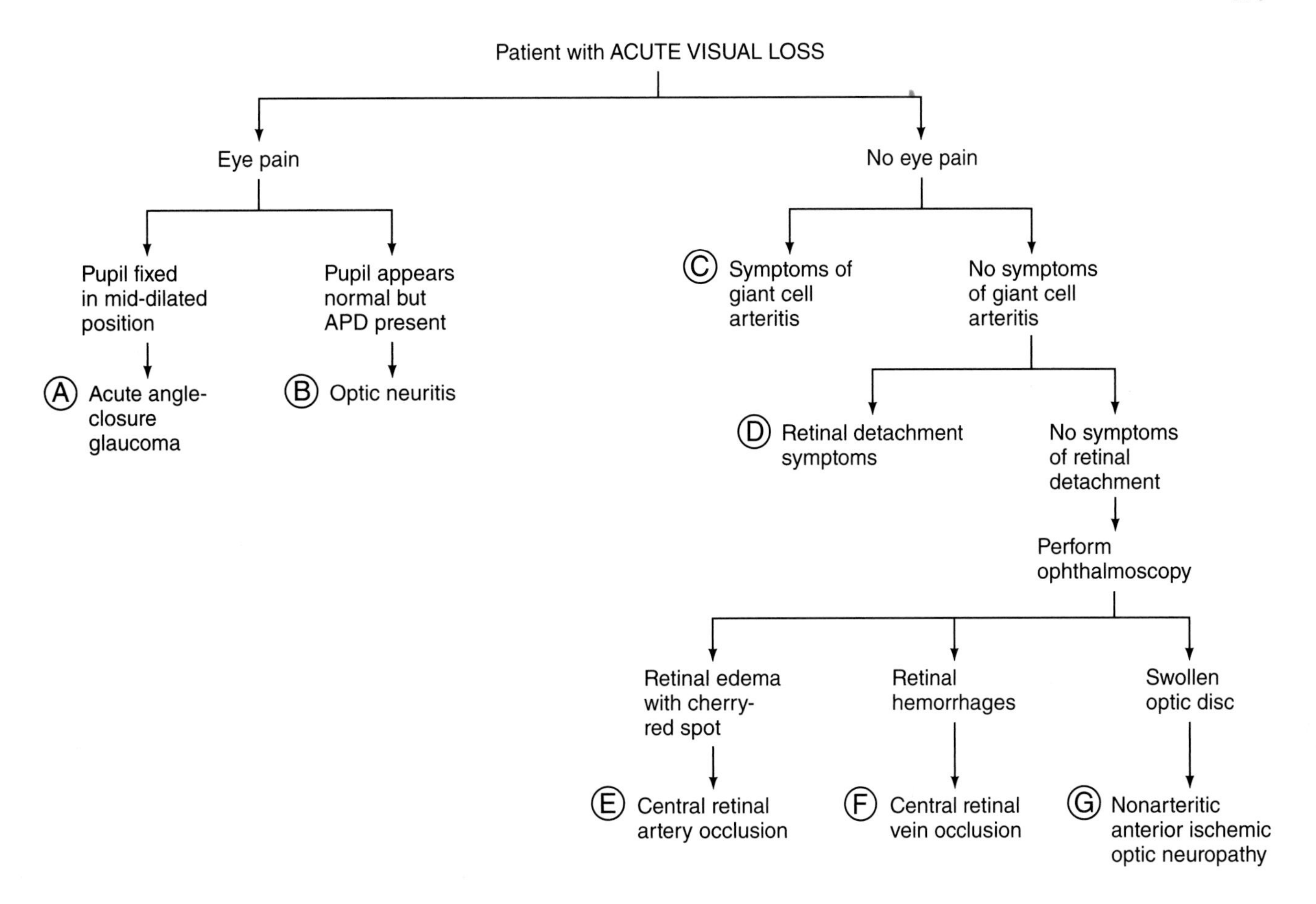

Patient with ACUTE VISUAL LOSS
Eye pain
No eye pain
Pupil fixed in mid-dilated position
Pupil appears normal but APD present
A Acute angle-closure glaucoma
B Optic neuritis
C Symptoms of giant cell arteritis
No symptoms of giant cell arteritis
D Retinal detachment symptoms
No symptoms of retinal detachment
Perform ophthalmoscopy
Retinal edema with cherry-red spot
Retinal hemorrhages
Swollen optic disc
E Central retinal artery occlusion
F Central retinal vein occlusion
G Nonarteritic anterior ischemic optic neuropathy

Pulmonary Disease

Patricia Kritek, MD
Section Editor

HEMOPTYSIS

Diana Gallagher, MD

Expectoration of blood from the respiratory tract, *hemoptysis,* is a common medical condition best managed through a stepwise evaluation. Hemoptysis can range from mild blood-tinged sputum to massive, life-threatening bleeding.

In the United States, the most common cause of hemoptysis is respiratory infection causing local trauma to airway mucosal surfaces and resulting in blood-tinged sputum. In the majority of cases, symptoms abate when the infection clears. Patients with chronic respiratory infections can develop bronchiectasis: airway dilation after recurrent inflammation and mucous plugging. These patients usually have chronic cough and phlegm, which can at times become bloody. Occasionally, in severe bronchiectasis as occurs in patients with cystic fibrosis, airways become markedly dilated and an adjacent bronchial artery ruptures with subsequent massive hemoptysis.

Patients with hemoptysis often worry that the cause is lung cancer. Less than 10% of patients with lung cancer will initially present with hemoptysis; as stated earlier, hemoptysis is much more likely to be caused by infection. Bronchogenic carcinoma should be a consideration in any patient with hemoptysis in the absence of infectious symptoms. Former or active smokers are of particular concern. Malignancies that metastasize to lung, such as renal cell, colon, melanoma, and breast cancer, should also be considered in proper context.

Less common etiologies include pulmonary infarction, mitral stenosis, congestive heart failure, tuberculosis, catamenial (menstrual), arteriovenous malformations, coagulopathy, foreign body, and vasculitis. Up to one third of cases of hemoptysis are "idiopathic," and most of these cases resolve on their own within 6 months.

A. A careful history and physical examination are imperative for evaluation. The first issue to clarify is the source of bleeding because "pseudohemoptysis" with blood from the nasooropharynx or GI tract can be confused with true hemoptysis.

B. Once it is clear that blood originates from the respiratory tract, it is important to clarify if it is a small amount of blood mixed with purulent phlegm or more substantive bleeding.

C. If the hemoptysis is only mild blood-streaked sputum and the patient is an otherwise healthy nonsmoker who is <40 years of age, a chest x-ray (CXR) to assess for infiltrate or mass followed by further conservative management is advised. If the patient has risk factors for malignancy, a bronchoscopy is recommended to rule out endobronchial lesions.

D. If frank blood is expectorated or repeated episodes of bleeding occur, an initial workup includes CXR, CBC, coagulation studies, and urinalysis (UA). This almost always warrants inpatient evaluation.

E. At this point, most patients are treated empirically for infection, but most warrant further evaluation. The next step is either a high-resolution chest CT or a bronchoscopy, depending on the most likely etiology for bleeding. Bronchoscopy is most useful to look for endobronchial masses. A high-resolution chest CT can reveal parenchymal abnormalities that could be missed by plain CXR. In most cases, a clinician will start with one test and if it is negative move to the other complementary test. A word of caution: Bronchoscopic evaluation with a normal CXR is usually low yield but deemed necessary, especially in men, smokers, those >40 years, and in cases of bleeding lasting ≥1 week.

F. Massive hemoptysis, conservatively defined as >200 ml in 24 hours, is a potentially life-threatening condition that requires urgent management. Airway stabilization is followed by evaluation for the source of bleeding. Interventional bronchial artery angiography offers diagnostic and therapeutic options because a bleeding vessel can be embolized. However, embolization carries a 10% risk of spinal artery embolization with paralysis and should be performed only by an experienced operator. Surgical resection is the usual alternative when embolization is too high risk or technically impossible. If the bleeding stops, evaluation as one would for nonmassive hemoptysis is appropriate.

G. In nonmassive hemoptysis, treatment is based on presumed etiology. Most of the time, this includes treatment of infection or definitive therapy for underlying malignancy. Recurrent nonmassive hemoptysis is also treated with embolization or resection if conservative management is unsuccessful.

References

Bidwell J, Pachner R. Hemoptysis diagnosis and management. Am Fam Physician 2005;72(7):1253–1260.

Lordan JL, Gascoigne A, Corris PA. Assessment and management of massive hemoptysis. Thorax 2003;58(9):814–819.

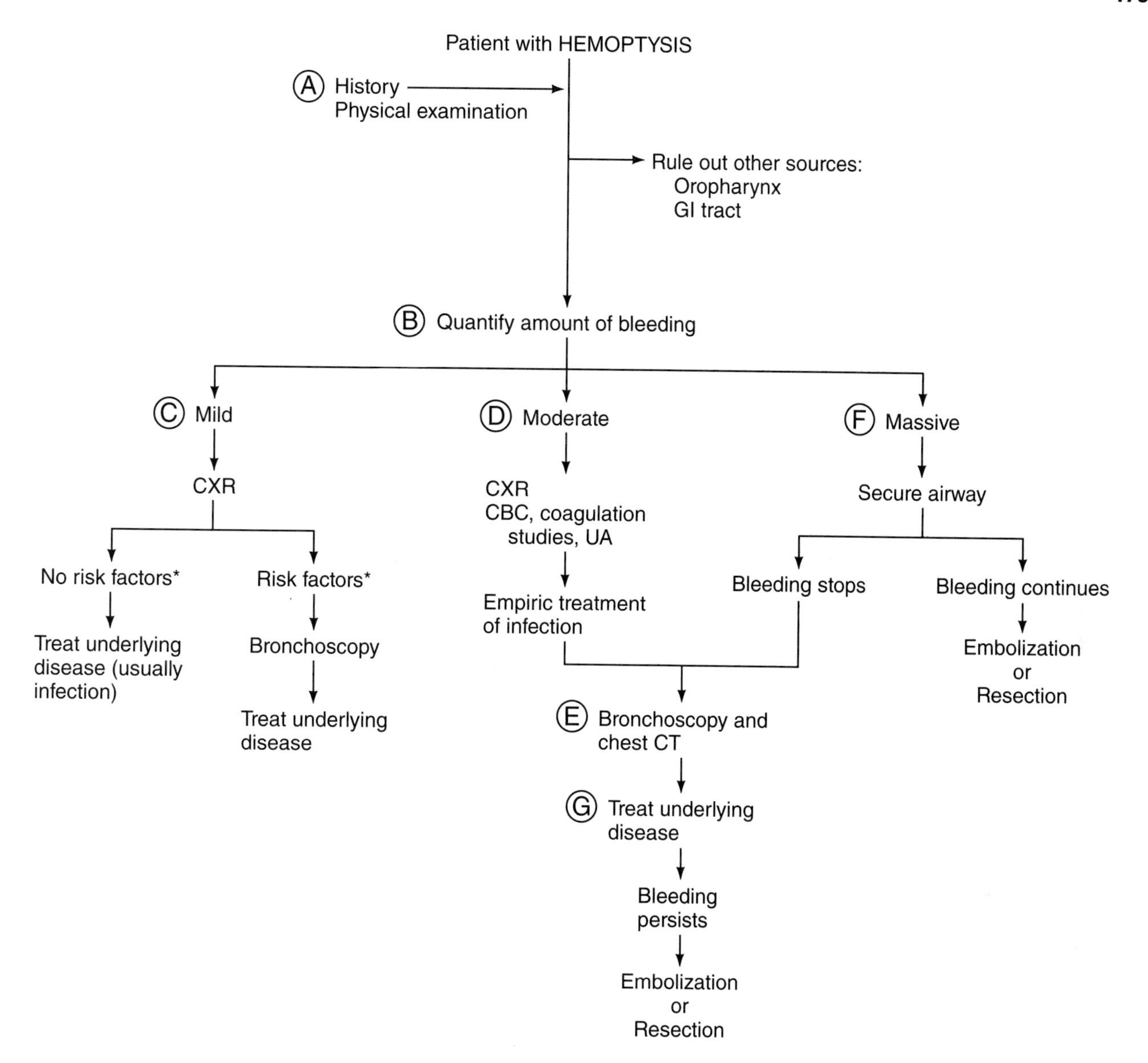
Patient with HEMOPTYSIS
(A) History
Physical examination
Rule out other sources:
Oropharynx
GI tract
(B) Quantify amount of bleeding
(C) Mild
CXR
No risk factors*
Treat underlying disease (usually infection)
Risk factors*
Bronchoscopy
Treat underlying disease
(D) Moderate
CXR
CBC, coagulation studies, UA
Empiric treatment of infection
(E) Bronchoscopy and chest CT
(G) Treat underlying disease
Bleeding persists
Embolization or Resection
(F) Massive
Secure airway
Bleeding stops
Bleeding continues
Embolization or Resection

*Risk factors: smoking, age >40, male

STRIDOR

Diana Gallagher, MD

Stridor, an audible high-pitched sound with respiration, is a common but serious symptom that requires immediate medical evaluation. It occurs when air is forced through a narrowed airway lumen. In general, narrowing superior to the vocal cords leads to inspiratory stridor, whereas narrowing below the vocal cords produces either expiratory or mixed stridor. Although much attention has been focused on the phase of stridor, the onset of symptoms also provides a useful approach to the management and differential diagnosis.

A. Patients who present with stridor should be triaged as having acute or chronic disease. The clinician should assess whether the symptoms occur with inspiration, expiration, or both and perform a focused history and physical examination. In patients who are stable, imaging can help characterize the airway lesion. The most important initial element of management is ensuring that the patient maintain a safe and patent airway.

B. Acute upper airway obstruction resulting in stridor classically presents with the sudden onset of dyspnea and respiratory distress. These patients should be brought immediately to the emergency department. Because of concern for impending airway closure, treatment for presumed anaphylaxis and laryngeal edema with epinephrine is appropriate in patients with acute stridor.

C. Laryngeal edema most often presents in cases of anaphylaxis or inhalational injuries. In anaphylaxis, a history of exposure to a known offending agent should be sought. Examination should include evaluation for swelling of the lips, tongue, or eyes and an urticarial rash. Rarely, patients will give a history of a hereditary form of angioedema from C1 esterase gene mutations. Thermal injury after smoke inhalation can cause delayed onset of airway edema, and patients require close ongoing monitoring for signs of distress.

D. Infection is another common cause of acute stridor. Although epiglottitis is the most concerning potential infection, the clinician should also consider bacterial tracheitis and retropharyngeal or peritonsillar abscess. Before widespread flu immunization, epiglottitis was a disease of childhood, but it is now increasingly recognized in adults. Adults present with fever, neck pain, and odynophagia and, as a late finding, stridor. If the stridor is subacute, lateral radiographs of the neck may be obtained and classically reveal swelling of the epiglottis (the so-called thumb sign), uvula, and prevertebral soft tissues. Epiglottitis can be a life-threatening condition requiring urgent tracheotomy in as many as 15% of adults; some series report a mortality rate as high as 7%.

E. Foreign body aspiration, although typically seen in children, can also occur in adults as a result of accidental inhalation or bulbar dysfunction as in amyotrophic lateral sclerosis (ALS), Parkinson's disease, or other neurologic diseases.

F. In the event of respiratory decompensation in the setting of acute stridor, a fiberoptic intubation in the hands of the most experienced operator is preferred, with backup in place for a surgical tracheotomy.

G. The clinician should consider a unique differential diagnosis for patients who present with subacute or chronic stridor. The first concern is for structural abnormalities in the upper airway resulting from neoplasms, benign cysts, or goiter. Additionally, tracheal stenosis can be seen resulting from protracted intubation with balloon cuff injury or in cases of severe gastroesophageal reflux disease (GERD). Vocal cord dysfunction with involuntary adduction of the cords will also produce intermittent stridor. More rarely, rheumatoid arthritis results in cricoarytenoid disease and subsequent stridor.

H. As part of the initial workup, flow-volume loops obtained by spirometry can suggest whether there is a fixed or variable obstruction and whether the obstruction is intrathoracic or extrathoracic in location. Most clinicians obtain a chest radiograph, although a CT scan with reconstructions of the airway highlights the nature and extent of the lesion more completely. Direct visualization with laryngoscopy in the hands of an otolaryngologist, or bronchoscopy by a pulmonologist, remains the gold standard and also allows for potential intervention.

References

Cordle R. Upper respiratory emergencies. In Tintinalli JE, Kelen GD, Stapczynski JS, et al, eds. Tintinalli's Emergency Medicine: A Comprehensive Study Guide, 6th ed. New York: McGraw-Hill, 2004:848–857.

Tierney LM Jr, McPhee SJ, Papadakis MA, eds; Gonzales R, Zeiger R, online eds., Current Medical Diagnosis and Treatment: Ear, Nose, and Throat: Dysphonia, Hoarseness, and Stridor. New York: McGraw-Hill, 2006.

Upper airway obstruction. In Fraser RS, Müller NL, Colman N, et al., Fraser and Pare's Diagnosis of Diseases of the Chest. Philadelphia: Elsevier, 1999:2021–2053.

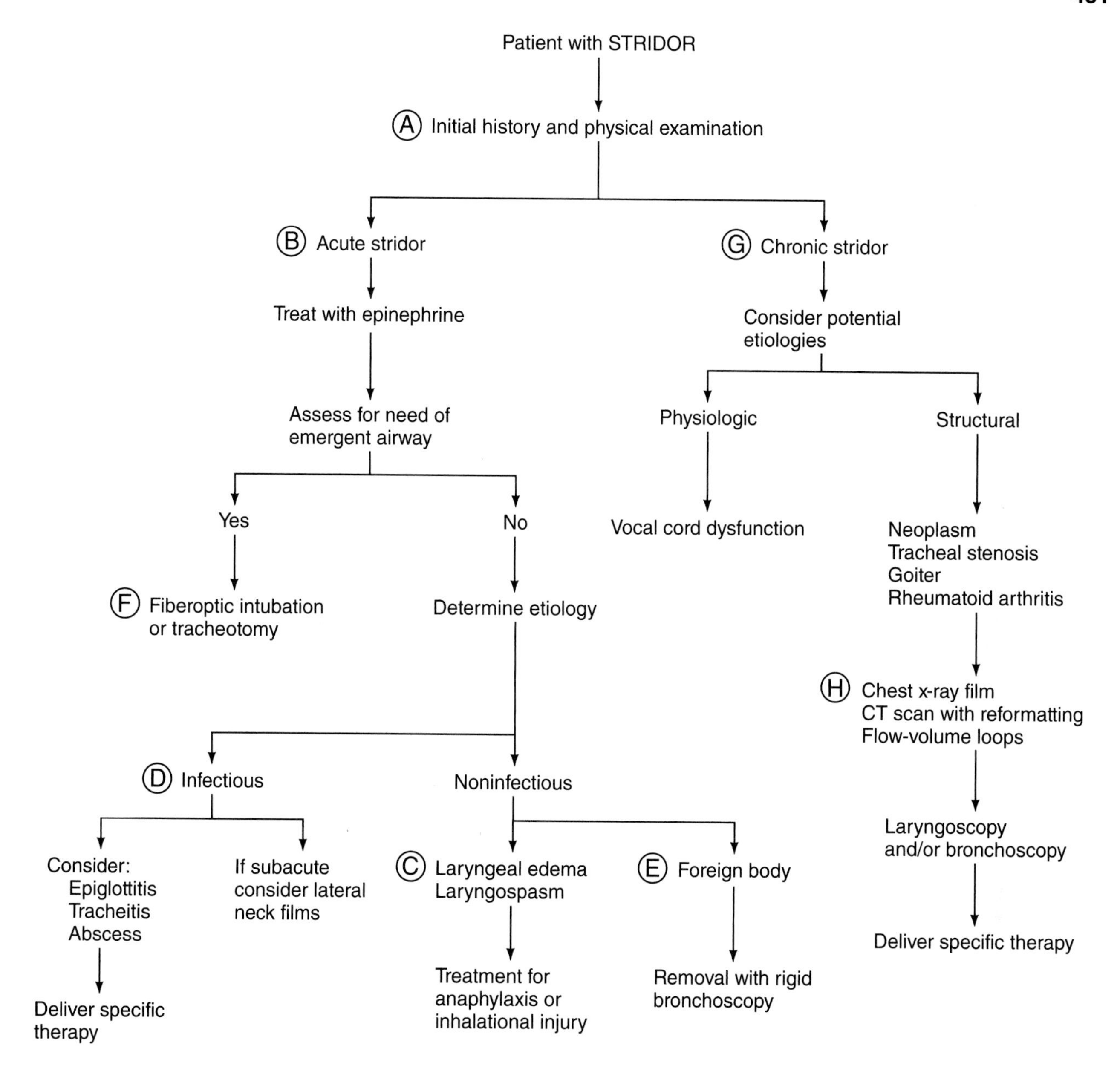
Patient with STRIDOR
(A) Initial history and physical examination
(B) Acute stridor
Treat with epinephrine
Assess for need of emergent airway
Yes
(F) Fiberoptic intubation or tracheotomy
No
Determine etiology
(D) Infectious
Consider:
Epiglottitis
Tracheitis
Abscess
Deliver specific therapy
If subacute consider lateral neck films
Noninfectious
(C) Laryngeal edema
Laryngospasm
Treatment for anaphylaxis or inhalational injury
(E) Foreign body
Removal with rigid bronchoscopy
(G) Chronic stridor
Consider potential etiologies
Physiologic
Vocal cord dysfunction
Structural
Neoplasm
Tracheal stenosis
Goiter
Rheumatoid arthritis
(H) Chest x-ray film
CT scan with reformatting
Flow-volume loops
Laryngoscopy and/or bronchoscopy
Deliver specific therapy

WHEEZING

Sunita Sharma, MD

Wheezes are continuous, high-pitched adventitious lung sounds that are superimposed on normal breath sounds. Wheezes are sounds that are produced by the oscillation of the airway walls with fluid within the airway lumen that occurs when airway caliber is narrowed to a critical value. The pitch of the wheeze is dependent on the elastic properties of the airway walls, the viscosity of the fluid in the airways, and the characteristics of the gas that pass through the narrowed airway. Although asthma is often considered the most common cause of wheezing, there are a number of nonasthmatic pulmonary conditions and nonpulmonary diseases associated with wheezing. A variety of diagnostic studies can be used to evaluate the patient with wheezing to determine the etiology of the wheeze.

A. The initial evaluation of a patient with wheezing should determine the degree of respiratory distress that the individual has incurred. Patients who exhibit signs concerning for impending respiratory failure, including tachypnea with accessory muscle use, hypoxemia, cyanosis, or severe acute respiratory acidosis, warrant emergent endotracheal intubation. Diagnostic studies to determine the etiology of wheezing can be performed after the initial stabilization of the patient. Because rapid therapy is essential, the diagnosis of anaphylaxis should be considered. If this is a probable cause of wheezing and/or stridor, immediate administration of epinephrine is required.

B. Respiratory failure resulting from severe asthma is a condition known as *status asthmaticus*. Early diagnosis of this condition is essential to initiate appropriate therapy. ABGs can be beneficial in the early assessment of patients with asthma flares but should not delay therapy. In the initial stages of an acute asthma exacerbation, it is common for a patient to have respiratory alkalosis as a result of tachypnea. Acute respiratory acidosis in a patient with known asthma is an ominous sign indicating impending respiratory failure and should warrant consideration of intubation. The mainstays of treatment for status asthmaticus include inhaled beta agonists and IV corticosteroids. Because it can take several hours for these therapies to have their optimal effect, the initial ventilator management in patients with status asthmaticus can be difficult and often requires specialized respiratory care services.

C. A detailed medical history including personal, family, and social history may provide clues that lead to an appropriate diagnosis. Personal history should include the age of onset of symptoms, triggers for wheezing, and aggravating and alleviating conditions. Past medical history including allergic rhinitis with postnasal drip symptoms, history of aspiration or conditions that predispose to aspiration, and a history of congestive heart failure (CHF) should be elicited as potential causes of wheezing. Smoking status and occupational and home exposures are also important in determining the cause of wheezing. A family history of asthma is also suggestive of a diagnosis of asthma. History of fever and new-onset sputum production raise the possibility of pneumonia or viral bronchitis.

D. Noninvasive tests such as radiographic studies and pulmonary function studies are useful in differentiating the disorders associated with wheezing. Chest radiographs are a simple way to initiate the evaluation of wheezing. Chest radiographs help diagnose large mass lesions causing airway obstruction and resulting in wheezing. Pulmonary function studies are another useful tool for the investigation of wheezing. Spirometry is used to identify obstruction, defined as FEV_1/FVC (forced expiratory volume in 1 second/forced vital capacity) $<70\%$. Additionally, flow-volume loops can identify upper airway obstruction and help differentiate among extrathoracic and intrathoracic, fixed and variable, and obstructive lesions.

(Continued on page 484)

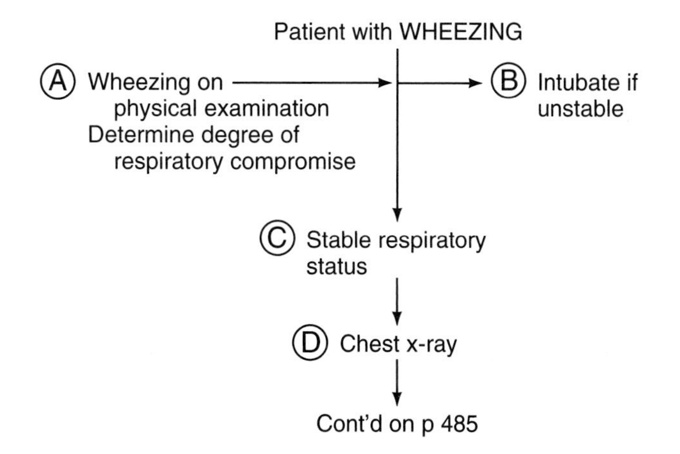
Patient with WHEEZING
Ⓐ Wheezing on physical examination
Determine degree of respiratory compromise
Ⓑ Intubate if unstable
Ⓒ Stable respiratory status
Ⓓ Chest x-ray
Cont'd on p 485

E. Asthma is the most common condition associated with wheezing. Asthma is a chronic obstructive pulmonary disease (COPD) that is associated with inflammation of the airways leading to *reversible* airflow obstruction. Asthma is commonly associated with an obstructive pattern on pulmonary function studies that is at least partially reversible with bronchodilators such as albuterol. Reversibility of airflow obstruction is defined as a 200 cc and 12% improvement in either FEV_1 or FVC after inhalation of albuterol. Patients who have a history consistent with asthma and normal pulmonary function studies can be further studied with a methacholine bronchoprovocation study. Patients who demonstrate a 20% decline in their FEV_1 with the inhalation of methacholine are diagnosed with asthma. The mainstays of treatment for asthma include inhaled corticosteroids, inhaled beta agonists, and leukotriene receptor blockers. Difficult-to-treat asthma may require systemic corticosteroids. Frequent use of systemic corticosteroids, nocturnal symptoms, emergency department visits, and previous intubations for asthma are all characteristics that suggest poorly controlled asthma and often portend a poorer prognosis for asthma outcomes.

F. Incompletely reversible airflow obstruction demonstrated by a reduction in the FEV_1/FVC ratio with minimal or no improvement after inhaled bronchodilator is suggestive of COPD such as chronic bronchitis and emphysema. A smoking history or chronic sputum production can suggest these conditions. Early-onset COPD or a family history of early-onset COPD raises the suspicion of alpha-1-antitrypsin deficiency. This can be evaluated by measuring alpha-1-antitrypsin levels. Poorly reversible airflow obstruction in a young patient with excessive sputum production and bronchiectasis on CT raises the possibility of cystic fibrosis. Cystic fibrosis is diagnosed by sweat-chloride testing or genetic studies. Fever and cough can suggest a viral etiology of wheezing in both patients with no history of lung disease and in individuals with preexisting COPD. The constellation of symptoms including wheezing, flushing, and profuse diarrhea is characteristic of carcinoid syndrome, which is characterized by an elevated urinary 5-hydroxyindoleacetic acid (5-HIAA) level. This is a rare cause of wheezing.

G. A variety of other atypical conditions can be associated with wheezing. The diagnosis of wheezing conditions other than COPD should be considered in all patients whose initial evaluation is inconsistent with asthma or when wheezing continues despite conventional asthma treatment. Postnasal drip is a common cause of wheezing. Postnasal drip causes wheezing from upper airway inflammation and airway narrowing that most commonly occurs at the level of the vocal cords. Treatment with inhaled corticosteroids is the treatment of choice for this condition. Gastroesophageal reflux disease (GERD) and aspiration are two other conditions often associated with wheezing. It is important to note that, whereas GERD has been associated with asthma exacerbations, reflux is also an independent cause of wheezing in patients without obstructive pulmonary diseases. Finally, a variety of interstitial lung diseases (ILDs) may have wheezing as a component of an atypical presentation. A CT scan can help with this diagnosis.

H. Pulmonary embolism (PE) is a less common cause of wheezing. Contrast-enhanced CT studies can help make this diagnosis. Patients typically present with acute-onset dyspnea, which may be associated with wheezing. Patients are typically found to have sinus tachycardia but can have patterns of right-sided heart strain on their echocardiogram. In patients in whom the diagnosis of pulmonary embolism is entertained and the renal function is impaired, ventilation/perfusion (V/Q) scans can help in making the diagnosis of pulmonary embolism.

I. The wheeze associated with CHF is commonly referred to as cardiac asthma because it mimics the wheeze associated with asthma. A history of orthopnea, paroxysmal nocturnal dyspnea, weight gain, and lower-extremity edema should raise the possibility of CHF as a potential etiology of wheezing in certain patients. A transthoracic echocardiogram is useful in the evaluation of cardiac function. Diuresis is the therapy for this cause of wheezing.

J. Invasive diagnostic testing should be reserved for patients in whom no alternative cause of wheezing has been determined. Invasive procedures such as bronchoscopy with bronchoalveolar lavage, transbronchial or endobronchial biopsies, Wang needle biopsies, mediastinoscopy, CT-guided biopsy, and open-lung biopsy can be performed when a diagnosis cannot be made by noninvasive means. The ideal invasive, diagnostic approach can be made in consultation with a pulmonologist, thoracic surgeon, and interventional radiologist.

References

American Thoracic Society. Committee on Pulmonary Nomenclature. Am Thorac Soc News 1977;3:6.

Holden DA, Mehta AC. Evaluation of wheezing in the nonasthmatic patient. Cleve Clin J Med 1990;57:345.

Irwin RS, Pratter MR, Holland PS, et al. Postnasal drip causes cough and is associated with reversible upper airway obstruction. Chest 1984;85:346.

McKean MC, Leech M, Lambert PC, et al. A model of viral wheeze in nonasthmatic adults: symptoms and physiology. Eur Respir J 2001;18:23.

Meselier N, Charbonneau G, Racineux JL. Wheezes. Eur Respir J 1995;8:1942.

Miller RD, Hyatt RE. Obstruction lesions of the larynx and trachea: clinical and physiologic characteristics. Mayo Clin Proc 1969;44:145.

Wong CY, Shum TT, Law GTS, et al. All that wheezes is not asthma. Hong Kong Med J 2003;9:39–42.

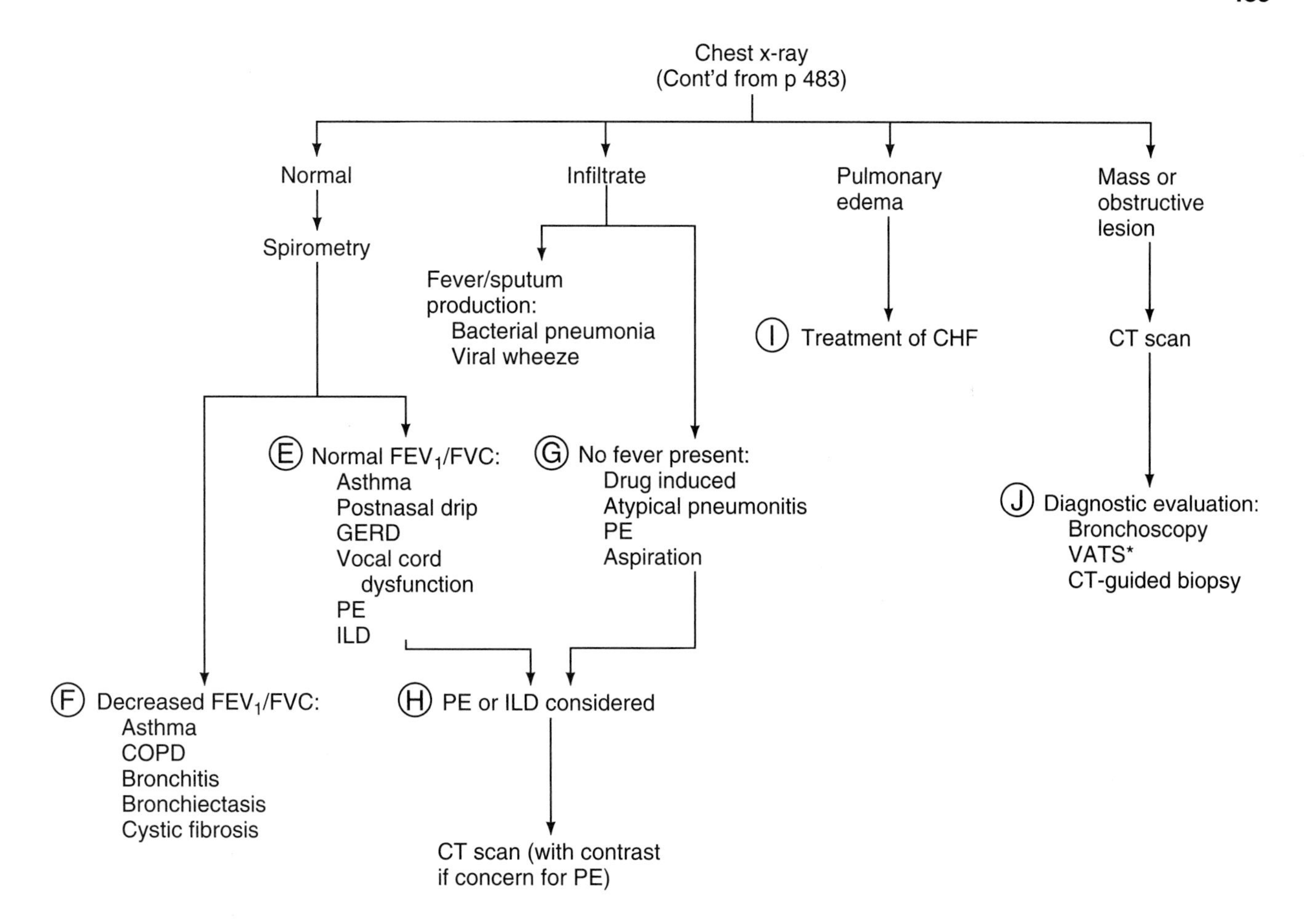
Chest x-ray
(Cont'd from p 483)
Normal
Infiltrate
Pulmonary edema
Mass or obstructive lesion
Spirometry
Fever/sputum production:
Bacterial pneumonia
Viral wheeze
I Treatment of CHF
CT scan
E Normal FEV_1/FVC:
Asthma
Postnasal drip
GERD
Vocal cord dysfunction
PE
ILD
G No fever present:
Drug induced
Atypical pneumonitis
PE
Aspiration
J Diagnostic evaluation:
Bronchoscopy
VATS*
CT-guided biopsy
F Decreased FEV_1/FVC:
Asthma
COPD
Bronchitis
Bronchiectasis
Cystic fibrosis
H PE or ILD considered
CT scan (with contrast if concern for PE)

*VATS, Video-assisted thoracoscopic surgery.

COUGH

Patricia Kritek, MD

Cough is one of the most common reasons that patients seek medical attention. Although it is one of the defense mechanisms protecting the respiratory system, it also contributes to the spread of airborne disease and can be bothersome to patients. Cough can result from infection, inflammation, and mechanical or chemical irritation. The majority of cases of cough can be diagnosed and treated by following a stepwise approach.

A. Obtaining a thorough history is the first step in the diagnosis and therapy of cough. Initial evaluation begins with categorizing the cough as acute (<3 weeks), subacute (3–8 weeks), or chronic (>8 weeks). This categorization is helpful because the majority of acute cough is infectious in nature, most commonly viral. Chronic cough has a more varied differential diagnosis (see later). Other important features of the history include current and past smoking history and occupational exposures. All patients with cough should be asked about the use of angiotensin-converting enzyme (ACE) inhibitors because cough is a common side effect of this class of medications. Review should also include potential infectious exposures such as tuberculosis, endemic fungi, and *Bordetella pertussis.*

B. Physical examination should focus on signs of underlying disease that would predispose to cough. These findings include cobblestoning of the posterior oropharynx or sinus tenderness suggesting postnasal drip, wheezing suggestive of asthma, or crackles consistent with interstitial lung disease. Many of the most common causes of cough, however, will have no localizing physical examination findings.

C. Acute cough is commonly caused by viral infections of the upper or lower respiratory tract. New-onset cough can also be a sign of an exacerbation of an underlying disease such as asthma, chronic obstructive pulmonary disease (COPD), or bronchiectasis or a response to a new allergen or irritant. Most causes of acute cough can be treated with an antihistamine and/or decongestant and do not require further evaluation. Although most acute coughs have a less serious cause, clinicians should remain vigilant to the possibility of life-threatening cough, including diagnoses such as pneumonia, congestive heart failure (CHF), and pulmonary embolism.

D. There are less data to guide the evaluation and management of subacute cough. Subacute cough that is not thought to follow an infection should be treated as chronic cough. Postinfectious cough can be from a variety of etiologies, including postnasal drip, exacerbation of underlying asthma, or bronchitis. Treatment should be guided by most likely cause of persisting cough.

E. The majority of chronic cough is the result of cough-variant asthma, upper airway cough syndrome (UACS), and gastroesophageal reflux disease (GERD). The most recent American College of Chest Physicians (ACCP) guidelines recommend the use of the term *UACS* in lieu of *postnasal drip* because it is more comprehensive. These guidelines also support the addition of nonasthmatic eosinophilic bronchitis (NAEB) as a common cause of chronic cough. NAEB consists of cough with normal spirometry without airway responsiveness and eosinophilic infiltration of the bronchial tree that resolves with steroid inhaler therapy.

F. All patients with chronic cough should have a chest x-ray (CXR) study to assess for mass lesions and infiltrates and other anatomic causes of cough.

G. Most algorithms, including that of the ACCP, recommend a strategy of empiric therapy after history, physical examination, and CXR. Initial therapy usually begins with UACS or asthma, but it can be guided by clinical impression based on history and physical examination. If UACS seems most likely, initiate empiric therapy with antihistamines and decongestants. If there is only a partial response, addition of nasal steroids or nasal anticholinergics should be considered. Further evaluation, including sinus films, is warranted in patients with persistent UACS symptoms after maximal therapy.

H. Patients in whom asthma is suspected should be treated with inhaled steroids and inhaled beta agonists. It is recommended that these patients initially undergo spirometry, with bronchodilator responsiveness testing. Some favor bronchoprovocation with methacholine to better assess for underlying asthma, but this is not needed in all patients. If patients respond partially, continued stepwise asthma therapy is indicated.

I. Treatment for NAEB entails inhaled steroids and patients usually respond within weeks of initiation of therapy. As stated previously, these patients have normal spirometry without bronchodilator responsiveness. The diagnosis can be confirmed by an examination of sputum for eosinophils.

J. If response is incomplete or there is no response to the initial empiric strategies, treatment for GERD is warranted. If patients have symptoms of reflux, it is reasonable to initiate a proton pump inhibitor (PPI) and lifestyle modifications to decrease reflux. Some recommend 24-hour esophageal pH monitoring to establish the diagnosis in patients without clear GERD symptoms.

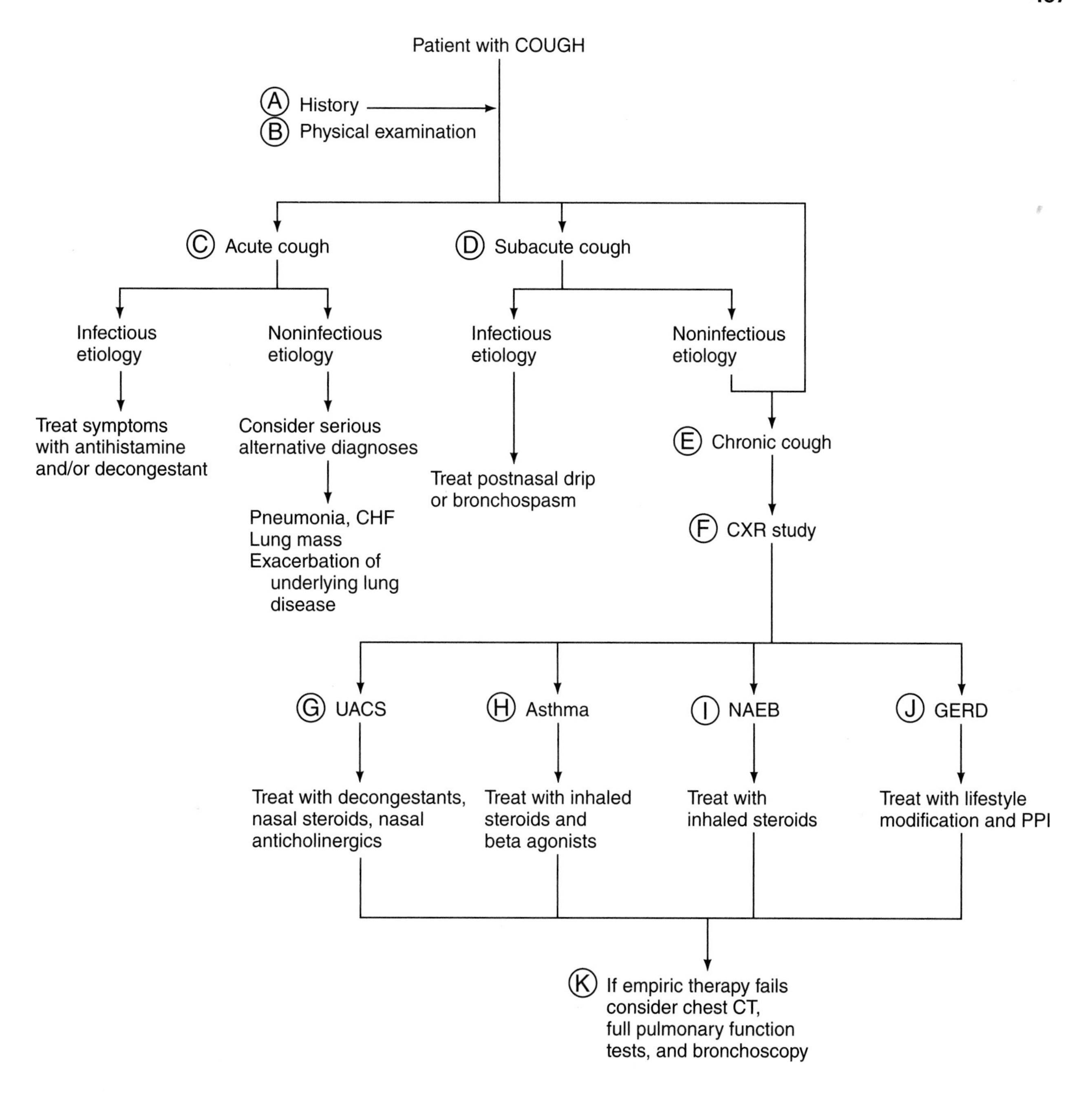

This therapy, at times, will take up to several months to have an impact on the patient's cough.

K. If all the previously mentioned empiric trials are ineffective, further diagnostic evaluation is appropriate. In most cases, CT scan of the chest, full pulmonary function testing (lung volumes, spirometry, DLCO [diffusing capacity of the lung for carbon monoxide]), and bronchoscopy are recommended.

References

Murray JF, Nadel JA. Textbook of Respiratory Medicine. Philadelphia: Saunders, 2000.

Pratter M. Overview of common causes of chronic cough: ACCP Evidence Based Clinical Practice Guidelines. Chest 2006;129: 59S–62S.

Pratter M, Brightling CE, Boulet LP, et al. An empiric integrative approach to the management of cough: ACCP Evidence Based Clinical Practice Guidelines. Chest 2006;129:222S–231S.

DYSPNEA

Essam Al-Ansari, MD

Dyspnea is the subjective sensation of shortness of breath, which may be discomfort or an abnormal awareness of breathing. Dyspnea can occur as a consequence of increased work of breathing or when there is stimulation of respiratory centers in the brainstem or receptors throughout the respiratory system. These receptors are located throughout the respiratory system, including the upper airway, the alveolar and interstitial space (juxtacapillary, or J, receptors), the airways, the respiratory muscles, and the chest wall. Dyspnea is often the most prominent symptom of pulmonary disease, but it can also be the primary manifestation of nonpulmonary disorders. Most notably, it is often difficult to distinguish between pulmonary and cardiac causes of dyspnea.

A. The initial assessment of a patient with dyspnea focuses on the history. Acute dyspnea should be evaluated urgently, often in the emergency department. More chronic dyspnea may be evaluated in a stepwise fashion in an outpatient setting. Key aspects of the history include smoking history or occupational/environmental exposures, symptoms associated with the dyspnea, and triggers of the dyspnea. The words the patient uses to describe the dyspnea can also be helpful. Common descriptions include "air hunger," "chest tightness," and "inability to get a full breath."

B. Physical examination helps guide further diagnostic studies. Inspection includes observation of pursed-lipped breathing (often associated with obstructive lung disease), the presence of Kussmaul's respirations (rapid and deep breaths, usually associated with severe metabolic acidosis), or Cheyne-Stokes respirations (a regularly irregular pattern, commonly seen in congestive heart failure [CHF]). Clubbing should raise suspicion of interstitial lung disease, bronchiectasis, or lung cancer. Cardiac examination can elicit signs of CHF such as S_3, S_4, and jugular venous distention. The findings of crackles, wheezes, or rhonchi also help distinguish between causes of dyspnea.

C. The first study in the evaluation of dyspnea is often a chest x-ray (CXR). This study can reveal underlying changes consistent with CHF, chronic obstructive pulmonary disease (COPD), or interstitial lung disease. It can also demonstrate pleural effusions, which may have been suspected based on the physical examination, and masses, which may have gone undetected. At the same time, initial studies should include a CBC to assess for anemia as a cause of dyspnea.

D. The most common nonpulmonary causes of dyspnea are cardiac in origin. These include CHF, cardiac ischemia, arrhythmias, and valvular disease. These different causes can be better distinguished by ECG, echocardiography, and possible cardiopulmonary exercise testing. Treatment should be guided by the individual diagnosis.

E. Other nonpulmonary causes include metabolic derangements and anemia and psychological causes of dyspnea such as anxiety, panic attacks, or depression. Psychological disorders are always a diagnosis of exclusion.

F. In a patient with presumed pulmonary disease and normal CXR, the next step is often pulmonary function testing (PFT). Initial spirometry can guide further studies, diagnose obstruction ($FEV_1/FVC <70\%$), and suggest restrictive physiology. Lung volumes will diagnose restriction, and additional PFT can help distinguish between interstitial lung disease, neuromuscular weakness, and results in disorders of the chest wall. The next step in patients with normal PFT and a normal CXR is often cardiopulmonary exercise testing and/or echocardiography.

G. An abnormal CXR usually prompts further radiograph studies, specifically a chest CT scan. A CT scan can reveal interstitial fibrosis, emphysema, pleural effusions, mass lesions, and pulmonary emboli. Further evaluation and therapy are guided by the findings on CT scan.

References

American Thoracic Society. Dyspnea. Mechanisms, assessment, and management: a consensus statement. Am J Respir Crit Care Med 1999;159:321.

Braunwald E, Fauci AS, Kasper DL, et al, eds. Harrison's Principles of Internal Medicine, 15th ed. New York: McGraw-Hill, 2001.

Michelson E, Hollrah S. Evaluation of the patient with shortness of breath: an evidence-based approach. Emerg Med Clin North Am 1999;17:221.

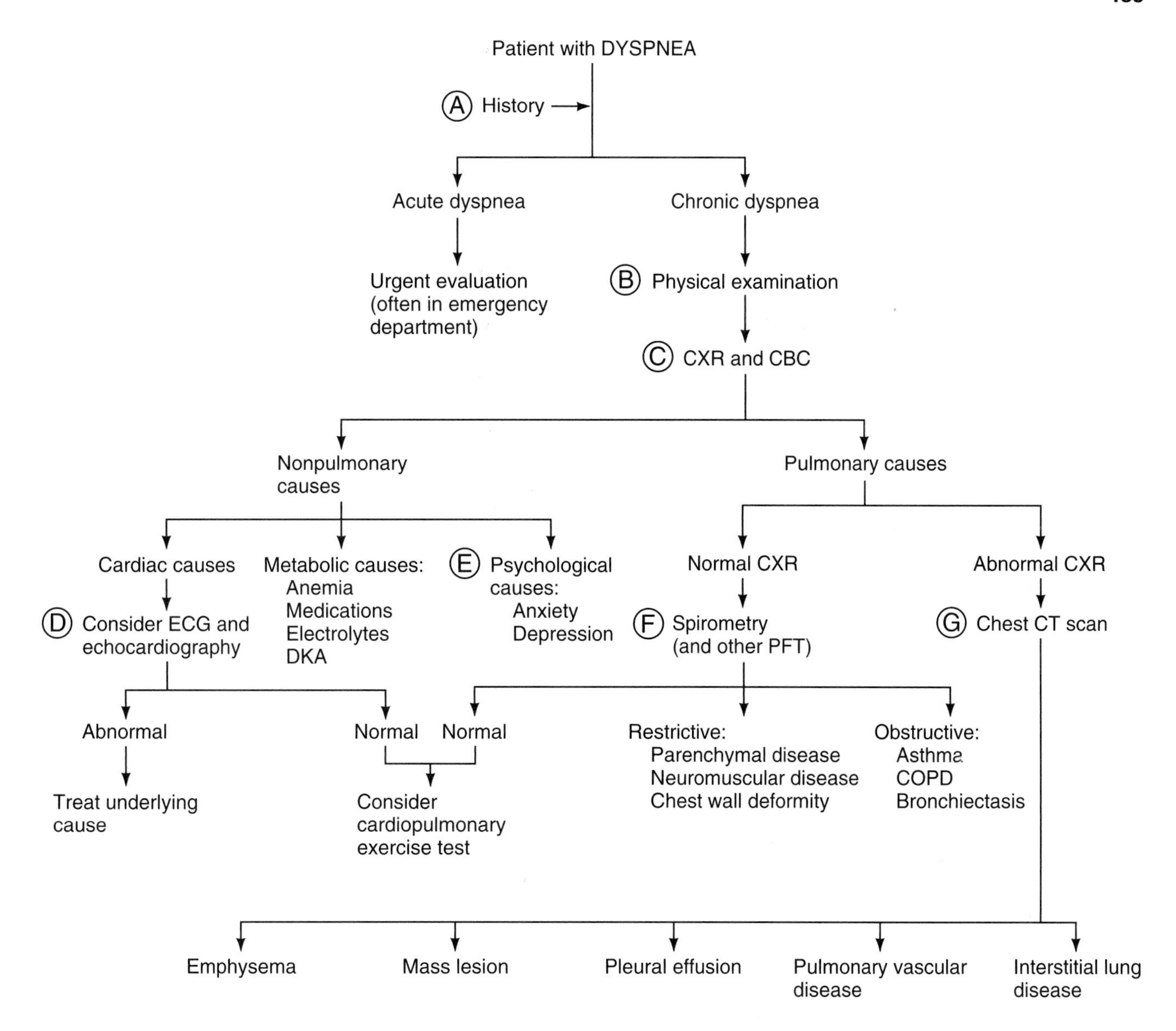
Patient with DYSPNEA
(A) History
Acute dyspnea
Chronic dyspnea
Urgent evaluation (often in emergency department)
(B) Physical examination
(C) CXR and CBC
Nonpulmonary causes
Pulmonary causes
Cardiac causes
Metabolic causes: Anemia Medications Electrolytes DKA
(E) Psychological causes: Anxiety Depression
Normal CXR
Abnormal CXR
(D) Consider ECG and echocardiography
(F) Spirometry (and other PFT)
(G) Chest CT scan
Abnormal
Normal
Normal
Restrictive: Parenchymal disease Neuromuscular disease Chest wall deformity
Obstructive: Asthma COPD Bronchiectasis
Treat underlying cause
Consider cardiopulmonary exercise test
Emphysema
Mass lesion
Pleural effusion
Pulmonary vascular disease
Interstitial lung disease

PLEURAL EFFUSION

Banu A. Karimi-Shah, MD

Many different clinical syndromes can result in accumulation of fluid in the pleural space. The most common causes of pleural effusion in the United States are congestive heart failure (CHF), pneumonia, and malignancy.

A. The differential diagnosis for the cause of a pleural effusion is large. Although sampling of the fluid for laboratory evaluation is necessary for diagnosis in most cases, history can help guide the diagnosis. Previous occupational and environmental exposures, travel outside the United States, presence of fever/constitutional symptoms, history of viral illness, CHF, and recent trauma are but a few of the points to ascertain during the interview.

B. Physical examination of the chest is characterized by diminished or absent breath sounds during auscultation, dullness to percussion, and decreased tactile fremitus. There is often an area of egophony superior to the effusion, reflecting adjacent atelectatic lung.

C. Conventional radiography is usually sufficient imaging to identify the presence of a pleural effusion. Lateral decubitus films can help to quantify the amount of fluid and determine whether it is free-flowing versus loculated. In some cases, ultrasound is required to localize and guide sampling of small fluid collections.

D. Thoracentesis is required in most cases to make a diagnosis. Presence of a >10-mm-thick stripe on a lateral decubitus film confirms that there is sufficient fluid to be obtained. The needle/catheter should be inserted one or two interspaces below the level of the percussed dullness, midway between the posterior-axillary line and the spine. Insertion should take place over the rib to avoid the neurovascular bundle that traverses the inferior costal margin. If the patient has dyspnea, a therapeutic thoracentesis should be performed. The clinician should be careful, however, to remove no more than 1500–1800 ml to avoid reexpansion pulmonary edema.

E. Pleural effusions fall into two broad categories based on Light's criteria: transudates and exudates. Light's criteria are fluid protein/serum protein >0.5, fluid lactate dehydrogenase (LDH)/serum LDH >0.6, and fluid LDH more than two thirds the upper limit of normal in the serum. Light's criteria are most sensitive for identifying exudates but have a lower specificity than other criteria.

F. Transudates accumulate as a result of an imbalance between hydrostatic and oncotic pressures in the pleural space. The leading causes of transudates are CHF and cirrhosis. For transudative pleural effusions, initial testing should be limited to total protein and LDH. Once a transudate is established, further testing may be misleading.

G. Exudates occur when local factors influencing the accumulation of pleural fluid are altered. An exudate is diagnosed when any *one* of Light's criteria is met. Further laboratory evaluation is warranted to specifically diagnose the cause of the exudates.

H. The gross appearance of the fluid can be helpful in specific situations: (1) hemothorax: grossly bloody, (2) anaerobic infection: putrid odor/pus, and (3) chylothorax: milky-white.

(Continued on page 492)

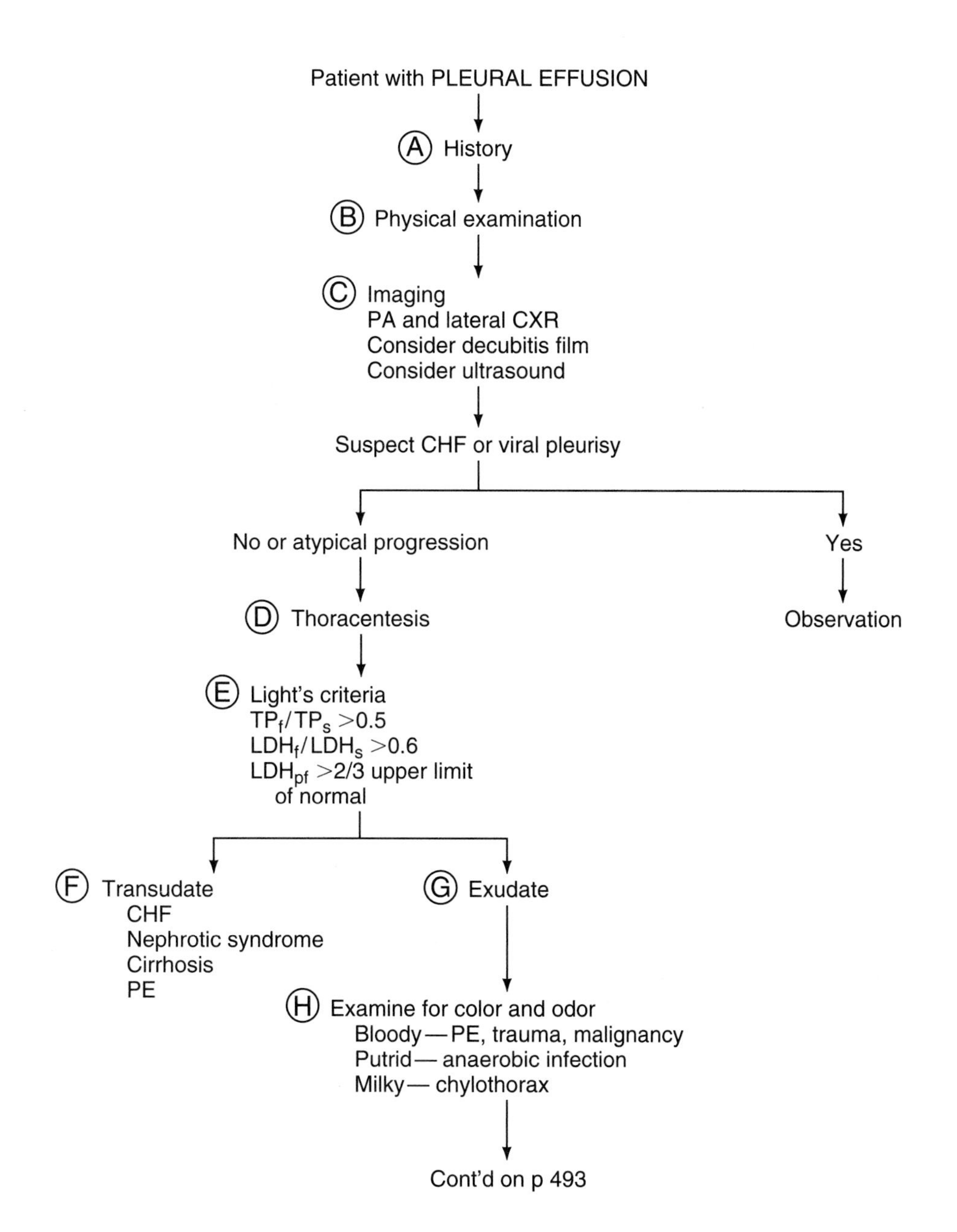
Patient with PLEURAL EFFUSION
(A) History
(B) Physical examination
(C) Imaging
PA and lateral CXR
Consider decubitis film
Consider ultrasound
Suspect CHF or viral pleurisy
No or atypical progression
Yes
Observation
(D) Thoracentesis
(E) Light's criteria
$TP_f/TP_s > 0.5$
$LDH_f/LDH_s > 0.6$
$LDH_{pf} > 2/3$ upper limit of normal
(F) Transudate
CHF
Nephrotic syndrome
Cirrhosis
PE
(G) Exudate
(H) Examine for color and odor
Bloody—PE, trauma, malignancy
Putrid—anaerobic infection
Milky—chylothorax
Cont'd on p 493

I. pH should be measured on most diagnostic pleural fluid samples. A pH <7.20 in the setting of an associated pneumonia indicates an empyema that will require chest tube placement/surgical drainage. Low pH can also be seen in effusions from rheumatoid arthritis, lupus, or malignancy. Malignant effusions with low pH are prognostic of low life expectancy. Glucose <60 mg/dl also suggests the presence of an empyema or a malignant effusion. Other classic causes of low glucose include effusions secondary to tuberculosis and rheumatoid arthritis.

J. A cell count of >50,000 suggests the presence of a complicated parapneumonic effusion/empyema. Chronic exudates are more likely to have low cell counts (<5000). Neutrophilic predominance suggests an acute process, whereas a fluid monocytosis is more likely in a chronic illness. Lymphocytosis in the pleural fluid is seen most commonly in lymphoma and tuberculosis. If mesothelial cells account for >5% of the cells, tuberculosis is an unlikely diagnosis, although not entirely ruled out.

K. Gram stain and culture of pleural fluid are done to rule out the presence of infection and to identify a specific organism. Inoculation of culture bottles at the bedside increases the yield of the test.

L. Cytology can be helpful in both the diagnosis and staging of malignancy. If lymphoma is suspected, flow cytometry should also be analyzed.

M. Additional studies that can be useful in specific clinical situations include triglyceride level (chylothorax) and amylase (esophageal rupture, malignancy, pancreatitis).

N. In more than 25% of cases, even after thorough testing of sampled pleural fluid, the cause of the pleural effusion remains an enigma. Observation versus more invasive procedures should be guided by the patient's clinical presentation and the pretest probability of a serious disease requiring treatment. In the latter group, surgical referral for thoracoscopy and pleural biopsy is warranted.

References

Light RW. Pleural effusion. N Engl J Med 2002;346:1971–1977.
Light RW. Pleural Diseases, 3rd ed. Baltimore: Lippincott Williams & Wilkins, 1995.

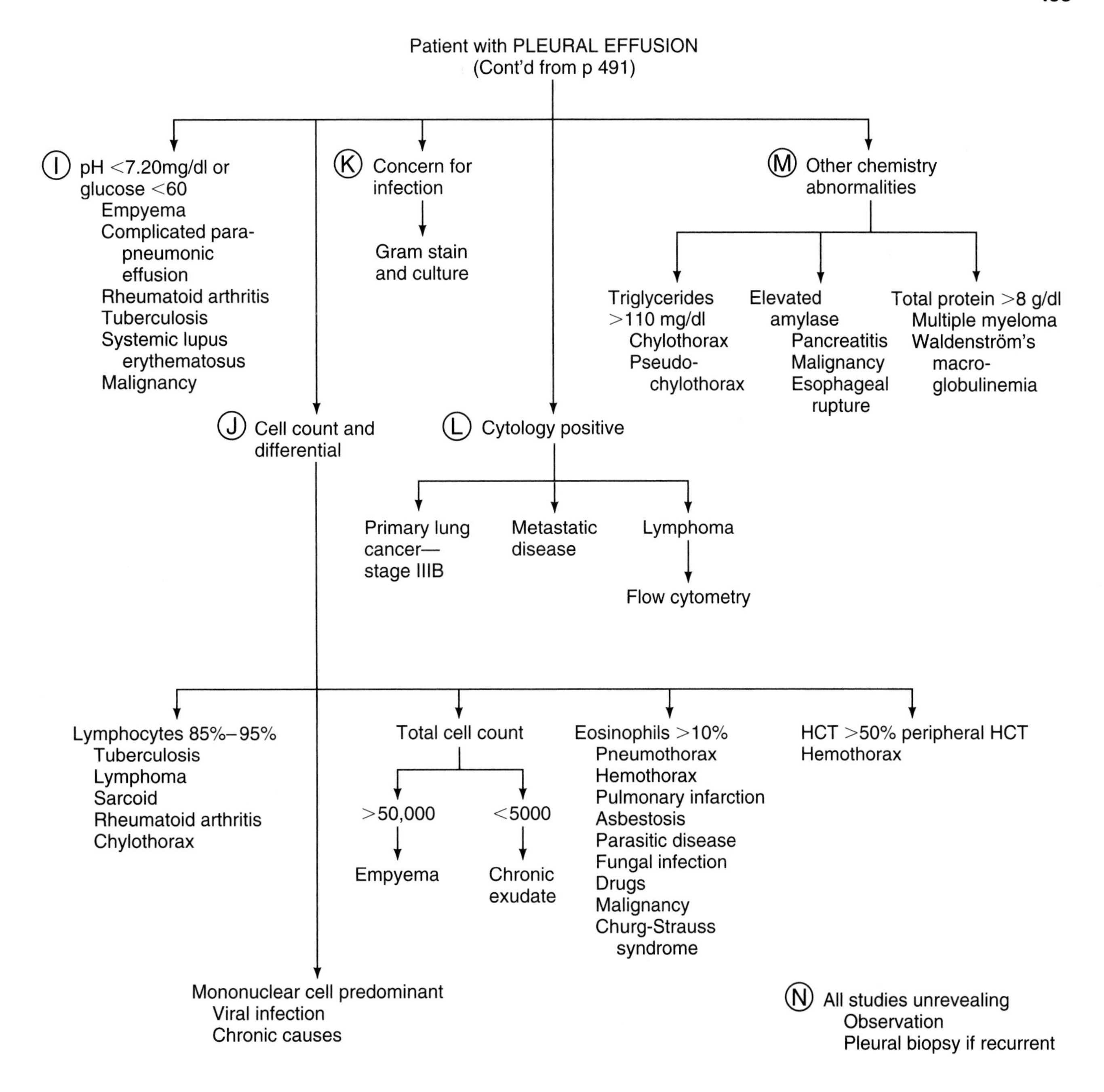
Patient with PLEURAL EFFUSION
(Cont'd from p 491)
Ⓘ pH <7.20mg/dl or glucose <60
Empyema
Complicated parapneumonic effusion
Rheumatoid arthritis
Tuberculosis
Systemic lupus erythematosus
Malignancy
Ⓚ Concern for infection
Gram stain and culture
Ⓜ Other chemistry abnormalities
Triglycerides >110 mg/dl
Chylothorax
Pseudo-chylothorax
Elevated amylase
Pancreatitis
Malignancy
Esophageal rupture
Total protein >8 g/dl
Multiple myeloma
Waldenström's macroglobulinemia
Ⓙ Cell count and differential
Ⓛ Cytology positive
Primary lung cancer—stage IIIB
Metastatic disease
Lymphoma
Flow cytometry
Lymphocytes 85%–95%
Tuberculosis
Lymphoma
Sarcoid
Rheumatoid arthritis
Chylothorax
Total cell count
>50,000
Empyema
<5000
Chronic exudate
Eosinophils >10%
Pneumothorax
Hemothorax
Pulmonary infarction
Asbestosis
Parasitic disease
Fungal infection
Drugs
Malignancy
Churg-Strauss syndrome
HCT >50% peripheral HCT
Hemothorax
Mononuclear cell predominant
Viral infection
Chronic causes
Ⓝ All studies unrevealing
Observation
Pleural biopsy if recurrent

MEDIASTINAL LYMPHADENOPATHY

Patricia Kritek, MD

Mediastinal lymphadenopathy, when found on a chest radiograph, merits further evaluation. These findings can be associated with either benign causes or malignant disease. As with most radiographic findings, comparison to old films can be helpful in the assessment of mediastinal lymphadenopathy. Patients with stable lymphadenopathy over several years often need no further evaluation.

A. The initial evaluation of a patient with mediastinal lymphadenopathy should be a thorough history. Because granulomatous disease is a common cause, a patient's travel history should be obtained with a focus on time spent in areas where histoplasmosis is endemic and on potential exposures to tuberculosis. Additionally, associated symptoms such as fever, night sweats, and weight loss should be elicited. Family history should focus on relatives with sarcoid, lymphoma, or other malignancies. The patient's smoking history is also relevant and should be reviewed.

B. Physical examination includes a thorough assessment for peripheral lymphadenopathy because often these lymph nodes are more easily accessible for biopsy. Although many patients will have a normal pulmonary examination, attention should be paid to signs of underlying lung disease. Additionally, a careful abdominal examination looking for hepatosplenomegaly should be performed.

C. For most patients, the next step in the evaluation of mediastinal lymphadenopathy is a chest CT scan. The CT scan allows better delineation of the lymphadenopathy and any associated parenchymal changes such as those associated with sarcoidosis. What may appear as lymphadenopathy on a chest radiograph may be found to be large pulmonary arteries or a distinct mass on CT imaging. Calcifications in the lymph nodes are more apparent on CT scan compared with chest radiograph. The CT scan can also help guide the approach for potential biopsy.

D. In patients with historical findings concerning for lymphoma (night sweats, weight loss, fevers) or metastatic malignancy, the next step is biopsy of the lymph nodes. If amenable, these nodes can be biopsied bronchoscopically; however, a mediastinoscopy is often necessary. Because the architecture of the lymph node is important, more than a fine needle aspiration should be performed if a diagnosis of lymphoma is entertained. Bronchoscopic biopsies can be used for the lymph node staging of lung cancers as well.

E. In patients in whom sarcoid is suspected, bronchoscopic biopsy of the lymph nodes and endobronchial and transbronchial biopsies are often all that is needed for a diagnosis. As discussed earlier, if there is concern for malignancy, a mediastinoscopy may be needed. Patients with concern for sarcoid should also have full pulmonary function tests (PFTs) obtained.

F. In patients with a history and physical examination results suggestive of infectious granulomatous disease, it is reasonable to place a purified protein derivative (PPD) skin test and send urine histoplasmosis antigen. Patients with parenchymal changes consistent with active tuberculosis (TB) should have three sputa evaluated for acid-fast bacilli. Once again, bronchoscopic biopsy can be attempted, but, if unrevealing, proceeding to mediastinoscopy may be necessary. This is particularly important when there is a question of tuberculosis because cultures with sensitivities will guide further therapy.

References

Duwe BV, Sterman DH, Musani AI. Tumors of the mediastinum. Chest 2005;128(4):2893–2909.

Sharafkhaneh A, Baaklini W, Gorin AB, et al. Yield of transbronchial needle aspiration in diagnosis of mediastinal lesions. Chest 2003;124(6):2131–2135.

Sharma A, Fidias P, Hayman LA, et al. Patterns of lymphadenopathy in thoracic malignancies. Radiographics 2004;24:419–434.

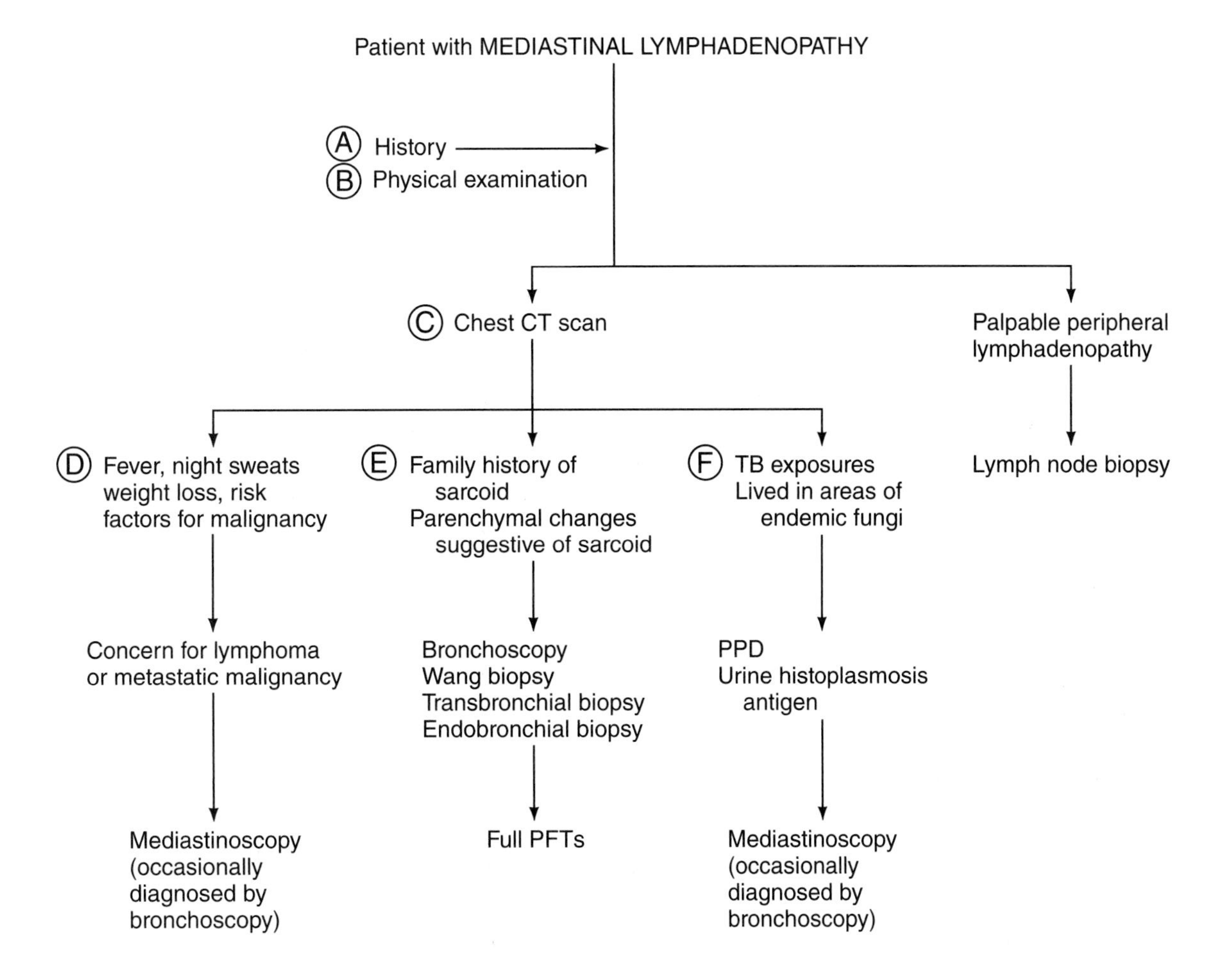
Patient with MEDIASTINAL LYMPHADENOPATHY
(A) History
(B) Physical examination
(C) Chest CT scan
Palpable peripheral lymphadenopathy
Lymph node biopsy
(D) Fever, night sweats weight loss, risk factors for malignancy
Concern for lymphoma or metastatic malignancy
Mediastinoscopy (occasionally diagnosed by bronchoscopy)
(E) Family history of sarcoid
Parenchymal changes suggestive of sarcoid
Bronchoscopy
Wang biopsy
Transbronchial biopsy
Endobronchial biopsy
Full PFTs
(F) TB exposures
Lived in areas of endemic fungi
PPD
Urine histoplasmosis antigen
Mediastinoscopy (occasionally diagnosed by bronchoscopy)

SOLITARY PULMONARY NODULE

Michael Cho, MD

A. A solitary pulmonary nodule (SPN) is a lesion <3 cm in diameter completely surrounded by pulmonary parenchyma and without other abnormalities. An incidental nodule is an uncommon finding in routine chest radiographs, but it is an increasingly common finding on CT scans. Although the majority of these lesions are benign, the possibility that the lesion represents a malignancy cannot be ignored. The 5-year survival for stage IA lung cancer with resection is 60%–80%, which contrasts with the dismal overall survival of lung cancer, which is 5%–16%. Despite these figures, screening has not been proved to reduce mortality from lung cancer and cannot be routinely recommended. Large-scale studies of the value of CT screening are currently ongoing and may lead to a different conclusion.

B. In addition to bronchogenic carcinoma, the differential diagnosis also includes other tumors such as carcinoid and metastatic disease. The most common benign cause of SPN in most series is granuloma, often resulting from prior infection from endemic fungi or mycobacterium. Other etiologies include chronic inflammation; fibrosis; benign neoplasms such as hamartomas and fibromas; infections such as pneumonia, round pneumonia, abscess, echinococcus, and *Dirofilaria*; inflammatory lesions such as Wegener's and rheumatoid nodules; and miscellaneous causes such as bronchogenic cysts, amyloid, intrapulmonary lymph nodes, rounded atelectasis, and mucoid impaction.

C. Standard practice dictates that stability over 2 years indicates the lesion is likely benign and no further follow-up is necessary. Previous stability in imaging does not always obviate the need for follow-up because some malignancies, such as bronchoalveolar cell carcinoma (BAC), can grow slowly. Thus, studies that are >2 years prior to the current film may be helpful, especially for lesions that do not appear entirely solid.

D. If the initial diagnosis was not made by a high-resolution chest CT, one should be obtained. A high-resolution CT scan allows better estimation of lesion size, calcification, and other characteristics. The addition of IV contrast is recommended by some experts because certain benign etiologies, such as arteriovenous fistulas, are more clearly identified. A CT scan may also reveal an alternative diagnosis. Commonly, multiple nodules are discovered and these should be approached differently than the SPN (see the section on multiple pulmonary nodules).

E. Risk assessment involves radiographic and patient factors. Larger lesions are usually malignant; very small (<5 mm) lesions are nearly always benign. Laminated, central, or popcorn calcification; smooth borders; and the presence of fat or cartilage are characteristic of benign lesions. The corona radiata sign, a spiculated appearance, thick-walled cavitation, and eccentric or stippled calcification are consistent with a malignancy. Clinical factors such as age, prior malignancy, hemoptysis, chronic obstructive pulmonary disease (COPD), certain environmental exposures, and history of lung cancer in a first-degree relative also increase the chances that the nodule represents cancer. Several studies have outlined approaches for risk stratification based on these characteristics; however, none have been universally accepted.

F. Patients at low risk (without any of the previously mentioned risk factors) can be followed clinically and radiographically. Historically, a repeat CT chest at 3, 6, 9, 12, and 24 months has been recommended. Recently published guidelines from the Fleischner Society suggest fewer CT scans may be feasible for lesions <8 mm. According to these recommendations, no repeat CT scan is necessary for lesions <5 mm in the absence of other risk factors.

G. Patients at moderate risk generally warrant further investigation. One exception may be when the clinician suspects an inflammatory or infectious etiology. In this case, a repeat CT scan in 4–6 weeks after appropriate therapy can demonstrate resolution and obviate further evaluation. For the remainder of the patients, options often depend on the specifics of the location of the lesion, patient characteristics, and the expertise at a given institution. Positron emission tomography (PET) scans have good sensitivity (>95% in some studies) and good specificity for lesions >1 cm. False-negative results can occur with slowly growing tumors, and false-positive results can occur in lesions with high metabolic activity, such as infection. CT-guided transthoracic needle aspiration may be especially useful in peripheral lesions, with a high sensitivity (approximately 90%) for malignancy, although it is less helpful for benign causes of SPN. Endobronchial lesions or lesions with a "feeding bronchus" may be best sampled by bronchoscopy. Finally, sputum cytology is noninvasive and is helpful if positive, although the sensitivity is quite low.

H. Most patients at high risk should have the SPN resected. This is usually feasible via video-assisted thoracic surgery (VATS) instead of standard thoracotomy, with less morbidity. In those in whom the risk of surgery is prohibitive or in those who decline surgery, alternatives for treatment of malignancy do exist and may include radiation, chemotherapy, and novel therapies such as radiofrequency ablation.

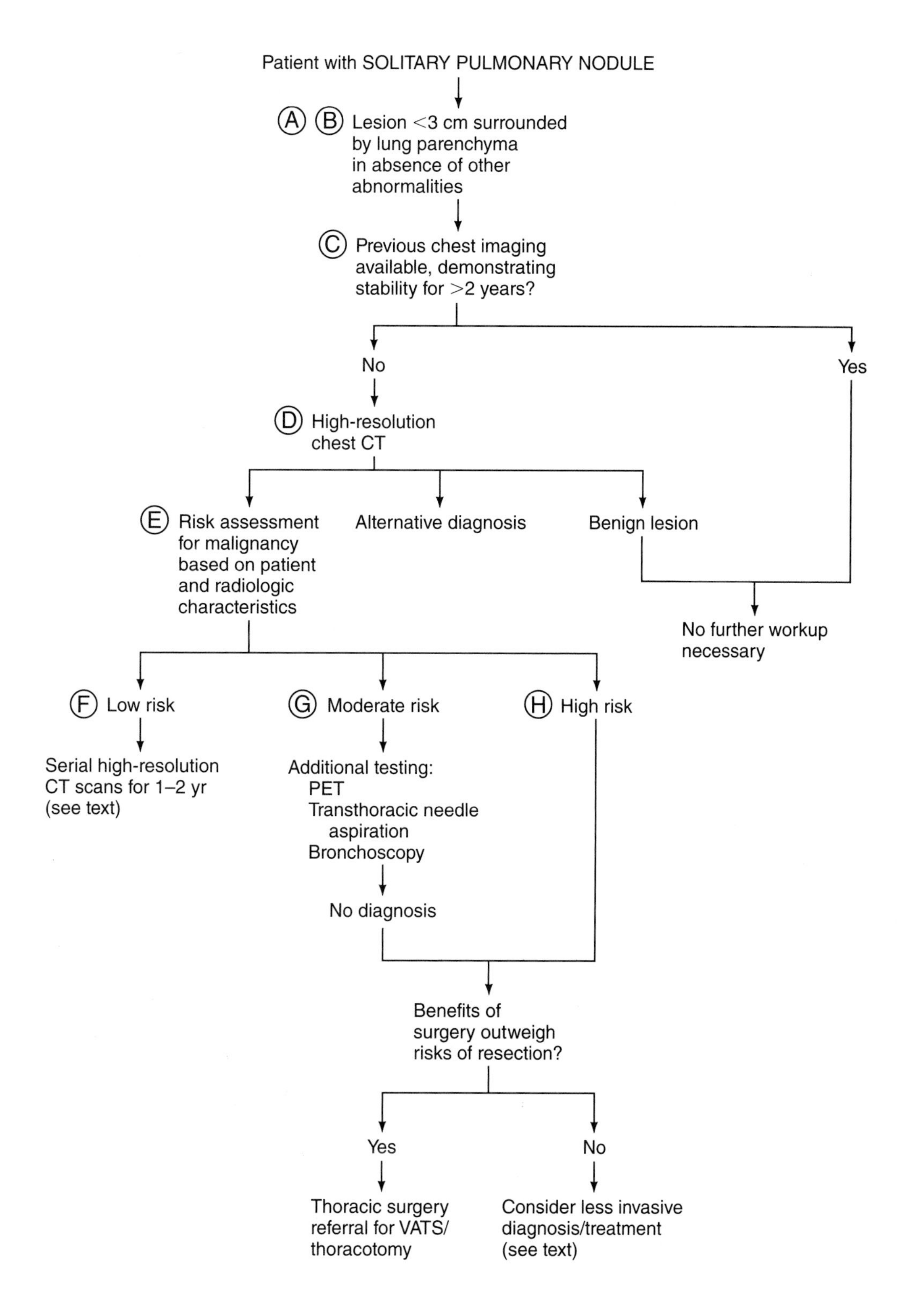

References

Benjamin MS, Drucker EA, McLoud TC, et al. Small pulmonary nodules: detection at chest CT and outcome. Radiology 2003;226(2):489–493.

Bielawski BC, Harrington D, Joseph E. A solitary pulmonary nodule with zoonotic implications. Chest 2001;119(4):1250–1252.

Henschke CI, Yankelevitz DF, Reeves AP, et al. CT screening for lung cancer: suspiciousness of nodules according to size on baseline scans. Radiology 2004;231(1):164–168.

Libby DM, Smith JP, Altorki NK, et al. Managing the small pulmonary nodule discovered by CT. Chest 2004;125(4):1522–1529.

MacMahon H, Austin JH, Gamsu G, et al. Guidelines for management of small pulmonary nodules detected on CT scans: a statement from the Fleischner Society. Radiology 2005;237(2):395–400.

Martini N, Bains MS, Burt ME, et al. Incidence of local recurrence and second primary tumors in resected stage I lung cancer. J Thorac Cardiovasc Surg 1995;109(1):120–129.

Ost D, Fein AM, Feinsilver SH. Clinical practice. The solitary pulmonary nodule. N Engl J Med 2003;348(25):2535–2542.

Schreiber G, McCrory DC. Performance characteristics of different modalities for diagnosis of suspected lung cancer: summary of published evidence. Chest 2003;123(1 Suppl):115S–128S.

Spiro SG, Silvestri GA. One hundred years of lung cancer. Am J Respir Crit Care Med 2005;172(5):523–529.

Tan BB, Flaherty KR, Kazerooni EA, et al. The solitary pulmonary nodule. Chest 2003;123(1 Suppl):89S–96S.

Yankelevitz DF, Henschke CI. Does 2-year stability imply that pulmonary nodules are benign? AJR Am J Roentgenol 1997;168(2):325–328.

MULTIPLE PULMONARY NODULES

Patricia Kritek, MD

A. It is increasingly common to find multiple small nodules on a CT scan that was done for other reasons. The initial evaluation should then include a comprehensive history and a physical examination. The history should focus on risks related to possible malignancy, infection, and underlying rheumatologic disease because these broad categories are responsible for the majority of these nodules. Specifically, determine whether the patient is immunocompromised because this broadens the differential greatly. Also explore recent exposures and recent travel. A past history of malignancy raises the possibility of metastatic disease, whereas associated symptoms of fever, weight loss, and night sweats may suggest lymphoma or infection.

B. As with a solitary pulmonary nodule, always seek out old radiographic images. Stability over months to years makes a benign process much more likely and rapid growth often favors infection. It should also be noted that with the increased use of CT scans, there are more patients who have multiple tiny (<5 mm) nodules. For the most part, in patients without high-risk factors, these can be followed with serial CT scans. Often, in a low-risk patient, one additional CT scan is all that is required.

C. If the history raises the concern for infectious etiologies, there are certain patterns on CT scan that suggest particular pathogens. Peripheral nodules, particularly those which cavitate, suggest septic emboli. Blood cultures and a search for a source of the emboli are appropriate. Lower lobe predominance is common with pulmonary abscesses, septic emboli, and infection with *Paragonimus westermani*. Whereas more common to cause a solitary pulmonary nodule, *Dirofilaria* (dog heartworm) can also cause multiple nodules. Multiple, small calcified nodules suggests prior granulomatous disease, including previous histoplasmosis infection or mycobacterial infection.

D. Other typical patterns include the "halo sign" of adjacent hemorrhage seen with angio-invasive aspergillosis and "tree-in-bud" changes of bronchiolitis classically seen with atypical mycobacterial infection. Innumerable, small nodules should make the physician consider miliary tuberculosis infection. Immunocompromised patients can present with nodules resulting from a variety of other organisms, including, but not limited to, nocardia, *Pneumocystis*, varicella, and other viruses. Also, common infections can present atypically in hosts with impaired immune systems, so the differential should be kept broad in this population. Sputum, bronchoscopy with bronchoalveolar lavage (BAL), serologies and more rarely a surgical lung biopsy may all play a role in determining a diagnosis.

E. In a patient with known malignancy, there should always be concern for metastatic disease presenting as multiple pulmonary nodules. Although many cancers can metastasize to the lung, certain types are more likely to do so. These include colon, breast, prostate, thyroid, renal, testicular, melanoma, and sarcoma. If the patient does not have known metastatic disease, it is reasonable to proceed with surgical biopsy of one of these lesions for guidance of future therapy.

F. Non-Hodgkin's lymphoma can present as multiple pulmonary nodules without associated lymphadenopathy. Primary lung cancer much more commonly presents as a solitary pulmonary nodule. That said, of the subtypes of lung cancer, bronchoalveolar cell carcinoma more often presents with multiple foci of disease. These lesions are often at least in part ground glass density on CT scan. If considering either lymphoma or lung cancer, a diagnosis should be aggressively pursued. Whereas a bronchoscopy with transbronchial biopsy and bronchial washings can be a first step, most of these lesions require surgical biopsy.

G. A variety of rheumatologic diseases can present with pulmonary nodules but the most common is rheumatoid arthritis. Pulmonary nodules are more common when the patient also has cutaneous nodules and are found more often in men than in women. Although atypical, sarcoid can also present as nodules in the lungs.

H. There are a variety of miscellaneous causes of multiple pulmonary nodules, most of which are suggested by history. A patient with an exposure to silica, talc, or coal dust may present with large, upper lobe predominant nodules often on a background of fibrosis. Patients with a history of IV drug abuse may also present with multiple nodules, which are a result of an inflammatory response to the talc used to "cut" the illicit drug. A vessel leading into a nodule or a lobular contour to a nodule should suggest arteriovenous malformations (AVMs), which can be confirmed by CT or traditional angiography. If multiple AVMs are found, consider a diagnosis of hereditary hemorrhagic telangiectasia (HHT).

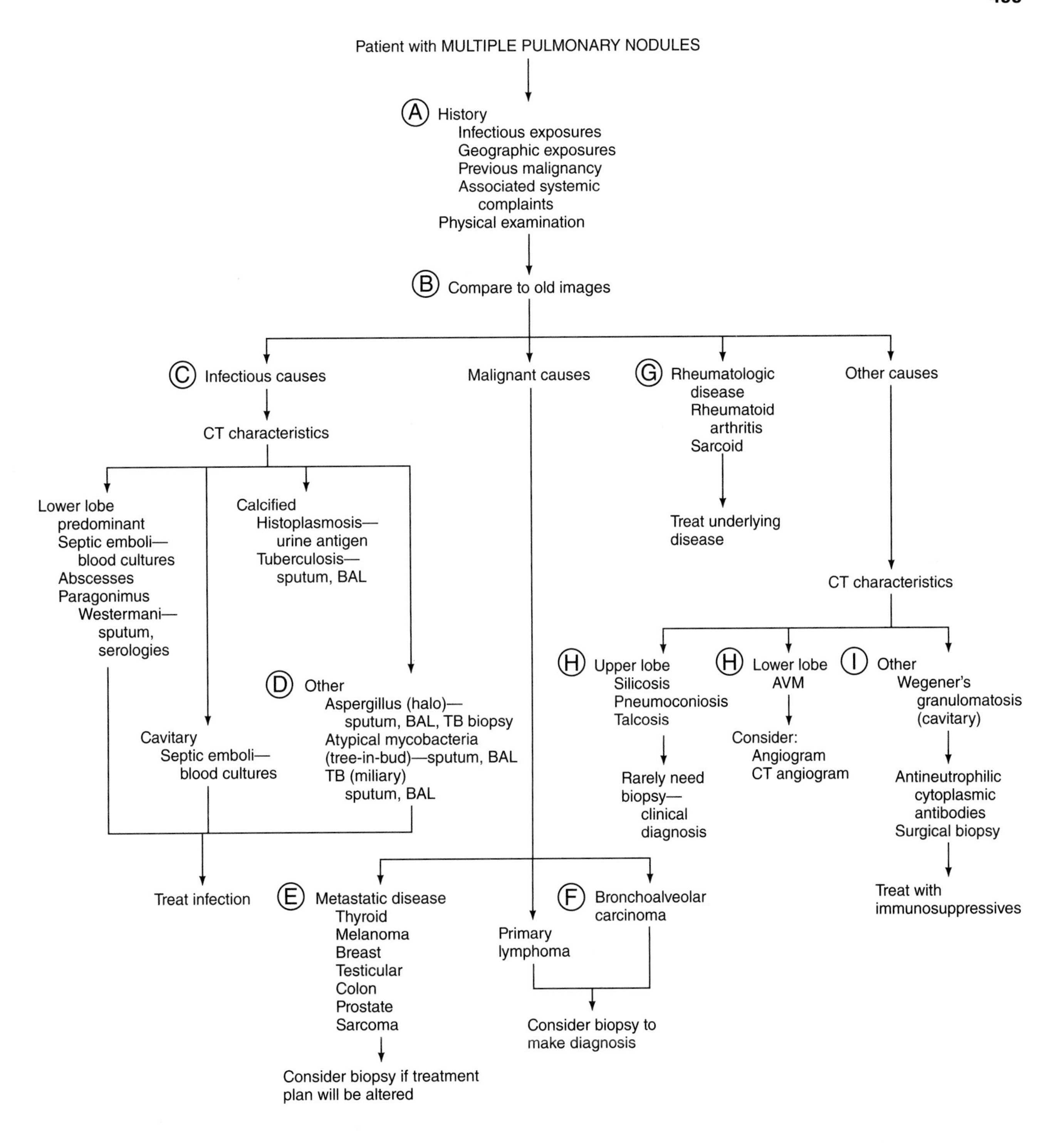

I. Wegener's granulomatosis can present as multiple pulmonary nodules, often cavitary in nature. Associated sinus disease, renal disease, or hemoptysis should raise the possibility of this diagnosis. A strongly positive ANCA is often present, but either a surgical lung or percutaneous kidney biopsy is commonly needed to make the diagnosis of Wegener's granulomatosis.

References

Fraser RS, Paré PD. *Fraser and Paré's Diagnosis of Diseases of the Chest*, ed 4, Philadelphia:W.B. Saunders, 1999.

Gould MK, Fletcher J, Iannettoni MD, et al. Evaluation of patients with pulmonary nodules: when is it lung cancer? ACCP evidence-based clinical practice guidelines (2nd edition). Chest 2007;132 (3 Suppl):108S–130S.

Lillington GA, Caskey CI. Evaluation and management of solitary and multiple pulmonary nodules. Clin Chest Med 1993;14(1):111–119.

Viggiano RW, Swensen SJ, Rosenow EC 3rd. Evaluation and management of solitary and multiple pulmonary nodules. Clin Chest Med 1992;13(1):83–95.

DIFFUSE INTERSTITIAL LUNG DISEASE

Paul Currier, MD

Diffuse interstitial lung disease (ILD) constitutes a broad variety of disease. Diagnosis can be a challenge, and in some cases surgical lung biopsy will ultimately be required. Treatment can also be challenging because of a lack of effective therapy for many of these diseases. A comprehensive guide to treatment of these diseases is outside the scope of this algorithm, which provides a general approach to diagnosis and treatment.

A. A comprehensive history is the first step in characterizing diffuse ILD. Initial questions should include a determination of the extent of the patient's dyspnea with particular emphasis on overall functional status and the impact of dyspnea on activities of daily living. Review the tempo and timing of the progression of symptoms, including dyspnea and cough. The presence of hemoptysis will guide further diagnostic evaluation. Because many interstitial lung diseases are related to collagen vascular diseases, a rheumatologic review of systems can be useful. Assess environmental exposures, including home and workplace. Because there are links between smoking and a variety of medications with ILD, review both of these histories. Include a family history because some ILDs have a genetic component.

B. The physical examination should include the patient's respiratory rate and observation for signs of respiratory distress. Oxygen saturation, at rest and with ambulation, should be measured. Classic pulmonary findings of diffuse ILD include bibasilar "Velcro-like" crackles, particularly in idiopathic pulmonary fibrosis (IPF). Other diseases, such as bronchiolitis obliterans organizing pneumonia (BOOP), may present with diffuse crackles, inspiratory squeaks and pops, and wheezes. Hypoxia can lead to pulmonary hypertension and cor pulmonale, which can result in an accentuated P_2 heart sound, elevated jugular venous pressure, and peripheral edema. A murmur of tricuspid regurgitation and fixed splitting of the second heart sound (as a result of the inability to decrease intrathoracic pressure during inspiration because of persistently elevated right-sided heart pressures) may be noted. Other peripheral signs may include clubbing and signs of rheumatologic disease, such as joint swelling or tight skin.

C. Laboratory values should include a CBC with differential (to look for signs of infection, eosinophilia, and anemia). Consider an ESR, ANA, antiglomerular basement membrane antibody, and possibly other rheumatologic laboratory tests based on suspicion of a specific illness. Antibodies for detection of hypersensitivity pneumonitis to environmental allergens should be sent if this is suspected. Peripheral blood eosinophilia ($>1 \times 10^9$ eosinophils) should raise the question of an eosinophilic pneumonia. For suspected sarcoidosis, a serum calcium level and angiotensin-converting enzyme level may be checked, although neither is diagnostic.

D. Pulmonary function tests (PFTs) should be obtained and often show a restrictive deficit as manifest by a decreased total lung capacity (TLC <80% predicted). Certain diffuse ILDs, such as pulmonary Langerhans' cell histiocytosis (PLCH), lymphomatoid granulomatosis, or sarcoidosis, may also have an obstructive component. It is often useful to have baseline lung function tests prior to beginning treatment to be able to monitor response to therapy.

E. A chest x-ray (CXR) should be obtained on all patients with suspected ILD. Historically, the sensitivity of a CXR to diagnose chronic diffuse ILD has been considered to be around 90%. The sensitivity of modern chest radiograph machines to diagnose chronic diffuse ILD may be even higher.

F. A normal CXR in a patient suspected of having disease should prompt a chest CT scan with high-resolution thin sections to allow for the greatest ability to diagnose early ILD. Signs of diffuse ILD on CXR should also be evaluated with CT scan to better characterize the disease process.

G. If the disease process is thought secondary to an environmental exposure or drug, eliminate the inciting agent. Depending on the time course of the disease, observation for clinical resolution of the disease process may be acceptable before proceeding to more invasive means of diagnosis.

H. A characteristic CT scan pattern and supporting clinical information may be sufficient to be diagnostic. The presence of honeycombing with basal and peripheral predominance is considered by some to be sufficient evidence for a diagnosis of IPF, whereas others believe that biopsy is required for diagnostic certainty. Other diseases with characteristic radiographic patterns, such as PLCH or lymphangioleiomyomatosis (LAM), may also be diagnosed radiographically when patient history is also consistent with the disease process and when biopsy may be difficult.

I. Bronchoscopy with bronchoalveolar lavage (BAL) alone may allow for a diagnosis in some of the diffuse ILDs. It should be performed in cases of suspected infection such as *Pneumocystis carinii* pneumonia (PCP) or in suspected cases of eosinophilic Pneumonia. A finding of

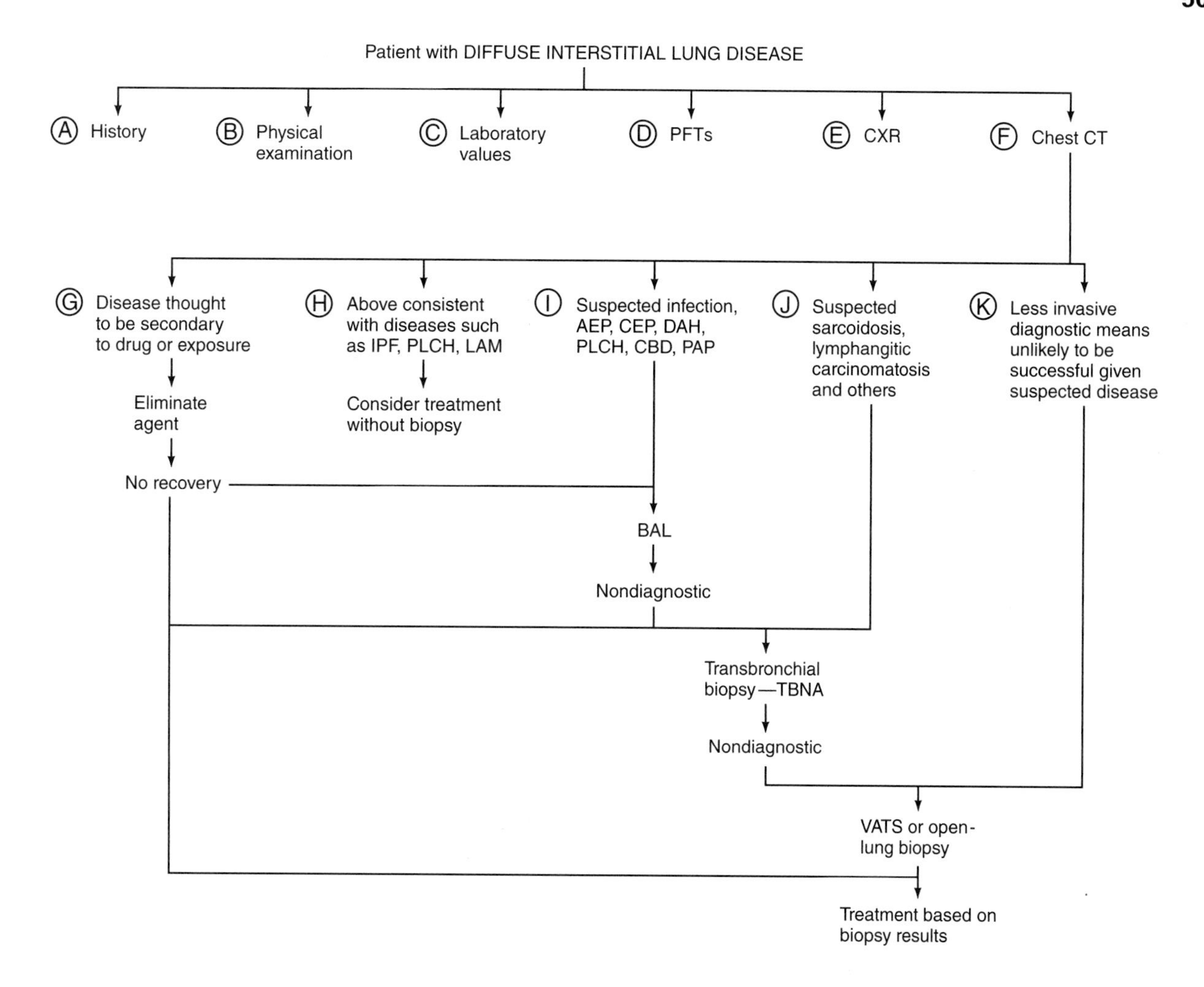

>25% eosinophils on BAL is generally considered consistent with acute idiopathic eosinophilic pneumonia (AEP), whereas >40% eosinophils is indicative of a diagnosis of chronic eosinophilic pneumonia (CEP). BAL should be performed in suspected cases of diffuse alveolar hemorrhage (DAH). Multiple lavage specimens in which bloody aspirate fails to clear and hemosiderin-laden macrophages are seen are characteristic of DAH. BAL may also be helpful in a variety of rarer diseases. These include PLCH (to look for >5% CDa1+ cells), chronic beryllium disease (CBD; to send cells from BAL for a beryllium lymphocyte proliferation test), and pulmonary alveolar proteinosis (PAP; to look for milky fluid and periodic acid–Schiff positive fluid.

J. Transbronchial biopsy performed via a flexible bronchoscope may be the diagnostic procedure of choice for a few ILDs. For suspected sarcoidosis, taking a minimum of four biopsies provides a sensitivity of >90%. Transbronchial needle aspiration (TBNA) of lymph nodes via bronchoscopy may also be helpful in making this diagnosis. Lymphangitic spread of cancer and hypersensitivity pneumonitis can be diagnosed by transbronchial biopsy. However, for most ILDs, diagnostic yield is often low and many clinicians would recommend proceeding directly to surgical biopsy.

K. For suspected disease processes in which less invasive studies have been unrevealing or are thought unlikely to reveal a diagnosis, surgical biopsy may be indicated. Surgical biopsy is now most often performed by video-assisted thoracoscopic surgical (VATS) biopsy. This form of biopsy is performed through three small incisions and is generally well tolerated. A chest tube is usually maintained for 1–2 days following the procedure with a short period of hospitalization. Mediastinoscopy should be performed if lymph nodes are enlarged. Open lung biopsy may occasionally be necessary based on the distribution of the disease process. The decision of which route of biopsy to pursue should be undertaken after thoughtful discussion with specialists and with the patient. Further therapy is then guided by the results of the biopsy.

References

Cottin V, Cordier JF. Eosinophilic pneumonias. Allergy 2005;60:841–857.

Epler GR, McLoud TC, Gaensler EA, et al. Normal chest roentgenograms in chronic diffuse infiltrative lung disease. N Engl J Med 1978;298(17):934–939.

King TE. Approach to the adult with interstitial lung disease. UpToDate Online. Available at: www.uptodate.com. Accessed March 20, 2006.

Lynch DA, Godwin JD, Safrin S, et al. High-resolution computed tomography in idiopathic pulmonary fibrosis. Am J Respir Crit Care Med 2005;172:488–493.

Schwarz MI, King TE. Interstitial Lung Disease, 4th ed. London: BC Decker, 2003.

POSITIVE TUBERCULIN SKIN TEST (PPD)

Ashwin Dharmadhikari, MD

Tuberculosis (TB) infection remains a leading cause of morbidity worldwide, making it an important area for public health prevention and treatment efforts. In the United States, its impact is seen in the 10–15 million individuals who are infected. Although annual rates of TB infection in the United States are declining, there are still cases in every state, and drug-resistant TB looms as the next hurdle in the care of patients with TB. One of the most important decision points in evaluating and treating patients for TB is to determine whether they have active TB disease or latent TB infection (LTBI). As part of that diagnostic evaluation, the tuberculin skin test (purified protein derivative; PPD) has historically been and continues to be an important tool.

A. Testing for TB or LTBI using the PPD is most useful when applied carefully in targeted populations. Random testing is of little utility and may unnecessarily expose patients to unneeded medications or health care evaluations. Knowledge of disease prevalence and patient risk are important factors in deciding who to test. The overall goals of PPD testing are to find people with LTBI who would benefit from prophylactic treatment and to find people with TB disease who would benefit from treatment. Individuals at low risk should not be routinely tested. PPD testing is safe in pregnancy.

B. Certain conditions place people into high-risk groups for exposure to TB. These conditions include close contact with a known or suspected case of TB, foreign-born individuals from endemic areas, residents of high-risk settings such as jails or nursing homes, health care workers, individuals who are medically underserved, injection drug users, or people in high-risk racial or ethnic populations. Once infected (i.e., patient has LTBI), individuals with HIV, substance abuse, diabetes, silicosis, prolonged immunosuppression, head and neck cancer, end-stage renal disease, hematologic malignancies, low body weight, gastrectomy or intestinal bypass, or malabsorption syndromes are at higher risk for progression to active disease.

C. The PPD skin test is a combination of low molecular weight proteins and carbohydrate components of the tubercle bacillus. It is administered intradermally on the volar forearm as 5 thousand units (TU) of PPD. Results are interpreted 48–72 hours later based on millimeters of skin induration, with predetermined thresholds for positivity based on patient demographics and risk factors to determine further treatment.

D. It is important that PPD results be read by health care professionals rather than by patients. The presence of induration meeting threshold criteria is termed *positive PPD* and generally represents infection with TB. False-positive PPD results may arise from nontuberculous mycobacterial infection or BCG (Bacille Calmette-Guérin) vaccination. False-negative PPD results may occur in the setting of anergy, recent TB infection, recent vaccination with live viruses, or overwhelming TB disease. Nonetheless, in immunocompetent individuals with latent TB infection, the PPD test approaches 100% sensitivity. On average, there is a 10% lifetime risk of developing TB disease from LTBI with a normal immune system. In patients who are HIV positive, this risk increases to a 7%–10% *annual* risk of developing TB disease. The greatest risk in all people occurs within the first 2 years after initial exposure to TB.

E. A result of 0–5 mm in any patient is read as "negative." Although there is a small risk of a false-negative result in patients who are anergic (usually as a result of immunosuppression), the current American Thoracic Society/Centers for Disease Control and Prevention/Infectious Diseases Society of America (ATS/CDC/ISDA) guidelines do not recommend routinely planting controls to test for anergy.

F. A PPD result is positive at ≥5 mm for patients who are HIV positive, recent contacts of those with TB, persons with chest radiographic findings of fibrotic changes, or patients who have received organ transplants or are immunosuppressed.

G. A threshold of ≥10 mm is used for people who have recently arrived from high prevalence areas, injection drug users, residents of nursing homes or jails, people who work with tuberculosis in a laboratory setting, health care workers, or children/adolescents exposed to adults at high risk.

H. A threshold of ≥15 mm is considered positive for people with no known risk factors for TB. As previously stated, for the most part, these patients should not have a PPD placed because LTBI testing should be targeted to those with increased risk of infection.

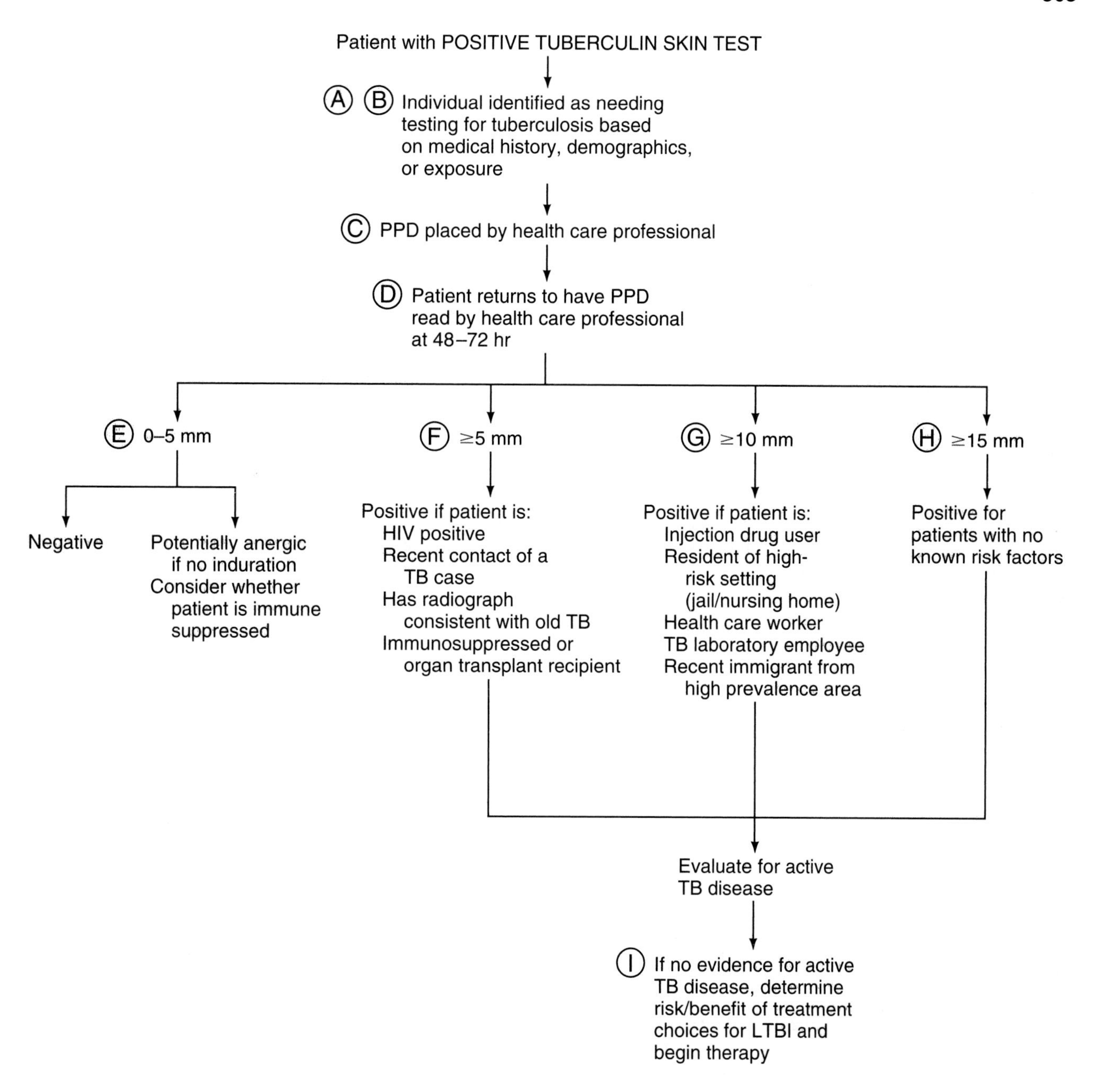

I. Once a patient is established as having a positive PPD, the next step involves using clinical and radiographic information to determine whether he or she has LTBI or active TB disease. For LTBI, the current ATS/CDC/ISDA guidelines recommend a course of isoniazid (also called INH) 300 mg daily for 9 months' duration, regardless of whether the patient is immunocompromised. Because patient compliance is often a challenge, there are three alternative regimens of one or two drugs of shorter duration.

References

American Thoracic Society Statement: Targeted tuberculin testing and treatment of latent tuberculosis infection. Am J Respir Crit Care Med 2000;161:5221–5247.

Blumberg HM, Burman WJ, Chaisson RE, et al. American Thoracic Society/Centers for Disease Control and Prevention/Infectious Diseases Society of America: Treatment of tuberculosis. Am J Respir Crit Care Med 2003;167:603.

Core curriculum on tuberculosis: What the clinician should know, 4th ed. Washington, DC: U.S. Department of Health and Human Services, Center for Disease Control and Prevention, National Center for HIV, STD, and TB Prevention, Division of Tuberculosis Elimination, 2000.

RESPIRATORY SYMPTOMS AND OCCUPATIONAL EXPOSURE TO ASBESTOS

Patricia Kritek, MD

A. The first step in any assessment is to take a comprehensive history with a focus on the exposure to asbestos. In the United States, the majority of exposure was to chrysolite, a serpentine fiber, which is thought to be less likely to cause disease. In contrast, the long rodlike fibers of amphibole asbestos (e.g., crocidolite, amosite, and tremolite) were much less commonly used. Specific occupations with the potential for high exposure to asbestos include plumbers, pipe fitters, insulation workers, electricians, boilermakers, and obviously those who worked mining asbestos. Shipyards, particularly in the 1940s, were a common place for occupational exposure. More recently, mechanics who specifically work on brakes are at risk for exposure to the asbestos found in brake linings. For the most part, symptomatic lung disease related to asbestos exposure manifests itself 15–20 years after the exposure. If symptoms occur much closer temporally to an exposure, the differential for the cause of dyspnea should be broadened.

B. A complete physical examination with particular emphasis on the lung examination should accompany history taking. The finding of crackles, decreased breath sounds, or dullness to percussion may suggest specific pathologies. In almost all cases, the next step should be a chest x-ray (CXR). Further evaluation is guided by what is found on imaging.

C. The most common finding in patients with asbestos exposure is pleural plaques—areas of pleural thickening and calcification. Plaques themselves are generally benign, although they may be seen in conjunction with other forms of asbestos-related lung disease. The clinician should obtain lung volumes to evaluate for restrictive physiology (total lung capacity <70% predicted) as a result of pleural disease if the patient presents with dyspnea. As plaques are associated with future asbestosis, these patients should be followed and monitored for future fibrosis.

D. Distinct from the parietal pleural plaques and much less common is diffuse visceral pleural thickening associated with asbestos exposure. This pathology is much more likely to result in restrictive physiology, which should be evaluated for with pulmonary function testing.

E. Although the majority of findings associated with asbestos are found many years after exposure, pleural effusions can be found after an acute exposure and more remotely. These effusions are exudative, often with a prominent eosinophilia. Although generally painless and often found incidentally, an acute asbestos pleural effusion may be painful and associated with fever and dyspnea. All of these effusions should be tapped. Chronic effusions warrant cytologic examination for malignancy and if there are any concerning features (e.g., loculation, associated irregular pleural thickening), a thoracoscopic pleural biopsy should be considered.

F. Malignant mesothelioma is strongly associated with asbestos; approximately 70% of patients with this disease have a known exposure. It is often difficult to diagnose and commonly requires pleural biopsy. Although in the past this may be have been done with needle biopsy, as the yield of this procedure is quite low, patients generally should proceed to thoracoscopic biopsy if pleural fluid cytology is unrevealing. Unfortunately, both surgical and chemotherapeutic options for mesothelioma are of limited benefit. Physicians should consider referral to a center that specializes in treatment of these rare cancers.

G. If the CXR reveals reticulonodular changes, the physician should have concern for asbestosis, which is often difficult to distinguish from idiopathic pulmonary fibrosis (IPF). Features that help distinguish these two diseases are a history of exposure to asbestos and associated pleural plaques. Although both diseases are generally lower lobe predominant, there is a subtype of asbestosis that is severe, upper lobe disease. Next steps in assessment include lung volumes and measurement of carbon dioxide diffusion in the lungs (DL_{CO}) to assess for restrictive physiology and abnormal gas exchange in addition to a CT scan of the chest to better characterize the infiltrates. A clinical diagnosis is usually made without the need for a lung biopsy, although at times this is undertaken to rule out alternative diagnoses. The finding of asbestos fibers or asbestos bodies adds to the diagnostic certainty but is not required and in itself is not pathognomonic of asbestosis. There is no specific therapy for asbestosis and care is generally supportive.

H. Cigarette smoking and asbestos have a synergistic effect in increasing the risk for primary lung cancer. If a mass is found on CXR, a CT scan should be obtained and further evaluation, as with any lung mass, should be pursued.

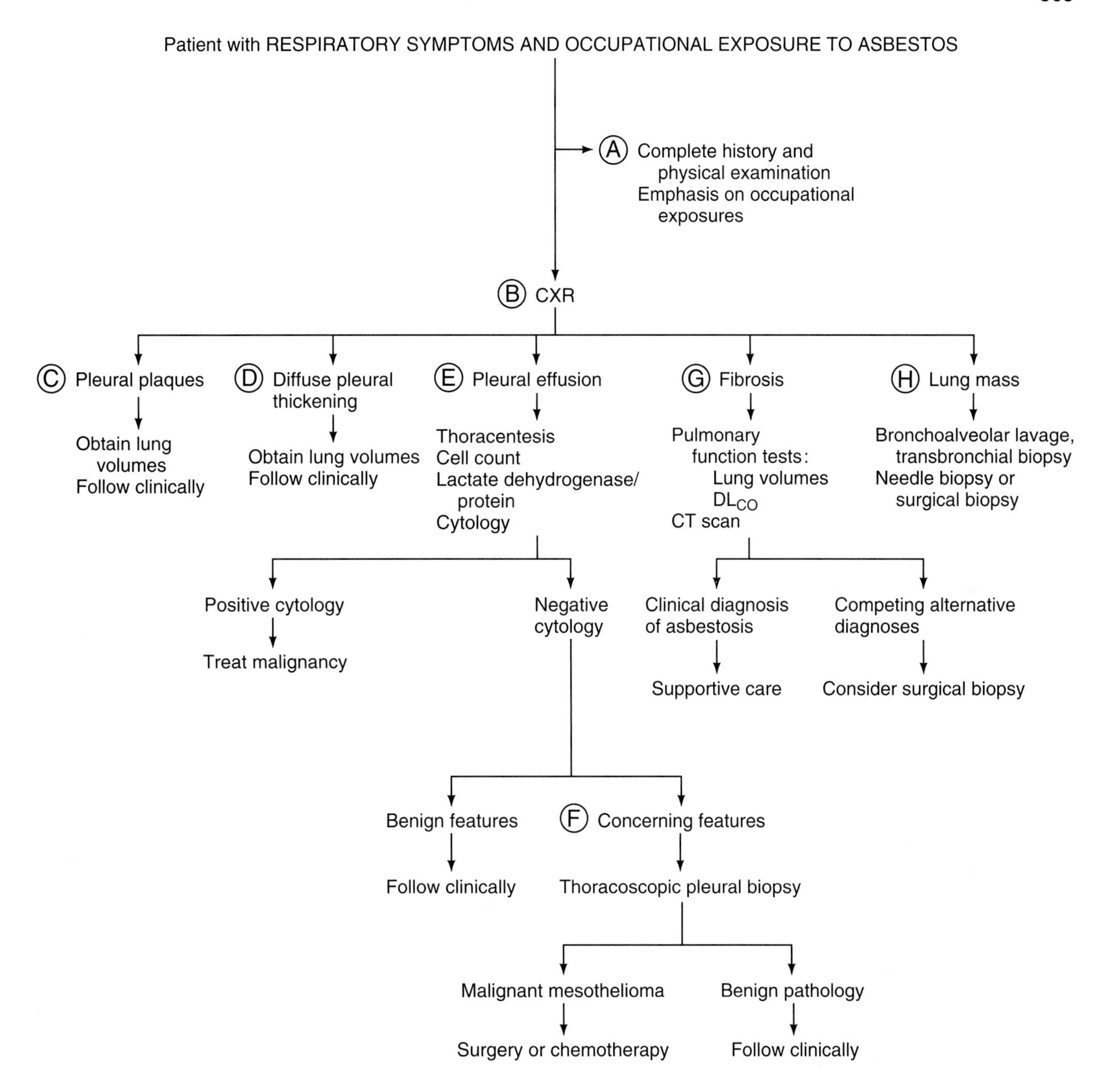

References

American Thoracic Society. Diagnosis and initial management of nonmalignant diseases related to asbestos. Am J Respir Crit Care Med 2004;170(6):691–715.

BTS statement on malignant mesothelioma in the UK, 2007. Thorax 2007;62(Suppl 2):ii1–ii19.

Chapman SJ, Philadelphia Cookson WO, Musk AW, et al. Benign asbestos pleural diseases. Curr Opin Pulm Med 2003;9(4):266–271.

Cugell DW, Kamp DW. Asbestos and the pleura: a review. Chest 2004;125(3):1103–1117.

Fraser RS, Paré PD. Fraser and Paré's Diagnosis of Diseases of the Chest, ed 4, Philadelphia: W.B. Saunders, 1999.

Gevenois PA, de Maertelaer V, Madani A, et al. Asbestosis, pleural plaques and diffuse pleural thickening: three distinct benign responses to asbestos exposure. Eur Respir J 1998;11(5):1021–1027.

Ghio AJ, Roggli VL. Diagnosis and initial management of nonmalignant diseases related to asbestos. Am J Respir Crit Care Med 2005;171(5): 527; author reply 528–530.

Ohar J, Sterling DA, Bleecker E, et al. Changing patterns in asbestos-induced lung disease. Chest 2004;125(2):744–753.

O'Reilly KM, Mclaughlin AM, Beckett S, et al. Asbestos-related lung disease. Am Fam Physician 2007;75(5):683–688.

Ross RM. The clinical diagnosis of asbestosis in this century requires more than a chest radiograph. Chest 2003;124(3):1120–1128.

Weill D, Weill H. Diagnosis and initial management of nonmalignant diseases related to asbestos. Am J Respir Crit Care Med 2005;171(5):527–528; author reply 528–530.

ASTHMA

Patricia Kritek, MD

A. Asthma is a chronic inflammatory lung disease characterized by episodes of increased airway inflammation resulting in airflow obstruction and dyspnea. The physician should consider a diagnosis of asthma in patients who have dyspnea on exertion, cough, or wheezing. As with any patient, the first step in evaluation is a thorough history, in this case with particular focus on conditions that trigger symptoms. Some examples of classic triggers of asthma include exercise, cold air, upper respiratory tract infections, animal dander, pollen, mold, and tobacco smoke. Because asthma is often associated with atopy, the physician should inquire about a personal history of eczema and seasonal allergies. Additionally, a family history of asthma or other atopic disease would support a diagnosis of asthma.

B. The physical examination in patients with asthma is often completely normal. That being said, one should listen for wheezing on lung examination and upper airway sounds (stridor) because this large airway obstruction can sometimes mimic asthma. In addition, the nares should be inspected for nasal polyps that can be found as part of a triad of asthma, nasal polyps, and aspirin sensitivity. The posterior oro-pharynx should be examined for "cobblestoning" associated with postnasal drip, a common exacerbating condition in asthma.

C. Although there is no single diagnostic test for asthma, spirometry with bronchodilator responsiveness is a common next step in the evaluation. Most patients with asthma will have normal pulmonary function when not having an exacerbation, so this finding does not exclude the diagnosis. If the patient is symptomatic, the spirometry should show an obstructive pattern with forced expiratory volume (FEV_1)/forced vital capacity (FVC) <70%. If either FEV_1 or FVC improves with the use of a bronchodilator, this would support the diagnosis of asthma because part of the definition of the disease is reversibility of airflow obstruction. The American Thoracic Society (ATS) criteria for "responsiveness" require an increase of 200 ml and 12% in either FEV_1 or FVC.

D. As already stated, a key aspect of asthma is variability in airflow obstruction. An alternative way to demonstrate this is with ambulatory peak flow monitoring. Peak flow meters are reasonably inexpensive and portable; however, the data are limited by the fact that the results are effort dependent. After being instructed in appropriate technique, patients should obtain peak flows at different times of day, when asymptomatic and when dyspneic or wheezy. Variability in peak flows >20% is consistent with asthma. Although useful diagnostically, the peak flow meter is generally more useful as a way to monitor for control of established disease.

E. If neither of these studies is revealing, it is reasonable to consider bronchoprovocation testing, traditionally done with methacholine. Patients are given progressively higher concentrations of inhaled methacholine, a muscarinic agonist that causes smooth muscle contraction, with repeated spirometry. The test is positive if there is a fall in FEV_1 of 20% from baseline. This test has a high negative predictive value, so it is most helpful as a way to rule out asthma. If a patient is unresponsive to methacholine, alternative diagnoses should be sought for the patient's dyspnea, cough, or wheeze.

F. Asthma is treated with a combination of quick relief and controller medications. The typical quick relief medication is a beta agonist inhaler, such as albuterol. Ideally, a patient's asthma is well enough controlled that there is only rare use of the reliever medication. If albuterol is required more than a few times a week, a controller medication should be initiated. For most patients, this means a steroid inhaler, although some patients respond well to leukotriene modifiers as first-line therapy. If symptoms are still not well controlled, higher-dose steroid inhalers or the addition of a long-acting beta agonist can be considered. If further escalation of therapy is required, it is appropriate to look for other causes of dyspnea and wheeze and refer the patient to a pulmonologist.

G. In addition to pharmacologic interventions, patients should be counseled to avoid triggers by minimizing allergen exposure and maintaining a clean living environment. If a patient with asthma is currently smoking, smoking cessation is essential. Clinicians should also create an "action plan" with patients based on peak flow measurements with thresholds for increasing therapy and seeking medical attention.

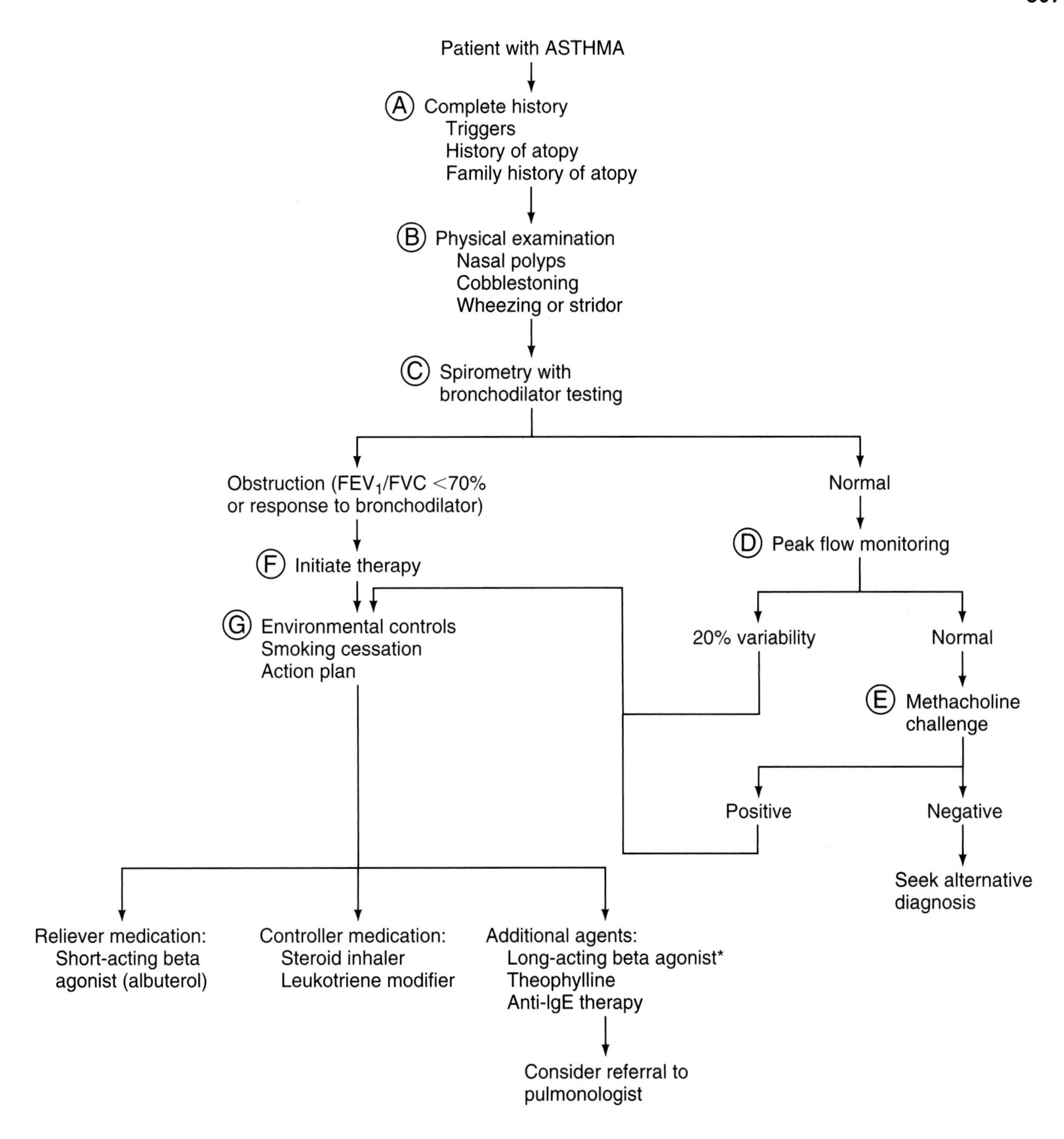

*Should not be used on its own because there is evidence of increased mortality with this use.

References

Chervinsky P, van As A, Bronsky EA, et al. Fluticasone propionate aerosol for the treatment of adults with mild to moderate asthma. The Fluticasone Propionate Asthma Study Group. J Allergy Clin Immunol 1994;94:676–693.

Global Initiative for Asthma (GINA). 2006. Available at: www.ginasthma.com.

National Heart, L.a.B.I., NHLBI. National Asthma Education and Prevention Program: Clinical treatment guidelines, 1997.

National Heart, L.a.B.I., NHLBI. National Asthma Education and Prevention Project: Update on selected topics, 2002.

Popa V. ATS guidelines for methacholine and exercise challenge testing. Am J Respir Crit Care Med 2001;163(1):292–293.

Sears MR. The definition and diagnosis of asthma. Allergy 1993;48 (17 Suppl):12-16; discussion 22–23.

Suissa, S, Dennis R, Ernst P, et al. Effectiveness of the leukotriene receptor antagonist zafirlukast for mild-to-moderate asthma. A randomized, double-blind, placebo-controlled trial. Ann Intern Med 1997;126(3):177–183.

RHEUMATOLOGY

Paul A. Monach, MD, PhD
Section Editor

MONOARTICULAR ARTHRITIS

Erika Noss, MD, PhD

A. A complete history and physical examination are crucial and are the most useful tools for making the correct diagnosis. Joint pain may result from abnormalities in the joint itself, in adjacent bone, or from surrounding ligaments, tendons, bursae, or soft tissues. Pain may also be referred from a neuropathic condition or pathology in another joint. Monarthritis of acute onset (hours to days) usually indicates trauma, infection, or a crystal-induced process. Rarely, it may represent an atypical presentation of a systemic inflammatory condition. Careful questioning may reveal prior joint symptoms, stiffness, or systemic symptoms such as fatigue. Monarthritis persisting >4–6 weeks may indicate a chronic condition such as atypical infection, osteoarthritis, tumor, or systemic inflammatory disease.

B. Aspiration of the affected joint for synovial fluid analysis is always indicated to evaluate monarthritis. Synovial fluid should be sent for WBC count with differential, Gram stain, culture, and crystal analysis. Additional tests do not generally improve diagnostic sensitivity. Synovial fluid WBC count is the single most important measurement to separate noninflammatory from inflammatory processes. With appropriate clinical correlation, a WBC count <2000 cells/mm^3 represents a noninflammatory process, whereas higher WBC counts represent inflammatory conditions. Polymorphonuclear leukocyte-predominant effusions (>75% cell count) also indicate an acute inflammatory process.

C. Acute bacterial arthritis is a medical emergency, and rapid treatment is warranted to prevent irreversible cartilage and bone destruction. Acute bacterial arthritis may be divided into nongonococcal and gonococcal causes. Gram-positive organisms, particularly *Staphylococcus aureus,* are the most common agents to cause nongonococcal bacterial arthritis. Nongonococcal infection is often associated with a primary focus of infection elsewhere. Therefore, an unexplained arthritis in the setting of bacteremia, pneumonia, or other infection should be presumed to represent septic arthritis. Disseminated gonococcal infection (DGI) may present as a painful monarthritis, polyarthritis (usually migratory [i.e., as one joint is improving, another is becoming inflamed]), or tenosynovitis. Subtle skin lesions, including macules, pustules, and vesicles, may also be present. Because synovial fluid cultures from patients with DGI are infrequently positive, evidence for infection should be sought from other sites (genitourinary, pharyngeal, rectal, skin lesions).

D. The diagnosis of gouty arthritis is established by the presence of intracellular needle-shaped, negatively birefringent crystals, whereas rhomboid-shaped, positively birefringent crystals indicate calcium pyrophosphate deposition disease (CPPD, also known as *pseudogout*). In patients <60 years of age, consider screening for associated disorders such as hemochromatosis, hyperparathyroidism, and hypothyroidism. Detection of calcium hydroxyapatite crystals is more difficult because it requires electron microscopy or Alizarin Red staining if clinically suspected. Although rare, identification of crystals does not negate the possibility of coexistent infection, so joint cultures should also be followed.

E. If analysis of synovial fluid does not reveal the diagnosis, radiographs of the affected joints and contralateral joints should be performed. Common findings include osteoarthritis and chondrocalcinosis (suggesting CPPD). Less often, unsuspected bony lesions such as fracture, malignancy, osteomyelitis, or Paget's disease may be detected. Repeat synovial fluid analysis should be done with additional cultures and smears for acid-fast bacteria and fungus. In endemic areas, a Lyme titer should be sent, especially if there is a history of rash, tick bite, or appropriate exposure. Rheumatoid factor (RF), anticyclic citrullinated antibody, and ANA may be sent to increase the sensitivity of detecting a systemic inflammatory disease such as an atypical presentation of rheumatoid arthritis or systemic lupus erythematosus.

F. If the diagnosis is still not clear, close observation is warranted. If symptoms remit, no further workup is necessary. Alternatively, additional axial or peripheral arthritic symptoms may develop to suggest evolution into a systemic inflammatory disease. If monarthritis persists for 4–6 weeks in the absence of a clear diagnosis, synovial biopsy should be considered to diagnose tuberculous or fungal infections, amyloid, pigmented villonodular synovitis, or other tumors.

G. Noninflammatory, nonbloody effusions should prompt joint radiography to examine for trauma, osteoarthritis, neuropathic arthritis, or avascular necrosis (AVN). Osteoarthritis may present with significant effusions with little inflammation compared to the degree of cartilage and bone destruction. Neuropathic arthropathy is most commonly associated with diabetes but may occur in a variety of neurologic diseases. Loss of pain and proprioceptive sensation allows joint movement to exceed normal range of motion, leading to significant joint instability. Ultimately, dislocation and deformity may occur. AVN is a common cause of shoulder, hip, or knee monarthritis in younger people requiring corticosteroids for

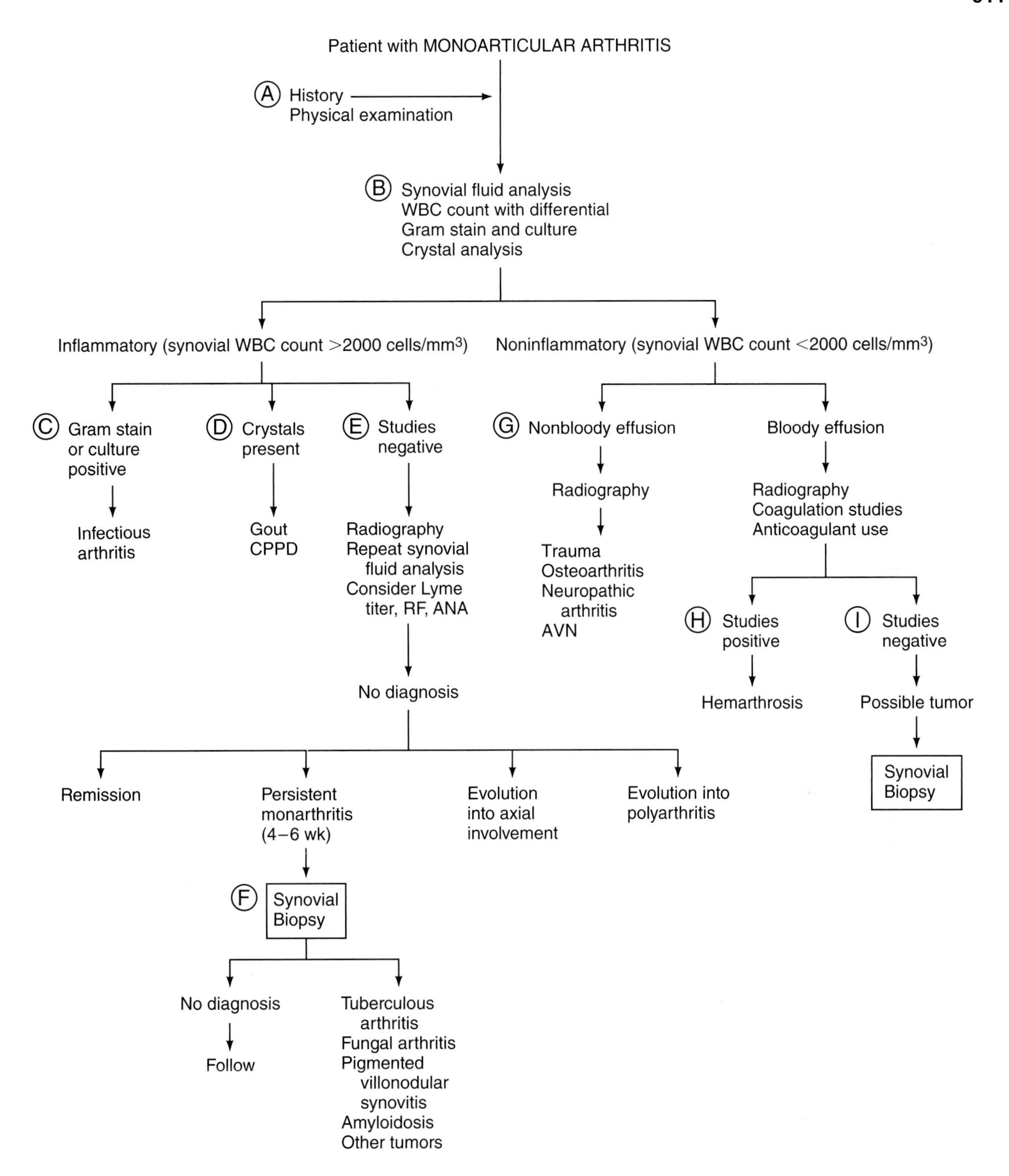

systemic diseases. If a high suspicion for AVN exists and radiographs are negative, MRI is more sensitive for detecting early changes associated with AVN. Similarly, if there is a history of trauma with persistent clicking, locking, or "give way" symptoms, MRI may be indicated to better evaluate joint soft-tissue structures.

H. Hemarthrosis may result from trauma, anticoagulant therapy, inherited coagulopathies, pigmented villonodular synovitis, or synovial hemangiomas. True hemarthrosis must be distinguished from a traumatic tap. Effusions from hemarthrosis are uniformly bloody and do not spontaneously clot.

I. Persistent bloody effusions in the absence of trauma or coagulopathy suggest tumor, particularly pigmented villonodular synovitis. In such cases, synovial biopsy is warranted for further diagnosis.

References

McCune WJ, Golbus J. Monarticular arthritis. In Harris ED, Budd RC, Genovese MC, et al, eds. Kelley's Textbook of Rheumatology, 7th ed. Philadelphia: Saunders, 2005.

Schumacher HR. Monarticular joint disease. In Klippel JH, Crofford LJ, Stone JH, Weyand CM, eds. Primer on the Rheumatic Diseases, 12th ed. Atlanta: Arthritis Foundation, 2001.

POLYARTICULAR ARTHRITIS

Peter Kim, MD

A. A thorough history and physical examination are required for the evaluation of polyarthritis. Historical features of interest include duration of symptoms; prior episodes of arthritis; and distribution, presence, and duration of morning stiffness. A complete review of systems is also required to assess for systemic illnesses with articular manifestations such as inflammatory bowel disease and psoriatic arthritis (PsA). The presence of rash, fevers, weight loss, night sweats, GI, Raynaud's phenomenon, lupus symptoms (in particular, alopecia, photosensitivity, pleurisy, oral ulcers), visual symptoms, antecedent illness, or infection should be sought. Patients should also be questioned about functional limitations (opening jars, holding or lifting objects, climbing stairs, dressing self). Laboratory tests should include CBC, ESR, C-reactive protein (CRP), chem-7, and rheumatoid factor (RF), and anticyclic citrullinated (anti-CCP) antibodies.

B. An important diagnostic feature of arthritis is inflammation. Features suggestive of an inflammatory arthritis include morning stiffness >30 minutes, increased pain or stiffness with prolonged immobility (gelling), fever or chills, and weight loss. Physical examination of involved joints will often reveal bogginess, erythema, warmth, diminished range of motion, and deformities. Features suggestive of a noninflammatory arthritis include pain predominantly with use or weightbearing. Physical examination will usually show cool, nonerythematous joints. There may be an effusion, crepitus, and pain to palpation along the joint line and osteophytes in smaller joints (e.g., Heberden's and Bouchard's nodes).

   If an effusion is present, arthrocentesis can be useful in establishing the diagnosis; the fluid should be sent for cell count with differential, crystal examination by polarized light microscopy, and culture with Gram stain. Cell counts of >2000 cells/mm^3 are consistent with an inflammatory effusion.

C. Inflammatory arthritis with a clear axial component is highly suggestive of a spondyloarthropathy: ankylosing spondylitis (AS), reactive (formerly Reiter's) arthritis, PsA, and enteropathic arthritis. Search for evidence of associated symptoms and signs: rash of psoriasis (especially along the hairline, around and inside the ears, gluteal cleft, lateral margins of the feet), nail pitting, dactylitis (sausage digit), diarrhea or abdominal pain, urethritis, pyoderma gangrenosum, uveitis, or keratoderma blennorrhagica. A radiograph of the pelvis may show sacroiliitis but only after years of disease activity. An MRI with short T1 inversion recovery (STIR) sequences will show evidence of sacroiliitis years before a plain radiograph.

D. Symmetry of joint involvement is a useful distinguishing characteristic of the polyarthritides, but it is not absolute. It is not unusual for a "symmetric arthritis" such as rheumatoid arthritis (RA) to present asymmetrically, especially early in its course. Similarly, an "asymmetric arthritis" can rarely present with complete symmetry.

E. RA typically presents as a symmetric polyarthritis with a predilection for the wrists and small joints of the hands and feet. Involvement of the distal interphalangeal (DIP) joints makes RA very unlikely and another diagnosis such as PsA or inflammatory osteoarthritis (OA) should be considered. The arthritis of lupus can be subtle, and the examination is often normal. Subacute bacterial endocarditis (SBE) and hepatitis C virus (HCV) infections can both cause a polyarthritis with a false-positive RF result. Postinfectious reactions can cause a polyarthritis that is difficult to distinguish from RA, but these usually last 4–6 weeks and resolve spontaneously. Peripheral edema and Raynaud's phenomenon can be the presenting symptoms of scleroderma. Remitting seronegative symmetric synovitis with pitting edema (RS3PE) is a seronegative synovitis with prominent edema thought to be in the clinical spectrum of polymyalgia rheumatica (PMR). A new laboratory test with greater specificity for RA than the RF is anti-CCP antibody.

F. All the spondyloarthropathies can also present as an asymmetric polyarthritis with or without axial involvement. Postinfectious reactions to a myriad of microbes can cause polyarthritis, especially streptococcal infections. Infectious arthritis should be considered in the appropriate settings: Lyme in endemic regions, HIV/AIDS and gonococcal if risk factor are present, and SBE if other signs and symptoms of SBE are present.

(Continued on page 514)

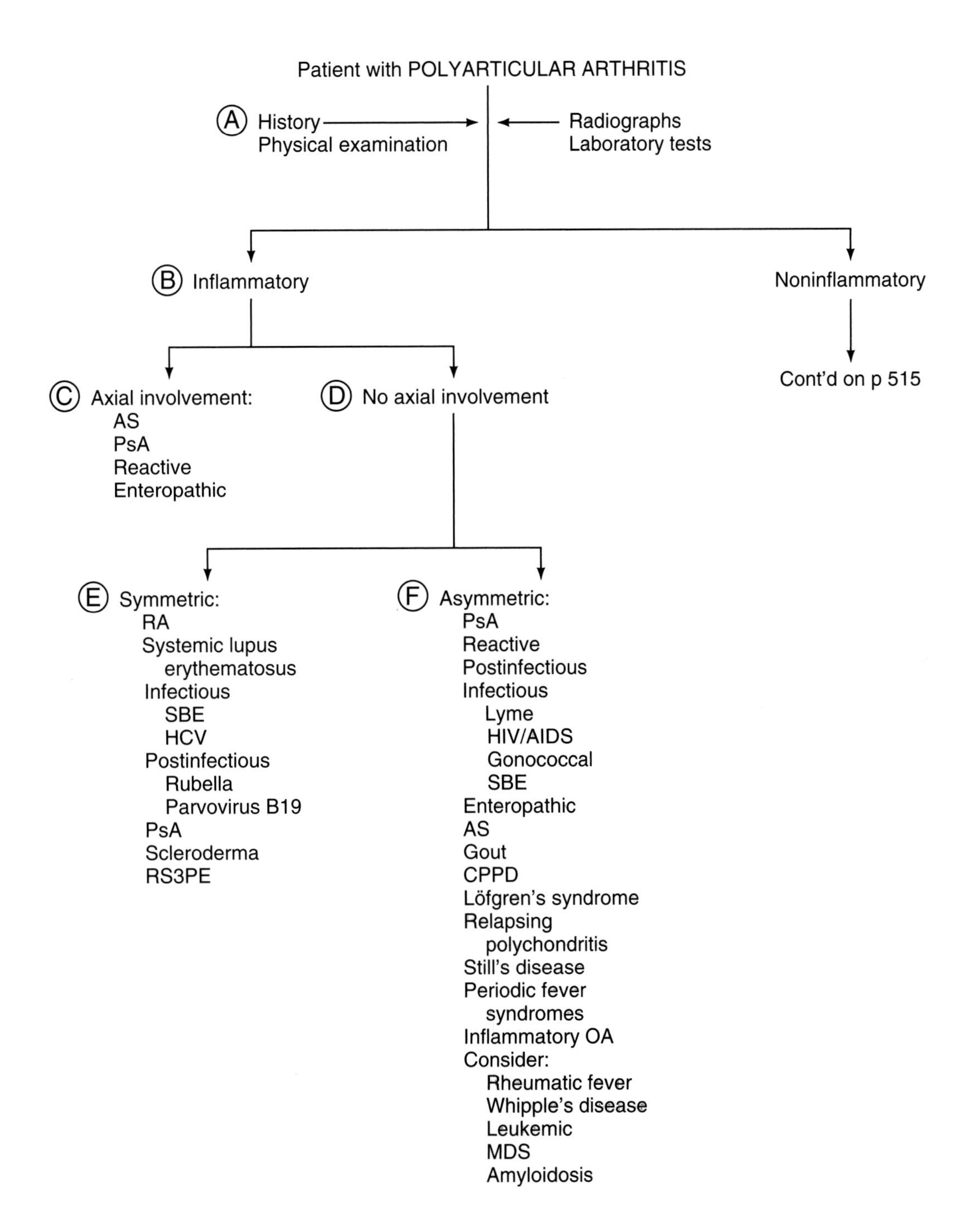

Patient with POLYARTICULAR ARTHRITIS
(A) History
Physical examination
Radiographs
Laboratory tests
(B) Inflammatory
Noninflammatory
Cont'd on p 515
(C) Axial involvement:
AS
PsA
Reactive
Enteropathic
(D) No axial involvement
(E) Symmetric:
RA
Systemic lupus
erythematosus
Infectious
SBE
HCV
Postinfectious
Rubella
Parvovirus B19
PsA
Scleroderma
RS3PE
(F) Asymmetric:
PsA
Reactive
Postinfectious
Infectious
Lyme
HIV/AIDS
Gonococcal
SBE
Enteropathic
AS
Gout
CPPD
Löfgren's syndrome
Relapsing
polychondritis
Still's disease
Periodic fever
syndromes
Inflammatory OA
Consider:
Rheumatic fever
Whipple's disease
Leukemic
MDS
Amyloidosis

G. Crystalline arthropathies (gout and calcium pyrophosphate dihydrate [CPPD]) are usually a monoarthritis but can present as a polyarthritis; a definitive diagnosis requires the demonstration of crystals in the joint fluid. Löfgren's syndrome (erythema nodosum, hilar adenopathy, periarthritis usually of the lower extremities) is an acute, self-limited form of sarcoidosis. Relapsing polychondritis can affect cartilage in joints, ears, nose, tracheobronchial tree, and proteoglycan-rich structures (eyes, heart, blood vessels, and inner ear). Still's disease causes daily fevers with a transient salmon-colored rash, elevated liver function test results, and ferritin. Recurrent attacks of fever and arthritis, especially in the setting of a positive family history, should prompt an evaluation for the periodic fever syndromes (familial Mediterranean fever, hyperimmunoglobulin D syndrome, tumor necrosis factor receptor–associated periodic syndrome, Muckle-Wells syndrome). Inflammatory OA should be considered if DIP joints are involved or if Heberden's or Bouchard's nodes are present. Rarer diagnoses include rheumatic fever, Whipple's disease, leukemic arthritis, and the arthritis associated with myelodysplastic syndromes (MDS).

Noninflammatory arthritis with a radiograph showing bony hypertrophy and cartilage space loss is consistent with a diagnosis of OA. OA can be primary or secondary to obesity, trauma, or injury. More importantly, OA can occur secondary to systemic illnesses such as hemochromatosis, ochronosis, hyperparathyroidism, Wilson's disease, acromegaly, and amyloidosis. Early age of onset, atypical distribution (metacarpophalangeal joints, wrists, elbows, shoulders, ankles), or unusual radiographs should prompt an evaluation for secondary causes.

H. Other causes of polyarthritis include avascular necrosis (AVN), which can have symptoms out of proportion to the examination. It is not uncommon to see a joint effusion with AVN. Clubbing, bone pain, and parostosis on radiographs are seen with hypertrophic pulmonary osteoarthropathy (HPOA).

References

Hoffiman GS. Polyarthritis: the differential diagnosis of rheumatoid arthritis. Semin Arthritis Rheum 1978;8:115–141.

Junnila JL, Cartwright VW. Chronic musculoskeletal pain in children: part II. Rheumatic causes. Am Fam Physician 2006;74:293–300.

Rindfleisch JA, Muller D. Diagnosis and management of rheumatoid arthritis. Am Fam Physician 2005;72:1037–1047.

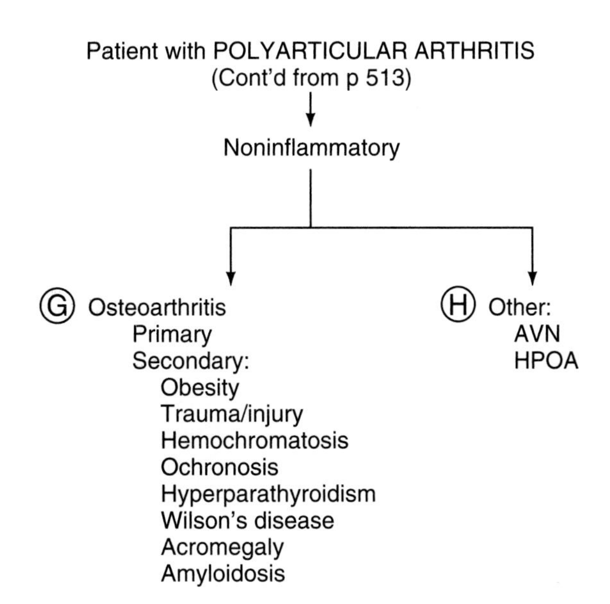
Patient with POLYARTICULAR ARTHRITIS
(Cont'd from p 513)
Noninflammatory
(G) Osteoarthritis
Primary
Secondary:
Obesity
Trauma/injury
Hemochromatosis
Ochronosis
Hyperparathyroidism
Wilson's disease
Acromegaly
Amyloidosis
(H) Other:
AVN
HPOA

SERONEGATIVE ARTHRITIS

Paul A. Monach, MD, PhD

A. The algorithm for this chapter starts at a point where a patient is suspected of inflammatory arthritis and serologic testing is negative for rheumatoid factor. Inflammatory arthritis is suggested by morning stiffness lasting >30 minutes, improvement rather than worsening with exercise, and soft-tissue swelling. Notable among the seronegative arthritides are the spondyloarthropathies, including ankylosing spondylitis, reactive arthritis, psoriatic arthritis, and arthritis associated with inflammatory bowel disease (IBD).

B. The distinction between inflammatory and degenerative disease, particularly of the spine, hip, and shoulder joints, is often difficult. Elevated ESR and C-reactive protein (CRP) are nonspecific and insensitive markers of seronegative arthritis but are nevertheless suggestive of inflammatory disease if elevated. The presence of effusion in a peripheral joint is suggestive of inflammatory arthritis, which can be documented by aspiration of synovial fluid having a WBC count of >2000 cells/mm^3. Human leukocyte antigen (HLA)-B27 is highly associated with ankylosing spondylitis and reactive arthritis syndromes that include the extraarticular manifestations described later (Reiter's syndrome). HLA-B27 is less strongly linked to arthritis associated with IBD or psoriasis unless the syndrome features spinal arthritis and/or anterior uveitis (iritis). Because HLA-B27 is common in populations at risk for seronegative arthritides, testing is only theoretically helpful when the pretest probability of ankylosing spondylitis is between 30% and 70%, a problematic estimation in routine practice. An infectious workup is indicated in the event of acute onset of seronegative arthritis with or without extracellular manifestations. Stool culture for *Salmonella, Shigella, Yersinia,* and *Campylobacter* should be considered, as should urethral swab or urine testing for *Chlamydia.* Streptococcal and other infections are also associated with reactive inflammatory syndromes involving arthritis, but these are not associated with HLA-B27 and do not present with the characteristic features of the spondyloarthropathies.

C. Spinal and/or sacroiliac (SI) involvement is suggested by low back pain and stiffness, neck pain and stiffness, or posterior thoracic pain with deep breathing or coughing. Schober's test is sensitive for lumbar spine disease but is nonspecific. With the patient standing, a mark is made at the L5 level ("dimples of Venus") and another 10 cm above. The patient is asked to flex the trunk forward with the arms hanging down toward the floor (and may bend the legs slightly so as to avoid a false-positive test result because of hamstring tightness), and the space between the points is measured. Expansion to <15 cm is abnormal. Chest expansion should be measured from forced expiration to full inspiration; expansion >5 cm is normal, and <2.5 cm is clearly abnormal. Physical examination tests for SI joint pathology are insensitive and nonspecific.

D. Radiography of the SI joints should be done to look for evidence of erosive disease suggestive of inflammation. An anteroposterior (AP) view of the pelvis is usually sufficient, although the Ferguson view is probably more sensitive. Radiography of the spine may show characteristic bony changes at the corners of the vertebral bodies (syndesmophytes). Radiographic changes usually occur only after several years of disease; earlier, CT, MRI, and bone scan are more sensitive, although bone scan does not distinguish between inflammatory and degenerative disease. All patients with ankylosing spondylitis have SI and/or spinal arthritis, but the spine is involved in a minority of patients with other spondyloarthropathies.

E. Peripheral joint involvement is often asymmetric; oligoarticular; and most common in proximal and lower extremity joints in ankylosing spondylitis, reactive arthritis, and IBD-associated arthritis. Patients with psoriatic arthritis can have symmetric polyarthritis that resembles rheumatoid arthritis, asymmetric oligoarthritis resembling the other spondyloarthropathies, or arthritis limited to several distal interphalangeal (DIP) joints. Often multiple joints and the intervening soft tissue are inflamed in a single digit, creating a "sausage digit" (dactylitis), particularly in psoriatic and reactive arthritis. Tenosynovitis is also common, particularly around the hand/wrist and foot/ankle, in these conditions.

F. The integumentary findings in psoriasis are most common on the extensor surfaces of the elbows and knees; other particularly common locations include the low back, hands and feet, scalp, umbilicus, gluteal cleft, and glans penis. Nail pitting and onycholysis are common and are associated with arthritis. Clinically and histologically similar lesions can occur acutely in reactive arthritis: keratoderma blennorrhagica of the feet, circinate balanitis, and nail pitting. Erythema nodosum is a syndrome of painful, red, cutaneous nodules on the lower legs and is common in IBD. Pyoderma gangrenosa is a more severe and less common neutrophilic dermatosis associated with IBD.

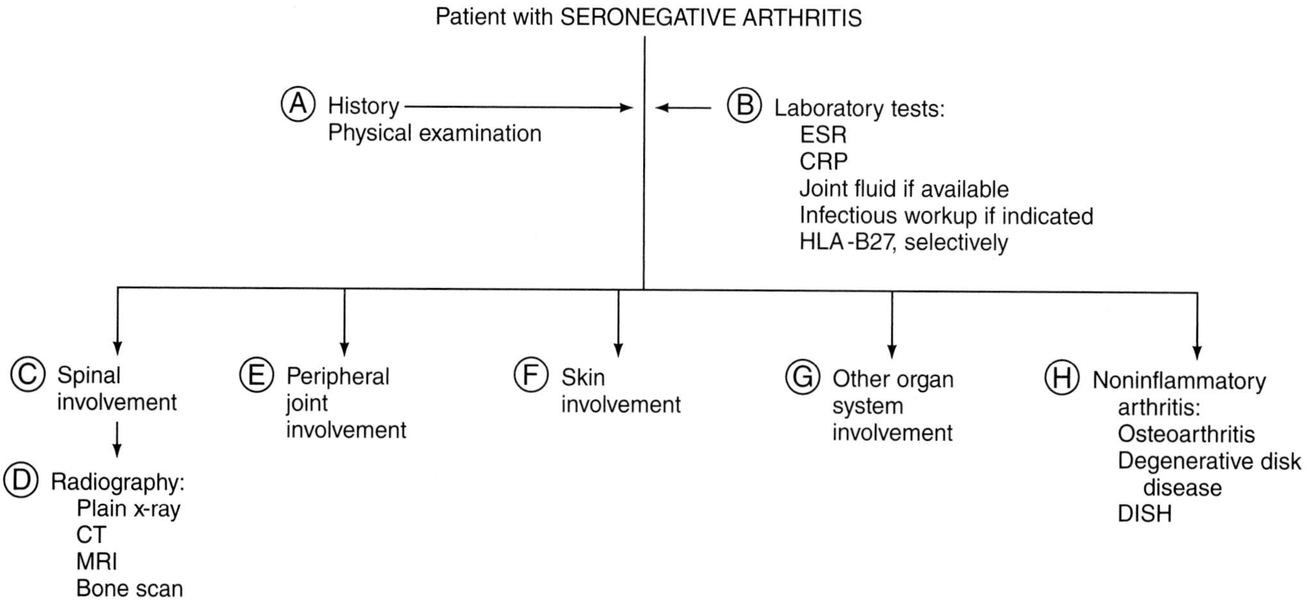

Patient with SERONEGATIVE ARTHRITIS

(A) History
Physical examination

(B) Laboratory tests:
ESR
CRP
Joint fluid if available
Infectious workup if indicated
HLA-B27, selectively

(C) Spinal involvement
(D) Radiography:
Plain x-ray
CT
MRI
Bone scan

(E) Peripheral joint involvement

(F) Skin involvement

(G) Other organ system involvement

(H) Noninflammatory arthritis:
Osteoarthritis
Degenerative disk disease
DISH

G. Conjunctivitis is part of the classic triad of Reiter's syndrome. However, anterior uveitis (iritis) is also common in reactive arthritis and in ankylosing spondylitis and IBD. A recent history of self-limited diarrhea and abdominal pain suggests a precipitating episode of gastroenteritis; a chronic history raises suspicion for IBD. Urethritis may suggest recent infection with *Chlamydia.* Patients with reactive arthritis may develop cardiac conduction defects that are generally not serious. Over the longer term, patients with ankylosing spondylitis may develop inflammation of the ascending aorta, leading to aortic valve insufficiency and/or aneurysm.

H. Noninflammatory disease of the spine is common. Degenerative disk disease and osteoarthritis of the spine and SI joints appear different on radiography, featuring disk shrinkage and marginal osteophytes rather than syndesmophytes. Diffuse idiopathic skeletal hyperostosis (DISH) is a noninflammatory disease that features exuberant ossification at sites of tendon and ligament attachment, including the spine, often in a patchy distribution and usually on the right side.

References

Kataria RK, Brent LH. Spondyloarthropathies. Am Fam Physician 2004;69:2853–2860.

Slobodin G, Rozenbaum M, Boulman N, Rosner I. Varied presentation of enthesopathy. Semin Arthritis Rheum 2007;37:119–126.

SOFT-TISSUE PAIN

Paul A. Monach, MD, PhD

A. "Soft-tissue rheumatism" is a spectrum of disorders that includes both focal pain associated with easily defined nonarticular musculoskeletal structures (tendonitis and bursitis) and generalized pain syndromes that may be manifestations of underlying diseases but more often are more commonly of idiopathic origin and no known pathology or pathophysiology.

B. Periarticular pain, in contrast to articular pain, is often reproduced on active but not passive joint movement, particularly in tendonitis or muscle strain. Pain with passive movement, if it occurs, should be with increasing stretch of the affected tendon. Even more suggestive of tendonitis or muscle strain is pain produced by isometric use of an involved muscle and tendon because the joint does not move. Irritated or damaged tendons are usually not visibly inflamed (no redness or swelling) unless in the setting of significant trauma or an inflammatory disease (especially the seronegative spondyloarthropathies), but there is often point tenderness. Bursitis features point tenderness and sometimes swelling and redness, at particular locations, including the front of the patella (prepatellar), the point of the elbow (olecranon), the lateral aspect of the shoulder (subdeltoid or subacromial), the medial aspect of the proximal tibia (anserine), the greater trochanter of the femur (trochanteric), and the ischial tuberosity (ischial). There is often a history of chronic or subacute trauma. Pain is usually but not always greater with active use of tendons near the bursa and is worsened by stretch (e.g., full flexion of the elbow in olecranon bursitis). The prepatellar and olecranon bursae are susceptible to infection and gout, so bursitis associated with swelling and redness at these sites should be aspirated to rule out infection and to evaluate for crystal deposition. Ligamentous sprain usually features a history of acute stretch injury, and examination features point tenderness and pain much greater with stretch of the ligament than with the opposite movement. Joint laxity may be apparent in a substantial or complete tear.

C. A generalized pain syndrome merits a comprehensive review of systems and physical examination to assess the likelihood of such diseases as systemic lupus, thyroid and parathyroid disease, metabolic myopathies (glycogen storage diseases and others), vitamin D deficiency, hepatitis C virus (HCV) infection, and multiple sclerosis. Practitioners differ greatly on how much laboratory evaluation to do related to these considerations. In our opinion, it is reasonable to measure thyroid-stimulating hormone (TSH), creatine kinase (CK), calcium, 25-OH vitamin D, and HCV antibodies; general laboratory testing of CBC, BUN, creatinine, electrolytes, and liver function is often done as well. ESR, C-reactive protein (CRP), and ANA are useful if they are negative, but moderately positive results are very common in the healthy population.

D. Fibromyalgia is a common idiopathic disorder with no known pathology, characterized by widespread pain and tenderness on examination in a number of characteristic areas, including the trapezii, the attachment of neck extensors to the occiput (and other areas of the neck and upper back), the joining of the second rib to the sternal cartilage, the upper outer buttock, the lateral elbow, the lateral hip near the greater trochanter, and the medial knee. Many patients are tender at other or all soft-tissue locations as well. There is often associated sleep disorder, depression, lack of exercise, chronic fatigue, headache, irritable bowel syndrome, and sometimes another, locally painful condition of definable cause. These factors may play a role in amplifying pain perception pathways, currently a popular working model for the disorder.

E. Intraarticular pain is usually experienced on both passive and active motion. Inflammatory arthritis is more likely than osteoarthritis to feature soft-tissue swelling, joint effusion, morning stiffness, and signs of inflammatory illness in other organ systems or systemically. Laboratory tests can be helpful as noted. See the chapters Monoarticular Arthritis and Polyarticular Arthritis polyarthritis and monoarthritis.

References

Chakrabarty S, Zoorob R. Fibromyalgia. Am Fam Physician 2007; 76:247–254.

Hwang E, Barkhuizen A. Update on rheumatic mimics of fibromyalgia. Curr Pain Headache Rep 2006;10:327–332.

Reilly PA. The differential diagnosis of generalized pain. Baillieres Best Prac Res Clin Rheumatol 1999;13:391–401.

Wilson JJ, Best TM. Common overuse tendon problems: a review and recommendations for treatment. Am Fam Physician 2005;72:811–818.

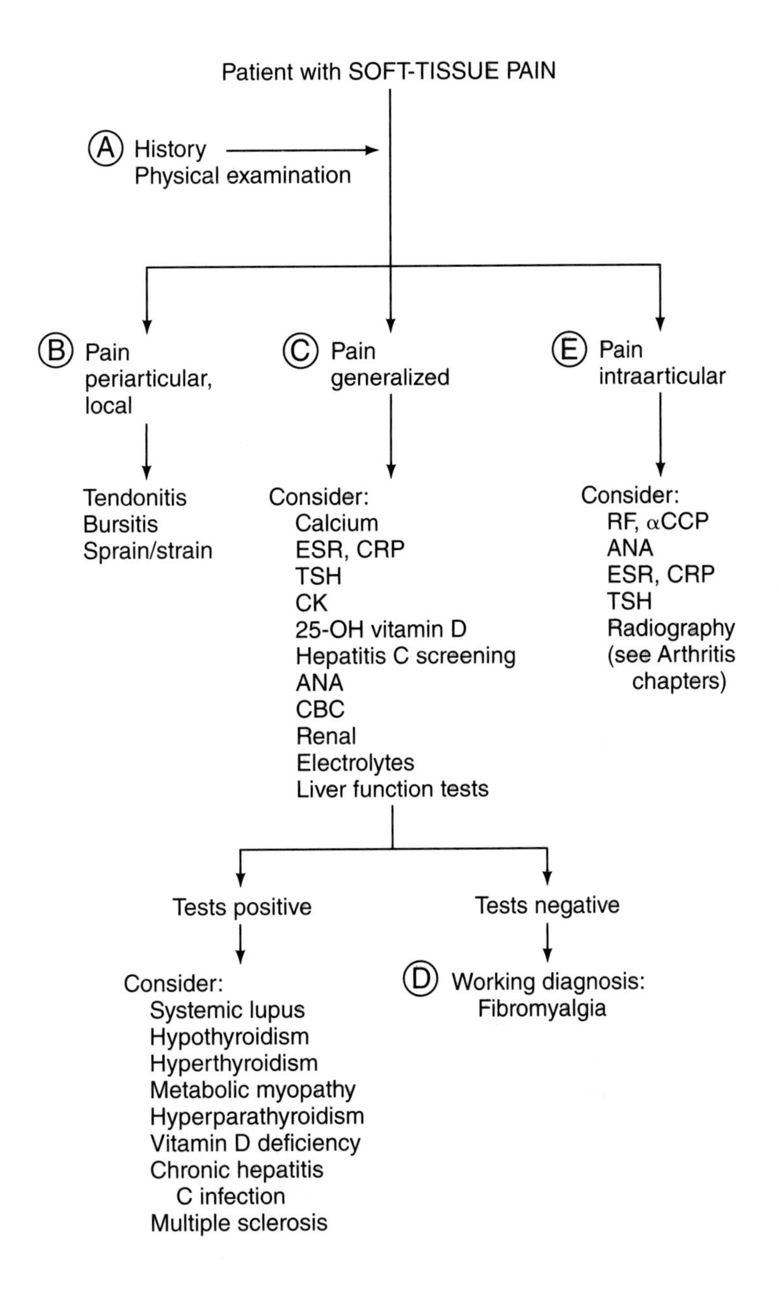
Patient with SOFT-TISSUE PAIN
(A) History
Physical examination
(B) Pain periarticular, local
Tendonitis
Bursitis
Sprain/strain
(C) Pain generalized
Consider:
Calcium
ESR, CRP
TSH
CK
25-OH vitamin D
Hepatitis C screening
ANA
CBC
Renal
Electrolytes
Liver function tests
(E) Pain intraarticular
Consider:
RF, αCCP
ANA
ESR, CRP
TSH
Radiography (see Arthritis chapters)
Tests positive
Consider:
Systemic lupus
Hypothyroidism
Hyperthyroidism
Metabolic myopathy
Hyperparathyroidism
Vitamin D deficiency
Chronic hepatitis C infection
Multiple sclerosis
Tests negative
(D) Working diagnosis: Fibromyalgia

NECK PAIN

Simon Helfgott, MD

Approximately 10% of the adult population complains of neck pain at some time. Unlike back pain, fewer patients require time away from work or claim disability, and very few develop permanent deficits. The cervical spine is composed of seven vertebrae that are supported by the cervical and trapezius muscles. In addition to supporting and providing movement for the head and neck, the seven vertebrae also serve to protect the spinal cord and spinal nerves whenever the spinal column is at risk for injury. This may explain why cervical strain is so common.

A. Neck pain is typically described at the base of the cervical spine or along the upper border of the trapezius muscle. This may be accompanied by headache. Physical or emotional stressors, poor sleeping habits, or poor posture can cause this pain. Some patients will also describe neck stiffness with lack of full neck motion. In older patients this might be a result of osteoarthritis of the cervical spine. Some patients develop numbness, tingling, or pain down an arm. This may be a result of disk herniation, especially at the level of C5-C6, producing pain in the shoulder tip and trapezius and radiating toward the anterior upper arm, radial forearm, and thumb. Lateral disk herniation at C6-C7 produces pain at the shoulder blade, pectoral area, and medial axilla with radiation toward the posterolateral upper arm, dorsal elbow and forearm, and palmar surface of the thumb and index finger. There may also be sensory impairment such as numbness or dysesthesia in these areas. Lateral herniation between C7 and T1 produces pain at the medial side of the forearm and sensory loss in the medial forearm and the ulnar nerve distribution of the hand. Central disk herniation at any cervical level can produce a syndrome of cervical myelopathy with bilateral long track signs in the extremities, gait dysfunction, and loss of coordination. In some of these patients neck pain may be minimal or even absent.

   Whiplash injury is the term used to describe cervical strain in the setting of an acute flexion/extension injury, often seen in car accidents involving rear-end collisions. Symptoms may include severe pain, spasm, and loss of motion in the neck and occipital headache.

B. The examiner should observe the movement of the head and neck, including rotation, lateral flexion, forward flexion, and extension. Palpation of the paraspinal and upper trapezius muscles can be performed to assess for tenderness and muscle spasm. Examination of motor strength and deep tendon reflexes and sensory findings in the arms and legs should be performed. The loss or asymmetry of upper extremity reflexes may identify the location of a disk herniation. However, deep tendon hyperreflexia in the upper or lower extremities might suggest spinal cord compression.

C. Imaging studies should be considered in patients who have severe, unrelenting pain that is not improving or presenting with abnormal peripheral nerve function. Plain films may document evidence for osteoarthritis, and in patients with acute injuries, they could identify an occult fracture. MRI and CT may be useful in identifying patients with disk herniations who might benefit from targeted epidural steroid injections or require referral to a surgeon. In most situations, MRI is preferred because it is more sensitive than CT in detecting disk herniations, tumor, infection, or fracture.

   Electromyography (EMG) should be considered only for those patients who continue to have persistent pain and whose imaging studies have not been helpful in identifying the source of the pain.

References

Alexander MP. Whiplash: chronic pain and cognitive symptoms. Neurology 2003;60:733.

Stiell IG, Clement CM, McKnight RD, et al. The Canadian C-spine rule versus the NEXUS low-risk criteria in patients with trauma. N Engl J Med 2003;349:2510.

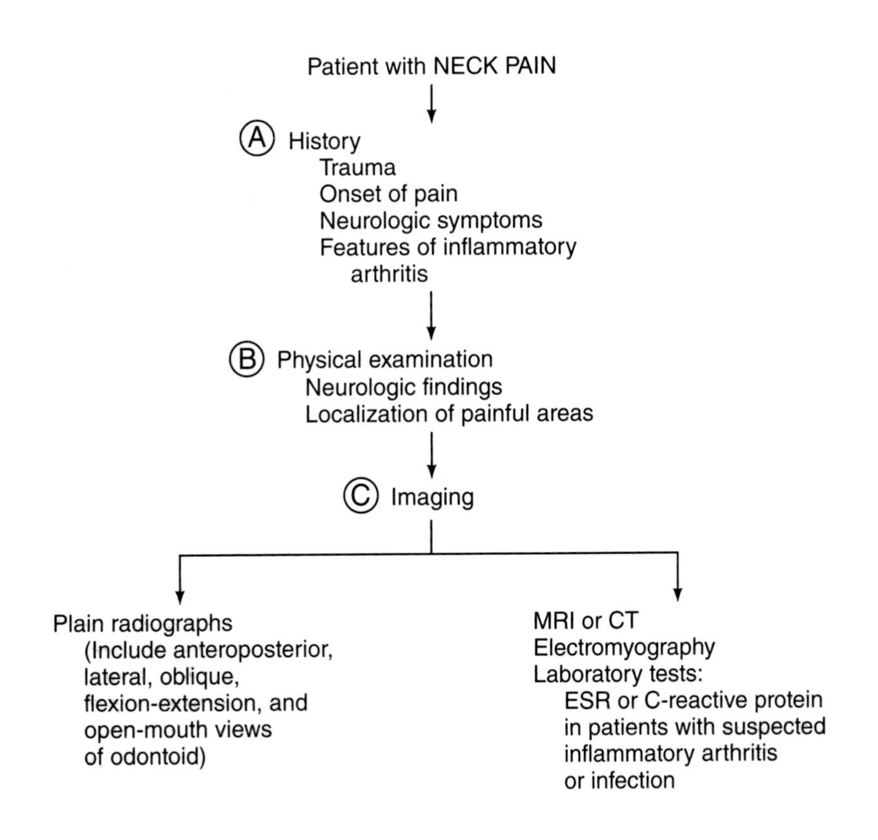
Patient with NECK PAIN
A History
Trauma
Onset of pain
Neurologic symptoms
Features of inflammatory arthritis
B Physical examination
Neurologic findings
Localization of painful areas
C Imaging
Plain radiographs
(Include anteroposterior, lateral, oblique, flexion-extension, and open-mouth views of odontoid)
MRI or CT
Electromyography
Laboratory tests:
ESR or C-reactive protein in patients with suspected inflammatory arthritis or infection

SHOULDER PAIN

Paul A. Monach, MD, PhD

A. Anterior glenohumeral dislocation, acromioclavicular (AC) separation, and rotator cuff tear are often strongly suggested by history and physical examination, with the former two conditions confirmable by radiography. Rotator cuff tear usually includes the supraspinatus tendon and as such, in a full tear, patients cannot initiate abduction of the arm from the vertical position without prominent recruitment of the deltoid and trapezius muscles. Rotator cuff tear can also occur insidiously, usually after a prolonged period of rotator cuff tendonopathy in older persons. Conversely, rotator cuff tendonopathy without tear of the tendon can occur with acute trauma but is more often idiopathic or from chronic overuse. Fractures of the humerus, clavicle, and scapula need to be considered in the setting of significant trauma. The more subtle "superior labrum anterior-posterior" (SLAP) lesion is a tear of the cartilaginous glenoid labrum that can occur after relatively minor trauma and requires more advanced imaging than plain radiography to diagnose conclusively.

B. Rotator cuff tendonitis and biceps tendonitis are both extremely common, and the diagnosis can often be made by physical examination. In evaluating the rotator cuff, it is valuable to check for pain with resisted external and internal rotation, but the most valuable tests are for impingement of the supraspinatus tendon. There are several variations of this test, but the common feature they have is resisted elevation of the arm with the thumb facing down. Subacromial (or subdeltoid) bursitis also produces a positive impingement sign, but there is usually more tenderness at the lateral edge of the acromion than in supraspinatus tendonitis. Tendonitis of the long head of the biceps is readily diagnosed by local tenderness of the tendon (located in a groove on the anterior shoulder, about halfway between the coracoid process and the lateral edge of the acromion) and pain with resisted elbow flexion or resisted elevation of the arm with the thumb facing up. Calcific tendonitis is an acute, self-limited disorder of unknown etiology that commonly affects the shoulder tendons, usually featuring severe pain and exquisite local tenderness and a characteristic radiographic appearance. Tendonopathies in general feature greater pain with active motion or isometric contraction than with passive motion. Adhesive capsulitis, also known as "frozen shoulder," is a painful disorder that often follows immobilization but is frequently idiopathic. It is characterized by limited motion of the shoulder joint in all directions, which is suggested by examination but cannot be definitively diagnosed without excluding frank arthritis. Primary osteoarthritis (OA) of the glenohumeral joint is uncommon, but OA following rotator cuff tear and OA of the AC joint are common. Inflammatory arthritis of the shoulder girdle is characteristic of polymyalgia rheumatica (PMR) and is common in the seronegative spondyloarthropathies, but other causes of monoarthritis and polyarthritis need to be considered. The shoulder examination, like the hip examination, is not sensitive for detecting joint effusion.

C. A thorough neurologic examination of the affected arm is important in the evaluation of shoulder pain because cervical radiculopathy from disk herniation or arthritis often presents as shoulder pain.

D. Plain radiography of the shoulder using three standard views is sufficient for most purposes: an anteroposterior (AP) view with the arm in internal rotation, an AP view in external rotation, and an axillary view. The AC joint and clavicle can usually be evaluated using these views as well. To evaluate for AC joint separation, a view with the patient standing and holding a weight in the hand and/or a frontal view allowing comparison of the AC joints may be helpful. Rotator cuff tear is inferred by a narrowing of the space between the acromion and the humeral head, and OA changes are often present at the corresponding surfaces if the condition is chronic. Even with a preserved acromiohumeral space, acromial spurring, which can contribute to chronic rotator cuff impingement, is commonly seen. Calcific tendonitis is apparent as an extraparenchymal radiodensity. Avascular necrosis, less common in the shoulder than in the hip and knee, is usually not apparent by plain radiography for about 6 weeks after onset. Cervical spine films are indicated if a neurologic deficit is detected; AP and lateral views may be sufficient to diagnose degenerative disease, but evaluation of neural foramina requires oblique views and, usually, more advanced imaging modalities.

E. CT and MRI are both more sensitive than plain radiography for diagnosing fractures, but there is less often need for using them for this purpose in the shoulder than in the hip and pelvis. MRI is the technique of choice for delineating rotator cuff pathology, but it needs to be done only if diagnosis is in doubt or surgery is being considered. Ultrasonography is used for

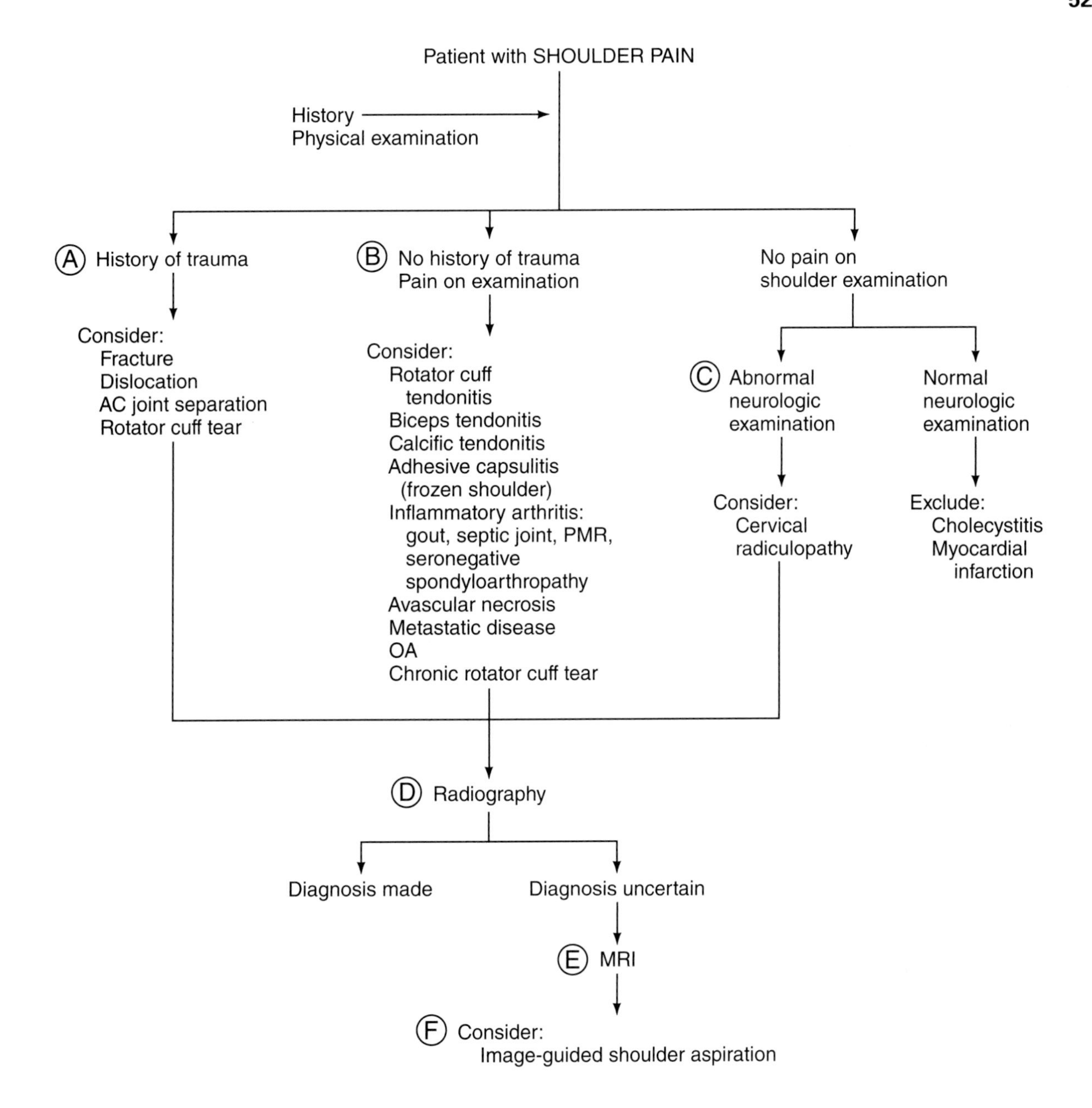

diagnosis of rotator cuff tears, but its value depends on the experience of the operator. MRI is the best technique for diagnosing nerve root compression, early avascular necrosis, and shoulder joint effusion.

F. Aspiration of the shoulder joint, under imaging guidance, is needed if there is suspicion of an infected joint. Such suspicion is increased by the presence of acute-onset, atraumatic, severe pain, particularly with physical examination, or radiographic evidence of effusion, and/or fever and other signs of infection.

References

Burbank KM, Stevenson JH, Czarnecki GR, Dorfman J. Chronic shoulder pain: part I. Evaluation and diagnosis. Am Fam Physician 2008; 77:453–460.

Burbank KM, Stevenson JH, Czarnecki GR, Dorfman J. Chronic shoulder pain: part II. Treatment. Am Fam Physician 2008;77:493–497.

Matsen FA III. Clinical practice: rotator-cuff failure. N Engl J Med 2008;358:2138–2147.

Quillen DM, Wuchner M, Hatch RL. Acute shoulder injuries. Am Fam Physician 2004;70:1947–1954.

LOW BACK PAIN

Simon Helfgott, MD

Most people will experience at least one episode of low back pain during their adult lifetime. Most of these are of short duration, lasting from days to a few weeks, and resolve with little if any therapeutic intervention. The challenge to the clinician is to identify those patients who may benefit from diagnostic interventions to further evaluate their pain.

A. When assessing the patient, the following questions should be considered.

Where does it hurt? Back pain is usually described as a dull steady ache over the lower lumbar spine that sometimes may radiate toward the buttocks. Patients usually do not complain of localized severe point tenderness except when there may be a fracture. Pain radiating down a leg may suggest nerve impingement from either disk herniation in a younger patient or osteophyte formation in an older individual.

When does it hurt? In patients with disk-related back pain, symptoms are often made worse by sitting or standing for extended periods. Coughing or sneezing may aggravate theses symptoms, which are generally related to a disk herniation that is impinging on a nerve root. In contrast, lying flat often alleviates this pain.

In patients with lumbar spinal stenosis, forward flexion of the back may "open up" the narrowed spinal canal foraminal spaces and improve the pain symptoms. Patients also describe relief when leaning forward to push a shopping cart ("shopping cart sign"). These patients note worsening of symptoms when standing for prolonged periods.

How does activity affect the pain? Generally, rest improves back pain symptoms, at least in the short term. This may be true for back pain from disk herniations or spinal stenosis from osteoarthritis. Symptoms are minimal on arising and worsen with activity. In contrast, patients with an inflammatory spondyloarthropathy (e.g., ankylosing spondylitis, psoriatic arthritis, or inflammatory bowel disease) note more stiffness and worsening of symptoms following periods of prolonged inactivity. These patients may also have nighttime symptoms and feel worse in the morning on arising.

Does the pain radiate? Radiation of pain down one leg (sciatica) may result from disk herniation or impingement caused by an osteophyte or a combination of both. The patient may describe pure leg pain without back pain, although most patients complain of both. Pain or dysesthesias in the perineum can result from cauda equina syndrome. These patients need to be identified promptly because surgical referral is urgently required.

What relieves the pain? By the time of their visit, patients may have self-treated with low doses of NSAIDs or acetaminophen. If there is benefit noted with these drugs, this information could be helpful in developing a management strategy for control of pain.

Application of heat or cold to the back may provide transient relief but does not aid in establishing a diagnosis.

B. Inspection of spine posture may demonstrate scoliosis or asymmetry. Forward flexion of the spine should be assessed for muscle spasm and ease of flexibility. Schober's test is a measure of lumbar flexibility used to evaluate patients with a spondyloarthropathy. A segment of the lumbar spine measuring 10 cm when standing should expand to about 15 cm or more when fully flexed. In cases of vertebral compression fracture, there may be localized tenderness on palpation. Persons with spinal stenosis generally have more pain with back extension rather than forward flexion. A straight leg raise (SLR) test should be performed with the patient supine and the uninvolved knee bent to 45 degrees and resting on the table. The examiner should hold the involved leg straight, cup the heel with the other hand, and gradually raise the leg. With a disk herniation impinging on a nerve root, the straight leg raise will stretch these roots and pain may radiate below the tested knee. Note that the SLR test is positive if the distal leg pain occurs with leg elevation <60 degrees.

When pain radiates down the nontested leg (crossed SLR) these findings are even more specific than pain going down the ipsilateral leg. Note that the SLR is more reliable in younger patients and loses diagnostic value in older patients. A detailed sensory and motor examination and assessment of deep tendon reflexes should be performed to identify specific dermatome involvement. This is very helpful when trying to ascertain the relevance of imaging findings noted on CT or MRI.

The most common areas for disk herniation and lumbar stenosis are at L4-L5 and L5-S1. At L4-L5 one might see loss of strength in the extensor hallucis longis and a dysesthesia over the big toe and medial foot. With L5-S1 disease, the toe flexors and ankle jerk are reduced and there are dysesthesia over the fifth toe and lateral foot. In the rare cauda equina syndrome, the S2, S3, and S4 roots may be involved and patients have bowel and bladder dysfunction with dysesthesia over the perineum.

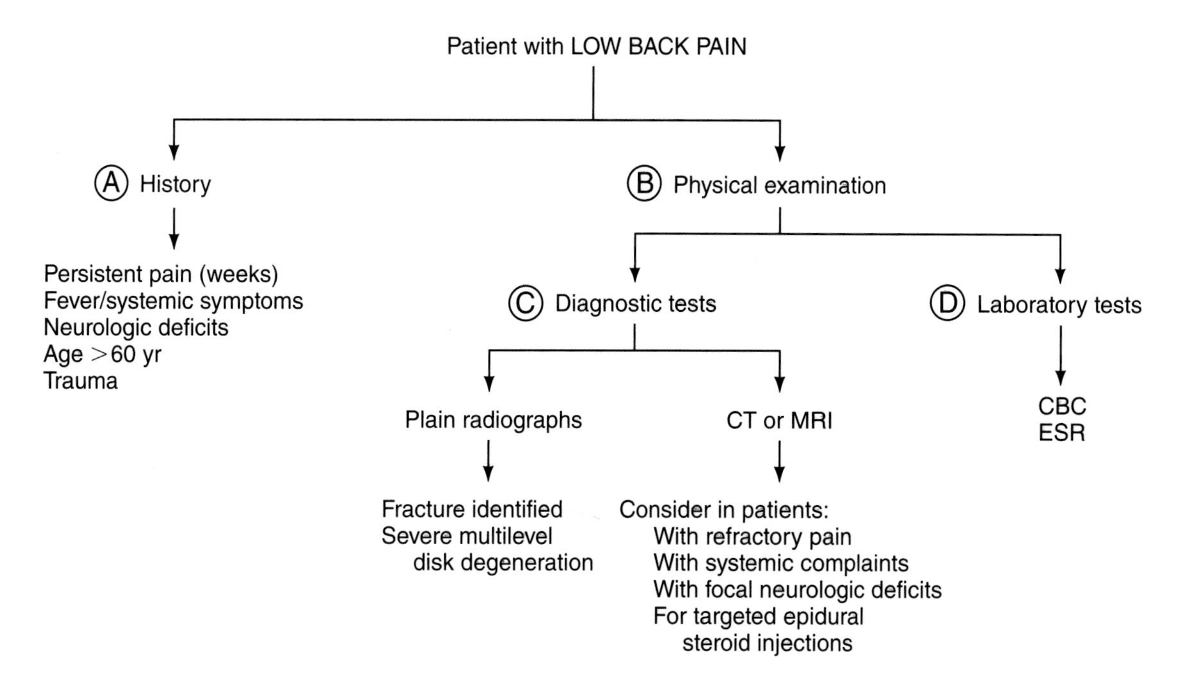

C. Current guidelines recommend obtaining plain radiographs in patients with fever, unexplained weight loss, neurologic deficits, IV drug abuse, or age >50 years. Radiographs are very useful in detecting structural abnormalities such as spondylolisthesis and scoliosis but are not sensitive for detecting cancer or infection. Imaging with CT or MRI should be reserved for the patient for whom there is a strong clinical suspicion of an infection, cancer, or presence of a persistent neurologic deficit. Imaging could be useful in determining whether targeted epidural injection of corticosteroid or surgical referral is appropriate.

Imaging needs to be interpreted carefully because a high percentage of patients with or without back pain symptoms will have abnormalities such as disk degeneration or bulging or protruding disks or even central or lateral canal stenosis. For example, it is highly unlikely that anyone >50 years will have a "normal" CT or MRI of the spine. Imaging is most useful when the clinical findings on physical examination correlate in a neuroanatomic fashion with the findings on MRI or CT. Radiologic findings that do not match the clinical examination should raise strong doubts about the value of MRI or CT in that particular patient.

D. Electromyography (EMG) is generally of limited value. CBC and ESR may be useful in the evaluation of patients suspected of having systemic disease such as infection, malignancy, or spondyloarthropathy.

References

Helfgott SM. Sensible approach to low back pain. Bull Rheum Dis 2001;50(3):1–4.

Jarvik JG, Deyo RA. Diagnostic evaluation of low back pain with emphasis on imaging. Ann Intern Med 2002;137:586–597.

Katz JN, Dalgas M, Stucki G, et al. Degenerative lumbar spinal stenosis. diagnostic value of the history and physical examination. Arthritis Rheum 1995;38:1236–1241.

HIP PAIN

Paul A. Monach, MD, PhD

A. Falls, especially in older persons, raise suspicion for hip fractures, particularly of the femoral neck and intertrochanteric region, but also of the acetabulum, elsewhere in the pelvis, or of the tip of the greater trochanter. Chronic overuse injuries from weightbearing exercise can produce stress fractures of the pelvis, and atraumatic pelvic "insufficiency" fractures can occur in older persons, particularly those with osteoporosis. Radiography and often more advanced imaging techniques are needed to rule out fracture.

B. Pain felt in the groin with examination of the hip is suggestive of hip joint disease. Groin pain with "log-rolling" the leg is probably the most specific finding because this maneuver does not stress the knee, back, or hip girdle musculature. A positive Thomas test to detect hip joint flexion contracture, in which a patient is unable to keep the affected leg on the examining table while the other leg is allowed to dangle off the table with the knee bent, is suggestive of serious disease. Pain of gradual onset is most suggestive of osteoarthritis (OA) but can occur with seronegative inflammatory arthritis (spondyloarthropathies) as well. Pain of rapid onset demands consideration of infection, avascular necrosis, or a noninfectious inflammatory arthritis. In some conditions, such as many cases of osteoarthritis and most of polymyalgia rheumatica, pain on motion of the hip joint is felt in a broader distribution down the thigh as far as the knee. Indeed sometimes patients complain of knee pain and the problem is only in the hip..

C. Isolated buttock pain is a less common presentation of hip arthritis but is a common presentation of degenerative disease in the lumbosacral (LS) spine (with or without spinal stenosis or nerve root impingement) or of degenerative or inflammatory disease of the sacroiliac (SI) joint. In the absence of neurologic deficit, the physical examination is usually nondiagnostic. Exquisite tenderness at the ischial tuberosity is suggestive of ischial bursitis, although in many cases pelvic fracture should still be ruled out.

D. An anteroposterior (AP) radiograph of the pelvis is often sufficient to diagnose osteoarthritis of the hip, degenerative or inflammatory arthritis of the SI joint, or pelvic fracture. However, depending on the location of symptoms, more detailed evaluation for fracture often includes AP and frog-leg views of the hip, anterior and posterior oblique views of the acetabulum, or Ferguson views of the SI joints. Excess fluid in the hip joint is often apparent from changes in soft-tissue planes. Avascular necrosis is generally not apparent on plain radiography until several weeks after onset. Evaluation of the LS spine by AP and lateral views is usually sufficient to establish degenerative disease; radiologically diagnosing nerve root and spinal cord impingement requires more advanced imaging.

E. Both CT and MRI are much more sensitive than plain radiographs for diagnosing fractures and should be considered if clinical suspicion is high despite normal plain films or if symptoms persist. Bone scans are also sensitive for fractures starting about 3 days after injury. MRI is sometimes needed to determine whether excess fluid is present in the hip joint or early in the course of avascular necrosis. CT and especially MRI are also more sensitive for detecting inflammatory disease of the SI joint but are often not clinically necessary. CT is an effective evaluation for lumbar spinal stenosis, and MRI is useful for both spinal stenosis and nerve root compression.

F. Aspiration of the hip joint, under imaging guidance, is needed if there is suspicion of an infected joint. Suspicion for such is increased by the presence of acute onset; atraumatic, severe pain, particularly with a positive Thomas test; radiographic evidence of hip effusion; and/or fever.

G. Lateral hip pain associated with tenderness over the greater trochanter is a common syndrome caused by either gluteus medius tendonitis or trochanteric bursitis. Patients with fibromyalgia usually have pain and tenderness in this region as well but usually bilaterally and in association with numerous other tender sites.

References

Adkins SB III, Figler RA. Hip pain in athletes. Am Fam Physician 2000;61:2109–2118.

Lane NE. Clinical practice: Osteoarthritis of the hip. N Eng J Med 2007;357:1413–1421.

Scialabba FA, DeLuca SA. Transient osteoporosis of the hip. Am Fam Physician 1990;41:1759–1760.

Toohey AK, LaSalle TL, Martienz S, Polisson RP. Iliopsoas bursitis: clinical features, radiographic findings, and disease associations. Semin Arthritis Rheum 1990;20:41–47.

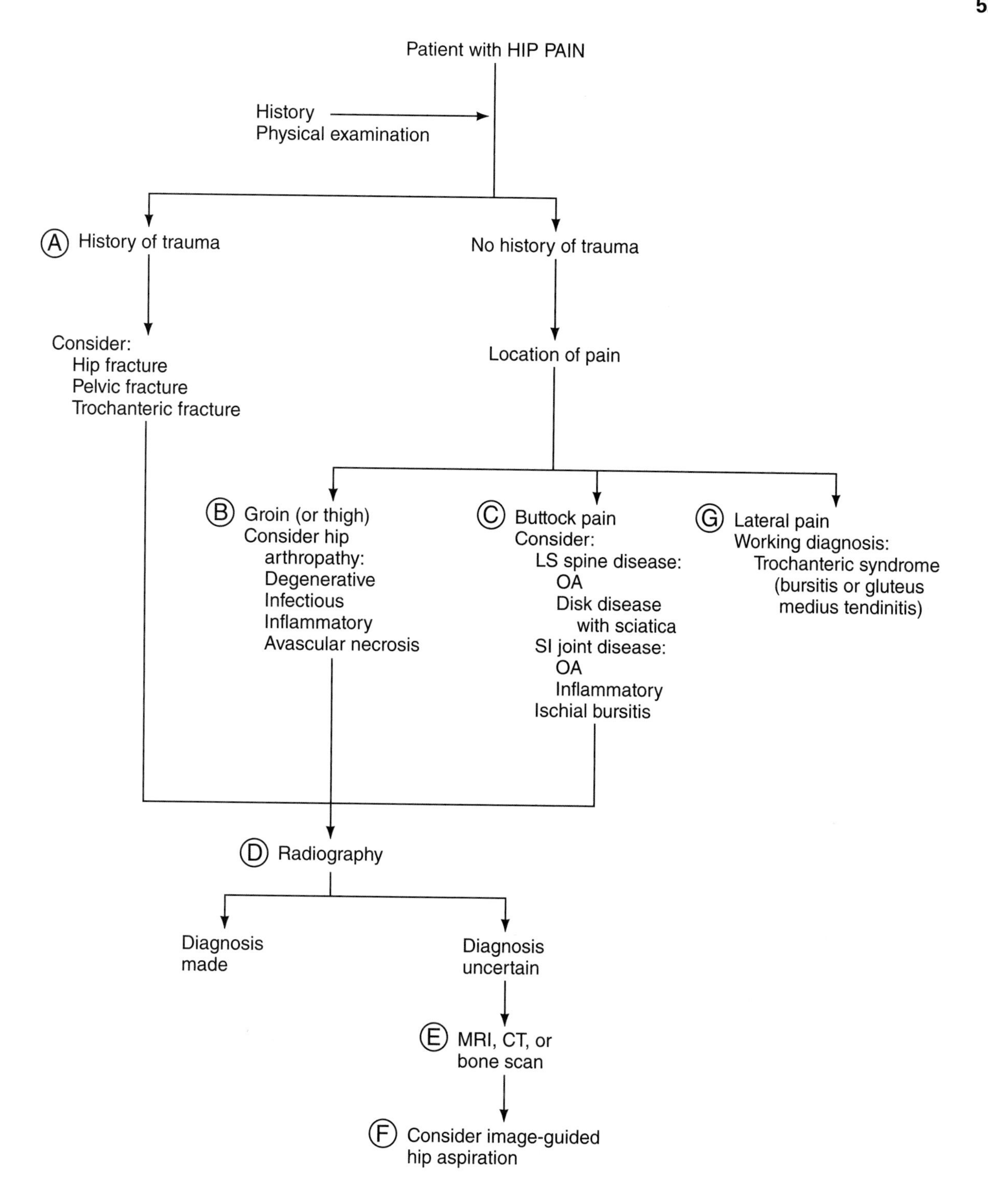
Patient with HIP PAIN
History
Physical examination
(A) History of trauma
No history of trauma
Consider:
Hip fracture
Pelvic fracture
Trochanteric fracture
Location of pain
(B) Groin (or thigh)
Consider hip
arthropathy:
Degenerative
Infectious
Inflammatory
Avascular necrosis
(C) Buttock pain
Consider:
LS spine disease:
OA
Disk disease
with sciatica
SI joint disease:
OA
Inflammatory
Ischial bursitis
(G) Lateral pain
Working diagnosis:
Trochanteric syndrome
(bursitis or gluteus
medius tendinitis)
(D) Radiography
Diagnosis
made
Diagnosis
uncertain
(E) MRI, CT, or
bone scan
(F) Consider image-guided
hip aspiration

HAND AND WRIST PAIN

Paul A. Monach, MD, PhD

A. With significant trauma, consider fracture or dislocation and begin assessment with radiography. Fracture of the distal radius (Colles' fracture) is a common complication of falls in patients with osteoporosis.

B. Articular involvement is suggested by swelling and/or tenderness over joints rather than between them and by similar degrees of pain with active and passive movement. Further workup of hand/wrist arthritis depends on acuity and the number of joints involved, in the hand/wrist and elsewhere.

C. Polyarthritis of the hand joints includes noninflammatory (osteoarthritis [OA]) and inflammatory (e.g., rheumatoid arthritis [RA], lupus, psoriatic arthritis) causes. OA affects the distal interphalangeal (DIP), proximal interphalangeal (PIP), and first carpometacarpal (CMC) joints. Wrist OA is uncommon in the absence of a history of acute or chronic trauma, and OA of the metacarpophalangeal (MCP) joints should raise suspicion for an underlying metabolic cause, such as hemochromatosis, hyperparathyroidism, or calcium pyrophosphate deposition disease (CPPD). Polyarticular gout can be either chronic (usually with asymmetrically distributed tophi detectable) or, less commonly, acute, but in both cases there is usually a prior history of monoarticular attacks in the great toe or midfoot. RA involves the metatarsal-phalangeals, PIP joints, and wrists in a symmetric distribution, and it seldom involves the DIP joints. Psoriatic arthritis can present like RA but more commonly is asymmetric and commonly involves the DIP joints. Suspicion for infection is low in a polyarticular presentation, so joint aspiration is indicated only to confirm suspected cases of acute gout. Radiography is often helpful in making the diagnosis and in assessing the degree of joint damage.

D. Monoarthritis requires consideration of infection and usually merits joint aspiration. Infection is much less common in the finger joints than in the wrist. Crystal disease often presents as monoarthritis, particularly in acute attacks of gout or pseudogout (acute inflammation associated with release of crystals formed during chronic CPPD disease). OA uncommonly presents as monoarthritis except after trauma. Among inflammatory arthritides, psoriatic arthritis and postinfectious reactive arthritis are the most likely to present as monoarthritis, with or without accompanying tenosynovitis.

E. Extraarticular disease is suggested by point tenderness over tendons or nodules and by pain greater with active/resisted than with passive motion. Tendon rupture features severe restriction on active movement of the affected finger. Tendonitis of the abductor pollicis tendon (de Quervain's tenosynovitis) is particularly common, and examination features local tenderness and pain with the Finkelstein test (passive medial displacement of the wrist while the thumb is tucked inside the fist). A flexor tendon nodule presents as a "trigger finger," with the bent finger transiently stuck in flexion of the PIP and DIP joints (reducible, with associated pain) and often with a tender nodule palpable over the palmar surface of the MCP joint. Ganglions and synovial cysts are common causes of focal swelling, with or without tenderness. Dupuytren's contracture is a chronic contracture of the palmar fascia associated with the fourth and fifth digits and has a strong genetic predisposition. People with diabetes often develop thickening, with or without contracture, of the palmar skin more diffusely and less severely.

F. Vascular disease from atherosclerosis is less common in the hand than in the foot, but vasospastic disease in association with cold exposure (Raynaud's phenomenon) is more common. When associated with underlying connective tissue disease, particularly scleroderma, Raynaud's phenomenon can be severe and threaten digital infarction and gangrene. Embolic disease and vasculitis must be considered in acute compromise of the circulation to the fingers.

G. Polyneuropathy usually presents symmetrically and with more severe disease in the feet than in the hands. Mononeuritis multiplex reflects damage, often from vasculitis, to peripheral nerves and usually begins in an asymmetric manner affecting multiple limbs. Compression of the median nerve in the carpal tunnel is common and presents with pain in the hand (often radiating), loss of sensation in the distribution of the median nerve (palmar aspect of the lateral three fingers and lateral palm), and weakness and atrophy of the thenar and hypothenar muscles. Chronic compression of the ulnar nerve leads to pain and sensory loss involving the lateral two fingers. Compression of the radial nerve, cervical nerve roots, and brachial plexus is a less common neurologic cause of isolated hand and wrist pain. Nerve conduction studies are often helpful in definitively diagnosing nerve compression and may be essential for diagnosing mononeuritis multiplex.

H. Thickening of the skin, particularly if the thickening is worse distally, should raise concern for scleroderma. A history of Raynaud's phenomenon is almost always obtained. Clubbing of the fingers should alert one to the development of hypertrophic osteoarthropathy (HOA), a painful bony enlargement of the distal extremities. Clubbing is associated with several chronic diseases, but severe HOA is particularly associated with lung cancer.

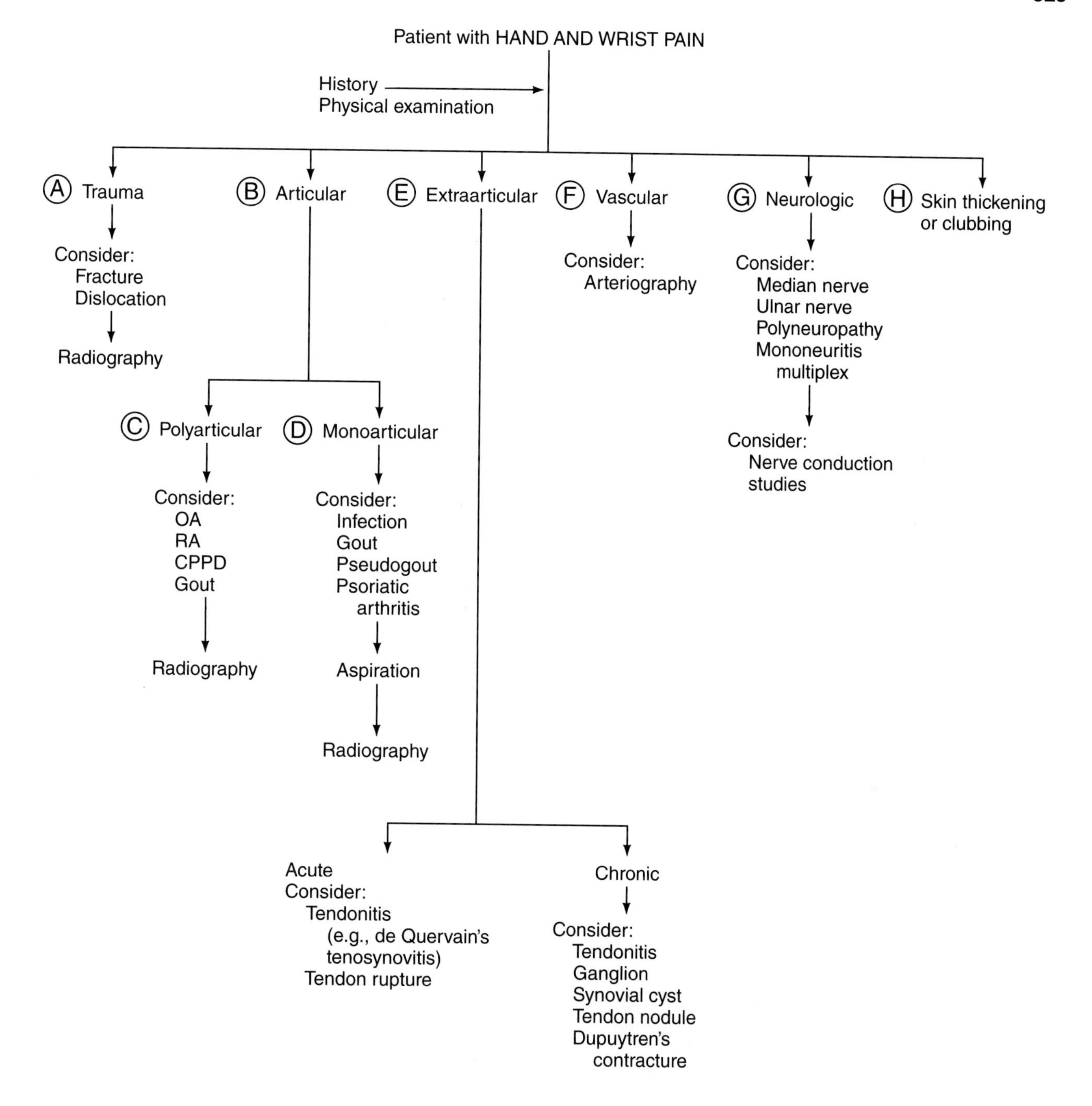

References

Caspi D, Flusser G, Farber I, et al. Clinical, radiologic, demographic, and occupational aspects of hand osteoarthritis in the elderly. Semin Arthritis Rheum 2001;30:321–331.

Forman TA, Forman SK, Rose NE. A clinical approach to diagnosing wrist pain. Am Fam Physician 2005;72:1753–1758.

Kassimos D, Creamer P. The hand x-ray in rheumatology. Hosp Med 2004;65:13–17.

Leggit JC, Meko CJ. Acute finger injuries: part II. Fractures, dislocations, and thumb injuries. Am Fam Physician 2006;73:827–834.

KNEE PAIN

Paul A. Monach, MD, PhD

A. Knee pain of intraarticular origin is suggested by joint effusion, pain with either active or passive motion, tenderness at the joint line, or evidence of compromise of the anterior or posterior cruciate ligament by positive anterior or posterior drawer test, respectively. Effusion is much more prominent, and much more likely to be tender, in inflammatory arthritis than in osteoarthritis and mechanical causes. Meniscal tears often produce locking and instability, and examination can reveal joint line tenderness (medial more often than lateral) and/or a positive McMurray's test (pain and palpable click at medial joint line during knee flexion and extension with ankle rotated laterally) or Apley's test (pain with compression of knee by pressing down on foot when patient is prone with affected knee bent at 90-degree angle). Tibial plateau fracture occurs in the setting of trauma, which can be minor in the setting of osteoporosis; point tenderness is a feature but can be difficult to distinguish from tenderness in other structures. Chondromalacia patella, a softening of articular cartilage, is a common condition presenting as a "patellofemoral syndrome" of anterior knee pain particularly with climbing and descending stairs. Recurrent hemarthrosis is a classic finding of hemophilia, but most cases currently are monophasic and associated with anticoagulation and/or trauma.

B. Acute knee pain associated with effusion should be evaluated by aspiration, with the fluid evaluated by Gram stain, culture, WBC count and differential, and examination for crystals. A large effusion in the setting of chronic knee pain of uncertain origin should also be aspirated. Knee effusion in the setting of a high suspicion for chronic degenerative disease or traumatic internal disruption does not require aspiration.

C. Chronic or acute articular knee pain generally merits radiography, using anteroposterior (AP), lateral, and "sunrise" (tangent to the patella) views. To evaluate for joint space narrowing, a weight-bearing AP view should be obtained. Avascular necrosis and osteomyelitis are often not apparent on plain radiography for about 6 weeks after onset.

D. MRI is the technique of choice to diagnose meniscal tear, anterior or posterior cruciate ligament tear, avascular necrosis, osteomyelitis, and most tumors. It also shows inflammation of the synovium (synovitis) well, although physical examination and laboratory workup usually make documentation of synovitis by MRI unnecessary. Bone scan is sensitive for infection, avascular necrosis, and most tumors but is also positive in osteoarthritis, so it is useful only when that is unlikely to be superimposed.

E. Extraarticular knee pain is revealed by the physical examination. Prepatellar bursitis features pain and tenderness of the anterior knee, often a well-defined area of redness and swelling anterior to and somewhat distal to the patella and pain with knee flexion but none with extension. Inflammation of the anserine bursa is apparent with focal tenderness at the medial aspect of the proximal tibia and pain with resisted knee flexion. Pain that is much greater with active than passive motion raises suspicion for tendonitis. Patellar tendonitis features pain with resisted knee extension and often tenderness between the patella and the tibia; quadriceps tendonitis is less common and features pain and tenderness above the patella with analogous maneuvers. Tendonitis of the hip adductors features medial pain elicited by resisted adduction of the leg. Tendonitis of the iliotibial band, analogously, features lateral pain elicited by resisted abduction. Pain in the lateral and medial collateral ligaments is elicited by stressing the ligaments with varus (holding the knee steady and moving the ankle medially) or valgus (holding the knee steady and moving the ankle laterally) movement, respectively. The examiner may also note ligamentous laxity with such maneuvers or focal tenderness over the affected ligament.

References

Calmbach WL, Hutchens M. Evaluation of patients presenting with knee pain: Part I. History, physical examination, radiographs, and laboratory tests. Am Fam Physician 2003;68:907–912.

Calmbach WL, Hutchens M. Evaluation of patients presenting with knee pain: Part II. Differential diagnosis. Am Fam Physician 2003;68:917–922.

Dixit S, DiFiori JP, Burton M, Mines B. Management of patellofemoral pain syndrome. Am Fam Physician 2007;75:194–202.

Felson DT. Clinical practice. Osteoarthritis of the knee. N Engl J Med 2006;354:841–848.

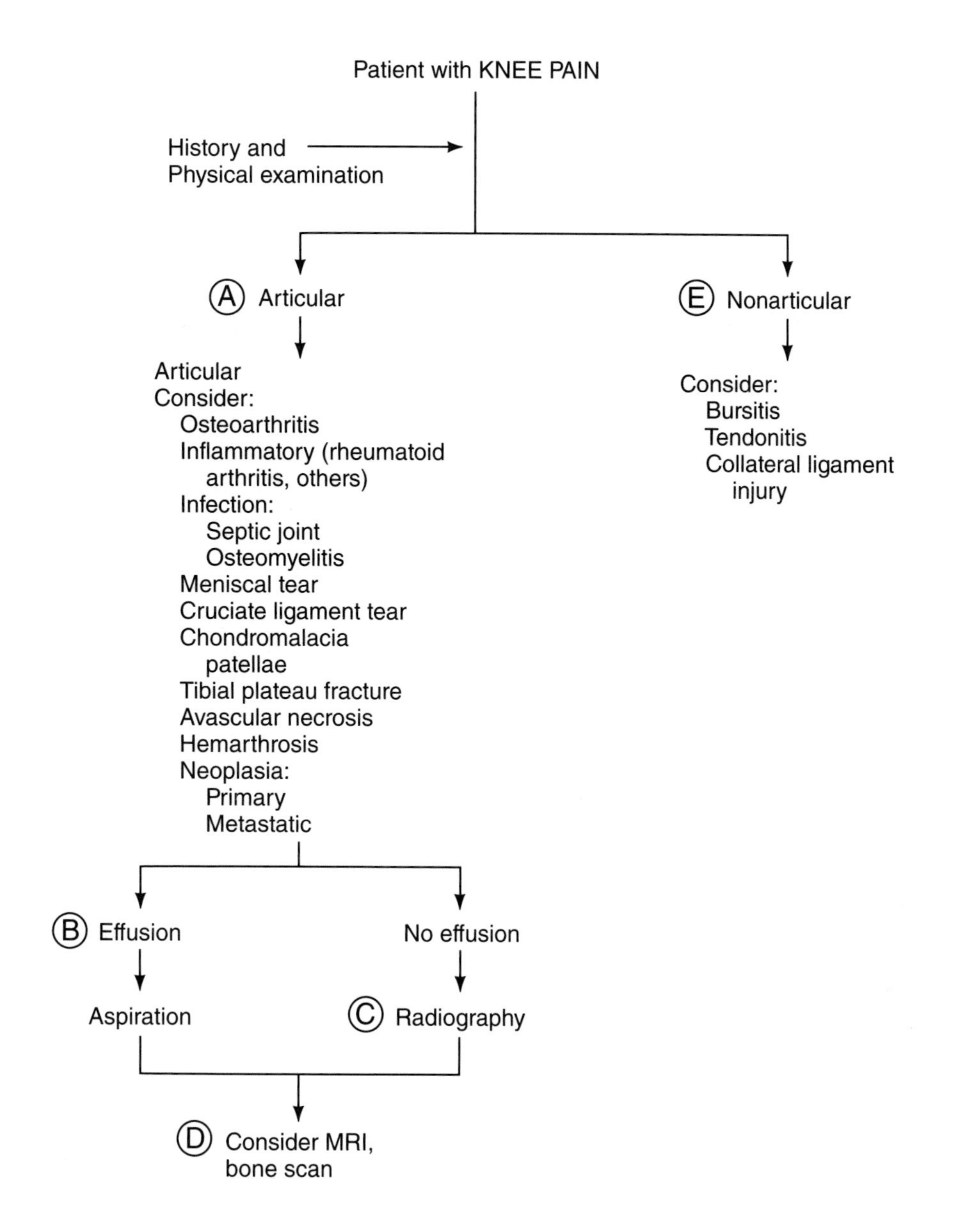
Patient with KNEE PAIN
History and
Physical examination
(A) Articular
(E) Nonarticular
Articular
Consider:
Osteoarthritis
Inflammatory (rheumatoid
arthritis, others)
Infection:
Septic joint
Osteomyelitis
Meniscal tear
Cruciate ligament tear
Chondromalacia
patellae
Tibial plateau fracture
Avascular necrosis
Hemarthrosis
Neoplasia:
Primary
Metastatic
Consider:
Bursitis
Tendonitis
Collateral ligament
injury
(B) Effusion
No effusion
Aspiration
(C) Radiography
(D) Consider MRI,
bone scan

FOOT PAIN

Paul A. Monach, MD, PhD

More than for any other part of the musculoskeletal system, pain in the foot must be approached with attention to possible musculoskeletal, vascular, neurologic, and dermatologic causes.

A. A history of foot trauma usually merits plain radiography using anteroposterior (AP), medial oblique, and lateral views. Even when the history is highly suggestive of a soft-tissue injury such as an ankle sprain, it is wise to rule out fracture as a component of the injury. Point tenderness over bony prominences, especially if it persists for more than a few days after injury, increases suspicion for fracture. Chronic, repetitive trauma commonly results in stress fractures in the foot, or tarsal sinus syndrome. Sometimes these conditions require MRI for diagnosis.

B. A musculoskeletal cause of foot pain is indicated by pain and tenderness associated with particular joints or tendons. Squeezing across the base of the toes is a good screening test for metatarsophalangeal (MTP) joint involvement. Squeezing across the foot at the highest point of the arch is a good screening test for midfoot (tarsal) joint involvement. A suggestion of arthritis by these tests merits workup for polyarthritis or monoarthritis, usually involving radiography and sometimes joint aspiration or laboratory testing.

C. There are numerous nonarthritic but nevertheless musculoskeletal causes of foot pain. Pes cavus, pes planus, malalignment of the ankle at the tibiotalar joint, hallux valgus (bunion), and hammertoe are readily detectable on examination, particularly with the patient standing. Morton's neuroma and synovial cysts are benign conditions presenting as painful nodules. Pain and tenderness of the plantar aponeurosis, especially at its insertion into the calcaneus, suggest plantar fasciitis. Tendonitis, especially of the Achilles tendon, tibialis posterior, peroneal, and tibialis anterior, is common and is apparent on examination by pain with resisted contraction of the relevant muscle group and often by passive stretching, point tenderness, or both.

D. Arterial flow should be assessed by palpation of the dorsalis pedis and posterior tibial pulses and by assessment of color, hair density, and capillary refill in the toes. Arterial insufficiency is usually caused by atherosclerosis, often with small vessel disease superimposed in people with diabetes and less commonly by embolic disease or vasculitis. Venous insufficiency presents with edema and is usually only painful during a phase of rapid increase or if associated with stasis dermatitis. A suggestion of arterial insufficiency by examination should lead to subsequent testing by Doppler ultrasound. Unilateral foot swelling should lead to Doppler testing to rule out deep venous thrombosis.

E. A generalized peripheral neuropathy, whether from diabetes or another cause, usually produces a symmetric loss of sensation beginning in the toes and slowly progressing proximally. Mononeuritis multiplex is a syndrome with asymmetric damage to peripheral nerves, often caused by vasculitis; confirmation by nerve conduction studies may be required. Small-fiber neuropathy often presents without evidence of damage to larger nerves, with absence of overt sensory loss or weakness. All neuropathies can present with hypersensitivity to painful stimuli (hyperalgesia) or perception of nonpainful stimuli as painful (allodynia). Tarsal tunnel syndrome is a syndrome of pain and paresthesia of the toes, sole, and medial foot resulting from compression of the posterior tibial nerve in the flexor retinaculum, located posterior and inferior to the medial malleolus. Confirmation of nerve compression by nerve conduction studies is often necessary.

F. Bacterial skin infection (cellulitis) of the foot is often difficult to distinguish from acute arthritis. Focal tenderness away from underlying joints is a helpful sign, especially if one can move nearby joints painlessly. Diffuse inflammation of the soft tissues of the ankle and foot (periarthritis) can be diagnosed analogously. This finding is particularly associated with a benign, self-limited subtype of sarcoidosis known as Löfgren's syndrome. Chronic edema in the feet can lead to stasis dermatitis, which is usually pruritic but sometimes painful.

References

Casellini CM, Vinik AI. Clinical manifestations and current treatment options for diabetic neuropathies. Endoct Pract 2007;13:550–566.

Van Wyngarden TM. The painful foot, Part I: common forefoot deformities. Am Fam Physician 1997;55:1866–1876.

Van Wyngarden TM. The painful foot, Part II: common rearfoot deformities. Am Fam Physician 1997;55:2207–2212.

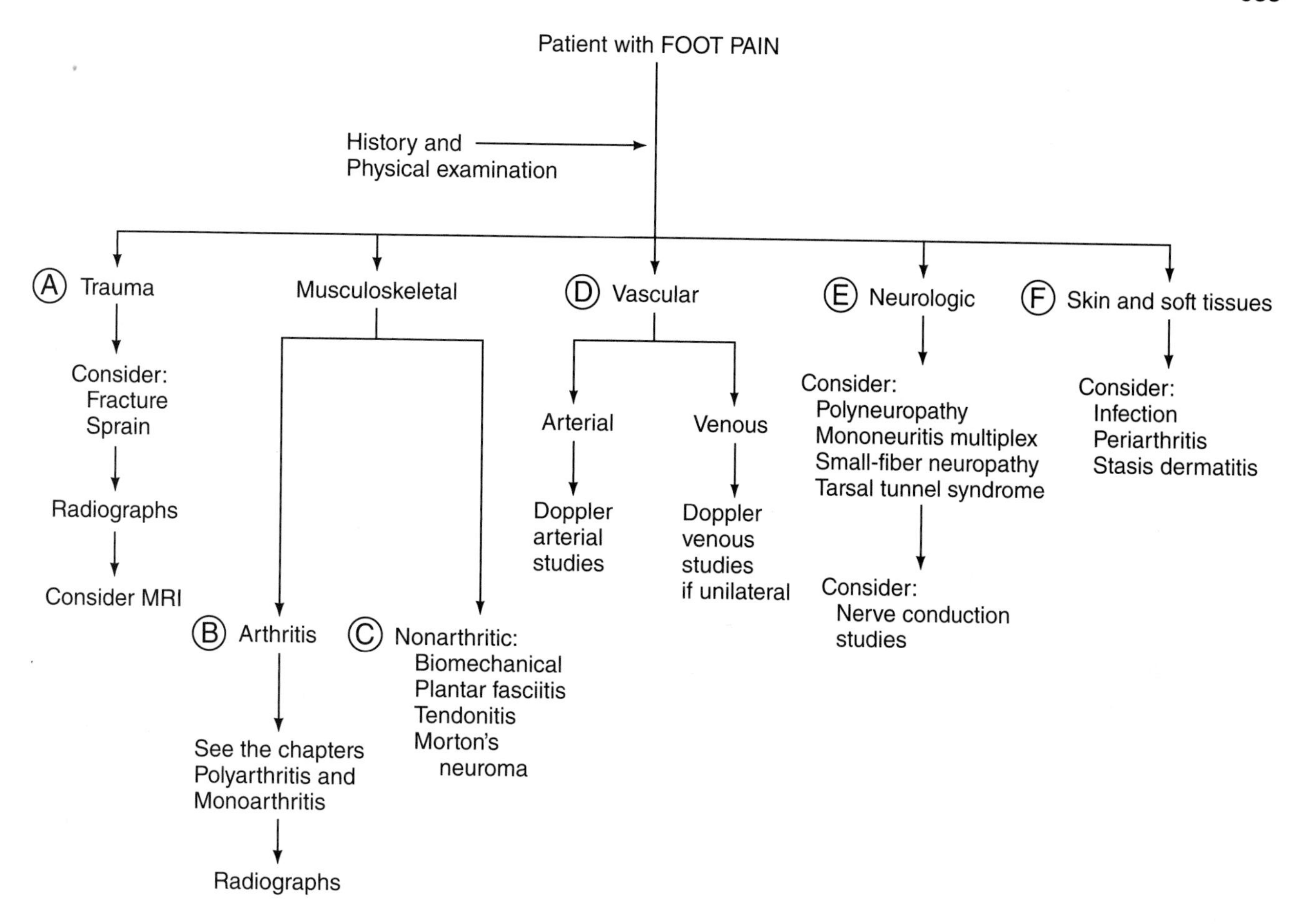
Patient with FOOT PAIN
History and
Physical examination
(A) Trauma
Consider:
Fracture
Sprain
Radiographs
Consider MRI
Musculoskeletal
(B) Arthritis
See the chapters
Polyarthritis and
Monoarthritis
Radiographs
(C) Nonarthritic:
Biomechanical
Plantar fasciitis
Tendonitis
Morton's
neuroma
(D) Vascular
Arterial
Doppler
arterial
studies
Venous
Doppler
venous
studies
if unilateral
(E) Neurologic
Consider:
Polyneuropathy
Mononeuritis multiplex
Small-fiber neuropathy
Tarsal tunnel syndrome
Consider:
Nerve conduction
studies
(F) Skin and soft tissues
Consider:
Infection
Periarthritis
Stasis dermatitis

SCLERODERMA

Sandeep K. Agarwal, MD, PhD

A. Scleroderma is a heterogeneous group of conditions associated with thickened, sclerotic skin, including diffuse cutaneous systemic sclerosis (DcSSc) and limited cutaneous systemic sclerosis (LcSSc, CREST syndrome [calcinosis, Raynaud's phenomenon, esophageal dysmotility, sclerodactyly, and telangiectasias]). It is more common in women than in men and usually presents between the ages of 30 and 50 years. The clinical course is highly variable, ranging from a self-limited to a progressive, fatal condition. Raynaud's phenomenon is a common presenting symptom. Skin thickening may be preceded by swelling with pitting edema and often progresses to ulceration and tethering of skin to underlying structures. Patients may have internal organ involvement of the GI tract, heart, lungs, and kidneys.

B. The initial approach to a patient with skin tightening should focus on determining the extent of cutaneous involvement and the presence of signs and symptoms of systemic involvement.

C. Patients with LcSSc, or CREST syndrome, have skin thickening limited to the hands and feet (sclerodactyly) but may also involve the face. Calcinosis is often noted over the hands, fingers, and olecranon bursa. Telangiectasias are seen on the palms, face, and lips. Patients often have a positive ANA in a centromere pattern. Patients should be evaluated and treated for esophageal dysmotility and pulmonary hypertension when present.

D. Patients with DcSSc have skin thickening of the hands and feet extending proximally and to the face, neck, and trunk. Skin tightening and tethering may cause joint contractures and ulcerations. Skin tightening around the mouth can limit the oral aperture, making eating and oral hygiene difficult. Raynaud's phenomenon, affecting >90% of patients, should be managed with behavior modification (i.e., avoiding exacerbating factors); however, pharmacologic or even surgical therapy may be necessary. Serologic evaluation is notable for the anti-Scl-70 antibody in 20% of patients. It is important to determine the extent of involvement to guide treatment.

E. Renal crisis, one of the most feared complications of DcSSc, presents with hypertension and acute renal failure. The urinary sediment contains mild proteinuria and few to absent cells and casts. High dosages of corticosteroids may increase the risk of renal crisis. Monitoring blood pressure may allow early detection. Angiotensin-converting enzyme (ACE) inhibitors are the primary treatment of renal crisis and may play a prophylactic role.

F. Pulmonary disease occurs in approximately 70% of patients with DcSSc in the form of interstitial lung disease with alveolitis and pulmonary hypertension. Patients usually present with dyspnea and a dry cough. Evaluation initially consists of chest x-ray, pulmonary function tests, and echocardiogram; and, if abnormal, high-resolution chest CT scan and bronchoscopy are useful. Treatment with immunosuppression is often begun, but prospective controlled trials are under way to determine whether they truly improve outcomes.

G. The most frequent internal organ system involved in scleroderma is the GI tract. Esophageal hypomotility and esophageal sphincter dysfunction result in gastroesophageal reflux disease (GERD). Patients should be evaluated for GERD and treated aggressively. Patients may have lower GI tract dysmotility, resulting in constipation and malabsorption. Promotility agents may be helpful.

H. Cardiac manifestations of scleroderma may include pericarditis, cardiomyopathy, and arrhythmias. Patients may require an ECG, Holter monitor, or echocardiogram if cardiac involvement is suspected.

I. Localized scleroderma (morphea and linear scleroderma) does not have internal organ involvement. It can occur virtually on any part of the body. Patients may have multiple plaques ranging in size from 1–30 cm. Facial involvement resulting in a depressed appearance is called *en coup de sabre* (the slash of the sword).

J. Eosinophilic fasciitis is a scleroderma-like disease characterized by inflammation and thickening of the deep fascia. The skin may have an "orange-peel" appearance. The CBC is notable for eosinophilia. Raynaud's phenomenon and internal organ involvement are absent. Scleredema and scleromyxedema should also be considered in the evaluation of skin thickening.

K. Skin thickening may be seen in several disorders, including diabetes, POEMS hypothyroidism (polyneuropathy, organomegaly, endocrinopathy, M protein, and skin changes), and chronic graft versus host disease (GVHD). Nephrogenic fibrosing dermopathy (NFD) is characterized by cutaneous fibrosis of the upper and lower limbs in patients receiving hemodialysis. Amyloidosis, bleomycin, and exposures to organic solvents may produce skin thickening as well.

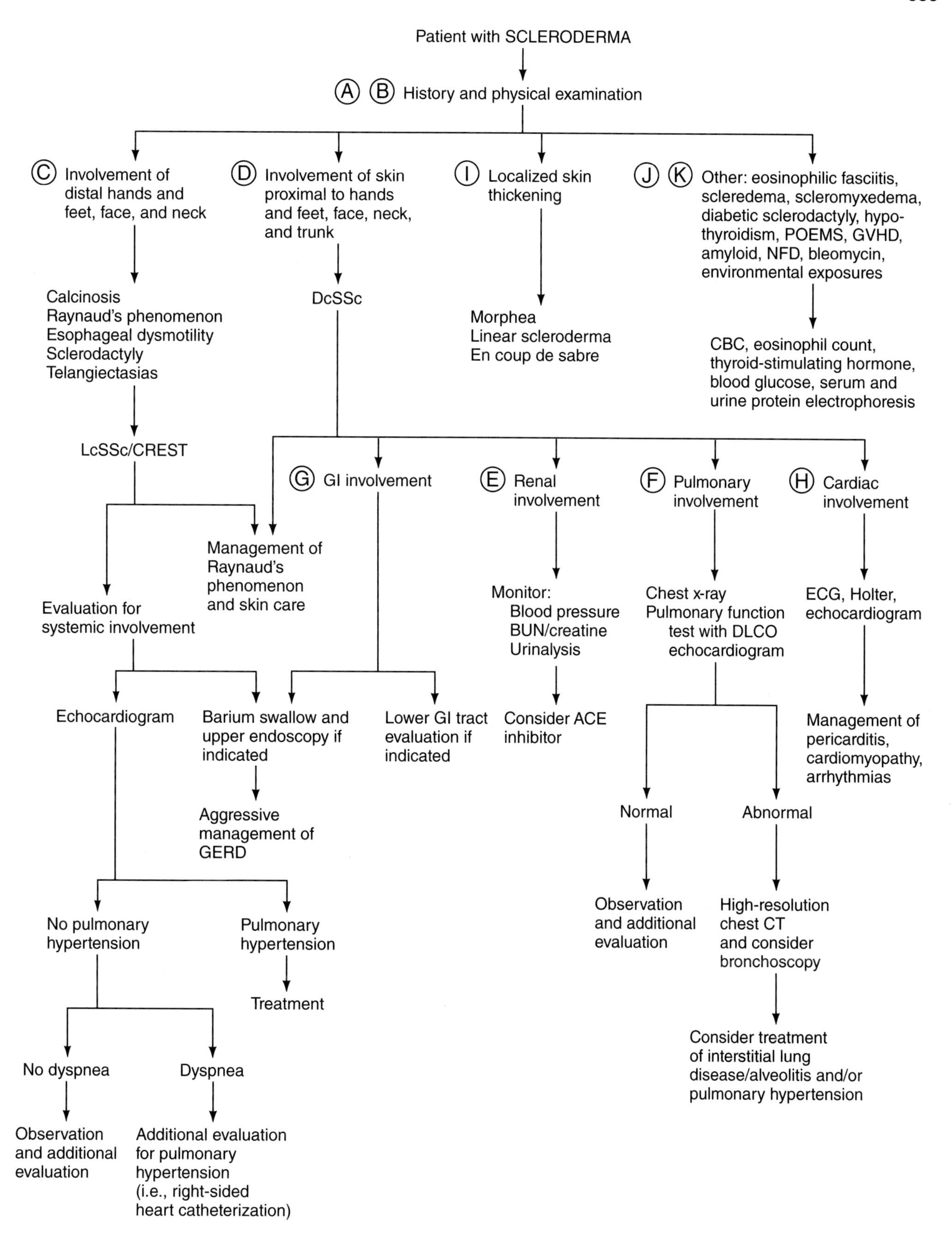

References

Highland KB, Silver RN. Clinical aspects of lung involvement: lessons from idiopathic fibrosis and the scleroderma lung study. Curr Rheumatol Rep 2005;7(2):135–141.

Shmerling RH. Diagnostic tests for rheumatic disease: clinic utility revisited. South Med J 2005;98(7):704–711.

Siebold JR. Scleroderma. In Harris ED, Budd RC, Firestein GS, et al, eds. Kelley's Textbook of Rheumatology, 7 ed. Philadelphia: Elsevier Saunders, 2005:1279–1308.

Steen VD. Systemic sclerosis. Rheum Dis Clin North Am 1990;16(3): 641–654.

Steen VD, Medsger TA Jr. Severe organ involvement in systemic sclerosis with diffuse scleroderma. Arthritis Rheum 2000;43(11):2437–2444.

DRY EYES AND DRY MOUTH (SJÖGREN'S SYNDROME)

Paul A. Monach, MD, PhD

A. Many patients complain of dry eyes and dry mouth that is nonpathologic and often changes with ambient humidity. Iatrogenic causes are also more common than inflammatory disease of the salivary and lacrimal glands (Sjögren's syndrome) and should be ruled out. Classes of medications that commonly cause symptoms of ocular and oral dryness (collectively called sicca symptoms) include those with anticholinergic affects (tricyclic antidepressants, older antihistamines), diuretics, and opioids.

B. Suspicion for Sjögren's syndrome is raised by certain elements in the history and physical examination. Ocular dryness is generally severe enough that conventional eyedrops are effective for only 1–2 hours, and patients often have problems with conjunctival irritation and are unable to wear contact lenses. Oral dryness often is severe enough that patients cannot swallow dry foods, such as crackers, without washing them down with liquid. There is often a history of severe dental disease (e.g., dental caries or periodontal disease). Routine examination of the eye is not particularly helpful because conjunctival redness is nonspecific and often absent; lacrimal glands are enlarged, tender, or both in a minority of cases. Examination of the mouth and salivary glands is somewhat more helpful. There may be no pooling of saliva under the tongue, dental caries are common, and salivary glands are more likely to be tender. Female patients with Sjögren's syndrome often suffer from vaginal dryness causing dyspareunia, a point of history that is often obtained only by specific questioning.

C. The majority of patients with Sjögren's syndrome have positive tests for ANAs, anti-Ro/SSA, and anti-La/SSB. The presence of anti-Ro or anti-La antibodies, or both, in the presence of characteristic symptoms is considered by some authorities to obviate more invasive testing.

D. Additional testing is often needed to diagnose Sjögren's syndrome. Tear production can be measured by Schirmen's test, in which a strip of Schirmer filter paper is placed with one end in the conjunctival sac. After 5 minutes, the strip is removed and the length of wetness is measured; <15 mm is abnormal. Slit-lamp examination after topical application of 1% rose bengal solution may demonstrate characteristic corneal or conjunctival damage. Salivary flow can also be measured, but this test is infrequently done. Biopsy of the interior lip to look for lymphocytic infiltration of minor salivary glands is a definitive procedure.

E. A patient diagnosed with Sjögren's syndrome warrants consideration of the presence of another connective tissue disease. Sjögren's syndrome is often a secondary phenomenon in patients with lupus, rheumatoid arthritis, or scleroderma. These diseases can generally be ruled out by history and physical examination, although in a patient who shows any signs of systemic illness, laboratory tests relevant to lupus (antibodies to ds-DNA, RNP, Sm, anti-cardiolipin, and lupus anticoagulant; CBC, BUN, and creatinine; urinalysis) should be considered. The majority of patients with Sjögren's syndrome also have positive results for rheumatoid factor, so this test is not helpful for assessing for superimposed rheumatoid arthritis. In patients without evidence of another systemic rheumatic disease (primary Sjögren's), it is still wise to evaluate organ systems that are often affected in addition to the eyes and mouth. Physical examination of the skin and peripheral nerves and joints is useful. Sjögren's syndrome is associated with lymphocytic infiltrations, which can occur in the kidneys. Therefore, it may be prudent to check for evidence of renal tubular acidosis or interstitial nephritis by urinalysis and urinary electrolytes. Sjögren's syndrome can also evolve into frank lymphoma, and a reasonable vigilance for this eventuality must be maintained. In this respect, quantitative immunoglobulins, CBC with differential, and a search for new lymph nodes may be productive.

References

Fox RI, Tornwall J, Michelson P. Current issues in the diagnosis and treatment of Sjogren's syndrome. Curr Opin Rheumatol 1999;11:364–371.

Ramos-Casals M, Brito-Zeron P, Font J. The overlap of Sjogren's syndrome with other systemic autoimmune disease. Semin Arthritis Rheum 2007;36:246–255.

Thanou-Stavaraki A, James JA. Primary Sjogren's syndrome: current and prospective therapies. Semin Arthritis Rheum 2008;37:273–292.

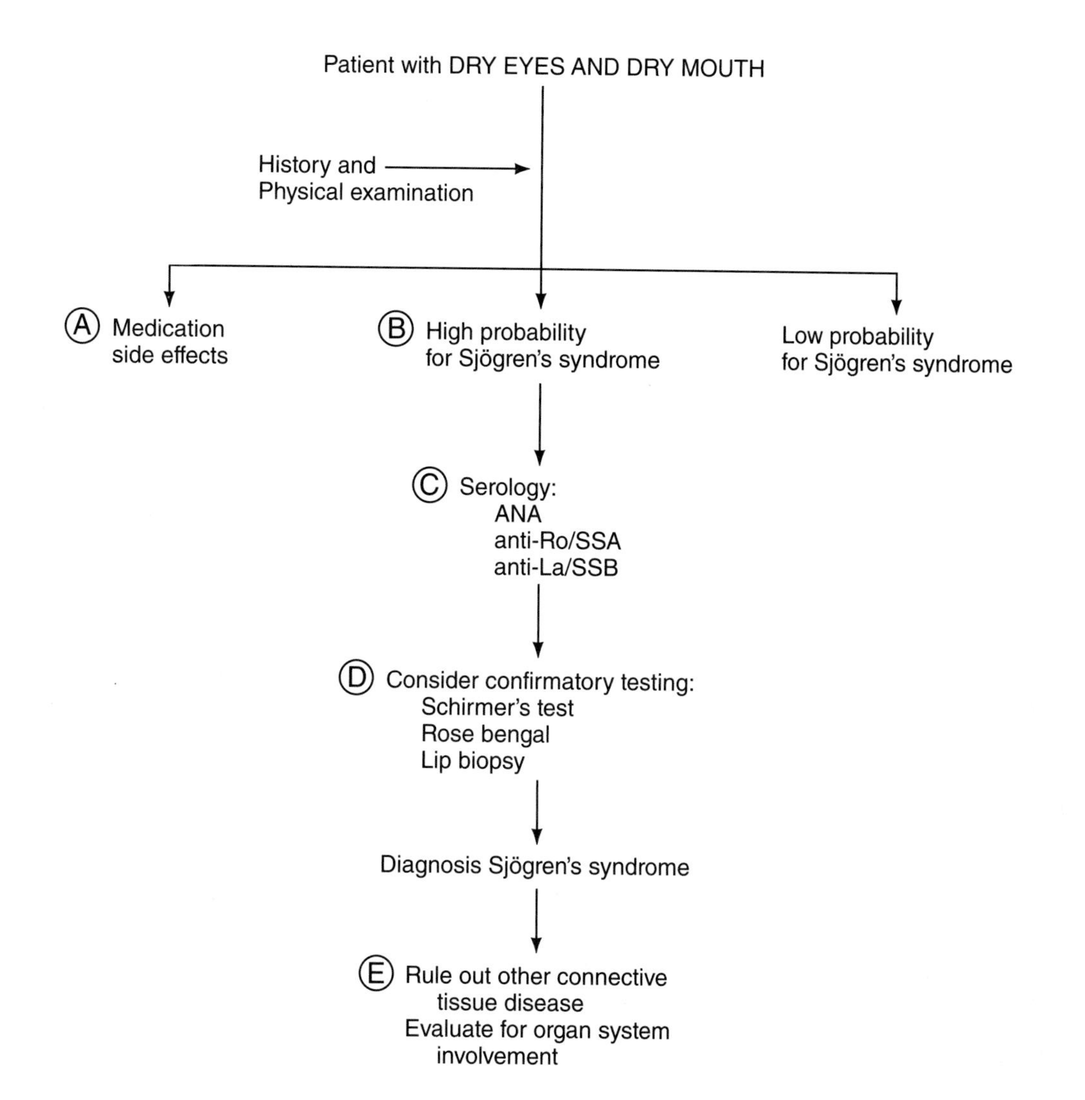
Patient with DRY EYES AND DRY MOUTH
History and Physical examination
(A) Medication side effects
(B) High probability for Sjögren's syndrome
Low probability for Sjögren's syndrome
(C) Serology:
ANA
anti-Ro/SSA
anti-La/SSB
(D) Consider confirmatory testing:
Schirmer's test
Rose bengal
Lip biopsy
Diagnosis Sjögren's syndrome
(E) Rule out other connective tissue disease
Evaluate for organ system involvement

RAYNAUD'S PHENOMENON

Alyssa Johnsen, MD, PhD

Raynaud's phenomenon is defined by episodic ischemia of the digits in response to cold or emotional stimuli. The three stages of Raynaud's include pallor, cyanosis, and rubor. Pallor is caused by vasospasm and loss of arterial blood flow, cyanosis reveals the deoxygenation of static venous blood, and rubor shows the reactive hyperemia following return of blood flow. Prevalence in the United States ranges between 4% and 11% in women and 3% and 8% in men, depending on the population studied. Severity can range from mild intermittent symptoms to severe persistent ischemia with ulceration of digits.

A. A thorough history should be obtained to differentiate true Raynaud's phenomenon from common cold intolerance. Classic Raynaud's is described as the sudden onset of cold fingers (or toes) in association with a sharply demarcated triphasic (white-blue-red) color change. It is usually symmetric, and asymmetry should prompt investigation of traumatic etiology or thrombotic/embolic phenomenon. In addition, symptoms of associated conditions should be sought by taking a complete review of systems. A complete medication history and an occupational exposure history are critical.

B. A complete physical examination is warranted to investigate for signs of an associated underlying condition. It is not necessary to perform provocative tests because they are often inaccurate. Nailfold capillary microscopy can be performed by placing a drop of grade B immersion oil on the patient's skin at the base of the fingernail and viewing the area with a handheld ophthalmoscope set at 10–40 diopters; capillaries of patients with an underlying rheumatic disease are frequently distorted and irregular.

C. Raynaud's phenomenon is considered primary if the symptoms occur without evidence of any associated disorder. Primary Raynaud's is more common in women than in men and usually starts at a younger age. The episodes are characterized by symmetric attacks with the absence of tissue necrosis, ulceration, or gangrene. For primary Raynaud's, the avoidance of cold temperatures and keeping the entire body warm is often sufficient therapy. In addition, avoiding vasoconstrictive medications, tobacco, and caffeine can be helpful. When conservative therapy is insufficient, long-acting calcium channel blockers can be tried.

D. Many medications have been implicated in Raynaud's phenomenon, including beta blockers, chemotherapeutic agents, interferon, estrogen, nicotine, narcotics, sympathomimetic agents, cyclosporine, cocaine, ergotamines, and clonidine. In addition, exposure to polyvinyl chloride and heavy metals has been associated with Raynaud's phenomenon. Withdrawal of offending medications and conservative therapy as for primary Raynaud's phenomenon should be attempted.

E. Raynaud's secondary to an underlying disease should be suspected in a patient with associated symptoms or signs, in those with new Raynaud's phenomenon after 40 years of age, or in those with severe ischemia or ulceration. In this population, guided by the history and physical examination, one could perform a CBC, general blood chemical analysis, urinalysis, ANA, C3, C4, ESR, C-reactive protein (CRP), and rheumatoid factor (RF). Further testing for cryoglobulins and serum protein electrophoresis (SPEP) can be ordered as well. As with primary Raynaud's, the avoidance of cold temperatures and keeping the entire body warm is recommended. In addition, avoiding vasoconstrictive medications, tobacco, and caffeine can be helpful. When conservative therapy is insufficient, long-acting calcium channel blockers can be tried. For cases of severe ischemia or digital necrosis, arterial studies should be performed and antiplatelet therapy and IV prostaglandins should be initiated.

F. Asymmetric Raynaud's should raise the suspicion for trauma or thrombotic or embolic phenomenon. Raynaud's secondary to trauma can occur when the ulnar artery is damaged as it courses the hook of the hamate bone in the wrist ("hypothenar hammer syndrome"). Hand-arm vibration exposure, as occurs with pneumatic hammer operators, can also cause a similar phenomenon. In asymmetric Raynaud's, thrombotic and embolic disease should also be considered. Allen's test should be performed. Doppler ultrasonography may be useful, but arteriography is the "gold standard."

References

De Angelis R, Del Medico P, Blasetti P, Cervini C. Raynaud's phenomenon: clinical spectrum of 118 patients. Clin Rheumatol 2003;22:279–284.

Suter LG, Murabito JM, Felson DT, Fraenkel L. The incidence and natural history of Raynaud's phenomenon in the community. Arthritis Rheum 2005;52:1259–1263.

Wigley FM. Raynaud's phenomenon. N Engl J Med 2002;347: 1001–1008.

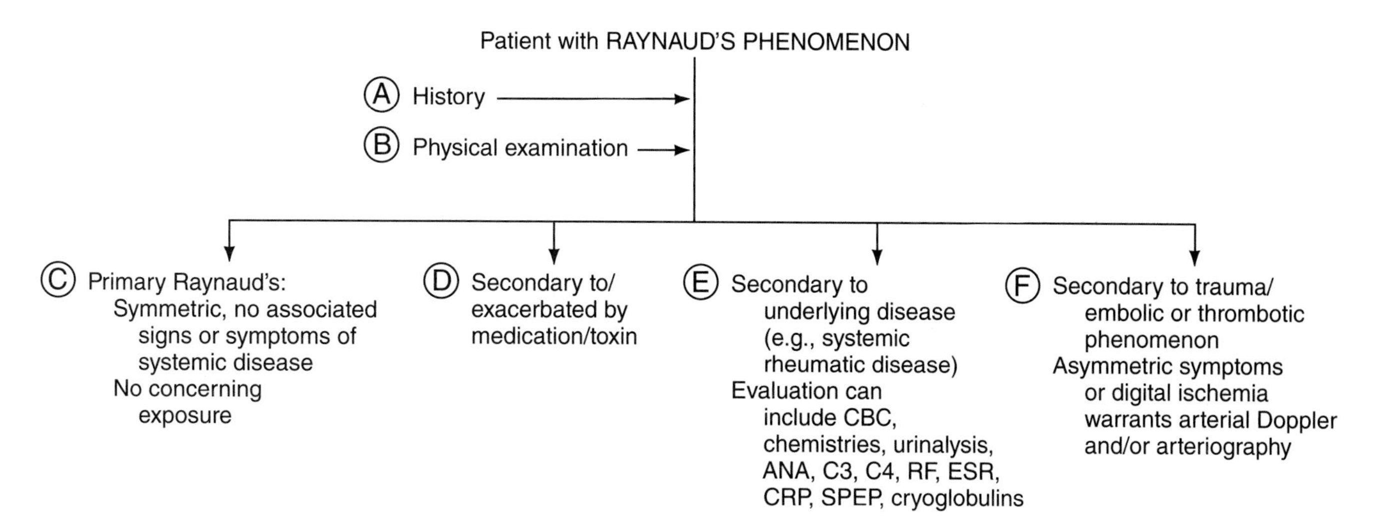
Patient with RAYNAUD'S PHENOMENON
(A) History
(B) Physical examination
(C) Primary Raynaud's:
Symmetric, no associated signs or symptoms of systemic disease
No concerning exposure
(D) Secondary to/ exacerbated by medication/toxin
(E) Secondary to underlying disease (e.g., systemic rheumatic disease)
Evaluation can include CBC, chemistries, urinalysis, ANA, C3, C4, RF, ESR, CRP, SPEP, cryoglobulins
(F) Secondary to trauma/ embolic or thrombotic phenomenon
Asymmetric symptoms or digital ischemia warrants arterial Doppler and/or arteriography

LOW BONE DENSITY

Alyssa Johnsen, MD, PhD

Low bone density is diagnosed by a bone mineral density (BMD) test and may be caused by osteoporosis (decreased bone mass with disrupted architecture), osteomalacia (disordered bone mineralization), or osteitis fibrosa cystica (characterized by marrow fibrosis).

A. In addition to a careful history and physical examination to identify potential underlying causes for low bone density, some experts also recommend a CBC, urinary calcium excretion, thyroid function, and serum chemistries (calcium, phosphorus, total protein, liver enzymes, alkaline phosphatase, creatinine, and electrolytes). If the history or evaluation suggests secondary causes, additional tests for serum 25-OH vitamin D, parathyroid hormone (PTH), ESR, and serum and urine protein electrophoresis can be considered.

B. In primary osteoporosis, laboratory study results should be normal. Abnormal study results may suggest an associated disorder.

The most common laboratory abnormalities in osteomalacia are hypophosphatemia and elevated serum alkaline phosphatase. A low alkaline phosphatase suggests hypophosphatasia. Hypophosphatemia with hypocalcemia usually indicates vitamin D deficiency, whereas isolated hypophosphatemia is most consistent with a renal tubular phosphate-wasting syndrome.

Primary hyperparathyroidism is diagnosed by a combination of hypercalcemia and an inappropriately elevated serum PTH. Secondary hyperparathyroidism as a result of renal failure will show a decreased serum calcium, increased serum phosphate, and increased serum PTH.

C. Vertebral fracture is the most common clinical presentation of osteoporosis. Primary osteoporosis is defined as the progressive loss of bone increasing with age.

D. Secondary osteoporosis can result from underlying medical conditions, including malabsorption; hypogonadism; hyperthyroidism; multiple myeloma; and the administration of certain medications, especially corticosteroids. Of the secondary causes, vitamin D deficiency and glucocorticoid use are among the most common.

E. The major symptom of osteomalacia is diffuse, dull, aching skeletal pain that is worsened by activity. Muscle weakness, usually involving the proximal musculature, is often present. Vitamin D deficiency accounts for the majority of cases of osteomalacia and can be caused by dietary deficiency or malabsorption resulting from GI disorders. Hypophosphatemia resulting from renal wasting is another important cause and can result from vitamin D deficiency, from primary renal tubular wasting, or as part of Fanconi's syndrome (e.g., as may be seen in multiple myeloma). Chronic renal failure can lead to decreased vitamin D metabolism and secondary hyperparathyroidism and can contribute to osteomalacia. Disorders of bone matrix such as hypophosphatasia, fibrogenesis imperfecta, and axial osteomalacia are rare causes of osteomalacia.

F. Osteitis fibrosa cystica is caused by hyperparathyroidism and is now rare. Many patients with hyperparathyroidism, however, do have low bone mineral density.

References

Crandall C. Laboratory workup for osteoporosis: which tests are most cost-effective? Postgrad Med 2003;114(3):35–38.

Favus MJ. Editorial: postmenopausal osteoporosis and the detection of so-called secondary causes of low bone density. J Clin Endocrinol Metab 2005;90(6):3800.

Tuck SP, Francis RM. Osteoporosis. Postgrad Med J 2002;78:526–532.

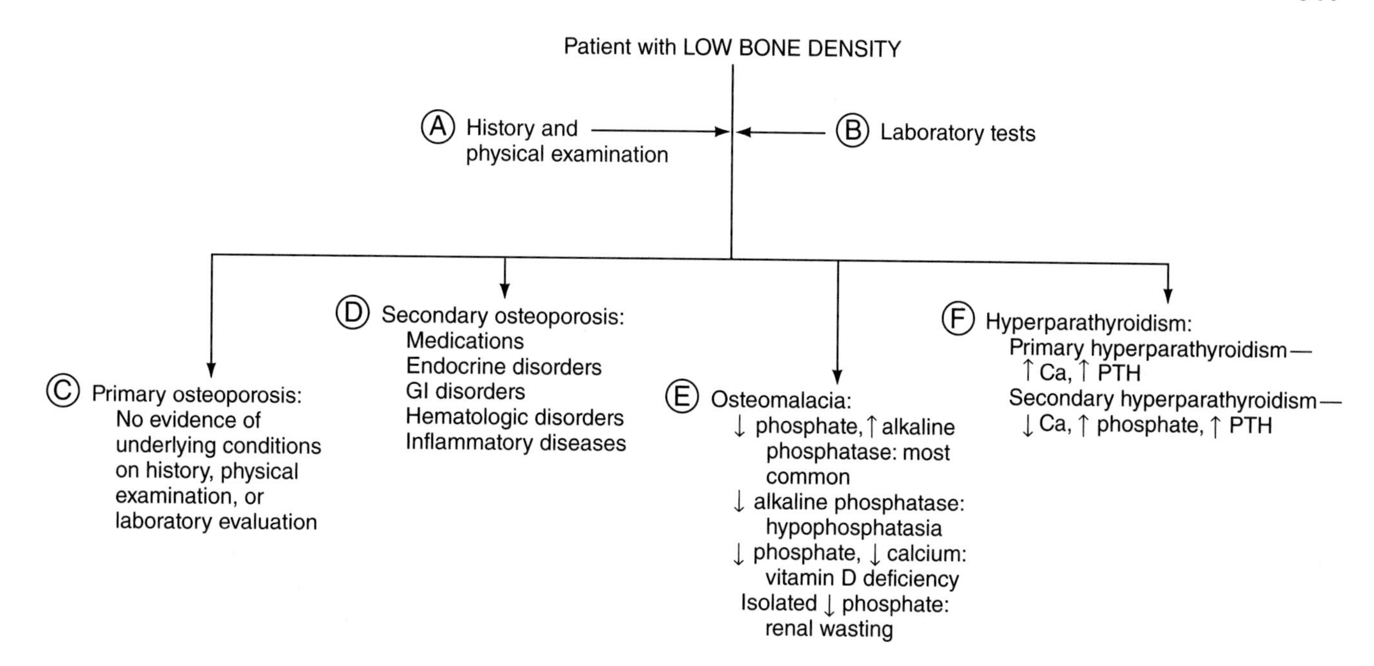

Patient with LOW BONE DENSITY
(A) History and physical examination
(B) Laboratory tests
(C) Primary osteoporosis:
No evidence of underlying conditions on history, physical examination, or laboratory evaluation
(D) Secondary osteoporosis:
Medications
Endocrine disorders
GI disorders
Hematologic disorders
Inflammatory diseases
(E) Osteomalacia:
↓ phosphate, ↑ alkaline phosphatase: most common
↓ alkaline phosphatase: hypophosphatasia
↓ phosphate, ↓ calcium: vitamin D deficiency
Isolated ↓ phosphate: renal wasting
(F) Hyperparathyroidism:
Primary hyperparathyroidism— ↑ Ca, ↑ PTH
Secondary hyperparathyroidism— ↓ Ca, ↑ phosphate, ↑ PTH

HYPERURICEMIA AND GOUT

Peter Kim, MD

A. Volume depletion, obesity, high metabolic turnover states (tumor lysis, myeloproliferative disorders, hemolysis), certain medications (ethanol, diuretics, salicylates, calcineurin inhibitors), and diets high in meat or seafood can cause an elevation of the serum uric acid level. Rare genetic disorders can also cause hyperuricemia. History should include a dietary history, drinking history, and lead exposure at work and home. Examination should search for evidence of arthritis in all joints, including asymptomatic ones, and for the presence of tophi on hands, feet, Achilles tendons, areas of minor trauma (olecranon bursa), and the ears (nodules on the pinna that do not transilluminate). Consider a radiograph of affected joint to look for tophi, joint destruction, and chondrocalcinosis.

B. The management of asymptomatic hyperuricemia is controversial, and there are insufficient data to guide management in most cases. The prevention of chronic urate nephropathy, nephrolithiasis, and gouty arthritis determines the decision to treat in asymptomatic cases. Chronic urate nephropathy is rare in the absence of tophaceous gout. Lead toxicity should be considered when uric acid levels are very elevated (>12 mg/dl). High urinary uric acid excretion increases the risk of urate nephrolithiasis, and allopurinol can be considered in this situation, especially if the patient only has a single kidney. If the hyperuricemia is iatrogenic, consider changes in therapy (change diuretics to another class of antihypertensives; losartan causes a modest reduction in serum uric acid). Many cases of renal insufficiency with hyperuricemia result from lead exposure. Weight reduction and reduction of purine-rich foods should be considered.

C. Although acute gout classically presents as a monoarthritis of the first toe (podagra) with marked inflammation, polyarticular and/or tophaceous presentations are not uncommon. They are seen especially in patients who are older or immunosuppressed (especially those with organ transplants). Septic arthritis always needs to be considered when dealing with monoarthritis or oligoarthritis. Other crystalline arthropathies should also be considered: calcium pyrophosphate dihydrate (calcium pyrophosphate deposition disease [CPPD] causing pseudogout), apatite, oxalate, and others. Arthrocentesis should be performed if possible to look for the presence of crystals and to rule out infection. If a crystal diagnosis cannot be made, the decision to treat can be made on the basis of a history and examination consistent with gout: prior episodes that resolved spontaneously within several days to a few weeks, development of maximal pain within 1 day, typical distribution (i.e., podagra), or evidence of tophi. Serum uric acid levels are lower during acute episodes of gouty arthritis, and the absence or presence of hyperuricemia should be used with caution in the diagnosis of arthritis. Atypical presentations include polyarthritis and indolent and chronic arthritis. Decisions to treat should be tailored to the individual patient.

D. The patient at low risk without renal, liver, or bone marrow impairment and no history of peptic ulcer disease can be treated with high-dose NSAIDs. NSAIDs work best when used at the first sign of symptoms and may be less effective for fully established arthritis.

E. In patients in whom NSAIDs are contraindicated, prednisone at doses of 10–60 mg can be used until the attack has resolved.

F. Alternative therapies include intraarticular steroids (particularly attractive option for monoarthritis of knee or ankle), colchicine, and narcotic analgesics. Oral colchicine (1.2 mg followed by 0.6 mg/hr for 6 doses) has a very narrow therapeutic window between symptom relief and GI upset (abdominal pain, nausea, vomiting, diarrhea). IV colchicine, although effective, is not recommended for the treatment of gout; rarely if ever do the benefits of treating a nonfatal and self-limited disorder outweigh the potential risks of IV colchicine (cardiovascular collapse, aplastic anemia, tissue necrosis). Narcotic analgesics can be used for symptomatic relief until the gout flare spontaneously resolves. In the rare patient in whom all therapies carry considerable risk, a viable option is to do nothing.

(Continued on page 544)

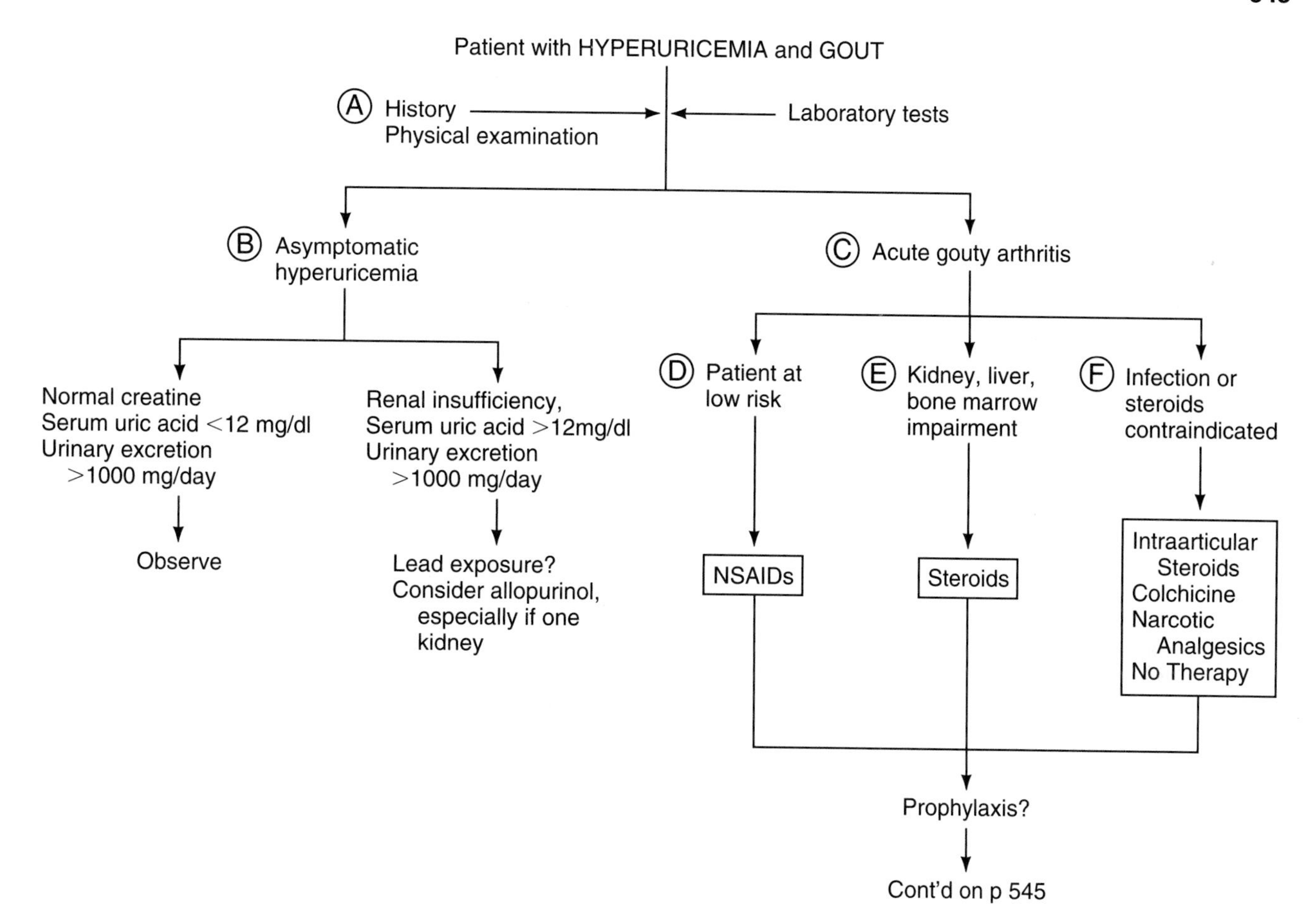
Patient with HYPERURICEMIA and GOUT
(A) History
Physical examination
Laboratory tests
(B) Asymptomatic hyperuricemia
(C) Acute gouty arthritis
Normal creatine
Serum uric acid <12 mg/dl
Urinary excretion >1000 mg/day
Observe
Renal insufficiency,
Serum uric acid >12mg/dl
Urinary excretion >1000 mg/day
Lead exposure?
Consider allopurinol, especially if one kidney
(D) Patient at low risk
NSAIDs
(E) Kidney, liver, bone marrow impairment
Steroids
(F) Infection or steroids contraindicated
Intraarticular Steroids
Colchicine
Narcotic Analgesics
No Therapy
Prophylaxis?
Cont'd on p 545

G. After the acute flare has resolved, prophylaxis can be considered. For patients with a first attack, especially with a clear inciting event such as binge drinking, prophylaxis is not indicated. Recurrent attacks or the presence of tophi are indications for uric acid–lowering therapy. Therapy should not be started for several weeks after the acute flare has resolved. Treatment that reduces uric acid can precipitate further flares of gout, so patients should be treated with colchicine prophylaxis (0.6 QD or 0.6 QOD if renal impairment) for the first year of therapy regardless of whether allopurinol or a uricosuric agent is used.
H. Patients in whom long-term prophylaxis is not indicated should be encouraged to avoid binge drinking, to reduce intake of purine-rich foods, and to lose weight if applicable. If the patient is taking a diuretic for hypertension, consider changing to another antihypertensive.
I. Allopurinol (a xanthine oxidase inhibitor) is the first-line therapy of many physicians in the treatment of gout regardless of whether the hyperuricemia results from overproduction or undersecretion; unfortunately, however, allopurinol does have a relatively high rate of hypersensitivity reactions. If the patient has a history of nephrolithiasis, uricosurics are contraindicated and allopurinol is the better choice. If the patient has renal impairment, uricosurics are usually ineffective and again allopurinol is a better choice but should be adjusted for glomerular filtration rate. Allopurinol inhibits the degradation of azathioprine and can cause toxicity; reduce the dose of azathioprine or switch to another agent.
J. If hyperuricemia is from underexcretion (<600 mg uric acid in 24 hours), probenecid can be used at a starting dose of 500 mg bid. Encourage adequate hydration to reduce the risk of nephrolithiasis.
K. Allopurinol and probenecid need to be titrated until the serum uric acid level is <6 mg/dl. Although the illness can flare while receiving therapy, this is not a reason to stop these medications; flares should be treated while continuing the uric acid–lowering medications. Prolonged therapy with colchicine can cause a myoneuropathy, especially for those taking calcineurin inhibitors. Follow deep tendon reflexes and motor strength while the patient is being treated.

References

Eggeneen AT. Gout: an update. Am Fam Physician 2007;76:801–808.
Pittman JR, Bross MH. Diagnosis and management of gout. Am Fam Physician 1999;59:1799–1806.
Schumacher HR Jr, Chen LX. The practical management of gout. Cleve Clin J Med 2008;75 (Suppl 5):S22–S25.

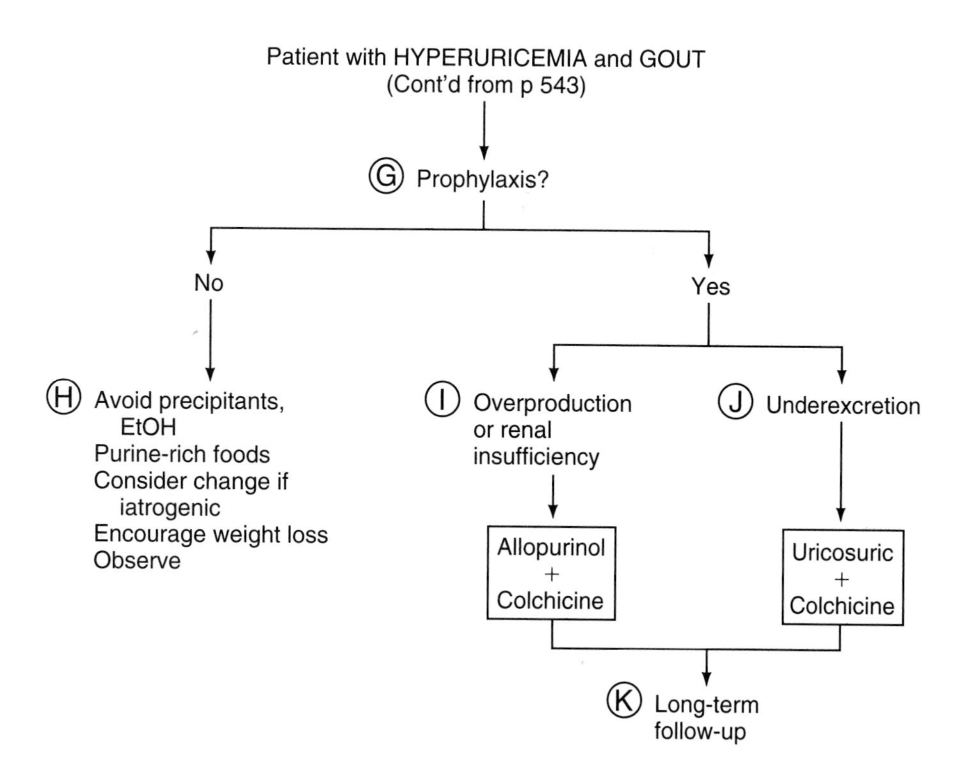
Patient with HYPERURICEMIA and GOUT
(Cont'd from p 543)
G Prophylaxis?
No
Yes
H Avoid precipitants,
EtOH
Purine-rich foods
Consider change if
iatrogenic
Encourage weight loss
Observe
I Overproduction
or renal
insufficiency
J Underexcretion
Allopurinol
+
Colchicine
Uricosuric
+
Colchicine
K Long-term
follow-up

DIFFUSE MUSCLE PAIN AND STIFFNESS: POLYMYALGIA RHEUMATICA AND GIANT CELL ARTERITIS

Peter Kim, MD

A. Diffuse muscle pain has multiple etiologies, including viral syndromes (especially influenza and coxsackie), polymyalgia rheumatica (PMR), drug-induced myopathies (e.g., fibrates and statins), and hypothyroidism. The inflammatory myopathies (dermatomyositis and polymyositis) are usually painless or minimally painful, but myalgias are not infrequently seen with these disorders. Laboratory tests should include a CBC, ESR, C-reactive protein (CRP), creatine kinase (CK), aspartate aminotransferase (AST), alanine aminotransferase (ALT), and thyroid-stimulating hormone (TSH).

B. Although weakness can be difficult to ascertain in the setting of pain, prominent weakness or elevation of muscle enzymes should prompt an evaluation directed toward disorders affecting muscle (muscular dystrophies, myositis, drug-induced myopathy) or other causes of weakness.

C. The typical presentation for PMR is an abrupt onset of bilateral shoulder and neck pain causing difficulty raising the arms over the head. Patients are almost without exception >50 years and usually >60 years. The lower back, pelvic girdle, and thighs can also be involved, and a few patients will present with pain starting in these areas. Most patients will describe more than half an hour of increased pain on waking, and constitutional symptoms (fever, weight loss, night sweats, anorexia) are not uncommon. Prominent synovitis or peripheral edema on examination can be seen with remitting seronegative symmetric synovitis with pitting edema (RS3PE), which some consider to be in the clinical spectrum of PMR. The inflammatory markers ESR and CRP are usually elevated, but a normal value does not exclude the diagnosis of PMR. Elevations in the muscle enzymes (CK, AST, ALT) are not consistent with the diagnosis of PMR and should be explained by alternative diagnoses. For patients with a more long-standing and insidious history of diffuse pain, consider fibromyalgia and vitamin D deficiency. Treatment of PMR usually requires modest dosages of steroids (e.g., 5 mg tid). Usually the patient improves dramatically within 48 hours; if not, the diagnosis should be questioned. Once symptoms are controlled, steroids are slowly tapered. The disease, an average, lasts for 18 months.

D. A critical distinction is to assess for giant cell arteritis (GCA). GCA should be considered a "can't miss" diagnosis because of the high risk of blindness and stroke with delay in therapy. All patients with a clinical history consistent with PMR should be specifically questioned for headache, scalp pain, jaw claudication, and visual symptoms (amaurosis fugax, blurring, or diplopia). Physical examination should also include palpation of the temporal arteries and comparison of pulses in the extremities. A funduscopic examination should be performed if visual symptoms are present. If GCA is suspected by history or physical examination, the patient should be started on high-dose (1 mg/kg of prednisone) steroids and a temporal artery biopsy should be arranged. If the patient has visual symptoms, pulse dose (1000 mg IV methylprednisolone QD for 3 days) steroids should be given followed by high-dose steroids. Treatment for up to 14 days with steroids will not affect the biopsy results.

References

Achkar AA, Lie JT, Hunder GG, et al. How does previous corticosteroid treatment affect the biopsy findings in giant cell (temporal) arteritis? Ann Intern Med 1994;120(12):987–992.

Plotnikoff GA, Quigley JM. Prevalence of severe hypovitaminosis D in patients with persistent, nonspecific musculoskeletal pain. Mayo Clin Proc 2003;78(12):1463–1470.

Salvarani C, Cantini F, Boiardi L, Hunder GG. Polymyalgia rheumatica and giant-cell arteritis. N Engl J Med 2002;347(4):261–271.

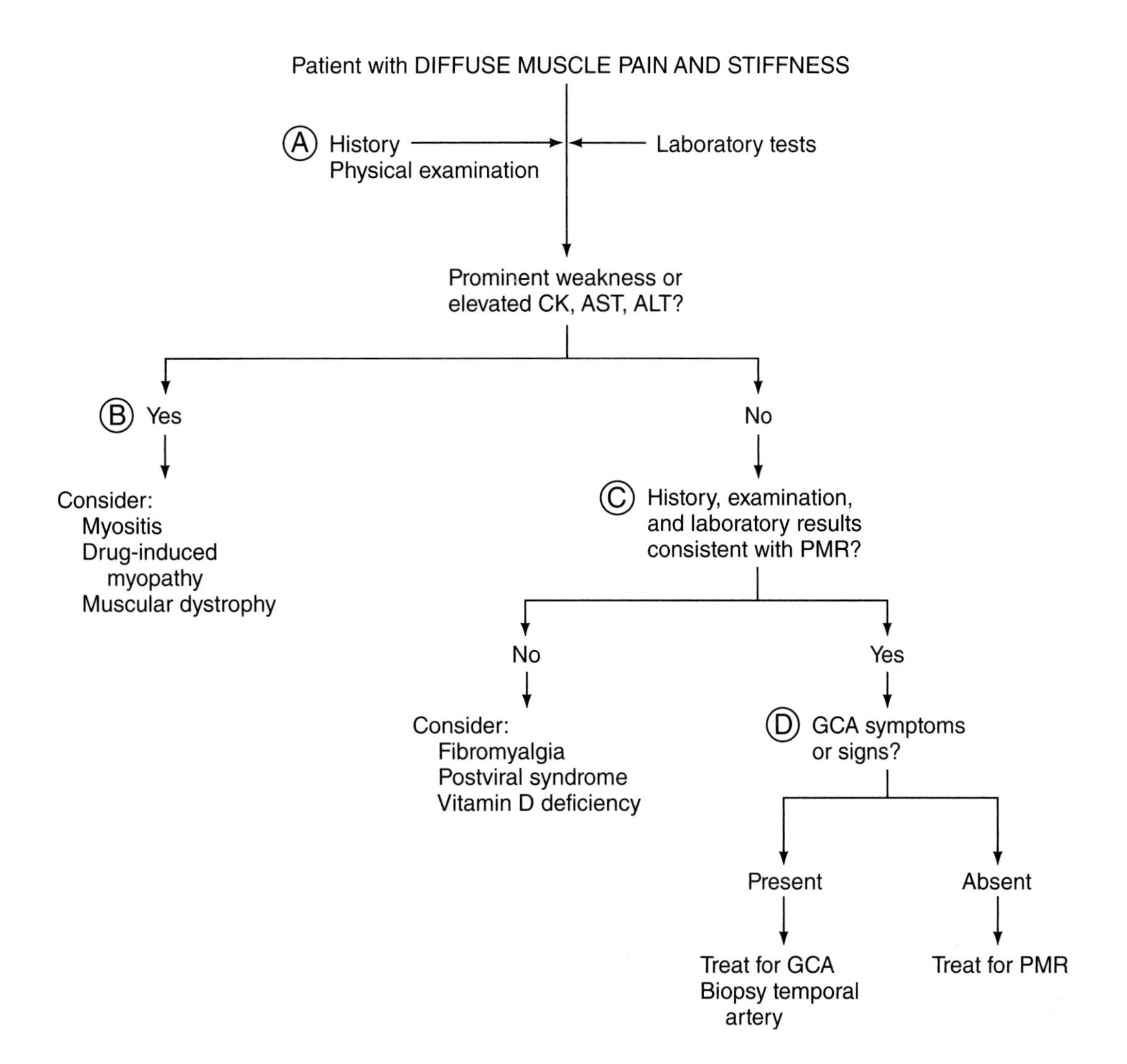
Patient with DIFFUSE MUSCLE PAIN AND STIFFNESS
A
History
Physical examination
Laboratory tests
Prominent weakness or
elevated CK, AST, ALT?
B
Yes
Consider:
Myositis
Drug-induced
myopathy
Muscular dystrophy
No
C
History, examination,
and laboratory results
consistent with PMR?
No
Consider:
Fibromyalgia
Postviral syndrome
Vitamin D deficiency
Yes
D
GCA symptoms
or signs?
Present
Treat for GCA
Biopsy temporal
artery
Absent
Treat for PMR

JOINT HYPERMOBILITY

Stuart B. Mushlin, MD, FACP, FACR

Joint hypermobility is a spectrum of disorders ranging from the benign to the severe. This chapter will discuss briefly the range of phenotypes and point out the medically serious complications that can arise in the more severe phenotypes.

Joint hypermobility is generally quantified by a scoring system, the Beighton score. One point is accorded for each of the following: extensibility of the elbow joint >10 degrees, extensibility of the knee joint >10 degrees, the ability to extend the fifth metacarpophalangeal (MCP) joint to 90 degrees, and the ability to oppose the thumb to the forearm. All of these generate 1 point each; if bilateral, they generate 2 points each. The last point (of a total of 9 possible points) is for the ability to place the palms on the floor with the knees straight (1 point). Approximately 12%–20% of a rheumatology population has a Beighton score of 5–9. Far fewer have a score ranging from 7–9.

A. A syndrome accompanies joint hypermobility, characterized in some patients by vague muscle aches, intermittent joint swellings without frank trauma or dislocation, and a typical fibromyalgia syndrome. Many patients have mitral valve prolapse (MVP) and associated palpitations. Many patients without a frank syndrome suffer from recurrent joint dislocations and in childhood have had frequent visits to orthopedists. Neonatologists and pediatricians encounter the severe genetic abnormalities causing joint hypermobility; the complete description of these is beyond the scope of this text.

   Two phenotypic syndromes—Marfan's syndrome and Ehlers-Danlos syndrome—may present with joint hypermobility and bear more extensive discussion here. Both of these syndromes may have medical emergencies requiring urgent management.

B. Marfan's syndrome is characterized by elongated body habitus, ectopia lentis (an upward displacement is characteristic), scoliosis, pes planus, high arched palate, dural ectasia (especially of the lumbosacral spine), and lung blebs. Vascular complications may be severe and include aortic dissection and dilation (usually DeBakey type I) and mitral valve prolapse and regurgitations. The scoliosis can be severe and cause chronic pain. The eye problems also can include retinal detachment. Adults (and probably children) should receive long-term prophylactic beta blockade to try to prevent aortic dilation and dissection. Counseling regarding the importance of low-impact physical activity is important, and ongoing aortic echocardiography is warranted. Particular problems may arise during pregnancy, and female patients wishing to conceive need to be counseled both on the genetic inheritance of Marfan's syndrome and the increased risk to the mother. One inherited disorder of connective tissue that can look phenotypically similar to Marfan's syndrome is homocystinuria. In that condition, the lens is dislocated in a downward fashion. Measurement of serum and urine homocysteine can confirm that diagnosis.

C. Ehlers-Danlos syndrome is a diverse grouping of abnormal collagen coding and transcription. An older classification (still used by many) defines up to 11 types. Many of these present very early after birth. Of importance in the differential diagnosis in adults is "type III," which can look like the hyperextensible joint syndrome. Unfortunately, there is no way currently to absolutely distinguish Ehlers-Danlos type III from mere hyperextensible joint syndrome. The distinction can become important because patients with type III Ehlers-Danlos syndrome may have severe mitral valve prolapse and mitral regurgitation. Patients with type IV Ehlers-Danlos syndrome have some joint hypermobility, but they are less hypermobile that the patients with type III. This phenotype is important to recognize because they can have spontaneous rupture of the colon, uterus (especially in pregnancy), and vascular tree. Other types of Ehlers-Danlos (especially I and II) have very thin skin that tends to scar like thin cigarette paper, especially over the elbows and knees. The skin is hyperdistensible and often nearly translucent. Hypermobility in these types is usually moderate.

   Management of the hypermobility joint syndrome involves splinting, physical therapy when appropriate, and counseling regarding activities. Occasionally nonsteroidal antiinflammatory drugs are useful. If the patient manifests fibromyalgia symptoms, then the customary fibromyalgia treatments are used.

   If Marfan's syndrome or Ehlers-Danlos syndrome is suspected, more rigorous investigations, especially echocardiograms, are warranted. In the case of Marfan's syndrome, beta blockade for adults (as yet not proved for children) is warranted. Detailed discussion of the genetic inheritance, gene abnormalities, and phenotypic syndromes for Ehlers-Danlos syndrome and Marfan's syndrome is available at the Online Mendelian Inheritance in Man website (www.ncbi.nlm.nih.gov/Omim/allresources.html).

References

El-Shahaly HA, el-Sherif AK. Is the benign hypermobility syndrome benign? Clin Rheumatol 1991:10:302.

Goldman L, Ausiello DA. Cecil Textbook of Medicine, 22nd ed. Philadelphia: Saunders, 2004:1637–1638.

Hakim AJ, Grahame R. Joint hypermobility syndrome: an update for clinicians. Int J Adv Rheumatol 2003;1:131.

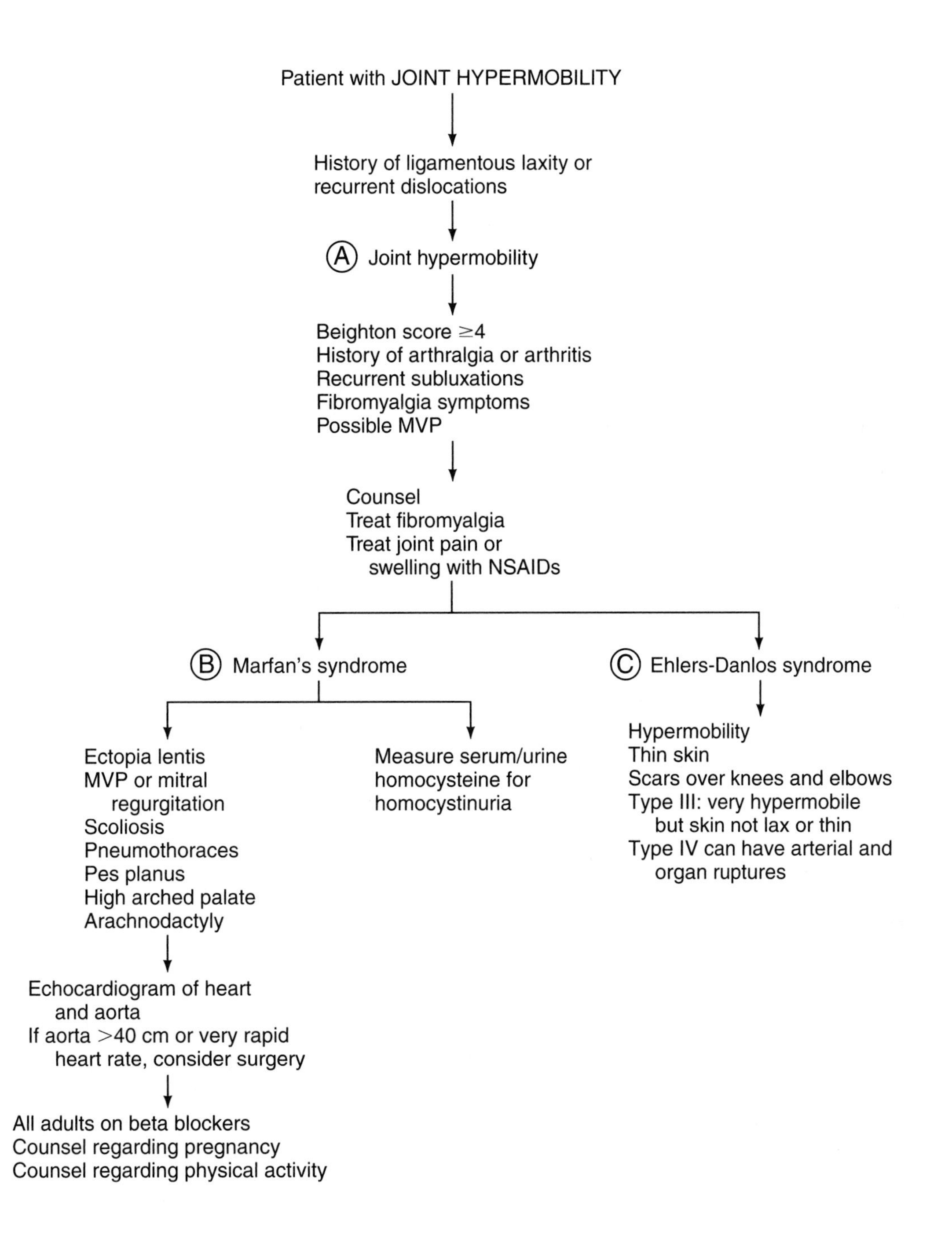
Patient with JOINT HYPERMOBILITY
History of ligamentous laxity or recurrent dislocations
(A) Joint hypermobility
Beighton score ≥4
History of arthralgia or arthritis
Recurrent subluxations
Fibromyalgia symptoms
Possible MVP
Counsel
Treat fibromyalgia
Treat joint pain or swelling with NSAIDs
(B) Marfan's syndrome
(C) Ehlers-Danlos syndrome
Ectopia lentis
MVP or mitral regurgitation
Scoliosis
Pneumothoraces
Pes planus
High arched palate
Arachnodactyly
Measure serum/urine homocysteine for homocystinuria
Hypermobility
Thin skin
Scars over knees and elbows
Type III: very hypermobile but skin not lax or thin
Type IV can have arterial and organ ruptures
Echocardiogram of heart and aorta
If aorta >40 cm or very rapid heart rate, consider surgery
All adults on beta blockers
Counsel regarding pregnancy
Counsel regarding physical activity

TEMPOROMANDIBULAR PAIN

Paul A. Monach, MD, PhD

A. History and physical examination are particularly helpful for identifying nonmusculoskeletal causes of pain near the temporomandibular joint (TMJ). Many nearby structures can become inflamed or infected. Otitis is often accompanied by ear pain, tinnitus, and hearing loss, and middle ear effusion and/or inflammation or damage to the tympanic membrane should be evident on otoscopy. Parotitis features tenderness and often swelling of the parotid gland, inferior to the TMJ, and observing the mouth while massaging the gland may reveal blocked flow or flow of purulent material from the orifice near the upper molars. Pain of dental origin is indicated by focal tenderness to palpation of the gums or percussion of the teeth. Sinusitis, particularly of the maxillary sinus, may feature purulent nasal drainage, tenderness over the sinus, and absence of exacerbation with minor movements of the jaw or with isometric use of the muscles of mastication. Temporal arteritis should be considered in a patient >50 years old with temporal headache and is often associated with fever, weight loss, jaw claudication (different from jaw pain apparent after initial movement), tenderness of the scalp and/or temporal artery, and (most ominously) transient or permanent monocular visual loss.

B. Trigeminal neuralgia is often suggested by a history of severe but transient episodes of pain over one side of the face, often worst at or seeming to originate from the preauricular region. Response to a trial of carbamazepine, which is generally ineffective for nonneuropathic causes of pain, may be more helpful diagnostically than the physical examination or diagnostic tests.

C. Pain in the TMJ itself is suggested by absence of the previously listed findings and by the presence of others. Pain with chewing or with tooth clenching is characteristic but nonspecific. Examination of the TMJ should include palpation both externally and internally (with the examiner's little finger in the patient's external auditory canal) while the patient is moving the jaw, paying attention to symmetry. Abnormalities on examination are, unfortunately, common in the asymptomatic population. Plain radiography is indicated as a first diagnostic test in chronic cases, unless the patient has evidence of a systemic inflammatory arthritic disease. Transcranial lateral views comparing the TMJs are generally used, and other views are available. CT and particularly MRI, however, are far more sensitive for appreciation of osseous changes, displacement of the articular disk, and detection of fractures and tumors. These techniques have largely replaced arthrography of the TMJ.

D. Osteoarthritis of the TMJ often features crepitus on examination. It usually follows internal derangement, so features of that disorder may coexist (see E). Imaging shows joint space narrowing and sclerosis and osteophyte formation of the adjoining bone.

E. Internal derangement is the most common disorder of the TMJ. It can be posttraumatic but usually results from ligamentous laxity and affects women more commonly than men. A history of chronic or transient inability to fully open the mouth (trismus) is common, and a palpable click may be noted during jaw movement on examination. MRI is the best diagnostic technique; CT is also effective.

F. Inflammatory arthritides such as rheumatoid arthritis, psoriatic arthritis and other seronegative spondyloarthropathies, and systemic lupus can all involve the TMJ, although involvement of the TMJ is usually of less consequence than that of other joints. TMJ involvement in gout or calcium pyrophosphate deposition disease (CPPD) is extremely rare. The TMJs are commonly involved in juvenile rheumatoid arthritis, however, and joint damage during skeletal growth can lead to a characteristic micrognathia.

G. The muscles of mastication are a frequent cause of temporomandibular pain, often in isolation and sometimes with coexisting features of internal derangement and/or osteoarthritis. A history of nocturnal teeth clenching and grinding (bruxism) may be obtainable from a patient's sleep companion (if available). Pain is often noted with isometric contraction of the muscles of mastication, and those muscles amenable to examination (masseter, temporalis) are often tender.

H. Facial pain of unknown etiology may occur in isolation or as part of a more widespread pain syndrome such as fibromyalgia. Tension headaches can include pain around the TMJ region in some patients. In both cases, pain is usually but not always bilateral. In the absence of a widespread pain syndrome, persistent unilateral pain of obscure origin merits imaging by MRI or CT to rule out neoplasm.

References

Marbach JJ. Temporomandibular pain and dysfunction syndrome. History physical examination, and treatment. Rheum Dis Clin North Am 1996;22:477–498.

Siccoli MM, Bassetti CL, Sandor PS. Facial pain: clinical differential diagnosis. Lancet Neurol 2006;5:257–267.

Wadhwa S, Kapila S. TMJ disorders: future innovations in diagnostic and therapeutics. J Dent Educ 2008;72:930–947.

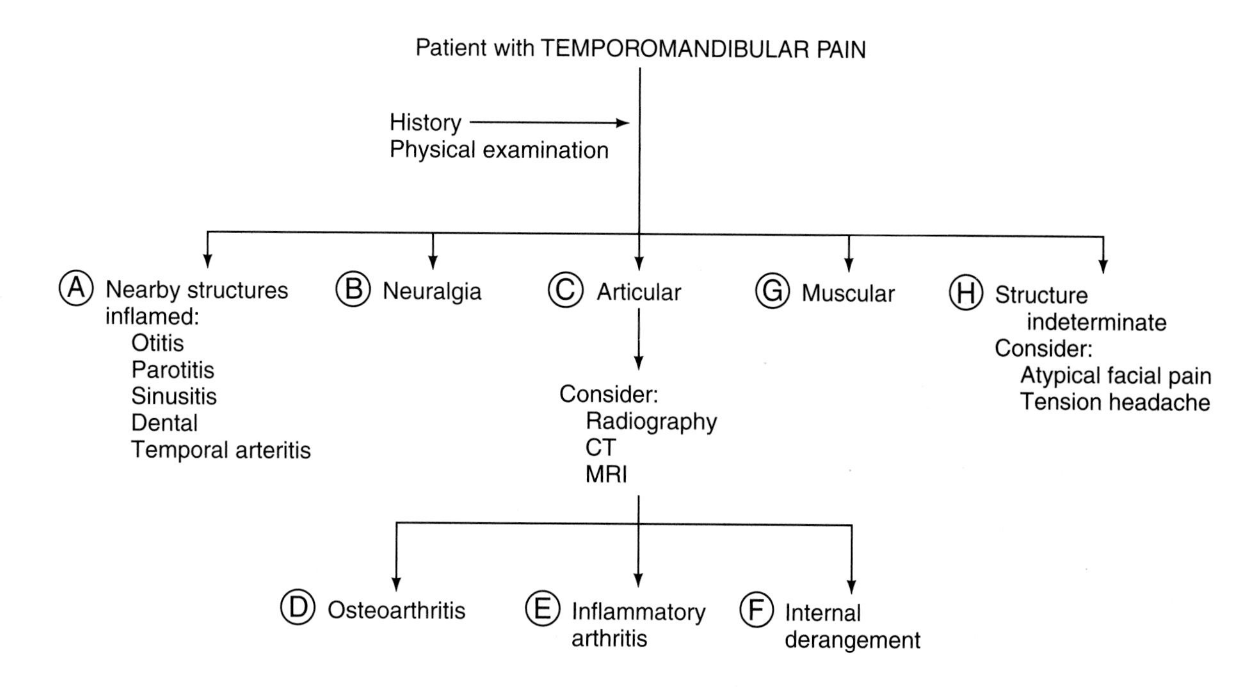
Patient with TEMPOROMANDIBULAR PAIN
History
Physical examination
(A) Nearby structures inflamed:
Otitis
Parotitis
Sinusitis
Dental
Temporal arteritis
(B) Neuralgia
(C) Articular
Consider:
Radiography
CT
MRI
(G) Muscular
(H) Structure indeterminate
Consider:
Atypical facial pain
Tension headache
(D) Osteoarthritis
(E) Inflammatory arthritis
(F) Internal derangement

ANTINUCLEAR ANTIBODY TEST

Alyssa Johnsen, MD, PhD

An ANA test is positive when a patient's serum recognizes components of the nucleus of a substrate cell. If the test is positive, a dilution ratio is given (e.g., 1:160 means the sample was diluted 160 times and was still positive). An ANA is most useful when ordered in a patient in whom autoimmune disease is strongly suspected. This test is often used to support a diagnosis of systemic lupus erythematosus (SLE).

A. Several features on history may make one suspect a diagnosis of SLE. A history positive for fever, fatigue, hair loss, rash, photosensitivity, Raynaud's phenomenon, oral ulcers, chest pain, shortness of breath, hematuria, arthritis or arthralgias, seizures, or mental status changes can be suggestive. None of these symptoms in isolation, however, is specific for SLE or any other rheumatic disease and could be caused by infectious or lymphoproliferative disorders.

B. A complete physical examination should be performed. Findings of rash, especially malar or discoid rash; oral ulcers; a pericardial friction rub; a pleural rub or effusion; or arthritis can be suggestive. If a pleural or pericardial effusion is suspected, further imaging, such as chest x-ray and echocardiogram is warranted. As with the historical features, none of these physical examination signs in isolation are specific for SLE or any rheumatic disease and could be caused by other diseases, including infectious or lymphoproliferative disorders.

C. If the history and physical examination are suggestive of SLE, further laboratory evaluation should be performed. A CBC, blood chemistries, liver function tests, and urinalysis with sediment should be ordered. Infection should be ruled out. In a patient who has a history and physical examination suggestive of SLE, an ANA can be a useful part of the evaluation.

D. A positive ANA is associated with many autoimmune diseases and some chronic infections and lymphoproliferative diseases. The estimated sensitivity and specificity of the ANA test for SLE are 100% and 86%, respectively. For other rheumatic diseases, it is 42% and 85%, respectively. The positive predictive value of the ANA is low—11% for SLE and 11% for other rheumatic diseases.

ANAs are also positive in the normal population, especially at low titers. Of healthy people, 32% have an ANA at 1:40, 13% at 1:80, and 3% present at >1:320. A higher titer (>1:640) is more suggestive of disease association.

If the ANA is determined by immunofluorescence, patterns of nuclear staining can be determined. These patterns are operator-dependent and have a low sensitivity and specificity, so they have largely been supplanted by specific tests. An anticentromere pattern should raise suspicion for scleroderma.

If an ANA is positive and the patient has symptoms suggestive of a systemic autoimmune disease, further specific antibody tests can be ordered. In addition, C3 and C4 levels are often low during an active lupus flare. ESR and C-reactive protein (CRP) are often high.

- Anti-dsDNA (double-stranded DNA)—specific for SLE, associated with disease activity and lupus nephritis.
- Anti-Sm (anti-Smith)—specific for SLE.
- Anti-RNP (anti-small nuclear ribonucleoprotein)—necessary for the diagnosis of mixed connective tissue disease, also associated with SLE, correlates.
- Anti-Ro (SSA)—associated with SLE and Sjögren's syndrome.
- Anti-La (SSB)—associated with SLE and Sjögren's syndrome.
- Antihistone—associated with SLE with a high specificity for drug-induced lupus.
- Anti-Scl-70 (anti-topoisomerase I)—associated with scleroderma.

References

Egner W. The use of laboratory tests in the diagnosis of SLE. J Clin Pathol 2000;53:424.

Slater CA, Davis RB, Shmerling RH. Antinuclear antibody testing: a study of clinical utility. Arch Intern Med 1996;156:1421.

Tan EM, Feltkamp TE, Smolen JS, et al. Range of antinuclear antibodies in "healthy" individuals. Arthritis Rheum 1997;40:1601.

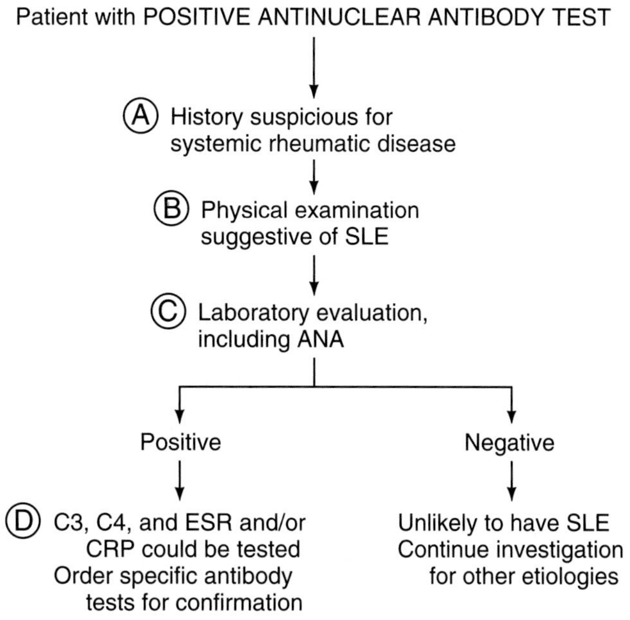

Patient with POSITIVE ANTINUCLEAR ANTIBODY TEST

↓

(A) History suspicious for systemic rheumatic disease

↓

(B) Physical examination suggestive of SLE

↓

(C) Laboratory evaluation, including ANA

- Positive
  - (D) C3, C4, and ESR and/or CRP could be tested
    Order specific antibody tests for confirmation
- Negative
  - Unlikely to have SLE
    Continue investigation for other etiologies

ELEVATED SERUM ALKALINE PHOSPHATASE LEVEL

Paul A. Monach, MD, PhD

A. An isolated alkaline phosphatase level is often encountered in asymptomatic patients, although a subsequent history and physical examination directed at the most common causes of such elevation often are revealing. The systems to consider are hepatobiliary and skeletal. An elevated alkaline phosphatase level is often the first sign of biliary tract disease in apparently healthy persons, although symptoms and signs of chronic liver disease may already be present. Skeletal conditions associated with elevation of alkaline phosphatase are usually painful. Serum alkaline phosphatase is also elevated in pregnancy, primarily as a result of placental production.

B. Additional laboratory tests help determine whether the elevation is of hepatobiliary origin. Serum gamma glutamyl transferase (GGT or GGPT) and 5'-nucleotidase (5'-NT) levels are usually also elevated in biliary tract disease, and other liver function tests (LFTs) may also be abnormal. The classic procedure of fractionating alkaline phosphatase by heat stability ("liver lives, bone burns") is infrequently performed and not well standardized in many laboratories.

C. Abnormal liver function tests require further workup, including imaging (ultrasound, CT, endoscopic retrograde cholangiopancreatography [ERCP]), viral and autoimmune serologies, and sometimes liver biopsy.

D. Elevated alkaline phosphatase of suspected skeletal origin should lead to evaluation of the calcium-phosphate hormonal system, with measurement of serum calcium, magnesium, phosphate, and 25-OH vitamin D. Elevation of parathyroid hormone (PTH) is unlikely unless calcium is also elevated, so its measurement is not necessary in the initial series of tests. Lung cancers often synthesize PTH-related polypeptide (PTHrp), so screening for this protein, and for lung cancer by imaging, is appropriate in at-risk patients with elevated calcium. Multiple myeloma is an uncommon cause of an elevated alkaline phosphatase, so testing of serum and urinary immunoglobulins for a monoclonal component is not usually indicated. Patients with significant chronic renal insufficiency present a special case: it is wise to measure PTH regardless of the calcium level because PTH can be markedly elevated even in the presence of normal or low calcium. It is also a good idea to measure 1,25-dihydroxyvitamin D because the kidney is required for the synthesis of this, the most active metabolite of vitamin D.

E. Elevated calcium and low phosphorus are characteristic of hyperparathyroidism, which should be confirmed with PTH, PTHrp testing, or both. Osteomalacia is characterized by normal calcium and low phosphorus. A vitamin D deficiency severe enough to raise the alkaline phosphatase level will usually be accompanied by this decline in phosphorus, regardless of whether symptoms and radiographic signs (e.g., osteoporosis and pseudofractures of the long bones around the knee) of osteomalacia are present. Bone metastases often increase serum calcium.

F. Paget's disease of bone features abnormal bone remodeling in sites that vary widely among patients but tend to remain constant in a patient over time. It is usually painful, and in some cases deformity is evident. Other bone diseases to consider in the setting of normal calcium-phosphate homeostasis include inflammatory arthritis and a healing fracture, both of which should be apparent by history and physical examination. As in the case of elevated calcium, metastases are an important consideration in the absence of another diagnosis.

G. Plain radiography directed at painful sites should be the initial imaging test. If these are normal, or if the patient is asymptomatic, then a radionuclide bone scan is a sensitive means of evaluating the entire skeleton for evidence of bone lesions from Paget's disease, metastases, or other (rare) infiltrative causes. Myeloma lesions are often invisible by bone scan but, as mentioned earlier, are uncommonly associated with elevated alkaline phosphatase. Any abnormality on bone scan should be followed by plain radiography or more advanced imaging (CT, MRI) of the site to assist in diagnosis.

References

Pratt DS, Kaplan MM. Evaluation of abnormal liver-enzyme results in asymptomatic patients. N Engl J Med 2000;342:1266–1271.

Reginato AJ, FALASCA GF, Pappu R, et al. Musculoskeletal manifestations of osteomalacia: report of 26 cases and literature review. Semin Arthritis Rheum 1999;28:287–304.

Whyte MP. Clinical practice: Paget's disease of bone. N Engl J Med 2006;355:593–600.

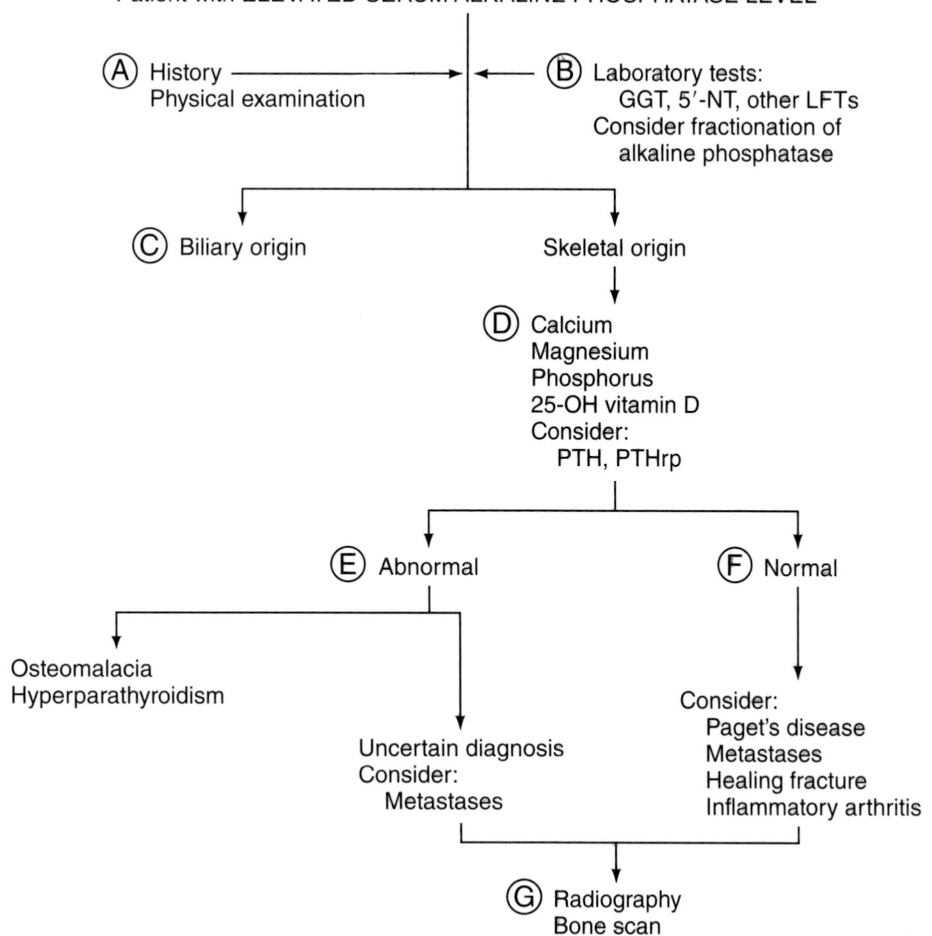
Patient with ELEVATED SERUM ALKALINE PHOSPHATASE LEVEL
(A) History
Physical examination
(B) Laboratory tests:
GGT, 5′-NT, other LFTs
Consider fractionation of
alkaline phosphatase
(C) Biliary origin
Skeletal origin
(D) Calcium
Magnesium
Phosphorus
25-OH vitamin D
Consider:
PTH, PTHrp
(E) Abnormal
(F) Normal
Osteomalacia
Hyperparathyroidism
Uncertain diagnosis
Consider:
Metastases
Consider:
Paget's disease
Metastases
Healing fracture
Inflammatory arthritis
(G) Radiography
Bone scan

ELEVATED CREATINE KINASE LEVEL

Sandeep K. Agarwal MD, PhD

A. Measurement of creatine kinase (CK) is the most common laboratory test used in the evaluation of skeletal and cardiac muscle disease. It is also often part of routine panel testing and should be considered in the evaluation of elevated transaminases when hepatic causes are less likely. This chapter focuses on the evaluation of CK in the workup of musculoskeletal complaints.

B. The initial approach to an elevated CK is a detailed history and physical examination focusing on determining the origin of CK (e.g., skeletal muscle, cardiac, brain). This may be readily apparent, as in a patient with acute chest pain and changes on ECG or with severe proximal muscle weakness.

C. If the cause is not clinically evident, the CK isoenzyme CK-MB and troponins should be obtained to determine if the elevated CK is of cardiac origin. CK-MB can be mildly elevated secondary to regenerating skeletal muscle, and cardiac troponins can be elevated in patients with myocardial involvement of inflammatory myositis. If the CK elevation is of cardiac origin, immediately pursue the appropriate cardiac evaluation and therapy.

D. Occasionally elevated CK levels result from cerebral causes (i.e., trauma), which are usually readily apparent based on the clinical history.

E. If the CK elevation is from skeletal muscle, the history should focus on ruling out medications (cholesterol-lowering agents, colchicine, antimalarials, zidovudine), drugs and alcohol, trauma, vigorous exercise, dystrophinopathies, inflammatory myopathies, infectious myopathies, endocrinopathies, and iatrogenic causes (intramuscular injections, postoperative). The physical examination should include a complete neurologic evaluation and musculoskeletal examination, including muscle strength testing.

F. The laboratory evaluation consisting of a CBC, electrolytes, and thyroid function tests is important to evaluate the patient for hypothyroidism, electrolyte abnormalities, and infectious causes. These should guide subsequent evaluation and treatment.

G. If the history, physical examination, and laboratory evaluation do not readily reveal a cause for the elevated CK, additional evaluation should be pursued. The role of skeletal muscle MRI is controversial and nonspecific but may be helpful to identify muscle groups for targeting biopsy. Electromyography (EMG) and nerve conduction studies (NCS) are useful to distinguish myopathic and neuropathic alterations. Unilateral EMG/NCS should be obtained, preserving the contralateral side for muscle biopsy.

H. If the EMG is completely normal, the patient may be followed closely. However, one must consider false-negative EMG results if clinical suspicion for an underlying disorder persists. Additional laboratory tests, ANA, rheumatoid factor, and myositis-specific antibodies (anti-Jo-1, anti-Mi-2, and antisignal recognition peptide) may be helpful. If the CK elevation persists or progresses, MRI and/or muscle biopsy should be considered.

I. If the EMG demonstrates myopathic changes, a muscle biopsy should be obtained to determine the underlying pathology. If the EMG demonstrates neuropathic changes, consider additional neurologic evaluation.

J. A muscle biopsy should be performed on clinically involved muscle on the contralateral side of the EMG to avoid possible artifact in the biopsy from the EMG needle. Routine histochemical analysis of biopsy may be sufficient to make a diagnosis, but special analysis is often necessary and should be obtained after discussion with the pathologist. If inclusion body myositis is suspected, the biopsy should be processed for electron microscopy.

K. If the muscle biopsy is normal, the patient may be followed closely. However, many muscle diseases are patchy, and a single biopsy may not detect the involved site. Therefore, if symptoms persist, a repeat muscle biopsy or MRI may be required. If symptoms progress, empiric therapy may be done but with caution.

L. If the muscle biopsy is consistent with an inflammatory myopathy, treatment of polymyositis or dermatomyositis consists of corticosteroids and other immunosuppressive medications. Patients with dermatomyositis should be evaluated for an underlying malignancy. Patients should also be evaluated for a possible connective tissue disease (CTD), including systemic lupus erythematosus, rheumatoid arthritis, or scleroderma.

M. The diagnosis of inherited and congenital myopathies often requires special tests on the muscle biopsy. Treatment is usually symptomatic. The patient should be evaluated by a neuromuscular specialist.

References

Dalakas MC, Hahlfeld R. Polymyositis and dermatomyositis. Lancet 2003;362(9388):971–982.

Shmerling RH. Diagnostic tests for rheumatic disease: clinic utility revisited. South Med J 2005;98(7):704–711.

Thompson PD, Clarkson P, Karas RH. Stain-associated myopathy. JAMA 2003;289(13):1681–1690.

Warren JD, Blumberg PC, Thompson PD. Rhabdomyolysis: a review. Muscle Nerve 2002;25(3):332–347.

Wortmann RL. Inflammatory diseases of muscle and other myopathies. In Harris ED, Budd RC, Firestein GS, et al, eds. Kelley's Textbook of Rheumatology, 7th ed. Philadelphia: Elsevier Saunders, 2005: 1309–1335.

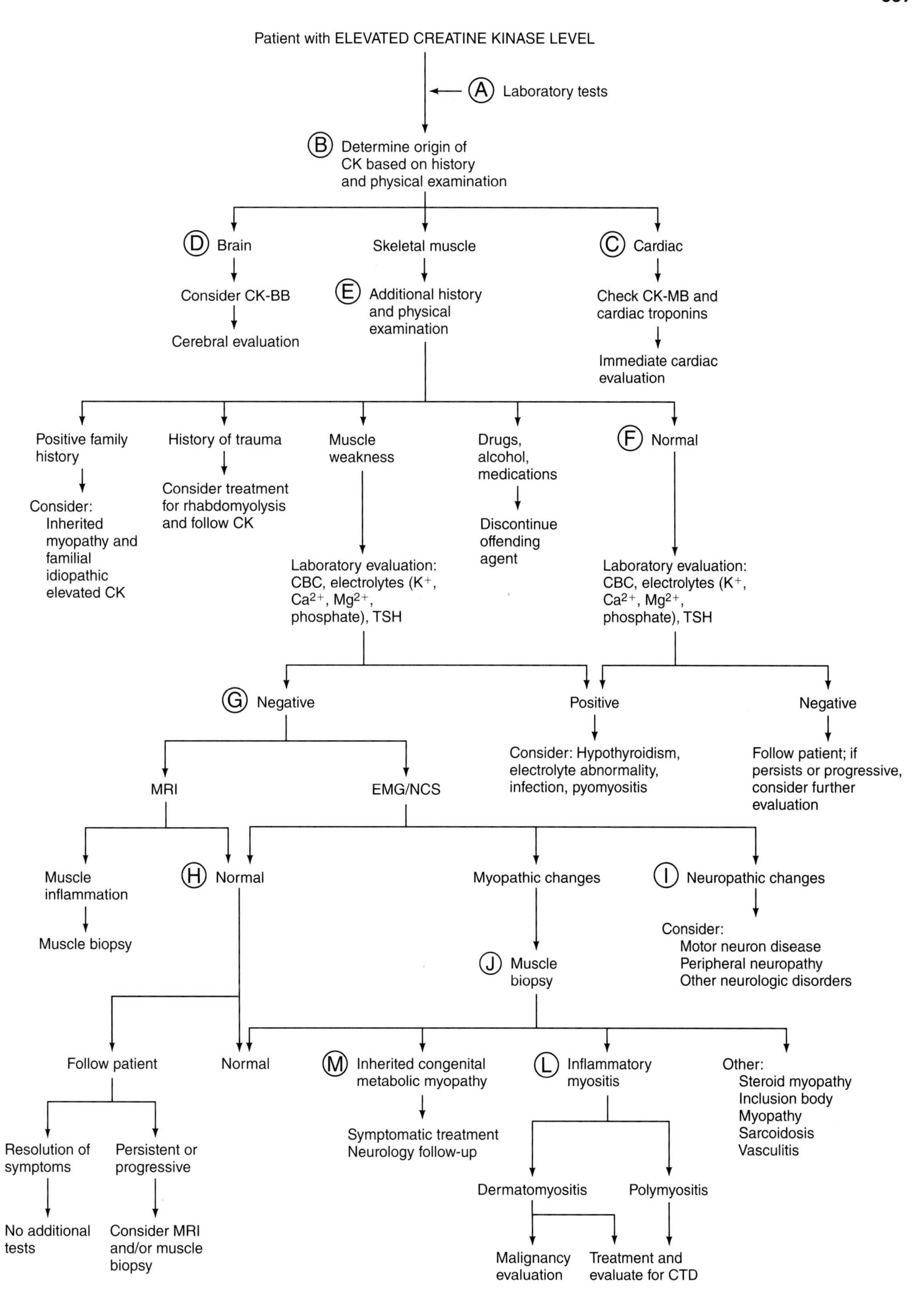

TSH, Thyroid-stimulating hormone.

Urology

Graeme Steele, MD, FCS, FACS
Section Editor

SCROTAL MASS

David McDermott, MD, and Graeme Steele, MD, FCS, FACS

Scrotal masses can present clinically as a result of tumor, trauma, and/or inflammation of the scrotal wall or its contents. The mass may be the result of an acute event or noted incidentally by the patient or a sexual partner. The key to diagnosis begins with consideration of the complete differential diagnosis and appropriate management based on clinical findings.

A. An accurate history of constitutional symptoms with characterization of the onset and duration of urologic symptoms allows the clinician to narrow the differential diagnosis of a scrotal mass considerably. A review of the patient's past medical history, family history, sexual history, and surgical history, with particular attention to genitourinary tract instrumentation, is important in the workup. Initial laboratory tests of value include urinalysis (UA), urine culture, and CBC. If there is a question of sexually transmitted disease, testing for *gonococcus* and chlamydia is indicated. If a solid scrotal mass is identified by examination or ultrasound (US) that raises concern for testicular neoplasm, serum alpha-fetoprotein (AFP), beta-human chorionic gonadotropin (hCG), and lactate dehydrogenase (LDH) should be obtained by the primary physician or the urologic consultant.

   Patients will present with either a painful or painless mass in the scrotum. Acute onset of pain with a scrotal mass is most frequently associated with acute epididymitis or torsion of the testicle or its appendages. A trauma history with marked testicular enlargement presents concern for organ rupture. Dull or chronic scrotal pain can be associated with noninflammatory conditions such as varicocele or hydrocele. In addition, approximately 30%–40% of patients with testicular cancer present with a chief complaint of a dull ache or a heavy sensation in the lower abdomen, anal area, or scrotum. Scrotal pain may be either primary or referred. Because of their embryologic relation to the testes, pathology in the kidneys or retroperitoneum can present as pain referred to the scrotum and is not associated with a mass. Scrotal edema is often a symptom of medical disease, which will cause generalized scrotal enlargement bilaterally, whereas other processes will localize to a hemiscrotum.

   Physical examination of the scrotum and its contents is performed by bimanual examination with the patient standing. First, the scrotal skin should be examined for sebaceous cysts, infected hair follicles, and other dermatologic abnormalities. Particularly in patients with diabetes or who are immunocompromised, cellulitis of the scrotal skin or abscess of the underlying soft tissue may present as a painful indurated mass associated with erythema and fluctuance. If the patient presents with a lateralizing complaint, begin the examination with the normal contralateral side. On testicular examination, this provides a baseline and allows the examiner to appreciate the relative size, contour, and consistency of the normal testis and the suspected gonad. Physical examination of the testis is performed by careful palpation of the testis between the thumb and first two fingers of the examining hand. The noral testis is homogeneous in consistency, freely movable, and separable from the epididymis. Any firm, hard, or fixed area within the substance of the tunica albuginea should be considered suspicious for tumor until proved otherwise. The epididymis lies posterior to the testicle and is palpable as a distinct ridge of tissue. The spermatic cord and inguinal canal should be palpated bilaterally to exclude involvement of cord structures or hernia. Transillumination with a flashlight is particularly helpful in determining whether a scrotal mass is solid or cystic. In patients in whom the diagnosis is unclear or in whom a hydrocele precludes adequate examination, imaging studies should be used as an important second step.

   Ultrasonography of the scrotum is essentially an extension of the physical examination. Any hypoechoic area within the tunica albuginea is suspicious for testicular cancer. Color flow Doppler ultrasonography will reveal decreased or absent blood flow to the gonad in torsion and typically will show increased flow in epididymoorchitis. Intrascrotal fluid collections are no barrier to the examination of the underlying testicular parenchyma by ultrasonography.

B. The differential diagnosis of a painless scrotal mass includes varicocele, hydrocele, and tumor. Less common diagnoses include hematoma and epididymal cyst (spermatocele). The differential diagnosis of a painful scrotal mass includes testicular torsion, epididymitis, and epididymoorchitis. Although rare, torsion of a testicular appendage can present with a painful scrotal mass. Inguinal hernias can present as a scrotal mass with or without pain.

(Continued on page 562)

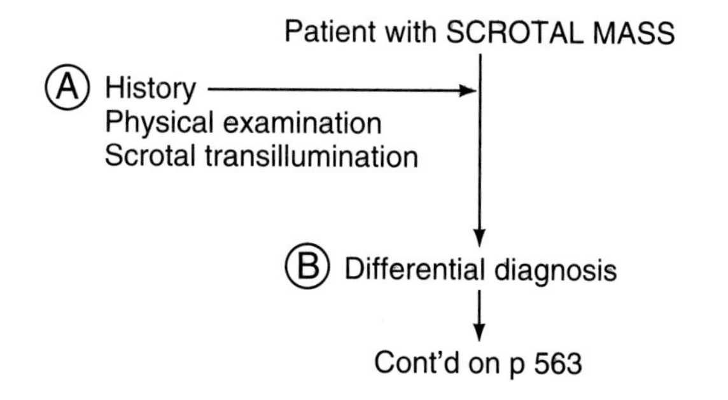
Patient with SCROTAL MASS
A
History
Physical examination
Scrotal transillumination
B
Differential diagnosis
Cont'd on p 563

C. Review of pathology:

Epididymitis: Epididymitis is inflammation of the epididymis as a result of an infection or a sterile process. Infectious epididymitis is secondary to an ascending infection commonly seen in conjunction with *Chlamydia trachomatis* or *Neisseria gonorrhoeae* infection in sexually active men <35 years or as a result of urinary tract infection (UTI), prostatitis, or urethral instrumentation in the elderly. *Escherichia coli* is the most common cause of infectious epididymitis in boys and the elderly. The typical presentation is acute or subacute onset of scrotal pain and swelling and may be associated with generalized constitutional symptoms. The amount of swelling may make localization of the epididymis difficult, in which case imaging to rule out torsion may be necessary. Reflux of sterile urine is thought to cause epididymal pain, which can be chronic and may be associated with a nodular texture or small mass in the epididymis. Sterile or chronic epididymitis is managed with NSAIDs and scrotal elevation; a 2- to 4-week course of a fluoroquinolone can be helpful. The current recommendation for treatment of epididymitis when chlamydia or gonococcus is suspected is ceftriaxone 250 mg IM once and doxycycline 100 mg PO bid for a 10-day course. Finally, a 10-day course of fluoroquinolone is appropriate for treatment of infectious epididymitis when coliform organisms are suspected.

Epididymoorchitis: Epididymoorchitis is the result of progression of an inflammatory process of the epididymis to involve the adjacent testicle. On examination, the testicle and epididymis will be tender and difficult to distinguish as two distinct structures. In severe cases, the overlying scrotal skin will be erythematous and indurated. US will show characteristic hypervascularity of both structures, making the diagnosis distinct from torsion, in which there will be low or absent blood flow. Supportive measures and antibiotic treatment are the same as for infectious epididymitis.

Varicocele: A varicocele is a dilated and tortuous vein or group of veins in the spermatic cord often described as feeling like a "bag of worms." Varicoceles occur in 15% of men, predominantly on the left side, and may become more obvious with the patient standing or with Valsalva and may disappear with the patient supine. Varicoceles are significant in that they are associated with infertility and can cause pain, in which case their management should be referred to a urologist.

Inguinal hernia: Herniation of bowel or omentum into the scrotum can produce a scrotal mass that may present with or without pain. Careful physical examination with auscultation of bowel sounds in the scrotum or successful hernia reduction can make the diagnosis. If physical examination and US are equivocal, a CT scan is warranted. If symptomatic or concerning for strangulation, referral to a general surgeon is warranted.

Epididymal cyst: An epididymal cyst is usually an incidental finding on routine physical examination in adolescents. Epididymal cysts are smooth, round, transilluminating structures generally found at the head of the epididymis. Rarely, epididymal cysts may enlarge enough to cause the patient pain, in which case surgical removal is necessary. Large epididymal cysts are referred to as spermatoceles.

Testicular torsion: Torsion must be the first consideration in any patient presenting with a painful scrotal mass because delay in diagnosis can result in loss of the testicle. Torsion refers to twisting of the spermatic cord with vascular compromise, resulting in sudden onset of pain and swelling of the affected testicle. A history of trauma may be present. Torsion occurs most commonly in men between the ages of 12 and 20 years. The characteristic high-riding position of the testicle along with swelling and tenderness can make examination difficult and distinguishing torsion from epididymitis a challenge. Color flow Doppler ultrasonography can easily make the diagnosis, but if torsion is seriously considered, immediate referral to a urologist for surgical exploration and detorsion is mandatory.

Hydrocele: A hydrocele is a fluid collection within the tunica vaginalis adjacent to the testes. The swelling is uniform, involving one hemiscrotum, and transilluminates. Hydroceles can present as primary lesions or as secondary phenomena. Of testicular tumors, 10% present with reactive hydroceles, which can make diagnosis of the tumor difficult. If there is any question as to whether transillumination is incomplete or a mass is palpable within a hydrocele, US is recommended.

Testicular tumor: The vast majority of testis tumors are germ cell tumors, which usually present as an enlarging testis, a testicular nodule, or testicular hardness and induration. The diagnosis is made clinically and confirmed with scrotal US. Treatment involves surgical removal of the testis via an inguinal incision, and further therapy depends on classification of the tumor and clinical stage.

References

Presti JC. Genital tumors. In Tanagho EA, McAninich JW, eds. Smith's General Urology. 16th ed. New York: McGraw-Hill, 2004.

Richie JP, Steele GS. Neoplasms of the testis. In Wein AJ, Kavoussi LR, Novick AC, et al, eds. Campbell-Walsh Urology, 9th ed. Philadelphia: WB Saunders, 2006.

Tanagho EA. Physical examination of the external male genitalia. In Tanagho EA, McAninich JW, eds. Smith's General Urology, 16th ed. New York: McGraw-Hill, 2004.

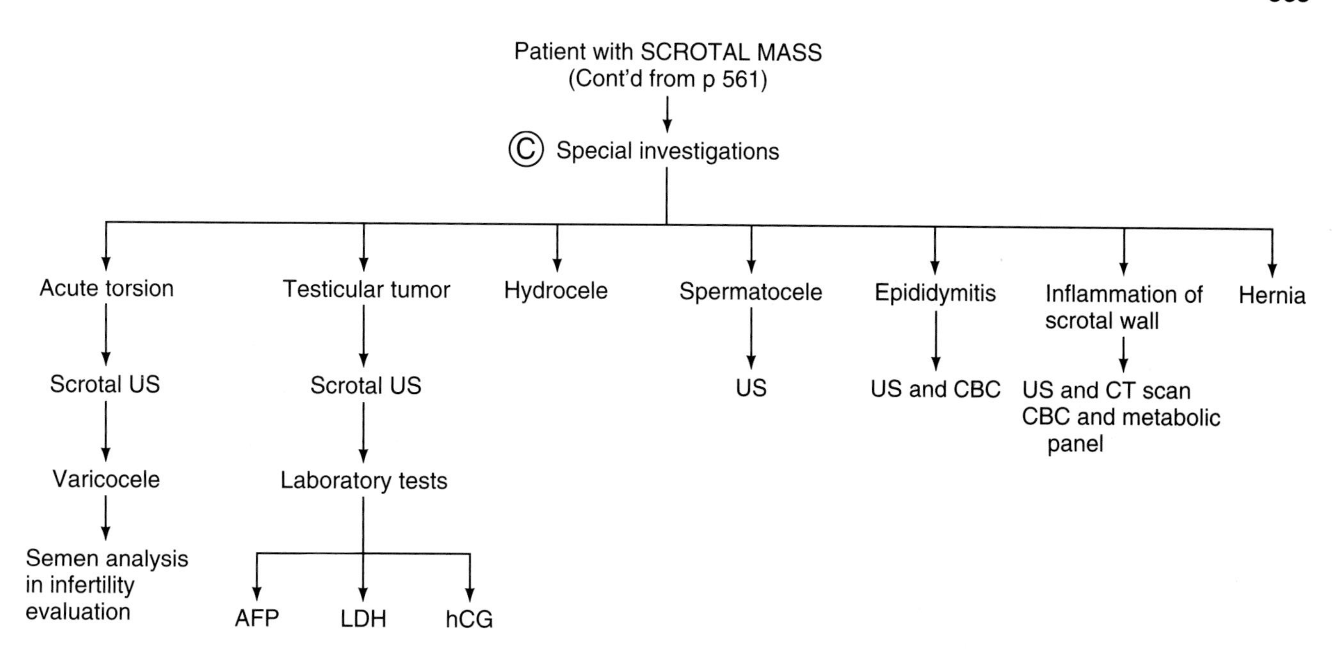
Patient with SCROTAL MASS
(Cont'd from p 561)
© Special investigations
Acute torsion
Scrotal US
Varicocele
Semen analysis in infertility evaluation
Testicular tumor
Scrotal US
Laboratory tests
AFP
LDH
hCG
Hydrocele
Spermatocele
US
Epididymitis
US and CBC
Inflammation of scrotal wall
US and CT scan
CBC and metabolic panel
Hernia

BENIGN PROSTATIC HYPERTROPHY

David Yeo, MD, and Graeme Steele, MD, FCS, FACS

A. The most common presentation for benign prostatic hypertrophy (BPH) is obstructive and irritative lower urinary tract symptoms (LUTS). Irritative symptoms of LUTS include frequency, nocturia, and urgency; obstructive symptoms of LUTS include hesitancy, incomplete bladder emptying, straining, weak stream, and dribbling. Assessment of LUTS begins with a focused history and physical examination, including onset and duration of urinary symptoms, medical and surgical history, sexual history, neurologic history, and rectal examination. The differential diagnosis includes BPH, prostate cancer, urinary tract infection (UTI), bladder cancer, bladder or ureteral calculi, urethral stricture, cystitis, prostatitis, polyuria, colovesical fistula, and neurogenic bladder.

B. Patients with a prostate-specific antigen (PSA) level >4.0 ng/ml, PSA velocity >0.75 ng/ml per year, or prostatic nodule palpated on rectal examination should undergo a prostate biopsy to assess for prostate cancer. When assessing risk for prostate cancer in patients who take 5-alpha reductase inhibitors, double the serum PSA value. PSA may be transiently elevated with prostatitis, UTI, ejaculation, urethral instrumentation, rectal manipulation, or extensive physical activity.

C. Irritative urinary symptoms with microhematuria warrant workup for ureteral calculi, bladder calculi, and malignancy of the urinary tract. Significant hematuria is defined as 3 RBCs per high-power field (hpf) on two of three voided urine specimens, >100 RBCs/hpf on any urinary specimen, or gross hematuria. Urine cytology is a useful screening tool for high-grade transitional cell carcinoma (TCC) of the urinary tract: negative or atypical cytology is considered negative for TCC; suspicious or TCC cytology is considered positive for TCC.

D. Use the American Urological Association Symptom Score and Quality of Life Questionnaire (AUASS/QOL) for a subjective measure of LUTS attributable to BPH. The AUASS/QOL is a validated questionnaire that quantifies common symptoms of LUTS, including incomplete bladder emptying, frequency, hesitancy, urgency, weak stream, straining, and nocturia, and an overall bother score from voiding symptoms. AUASS/QOL ≤7 indicates mild or nonbothersome symptoms; AUASS/QOL ≥8 indicates moderate/severe or bothersome symptoms. Objective measures for BPH include postvoid residual (PVR) volume, uroflowmetry, and urodynamics. In patients with normal bladder function, PVR >50 cc or urine flow <10 cc/sec suggest lower urinary tract obstruction.

E. Medical therapy generally is used as the initial treatment for patients with moderate to severe LUTS from BPH. Medical therapy consists of two major classes: selective alpha-1 antagonists and type II 5-alpha reductase inhibitors. Alpha-1 antagonists relax the smooth muscle in the prostate and bladder neck to improve urinary flow. Symptomatic improvement begins 1 week after starting alpha blockers. Hypotension and retrograde ejaculation are common side effects that limit the use of alpha blockers. Both therapeutic and undesired effects of alpha blockers are dose dependent. Type II 5-alpha reductase metabolizes testosterone to dihydrotestosterone (DHT); DHT stimulates prostate growth. 5-Alpha reductase inhibitors decrease prostate size by inducing prostate apoptosis and inhibiting the conversion of testosterone to DHT. These medications are indicated in patients with a large prostate (>40 g). Therapeutic effects of 5-alpha reductase inhibitors begin in 4–6 weeks with maximal results at 6–9 months. The major side effects are decreased libido, impotence, and ejaculatory dysfunction. Of note, 5-alpha reductase inhibitors reduce PSA by 50% after 6 months without reducing the risk of prostate cancer.

F. Surgical intervention is reserved for patients who fail or do not tolerate medical therapy and for patients with complications related to BPH, such as refractory urinary retention, bladder calculi, renal insufficiency from lower urinary tract obstruction, or recurrent UTIs. Transurethral resection of the prostate (TURP) or laser vaporization of the prostate (PVP) is the first-line surgical treatment for BPH. Open or laparoscopic prostatectomy is an option for patients with extremely large prostates (>75 g) or for those with concomitant bladder stones or bladder diverticulum. Various minimally invasive therapies have been developed that use energy sources low in heat to cause prostate necrosis, including microwave thermotherapy, radiofrequency waves, and ultrasound waves. Minimally invasive therapies for BPH provide symptomatic improvement superior to medical therapy but inferior to TURP.

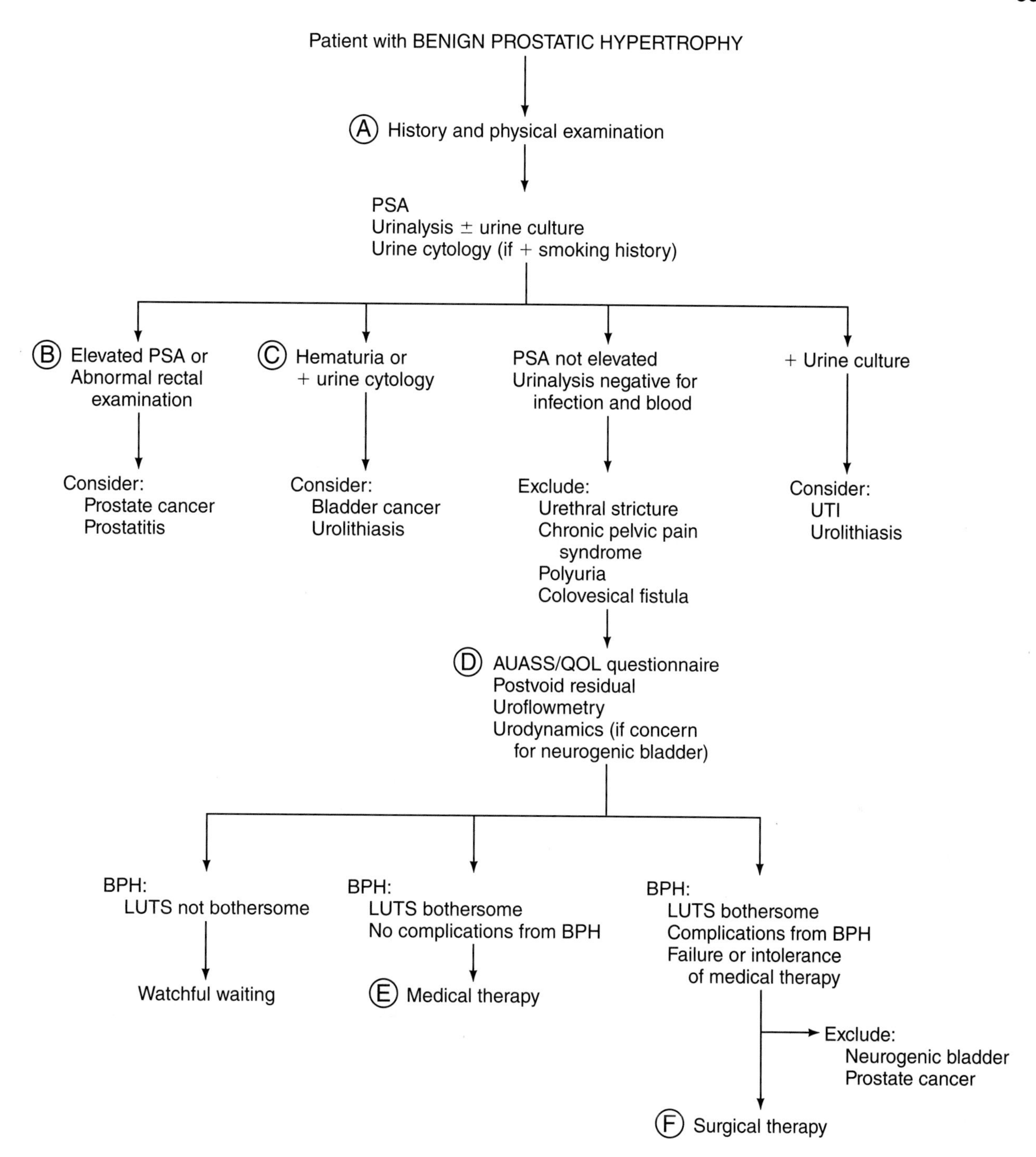

References

Abrams PH, Griffiths DJ. The assessment of prostatic obstruction from urodynamic measurements and from residual urine. Br J Urol 1979;51:129.

Barry MJ, Fowler FJ Jr, O'Leary MP et al. The American Urological Association Symptom Index for benign prostatic hyperplasia: J Urol 1997;148:1549–1557.

McConnell JD. Benign prostatic hyperplasia: treatment guidelines and patient classification. Brit J Urol 1995;76 Suppl. 1:29.

PROSTATITIS

David Yeo, MD, and Graeme Steele, MD, FCS, FACS

A. Prostatitis is inflammation of the prostate gland that encompasses a spectrum of clinical disease. The most common presentation is recurrent dysuria with irritative and obstructive urinary symptoms in the absence of bacterial infection. Specific complaints may include perineal pain, low back pain, suprapubic pain, dysuria, frequency, urgency, nocturia, straining, weak stream, hesitancy, and a sense of incomplete bladder emptying. The differential diagnosis for prostatitis includes sexually transmitted diseases (STDs), urinary tract infections, genitourinary malignancy, urolithiasis, urethral stricture, and neurogenic bladder. Workup for all cases of prostatitis begins with a focused history and physical examination, including sexual history, urinalysis, and urine culture. Based on a patient's risk factors, further studies may include urethral cultures for gonorrhea and chlamydia, testing for herpes and HIV, serum creatinine, serum prostate-specific antigen (PSA), postvoid residual recording, voided urine cytology, CT scan, cystoscopy, transrectal ultrasound of the prostate (TRUS), and urodynamics.

B. Hematuria warrants workup for urolithiasis, genitourinary malignancy, and urinary tract infection. Significant hematuria is defined as ≥3 RBCs per high-power field (hpf) on two of three voided urine specimens, >100 RBCs/hpf on any urinary specimen, or gross hematuria.

C. Acute bacterial prostatitis, a bacterial infection of the prostate of sudden onset, represents 2%–5% of prostatitis cases. Typically, patients are sexually active men <35 years, presenting with perineal or suprapubic pain, urethral discharge, obstructive urinary symptoms, and systemic signs of infection. Transmission can be sexual from *Neisseria gonorrhoeae* and *Chlamydia trachomatis* or by direct extension of *Escherichia coli* from the lower urinary tract or rectum.

D. Chronic bacterial prostatitis, a recurrent or persistent bacterial infection of the prostate, represents 2%–5% of prostatitis cases. Typically, patients are older men, presenting with intermittent and milder symptoms of dysuria than those with acute bacterial prostatitis. On examination, the prostate is tender and boggy with suprapubic tenderness during acute episodes of prostatitis. The most common causative organism is *E. coli*; other organisms include Enterobacteriaceae, enterococci, and *Pseudomonas aeruginosa*. Start empiric treatment with 8–16 weeks of trimethoprim/sulfamethoxazole (TMP) or quinolone antibiotics. Symptomatic control may be achieved with alpha blockers, anticholinergics, NSAIDs, and sitz baths. Consider surgical management with transurethral resection of the prostate (TURP) in men with prostate calculi, prostatic abscess, or persistent prostatitis after extensive medical management.

E. Chronic pelvic pain syndrome represents 90%–95% of prostatitis cases and is a diagnosis of exclusion. This syndrome is defined as genitourinary pain in the absence of identifiable infection, malignancy, urethral structure, and neurologic dysfunction. Proposed mechanisms include nonbacterial infection, reflux of urine into the ejaculatory ducts, and autoimmune disease. Possible infectious agents include *Trichomonas vaginalis, Chlamydia trachomatis, Ureaplasma urealyticum*, cytomegalovirus, and *Mycobacterium tuberculosis.* Empiric treatment begins with trimethoprim/sulfamethoxazole or quinolone antibiotics for 6–8 weeks. If there is no response, consider 4–6 weeks of doxycycline or metronidazole. For severe symptoms, patients can be started with some combination of alpha blockers, anticholinergics, narcotics, NSAIDs, tricyclics, and allopurinol. Other supportive measures include sitz baths, avoidance of alcohol and caffeine, prostatic message, pelvic floor exercises, stress reduction, and biofeedback.

Refrences

Meares EM Jr: Prostatitis and related disorders. In Walsh PC, Retik AB, Vaughan ED, Wein AJ (eds): Campell's Urology, 7th ed. Philadelphia, WB Saunders, 1998, pp 615–530.

Nickel JC: Effective office management of chornic prostatitis. Urol Clin North Am 1998;25:677–684

Nickel JC, Moon T: Chronic bacterial prostatitis: an evolving clinical enigma. Urology 2005;66:2–8.

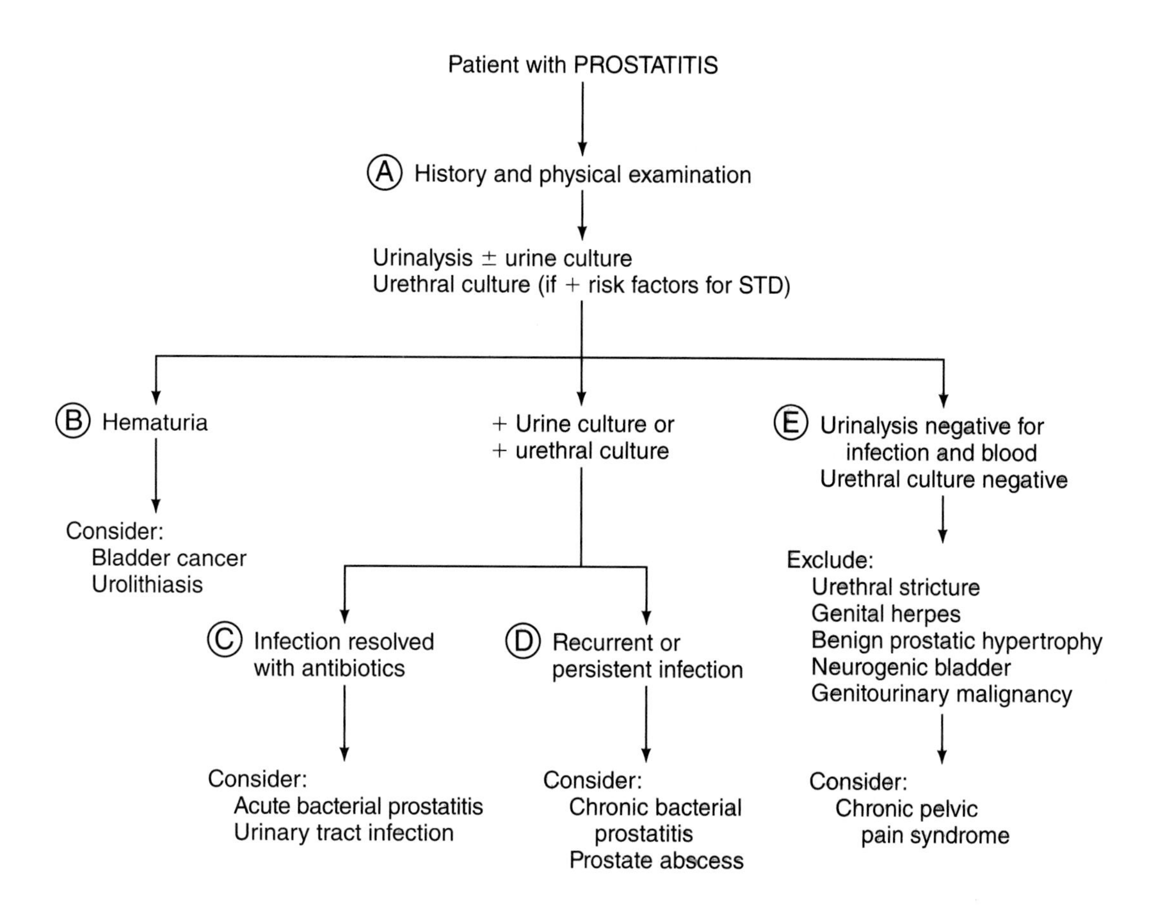
Patient with PROSTATITIS
(A) History and physical examination
Urinalysis ± urine culture
Urethral culture (if + risk factors for STD)
(B) Hematuria
Consider:
Bladder cancer
Urolithiasis
+ Urine culture or
+ urethral culture
(C) Infection resolved
with antibiotics
Consider:
Acute bacterial prostatitis
Urinary tract infection
(D) Recurrent or
persistent infection
Consider:
Chronic bacterial
prostatitis
Prostate abscess
(E) Urinalysis negative for
infection and blood
Urethral culture negative
Exclude:
Urethral stricture
Genital herpes
Benign prostatic hypertrophy
Neurogenic bladder
Genitourinary malignancy
Consider:
Chronic pelvic
pain syndrome

URINARY INCONTINENCE

Stephen B. Williams, MD, and Graeme Steele, MD, FCS, FACS

Urinary incontinence is an important health problem and affects 10 million patients to some degree. Approximately 50% of patients in nursing homes are affected by urinary incontinence, and >$15–$20 billion is spent annually on management of this problem. There are four types of urinary incontinence: stress, urge, overflow, and mixed.

When approaching a patient with questionable urinary incontinence it is imperative to obtain a thorough history and physical examination. Cystometry may help confirm your clinical suspicion but is not absolute, especially if the urinary symptoms are not reproduced during the study. Treatment differs between each type of urinary incontinence; therefore, it is imperative to make the correct diagnosis.

A. Stress incontinence results from an anatomic defect or weakness in the pelvic floor that results in poor support and hypermobility of the urethra. The sphincteric mechanism itself is intact (usually). The defect arises when the bladder undergoes filling/storage and the intravesical pressure exceeds intraurethral pressure as a result of excessive mobility of the urethra. The stages of stress urinary incontinence ascend from I and II depending on the degree of urethral hypermobility; stage III involves an associated defect in the intrinsic sphincter.

   Diagnosis starts with the history and physical examination with patients reporting urinary leakage on activities that results in increased intraabdominal pressure. Leakage tends to occur with coughing, sneezing, and/or Valsalva. Information about routine past medical/surgical history, medications, and diet may be useful. As with most patients with urinary symptoms, we recommend sending the serum for basic chemistry if one is not on file and the urine for urinalysis and urine culture to rule out any associated urinary tract infection. Physical examination is important to rule out any associated cystocele, rectocele, or prolapse. Neurologic examination also may be helpful. If there is continued suspicion for stress incontinence, the patient should undergo cystometry, which should include a cystogram and urodynamic analysis. Cystometry will help look at the anatomy and the physiology of both the urethra and sphincteric mechanism.

   Treatment for stress urinary incontinence is surgical and is centered around restoring the normal integrity of the pelvic floor support. This can be accomplished by the Marshall-Marchetti-Krantz suprapubic approach and the modified Burch procedure, which fixes the anterior vaginal wall to Cooper's ligament. Other techniques include a variety of vaginal suspension procedures that tend to rely on sutures placed paravaginally, which are secured in the suprapubic area and tied over the rectus sheath. Sling procedures have become popular; they use either cadaveric tissues for support or, most commonly, synthetic material. The sling procedures may be used with sphincter damage and combined cystocele repair, depending on the type of system used. Of mention, another less invasive tool in patients not suitable for surgery is the pessary.

B. True urge incontinence is defined as detrusor instability with normal intrinsic sphincter function, no neuropathy, and normal anatomy. As with stress incontinence, history and physical examination supported by cystometry will help elucidate urge urinary incontinence. The patient usually reports inability to hold urine long enough to void in an appropriate place on a repetitive basis. The most common causes of urge incontinence include age, inhibition of neurologic control of micturition (spinal abnormality, stroke), and bladder irritation (infection, inflammation, cancer, hematuria, stones). If urinalysis shows microscopic hematuria, then an evaluation, which should include urine cytology, imaging, and cystoscopy to identify the source of bleeding, should be initiated. Based on urodynamics and pressure/flow studies, one may sometimes find uninhibited detrusor contractions during bladder filling.

   On the results of the urodynamic study, treatment focuses on decreasing these uninhibited contractions, most commonly with antimuscarinic agents. Side effects differ among different medications, and the physician and patient must tailor which medication and dose provide the best symptomatic relief with the fewest side effects. The final treatment for urge incontinence may include surgery with either sacral nerve modulation or augmentation cystoplasty.

C. Overflow incontinence is not true incontinence and usually results from an obstructive or neuropathic lesion. History and physical examination usually reveal impaired detrusor contraction, bladder outlet obstructive symptoms (decreased force of stream, urgency, terminal dribbling), or both, but also may reveal irritative symptoms (frequency, nocturia, dysuria). Uroflow and postvoid residual will guide the suspicion for bladder outlet obstruction; however, urodynamics will help confirm the diagnosis.

   Treatment of the underlying cause of the obstruction will treat the overall incontinence. For example, classically the patient will have an enlarged prostate, and treatment for the enlarged prostate (type I alpha blocker and type II 5-alpha reductase inhibitors) will help resolve the overflow incontinence. Agents that decrease bladder contractility should be avoided.

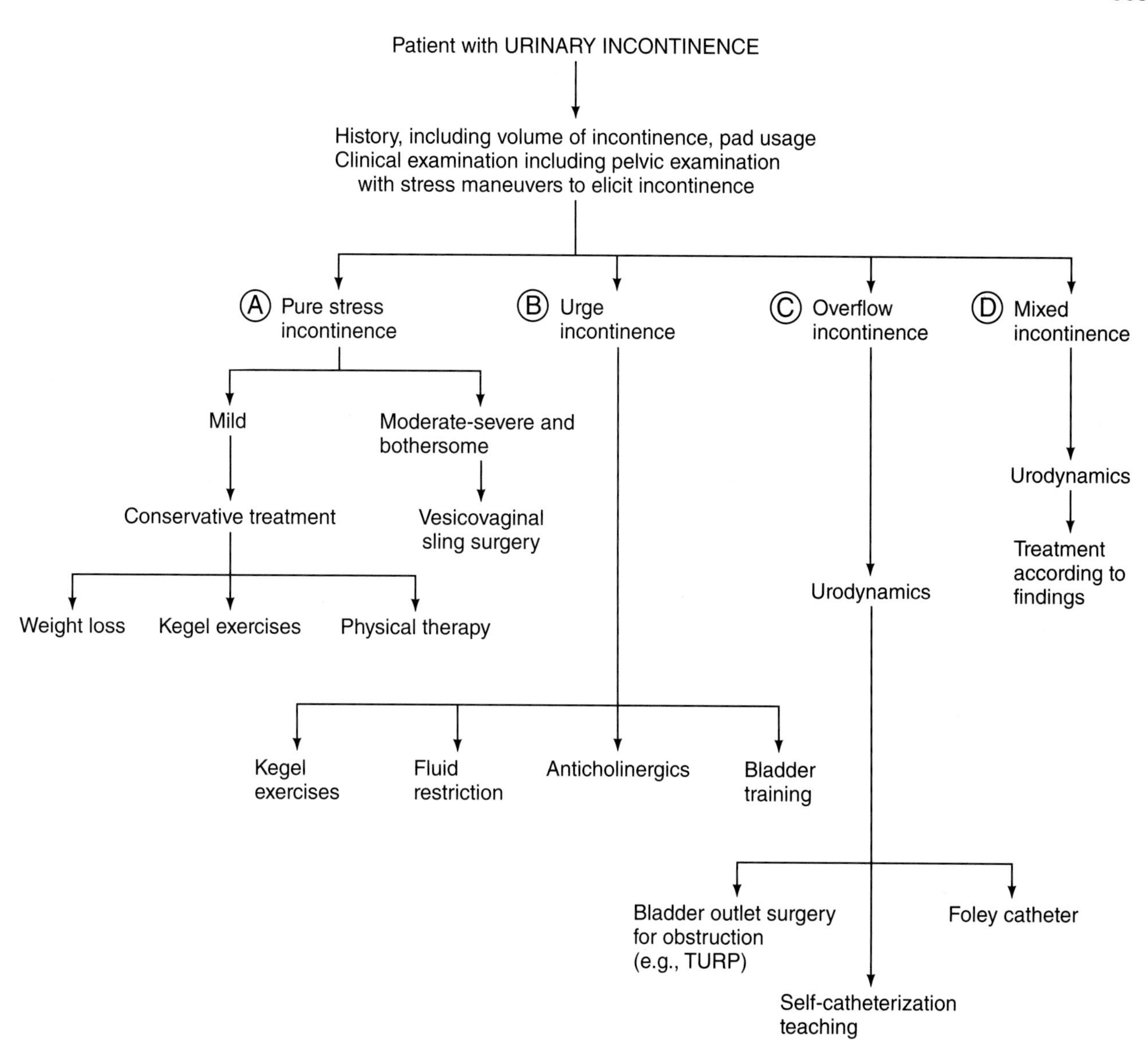

TURP, Transurethral resection of the prostate.

D. Mixed incontinence often involves detrusor overactivity (urgency) associated with urethral hypermobility/ urethral intrinsic sphincter dysfunction (stress). History and physical examination supported by cystometry will help elucidate the severity of mixed incontinence and what is likely contributing to the overall incontinence. Treatment is based on the severity and type of symptoms.

References

Abrams P, Cardozo L, Fall M, et al. The standardisation of terminology of lower urinary tract function: Report from the Standardisation Subcommittee of the International Continence Society. Neurourol Urodyn 2002;21:167.

Burgio KL, Goode PS, Locher JL, et al. Behavioral training with and without biofeedback in the treatment of urge incontinence in older women: a randomized controlled trial. JAMA 2002;288:2293.

Diokno AC. Diagnostic categories of incontinence and the role of urodynamic testing. J Am Geriatr Soc 1990;38:300.

DuBeau CE. Interpreting the effect of common medical conditions on voiding dysfunction in the elderly. Urol Clin North Am 1996;23:11.

Harris SS, Link CL, Tennstedt SL, et al. Care seeking and treatment for urinary incontinence in a diverse population. J Urol 2007;177:680.

Resnick NM. Voiding dysfunction in the elderly. In Yalla SV, McGuire EJ, Elbadawi A, et al, eds. Neurourology and urodynamics: principles and practice. New York: MacMillan, 1984:303.

Sze EH, Jones WP, Ferguson JL, et al. Prevalence of urinary incontinence symptoms among black, white, and Hispanic women. Obstet Gynecol 2002;99:572.

Taub DA, Hollenbeck BK, Wei JT, et al. Complications following surgical intervention for stress urinary incontinence: a national perspective. Neurourol Urodyn 2005;24:659.

URINARY RETENTION

Glen W. Barrisford, MD, and Graeme Steele, MD, FCS, FACS

Acute urinary retention (AUR) is urinary retention that develops in a rapid manner. Among urologic emergencies, AUR is the most commonly encountered. The most frequent etiology is benign prostatic hyperplasia (BPH), and the typical patient is >60 years. The typical clinical course of BPH is progression over time. In men >70 years, approximately 1 in 10 will develop AUR over a 5-year period.

Increased life expectancy among men has resulted in a similarly increased incidence of BPH and related disorders. As a consequence, it is important for medical professionals to become familiar with the risk factors/etiology associated with and the initial management of AUR. Risk factors, acute management, and medical and surgical therapy will be reviewed.

Most commonly, retention of urine develops secondary to an obstructive process. Obstructive pathology includes BPH, malignancy, urethral stricture, urolithiasis, phimosis, and paraphimosis. However, the use of medications, trauma, neurologic disease, infection, and (infrequently) psychological pathology can be the source of urinary retention.

A great deal of research has focused on the identification of risk factors associated with the development of urinary retention. The following factors are considered the most well established.

- Age: Age >70 years carries a relative risk (RR) of 7.8 for the development of urinary retention.
- Symptom score: The American Urological Association (AUA) symptom score is a method used to quantify one's symptoms. This questionnaire is easy to complete and considers seven components (frequency, urgency, nocturia, weak stream, intermittency of stream, straining to void, and incomplete emptying). Each component is scored from 0 to 5 (5 being the most severe). A maximum score of 35 can be obtained. A score of 7 represents an RR of 3.2 for the development of urinary retention. Repeated administrations of this survey can be used to follow progression over time.
- Prostate volume: Prostatic volumes >30 ml as measured by transrectal ultrasound have been associated with an RR of 3.0.
- Urinary flow rate: Urinary flow rate of <12 ml/sec carries an RR of 3.9.

A. AUR commonly presents with the inability to pass urine and lower abdominal/suprapubic discomfort. Patients can present with notable distress. Conversely, chronic urinary retention can develop over a substantial period of time with progressive obstruction or bladder dysfunction. These patients are often less severely affected and are often without discomfort.

Patients with urinary retention often will present to the emergency department or to the office of a primary physician. Patients are unlikely to present initially to a urologist, so it is imperative for health care professionals to be familiar with the initial management.

The initial evaluation should focus on relevant medical and surgical history with particular attention to a history of prior episodes of retention, prior urologic surgery, prior radiation, or trauma. Additional relevant information includes hematuria, dysuria, fever, back pain, and a list of medications. The physical examination should focus on the following elements:

- Abdominal palpation: Palpation of the lower abdomen can reveal a palpable bladder and often can provoke great discomfort.
- Rectal examination: Rectal masses, impaction of stool, and perineal sensation/reflexes should be evaluated. Examination of the prostate gland to evaluate for malignancy or prostatitis should be performed. However, a prostate with a normal consistency and size does not rule out obstructive pathology.
- Pelvic examination: Urinary retention in females can be a sign of pelvic malignancy or severe pelvic floor weakness.
- Laboratory evaluation: Urine should be sent for routine urinalysis and culture (usually after catheter placement). Additionally, studies should be performed according to the clinical scenario.

B. The initial management of AUR involves prompt bladder decompression. This can be accomplished with urethral or suprapubic catheterization. Although there are no uniform guidelines for bladder decompression, most urologists prefer urethral catheterization for the initial management of AUR. Because patients with AUR more often present to a medical office or emergency department than to a urology office, clinician comfort with urethral catheterization is likely to greatly exceed suprapubic (SP) catheterization.

Placement of an SP catheter is sometimes necessary in patients with urethral stricture disease, severe BPH, or other anatomic abnormalities that preclude Foley catheter placement per urethra. SP catheters are usually placed by an urologist, but they may be placed by others on an emergency basis. Ultrasound guidance may be indicated when adhesions are possible from prior abdominal surgery.

We prefer SP catheters in patients, especially females, who are expected to require long-term bladder drainage. SP catheters prevent bladder neck and urethral dilation and therefore prevent urinary incontinence resulting from sphincter dysfunction. Furthermore, SP catheters for men avoid the risk of subsequent urethral stricture, a common complication in men requiring long-term urethral catheterization.

(Continued on page 572)

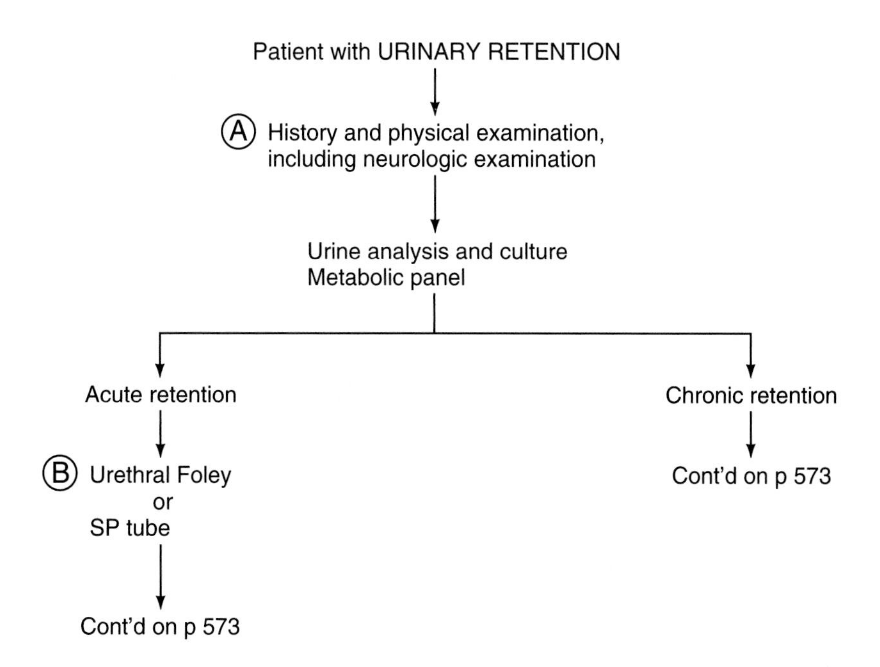
Patient with URINARY RETENTION
(A) History and physical examination, including neurologic examination
Urine analysis and culture
Metabolic panel
Acute retention
Chronic retention
(B) Urethral Foley
or
SP tube
Cont'd on p 573
Cont'd on p 573

C. Clean intermittent catheterization (CIC) as a decompression strategy has been advocated, with data suggesting improvement in the rate of spontaneous voiding and reduction in urinary infections when compared to indwelling catheters. Although this option is associated with a reduction in complications when compared to indwelling catheter placement, it is associated with certain disadvantages including patient preference, nursing time (inpatients/nursing home), and ongoing care and management (supplies, etc.). However, this option still represents a solution superior to an indwelling catheter and should be advocated when possible.

In the past, it was recommended that initial urine drainage be limited to 500–1000 ml to reduce the complications of transient hematuria, hypotension, and postobstructive diuresis. Current practice has recognized that partial drainage and clamping are not necessary with AUR and may increase the risk for urinary tract infection. Rapid complete bladder decompression can be conducted safely, provided prudent supportive care is available and special attention is given to patients who are elderly or infirm.

Once the bladder is safely decompressed, consideration must be given to hospital admission versus outpatient management. Hospitalization is indicated for patients who are uroseptic or have obstruction related to malignancy or spinal cord compression. The majority of patients can be managed on an outpatient basis after bladder drainage. Prophylactic antibiotics are not routinely indicated unless suspicion exists for a urinary infection at the time of drainage. Additional instructions regarding catheter and drainage bag management should be given prior to discharge.

Emergent surgical therapy rarely is recommended because it tends to be associated with a greater risk of complication or death as compared to bladder decompression and delayed surgical intervention. In rare instances, a prostatic abscess is diagnosed and drained via transurethral resection or transrectal ultrasound guidance. This will often relieve both urinary retention and septic sequelae.

D. Following an initial episode of urinary retention, a patient can be given a trial without a catheter ("voiding trial"). This usually occurs 2–3 days following catheter placement. Successful voiding is reported in 20%–40% of patients. The optimal duration of catheterization prior to removal has been evaluated with contradictory findings. A detailed discussion is beyond the scope of this section. However, in practice we often use an interval between 3 and 14 days, depending on the clinical circumstances.

Several factors favor voiding after catheter removal. These factors include age <65 years, detrusor pressure >35 cm H_2O, a drained volume of <1 L at initial bladder decompression, and the identification of a precipitating event. Prior to the era of medical intervention for obstructive voiding, studies determined that 50% of patients who initially voided on catheter removal developed another episode of AUR within 1 week and 67% would develop a second episode within 1 year.

E. The two main classes of drugs used in the treatment of BPH are alpha blockers and 5-alpha reductase inhibitors. Alpha blockers function to relieve the mechanical obstruction associated with BPH by relaxation of the smooth muscle at the bladder neck and the prostatic capsule. The use of alpha blockers in patients with AUR prior to catheter removal has a beneficial effect on a voiding trial. A variety of alpha blockers (terazosin, doxazosin, tamsulosin) are presently available with similar efficacy and side effect profiles. 5-Alpha reductase inhibitors (finasteride, dutasteride) provide selective blockade for the conversion of testosterone to dihydrotestosterone. This effectively reduces the prostatic volume over time. Medications in this category decrease the incidence of AUR in men with BPH. Additionally, 5-alpha reductase inhibitors do not have a role in the acute management of AUR because several weeks of therapy are required before optimal efficacy.

F. Surgical therapy remains the definitive treatment of AUR. Among symptomatic patients with BPH, transurethral resection of the prostate (TURP) reduces the risk of developing AUR by 85%–90%. TURP remains the gold standard, although a variety of other modalities are available. The common goal remains the endoscopic ablation of prostatic tissue thought to be the source of the obstruction.

With respect to the timing of surgery, the general recommendation is to wait ≥30 days following an episode of AUR. Patients who undergo TURP immediately following an episode of AUR are at a greatly increased risk of complications, including intraoperative bleeding and sepsis.

In our view, all patients being evaluated for surgical intervention following an episode of AUR require urodynamic evaluation to determine whether retention is directly related to outlet obstruction, with concomitant elevation in bladder pressures or to an inefficient bladder muscle. Patients with bladder impairment are unlikely to benefit from a surgical procedure aimed at reducing outlet resistance.

The use of urethral stenting provides only modest improvement and is associated with a variety of complications, including stent migration, infection, encrustation, and calculus formation. This modality is presently reserved for patients unfit for more invasive surgical intervention.

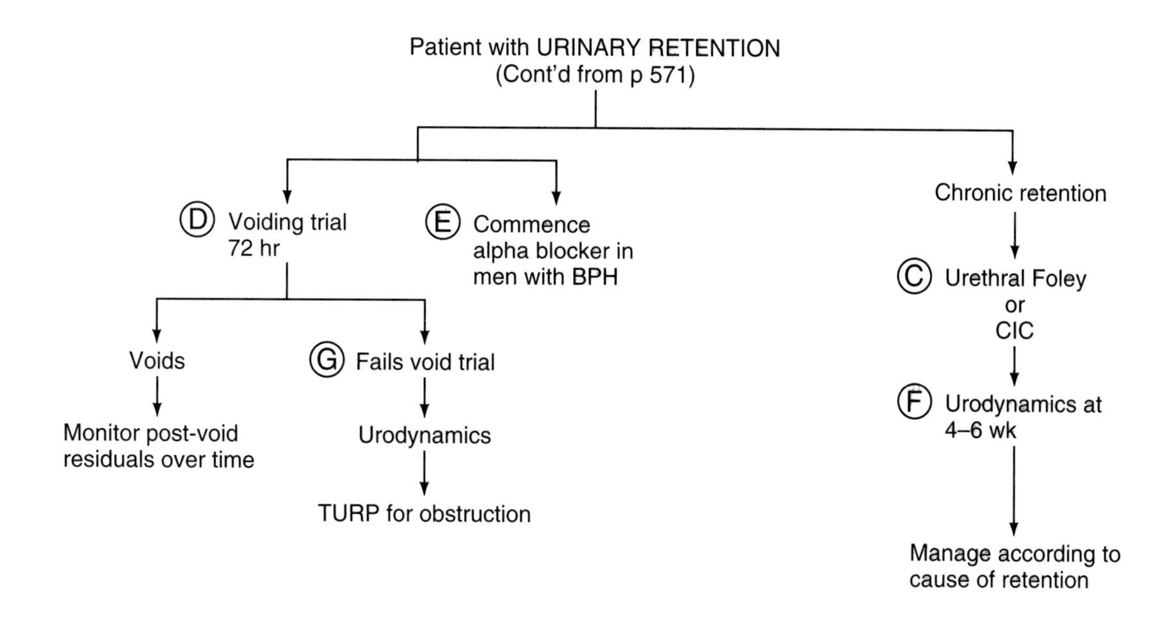

References

Choong S, Emberton M. Acute urinary retention. BJU Int 2000;85(2):186–201.

Contemporary Urology. Urology Times 2005 Fact Book. 2005. Advanstar Medical Economics Healthcare Communications Secondary Research Services.

Curtis LA, Dolan TS, Cespedes RD. Acute urinary retention and urinary incontinence. Emerg Med Clin North Am 2001;19(3):591–619.

Emberton M, Anson K. Acute urinary retention in men: an age old problem. BMJ 1999;318(7188):921–925.

Fong YK, Milani S, Djavan B. Natural history and clinical predictors of clinical progression in benign prostatic hyperplasia. Curr Opin Urol 2005;15(1):35–38.

Jacobsen SJ, Jacobson DJ, Girman CJ, et al. Natural history of prostatism: risk factors for acute urinary retention. J Urol 1997;158(2):481–487.

Murray K, Massey A, Feneley RC. Acute urinary retention—a urodynamic assessment. Br J Urol 1984;56(5):468–473.

Powell PH, Smith PJ, Feneley RC. The identification of patients at risk from acute retention. Br J Urol 1980;52(6):520–522.

Thomas K, Chow K, Kirby RS. Acute urinary retention: a review of the aetiology and management. Prostate Cancer Prostatic Dis 2004;7(1):32–37.

WOMEN'S HEALTH

Stuart B. Mushlin, MD, FACP, FACR
Section Editor

VAGINAL DISCHARGE

Amir Nasseri, MD

A. Vulvovaginitis is the most common complaint necessitating a gynecologic examination. It commonly is defined as inflammation of the vulva and vagina. The diagnosis is often evident from the history. Upon initial evaluation, obtain a thorough history of previous episodes; possible sexual exposure; odor, color, and consistency of the discharge; and whether the discharge is causing itching. Pay particular attention to factors that can change vaginal flora, thus leading to vaginitis (recent use of antibiotic, oral contraceptives, or spermicides; douching). Also consider systemic conditions (poorly controlled diabetes, menopause, AIDS).

B. The cause of the vaginitis often can be determined at the time of speculum examination. Prepare two wet mounts using 10% potassium hydroxide (KOH) and normal saline and view them under low and high power. Appearance of the discharge often can be helpful in diagnosis: bacterial vaginosis (BV) gives a gray-white appearance; *Trichomonas vaginalis,* a profuse, watery, white green or yellow appearance; and *Candida,* a white cheesy discharge. Determining the pH of the vaginal discharge using pH indicator paper can be most useful. Normal physiologic discharge and yeast usually are <4.5; >5.0 may indicate *Trichomonas* or bacterial vaginosis.

C. If wet mount is nondiagnostic, consider allergic reaction to chemical or physical irritants. These possibilities are numerous and include tight clothing, deodorants, laundry detergent, soaps, tampons, and spermicides. Obtain culture for *Neisseria gonorrhoeae* and *Chlamydia trachomatis* in sexually active patients, and base treatment on subsequent results. Viral causes of vulvovaginitis include human papillomavirus (HPV) and herpes simplex virus (HSV). These often are diagnosed by appearance but can be confirmed by biopsy and culture. Aphthous ulcers can also occur on the vulva with an appearance similar to HSV.

D. The appearance of the unicellular protozoan *T. vaginalis* is diagnostic. Culture is not necessary for confirmation. The appearance under high power is of mobile flagellated organisms slightly larger than a white blood cell. The smear also may have many inflammatory cells and vaginal epithelial cells.

Both the patient and sexual partner must be treated with metronidazole given as a one-time 2-g dose or 500 mg twice a day for 7 days. Patients who are compliant, not reexposed to male partners, and fail initial therapy may be given 1 g of metronidazole twice a day orally along with 500 mg of metronidazole twice a day intravaginally for 7–14 days. (The 2-g dose is contraindicated in the first trimester of pregnancy.) Patients should avoid alcohol ingestion while taking metronidazole.

E. A thin gray-white discharge with an unpleasant odor ("musty" or "fishy") often is caused by *Gardnerella vaginalis,* a gram-variable coccobacillus. The normal saline wet mount often shows "clue cells": stippled epithelial cells (*Gardnerella* organisms adhered to the epithelial cells). Treatment consists of oral metronidazole 500 mg twice daily for 7 days or oral clindamycin 300 mg twice daily for 7 days. Local regimens provide similar response and are associated with fewer systemic side effects; these consist of 0.75% metronidazole gel inserted twice daily for 5 days or 2% clindamycin cream nightly for 7 nights. In cases of recurrence, empirically switch to a different agent (e.g., from metronidazole to clindamycin). If recurrence persists, extended intravaginal therapy with either metronidazole or clindamycin daily for 3 weeks followed by intravaginal therapy every third day for an additional 3 weeks may be warranted, allowing lactobacilli to recolonize the vagina. Treatment of the partner is controversial.

F. Significant vulvar pruritus is the usual presenting symptom of vaginal yeast infections. The appearance of filamentous forms (pseudohyphae, which are thin, greenish, segmented, and branched) and blastospores on KOH wet mount can confirm clinical suspicion. Many equally effective topical treatment regimens are available, including clotrimazole 1% cream, one applicator (5 g) per vagina every night for 7 nights or miconazole, 200-mg suppositories at bedtime for 3 nights. The cream should also be applied to the vulva for pruritus. An alternative to topical therapy is a one-time dose of 150 mg oral fluconazole. If necessary, this dose can be repeated in 1 week. Studies show a single dose of oral fluconazole to be as effective as intravaginal suppositories. Some patients prefer this single oral dose because of its low rate of side effects, route of administration, and cost-effectiveness.

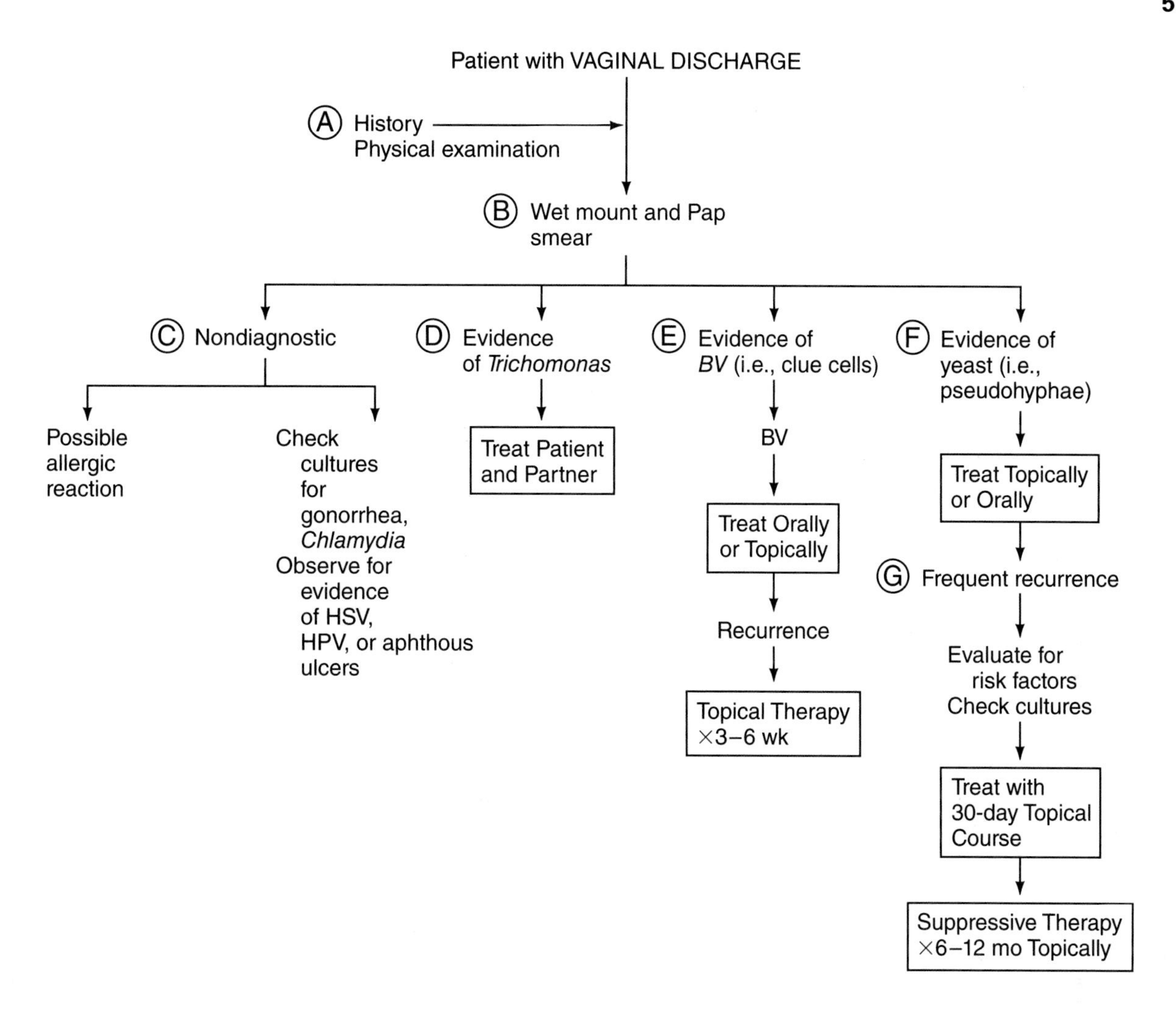

G. Recurrent yeast infection can be frustrating for both practitioner and patient. Obtain culture of the discharge on Sabouraud's or Nickerson's medium to confirm the cause as yeast. Evaluate for other complicating factors, including evidence of diabetes, immunodeficiency (AIDS), or reinfection from partner (10%–15% of male sexual partners of women with yeast infections have had positive oral, rectal, and seminal cultures). Treatment options are varied and include topical therapy for 30 days, and 200 mg of ketoconazole by mouth twice daily for 14 days. *Candida albicans* is the cause of monilial vulvovaginitis in >90% of cases, but occasionally *Torulopsis glabrata* can be a cause of resistant yeast. A 3- to 7-day course of terconazole often eliminates the organism.

In many cases, however, suppressive rather than curative therapy is in order. A daily 100-mg dose of ketoconazole orally for 6 months may be used, but this must be weighed against the possibility of liver toxicity. Alternatively, topical therapy for 6–12 months using biweekly application of boric acid or an azole may decrease the frequency of recurrence. (Boric acid, oral fluconazole, and ketoconazole should not be used during pregnancy.)

References

American College of Obstetricians and Gynecologists. Vulvovaginitis. ACOG Technical Bulletin No. 135. Washington, DC, 1989, American College of Obstetricians and Gynecologists.

Quilligan EJ, Zuspan FP. Current Therapy in Obstetrics and Gynecology, 5th ed. Philadelphia:WB Saunders, 1999.

Sobel JD. Vaginal infections in adult women. Med Clin North Am 1990;74:1573.

Sobel JD, Brooker D, Stein GE, et al. Single dose fluconazole compared with conventional clotrimazole topical therapy of *Candida* vaginitis. Am J Obstet Gynecol 1995;172:1263.

Stenchever MA. Office Gynecology, 2nd ed. St. Louis:Mosby, 1996.

CERVICITIS

Hugh S. Miller, MD

A. Although acute cervicitis can result from trauma, malignancy, or systemic collagen vascular conditions, it is most commonly caused by infectious agents, notably *Neisseria gonorrhoeae, Chlamydia trachomatis,* and to a lesser extent herpes simplex virus (HSV). The epidemiology of these pathogens is similar, and 25%–45% of patients have concomitant infections. Assessing a patient's risk for cervical infection involves taking a careful history, including age at first sexual contact, number of sex partners, and history of previous sexually transmitted diseases (STDs) or pelvic inflammatory disease (PID). It is important to distinguish infections of the lower genital tract limited to the cervix (cervicitis) from those occurring in the vagina (vaginitis) or vulva (vulvitis) and from upper genital tract disease, such as PID. When cervicitis is associated with signs or symptoms of systemic disease, including fever, lower abdominal pain, or pelvic pain, consider PID as an additional diagnosis. Cervicitis generally is associated with mucopurulent discharge collected from the cervix and posterior vaginal fornix. Because the vaginal discharge associated with vaginitis often appears similar, it is prudent to evaluate the discharge for the common vaginal pathogens (candidal vaginitis, bacterial vaginosis, and *Trichomonas vaginalis*). For patients with a confirmed diagnosis of cervicitis who are at risk for STDs, offer screening for other STDs, including syphilis, HIV, and human papillomavirus (HPV), and Pap smear with reflexive HPV testing, if not screened in the past year.

B. Too often, lower abdominal pain in sexually active women prompts the diagnosis of PID without application of criteria to substantiate the diagnosis. Hager's criteria for diagnosing acute salpingitis are listed in Table 1. The severity of the illness determines whether outpatient care or hospitalization is appropriate. Inpatient parenteral regimens combine a broad-spectrum cephalosporin (cefoxitin or cefotetan) with tetracycline (doxycycline) or clindamycin with an aminoglycoside. The preferred outpatient regimen combines ceftriaxone with tetracycline (doxycycline), but quinolones (ofloxacin) can be combined with either metronidazole (Flagyl) or clindamycin. If pregnancy is possible, avoid tetracyclines and quinolones.

Table 1 Criteria for Diagnosing Acute Salpingitis

History of lower abdominal pain or tenderness, cervical motion tenderness, and adnexal tenderness

Plus one of the following objective findings:

- Fever (body temperature >38° C)
- Leukocytosis (WBC count >10,500/mm^3)
- Culdocentesis fluid containing WBCs or bacteria
- Inflammatory mass on pelvic examination or sonography
- Erythrocyte sedimentation rate >20 mm/hr
- Evidence of gonococcus or *Chlamydia* on cervical Gram stain

C. Cervical ulcerations often are accompanied by inguinal or vulvar adenopathy. Pain distinguishes HSV from syphilitic lesions in primary outbreaks. Primary genital HSV often involves the vulva, urethra, and cervix, progressing from multiple painful vesicles to ulcers in the presence of a systemic viremia. Recurrent HSV occurs in the presence of circulating antibodies and is associated with an infection of muted duration and intensity. Acyclovir is the mainstay of treatment and is particularly effective in primary infections in which early intervention significantly reduces viral shedding, accelerates healing, and hastens recovery. Because acyclovir therapy has been changed to less frequent dosing (400 mg three times a day) with proven efficacy, compliance is favored. Valacyclovir and famciclovir, two newer acyclic nucleoside derivatives, also may be considered for primary treatment of genital HSV. Syphilis, by contrast, usually manifests on the cervix in a primary infection; however, because it usually is asymptomatic, it is rarely diagnosed at this stage. Identification of the stage of infection plays a major role in determining the duration of treatment. Penicillin is the drug of choice, with almost no reported resistant strains.

D. When a growth is noted on the cervix in association with cervicitis and discharge, obtain a cervical biopsy specimen from the leading edge of the lesion to exclude endophytic cervical neoplasia. More commonly, a whitish exophytic lesion is associated with genital warts or HPV. These lesions by themselves usually represent an infectious process involving HPV serotypes 6 and 11. The HPV serotypes (16, 18, 31, 33, and 35) are recognized for their contribution to the neoplastic transformation that can promote cervical cancer. Application of 3% acetic acid to the cervix, along with colposcopically directed biopsies, enables distinction between infectious and neoplastic lesions. This distinction influences the choice of treatment. In rare instances tuberculous cervicitis manifests as a mucopurulent discharge or fungating mass. Diagnosis is made by cervical biopsy demonstrating caseating granulomas or acid-fast bacilli stain or culture.

(Continued on page 580)

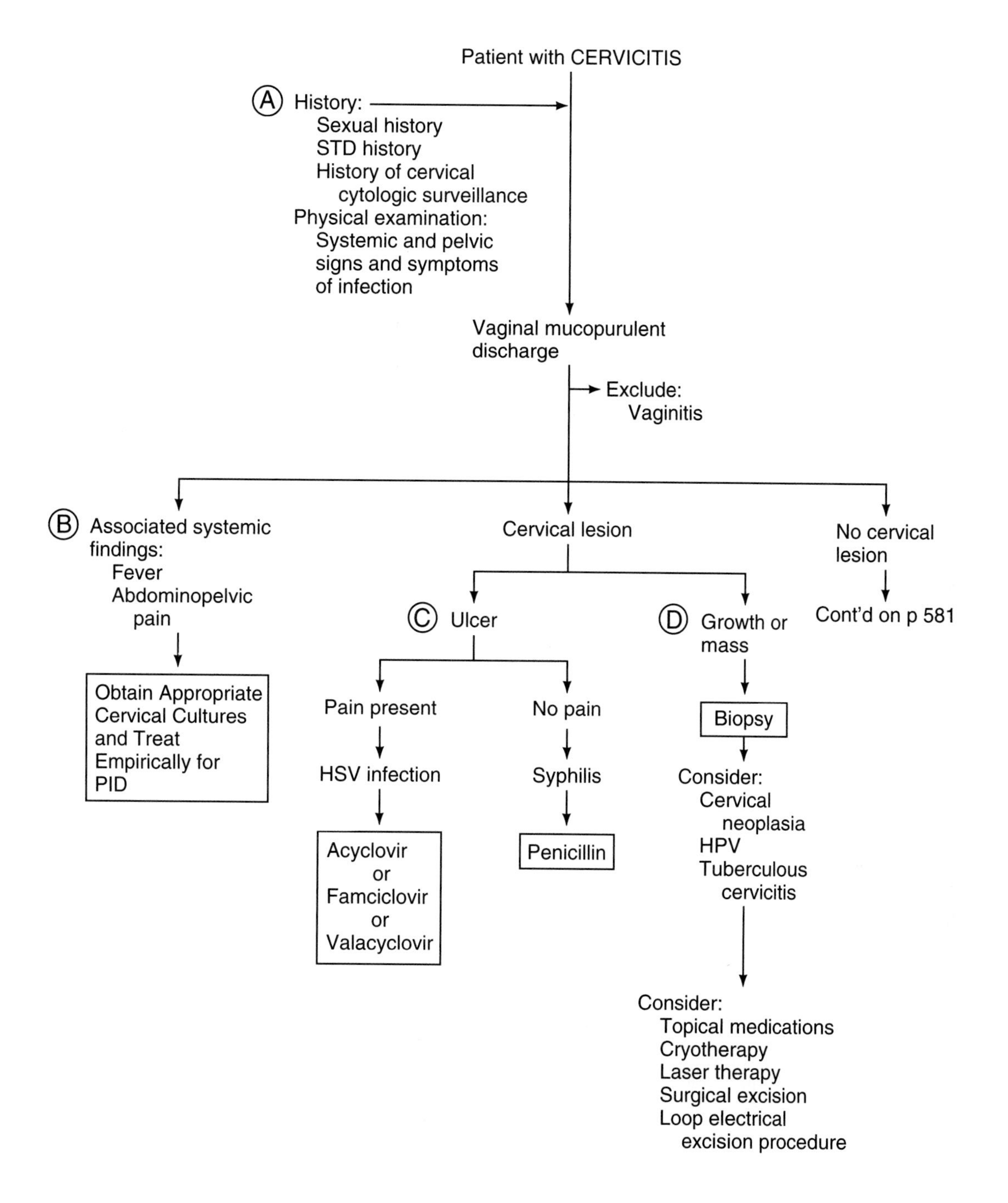
Patient with CERVICITIS
(A) History:
Sexual history
STD history
History of cervical cytologic surveillance
Physical examination:
Systemic and pelvic signs and symptoms of infection
Vaginal mucopurulent discharge
Exclude: Vaginitis
(B) Associated systemic findings:
Fever
Abdominopelvic pain
Obtain Appropriate Cervical Cultures and Treat Empirically for PID
Cervical lesion
(C) Ulcer
Pain present
HSV infection
Acyclovir or Famciclovir or Valacyclovir
No pain
Syphilis
Penicillin
(D) Growth or mass
Biopsy
Consider:
Cervical neoplasia
HPV
Tuberculous cervicitis
Consider:
Topical medications
Cryotherapy
Laser therapy
Surgical excision
Loop electrical excision procedure
No cervical lesion
Cont'd on p 581

E. Gonococcal endocervicitis manifests symptoms, including mucopurulent vaginal discharge, uterine bleeding, and dysuria, in 40%–60% of infections. The gold standard for the diagnosis is an endocervical culture plated on modified Thayer-Martin medium. More practical are newer rapid-assay techniques, such as Gonozyme. Also, DNA probes are now available that have similar accuracy to culture but have the convenience of not needing to be processed immediately, as do the cultures. Although procaine penicillin G, ampicillin, and amoxicillin continue to be effective, ceftriaxone 250 mg intramuscularly is preferred. The single treatment ensures compliance while simultaneously covering penicillinase-producing and chromosomally mediated resistant *N. gonorrhoeae.* Alternative treatments include fluoroquinolones (a single intramuscular dose of ciprofloxacin 500 mg, ofloxacin 400 mg, or levofloxacin 250 mg), although it must be noted that there is a rising incidence of quinolone-resistant strains. Although *Chlamydia* is the most prevalent sexually transmitted organism in the United States, acute cervical infection often is asymptomatic. *Chlamydia* is readily diagnosed by nucleic acid amplification. Direct culture, fluorescent monoclonal antibody staining, or enzyme-linked immunoassay (ELISA) is an alternative method of diagnosis. Both of these methods are comparable to culture in their specificity and sensitivity and are less expensive. Azithromycin 1 g as a single, observed dose is the preferred therapeutic regimen. Doxycycline 100 mg twice daily for 7 days is an alternative choice, although it is less preferred as a result of the problems with compliance and should be avoided in pregnancy. When both *N. gonorrhoeae* and *Chlamydia* are present, azithromycin 2 g as a single dose can be used alone. Because both *N. gonorrhoeae* and *Chlamydia* are reportable STDs, encourage patients to facilitate the evaluation and treatment of their sex partners. In some cases it may be helpful to obtain a test of cure to verify both patient compliance and microbial sensitivity.

References

ACOG Technical Bulletin. Gonorrhea and chlamydial infections. No. 19a. March 1994.

Drugs for sexually transmitted diseases. Med Lett Drugs Ther 1995;37:117.

Sweet RL, Gibbs RS. Infectious Diseases of the Female Genital Tract, ed 4. Philadelphia: Lippincott Williams & Wilkins, 2002.

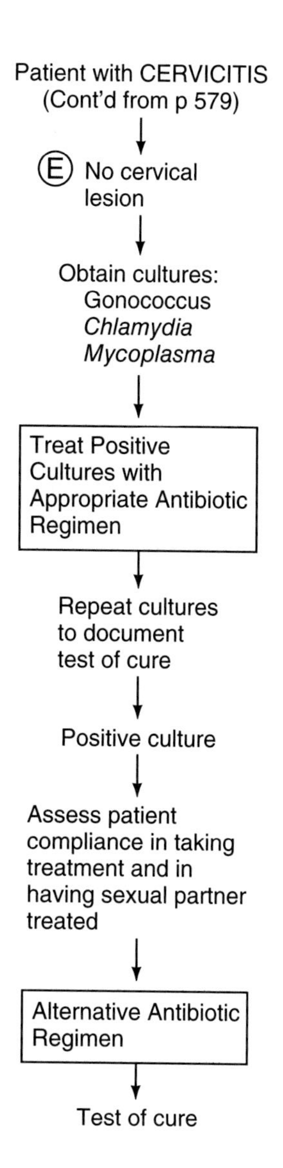
Patient with CERVICITIS
(Cont'd from p 579)
E
No cervical lesion
Obtain cultures:
Gonococcus
Chlamydia
Mycoplasma
Treat Positive Cultures with Appropriate Antibiotic Regimen
Repeat cultures to document test of cure
Positive culture
Assess patient compliance in taking treatment and in having sexual partner treated
Alternative Antibiotic Regimen
Test of cure

SECONDARY AMENORRHEA

Nancy A. Curosh, MD

Secondary amenorrhea is arbitrarily defined as the absence of menses for 6 months or the equivalent of three previous cycle intervals, whichever is longer, in women who previously had menses. Exclude physiologic amenorrheas, such as pregnancy, the immediate postpartum state, lactation, and menopause. It is helpful to consider secondary amenorrhea as an abnormality in one of four areas: the outflow tract, including the uterus, cervix, and vagina; the ovaries; the anterior pituitary; and the hypothalamus. Take a careful history, including questions concerning menstrual history, surgical procedures, medication use, changes in weight or diet, exercise patterns, a history of hot flashes, and medical illnesses. On physical examination, pay attention to body habitus, secondary sexual characteristics, evidence of androgen excess, galactorrhea, visual fields, and evidence of endocrinopathies, and do a thorough pelvic examination. If localizing signs or symptoms are found, the investigation can be channeled as appropriate.

A. About 20% of cases of secondary amenorrhea are caused by hyperprolactinemia. Although galactorrhea may indicate this diagnosis, its absence is not reassuring, and all patients should be screened with a serum prolactin level. A number of physiologic and pharmacologic events can alter prolactin levels. Elevation can occur from any stress—physical or emotional. In fact, the stress of a blood draw may increase the level slightly. Levels should not be drawn after a recent breast examination because breast stimulation can increase prolactin. Prolactin also can be increased by many medications, including oral contraceptives, estrogens, phenothiazines, tricyclic antidepressants, metoclopramide, and benzodiazepines. The serum prolactin usually is <100 ng/ml if from one of these causes. If levels remain elevated after excluding these, investigate further.

B. The progestin challenge test is used to assess the endogenous estrogen level and the competence of the outflow tract; 10 mg medroxyprogesterone acetate (Provera) is given by mouth for 5 days. Withdrawal bleeding should occur within 2 days to 2 weeks if there is a sufficient estrogen level and a competent outflow tract. Any amount of bleeding is considered a positive test, but mild spotting implies low estrogen levels, and an evaluation for causes of hypoestrogenism is warranted. The presence of estrogen suggests that the major components of the hypothalamic, pituitary, ovarian, and uterine pathways are at least minimally functioning. The diagnosis of anovulation is made. Management of anovulation depends on whether the patient currently desires pregnancy or contraception. Because chronic unopposed estrogen can induce endometrial hyperplasia, the patient should receive progestin therapy (either in the form of oral contraceptive pills or cyclical progestin) to induce endometrial shedding on a regular basis.

C. If there is no withdrawal bleeding after a progestin challenge, there is either an outflow tract problem or insufficient estrogen. An estrogen-progestin challenge test can help differentiate between these two problems. Orally active estrogen is given to stimulate endometrial proliferation. An appropriate dose is 2.5 mg of conjugated estrogens daily for 21–25 days. A progestational agent (10 mg Provera) is given for the last 5–10 days to induce withdrawal. If no withdrawal bleeding occurs, there is a problem with the outflow tract, such as Asherman's syndrome or active endometritis. In a patient with a normal pelvic examination and no history of pelvic infections or trauma, including curettage, the estrogen-progestin challenge test may be eliminated.

D. Hypothalamic amenorrhea is the most common cause of secondary amenorrhea, occurring in approximately 60% of cases. It is most likely caused by a defect in the pattern of pulsatile gonadotropin-releasing hormone (GnRH) secretion. Hypothalamic amenorrhea is a diagnosis of exclusion, but clearly there are groups in which this occurs frequently, such as in patients with anorexia nervosa, strenuous exercisers, and patients under stress. If possible, the precipitating circumstances should be dealt with and eliminated. Often, reassurance and time is all that is needed. Follow these patients closely to ensure that nothing has been overlooked. If there is no evidence for an eating disorder, weight loss, or stress, MRI should be ordered to rule out a pituitary tumor. Consider estrogen replacement if the amenorrhea is not resolved in a reasonable time. If fertility is desired, clomiphene, Pergonal, and GnRH are often effective.

E. If luteinizing hormone (LH) and follicle-stimulating hormone (FSH) levels are high, ovarian failure is the most likely explanation. Patients <35 years should undergo karyotyping. If any portion of a Y chromosome is found, the chance of a gonadal malignancy is greatly increased. In rare circumstances, LH and FSH are elevated but the ovaries contain follicles (resistant ovary syndrome). However, in most cases, if the gonadotropins are elevated, premature ovarian failure can be diagnosed. Premature ovarian failure can be caused by autoimmune disease; consider and investigate this as appropriate. If the etiology of the ovarian failure is autoimmune, adrenal and thyroid function should also be tested. If there are no contraindications, hormonal replacement therapy should be used in premature ovarian failure to avoid the long-term sequelae of estrogen deficiency.

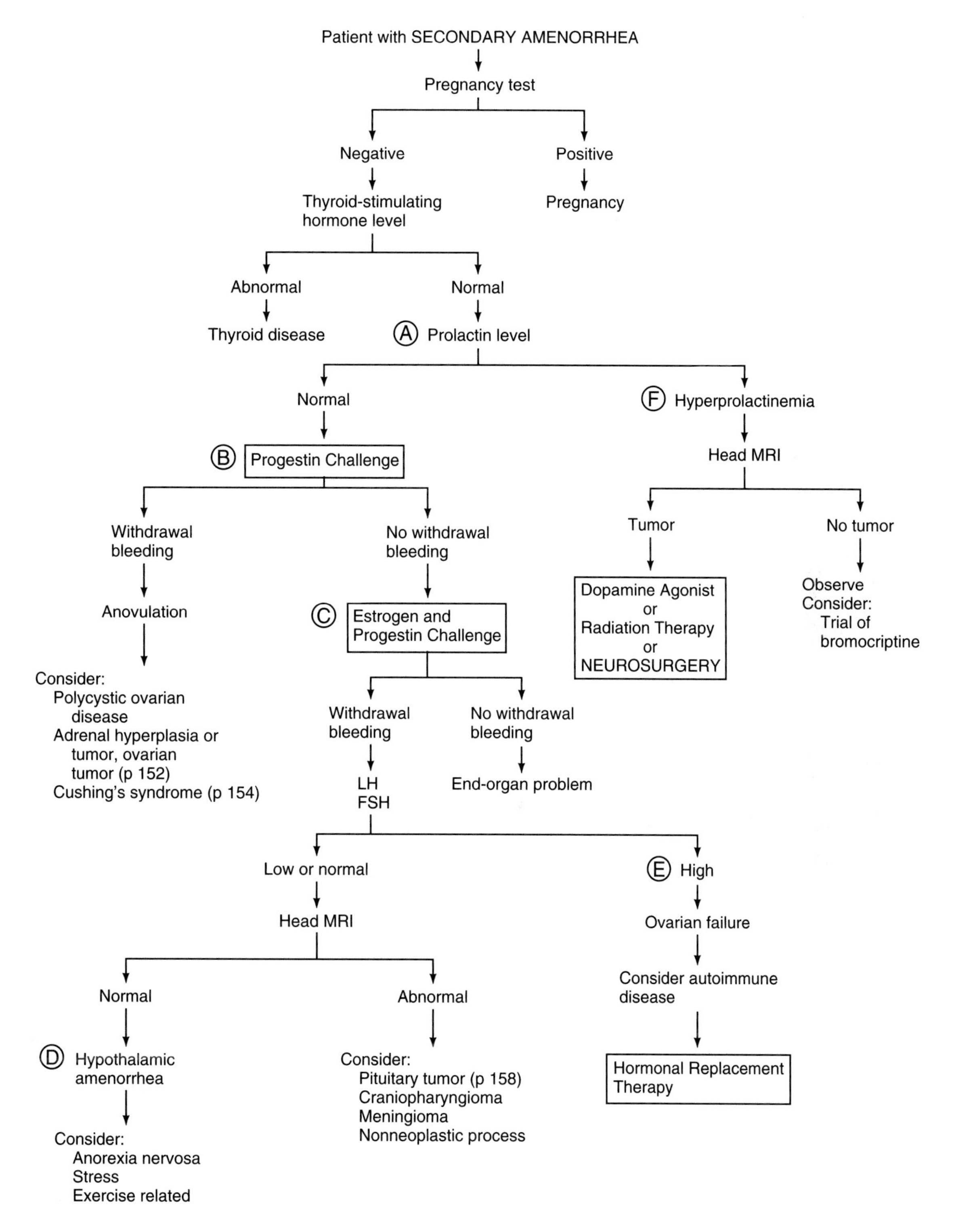

F. Hyperprolactinemia warrants MRI of the head. Various tumors, such as craniopharyngiomas and meningiomas, may cause hyperprolactinemia, but pituitary adenomas are the most common. Dopamine agonists, radiation therapy, and neurosurgery are therapeutic options for pituitary adenomas, depending on the size and extension of the tumor and the presence of symptoms. Excellent results usually are obtained with bromocriptine. Often, no tumor is found and careful observation is warranted. Consider a trial of bromocriptine, particularly if fertility is desired.

References

Malo JW, Bezdicek BJ. Secondary amenorrhea: a protocol for pinpointing the underlying cause. Postgrad Med 1986;79:86.

Scommegna A, Carson SA. Secondary amenorrhea and the menopause. In Gold JJ, Josimovich JB, eds. Gynecologic Endocrinology, ed 4. New York: Plenum, 1987:369.

Soulez B, DeWailly D, et al. Polycystic ovary syndrome: a multidisciplinary challenge. Endocrinologist 1996;6:1.

Speroff L, Glass RH, Kase NG. Clinical Gynecologic Endocrinology and Infertility, ed 6. Philadelphia: Lippincott Williams & Wilkins, 1999.

Warren MP. Amenorrhea in endurance runners. J Clin Endocrinol Metab 1992;75:6.

ABNORMAL VAGINAL BLEEDING

Hugh S. Miller, MD

A. Significant abnormal vaginal bleeding not emanating from the uterus is uncommon and usually is discerned from a careful history and physical examination. The initial assessment should exclude genitourinary (hematuria) and GI (hematochezia) etiologies, allowing one to concentrate on genital etiologies, predominantly uterine. Abnormal perimenarchal and early perimenopausal bleeding usually is hormonally mediated, although bleeding characteristics may vary widely. Conversely, late perimenopausal and postmenopausal bleeding is more likely to be related to a neoplastic process that is not necessarily malignant. Women at high risk for genital tract cancer can be identified through a detailed obstetric, gynecologic, and medical history (endocrine disorders, pituitary tumors, and blood dyscrasias) that includes menstrual history, contraceptive use, exposure to sexually transmitted diseases (STDs), history of premalignant conditions of the cervix or uterus, human papillomavirus (HPV) infection, obesity, and preexisting malignancy.

B. The complete physical examination permits exclusion of extragenital tract etiologies, although they lend further support to a potential endocrine or hematologic cause if thyromegaly or diffuse petechiae are present. Pelvic examination is essential to localize the source of bleeding through identification of lesions or other significant pathologic conditions (i.e., polyps, uterine fibroids, or pelvic masses). The Pap smear, obtained before bimanual examination, is essential in screening for cervical cancer and occasionally suggests the presence of cervicitis or higher genital tract neoplasias. Collect appropriate cultures in patients identified by history to be at significant risk for STDs. Test all women of reproductive age for pregnancy, regardless of menstrual history, by urine human chorionic gonadotropin (hCG) testing because pregnancy is the most common cause of abnormal vaginal bleeding. When bleeding is significant or persistent, obtain a CBC to determine anemia and rule out coagulopathies or occult hematologic malignancies. Other testing is dictated by the history and physical examination, including various endocrine, coagulation, and imaging studies. Transvaginal ultrasound is invaluable in the evaluation and management of these patients. In addition to adnexal and ovarian assessment, evaluate the myometrium for fibroids and the endometrium for its thickness. In postmenopausal women, an endometrial thickness of <5 mm generally is considered the upper limit of normal. In premenopausal women, endometrial thickness varies from 4–8 mm in the follicular phase and 7–14 mm in the secretory phase. Saline infusion sonohysterography, in which saline is infused into the endometrial cavity before sonography, has led to better definition of cavitary lesions (e.g., submucosal fibroids, uterine polyps) and is further expanding the indications for pelvic sonography.

C. Focus first on the source of the bleeding. The necessary equipment (including specula of various sizes and shapes), flexible lighting, and adequate assistance must be available. If a lesion is identified in the genital tract, obtain a biopsy regardless of the patient's age.

D. Abnormal bleeding in premenopausal women often is attributable to contraceptive methods. In addition to oral contraceptive pills, Depo-Provera is associated with abnormal bleeding in the first 3–9 months of use. In the absence of an obvious cause, the etiology is most likely "dysfunctional uterine bleeding," a diagnosis of exclusion. The cause of bleeding in patients using hormonal contraception is excess or insufficient estrogen or progesterone. Depending on the patient's wishes, therapeutic options include receiving no additional therapy, discontinuing or changing to a new contraceptive method, or adding some hormonal manipulation. Lack of an organic explanation for persistent abnormal bleeding refractory to hormonal manipulation should prompt further evaluation of the uterine cavity, in the form of transvaginal sonography with or without saline infusion, office hysteroscopy, or endometrial biopsy (EMB). In patients at risk for hyperplasia, EMB may be sufficient, although more and more physicians choose direct visualization by sonography or hysteroscopy.

E. The incidence of adenocarcinoma of the uterus in women >40 years is about 5%. The incidence increases with age. Therefore, abnormal bleeding in women who are 40 years must be evaluated by EMB. Women at increased risk because of obesity, chronic anovulation, exogenous unopposed estrogen, or preexisting cancer (particularly breast cancer) may warrant EMB regardless of age. In postmenopausal women who use hormone replacement therapy, a diligent evaluation is indicated to rule out occult carcinoma. When histopathologic study reveals hyperplasia with cellular atypia, medical or surgical treatment is necessary. Treatment of endometrial carcinoma should involve consultation with a gynecologist or oncologist to determine the best course of therapy. Reevaluate patients diagnosed with hyperplasia with atypia for persistent or worsening hyperplasia within 3–6 months of treatment.

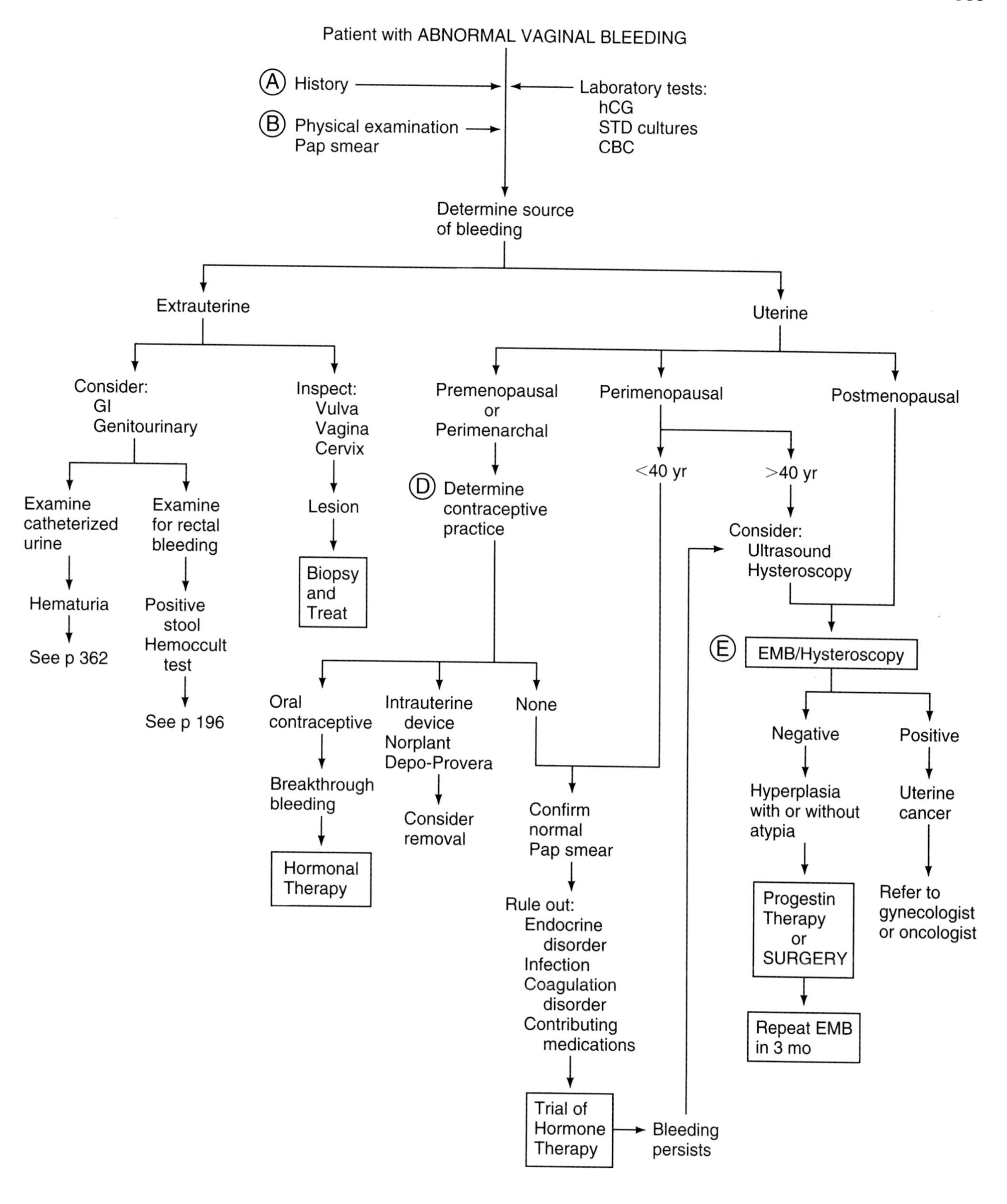

References

ACOG Technical Bulletin. Dysfunctional uterine bleeding. No. 134, October 1989.

ACOG Technical Bulletin. Gynecologic ultrasonography. No. 215, November 1995.

Mischell DR Jr. Abnormal uterine bleeding. In Herbst AL, Mishell DR Jr, Stenchever MA, et al, eds. Comprehensive Gynecology, ed 4. St. Louis: Mosby, 2001:1079.

Wathen PI, Henderson MC, Witz CA. Abnormal uterine bleeding. Med Clin North Am 1995;79:329.

VAGINAL BLEEDING IN PREGNANCY

Janet Moore, MD

Bleeding in pregnancy may have a number of causes, including obstetric, gynecologic, and nongynecologic causes. It is relatively common, complicating up to 5% of term pregnancies. Rapidly determining the cause is of utmost importance to ensure maternal and fetal well-being.

A. Initial management, regardless of gestational age, includes stabilization of the patient followed by thorough history and physical examination, with determination of the amount and rate of bleeding. Once the patient is hemodynamically stable, investigate the cause of the bleeding.

B. Gestational age can be estimated by date of last menstrual period, fundal height, or sonography. The main differential diagnosis for bleeding in early pregnancy is spontaneous abortion (SAb) and ectopic pregnancy. Proceed immediately to speculum examination.

C. SAb is termination of pregnancy before 20 weeks (<500 g). Bleeding in SAb is caused by hemorrhage into the decidua basalis and necrotic changes in the tissue. If when the speculum is placed there is blood in the vagina but the cervical opening (os) is closed, threatened abortion is the diagnosis. About half of women who bleed in the first trimester go on to abort. If the bleeding is associated with pain and cramping, the prognosis is worse. However, if fetal cardiac activity is demonstrated, only 10% proceed to abortion (fetal cardiac activity can be documented by transvaginal ultrasound [US] at 5 weeks). Management is complete pelvic rest; bed rest is not warranted.

D. Bleeding is the most common sign of a molar pregnancy and can be intermittent or continuous, lasting weeks to months. The bleeding usually is brown, rarely bright red. Other signs include uterine size greater than expected for gestational age, intractable nausea and vomiting, highly elevated levels of beta-human chorionic gonadotropin (β-hCG), or high blood pressure. The diagnosis is confirmed by US, which may show a complete mole or a partial mole with coexisting viable pregnancy. Treatment is evacuation, with serial β-hCG determinations until undetectable, and delaying conception for at least 1 year. Chemotherapy may be required if β-hCG remains elevated.

E. Cervicitis from chlamydial infection or gonorrhea can present with spotting and increased vaginal discharge. On speculum examination there are signs of inflammation and purulent discharge. Vaginitis most commonly is caused by bacterial vaginosis, trichomoniasis, or candidiasis. Vaginitis tends to present with serosanguineous discharge, especially after intercourse. Cervical polyps and cervical cancer also can present with bleeding. On speculum examination, polyps appear to be hanging out of the cervical canal and are smooth, soft, and red to purple. They bleed readily when touched. Cervical cancer often has a cauliflower-like, necrotic appearance. Both cause bleeding after intercourse or vaginal examination.

F. Nongynecologic causes include urinary tract infection, GI bleeding, lymphoma, and thrombocytopenia.

G. If on speculum examination the os is closed and there is no blood in the vagina but fetal cardiac activity is absent on US or fetal Doppler (present after about 10 weeks), a *missed abortion* has occurred; that is, the fetus has died but has been retained, often for weeks. Management generally is elective evacuation to decrease the risk of sepsis or DIC.

H. In ectopic pregnancy implantation occurs at a site other than the endometrium, most commonly (96%) in the tubes. Bleeding is thought to be the result of the pregnancy outgrowing its blood supply, which leads to declining endocrine function of the placenta, resulting in inadequate endometrial support with subsequent breakthrough bleeding. Bleeding usually is scant and associated with abdominal pain, often unilateral. Diagnosis is made by serial β-hCG determinations and sonography. The β-hCG level doubles every 48 hours in a normal pregnancy. Ectopic pregnancies have impaired production of β-hCG and thus have a prolonged doubling time. Transvaginal US allows visualization of a gestational sac once the β-hCG is >1500 mIU/ml, whereas transabdominal US can detect the sac if β-hCG is >6000 mIU/ml. If no sac is seen in the uterus, ectopic pregnancy is presumed. Treatment is laparoscopic salpingostomy, laparotomy if the patient is hemodynamically unstable, or intramuscular injection of methotrexate if the sac is <4 cm and unruptured. Regardless of treatment modality, β-hCG level is followed until undetectable.

I. If the os is open on speculum examination, inevitable abortion is the diagnosis. Bleeding in an inevitable abortion usually is associated with cramping. Management may be expectant or may consist of evacuation of the products of conception (POC).

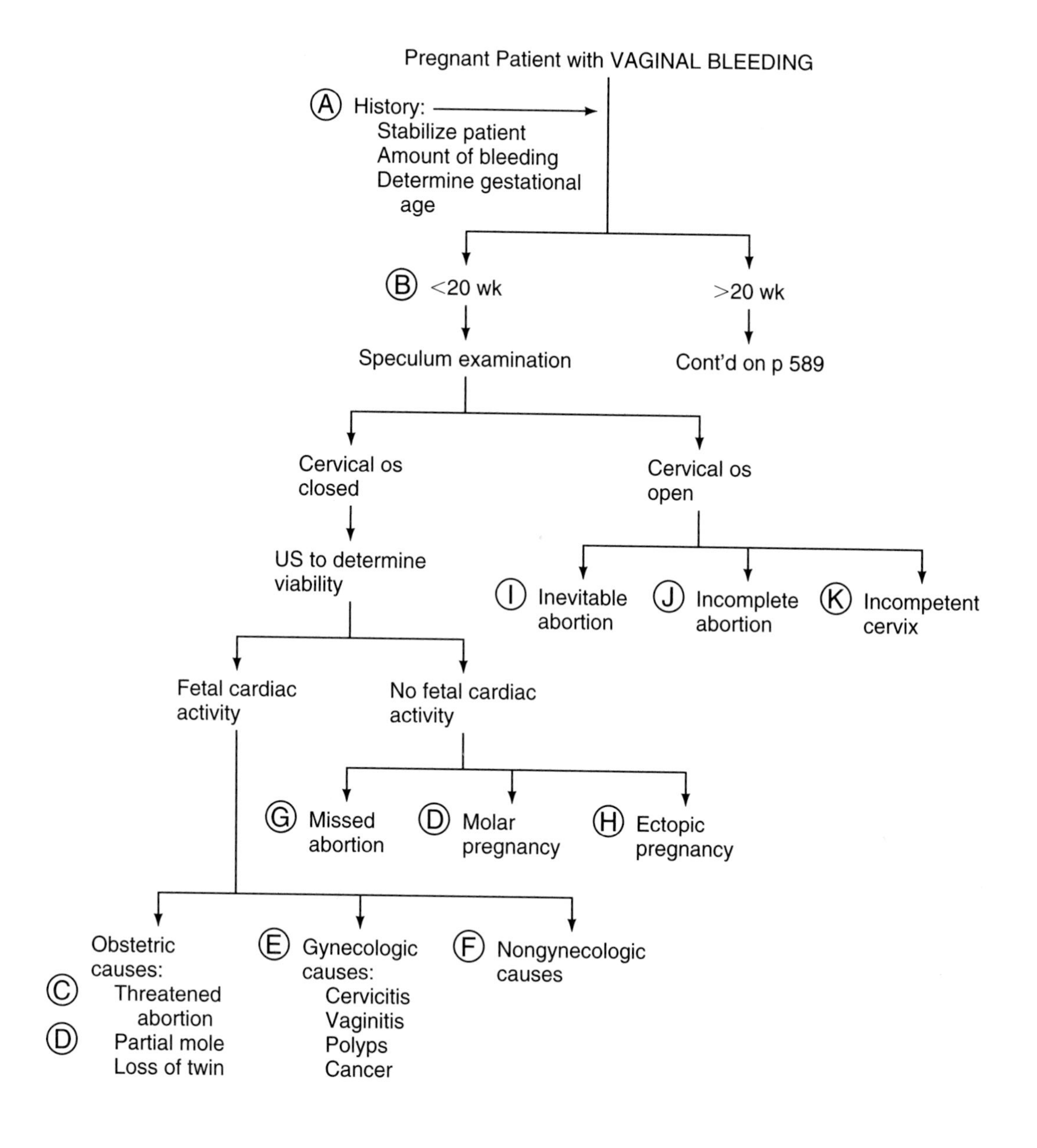

J. An incomplete abortion has occurred when the os is open and there has been partial passage of the POC. Bleeding can be significant because the retained POC do not allow complete myometrial contraction and uterine involution. Evacuation is mandated to prevent significant hemorrhage and sepsis.

K. In incompetent cervix the os is open with symptoms of pelvis pressure, low back pain, and increased vaginal discharge. Risk factors include previous cervical laceration or surgery and exposure to diethylstilbestrol (DES). Treatment is attempted emergency cerclage in the existing pregnancy and elective cerclage in future pregnancies at 10–14 weeks.

L. Vaginal bleeding in the third trimester is an absolute contraindication to pelvic examination until the location of the placenta can be determined. Therefore US must be performed to rule out placenta previa before further examination. Speculum or digital examination in the presence of placenta previa can lead to life-threatening obstetric hemorrhage.

M. Placenta previa is abnormal implantation of the placenta over the cervical os. Complete placenta previa covers the os; partial incompletely covers the os; marginal is directly adjacent to the os. Placenta previa complicates 1 of 200 term pregnancies and usually presents as painless vaginal bleeding. Incidence is increased with advanced maternal age, increased parity, and previous uterine surgery. Management from 24–36 weeks includes stabilization of the patient, fetal monitoring, blood typing and screening, and RhoGAM injection if indicated. Once maternal and fetal well-being are ensured, the patient should remain hospitalized on bed rest with maintenance of hematocrit at 30% in case of future large hemorrhage. Of those, 20% are complicated with uterine activity because blood acts as an irritant. However, cervical dilation cannot be determined directly, so tocolysis may be started empirically.

N. Placental abruption results from premature separation of the placenta before delivery. The cause in most cases is unknown, but there is an association with increased maternal age and parity, abdominal trauma, cocaine use, and smoking. Abruption presents with a clinical triad of bleeding, uterine hyperactivity/hypertonicity, and fetal distress. Diagnosis generally is clinical, although US may support the diagnosis in 50% of cases with evidence of retroplacental clot or other hemorrhage. Maternal complications include shock, DIC, and ischemic necrosis. Therefore, in addition to a hemoglobin, hematocrit, and blood type and screen, evaluation for consumptive coagulopathy should include fibrinogen and fibrin split products, platelets, and prothrombin time/partial thromboplastin time. RhoGAM should be given to the Rh(−) mother. A Kleihauer-Betke test will determine whether >30 ml of fetal blood has entered the maternal circulation, necessitating additional RhoGAM therapy in the Rh(−) mother.

O. Rupture of a fetal blood vessel is a rare occurrence that can happen in association with a velamentous insertion of the umbilical cord. Fetal monitoring shows signs of fetal distress, most often alternating fetal tachycardia-bradycardia as the fetus attempts to compensate for acute blood loss.

P. In preterm labor with cervical dilation, cervical change can cause spotting secondary to dilation and effacement. Other symptoms include pelvic pressure, vaginal discharge, and backache, with or without frank contractions. Rule out premature rupture of membranes with sterile speculum examination looking for pooling of amniotic fluid in the vagina, positive Nitrazine test, and ferning. If gestation is 34 weeks, management includes betamethasone injection for fetal lung maturity, antibiotic prophylaxis for group B streptococcus, and tocolysis. If <34 weeks, expectant management with bed rest and pelvic rest is recommended.

Q. Normal labor with bloody show is a final possibility.

References

Abortion. In Cunningham FG, MacDonald PC, Leveno KJ, et al, eds. Williams Obstetrics, ed 20. Norwalk, CT: Appleton & Lange, 1996:579.

Benedetti T. Obstetric hemorrhage. In Gabbe SG, Niebyl JR, Simpson JL, eds. Normal and Problem Pregnancies, ed 4. New York: Churchill Livingstone, 2002:503.

Droegemueller W. Benign gynecological lesions. In Mishell DR Jr, Stenchever MA, Droegemueller W, et al, eds. Comprehensive Gynecology, ed 4. St. Louis: Mosby, 2001:846.

Herbst AL. Malignant diseases of the cervix. In Mishell DR Jr, Stenchever MA, Droegemueller W, et al, eds. Comprehensive Gynecology, ed 4. St. Louis: Mosby, 2001:889.

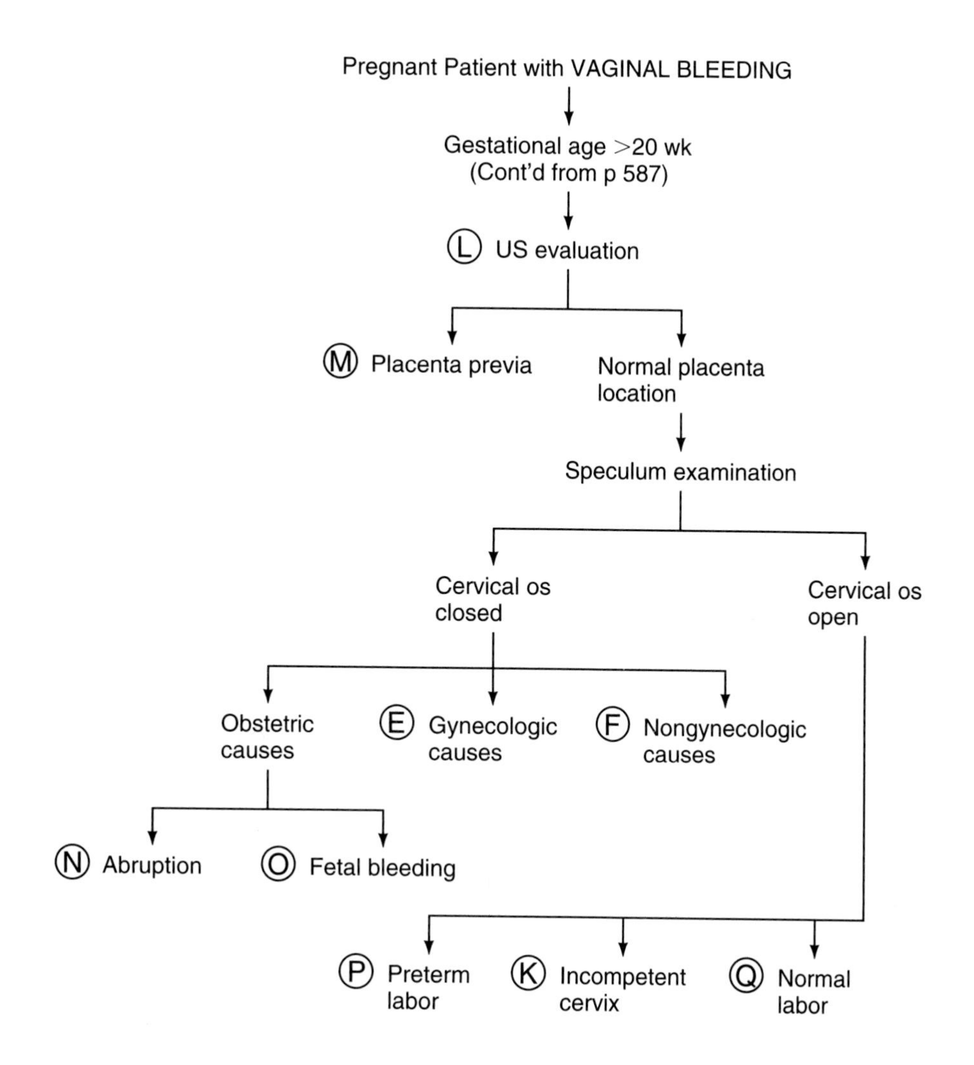
Pregnant Patient with VAGINAL BLEEDING
Gestational age >20 wk
(Cont'd from p 587)
Ⓛ US evaluation
Ⓜ Placenta previa
Normal placenta location
Speculum examination
Cervical os closed
Cervical os open
Obstetric causes
Ⓔ Gynecologic causes
Ⓕ Nongynecologic causes
Ⓝ Abruption
Ⓞ Fetal bleeding
Ⓟ Preterm labor
Ⓚ Incompetent cervix
Ⓠ Normal labor

ACUTE ABDOMINAL PAIN IN WOMEN

Robert N. Samuelson, MD

A. The acute abdomen refers to any condition requiring an "acute" medical decision. The potential causes of acute abdominal pain in women are multiple. A thorough history can quickly eliminate a number of these. Information about menstrual cycles, previous episodes of similar pain, sexual activity, contraception, vaginal discharge, and changes in bowel, bladder, or appetite can quickly narrow the differential diagnosis. Findings in the acute abdomen often include severe pain, which may be caused by infection, bleeding, infarction of tissue, or obstruction of a hollow viscus (bowel, fallopian tube, or ureter). Any of these conditions can irritate and inflame the peritoneum, making it sensitive to movement. Loss of appetite, nausea, and vomiting often accompany the pain and tenderness. Laboratory studies necessary for adequately evaluating an acute abdomen include a CBC with differential, ESR, pregnancy test (urine or serum), urinalysis, and occasionally an amylase or lipase. Obtain cervical cultures for *Neisseria gonorrhoeae* and *Chlamydia trachomatis* at initial evaluation if the history warrants.

B. If the pregnancy test is positive, the differential diagnosis can be narrowed considerably. It is important to recognize that conditions other than pregnancy can be the source of the pain. If gestational age is <10–12 weeks, consider ectopic pregnancy, rupture or torsion of ovarian cyst, or septic or threatened abortion. If gestational age is >12–14 weeks, ectopic pregnancy becomes less likely; consider other entities, such as ruptured or torsed adnexa, appendicitis, septic abortion, ureteral colic, and pyelonephritis.

C. Ultrasonography continues to expand its role in the evaluation of obstetric and gynecologic patients with abdominal pain. Its use in conjunction with quantitative beta-human chorionic gonadotropin (β-hCG) can be important. With normal pregnancy, a gestational sac often is seen at 5–6 weeks of gestation. When the β-hCG level reaches 6500 mIU/ml, an abdominal scan can visualize a gestational sac; at 1500 mIU/ml a transvaginal probe often visualizes the pregnancy. If, on the basis of sonographic findings and quantitative β-hCG values, the possibility of an ectopic pregnancy still exists, the patient needs referral for possible surgical management (laparoscopy/laparotomy) or medical management (e.g., methotrexate) for an ectopic pregnancy. If an early intrauterine pregnancy is confirmed by sonography, other sources for the pain must be determined. Ruptured or torsed ovarian cysts, appendicitis, or an infected abortion also can present with abdominal pain.

D. If the pregnancy test is negative, history again plays an important role. Patients with a history of recurrent cyclic pain related to menses and who now have an acute exacerbation may have a ruptured endometrioma. Patients with a history of fever, chills, and vaginal discharge with a recent change in sexual partners are at risk for pelvic inflammatory disease (PID). (Patients taking oral contraceptives are at decreased risk for ovarian cyst formation.) If an infectious cause is determined, admit the patient for IV antibiotics; if no improvement is seen in 24–48 hours, consider laparoscopy. CT may be helpful in the evaluation of the patient because it is both specific and sensitive for appendicitis. On occasion, however, the determination of PID versus appendicitis often is not resolved until laparoscopy or laparotomy is performed. Other entities that must always be considered are adnexal torsion, ovarian cyst rupture, exacerbation of endometriosis, degenerating fibroid, renal calculi, and mesenteric lymphadenitis.

E. Although many imaging modalities are available to the practitioner, the choice may need to be made in concert with the radiologist. A thin pregnant patient can be evaluated well with ultrasound; in obese postmenopausal patients more information may be obtained by CT. The need for surgical exploration often takes precedence over imaging studies. Many of the disorders in premenopausal patients apply also to postmenopausal patients. Cyst formation occurs infrequently in elderly patients, but its appearance must be evaluated carefully for the possibility of malignancy. Other processes that can cause acute pain include colonic diverticulitis (75% of these resolve with proper attention and antibiotics), bowel obstruction (most of these need exploration), and vascular lesions (mesenteric thrombosis), dissecting or leaking aneurysm, and acute cholecystitis or pancreatitis.

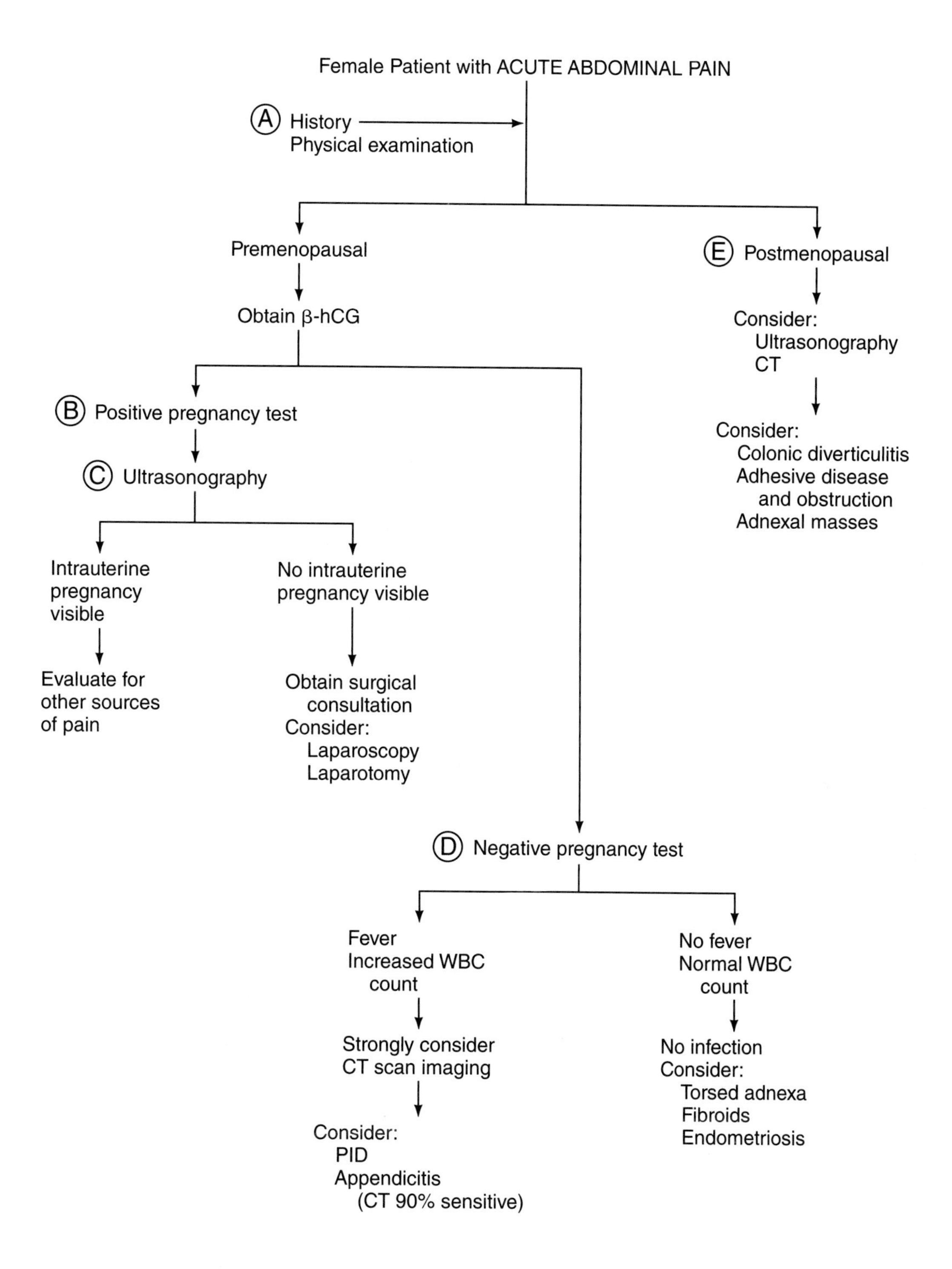

References

Epstein FB. Acute abdominal pain in pregnancy. Emerg Med Clin North Am 1994;12:151.

Jeffrey RB, Ralls PW. CT and Sonography of the Acute Abdomen, ed 2. Philadelphia: Lippincott-Raven, 1996.

Kiernan GV, Cales RH. Acute abdominal disorders. Emerg Med Clin North Am 1989;7:30.

Merrell RC. Gastroenterological emergencies. Gastroenterol Clin North Am 1988;17:75.

Wagner JM, McKinney WP, Carpenter JL. Does this patient have appendicitis? JAMA 1996;276:1589.

CHEST PAIN IN WOMEN

Dawn Lemcke, MD

The evaluation of chest pain in women is an important step in the diagnosis of coronary artery disease (CAD). The diagnosis of CAD in women is problematic because most of the diagnostic pathways and outcomes are based on research in men. Epidemiologic studies show that CAD is a significant cause of morbidity and mortality in women and that women have a worse prognosis than men with myocardial infarction. Improved diagnosis of CAD in early stages is critical to prevent complications in women. This chapter's algorithm includes not only the pretest likelihood of disease but also guidelines for choosing the best tests for women.

A. There are clear gender differences in presenting symptoms of chest pain and in risk factor stratification. Women may have more atypical sites of pain, such as neck, shoulder, and intrascapular pain, and may have more associated symptoms of exertional dyspnea or decreased exercise tolerance. It is thus important to ask not only the usual historical questions to try to determine whether the patient has angina but also to ask about atypical characteristics. Risk factor assessment can be divided into major, intermediate, and minor determinants (Table 1). These, along with the character of the pain, can be used to place women in categories of likelihood of CAD. This stratification makes testing for CAD more cost effective and informative. Risk factor assessment is more likely to predict CAD in women (54.5% of cases, compared with 39.3% of cases in men). Stronger predictive value exists, particularly in younger women with risk factors.

Table 1 **Risk Factor Determinants of Coronary Artery Disease in Women with Chest Pain**

Major
Typical angina
Postmenopausal status
Diabetes (twice the risk of CAD of male diabetic patients)
Peripheral vascular disease
Intermediate
Hypertension
Smoking, especially in premenopausal women
Lipid abnormalities, including high-density lipoprotein <35 mg/dl and triglycerides >400 mg/dl
Minor
Age >65 years
Central obesity (waist/hip ratio >0.85 or waist >38 cm)
Sedentary lifestyle
Family history of CAD (2.8 times increase in relative risk of nonfatal myocardial infarction and 5 times increase in CAD)
Other risk factors (hemostatic, psychosocial)

B. Evaluate a baseline electrocardiogram (ECG) before conducting other tests in women. Because exercise tolerance testing (ETT) in women may be flawed by false-positive results, having a normal resting ECG improves the diagnostic yield of testing. If the resting ECG is abnormal, with left ventricular hypertrophy, bundle branch block, or an early J point elevation, it may increase the likelihood of a false-positive result, and therefore an imaging ETT may be the most cost-effective test in this group. The use of stress echocardiography as an initial test in all women with chest pain has been proposed as a cost-effective approach, achieving a diagnostic accuracy similar to that of stress thallium ETT. Stress echocardiography is less costly than stress thallium ETT but is technically demanding for the average echo laboratory and thus may not be widely available.

C. High likelihood of disease or definite angina is predicted by two or more major determinants or by one major plus more than one intermediate or minor determinant. This group of women has a pretest likelihood of CAD of 80%. In this group, ETT without imaging is the initial test of choice (unless the patient has clinical characteristics other than being female that necessitate imaging). Studies show that 60%–75% of women in this group had significant CAD at angiography, and 29%–53% had multivessel disease. The specificity of ETT in this setting is 57%, with a sensitivity of 80%. Women with single-vessel disease may be missed by ETT; only 43% of them will have abnormal findings. When following women with characteristics suggestive of angina, remember that single-vessel disease is more common in women than in men. Nonetheless, despite its limitations, a maximal negative ETT should not be overlooked, because it largely rules out exercise-induced ischemia associated with multivessel disease. If symptoms persist despite a negative maximal ETT, raising concern of single-vessel disease, stress echocardiography or pharmacologic stress echocardiography may be appropriate. This technique has a sensitivity and specificity of 80%–90% for single-vessel disease in women.

D. The most cost-effective approach in women with typical angina and a normal baseline ECG is ETT. Women in this group are unlikely to have false-positive results, and the likelihood of false-negative results is much less than in their male counterparts if they achieve maximal heart rate. Imaging ETT increases the cost of this test and adds little clinically useful information.

(Continued on page 594)

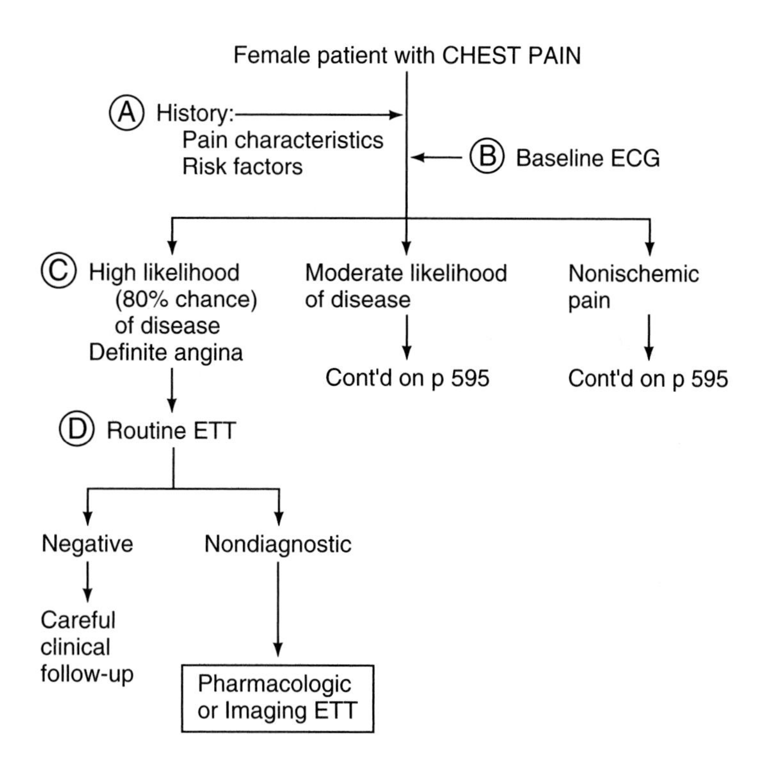
Female patient with CHEST PAIN
A History:
Pain characteristics
Risk factors
B Baseline ECG
C High likelihood
(80% chance)
of disease
Definite angina
Moderate likelihood
of disease
Nonischemic
pain
Cont'd on p 595
Cont'd on p 595
D Routine ETT
Negative
Nondiagnostic
Careful
clinical
follow-up
Pharmacologic
or Imaging ETT

E. If the ETT is negative, the patient can be followed closely. A decision about management may be difficult for the woman with a positive test result. The literature holds convincing evidence of the gender differences in further testing after a positive ETT result. It is unclear whether this gender difference represents patient preference (women perceive their risk of heart disease as low); physician perception of the "benign" nature of CAD in women, based on the Framingham and CASS studies; or overtreatment of men. A woman should be referred for coronary angiography for the same reasons as her male counterpart (i.e., unstable angina or markedly positive ETT at low workload). Some advocate angiography for women with a positive ETT at high workload. Some studies show a higher incidence of cardiac events in women regardless of initial ETT response: 14.3% of women with an abnormal ETT result will have a cardiac event, versus 6% of men with a positive ETT. Because most of the coronary events occurred in patients who did not undergo revascularization procedures, one can make an excellent case for complete evaluation and treatment, including catheterization, for all women with positive tests. This strategy may actually be of greater benefit to women than similar care is to men.

F. Moderate likelihood of disease is predicted by one major or by multiple indeterminate and minor determinants. This group has the widest pretest probability of CAD, ranging from 20%–80%. Most women in actual practice are in this category. The prevalence of CAD in this group is about 30%–40%, with 4%–22% having multivessel disease. These women clearly need further examination, but the best test to use is unclear. The sensitivity and specificity of routine ETT in this group are about 65%. Therefore, a test result has a reasonable chance of being either a false positive or a false negative. Because this may not add to the diagnostic certainty, it may be more prudent to proceed with either a thallium/sestamibi ETT or stress echocardiography. Although the sensitivity of these tests does not add significantly to the ETT, the addition of imaging improves specificity in women to 80%–90%. In particular, stress echocardiography may dramatically improve the sensitivity and specificity for single-vessel disease.

G. Women with nonischemic pain are in the lowest risk group, with >20% likelihood of CAD. This group is defined as those with no major determinants, no or one intermediate determinant, and two or fewer minor determinants. On further analysis, the nonischemic pain group will have a 2%–7% incidence of CAD and virtually no multivessel disease. Because of the low prevalence of significant disease in this group, any test that might show an abnormality is of little value, or more likely a false positive. Look for noncardiac causes of pain (e.g., cholecystitis, gastroesophageal reflux, chest wall pain, pulmonary etiologies, or anxiety) in this group before proceeding with evaluation.

H. If the patient continues to have symptoms that limit her lifestyle, further evaluation with imaging, ETT, or even angiography may be needed to refute or confirm the existence of CAD, particularly in postmenopausal women.

References

DeSanctis R. Clinical manifestations of coronary artery disease: chest pain in women. In: Wenger N, Speroff L, Packard B, eds. Cardiovascular health and disease in women. Proceedings of an NHLBI Conference. LeJacq Communications, 1993.

Douglas P, Ginsburg G. The evaluation of chest pain in women. N Engl J Med 1996;334:1311.

Gibbons EF. Evaluation of chest pain. In Lemcke D, Pattison J, Marshall L, et al., eds. Primary care of women, Norwalk, CT: Appleton-Lange; 1995.

Gibbons EF. Risk factors for coronary artery disease and their treatment. In Lemcke D, Pattison J, Marshall L, et al., eds. Primary care of women, Norwalk, CT: Appleton-Lange; 1995.

Judelson D. Coronary heart disease in women: risk factors and prevention. JAMA 1994;49:186.

Wenger N. Coronary heart disease in women: gender differences in diagnostic evaluation. JAMA 1994;49:181.

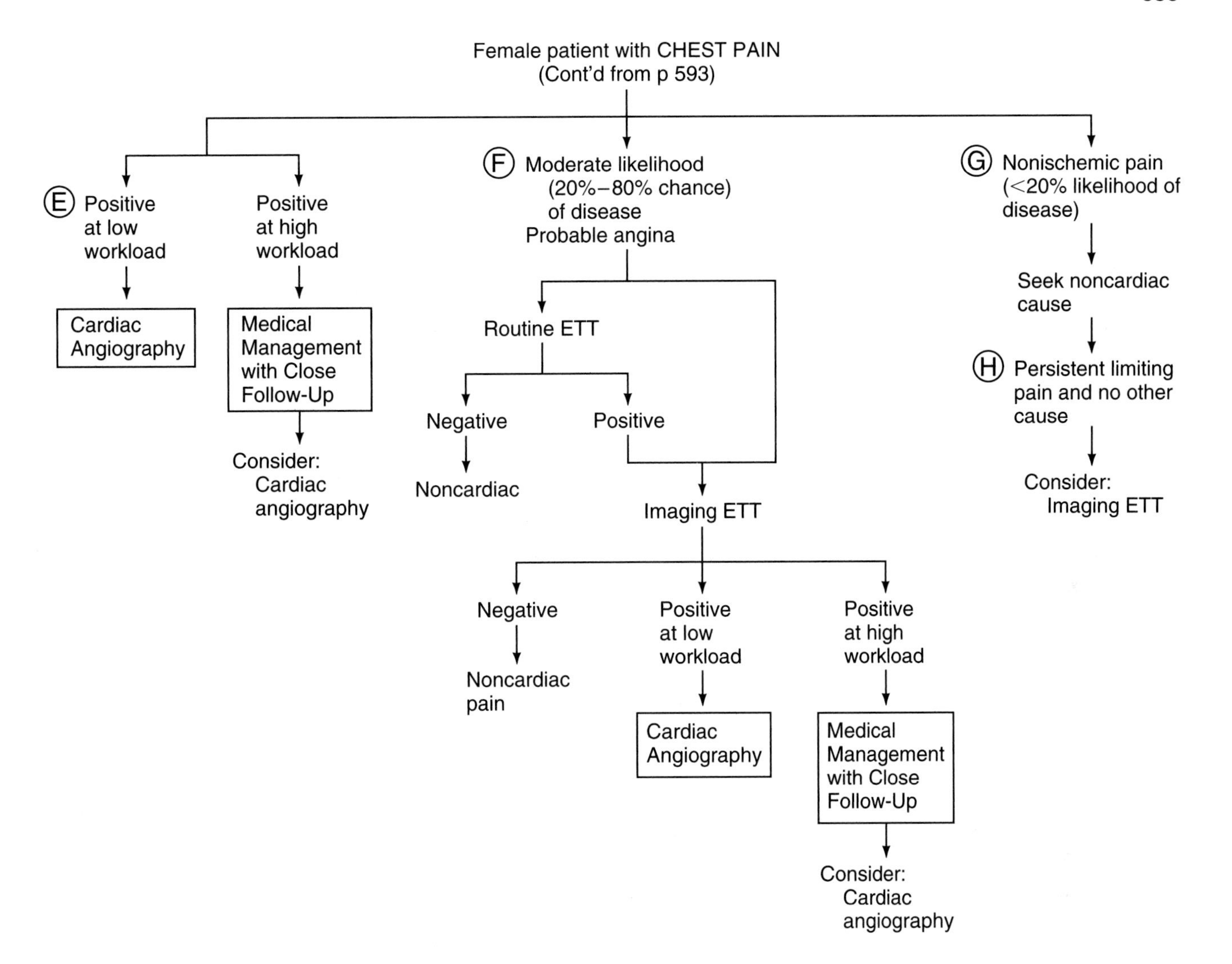
Female patient with CHEST PAIN
(Cont'd from p 593)
E Positive at low workload
Cardiac Angiography
Positive at high workload
Medical Management with Close Follow-Up
Consider: Cardiac angiography
F Moderate likelihood (20%–80% chance) of disease Probable angina
Routine ETT
Negative
Noncardiac
Positive
Imaging ETT
Negative
Noncardiac pain
Positive at low workload
Cardiac Angiography
Positive at high workload
Medical Management with Close Follow-Up
Consider: Cardiac angiography
G Nonischemic pain (<20% likelihood of disease)
Seek noncardiac cause
H Persistent limiting pain and no other cause
Consider: Imaging ETT

URINARY TRACT INFECTION IN WOMEN

Michael D. Katz, PharmD

A. Patients with lower urinary tract infection (UTI) or cystitis complain primarily of dysuria. Frequency, nocturia, urgency, and suprapubic tenderness also may be present. About one third of patients with only lower tract symptoms have an occult renal infection. Patients with overt upper tract infection or acute pyelonephritis usually have flank, low back, or abdominal pain; fevers; chills; malaise; and nausea and vomiting. Concomitant lower tract symptoms also may be present.

B. Individuals with pyelonephritis (PN) often can be successfully treated as outpatients. However, patients with nausea and vomiting who are unable to take oral fluids and medications should be hospitalized. Enterobacteriaceae are the most common pathogens associated with acute pyelonephritis. A wide variety of antimicrobial regimens is available. Initial outpatient therapy may include trimethoprim/sulfamethoxazole (TMP/SMX), a cephalosporin, or a fluoroquinolone. The conventional IV regimen of ampicillin and gentamicin is effective, although TMP/SMX, fluoroquinolones, and cephalosporins also may be considered. The initial choice of therapy must be based on the most likely organisms present and local susceptibility patterns. Definitive therapy must be guided by results of culture and sensitivity tests.

C. In patients with acute cystitis, certain risk factors increase the chance of an occult renal or complicated UTI. Such risk factors include nosocomial infection, pregnancy, known urinary tract abnormality or stone, indwelling catheter or recent instrumentation, previous relapse after therapy for UTI, previous UTI before 12 years of age, acute PN or more than three UTIs in the past year, symptoms for >7 days before therapy, recent antibiotic use, diabetes, and other immunosuppressing conditions. Treat patients with one or more of these risk factors as having an upper tract infection.

D. In acute, uncomplicated cystitis, 3-day antibiotic therapy can be given without obtaining a culture. Seven-day regimens are effective but are associated with a higher incidence of adverse drug reactions, noncompliance, and increased cost. Highly effective 3-day regimens include TMP/SMX 160 mg/800 mg twice daily, amoxicillin/clavulanate 500 mg/125 mg every 12 hours, ciprofloxacin 250 mg every 12 hours, and norfloxacin 400 mg every 12 hours. Because of widespread *Escherichia coli* resistance, ampicillin/amoxicillin alone may not be as effective as other regimens. Studies with cephalosporins in 3-day regimens have shown conflicting results. Posttherapy urine cultures are needed only in patients with persisting symptoms, complicating factors, or pregnancy. In patients who are pregnant, or whose pregnancy status is unknown, nitrofurantoin is the preferred agent.

E. Sexual intercourse and use of diaphragms or spermicide use alone have been associated with an increased risk of UTI. Urination after intercourse may reduce the frequency of relapse. Postcoital antibiotic therapy also is effective. Regimens include TMP/SMX 1/2 SS tablet, cephalexin 250 mg, or nitrofurantoin 50 mg within 2 hours after intercourse. Discontinuing use of a diaphragm for contraception also may reduce the frequency of relapse.

F. In patients with dysuria, a positive urine culture is considered to be $>10^2$ CFU/ml growth. Treat patients with a positive culture for 7–14 days. In acute cystitis, >90% of cases are caused by *E. coli* and other Enterobacteriaceae, *Staphylococcus saprophyticus,* and *Enterococcus.* Unless a highly resistant pathogen is present, an inexpensive agent, such as TMP/SMX, should be adequate. Reserve more expensive agents, such as the fluoroquinolones, cephalosporins, and amoxicillin/clavulanate, for resistant infections.

G. In patients with frequent recurrences, chronic suppression can reduce this frequency by 95%. Many regimens have been evaluated. If possible, choose the least toxic, least expensive agent. Effective daily regimens include nitrofurantoin 50–100 mg, TMP/SMX 40–80 mg/200–400 mg, and trimethoprim 100 mg. Thrice-weekly administration of TMP/SMX 40 mg/200 mg also has proved effective. Cranberry juice, 300 ml/day, has significantly reduced bacteriuria in postmenopausal women.

References

Bacheller CD, Bernstein JM. Urinary tract infections. Med Clin North Am 1997;81:719.

Hooton TM, Stamm WE. Diagnosis and treatment of uncomplicated urinary tract infection. Infect Dis Clin North Am 1997;11:551.

Stapleton A, Stamm WE. Prevention of urinary tract infection. Infect Dis Clin North Am 1997;11:719.

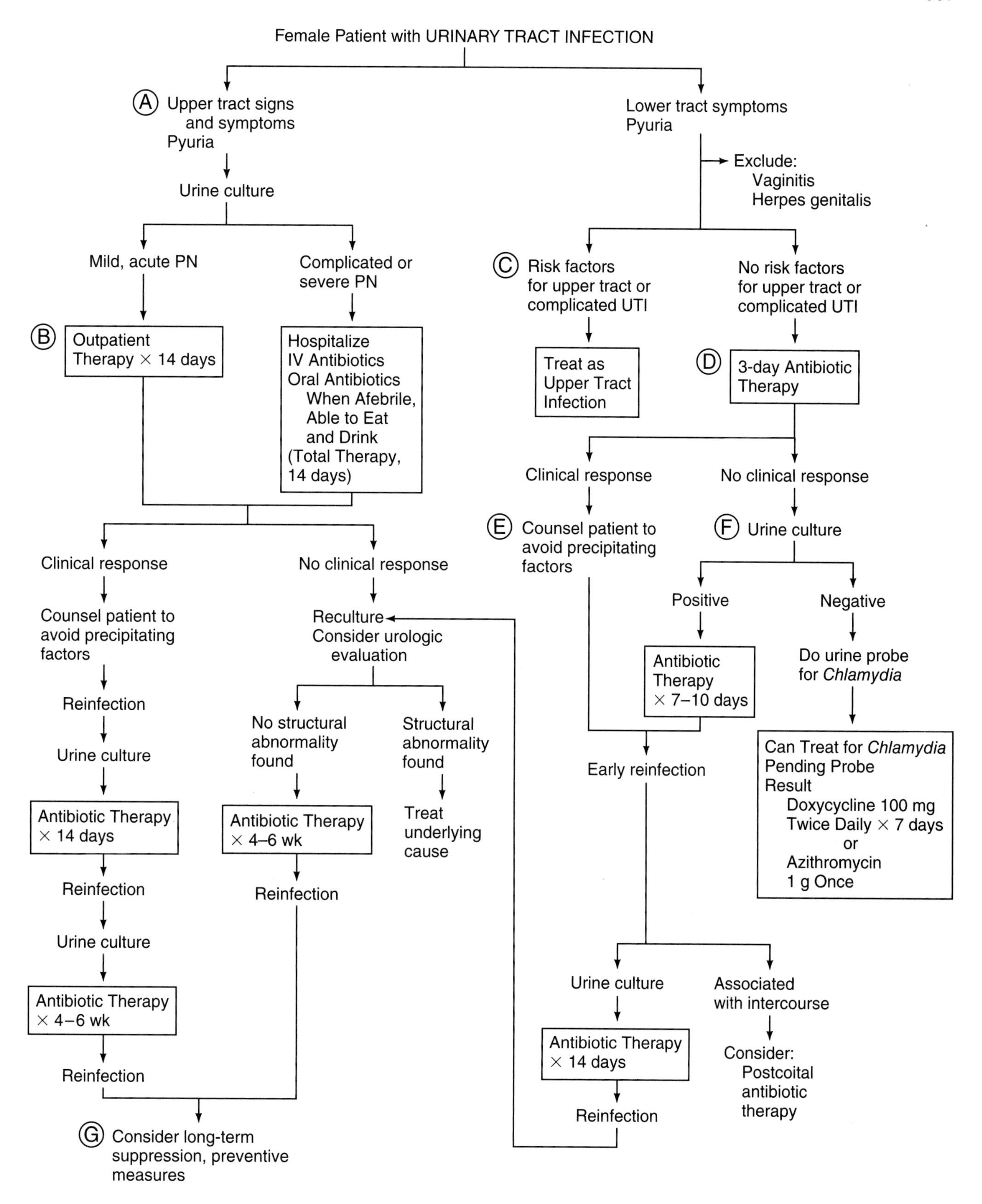

Female Patient with URINARY TRACT INFECTION
(A) Upper tract signs and symptoms Pyuria
Urine culture
Mild, acute PN
Complicated or severe PN
(B) Outpatient Therapy × 14 days
Hospitalize
IV Antibiotics
Oral Antibiotics When Afebrile, Able to Eat and Drink
(Total Therapy, 14 days)
Clinical response
Counsel patient to avoid precipitating factors
Reinfection
Urine culture
Antibiotic Therapy × 14 days
Reinfection
Urine culture
Antibiotic Therapy × 4–6 wk
Reinfection
No clinical response
Reculture
Consider urologic evaluation
No structural abnormality found
Antibiotic Therapy × 4–6 wk
Reinfection
Structural abnormality found
Treat underlying cause
(G) Consider long-term suppression, preventive measures
Lower tract symptoms Pyuria
Exclude:
Vaginitis
Herpes genitalis
(C) Risk factors for upper tract or complicated UTI
Treat as Upper Tract Infection
No risk factors for upper tract or complicated UTI
(D) 3-day Antibiotic Therapy
Clinical response
(E) Counsel patient to avoid precipitating factors
No clinical response
(F) Urine culture
Positive
Antibiotic Therapy × 7–10 days
Negative
Do urine probe for Chlamydia
Can Treat for Chlamydia Pending Probe Result
Doxycycline 100 mg Twice Daily × 7 days
or
Azithromycin 1 g Once
Early reinfection
Urine culture
Antibiotic Therapy × 14 days
Reinfection
Associated with intercourse
Consider:
Postcoital antibiotic therapy

BREAST MASS

Laurie L. Fajardo, MD

Breast cancer is the most common malignancy and the second leading cause of cancer-related death among U.S. women. The most effective means for diagnosing early breast cancer is screening mammography in combination with physical examination. Nonpalpable breast lesions (detectable only by mammography) may represent small, early, and potentially curable cancers. Because mammography cannot provide a specific diagnosis for breast lesions, biopsies are often required to determine whether a mass is benign or malignant. More than 1 million breast biopsies are performed in the United States annually; 11%–36% of biopsies performed for mammographically identified nonpalpable abnormalities are positive. The use of percutaneous fine needle aspiration (FNA) or core needle biopsy (CNB) for palpable breast masses, or stereotactic- or sonography-guided CNB for nonpalpable masses, may reduce the expense and morbidity associated with the diagnostic workup of breast lesions and decrease the number of open breast biopsies for benign lesions (see also Gynecomastia, p 162).

A. Needle aspiration of breast masses that feel benign should be a routine part of the evaluation of breast masses. It is safe, is cost-effective, and immediately helps distinguish cystic from solid masses. It can be performed with an 18- to 22-gauge needle with local anesthesia. Nonbloody fluid can be discarded without being sent to the laboratory for pathologic study. A persistent mass or bloody fluid mandates excisional biopsy to rule out malignancy.

B. Diagnostic mammography is indicated (1) for breast signs or symptoms (pain, mass, discharge, thickening, skin or nipple retraction, nipple eczema), (2) before breast surgery (biopsy, augmentation, reduction), (3) as routine follow-up of a patient with previous breast cancer (all remaining breast tissue), and (4) for metastatic cancer of unknown primary site. Preoperative mammography is performed (1) to characterize a lesion as obviously benign (lipoma, oil cyst, calcified fibroadenoma) or malignant (to plan the surgical approach), (2) to determine the size and extent of the lesion for adequate excision and treatment selection (especially important in a patient for whom conservative surgery and irradiation are being considered because multicentric disease in the affected breast is a contraindication to this procedure), (3) to detect additional lesions in the ipsilateral or contralateral breast, and (4) to obtain a baseline for comparison with follow-up mammography. It is important to recognize that mammograms may be negative even when breast cancer is obviously present. Thus a negative mammogram does not replace the need for biopsy of a palpable mass.

C. For palpable breast masses, percutaneous FNA or CNB can be performed with local anesthesia. To evaluate nonpalpable masses, CNB can be guided with stereotactic mammography or sonographic images. The accuracy of these procedures is >90%. If needle biopsy shows a breast mass to be benign, conservative follow-up with physical examination and mammography can be instituted, obviating the need for further surgical intervention. If a needle biopsy is positive, surgical excision can be planned to cure or stage the patient with a single surgical procedure.

D. Many authors have suggested that because of the possibility of a false-negative FNA, *all* palpable masses should undergo excisional biopsy. In one study using physical examination, mammography, and FNA followed by excisional biopsy for confirmation of pathology, patients who had negative or benign findings on all three clinical tests (physical examination, mammography, and FNA) also had benign surgical pathologic conditions. This has led to the recommendation for clinical and mammographic observation rather than surgical excision when these criteria are fulfilled.

E. When breast malignancy is confirmed histologically, a routine outpatient workup to exclude distant metastasis is indicated. Complete physical examination, CBC, liver function tests (LFTs), and chest x-ray (CXR) are routinely performed. A preoperative bone scan is indicated only if the patient has symptoms that are suspicious for bony metastasis. CT of the liver is indicated only if the LFT results are abnormal. The AJC-UICC staging system for breast cancer has been modified recently. Clinical staging includes careful inspection and palpation of the skin, breast, and lymph nodes (axillary, supraclavicular, and cervical) and pathologic examination of the breast or other tissues to establish the diagnosis of breast carcinoma. Pathologic staging includes data used for clinical staging, surgical resection, and a pathologic examination of the primary carcinoma. Pathologic staging can now be performed if the primary tumor is removed with no growth tumor in the margins and, in addition, if at least the lowest level (1) of axillary lymph nodes is resected, rather than all three levels.

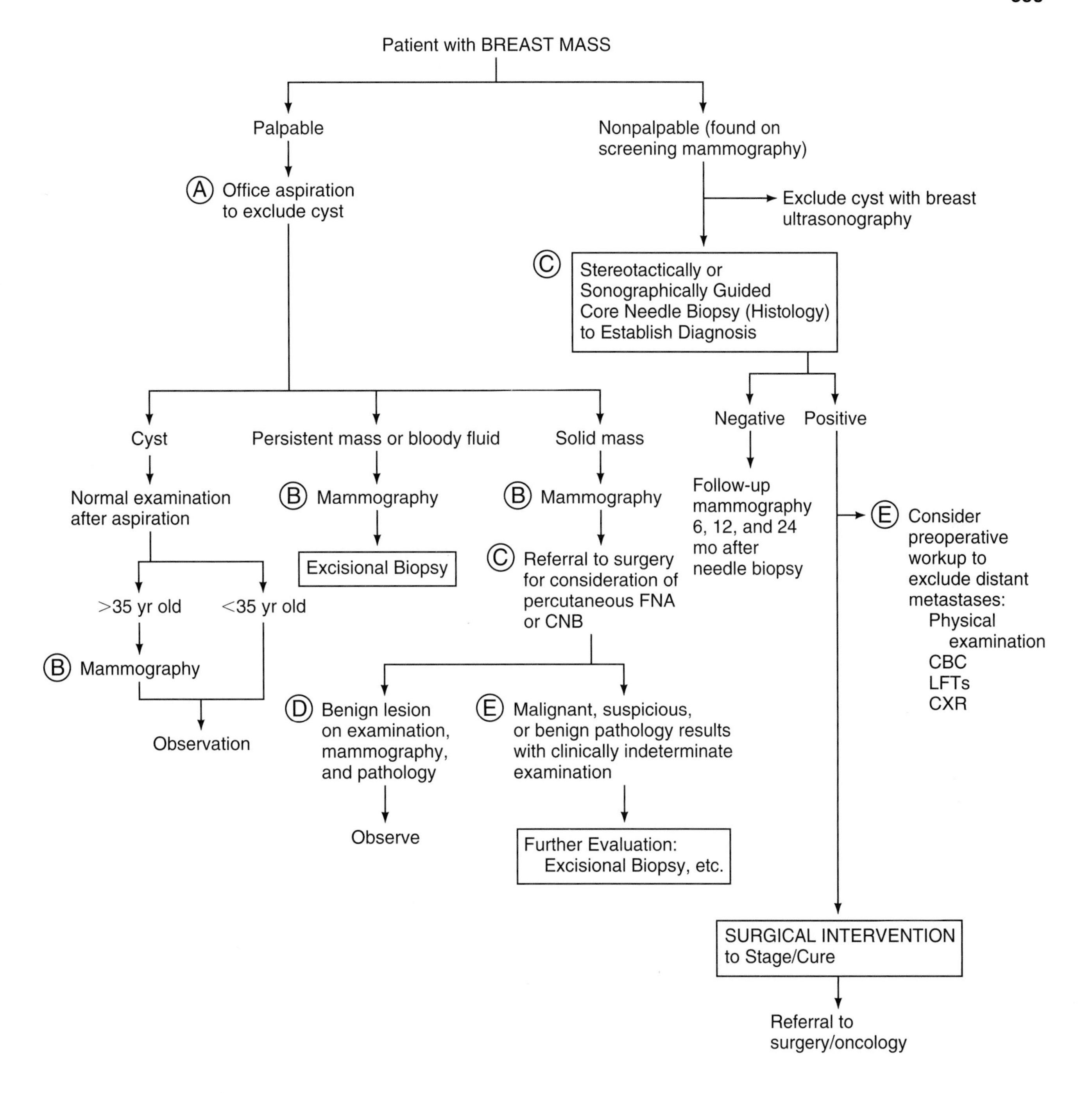

References

Bigelow R, Smith R, Goodman PA, et al. Needle localization of nonpalpable breast masses. Arch Surg 1985;120:565.

Brenner RJ, Fajardo LL, Fisher PR, et al. Percutaneous core biopsy of the breast: effect of operator experience and number of samples on diagnostic accuracy. AJR 1996;166:341.

Donegan WL. Evaluation of a palpable breast mass. N Engl J Med 1992; 327:937.

Fajardo LL. Cost-effectiveness of stereotactic breast core needle biopsy. Acad Radiol 1996;3(Suppl 1):S21.

Fajardo LL, Davis JR, Wiens JL, et al. Mammography-guided stereotactic fine needle aspiration cytology of nonpalpable breast lesions: prospective comparison with surgical biopsy results. AJR 1990;155:977.

Fajardo LL, DeAngelis GA. The role of imaging guided breast biopsy in the evaluation of mammographically detected abnormalities. Surg Oncol Clin North Am 1997;6(2):285.

Greene FL, Page DL, Fleming ID, et al., eds. *AJCC Cancer Staging* Manual, ed 6. New York: Springer-Verlag, 2002.

Hillner BE, Bear HD, Fajardo LL. Estimating the cost-effectiveness of stereotactic biopsy for nonpalpable breast abnormalities: a decision analysis model. Acad Radiol 1996;3:351.

Howard J. Using mammography for cancer control: an unrealized potential. CA 1987;37:33.

Silverberg E, Borring CC, Squires TS. Cancer statistics, 1990. Cancer J Clin 1990;40:9.

ADJUVANT THERAPY CHOICES IN BREAST CANCER

Alexi Wright, MD, and Ann Partridge, MD, MPH

Adjuvant systemic treatment refers to chemotherapy, endocrine therapy, or biologic agents given with curative intent in addition to local treatment for breast cancer (i.e., surgery with or without radiation). The goal is to eliminate clinically occult micrometastatic disease that might result in disease recurrence. Systemic treatment given before definitive surgery, often done in the setting of locally advanced disease, is termed *neoadjuvant* therapy.

A. Decision making: The decision to use adjuvant therapy requir es balancing a patient's risk of disease recurrence, expected benefits from systemic therapy, and toxicities associated with treatment. Important prognostic features include age, medical comorbidities, histologic subtype, tumor size, tumor grade, angiolymphatic invasion, number of lymph nodes involved, and hormone receptor and human epidermal growth factor receptor 2 (HER2) status. A validated computer-based algorithm, Adjuvant! Online (www.adjuvantonline.com), estimates a patient's 10-year risk of recurrence and mortality based on these factors (except HER2) and estimates the impact that adjuvant treatments will have. Increasingly, oncologists are incorporating information from genomic tests (e.g., Oncotype Dx) into prognostication and decision making, particularly for patients with estrogen receptor-positive (ER+) lymph node–negative disease.

B. Chemotherapy: Overall, modern adjuvant chemotherapy reduces breast cancer mortality by approximately 50% in women <50 years and 33% in women 50–69 years of age. Benefits are greatest in patients with estrogen and progesterone receptor–negative tumors. In the United States, guidelines suggest consideration of adjuvant chemotherapy for tumors equal to 1 cm or any tumor with lymph node involvement. Patients' with high risk features and tumors 0.6–1.0 cm should also consider treatment. Conventional chemotherapy has significant toxicities, however, including alopecia, nausea, bone marrow suppression, cardiomyopathy, neuropathy, and hypersensitivity reactions. Recent evaluations using genomic testing suggest that some patients may be spared the toxicity of chemotherapy even when conventional prognostic factors suggest higher-risk disease.

There are many different regimens to choose from because no combination of chemotherapy has been shown to be superior in all situations. In the United States, anthracycline-containing regimens (doxorubicin and cyclophosphamide, or "AC"-type regimens) have conventionally formed the backbone of adjuvant treatment. A large meta-analysis showed that these regimens lower the annual odds of recurrence and death significantly more than cytoxan methotrexate 5-fluoracil (CMF). The addition of paclitaxel is associated with a further reduction in the risk of disease recurrence and death (by 17% and 18%, respectively). Treatment schedules also matter in this setting; patients following an AC-type treatment with paclitaxel in a "dose-dense fashion," every 2 weeks, have better outcomes than those treated every 3 weeks. Recent evidence suggests that docetaxel and cyclophosphamide (or "TC") chemotherapy is an effective alternative regimen that avoids the risk of cardiotoxicity associated with anthracyclines.

C. Endocrine therapy: Adjuvant hormonal therapy benefits patients who have hormone receptor–positive (HR+) tumors, including tumors that are ER+ or progesterone receptor positive (PR+), but not patients with hormone-resistant tumors. In women with HR+ disease, adjuvant tamoxifen decreases the annual odds of recurrence and death (by 39% and 31%, respectively) independent of age, menopausal status, lymph node involvement, or the use of adjuvant chemotherapy. Premenopausal women with HR+ breast cancers should receive tamoxifen for at least 5 years, and ongoing studies are evaluating the risks and benefits of the addition of ovarian suppression or extended duration of tamoxifen. In recent years, several prospective randomized trials have shown increased disease-free survival and lower rates of ipsilateral, contralateral, and metastatic breast cancer in postmenopausal women treated with aromatase inhibitors (e.g., letrozole, anastrozole, and exemestane) compared to tamoxifen. Extended treatment with letrozole after 5 years of tamoxifen has also been shown to further improve these results, but the optimal duration of aromatase inhibitor treatment and sequence of therapy (i.e., when and whether to include tamoxifen) is under active investigation. All endocrine therapies are associated with menopausal symptoms, including hot flashes and night sweats. Tamoxifen confers an additional increased risk of uterine cancer and deep venous thrombosis, whereas aromatase inhibitors are associated with vaginal dryness, musculoskeletal symptoms, osteoporosis, and a higher risk of bone fracture.

(Continued on page 602)

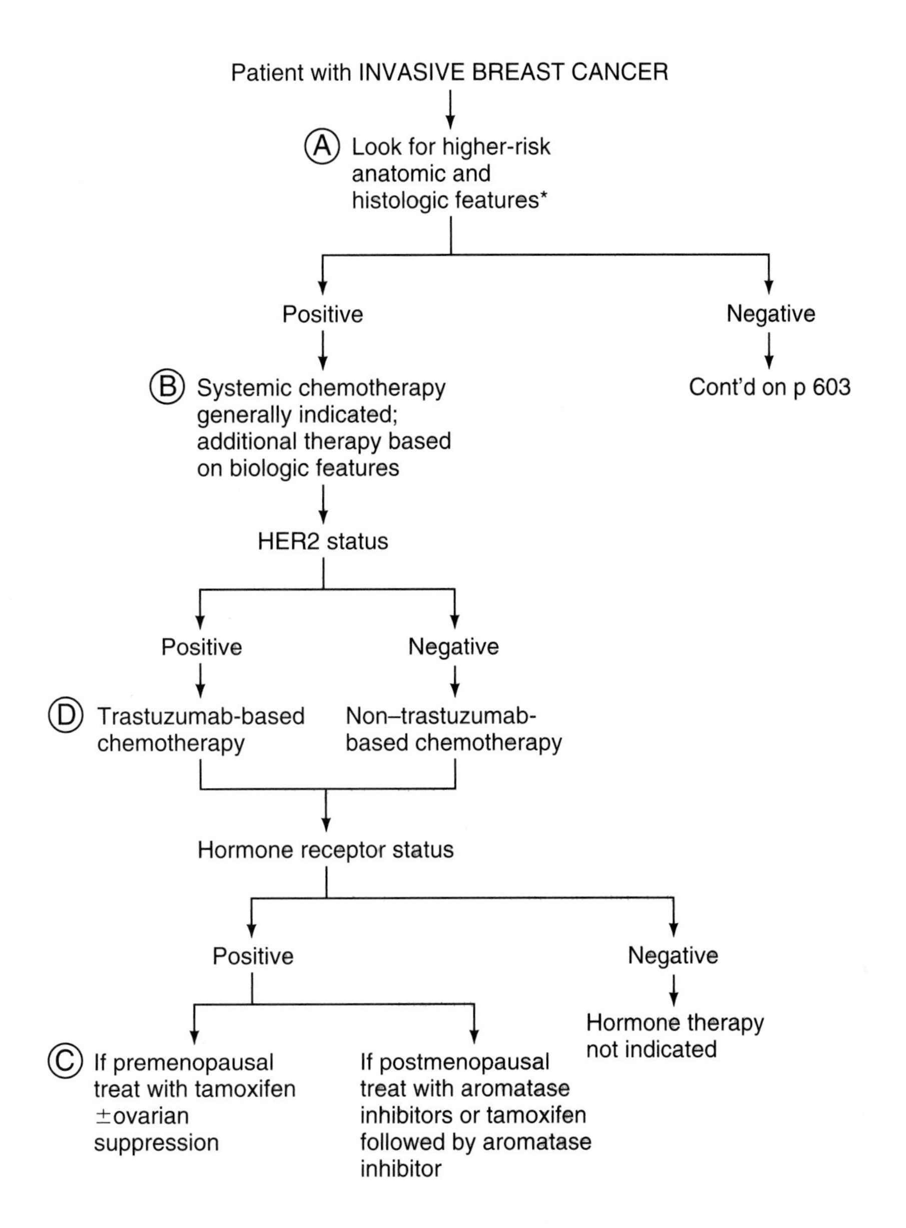
Patient with INVASIVE BREAST CANCER
(A) Look for higher-risk anatomic and histologic features*
Positive
Negative
(B) Systemic chemotherapy generally indicated; additional therapy based on biologic features
Cont'd on p 603
HER2 status
Positive
Negative
(D) Trastuzumab-based chemotherapy
Non–trastuzumab-based chemotherapy
Hormone receptor status
Positive
Negative
Hormone therapy not indicated
(C) If premenopausal treat with tamoxifen ±ovarian suppression
If postmenopausal treat with aromatase inhibitors or tamoxifen followed by aromatase inhibitor

*Large tumor, multiple positive lymph nodes, high-grade disease.

D. Biologic agents: Nearly one fifth of breast cancers overexpress HER2, a cell surface tyrosine kinase receptor, which is associated with a poor prognosis unless treated with trastuzumab, a humanized, monoclonal antibody. Two parallel trials, analyzed together, showed a dramatic reduction in disease recurrence and death (by 52% and 33%, respectively) associated with 1 year of treatment with trastuzumab following an anthracycline-based chemotherapy regimen. Other trials have tested trastuzumab in patients treated with a variety of chemotherapeutic regimens and have confirmed significantly improved disease-free survival. Treatment with trastuzumab is associated with up to a 4.1% risk of severe cardiomyopathy, so concurrent treatment with anthracyclines should be avoided, and patients should be closely monitored for signs of cardiac dysfunction. Other novel biologic therapies, including lapatinib and bevacizumab, are currently under active investigation in women with early breast cancer.

References

Albain K, Barlow W, Shak S, et al. Prognostic and predictive value of the 21-gene recurrence score assay in postmenopausal, node-positive, ER-positive breast cancer. [meeting abstract]. San Antonio Breast Cancer Symposium 2007, abstract 10.

Berry DA, Cirrincione C, Henderson IC, et al. Estrogen-receptor status and outcomes of modern chemotherapy for patients with node-positive breast cancer. JAMA 2006;295:1658–1667.

Boccardo F, Rubagotti A, Puntoni M, et al. Switching to anastrazole versus continued tamoxifen treatment of early breast cancer: preliminary results of the Italian Tamoxifen Anastrozole Trial. J Clin Oncol 2005;23:5138–5147.

Citron ML, Berry DA, Cirrincione C, et al. Randomized trials of dose-dense versus conventionally scheduled and sequential versus concurrent combination chemotherapy as postoperative adjuvant treatment of node-positive primary breast cancer: first report of Intergroup Trial C9741/Cancer and Leukemia Group B Trial 9741. J Clin Oncol 2003;21:1431–1439.

Early Breast Cancer Trialists' Collaborative Group. Effects of chemotherapy and hormonal therapy for early breast cancer on recurrence and 15-year survival: an overview of the randomized trials. Lancet 2005;365:1687–1717.

Early Breast Cancer Trialists' Collaborative Group. Polychemotherapy for early breast cancer: an overview of the randomized trials. Lancet 1998;352:930–942.

Fan C, Oh DS, Wessels L, et al. Concordance among gene-expression based predictors for breast cancer. N Engl J Med 2006;355:560–569.

Goss PE, Ingle JN, Martino S, et al. A randomized trial of letrozole in postmenopausal women after five years of tamoxifen therapy for early-stage breast cancer. N Engl J Med 2003;349:1793–1802.

Henderson IC, Berry DA, Demetri GD, et al. Improved outcomes from adding sequential paclitaxel but not from escalating doxorubicin dose in an adjuvant chemotherapy regimen for patients with node-positive primary breast cancer. J Clin Oncol 2003;21:976–983.

Howell A, Cuzick J, Baum M, et al. Results of the ATAC (Arimidex, Tamoxifen, Alone or in Combination) trial after completion of 5 years' adjuvant treatment for breast cancer. Lancet 2005;365:60–62.

Joensuu H, Kellokumpu-Lehtinen PL, Bono P, et al. Adjuvant docetaxel or vinorelbine with or without trastuzumab for breast cancer. N Engl J Med 2006; 354(8): 809–820.

Jones SE, Savin MA, Holmes FA, et al. Phase III trial comparing doxorubicin plus cyclophosphamide with docetaxel plus cyclophosphamide as adjuvant therapy for operable breast cancer. J Clin Oncol 2006;24:5381–5387.

National Comprehensive Cancer Network (www.nccn.org). Outside of the United States, many physicians follow practice guidelines from the International Consensus Panel.

Paik S, Shak S, Tang G, et al. A multigene assay to predict recurrence of tamoxifen-treated, node-negative breast cancer. N Engl J Med 2004;351:2817–2826.

Peto R, for the Early Breast Cancer Trialists' Collaborative Group. The worldwide overview: new results for systemic adjuvant therapies. San Antonio Breast Cancer Symposium, plenary lecture one, 12/13/07.

Peto R, Davies C. ATLAS (Adjuvant Tamoxifen, Longer Against Shorter): international randomized trial of 10 versus 5 years of adjuvant tamoxifen among 11,500 women-preliminary results [meeting abstract]. San Antonio Breast Cancer Symposium 2007, abstract 48.

Piccart-Gebhart MJ, Procter M, Leyland-Jones B, et al. Trastuzumab after adjuvant chemotherapy for HER2-positive breast cancer. N Engl J Med 2005;353:1659–1672.

Romond EH, Perez EA, Bryant J, et al. Trastuzumab plus adjuvant chemotherapy for operable HER2-positive breast cancer. N Engl J Med 2005;353:1673–1684.

Thurlimann B, Keshaviah A, Coates AS, et al. A comparison of letrozole and tamoxifen in postmenopausal women with early breast cancer. N Engl J Med 2005;353:2747–2757.

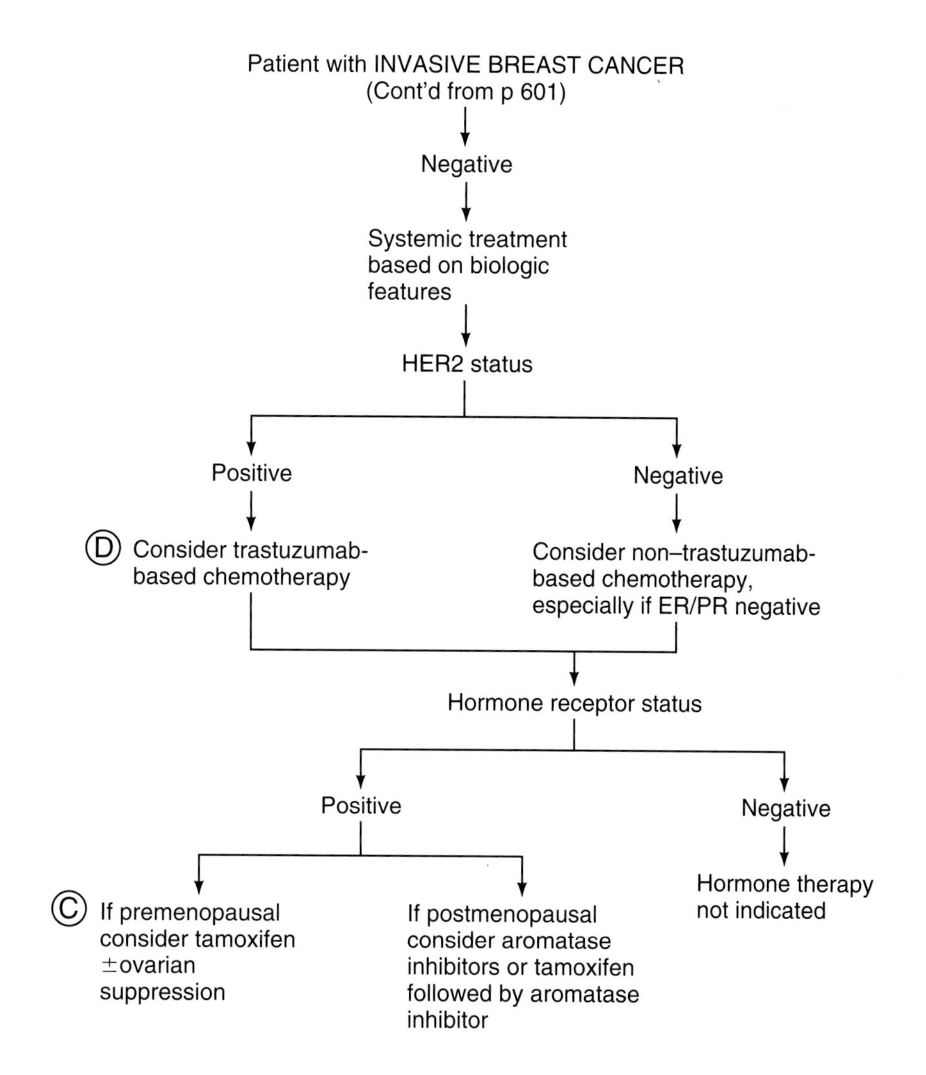
Patient with INVASIVE BREAST CANCER
(Cont'd from p 601)
Negative
Systemic treatment based on biologic features
HER2 status
Positive
Negative
D Consider trastuzumab-based chemotherapy
Consider non–trastuzumab-based chemotherapy, especially if ER/PR negative
Hormone receptor status
Positive
Negative
C If premenopausal consider tamoxifen ±ovarian suppression
If postmenopausal consider aromatase inhibitors or tamoxifen followed by aromatase inhibitor
Hormone therapy not indicated

NIPPLE DISCHARGE

Homeira Baghdadi, MD

A. Although nipple discharge is more commonly associated with benign than malignant lesions, cancer needs to be ruled out as the cause. As an initial step a careful medical history and examination is of paramount importance. To be significant, any type of nipple discharge should be true, spontaneous, persistent, and nonlactational. Question the patient for any medication, recent pregnancy, and evidence of amenorrhea. Pharmaceuticals that can cause galactorrhea include estrogens, phenothiazines, opiates, tricyclic antidepressants, dopamine antagonists, and many others by different mechanisms.

There are seven basic types of nipple discharge. Milky, multicolored, and purulent secretions are treated medically except for an abscess concomitant with a purulent discharge that requires surgical drainage. The remaining four types are yellow or serous, pink or serosanguineous, bloody or sanguineous, and clear or watery. These four types can be the result of cancer and often require surgery to obtain tissue for histologic study.

B. It is important to differentiate between galactorrheal and nongalactorrheal discharge. Galactorrhea may occur bilaterally or unilaterally. Secretions may be thick or thin, or pure white or close to colorless, or they may have a grayish or greenish hue. Fat stain is highly sensitive for determining presence of milk. Galactorrhea usually is of hormonal or pharmacologic origin. Measure serum prolactin and thyroid-stimulating hormone (TSH) in all patients with galactorrhea. If prolactin is elevated, obtain an MRI to determine whether the patient has a pituitary mass. If the prolactin and TSH are normal, follow the patient yearly or as indicated clinically. Human growth hormone (GH) binds to and activates prolactin receptors and GH receptors. Thus, galactorrhea may be an early sign of acromegaly. If clinically warranted, obtain a GH measurement. If the TSH is high, evaluate the patient for hypothyroidism. Patients with galactorrhea caused by hypothyroidism may have normal, high normal, or moderately elevated concentrations of prolactin. The majority of women with galactorrhea do not have an underlying, pathologic cause. At least half of women who have ever lactated can have galactorrhea at some time in their lives. Moreover, women who manipulate their breasts, or whose partners do so, can also experience galactorrhea. When galactorrhea is bilateral, a neoplastic process is particularly unlikely. Therefore, galactorrhea rarely requires treatment, unless an underlying cause is identified.

C. In patients with nongalactorrheal discharge, first perform a careful and thorough breast examination. Palpation of a mass requires immediate and complete evaluation to rule out a malignant process. If no mass is palpable, consider cytology and mammography. Although a mass usually is present when the discharge is caused by cancer, there is no palpable mass in 13% of cancers with nipple secretions. Do not rely solely on the cytology of the discharge. There is a reported 18% false-negative rate and 2.6% false-positive rate with standard cytology alone. Mammography has a 9.5% false-negative rate and 1.6% false-positive rate for detecting cancer in patients with a nipple discharge. The ability of soft-tissue mammography to identify and localize intraductal papillomas is limited. A number of authors have suggested that galactography (a contrast mammogram obtained by injecting a radiopaque dye into the discharging duct) is the diagnostic procedure of choice for nipple discharge. It is better than soft-tissue mammography in its ability to visualize and localize small intraductal papillomas. However, its ability to differentiate benign from malignant lesions is limited, and it is a time-consuming procedure that can be uncomfortable to the patients. Because diagnostic tests are not 100% accurate, surgically significant discharges should be evaluated with biopsy and histologic tissue examinations. Although rare, a watery discharge must be considered with concern. There is an increasing likelihood of cancer when the discharge is (in order of increasing frequency) serous, serosanguineous, sanguineous, or watery; when it is accompanied by a lump; when there are adverse cytologic and mammographic findings; and when the patient is >50 years of age.

References

Dickey, Richard P. Drugs that affect the breast and lactation. Clin Obstet Gynecol 1975;18:95.

Fiorica JV, James V. Nipple discharge. Obstet Gynecol Clin North Am 1994;21:453.

Gulay H, Bora S, Kilicturgay S, et al. Management of nipple discharge. J Am Coll Surg 1994;178:471.

Haney AF. Galactorrhea. In Bardin CW, ed. Current Therapy in Endocrinology and Metabolism, ed 6. St. Louis: Mosby, 1997:393.

Leis HP Jr. Management of nipple discharge. World J Surg 1989;13:736.

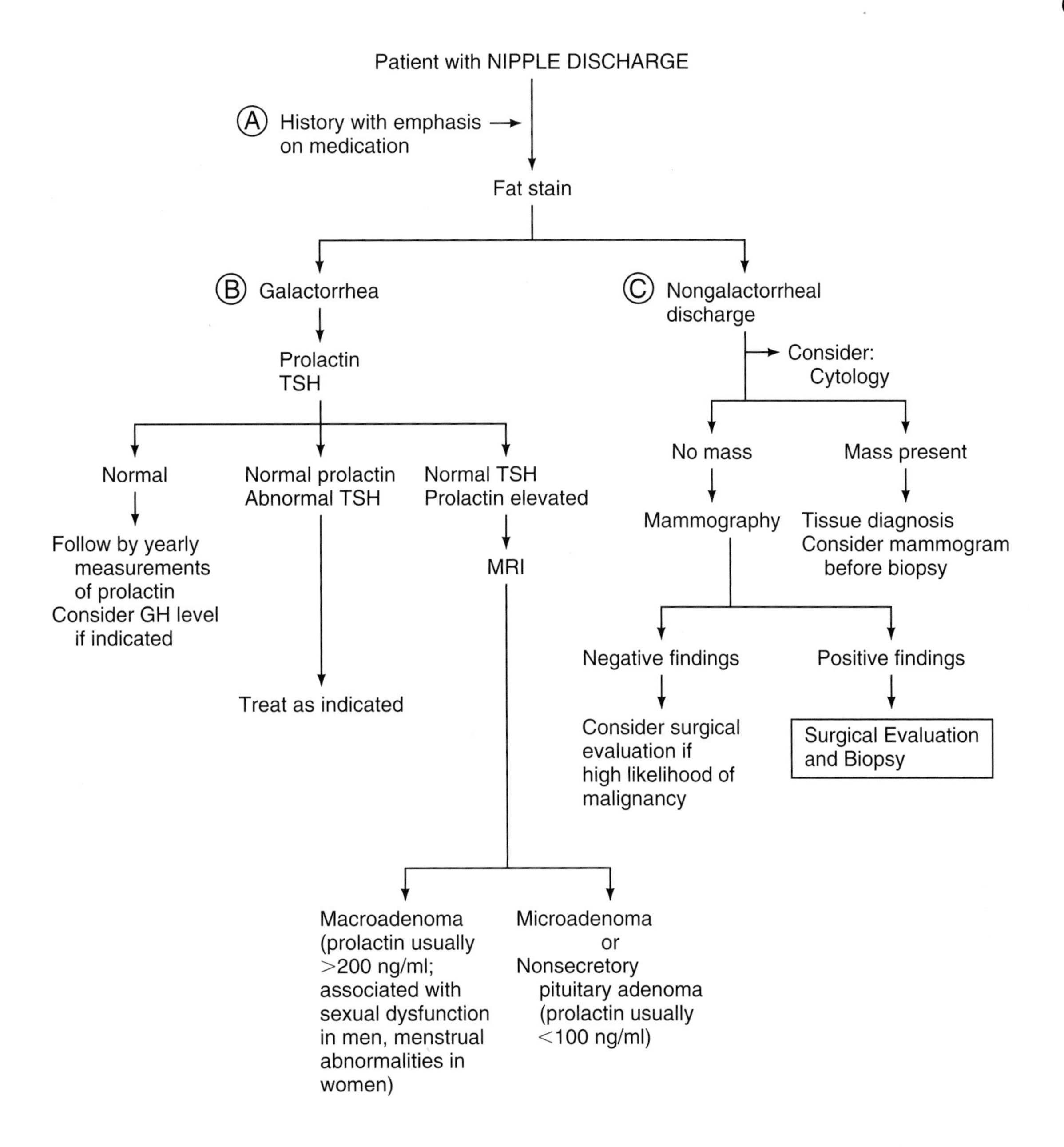
Patient with NIPPLE DISCHARGE
(A) History with emphasis on medication
Fat stain
(B) Galactorrhea
Prolactin
TSH
Normal
Follow by yearly measurements of prolactin
Consider GH level if indicated
Normal prolactin
Abnormal TSH
Treat as indicated
Normal TSH
Prolactin elevated
MRI
Macroadenoma (prolactin usually >200 ng/ml; associated with sexual dysfunction in men, menstrual abnormalities in women)
Microadenoma or Nonsecretory pituitary adenoma (prolactin usually <100 ng/ml)
(C) Nongalactorrheal discharge
Consider: Cytology
No mass
Mammography
Negative findings
Consider surgical evaluation if high likelihood of malignancy
Positive findings
Surgical Evaluation and Biopsy
Mass present
Tissue diagnosis
Consider mammogram before biopsy

ABNORMAL PAP SMEAR

Hugh S. Miller, MD

The decline in cervical cancer from the first to the seventh most common cancer among women in the United States is directly attributable to the use of screening Pap smears. The Pap smear is both sensitive and specific for pathology of the genital tract, including the vagina, cervix, uterus, and occasionally, even fallopian tubes and ovaries. The Bethesda System (TBS) was adopted in 1988 (revised in 1991) in an attempt to establish national standards for an industry that had been heavily criticized for its lack of standards and inadequate quality assurance. Its creation established the cytopathology report as a medical consultation and displaced the former Papanicolaou classification. With TBS cytopathologists must first determine the adequacy of the sample and then distinguish among inflammatory, infectious, and neoplastic processes. TBS adopted two new terms, *low-* and *high-grade squamous intraepithelial lesions* (SIL), to replace the previous terminology, exclusive of invasive carcinoma. Some cytopathologists may still use the former classifications of dysplasia, cervical intraepithelial neoplasia (CIN) 1–3. The new descriptive nomenclature, which includes the classifications of atypical squamous cells of undetermined significance (ASC-US) and low-grade squamous intraepithelial lesion (LSIL), has caused management controversy equal to that of the previous system.

A. Cervical cytopathology is strongly associated with sexual activity and human papillomavirus (HPV) infection, which is considered a sexually transmitted disease (STD). A complete gynecologic history, including STD history, age at first coitus, number of sexual partners, use of tobacco products, and previous abnormal cervical cytopathology with concomitant diagnostic procedures and treatment, is important in the evaluation of a patient with an abnormal Pap smear.

B. Evaluation of the female genital tract requires the best illumination and the proper size and shape of speculum to optimize visualization. Initially, examine the unprepared vulvar, vaginal, and cervical epithelium for whitish patches, growths, or ulcerations. Remember that the use of bactericidal or bacteriostatic lubricants compromises the culture and cytopathology results. Cervical friability, with or without an associated lesion, can represent an infectious condition or a neoplastic one. When a Pap smear is judged unsatisfactory, it usually is because of either the absence of endocervical cells or drying artifact. A properly obtained Pap smear contains exophytic and endophytic cervical cells to maximize the probability of sampling the transformation zone. A moistened cotton-tipped applicator and a spatula generally suffice. The endocervical brush collects a better endocervical sampling at an increased cost, with greater patient discomfort, and a higher risk of provoking bleeding that can obscure the cervical field. HPV DNA identification and cervicography are newer techniques developed to better identify patients at risk for invasive carcinoma by improving sensitivity and specificity. Papnet and the ThinPrep Pap Test, a liquid-based test, are newer screening technologies that may replace the conventional Pap smear. An advantage of the liquid-based Pap test is that it allows for "reflexive HPV testing" if the result is ASC-US. If HPV is present in the sample, the patient can proceed directly to colposcopy and not have to undergo several repeat tests to confirm the finding.

C. Consider the finding of ASC-US in a "satisfactory" Pap smear in the context of the patient's individual risk factors. For patients at risk or those with straightforward SIL, proceed with colposcopy and colposcopically directed biopsies. Loop electroexcision procedure (LEEP) has led some experienced colposcopists to collect a surgical specimen for diagnosis simultaneous with definitive surgical treatment. Patients exhibiting primary ASC-US associated with HPV derive minimal benefit from ablative therapy. Even many patients diagnosed with LSIL (60%) have spontaneous regression of their lesions without treatment. From the standpoint of infectious disease, patients with identifiable lesions benefit from ablative therapy, as do those with significant dysplasia. Cryoablation is preferred, but various topical preparations, laser therapy, LEEP, and cold-knife conization continue to be used. Management of patients with LSIL must be individualized to include the assessment of patient compliance with follow-up. After each specific intervention, reassess the cervix at 4- to 6-month intervals for 2 years, or until there have been three consecutive negative Pap smears. Annual surveillance may then resume.

D. Because abnormal Pap smears are strongly associated with HPV, consider other STDs in the evaluation of these patients. Cervicitis (see p 578) may be caused by more than one genital tract pathogen and may require collection of cultures and initiation of antibiotic therapy. Recurrent dysplasia should prompt further assessment of risk factors, such as smoking, chronic disease, and HIV status.

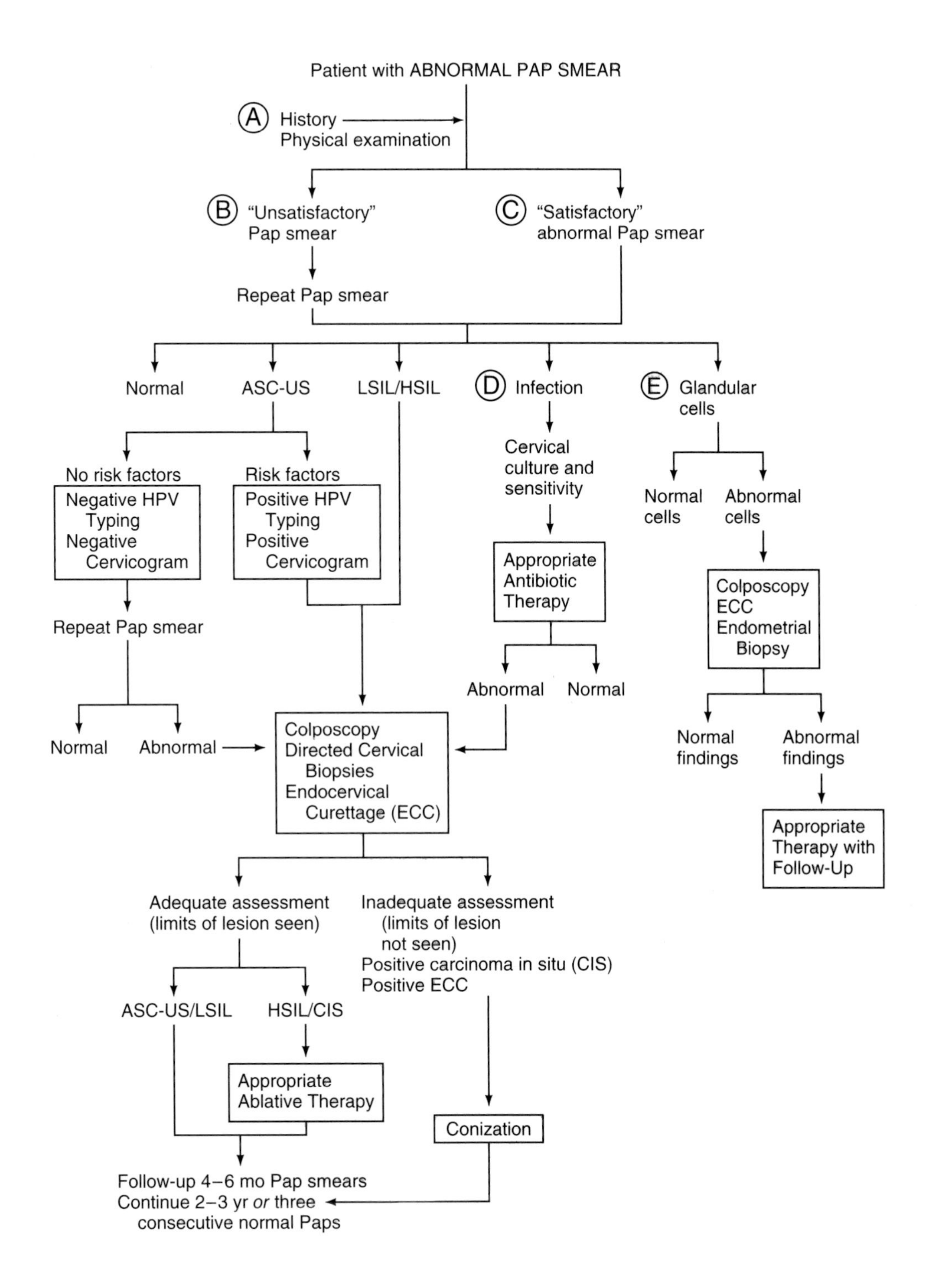

E. The cervix regularly rests in the posterior vaginal fornix, contributing to its exfoliated cells and those arising from the upper genital tract (endocervix, uterus, fallopian tube, and rarely, ovary). When normal endometrial or glandular cells are reported on the routine Pap smear, no further evaluation is needed. However, TBS allows a more precise characterization of the cell type and its morphology. In cases of atypical or neoplastic glandular cells, there is a high risk that a malignancy is present and further evaluation and treatment of the upper genital tract by an oncologic gynecologist is required.

References

American College of Obstetricians and Gynecologists. Cervical cytology: evaluation and management of abnormalities. Washington, DC: American College of Obstetricians and Gynecologists, ACOG Technical Bulletin No. 183, August 1993.

American College of Obstetricians and Gynecologists. Genital human papillomavirus infections. Washington, DC: American College of Obstetricians and Gynecologists, ACOG Technical Bulletin No. 193, June 1994.

Kurman RJ, Henson DE, Herbst AL, et al. Interim guidelines for management of abnormal cervical cytology. JAMA 1994;271:1866.

PREMENSTRUAL DYSPHORIC DISORDER

Jessica Byron, MD

A. More than 40% of women experiencing cyclic menstruation report premenstrual symptoms, ranging from negligible in many women to disabling in up to 15%. Many symptoms and signs have been described as part of premenstrual syndrome (PMS), including bloating, edema, weight gain, breast pain, acne, appetite changes, headaches, joint pain, diarrhea, constipation, anger or irritability, increased interpersonal conflicts, anxiety, aggression, depression, lethargy, fatigue, sleep disorder (hypersomnia, insomnia), difficulty concentrating, and restlessness. None of these symptoms is pathognomonic. It is the cyclic occurrence of symptoms beginning near or after ovulation and resolving soon after the onset of menses that is of diagnostic significance. In addition, the premenstrual changes must be significant enough to interfere with work, school, or usual social activities or relationships with others. The role of ovarian steroids, prolactin, prostaglandins, mineralocorticoids, neurotransmitters, endogenous opiates, vitamin and mineral deficiencies, and psychological factors is unclear.

B. Diagnostic evaluation of PMS involves clinical evaluation and review of the patient's prospective daily charting of the timing, type, and rating of severity of symptoms for at least two menstrual cycles. Take a medical history to rule out cardiac, renal, or thyroid disease, collagen vascular disease, and diabetes. Also exclude other problems, including anemia, breast disease, dysmenorrhea, endometriosis, perimenopausal changes, or premenstrual exacerbation of allergies, arthritis, asthma, diabetes, irritable bowel syndrome, migraine, and seizure disorders. Determine whether the patient has premenstrual dysphoric disorder (PMDD), which affects 5%–10% of normally cycling women. Many women with severe PMS meet the diagnostic criteria for PMDD. PMS/PMDD must be differentiated from other psychiatric disorders (anxiety, depression, eating or personality disorders) because these disorders also cause symptoms in the follicular phase. Perform physical examination and laboratory testing as needed. Investigators have been unable to document specific changes in hormone levels, prolactin, aldosterone, endorphins, and glucose tolerance. There are no laboratory tests to diagnose PMS.

C. It is essential to review the patient's daily symptom chart, which has tracked symptoms for two complete menstrual cycles. A variety of forms are available. One way is to ask the patient to list the symptoms that affect her most. The checklist is started on the first day of the period and each evening the symptoms are rated on a scale of 0–4 (0 = symptom is absent; 4 = symptom is severe and patient cannot function). At least five symptom scores during the luteal phase must show a marked change from scores in the follicular phase for PMS to be diagnosed. For severe PMS and PMDD, the questionnaire developed by Endicott and Harrison is helpful.

D. Review of treatment research fails to demonstrate consistently effective therapy, and the rate of response to placebo appears to be 50%. Numerous treatments have been advocated. Initial interventions are education and support, stress reduction, healthy nutrition, and regular exercise. Many women are reassured by chart review and can plan their schedules according to symptom severity, use relaxation exercises, join a support group, or participate in an exercise program to relieve stress. Eating complex carbohydrates (whole grains, beans, fresh fruits, vegetables) and low-protein foods and tapering caffeine intake, especially during the luteal phase, may diminish symptoms but efficacy remains unproved. Neither natural progesterone (in suppository or micronized oral preparations) nor synthetic progestins are effective for PMS.

E. Offer medical treatment or referral to women who meet the diagnostic criteria for PMDD. Consider prescribing a selective serotonin reuptake inhibitor (SSRI) if there are symptoms of PMDD or if PMS is severe and symptoms include psychosocial difficulties. When SSRIs do not work, an anxiolytic agent may be the next choice. Anovulation therapy with oral contraceptives (OCPs), danazol, and gonadotropin-releasing hormone (GnRH) agonists (goserelin acetate, leuprolide acetate, nafarelin acetate) can relieve symptoms of severe PMS, but unpleasant side effects are common and lead to discontinuance. OCPs appear to relieve PMS symptoms in about one third of women. Consider further evaluation or referral when the diagnosis is uncertain, another medical or psychiatric disorder is suspected, the patient is a risk to herself or others, or standard dosages of medications are ineffective in reducing symptoms.

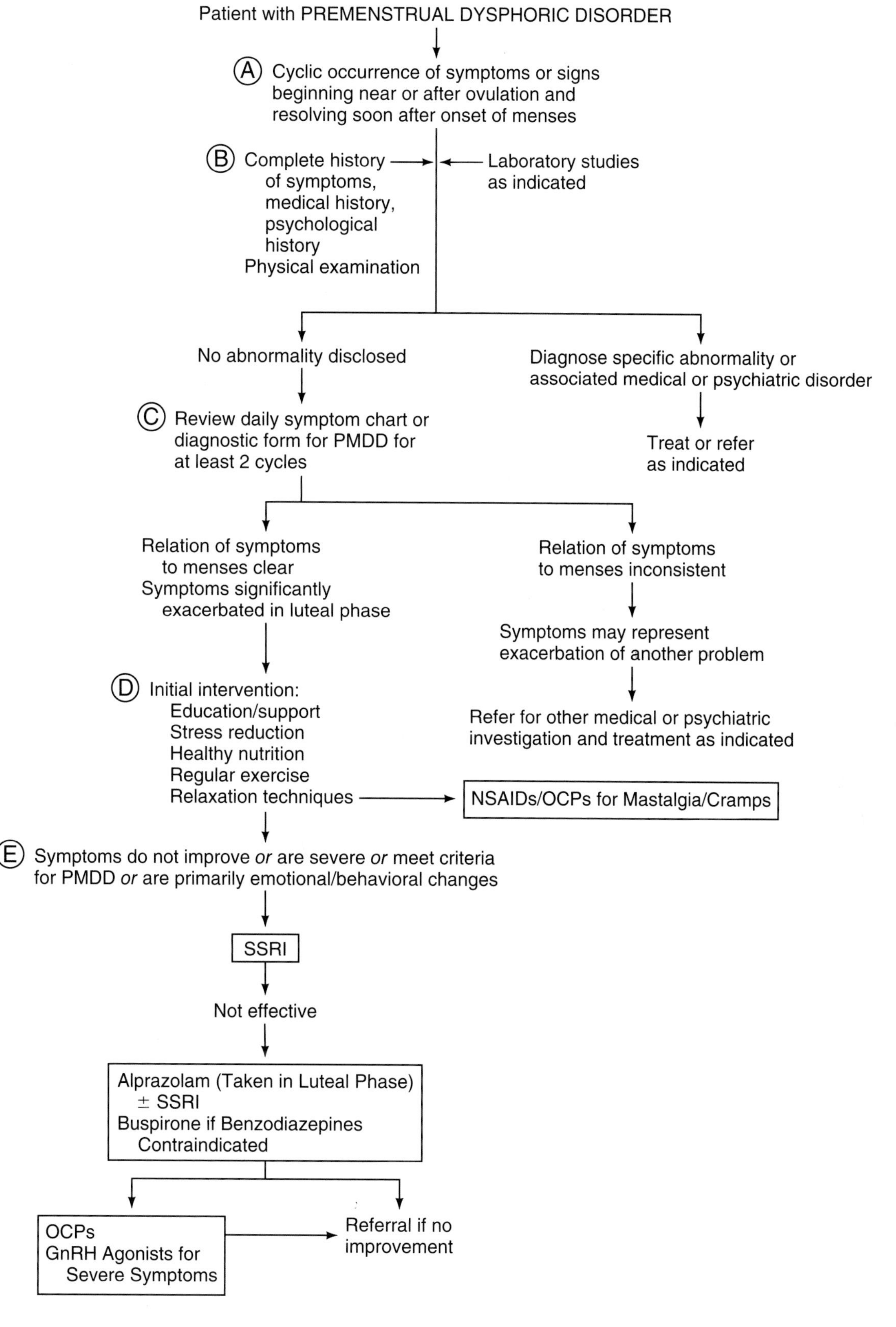

References

Barnhart KT, Freeman EW, Sondheimer SJ. A clinician's guide to the premenstrual syndrome. Med Clin North Am 1995;79:1457.

Endicott J, Freeman EW, Kielich A, et al. PMS: new treatments that really work. Patient Care 1996;April:88.

Goodale IL, Domar AD, Benson H. Alleviation of premenstrual syndrome with the relaxation response. Obstet Gynecol 1990;75:649.

Rubinow DR, Schmidt PJ. The treatment of premenstrual syndrome: forward into the past (editorial). N Engl J Med 1995;332:1574.

Sayegh R, Schiff I, Wurtman J, et al. The effect of a carbohydrate-rich beverage on mood, appetite and cognitive function in women with premenstrual syndrome. Obstet Gynecol 1995;86:520.

Severino SK, Moline ML. Premenstrual syndrome: identification and management. Drugs 1995;49(1):71.

CONTRACEPTIVE CHOICES

Ana Maria López, MD, MPH, FACP

The decision to conceive or not to conceive is a complicated one, dependent on multiple factors. It also is one in which many patients request physician participation. To facilitate this process, the physician must be well versed in biologic factors that may influence this decision and must be sensitive to patient concerns. Biologic factors that affect contraceptive choice include age, tobacco use, history of pelvic inflammatory disease (PID), and history of cardiovascular disease. Important patient issues that must be clarified include plans for future fertility, current sexual lifestyle, impact of unplanned pregnancy, history of compliance, and role of partner in birth spacing. Patients often have questions about efficacy (Table 1), safety, cost, and noncontraceptive benefits and the need to access the health care system to obtain or continue use of a specific birth control method (BCM). By applying active listening skills to the patient-physician interaction, the physician can help the patient make an informed choice.

Table 1. **Contraceptive Effectiveness in First Year in the United States***

BCM	Effectiveness: Theoretical (%)†	Typical (%)‡
Vasectomy	99.9	99.85
BLTL	99.8	99.6
Norplant	99.96	99.96
Depo Provera	99.7	99.7
OCs		
Combined	99.1	97
Mini-pill	99.5	80
IUD		
Cu-T 380A	99.2	97
Progestasert	98.0	93
Condom	98	88
Diaphragm	96	82
Cervical cap	94	82
Sponge		
Parous patient	91	72
Multiparous patient	94	82
Spermicides	97	80
Fertility awareness methods		
Calendar	90	80
With BBT, postovulation coitus only	98	97
Lactation		
Breast feeding on demand with amenorrhea, first 6 months postpartum	99	96
Chance	15	15

*Based on data in Hatcher et al, Trussel et al (1987), and Trussel et al (1990).

†Theoretical effectiveness attempts to predict the percent of contraceptive failures expected among couples using the BCM perfectly, consistently, and correctly for an entire year.

‡Typical effectiveness attempts to predict the percent of contraceptive failures expected among typical couples using the BCM for an entire year.

A. Vasectomy is simple, inexpensive, and safe but does not confer immediate sterility. Sperm usually are not present after 25 ejaculations, but this can be confirmed only by microscopic examination of the semen. Although antibody formation to sperm has been noted after vasectomy, clinically adverse implications have not been fully elucidated. Bilateral tubal ligation (BLTL) is the most common BCM in the world. It is an outpatient procedure with a lower mortality rate than childbirth (3:100,000 versus 14:100,000). If BLTL fails, the risk of ectopic pregnancy is increased. Vasectomy and BLTL may be reversed by microsurgical techniques. The success of reversals is inversely related to the amount of tissue originally damaged. Patients must be counseled that these are permanent BCMs and that their potential reversibility does not guarantee fertility.

B. Combination oral contraceptives (OCs) are second only to BLTL as the most common BCM in the world today. OCs were the first BCM to separate contraceptive use from sexual activity. They contain either estrogen and progesterone in fixed or variable combination or progesterone alone, the "mini-pill." The latter contains low-dose progesterone and is an option in women for whom estrogen is contraindicated (e.g., older women with cardiovascular risk factors) or in women who are lactating. Its efficacyis less than that for the combination OCs. In the former, the estrogen and progesterone hormone combination may be fixed (monophasic) or variable (phasic). In phasic preparations, the pills within a pack contain variable doses of the progestin and occasionally of the estrogen to decrease the overall hormonal doses while maintaining contraceptive effects and decreasing metabolic side effects.

OCs act by preventing ovulation. If ovulation should occur, implantation is prevented by changes in the cervical mucus and endometrium.

Patients should be instructed to start the pack of pills at the onset of the menses or on the first Sunday after the start of menstruation. Contraceptive efficacy requires about 2–4 weeks to develop. During these initial first few weeks another BCM should also be used. In a 28-day pack, 21 pills contain active hormone preparation and 7 are placebo pills that serve to facilitate daily pill taking. Some packs containing 21 pills and no placebos are available in some brands. If a pill is missed, the woman should take one pill every 12 hours until all the forgotten pills have been taken. A back-up BCM is advised for

(Continued on page 611)

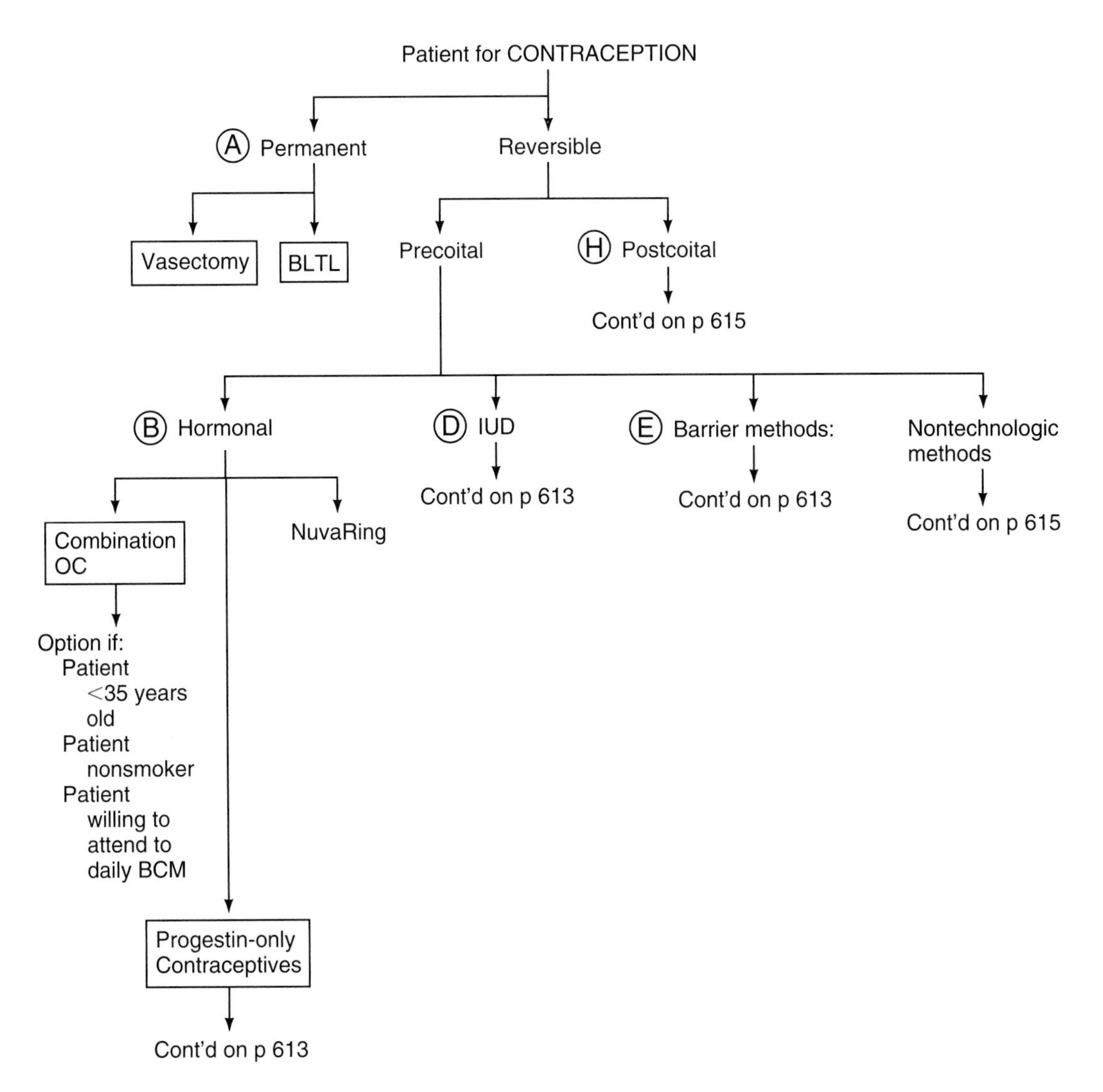

the remainder of the month. If three or more pills are missed repeatedly, another BCM should be considered. In the case of the mini-pill, even a 3-hour delay in pill taking may result in compromised antifertility activity; therefore a back-up BCM is recommended for 48 hours for such a delay. Patients should be counseled that OCs only prevent pregnancy, not sexually transmitted diseases. Condoms are still needed to prevent sexually transmitted diseases while one is taking OC.

Absolute contraindications to OC use include history of thrombophlebitis or thromboembolic events, cigarette smoking (1 pack/day or more), and age >35 years; hypertension; history of estrogen-dependent malignancy, such as breast or endometrial cancer; undiagnosed abnormal vaginal bleeding; and impaired liver function with history of cholestatic jaundice with prior pill use or with pregnancy or history of hepatic adenomas or carcinomas. Relative contraindications to OC use: smoker (1 pack/day or more) and history of migraines, severe headaches, seizures, severe depression, hyperlipidemia, ovarian dysfunction, gallbladder disease, diabetes mellitus, gestational diabetes, melanoma, obesity (550% overweight), or lactation.

Estrogen-related side effects include nausea, breast tenderness, cyclic weight gain, thrombophlebitis and thromboembolic events particularly in smokers, leukorrhea, cervical ectopy, headaches, hypertension, and benign or malignant hepatic neoplasias. Progesterone-related side effects include weight gain, depression, fatigue, decreased libido, acne, carbohydrate intolerance, and hyperlipidemia. OCs should be prescribed after a thorough history and physical examination have been performed. Once the patient is placed on OC therapy, close follow-up is necessary.

Hormonal contraception is also available as a vaginal ring (NuvaRing). This ring is inserted into the vagina and is removed after 3 weeks, allowing for menses to occur, before it is replaced again after one week. The ring contains ethinyl estradiol and etonogestrel. The principle advantage is that the patient does not need to remember to take daily pills, therefore increasing compliance.

With all the oral contraceptive methods and NuvaRing, the option exists to avoid menses by taking pills continuously and omitting the 1 week off. Some preparations are marketed as such (Seasonale), but any preparation can be modified to prevent menses. It is recommended that if patients choose the continuous method of oral contraception, menses should be allowed to occur quarterly, by omitting pills (or the ring) for 1 week.

C. Long-acting progestin-only contraceptives include Depo Provera. Norplant, the implantable progestin device, is no longer commonly used in this country since questions regarding its efficacy were raised (and subsequently dismissed) in 2000. The advantage of these progestin-only methods is that the estrogen-associated thromboembolic complications are avoided. Women most at risk for estrogen-related side effects are 35 years old or older, smokers, hypertensive patients, and those with a history of hypercoagulability. Progesterone-related side effects include increased low-density lipoprotein and decreased high-density lipoprotein with increased carbohydrate intolerance, possibly leading to diabetes. These methods act by inhibiting ovulation, maintaining thick cervical mucus inhospitable to sperm, and producing thin atrophic endometrium subject to premature luteolysis. Depo Provera, "the shot," consists of 150 mg of medroxyprogesterone given intramuscularly every 3 months. Although women often experience irregular vaginal bleeding in the first 12 months, the most common side effect after the first year is amenorrhea.

D. Intrauterine devices (IUDs) have a long history, but currently only two are available in the United States: Cu-T 380A and Mirena (a levonorgestrel-eluting IUD), with the former being more widely used. Cu-T 380A is FDA approved for 10-year use; however, Progestasert must be replaced every 5 years. IUDs are thought to act by inhibiting fertilization and implantation through local foreign body inflammation and because of the copper or progesterone effect of producing an atrophic endometrium. IUDs are contraindicated in patients with a known history of PID or ectopic pregnancy. They are inserted at the time of a woman's menses. Side effects for the copper IUD include menorrhagia, which may result in anemia; dysmenorrhea; and uterine perforation secondary to a wandering IUD. The Mirena IUD reduces menstrual bleeding and is ideal for patients who have heavy vaginal bleeding or for perimenopausal women who are experiencing dysfunctional uterine bleeding. Instruct the woman to ascertain IUD placement by checking for the IUD string.

E. Barrier methods require active patient participation. The diaphragm and cervical cap have been available for about 100 years and require fitting by a health care practitioner. Diaphragm use requires spermicide application before each episode of intercourse. It can be inserted up to 2 hours before intercourse and must remain in place 6–8 hours after coitus. Refitting must take place after pregnancy, pelvic surgery, or weight change of 10 pounds or more. In the United States, the Prentif cap is the only cervical cap available. It is inserted no less than half an hour before intercourse with a small amount of spermicide within the dome and can remain in place for 72 hours. A 24-hour limit is recommended to decrease cervical irritation and risk of toxic shock syndrome (TSS). Repeated spermicide applications are not required. The cervical cap cannot be used during menses. The cervical sponge is no longer available in the United States but is available abroad. It does not require health practitioner fitting and contains 1 gram of nonoxynol-9. It is available without a prescription and can be used continuously for 24 hours after moistening with tap water. All the aforementioned methods carry the risk of TSS. Spermicides can be used alone, although their efficacy is greatest when used in combination with condoms. Noncontraceptive benefits of nonoxynol-9 include prevention of STDs and PID. Condoms are the only male form of contraception. Problems with efficacy are associated with improper use (i.e., not leaving a 1/2-inch reservoir at the tip or not withdrawing carefully immediately after coitus). The Reality female condom has been developed and is commercially available. Recent studies in male contraception confirm the contraceptive efficacy of hormone-induced oligospermia.

(Continued on page 614)

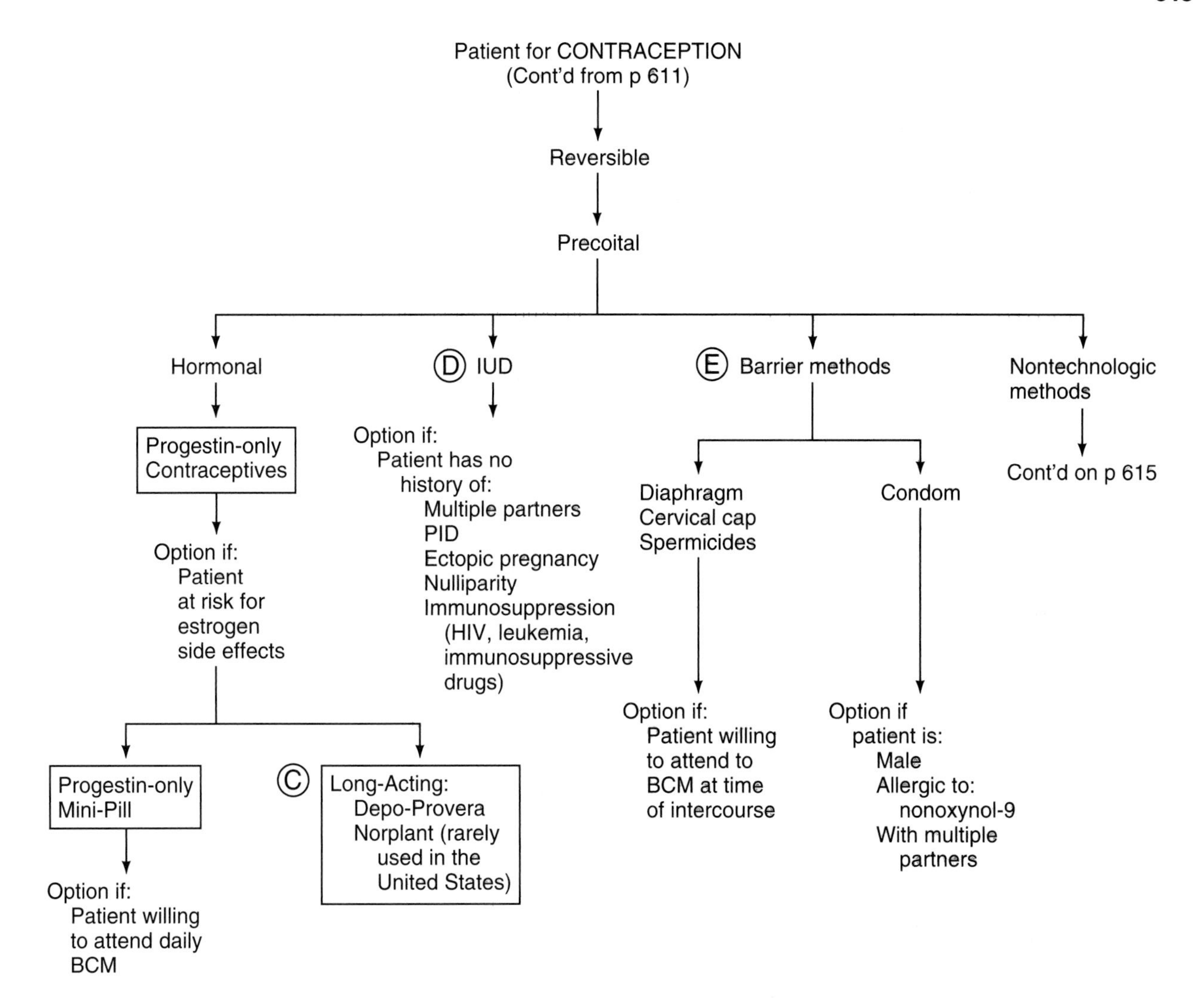
Patient for CONTRACEPTION
(Cont'd from p 611)
Reversible
Precoital
Hormonal
Progestin-only Contraceptives
Option if: Patient at risk for estrogen side effects
Progestin-only Mini-Pill
Option if: Patient willing to attend daily BCM
C Long-Acting: Depo-Provera Norplant (rarely used in the United States)
D IUD
Option if: Patient has no history of: Multiple partners PID Ectopic pregnancy Nulliparity Immunosuppression (HIV, leukemia, immunosuppressive drugs)
E Barrier methods
Diaphragm Cervical cap Spermicides
Option if: Patient willing to attend to BCM at time of intercourse
Condom
Option if patient is: Male Allergic to: nonoxynol-9 With multiple partners
Nontechnologic methods
Cont'd on p 615

F. Fertility awareness methods (FAMs) can be as effective as OCs in preventing pregnancy if used appropriately, with intercourse restricted to the postovulatory period. Efficacy is directly related to the use of multiple factors to detect fertility. Because of the complexity of these factors, formal instruction is advised before attempting use for either contraception or conception. Basal body temperature (BBT) is recorded daily to detect a temperature rise of 0.4°–0.8° F, indicating ovulation. Cervical mucus also must be examined daily because wet, thin mucus (as opposed to thick, dry mucus) facilitates sperm mobility. A record of the length of the patient's cycles is maintained. From this historical information and awareness that ovulation usually takes place 14 days before the onset of menses, a period of high-risk days can be defined. Some patients also note changes in cervical position and texture throughout the menstrual cycle. Finally, mittelschmerz (mid-cycle pain) is a sign of ovulation that some women consistently recognize. This method is not recommended for women who do not have regular periods.

G. Worldwide, lactation is a successful BCM. Recent data reveal that breastfeeding on demand while remaining amenorrheic in the first 6 months postpartum is 98% effective as a BCM. Unfortunately, most U.S. patients are unable or do not desire to breastfeed on demand for 6 months. During the first 6 months of lactation, prolactin levels are high and inhibit ovulation. After this time, however, prolactin levels decline and ovulation recurs. Because women cannot predict when ovulation will recur, lactation as a sole means of birth control is unreliable.

H. Postcoital hormonal approaches include the use of levonorgestrel (0.75 mg every 12 hours for two doses) or ethinyl estradiol-levonorgestrel (100 mcg–0.5 mg every 12 hours for two doses) within 72 hours of the episode of unprotected intercourse: Postcoital IUDs have also been used. The Cu-T may be inserted up to 5 days after intercourse; however, it is contraindicated in rape cases, in women with multiple partners, and in nulliparous patients. In prescribing postcoital OCs or IUDs, take care to screen for potential contraindications. Although these methods are part of clinical practice and are prescribed for postcoital contraception, the FDA has not approved their postcoital use, nor has it approved them for nonprescription availability. RU486 (mifepristone), a progesterone antagonist, 600 mg as a single dose, has been shown to be 100% effective in preventing pregnancy, even if taken up to 120 hours after coitus. It is widely used in Europe but is not approved for this purpose in the United States.

References

Affandi B, Santoso SS, Djajadilaga, et al. Five-year experience with Norplant. Contraception 1987;36:429.

Albertson BD, Zinaman MJ. The prediction of ovulation and monitoring of the fertile period. Adv Contracept 1987;3:263.

Alderman P. The lurking sperm. JAMA 1988;259:3142.

Burnhill MS. The rise and fall and rise of the IUD. Am J Gynecol Health 1989;III(3):6.

Choice of contraceptives. Med Lett Drugs Ther 1995;37:9.

Gallen ME. Men—new focus on family planning. Pop Rep 1987;Series J:890.

Geerling JH. Natural family planning. Am Fam Physician 1995;52:1749.

Haspels AA. Emergency contraception: a review. Contraception 1994. 50:101.

Hatcher RA, Stewart F, Trussell J, et al. Contraceptive Technology, ed 16, New York, 1994, Irvington.

Kaunitz AM, Illions EH, Jones HL, et al. Contraception: a clinical review for the internist. Med Clin North Am 1995;79:1377.

Kennedy KI, Rivera R, McNeilly AS. Consensus statement on the use of breastfeeding as a family planning method. Contraception 1989;39:477.

Topical spermicides. Med Lett Drugs Ther 1980;22:90.

Trussell J, Hatcher RA, Cates W Jr, et al. Contraceptive failure in the United States: an update. Stud Fam Plann 1990;21:51.

Trussell J, Kost K. Contraceptive failure in the United States: a critical review of the literature. Stud Fam Plann 1987;18:237.

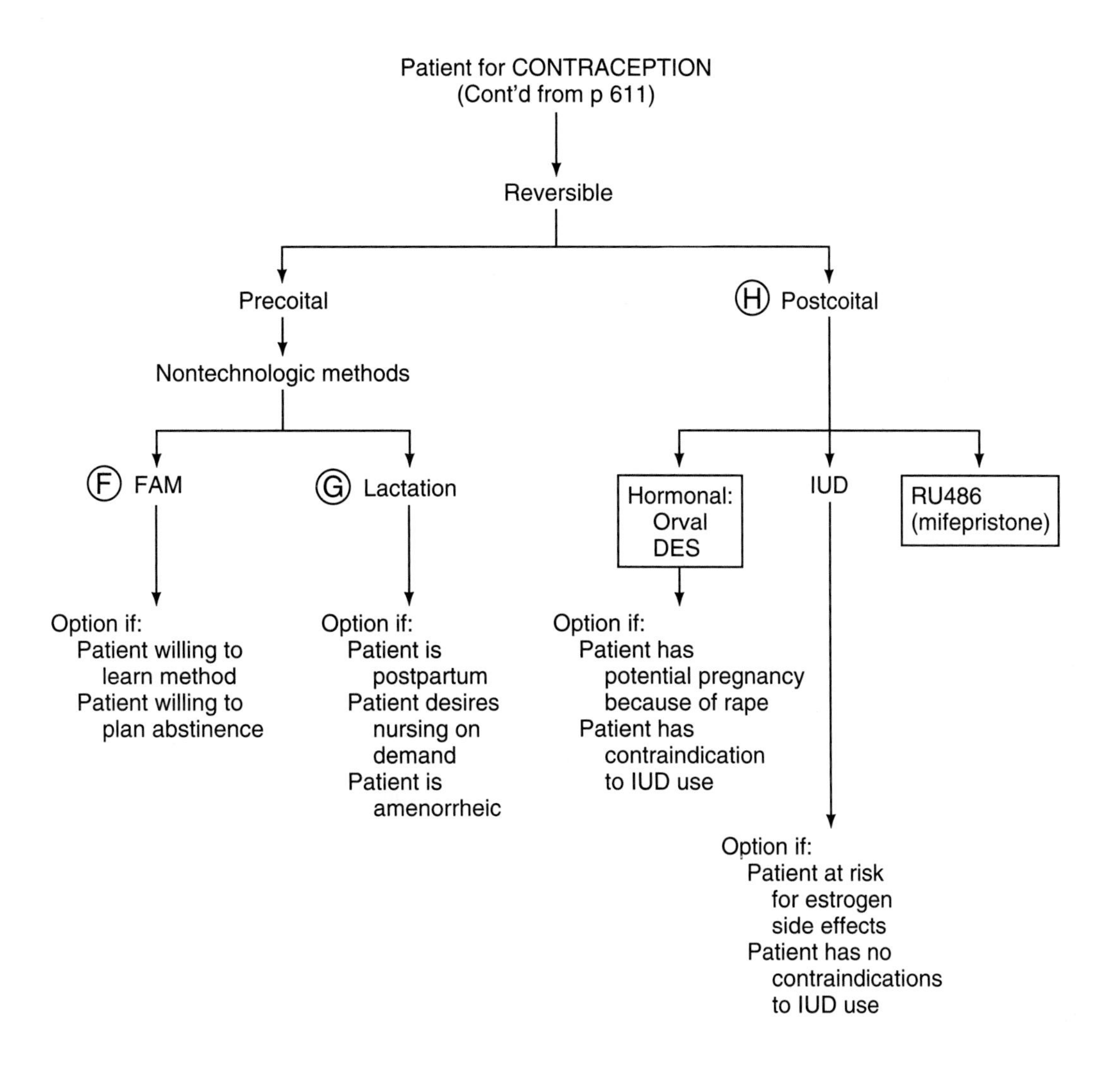
Patient for CONTRACEPTION
(Cont'd from p 611)
Reversible
Precoital
Nontechnologic methods
(F) FAM
(G) Lactation
(H) Postcoital
Hormonal:
Orval
DES
IUD
RU486
(mifepristone)
Option if:
Patient willing to learn method
Patient willing to plan abstinence
Option if:
Patient is postpartum
Patient desires nursing on demand
Patient is amenorrheic
Option if:
Patient has potential pregnancy because of rape
Patient has contraindication to IUD use
Option if:
Patient at risk for estrogen side effects
Patient has no contraindications to IUD use

USE OF ORAL CONTRACEPTIVES

Terra A. Robles, PharmD

Early studies found that oral contraceptives (OCs), which had a greater amount of estrogen, were associated with serious adverse outcomes. Today's low-dose formulations retain efficacy while minimizing side effects and have an overall lower risk of cardiovascular disease. OCs contain synthetic estrogens and progestins. They differ in dosage, proportion of active ingredients, and prescribed regimens. Effectiveness, safety, and patient acceptability are important in selection of OC products. Provide a product that offers the lowest effective dose of both hormones and minimizes side effects. Data are not available for determining which OC is "better"; cost considerations should be included in product selection.

A. Before prescribing an OC, obtain a complete history, including history of previous contraceptive use and failures or adverse effects of previously used methods; menstrual history, focusing on patterns and problems; history of blood clots and tobacco use; gynecologic and obstetric history; family history of coagulopathy; and general medical history. Perform a complete physical examination in which risk factors are assessed and contraindications to OC use determined. Order appropriate laboratory tests as necessary.

B. Monophasic pills contain a constant estrogen and progestin dose. Biphasic products contain a constant dose of estrogen, with a lower progestin dose on days 1–10 than on days 11–21. Triphasic pills have varied amounts of hormones; Ortho-Novum 777, Tri-Levlen, Tri-Cyclen, and Triphasil have an increase of progestin at midcycle and end cycle; Tri-Norinyl has increased progestin only at midcycle. Ortho-Novum 777, Tri-Cyclen, and Tri-Norinyl have fixed amounts of estrogen; Triphasil and Tri-Levlen have increased estrogen at midcycle. These differences in triphasic pills are generally insignificant in most women who do not have specific problems or menstrual irregularities.

   Ethinyl estradiol (EE) and mestranol are the two estrogen agents used in OCs. EE is pharmacologically active and mestranol is hepatically converted to EE. Progestins used in OCs include norethindrone, norethindrone acetate, ethynodiol diacetate, dl-norgestrel, norethynodrel, levonorgestrel, desogestrel, and norgestimate. Norethindrone acetate and ethynodiol diacetate are metabolized to norethindrone and offer no significant advantage over norethindrone. dl-Norgestrel and levonorgestrel are isomers, levonorgestrel being the active component. Some studies suggest that dl-norgestrel has little pharmacologic activity, but others state that it prevents breakthrough bleeding (BTB) more effectively. Norgestrel, levonorgestrel, and desogestrel have the highest progestational effects. Norethynodrel has the highest estrogenic effects with all others having minimal to no estrogenic effects. The greatest androgenic effects are seen by norgestrel and levonorgestrel.

   Estrogen is the major determinant for inducing increases in blood pressure (BP); however, progestins also may be associated. Carbohydrate and lipid alternations are caused by the progestin component in OCs. Desogestrel, norgestimate, and low doses of norethindrone have little if any effects on carbohydrate metabolism. Progestins decrease high-density lipoproteins (HDLs) and increase low-density lipoproteins (LDLs); estrogens have the opposite effect.

   A back-up method of birth control is recommended with the first cycle of OCs. Compliance is important for low-dose OCs because missed pills often lead to breakthrough ovulation.

C. The American College of Obstetricians and Gynecologists states that nonsmoking healthy women aged 35–44 years may continue using OCs. However, women with preexisting diseases that affect the cardiovascular system should not use OCs. Use clinical judgment in deciding whether any woman with cardiovascular disease risk factors (e.g., hypertension, diabetes mellitus, or hypercholesterolemia) should use OCs. Some studies of low-dose OCs show no increased risk of cardiovascular complications; however, OCs are currently considered synergistic in increased risk, and each patient must be carefully evaluated for OC use. Follow and monitor patients closely, and offer alternative contraceptive methods when indicated, especially for smokers >35 years of age.

D. Progestin-only pills, or "mini-pills," have lower effectiveness than combination OCs (COCs) because ovulation is not consistently inhibited. Progestin-only pills are taken every day of the month, without a break for withdrawal bleeding. Up to two thirds of users experience menstrual irregularities, BTB, and amenorrhea. Mini-pills also are used in lactating women.

(Continued on page 618)

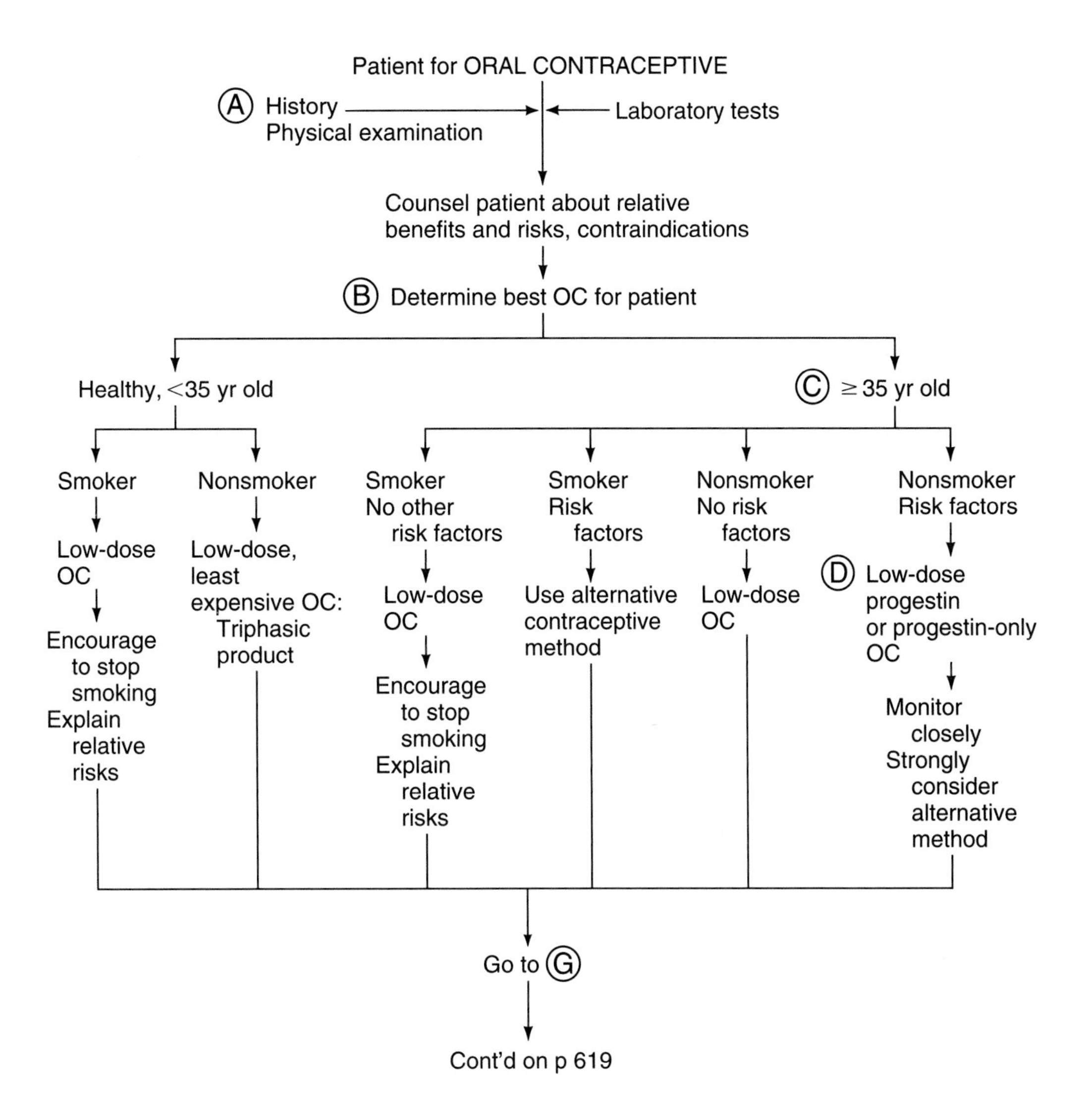

Patient for ORAL CONTRACEPTIVE
(A) History
Physical examination
Laboratory tests
Counsel patient about relative benefits and risks, contraindications
(B) Determine best OC for patient
Healthy, <35 yr old
(C) ≥35 yr old
Smoker
Nonsmoker
Smoker No other risk factors
Smoker Risk factors
Nonsmoker No risk factors
Nonsmoker Risk factors
Low-dose OC
Low-dose, least expensive OC: Triphasic product
Low-dose OC
Use alternative contraceptive method
Low-dose OC
(D) Low-dose progestin or progestin-only OC
Encourage to stop smoking Explain relative risks
Encourage to stop smoking Explain relative risks
Monitor closely Strongly consider alternative method
Go to (G)
Cont'd on p 619

E. There is some concern about infant exposure to estrogens. Some believe this exposure is not clinically significant; others advocate waiting until an infant is weaned before instituting OC use. The pill may diminish the protein content and volume of breast milk. The FDA recommends deferring the use of OCs until a baby is weaned.

F. Diabetic patients whose diabetes is controlled may take low-dose OCs. Products with norethindrone, desogestrel, or norgestimate are least likely to alter glucose tolerance. Pregnancy prevention needs to be weighted against the risk of pregnancy, and the risk of fetal malformations in poorly controlled diabetic pregnancies.

G. ACHES is a mnemonic commonly used to help remember possible adverse effects of OCs: *A*, abdominal pain (gallbladder disease, hepatic adenoma, pancreatitis, blood clot); *C*, chest pain (pulmonary embolism, myocardial infarction); *H*, headaches (stroke, migraines, hypertension); *E*, eye problems (hypertension, stroke); *S*, severe leg pain (venous thromboembolism). COCs have relative estrogen dominance, and estrogen-related side effects can be expected to predominate. Familiarization with symptoms of estrogen/progestin excess/deficiency will aid in OC adjustments. Symptoms of estrogen excess include nausea, breast tenderness, fluid retention, cervical mucorrhea, and cyclic headaches, whereas estrogen deficiency is suggested by early or midcycle BTB, increased spotting, and hypomenorrhea. Symptoms of progestin excess are increased appetite, depression, fatigue, acne, diabetogenic effects, and decreased libido; symptoms of progestin deficiency include late-cycle BTB, amenorrhea, and hypermenorrhea. An excess of both hormones can cause headaches, weight gain, and hypertension. Many symptoms occurring in the first cycle of OC use improve by the second or third cycle.

H. Lowering the potency of OCs for greater safety has led to an increased incidence of BTB. BTB is common in the first few cycles of OC use.

I. Estrogens are conjugated in the liver and hydrolyzed by intestinal bacteria. Any drug that affects these two systems may lead to decreased OC efficacy.

J. The absence of withdrawal bleeding may be the result of insufficient endometrial development. Switching to an OC with greater progestin content may resolve the problem.

K. An increase in BP may be seen even in normotensive patients. Increases can occur 1–36 months after initiation of the OC. The risk is lower with low-dose OCs. Patients who are started on OCs should be checked for BP changes within the first month. When hypertension is associated with an OC, it is reversible. Monitor any patient who develops hypertension while taking OCs closely for the development of OC-associated complications. A return to normal BP after discontinuation of OC may take 3–6 months.

L. Breast tenderness usually is caused by cyclic fluid retention or growth of breast tissue. An OC with lower estrogenic activity or greater progestational activity or an OC with less estrogen *and* less progestin may alleviate the tenderness. If tenderness persists, a progestin-only pill may be tried.

M. Nausea may occur often during the first few cycles of OC use or may occur with the first few pills of each cycle. Many patients can prevent nausea by taking the pill with food or at bedtime. If nausea persists, an OC with lower estrogenic activity (as little as 20 μg in severe cases) may bring relief. Vomiting is rare. If vomiting occurs within 2 hours after taking the OC, the dose should be repeated to ensure contraception.

N. Weight loss and gain occur with equal frequency in OC users. Most weight changes are unrelated to OC use. However, estrogen can cause cyclic weight gain as a result of fluid retention, and progestins can stimulate appetite and insulin release.

O. There is an increased risk of stroke in OC users with a history of migraine. Cerebrovascular accident (CVA) must be ruled out in all OC users who have migraine headaches. Vascular (migrainelike) headaches generally do not improve with a change in OC; these patients need to consider alternative contraceptive methods. Headaches accompanied by fluid retention (edema, breast enlargement, cyclic weight gain) may be caused by both estrogens and progestins. Prescribe an OC with lower estrogenic or progestational activity and follow the patient closely to ensure resolution of symptoms after one or two cycles.

P. Depression may be caused by an excess of estrogen or progestin or by a deficiency of estrogen. If switching to an OC with lower estrogenic or progestational activity does not alleviate the depression, the pill should be discontinued for three to six cycles and reevaluation performed at that time.

References

Casper RF, Powell AM. Evaluation and therapy of breakthrough bleeding in women using a triphasic oral contraceptive. Fertil Steril 1991;55:292.

Ellsworth AJ, Leversee JH. Oral contraceptives. Primary Care 1990;17:603.

Hatcher RA, Stewart F, Trussell J, et al. Contraceptive Technology, ed 16. New York:Irvington, 1994.

Heath CB. Helping patients choose appropriate contraception. Am Fam Physician 1993;48:1115.

Orife J. Benefits and risks of oral contraceptives. Adv Contracept 1990;6(Suppl):15.

Wall DM, Roos MP. Update on combination oral contraceptives. Am Fam Physician 1990;42:1037.

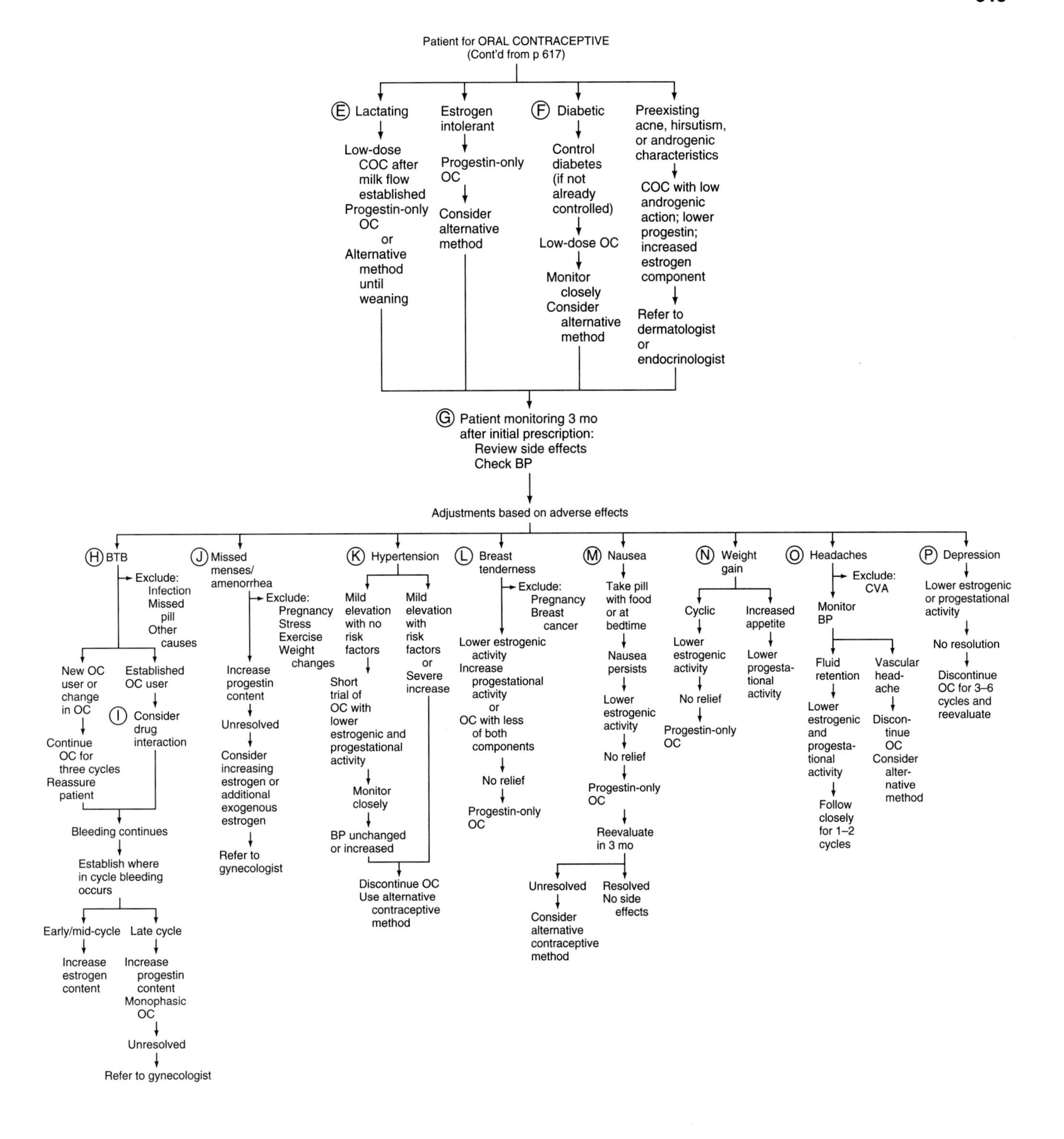
Patient for ORAL CONTRACEPTIVE
(Cont'd from p 617)
E Lactating
Low-dose COC after milk flow established
Progestin-only OC
or
Alternative method until weaning
Estrogen intolerant
Progestin-only OC
Consider alternative method
F Diabetic
Control diabetes (if not already controlled)
Low-dose OC
Monitor closely
Consider alternative method
Preexisting acne, hirsutism, or androgenic characteristics
COC with low androgenic action; lower progestin; increased estrogen component
Refer to dermatologist or endocrinologist
G Patient monitoring 3 mo after initial prescription:
Review side effects
Check BP
Adjustments based on adverse effects
H BTB
Exclude:
Infection
Missed pill
Other causes
New OC user or change in OC
Continue OC for three cycles
Reassure patient
Established OC user
I Consider drug interaction
Bleeding continues
Establish where in cycle bleeding occurs
Early/mid-cycle
Increase estrogen content
Late cycle
Increase progestin content
Monophasic OC
Unresolved
Refer to gynecologist
J Missed menses/ amenorrhea
Exclude:
Pregnancy
Stress
Exercise
Weight changes
Increase progestin content
Unresolved
Consider increasing estrogen or additional exogenous estrogen
Refer to gynecologist
K Hypertension
Mild elevation with no risk factors
Short trial of OC with lower estrogenic and progestational activity
Monitor closely
BP unchanged or increased
Mild elevation with risk factors
or
Severe increase
Discontinue OC
Use alternative contraceptive method
L Breast tenderness
Exclude:
Pregnancy
Breast cancer
Lower estrogenic activity
Increase progestational activity
or
OC with less of both components
No relief
Progestin-only OC
M Nausea
Take pill with food or at bedtime
Nausea persists
Lower estrogenic activity
No relief
Progestin-only OC
Reevaluate in 3 mo
Unresolved
Consider alternative contraceptive method
Resolved
No side effects
N Weight gain
Cyclic
Lower estrogenic activity
No relief
Progestin-only OC
Increased appetite
Lower progestational activity
O Headaches
Exclude:
CVA
Monitor BP
Fluid retention
Lower estrogenic and progestational activity
Follow closely for 1–2 cycles
Vascular headache
Discontinue OC
Consider alternative method
P Depression
Lower estrogenic or progestational activity
No resolution
Discontinue OC for 3–6 cycles and reevaluate

FEMALE INFERTILITY

Lorna A. Marshall, MD

Infertility is failure to conceive after 1 year of unprotected intercourse. It is a common problem, estimated to affect 8%–15% of married couples. Even before a couple is considered infertile, counseling should include a discussion of the menstrual cycle and appropriate timing of intercourse. In general, intercourse should occur about every 36–72 hours from 3–4 days before until 2 days after ovulation. It is important that sperm be available before ovulation. Ovulation usually occurs about 14 days before the subsequent menses or on about day 14 of a 28-day cycle. Encourage couples who wish to time intercourse more precisely to use prospective methods to detect ovulation, such as home ovulation predictor kits that detect a surge in luteinizing hormone (LH). Basal body temperature charts may identify the day of ovulation retrospectively, so they are not as useful in timing intercourse.

Considerable controversy remains about what constitutes a basic and complete fertility evaluation. Cost-effectiveness is an important part of the decision-making process because many insurance plans cover little or none of the evaluation and treatment of infertility. The current trend is to minimize testing and to move more quickly through a treatment plan. For example, laparoscopy was once a standard part of a fertility evaluation; now its considerable expense is often avoided in favor of using resources for treatments, such as reproductive technologies. Often it is more cost-effective to refer the patient to a specialist before expensive testing is performed so that the remainder of the evaluation can be integrated into the overall treatment plan.

A. The couple should be present for the initial fertility evaluation. Take a complete reproductive history of the female partner, including past and current menstrual pattern, contraceptive use, sexually transmitted diseases (STDs), prior pregnancies, pelvic pain or dysmenorrhea, in utero exposure to diethylstilbestrol, and past gynecologic procedures. Review medical and family histories, use of medications, and coital pattern.

B. A complete physical examination includes body habitus, abnormal hair growth patterns, a careful thyroid examination, and exclusion of galactorrhea. Perform careful pelvic examination, ruling out pelvic masses. Tender nodularity in the posterior cul de sac or a fixed uterus suggests endometriosis.

C. Advanced age of the female partner (>35 years) is a strong risk factor for infertility. Initiate an evaluation after 6 months of unprotected intercourse and proceed more quickly than in younger women. Obtain a cycle day 3 follicle-stimulating hormone (FSH) level to provide information on the success of various therapies, and quickly perform a basic evaluation. Consider an early referral to a specialist. Many women >40 years and those with elevated FSH levels may conceive only with eggs donated from younger women.

D. Ovulation may be evaluated in many ways. If the menstrual interval is >35 days, anovulation is likely. Obtain thyroid-stimulating hormone (TSH), FSH, and prolactin levels, and initiate treatment with clomiphene citrate. In women with normal menses, ovulation is likely if two to three cycles of basal body temperature charts are biphasic or if a LH surge is detected. A temperature elevation should be maintained for ≥11 days. Ovulation can be confirmed with a midluteal (usually day 21) progesterone level of >5 ng/ml. Use other laboratory tests sparingly; many physicians measure TSH and prolactin levels on all infertile women, regardless of ovulatory status. Serial ultrasound studies of ovulation add considerable expense and usually little information to a basic evaluation. A timed endometrial biopsy will document normal ovulation but adds expense and rarely influences decision making.

E. In general, a day 3 FSH level of >15 mIU/ml and estradiol >50 pg/ml predict a low success rate with reproductive technologies, and probably with most other fertility treatments. These values may vary considerably between laboratories.

F. If the female partner is anovulatory or oligomenorrheic and laboratory test results are normal, clomiphene citrate may be prescribed for up to three ovulatory cycles. After a spontaneous or progestin-induced menstrual cycle, the starting dosage is 50 mg for 5 days, starting on day 3, 4, or 5 of the cycle. Use basal body temperature charts to monitor ovulation. The dosage may be increased to 100 mg if anovulation persists, if basal body temperature rises after day 20, or if the luteal phase is <11 days. Of patients who will conceive, 80% do so within the first three ovulatory cycles.

(Continued on page 622)

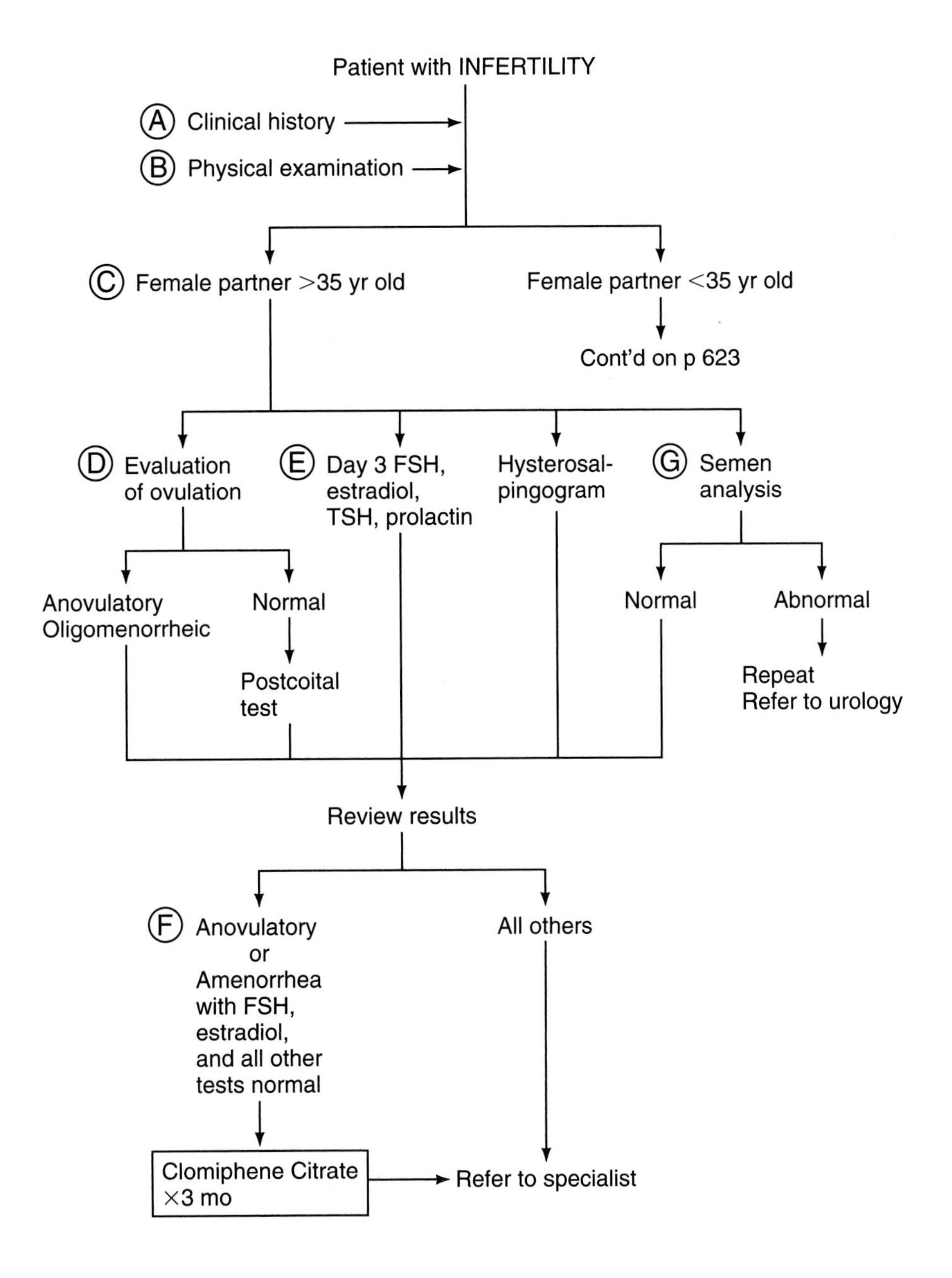
Patient with INFERTILITY
(A) Clinical history
(B) Physical examination
(C) Female partner >35 yr old
Female partner <35 yr old
Cont'd on p 623
(D) Evaluation of ovulation
(E) Day 3 FSH, estradiol, TSH, prolactin
Hysterosal-pingogram
(G) Semen analysis
Anovulatory Oligomenorrheic
Normal
Postcoital test
Normal
Abnormal
Repeat
Refer to urology
Review results
(F) Anovulatory or Amenorrhea with FSH, estradiol, and all other tests normal
All others
Clomiphene Citrate ×3 mo
Refer to specialist

Treatment of the female partner should not be initiated before a thorough evaluation of the male partner, including semen analysis, has taken place.

References

Glatzstein IZ, Harlow BL, Hornstein MD. Practice patterns among reproductive endocrinologists: the infertility evaluation. Fertil Steril 1997;67:443.

Jaffe SB, Jewelewicz R. The basic infertility investigation. Fertil Steril 1991;56:599.

Marshall L. Infertility. In Lemcke DP, Pattison J, Marshall LA, et al, eds. Primary Care of Women. Norwalk, CT: Appleton & Lange, 1995:499.

Speroff L, Glass RH, Kase NG. Clinical Gynecologic Endocrinology and Infertility, ed 5. Baltimore: Williams & Wilkins, 1994:809.

Toner JP, Hilput CB, Jones GS, et al. Basal follicle-stimulating hormone level is a better predictor of in vitro fertilization performance than age. Fertil Steril 1991;55:784.

Wilcox AJ, Weinberg CR, Baird DD. Timing of sexual intercourse in relation to ovulation: effects on the probability of conception, survival of the pregnancy, and sex of the baby. N Engl J Med 1995;338:1517.

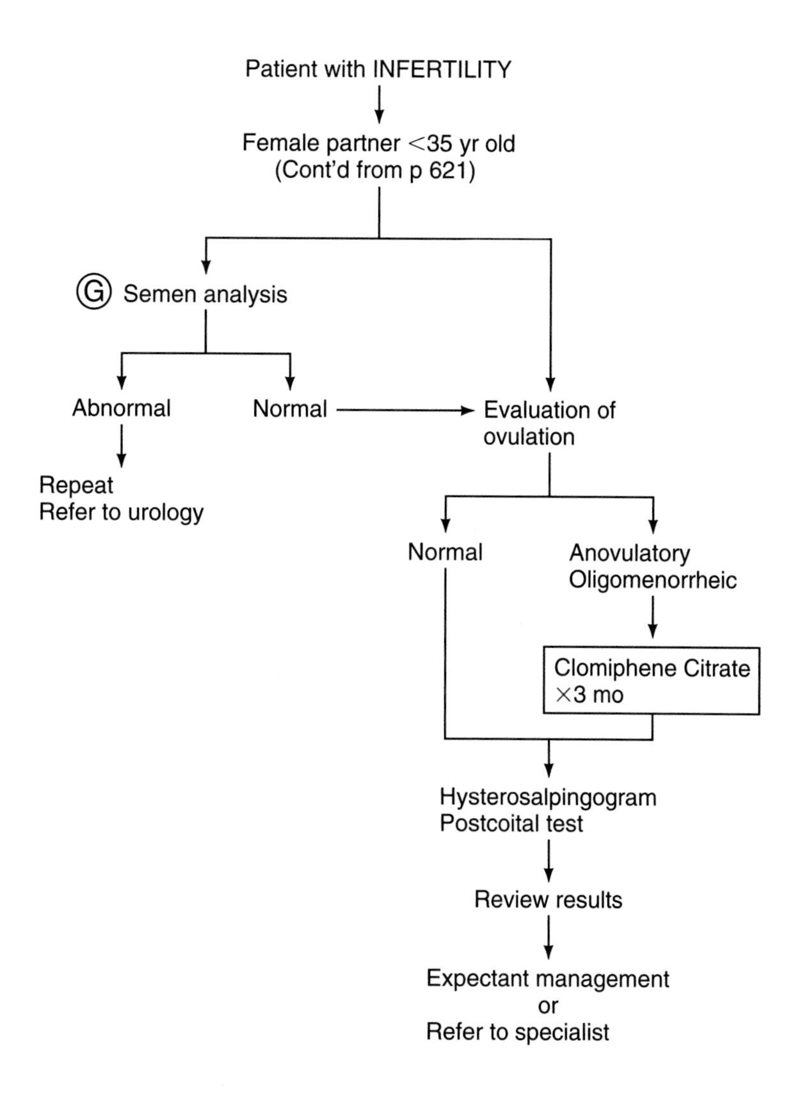
Patient with INFERTILITY
Female partner <35 yr old
(Cont'd from p 621)
G Semen analysis
Abnormal
Normal
Repeat
Refer to urology
Evaluation of ovulation
Normal
Anovulatory
Oligomenorrheic
Clomiphene Citrate ×3 mo
Hysterosalpingogram
Postcoital test
Review results
Expectant management
or
Refer to specialist

DOMESTIC VIOLENCE

Elaine J. Alpert, MD

Domestic violence (DV) is a pattern of assaultive and coercive behaviors used in the context of dating or intimate relationships. This recently recognized problem in medicine affects 8%–12% of U.S. women per year, with lifetime prevalence approaching 30%. One in nine women seen for emergency care for any stated reason is actually there because of the acute or chronic effects of DV, and >50% of all women who seek emergency care have, at some time in their lives, been victims of DV. Fully one third of all women who visit emergency facilities for trauma are there for treatment of injuries caused by DV.

The spectrum of DV includes physical injury, sexual assault, social isolation, verbal abuse, threats, humiliation, economic deprivation, and restriction of access to transportation and other resources. DV has devastating short- and long-term effects on the life, health, and functioning of victims, their children, and other dependents. Of abused persons, 95% are adolescent or adult women in heterosexual relationships; however, DV also occurs in same-sex relationships and, in a small proportion of cases, by women perpetrators against male victims. Although women who are young, poor, and unmarried are most likely to experience DV, the condition affects every age, income level, and geographic area. Rates of DV are consistent across racial and ethnic categories when age, income, and education are controlled for.

Physicians in every specialty and practice setting have patients who are current, former, or potential victims of abuse. Asking questions about the possibility of DV must be done in a compassionate, nonjudgmental manner, preserving the patient's privacy and focusing on safety and empowerment. All patients should be routinely screened for DV in emergency, primary care, and specialty settings. Because of the prevalence, varied presentation, and consequences of DV, core competence in screening, assessment, and intervention is now part of the standard of care for all practicing physicians.

A. Taking a careful history is vital to diagnosis and the first step toward assessment and intervention. Ask every patient about current or former abuse at the first visit and periodically thereafter. Because of the high prevalence of DV in the emergency setting, every patient should be screened at every visit. Ask questions in a respectful, nonjudgmental manner. Direct questions usually are best. You can ask, "At any time (or, since I last saw you) has your partner (or ex-partner) hit, kicked, or otherwise hurt or frightened you?" Even if your patient is being abused, she may choose not to disclose this to you at this time. If your index of suspicion is high, it is acceptable to follow your initial screening question with, "When I see a patient with an injury (or illness) such as yours, often it is because someone has hurt her. Has someone been hurting you?" Follow-up questions are indicated if the patient discloses (see E).

B. A careful physical examination with a high index of suspicion is vital in diagnosing DV. Physical injuries often are multiple, bilateral, and occur over time; thus they may be in different stages of healing at the time of your evaluation. The explanation given for trauma may be inconsistent with the injury pattern. If this is the case, use the follow-up question noted in A. Other suspicious findings include psychological distress (including suicide attempts and substance abuse) and evidence of sexual assault.

(Continued on page 626)

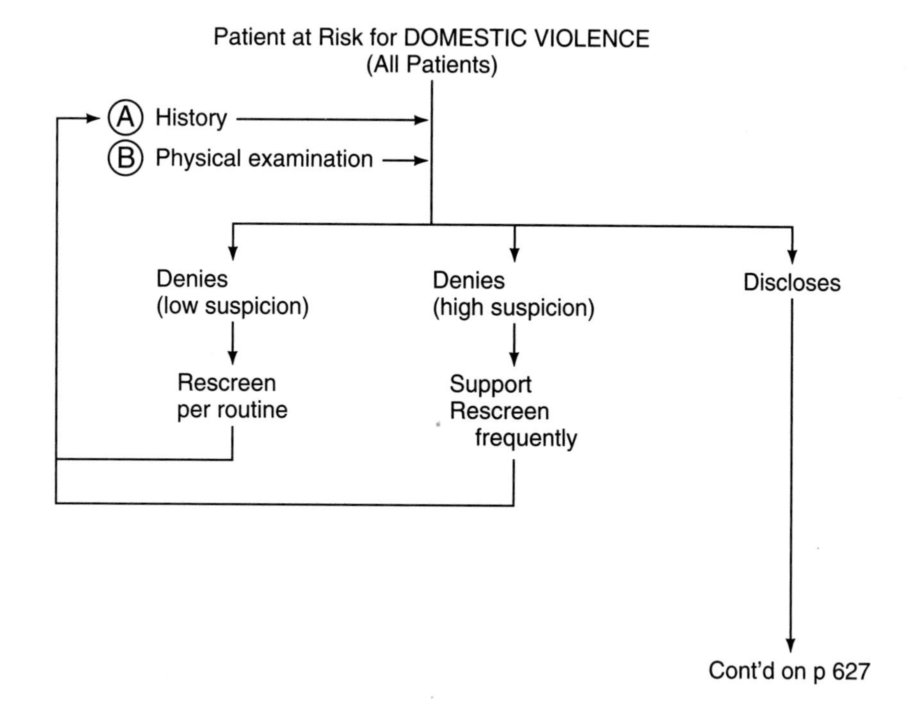
Patient at Risk for DOMESTIC VIOLENCE
(All Patients)
(A) History
(B) Physical examination
Denies
(low suspicion)
Rescreen
per routine
Denies
(high suspicion)
Support
Rescreen
frequently
Discloses
Cont'd on p 627

C. Begin intervention as soon as the diagnosis of DV is established. It is crucial to validate and support the patient, who in all likelihood is fearful and ashamed. You can say, "I am glad you chose to share this difficult issue with me," "I am concerned for your safety and well-being," and "Help is available."

D. Careful documentation is vital to appropriate care. Record the patient's statements without bias or judgment. After obtaining the patient's consent, sketch or photograph evidence of trauma and include it in the chart. Include the patient's face in at least one photo and a notation of the exact date and time of the photo. Take follow-up photos if possible. Reporting requirements vary from state to state; thus all documentation should be undertaken with the patient's knowledge and consent and with the patient's immediate and long-term safety kept foremost in importance.

E. Risk assessment is also known as lethality assessment. Nationwide, approximately one third of all women murder victims whose assailant can be identified have been killed by a current or former intimate partner. Thus the patient's safety is the top priority in evaluation and intervention. Ask the patient, "Has your partner (or ex-partner) ever threatened or tried to kill you or your children?" "Do you feel you are in danger now?" "Is it safe for you to return home?" Indicators of potential lethality include an increase in the frequency or severity of the abuse, threats of homicide or suicide by the partner, the availability of a firearm, the abuser's knowledge of the victim's plan to leave or to get help, and a history of violent criminal behavior by the abuser.

F. Helping victims learn how to stay safe, defining and making accessible available resources, and providing options and referrals are the key interventions in DV. However, there is no medical magic to offer victims. Empowerment is vital because disempowerment of victims is necessary for abusers to maintain the cycle of abuse. In addition to the validating and supporting statements suggested in C, convey to the patient that she deserves better and that the abuse is not her fault. Make the patient feel that choices and help are available. Offer information such as, "Domestic violence is common," "Physical violence is only one part of the spectrum of domestic violence," "Domestic violence often increases in frequency and severity over time," and "Services for battered women include, in addition to shelter, support groups, community outreach, services for children, legal assistance, immigration assistance, and so on."

G. Necessary medical care, referrals, and follow-up can be provided in the office setting using posters, pamphlets, and a trusted office staff member or consultant (e.g., from social work or the local sheltering organization) to ensure follow-up for safety-related issues. Medical follow-up is also indicated to ensure improving physical and psychological health.

H. Initiate safety planning for every patient who is a victim of DV. Make the plan in concert with the patient according to the individual's resources and needs. Components of a safety plan include (1) a "crisis" plan to be followed in case of emergency, (2) identification of a safe place to go and a way to get there, and (3) logistical issues concerning finances, children, and housing. Life decisions should be made by the victim of DV. Physicians should provide information, support, resources, and follow-up, but they should not tell the patient what to do. The victim knows best what needs to take place to stay alive. The decision may be to remain in the house with the abuser still present, to remain in the house and obtain police or judicial assistance to have the abuser vacate the house, or to leave entirely, to a known or an undisclosed location. Regardless of the immediate decisions, the victim's situation will evolve over time, as will the readiness to change the situation and safety plan.

References

Abbott J, Johnson R, Koziol-McLain J, et al. Domestic violence against women: incidence and prevalence in an emergency department population. JAMA 1995;273:1763.

Alpert EJ. Violence in intimate relationships and the practicing internist: new "disease" or new agenda? Ann Intern Med 1994;123:774.

Bachman R, Saltzman L. Violence against women: estimates from the redesigned survey. Washington, DC: US Department of Justice, Office of Justice Programs, Bureau of Justice Statistics. NCJ-154348, August 1995.

Flitcraft A, Hadley S, et al. Diagnostic and Treatment Guidelines on Domestic Violence. Chicago: American Medical Association, 1992.

Ganley A. Understanding domestic violence. In Ganley A, Warshaw C, Salber P, eds. Improving the Health Care Response to Domestic Violence: A Resource Manual for Health Care Providers. San Francisco:Family Violence Prevention Fund, 1995:15.

Wilt S, Olson S. Prevalence of domestic violence in the United States. J Am Med Women's Assoc 1996;51:77.

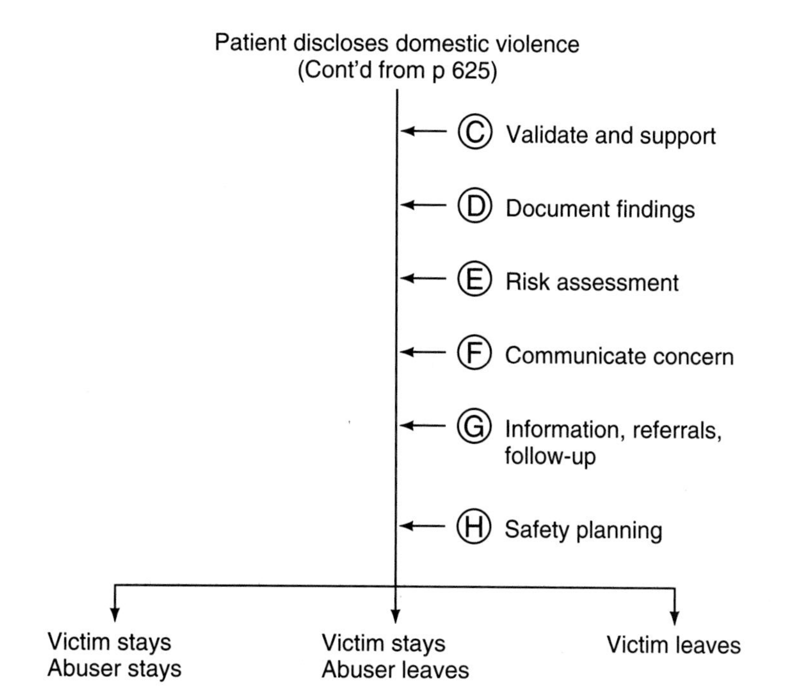
Patient discloses domestic violence
(Cont'd from p 625)
Ⓒ Validate and support
Ⓓ Document findings
Ⓔ Risk assessment
Ⓕ Communicate concern
Ⓖ Information, referrals, follow-up
Ⓗ Safety planning
Victim stays Abuser stays
Victim stays Abuser leaves
Victim leaves

ECTOPIC PREGNANCY

Daniela Carusi, MD, MSc

Ectopic pregnancies are those implanted outside of the uterine cavity, the majority of which are in the fallopian tube. Such a pregnancy may lead to tubal rupture and intraabdominal hemorrhage and represents the major cause of maternal death in the first trimester. Early intervention for an ectopic pregnancy may reduce morbidity, and early suspicion and evaluation are critical. *Thus any reproductive-age woman presenting with abdominal pain, pelvic pain, hemodynamic instability, or abnormal vaginal bleeding should have a pregnancy test. If the test is positive, she should be considered to have an ectopic pregnancy until proved otherwise.*

A. A ruptured ectopic pregnancy can lead to catastrophic intraabdominal hemorrhage. Therefore, the patient's initial evaluation should focus on the severity of her symptoms, vital signs, and abdominal examination. Young women may lose a large volume of blood before becoming hypotensive, so any signs of orthostasis or significant tachycardia should be taken seriously. Severe abdominal pain, abdominal distention, rebound, or abdominal guarding should also raise suspicion for major bleeding. Patients with these findings should be referred for emergency care and surgical consultation.

B. A stable patient should have a history and physical examination, with attention paid to the abdominal examination, assessment of active vaginal bleeding and cervical dilation, and careful pelvic examination to evaluate uterine enlargement and presence of an adnexal mass. Laboratory testing should include a quantitative serum beta-human chorionic gonadotropin (β-hCG) level, hemoglobin concentration, and blood type (patients who are Rhesus negative and have vaginal bleeding should receive Rh immune globulin). If available, a serum progesterone level can be helpful as well. All patients should undergo a pelvic ultrasound (US) examination regardless of the hCG level; even with a low serum hCG, an adnexal mass or hemoperitoneum may still be visualized.

C. Pelvic US findings may be extremely useful but also need to be interpreted very carefully. Accurate US diagnosis is highly dependent on the skill of the ultrasonographer, patient habitus, presence of uterine fibroids or other obstructive lesions, and ability of the patient to tolerate a vaginal ultrasound probe. An intrauterine pregnancy is confirmed when one visualizes a gestational sac and embryo surrounded by myometrium, above the level of the cervix. Similarly, an ectopic pregnancy is confirmed when an indisputable embryo is viewed outside of the endometrial cavity. Individual ultrasonographers may make one of these diagnoses with lesser criteria. However, the stakes of misdiagnosis (unnecessary surgery, interruption of a normal pregnancy, or tubal rupture) are high. Therefore, it is prudent to discuss the certainty of the US findings with the sonographer before acting on this information. If there is any doubt in the diagnosis, further diagnostic steps should be taken.

D. In the majority of cases, a diagnosis cannot be confirmed with ultrasound alone. At this point one needs to determine whether this is an abnormal pregnancy (either intrauterine or ectopic), in which case more invasive testing can be performed. A normal intrauterine pregnancy may be seen on transvaginal US when the hCG level is >1500–2000. Again, this will depend on the skill of the radiologist, the quality of the ultrasound study, and possible variances with the laboratory assay, so a higher hCG "discriminatory zone" (in the range of 2000–4000) may be used if there is any doubt about the findings. The serum progesterone level can help here as well because a level <5 correlates with an abnormal pregnancy.

E. If the location of the pregnancy remains unknown and the gestation is not clearly abnormal, the serum β-hCG level should be repeated in 48 hours. An increase of <50% or a decrease in the level is indicative of an abnormal pregnancy. If the hCG level increases appropriately, the patient should be followed closely until the level exceeds 2000, at which time the ultrasound is repeated. Patients who wait for further testing must be pain free and hemodynamically stable and must be able to return for further testing or emergency care until the situation is resolved. They must understand and accept the possibility of tubal rupture and intraabdominal bleeding. Patients who do not meet these criteria may require hospital admission while undergoing further evaluation.

F. Once an abnormal pregnancy has been confirmed with correlation of US and hCG or progesterone levels, the uterine cavity should be sampled. This is usually accomplished with dilation and curettage (D&C) of the uterus or by evacuation with a manual vacuum aspirator in the office. The removed tissue can be examined both grossly and microscopically for the presence of trophoblastic tissue or chorionic villi. Such findings confirm that the abnormal pregnancy was intrauterine. If no products of conception are identified, the pregnancy is most likely ectopic and should be treated as such. In some cases placental tissue can be missed during sampling and histologic evaluation. In these cases the evacuation

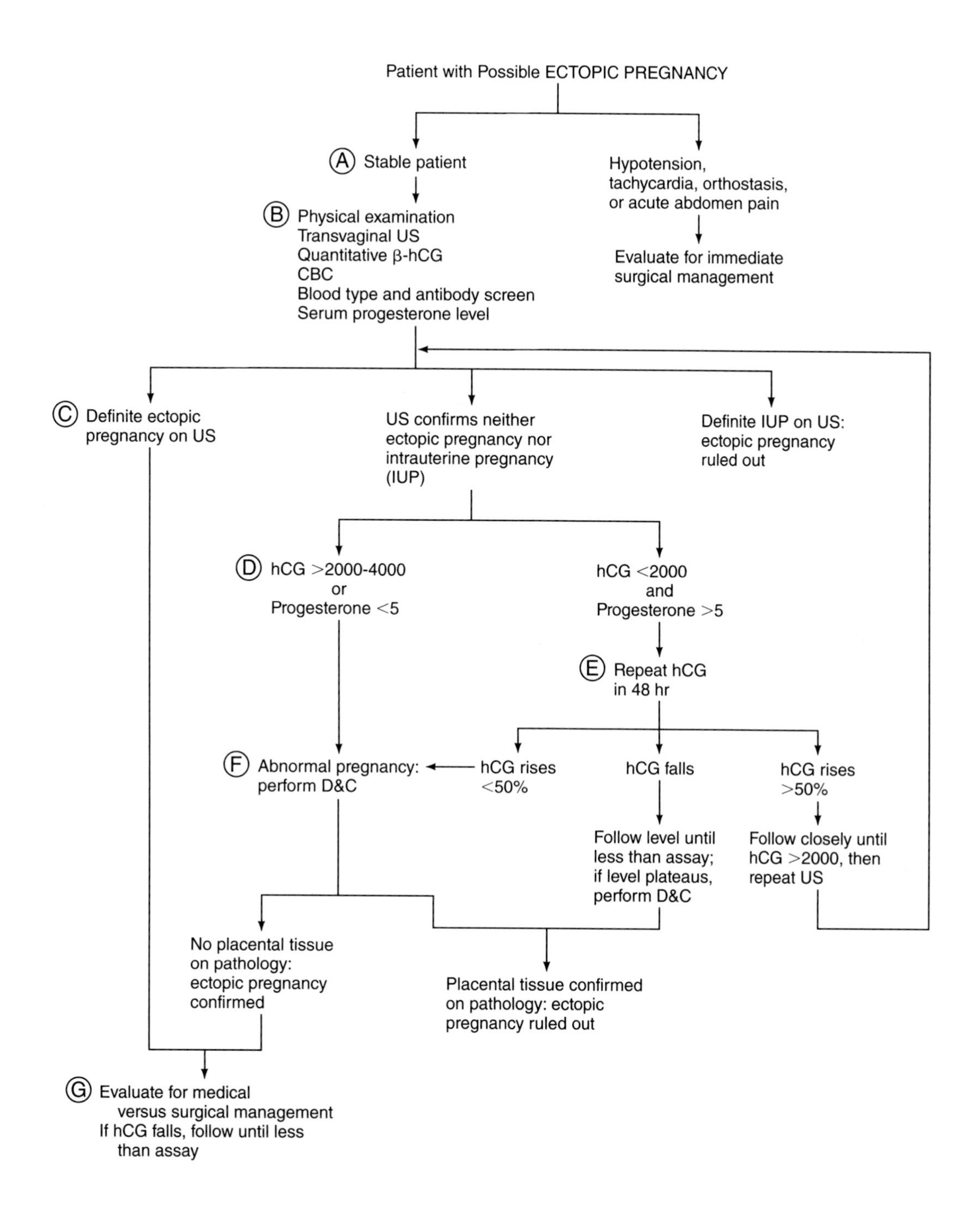

procedure will be followed by a sharp decrease in serum hCG level (>15% in 12–24 hours).

G. Once an ectopic pregnancy is confirmed, the patient must be evaluated for medical or surgical management. The former involves intramuscular methotrexate injection, whereas the latter may be accomplished via laparoscopy or laparotomy. The proper treatment should be determined with the help of a gynecologic surgeon and after careful counseling of the patient. If the serum hCG level is decreasing spontaneously, a patient who is reliable may be followed with serial hCG levels alone. The ectopic pregnancy is considered resolved when the serum hCG level is below the threshold of the assay, which may require weeks of careful follow-up. If the level plateaus or begins to increase, the patient must be reevaluated for interventional therapy.

References

Barnhart KT, Sammel MD, Rinaudo PF, et al. Symptomatic patients with an early viable intrauterine pregnancy: HCG curves redefined. Obstet Gynecol 2004;104(1):50–55.

Barnhart KT, Simhan H, Kamelle SA. Diagnostic accuracy of ultrasound above and below the beta-hCG discriminatory zone. Obstet Gynecol 1999;94(4):583–587.

Stovall TG, Ling FW, Carson SA, et al. Serum progesterone and uterine curettage in differential diagnosis of ectopic pregnancy. Fertil Steril 1992;57(2):456–457.

Stovall TG, Ling FW, Gray LA, et al. Methotrexate treatment of unruptured ectopic pregnancy: a report of 100 cases. Obstet Gynecol 1991;77(5): 749–753.

OSTEOPOROSIS AND OSTEOPENIA

Maria A. Yialamas, MD

A. The initial evaluation for osteoporosis begins with a careful history and physical examination for risk factors for bone loss. Patients at risk for osteoporosis include postmenopausal women >65 years, postmenopausal women of any age with additional risk factors (personal history of fracture as an adult, fracture in a first-degree relative, current smoker, use of steroids, more than two alcoholic drinks per day, low weight, menopause before age 45, recent falls, low physical activity, lifelong low calcium intake, impaired vision, dementia), men and premenopausal women with low-impact fractures, and anyone with known secondary causes of osteoporosis. Patients in any of these categories should obtain a bone mineral density (BMD) scan.

B. Bone density scans measure a given individual's bone mass. The World Health Organization (WHO) defines osteopenia as a T score (standard deviations below or above the mean for young adults) of <-1.0 but >-2.5. Osteoporosis is defined as a T score ≤ -2.5.

C. Lifestyle interventions should be recommended to all patients who have osteoporosis or osteopenia. These include calcium supplements of 1200–1500 mg daily, vitamin D supplementation of 800 IU daily, weight-bearing exercise, smoking cessation, and limiting alcohol intake to no more than two drinks per day.

D. Initial laboratory evaluation for patients with osteoporosis and osteopenia should include a calcium, albumin, phosphorus, and alkaline phosphatase test to assess for possible hyperparathyroidism, osteomalacia, or other calcium and phosphate disorders. Renal function should be assessed with a BUN and creatinine, and a thyroid-stimulating hormone (TSH) test should be ordered to exclude hyperthyroidism. A 25-OH vitamin D level should be ordered to assess for possible vitamin D deficiency. In men with osteoporosis, a total testosterone level should be measured.

E. Renal insufficiency can cause low BMD. The etiology is multifactorial and includes secondary hyperparathyroidism from low 1,25-dihydroxyvitamin D levels.

F. Vitamin D deficiency may contribute to bone loss. Vitamin D deficiency is defined as levels <15 ng/ml. The goal vitamin D level for optimal bone health is >30 ng/ml.

G. Hyperthyroidism increases bone turnover and, as a result, decreases bone mass. Studies have demonstrated that even subclinical hyperthyroidism (specifically when the TSH is <0.1 mU/L) can place patients at increased risk for osteoporosis.

H. If calcium is increased and/or phosphorus is decreased, the patient may have hyperparathyroidism. If this pattern is seen, an intact parathyroid hormone (iPTH), calcium, albumin, and phosphorus level should be drawn simultaneously to assess for this possibility.

I. If the patient has a Z score (standard deviations above or below the mean for age-matched controls) that is <-2.0, a thorough evaluation for secondary causes of osteoporosis should be performed. This additional testing may include a serum protein electrophoresis (SPEP), urine protein electrophoresis (UPEP) to exclude multiple myeloma, iPTH to definitively exclude hyperparathyroidism, 24-hour urine calcium and creatinine to evaluate for hypercalciuria, and overnight dexamethasone suppression test to assess for Cushing's syndrome.

J. Treatment of osteoporosis and osteopenia should be focused on treating the underlying secondary cause, if present, and appropriate calcium and vitamin D intake. Other therapies that should be considered include bisphosphonates (oral or IV) and raloxifene. For patients with very severe osteoporosis, PTH injections should be considered. All patients should have repeat BMD scans in 1–2 years to assess effectiveness of treatment.

References

Kanis JA, Borgstrom F, De Laet C, et al. Assessment of fracture risk. Osteoporos Int 2005;16:581.
Khosla S, Melton LJM. Osteopenia. N Engl J Med 2007;356:2293.
National Osteoporosis Foundation. Physician's guide to prevention and treatment of osteoporosis. www.nof.org/physguide/index.htm. 2003.
Raisz LG. Screening for osteoporosis. N Engl J Med 2005;353:164.

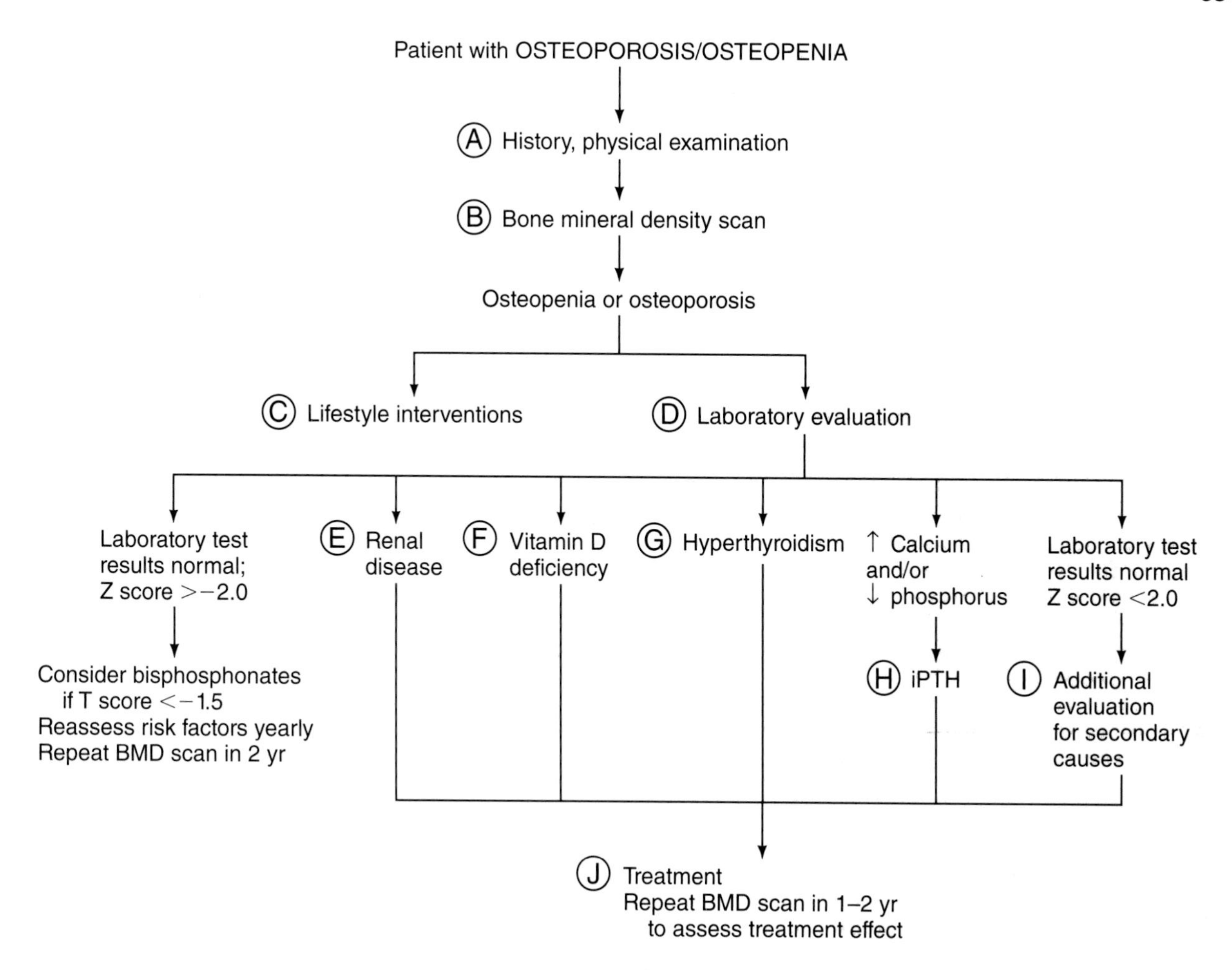

Patient with OSTEOPOROSIS/OSTEOPENIA
(A) History, physical examination
(B) Bone mineral density scan
Osteopenia or osteoporosis
(C) Lifestyle interventions
(D) Laboratory evaluation
Laboratory test results normal; Z score >−2.0
Consider bisphosphonates if T score <−1.5
Reassess risk factors yearly
Repeat BMD scan in 2 yr
(E) Renal disease
(F) Vitamin D deficiency
(G) Hyperthyroidism
↑ Calcium and/or ↓ phosphorus
(H) iPTH
Laboratory test results normal Z score <2.0
(I) Additional evaluation for secondary causes
(J) Treatment
Repeat BMD scan in 1–2 yr to assess treatment effect

Emergency Medicine

Richard D. Zane, MD, FAAEM
Section Editor

ACUTE PULSELESS EXTREMITY

Richard D. Zane, MD, FAAEM

A. In the evaluation of a patient with potential vascular emergency, the history and physical examination are extremely important because time of onset and situation leading to the ischemia often influence the type and urgency of treatment. In the absence of trauma, acute lower extremity ischemia may occur for myriad reasons, including myocardial infarction (MI), ventricular aneurysm, valvular heart disease, arrhythmia, or arterial occlusive disease. It is important to establish any history of vascular disease, including cardiac, and whether previous vascular occlusive disease has been diagnosed or vascular reconstructive operations have been performed in the past.

B. Abrupt onset of severe unremitting pain is the classic symptom of acute ischemia, although in patients with a known history of vascular occlusive disease of the lower extremities, pain may be less severe if collaterals have formed. In general, ischemic pain is severe and requires copious opioid analgesia for even moderate relief. The classic physical finding is of a cool pale extremity with absent or extremely weak pulses. Although pulselessness can often be obvious in its presentation, patients may present with progressive symptoms of claudication that has led to acute ischemia. These patients may present in a quiescent manner with minimal physical findings. The findings of paresthesia and paralysis are late findings and usually predict a poor outcome.

C. The etiology of true acutely absent pulses is usually trauma, embolism, or thrombosis. In patients with a history of a revascularization procedure, thrombosis of the bypass conduit or stent is the most common cause of acute ischemia.

D. In a patient with acutely absent pulse and the sudden onset of symptoms, it may be difficult to differentiate thrombosis from embolism as the cause of the ischemia. Thrombosis tends to occur more often in younger patients than in patients with embolism and in patients with a known history of vascular occlusive disease or previous vascular surgery. Embolism usually occurs more commonly in patients with known heart disease (mitral stenosis or regurgitation, atrial fibrillation, acute MI). Patients with embolism may have had an earlier embolic event but usually have no history of chronic circulatory impairment.

E. The hallmark of treatment for limb ischemia is anticoagulation and revascularization. Early anticoagulation with heparin preserves the patency of needed collateral blood vessels. The typical adult dose of heparin is an IV bolus of 10,000 U followed by a minimum dosage of 1000 U/hr to prolong the activated partial thromboplastin time to >2½ times control.

F. Patients with acute limb ischemia require emergency evaluation by a vascular surgeon. Many patients will require emergency angiography to determine the level of the occlusion and the extent of vascular injury of disease. The decision to perform angiography should be done in consultation with a vascular surgeon.

G. If the limb is viable, fibrinolytic therapy may be an option if thrombosis or embolic disease is suspected. Although there is no agreed-upon window when intra-arterial fibrinolytic therapy is no longer useful, most authors agree that 12 hours, depending on the size of the clot and precipitousness of the occlusion, is the maximum window of opportunity to restore arterial flow. The catheter is placed directly in the clot by the radiologist, and a bolus infusion fibrinolytic is given directly into the clot.

H. If paresthesia or paralysis is present, the limb may soon become unsalvageable without prompt operative intervention. It is important to distinguish sensitivity to light touch from that of pressure, pain, and temperature. Pressure, pain, and temperature sensations are carried by larger nerves that are more resistant to ischemia and therefore may remain intact when sensation to light touch has diminished. After the abrupt onset of perfusion impairment, the clock begins ticking. If the collateral circulation is not well developed, one usually has <4–6 hours to restore the circulation. Attempts to provide revascularization after 12 hours are seldom successful.

References

Aufderheide TP. Peripheral arteriovascular disease. In Marx JA, Hockberger RS, Walls RM, eds. Rosen's Emergency Medicine: Concepts and Clinical Practice, 5th ed. St. Louis: Mosby, 2002:1187.

Creager MA. Peripheral arterial disease. In Braunwald E, Zipes DP, Libby P, et al, eds. Braunwald's Heart Disease: A Textbook of Cardiovascular Medicine, 7th ed. St. Louis: Saunders, 2005:1437.

Lipsitz EC. Antithrombotic therapy in peripheral arterial disease. Clin Geriatr Med 2006;22(1):183–198.

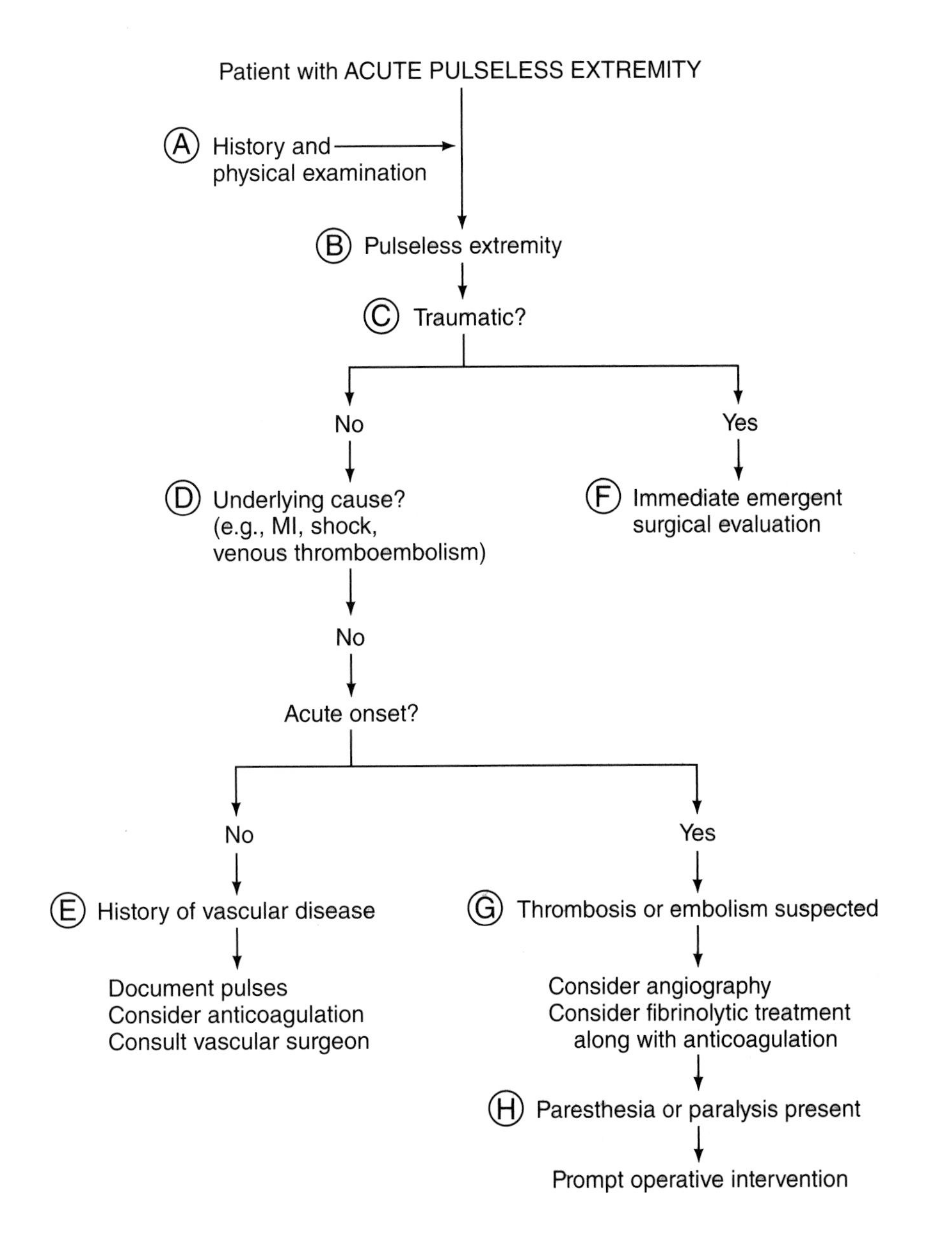

Patient with ACUTE PULSELESS EXTREMITY
Ⓐ History and physical examination
Ⓑ Pulseless extremity
Ⓒ Traumatic?
No
Yes
Ⓓ Underlying cause? (e.g., MI, shock, venous thromboembolism)
Ⓕ Immediate emergent surgical evaluation
No
Acute onset?
No
Yes
Ⓔ History of vascular disease
Document pulses
Consider anticoagulation
Consult vascular surgeon
Ⓖ Thrombosis or embolism suspected
Consider angiography
Consider fibrinolytic treatment along with anticoagulation
Ⓗ Paresthesia or paralysis present
Prompt operative intervention

FOREIGN BODY INGESTION

Richard D. Zane, MD, FAEEM

The majority of foreign body ingestions pass asymptomatically through the GI tract, with most occurring in the pediatric patient population. In adults the majority of foreign body ingestions causing esophageal impaction result from food (meat and bones); in children, coins are most common. Patients with preexisting esophageal stricture or those who use dentures, have psychiatric disease, or have mental retardation are particularly susceptible to esophageal impaction.

A. The vast majority of foreign body ingestions can be managed expectantly. The approach to an ingested foreign body depends greatly on the patient's past medical history, the time of ingestion, and what was ingested. If the ingestion results in obstruction, determining anatomic point of obstruction is important.

   Certain foreign bodies deserve special attention: button or disk batteries may contain the alkaline potassium hydroxide and a number of heavy metals such as lithium, nickel, zinc, cadmium, or mercury. Most batteries are not biologically sealed. Batteries in the esophagus must be removed urgently because of the possibility of liquefaction necrosis from the alkaline solution and subsequent perforation and/or pressure necrosis of the esophageal wall. Once the battery passes into the stomach, spontaneous passage from the body is likely to follow and may be documented by repeat radiographs. Lack of passage from the stomach after 48 hours or lack of progression below the stomach after 72 hours may necessitate surgical or endoscopic intervention. If a radiograph shows the battery integrity has been violated, consider GI tract decontamination with lavage, charcoal, and cathartic; consult the local poison control center for consideration of chelation therapy.

   Sharp objects (e.g., fish or chicken bones, pins, needles) lodged in the esophagus must be urgently removed. If an object is above the cricopharyngeal muscles, direct laryngoscopy is the simplest initial approach, whereas immediate esophagoscopy is applied for objects below this point. Although most sharp objects that reach the stomach pass spontaneously through the rest of the digestive tract, there is a 35% complication rate.

   History and physical examination are brief and directed with careful attention to airway compromise. A detailed examination of the oral and nasal pharynx for erythema, edema, abrasions, and cuts may guide the clinician to the foreign body. Evaluate the neck and soft tissues for subcutaneous emphysema. Auscultate and percuss the neck and chest for stridor, breath sounds, wheezing, hyperresonance, or dullness to percussion.

B. Use of topical anesthesia such as Cetacaine or viscous lidocaine for the mucosa will facilitate examination of the pharynx and hypopharynx with direct or indirect laryngoscope. If the object is visualized and no sharp or jagged edges are known to be present, remove it with Magill forceps.

C. Plain radiographs may be able to demonstrate the foreign body if it is radiopaque. Many foreign bodies, such as food and fish bones, will not show up on radiographs. Soft-tissue neck films may show air in the subcutaneous tissues, indicating perforation, and may be able to detect if the foreign body is in the trachea or the esophagus. Coins lodged in the trachea tend to align in the sagittal plane; those in the esophagus usually appear in the coronal alignment. An anteroposterior view of the chest may show a pneumothorax, the foreign body, a lung abscess, or lobar atelectasis. Finally, if indicated by the lack of findings on the first two radiographs, obtain a flat and upright plate of the abdomen to determine whether the foreign body is indeed radiolucent and has already passed beyond the pylorus. If the patient complains of abdominal pain, look for signs of obstruction or perforation such as free air under the diaphragm.

D. If the foreign body was aspirated, symptoms may range from throat pain, cough, or stridor to episodes of cyanosis or apnea and acute respiratory distress or collapse. Rarely, a patient may present late with signs and symptoms of postobstructive infection. In cases of complete airway obstruction, do an oropharyngeal sweep, Heimlich maneuver, and direct laryngoscopy as indicated and have Magill forceps on hand to remove the object if it is visualized. If unsuccessful, prepare for cricothyrotomy.

E. If a foreign body acts as a one-way valve in a mainstem bronchus, air can get in but not out. Expiratory wheezes are present on physical examination, and the involved, partially obstructed lung may appear overexpanded and hyperlucent on an expiratory chest radiograph. The diaphragm may appear fixed and flat, and the heart and mediastinum may be shifted to the opposite, uninvolved side. When the obstruction becomes complete, air cannot get in or out and the involved lung may appear atelectatic on radiographs, with the heart and mediastinum shifted to the involved side.

(Continued on page 638)

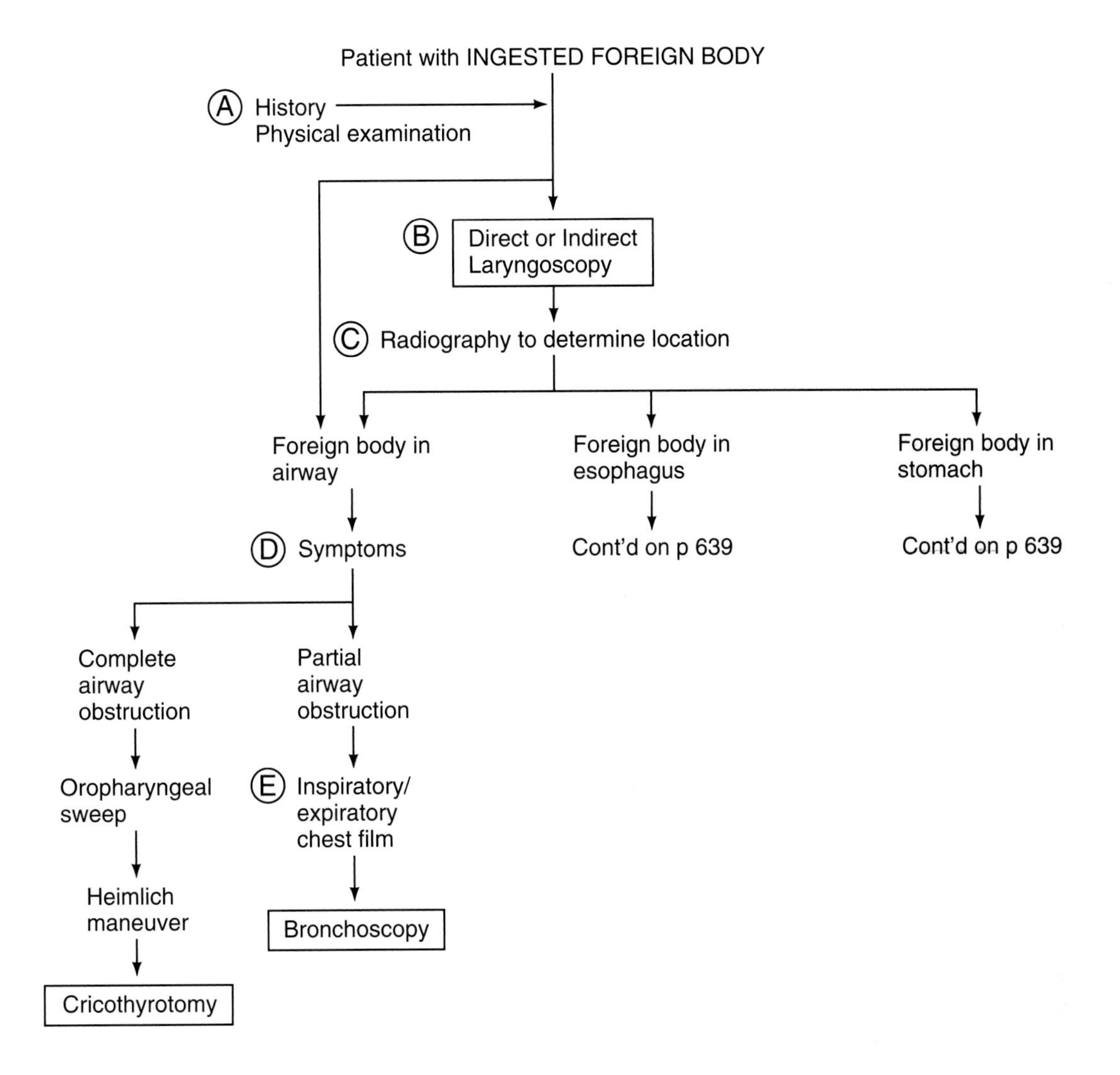
Patient with INGESTED FOREIGN BODY
A History
Physical examination
B Direct or Indirect Laryngoscopy
C Radiography to determine location
Foreign body in airway
Foreign body in esophagus
Foreign body in stomach
D Symptoms
Cont'd on p 639
Cont'd on p 639
Complete airway obstruction
Partial airway obstruction
Oropharyngeal sweep
E Inspiratory/ expiratory chest film
Heimlich maneuver
Bronchoscopy
Cricothyrotomy

F. Inability to swallow, trouble with secretions, and refusal to eat are common symptoms of an esophageal obstruction. Patients also may be vomiting or gagging and may complain of neck, throat, or chest pain. The most common sites of obstruction are those where physiologic narrowing occurs (e.g., the level of the cricopharyngeal muscle, the aortic arch, the gastroesophageal junction, Schatzki's ring).

G. The patient may be given a suction catheter to manage and control secretions.

H. After spontaneous passage of a known esophageal foreign body, perform nonemergent esophagoscopy to evaluate the esophagus for possible perforation and/or an underlying pathologic condition. No foreign body should remain in the esophagus for >24 hours because of the increased risk of perforation into the trachea or heart, fistula formation, and mediastinitis. Endoscopy is the procedure of choice for visualization of the esophagus and removal of foreign bodies.

I. Anticipate vomiting after the foreign body is dislodged; be prepared to deal with subsequent complications. Prior to the advent of endoscopy, foreign body removal with nasogastric tubes, Foley catheters, and ring magnets were not uncommon but are now considered contraindicated.

J. If esophageal obstruction is considered to result from a food impaction in the lower esophagus, IV glucagon may be administered to attempt to relax the smooth muscles and the lower gastroesophageal sphincter without inhibiting peristalsis. After a test dose to exclude hypersensitivity to the drug, give a 1-mg dose of IV glucagon with the patient in the upright position. Repeat with a second dose of 2 mg if the patient experiences no relief 20 minutes after the first injection. Each dose should be followed by an oral challenge with water. If the obstruction is relieved, perform esophagoscopy to evaluate for damage or an underlying pathologic condition. Although carbonated beverages were once thought to be useful for esophageal obstruction, they have not been shown to have any role in relieving esophageal food impaction. Administering meat tenderizer, papain, is contraindicated because it may cause esophageal erosion and perforation.

K. Consider endoscopic removal for all potentially sharp objects in the stomach. Objects thicker than 2–2.5 cm have a high likelihood of requiring endoscopic removal because they tend to get stuck at the pylorus, and those longer than 10 cm tend to get stuck at the duodenal sweep. Failure to progress as documented by radiographs is an indication to intervene and remove the object by endoscopic means.

L. Most foreign bodies that pass the pylorus are excreted per rectum in 24–72 hours without complications. Antacids and cathartics have not proved to be of value. Expectant observation may or may not include repeat radiographs to document advancement of the foreign body. If there is abdominal pain, nausea, or vomiting, obtain a radiograph to determine the presence of an obstruction or perforation. Surgical consultation and intervention may be indicated.

References

Duncan M, Wong RK. Esophageal emergencies: things that will wake you from a sound sleep. Gastroenterol Clin 2003;32(4):1035–1052.

Lowell M. In Marx JA, Hockberger RS, Walls RM, eds. Rosen's Emergency Medicine: Concepts and Clinical Practice, 5th ed. St Louis: Mosby, 2002:1234.

Uyemura MC. Foreign body ingestion in children. Am Fam Physician 2005;72(2):287–291.

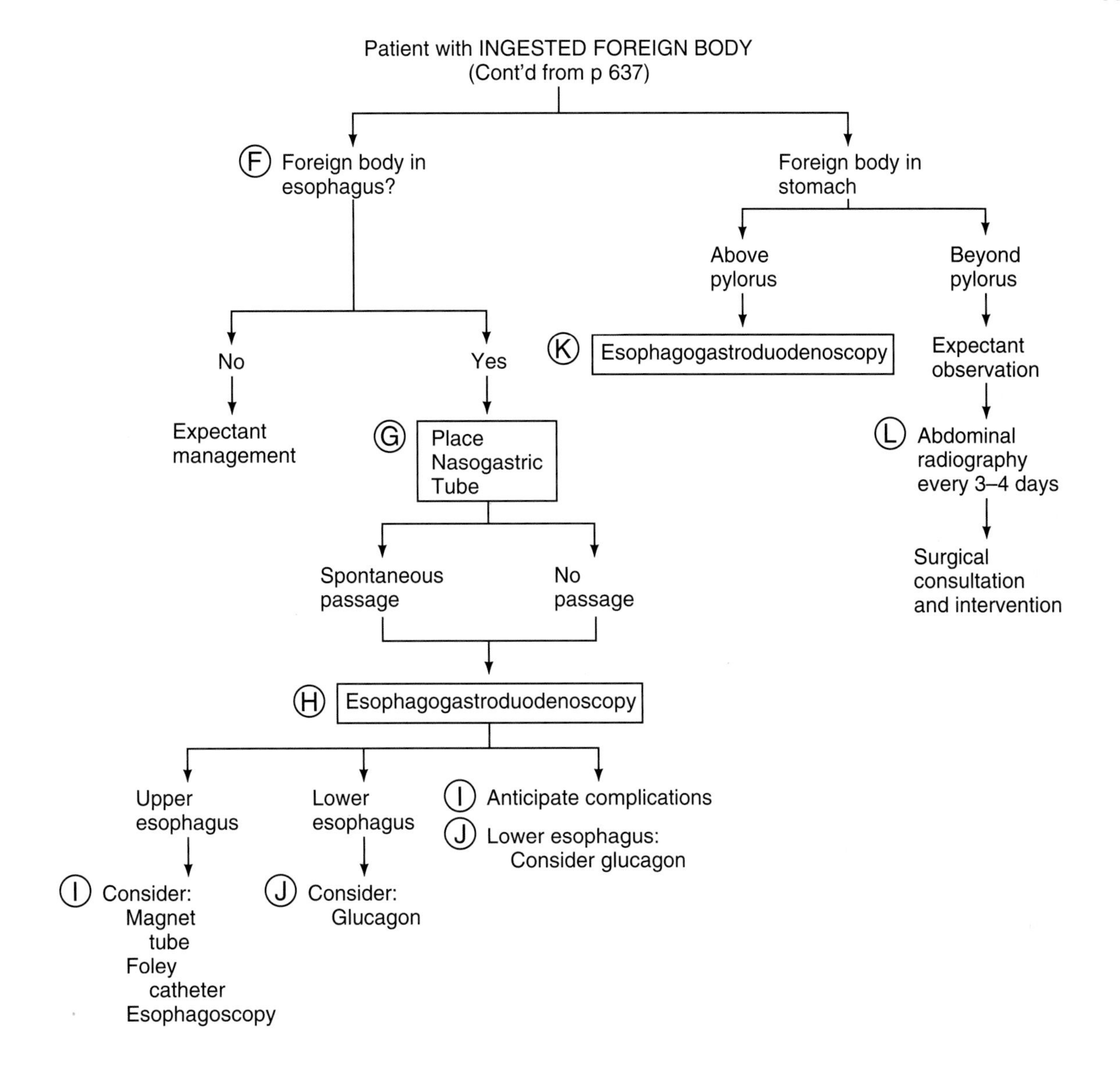
Patient with INGESTED FOREIGN BODY
(Cont'd from p 637)
F Foreign body in esophagus?
No
Expectant management
Yes
G Place Nasogastric Tube
Spontaneous passage
No passage
H Esophagogastroduodenoscopy
Upper esophagus
I Consider: Magnet tube Foley catheter Esophagoscopy
Lower esophagus
J Consider: Glucagon
I Anticipate complications
J Lower esophagus: Consider glucagon
Foreign body in stomach
Above pylorus
K Esophagogastroduodenoscopy
Beyond pylorus
Expectant observation
L Abdominal radiography every 3–4 days
Surgical consultation and intervention

CAUSTIC INGESTION AND EXPOSURE

Richard D. Zane, MD, FAAEM

Caustics, a category of chemicals, have the potential to cause tissue injury or burn on contact, with the most commonly ingested caustic agent being an alkali. Most caustic ingestions occur in children and are unintentional. When they do occur in adults, they are typically the result of a suicide attempt, psychiatric illness, or intoxication. Storage of caustic agents in atypical containers such as soda cans or water bottles is the cause of many ingestions. Although the severe mouth pain caused by ingesting caustics often limits ingestions to small quantities, one mouthful can be enough to cause serious injury or even death.

The most significant and acute emergency is the development of laryngeal edema, which may necessitate tracheal intubation for airway protection, and esophageal or gastric perforation, which can rapidly progress to systemic shock.

Caustic exposure to skin most typically results in a burn and is commonly referred to as a chemical burn. Most chemical burns are the result of direct damage to the skin from a chemical reaction, although some may cause a burn secondary to an exothermic chemical reaction often precipitated by exposure to water.

A. An important component of the initial evaluation, after airway, breathing, and circulation, is to note the time of ingestion in relation to the last meal and the type, form, and concentration of substance ingested if possible. Alkali are commonly found in lye, drain cleaners, oven cleaners, Clinitest tablets, and button batteries; acids are found in swimming pool cleaners, rust removers, and battery acid.

   Almost half of patients with caustic ingestion will report ingesting only a very small amount of chemical, yet up to 20% of these patients will have esophageal injury on endoscopy. Larger ingestions may present with signs and symptoms of airway and respiratory compromise and esophageal perforation and may present with the relatively late findings of mediastinitis: respiratory distress, subcutaneous emphysema, and shock.

B. Alkali burns cause liquefaction necrosis in the esophagus, involving the mucosa, submucosa, and longitudinal muscle. The stomach is affected in 20% of cases.

C. Alkali burns to the cornea are an ophthalmologic emergency and require continuous irrigation for at least 3 hours, instillation of antibiotics, and emergent ophthalmologic consultation.

D. If the patient has ingested a battery, or if there is any suspicion that a battery has been ingested, the entire GI tract should be evaluated with radiographs. Symptoms of battery ingestion include vomiting, refusal to eat, increased salivation, and pain on swallowing. Emetics are contraindicated.

E. Cathartics may be administered to facilitate evacuation; emesis should not be attempted. Endoscopic removal is indicated if the battery does not pass in 36–48 hours or if the patient develops symptoms.

F. Acids cause coagulation necrosis with eschar formation and mainly affect the stomach, leading to pylorospasm and eventual full-thickness necrosis and perforation.

G. Patients who have ingested an alkali or battery and have a reliable history, no symptoms, and a normal physical examination can be monitored in the emergency department or observation unit and discharged after 3–4 hours as long as they remain asymptomatic. Acid ingestion poses a higher risk of perforation, and all such patients should be admitted.

H. First-degree burns cause hyperemia with superficial mucosal desquamation; second-degree burns cause blistering and shallow ulcers; third-degree burns suggest total loss of esophageal epithelium.

I. Treatment of esophageal burns with steroids is not universally agreed to result in better outcomes, but many centers advocate using steroids in second-degree esophageal burns. It generally is accepted that patients with first-degree burns rarely develop esophageal strictures; patients with third-degree burns develop strictures regardless of steroid treatment. Steroids may delay stricture development in those with second-degree burns and should be used with an antibiotic to offset the increase in infection rate caused by steroid use. The dose of methylprednisone is 2 mg/kg/day; 1 g ampicillin every 6 hours or 100 mg/kg every 24 hours in children may be used.

J. Hydrofluoric (HF) acid deserves special mention. It is an agent that rarely can be found in household substances but is commonly used in industry. Minimal exposures can cause very significant morbidity and

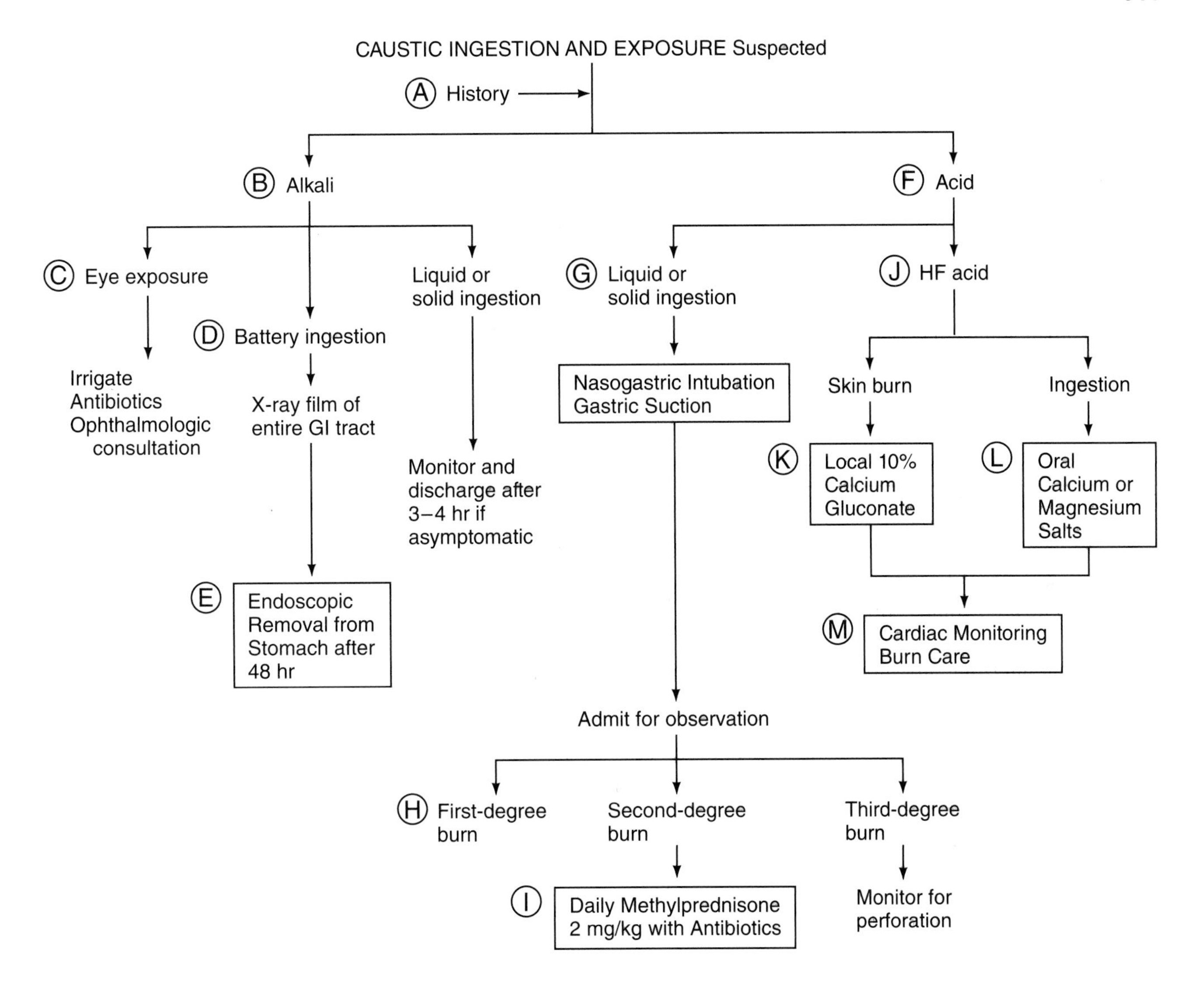

mortality because it dissociates in tissue and affects metabolism by liquefaction necrosis, bone destruction, and production of insoluble salts. Inhalation exposures to concentrated HF for 5 minutes usually are fatal.

K. Initial management for HF burns after decontamination is directed at deactivating the fluoride ion. For severe burns, inject intradermally 10% calcium gluconate into, and for a distance of 0.5 cm around, the burn. For mild to moderate burns, apply calcium gluconate gel locally. For more diffuse burns, arterial injection of calcium gluconate may be indicated.

L. For unknown amounts of HF acid ingestion, administer 300 ml magnesium citrate. If the concentration of HF acid is known, administer oral magnesium on a milliequivalent-for-milliequivalent basis.

M. Monitor the QT interval for signs of hypocalcemia and make frequent evaluations of acid-base status, electrolytes, and calcium.

References

Mandell DL. Traumatic emergencies involving the pediatric airway. Clin Pediatr Emerg Med 2005;6(1):41–48.

Newton E. Surgical complications of selected gastrointestinal emergencies: pitfalls in management of the acute abdomen. Emerg Med Clin North Am 2003;21(4):873–907, viii.

Poley JW. Ingestion of acid and alkaline agents: outcome and prognostic value of early upper endoscopy. Gastrointest Endosc 2004;60(3): 372–377.

Wax PM, Schneider SM. In Marx JA, Hockberger RS, Walls RM, eds. Rosen's Emergency Medicine: Concepts and Clinical Practice, 6th ed. St Louis: Mosby, 2002:2115.

MAMMAL BITES

Richard D. Zane, MD, FAEEM

It is difficult to determine the incidence of animal bites because the vast majority of people bitten do not seek medical treatment. Most patients with bites who present for emergency care have been bitten by dogs, cats, or rodents. Most animal bites can be managed safely as outpatient procedures, except for those patients requiring surgical reconstruction or IV antibiotics for postbite infections. Treatment of bite injuries follows that for traumatic injury and laceration care, with special attention to wound irrigation and debridement and prophylaxis of potential infectious complications, including rabies and tetanus.

A. Initial treatment of bite injury requires aggressive wound cleansing with soap and water and copious irrigation. Wound cleansing within 3 hours of a bite injury substantially reduces the risk of rabies transmission. In most areas with a municipal water supply, tap water is perfectly sufficient for high-volume wound irrigation.

B. Patients should receive tetanus immunization for any bite with potential skin breakage if the patient has not been immunized within the previous 5 years.

Rabies treatment differs for different animal bites, and prevalence of rabies in specific animals may differ depending on the region of the country. Most rabies exposures in the United States occur from wild animals, with skunks, foxes, raccoons, and bats being the primary culprits. This varies greatly by region and country; one must contact the local heath department to determine whether a bite carries a risk for rabies. Once a patient is infected with rabies, the infection is almost universally fatal. If a patient is bitten by a dog, cat, or ferret, rabies prophylaxis should be held unless the animal develops signs or symptoms of rabies. If the animal is unavailable, then consult the local health department. Bites by skunks, foxes, bats, raccoons, and any wild carnivores should be considered rabid, and the patient should be given prophylaxis for rabies. Any contact with any bat, including a scratch, should be considered a rabid bite, and prophylaxis should be administered. Other animals need to be considered individually.

C. Animal bites have different rates of infectious potential depending on the animal, the area of the wound, the extent of the wound, and the comorbidities of the patient (Table 1).

Table 1 **Infectious Potential of Mammal Bites**

Factor	High Risk	Low Risk
Species	Cat	Dog
	Human	Rodent
	Probably primate	
	Pig	
Location of wound	Hand	Face
	Below knee	Scalp
	Through-and-through oral	Mucosa
	Over joint	
Wound type	Puncture	Large
	Extensive crush	Superficial
	Contaminated	Clean
	Old	Recent
Patient	Elderly	
	Diabetic	
	Prosthetic valve	
	Peripheral vascular disease	
	Asplenic	
	Alcoholic	
	Steroids, cytotoxic drugs	

From Weber EJ. Mammalian bites. In Marx JA, Hockeberger RS, Walls RM, eds. Rosen's Emergency Medicine: Concepts and Clinical Practice, 5th ed. St. Louis: Mosby, 2002:774.

(Continued on page 644)

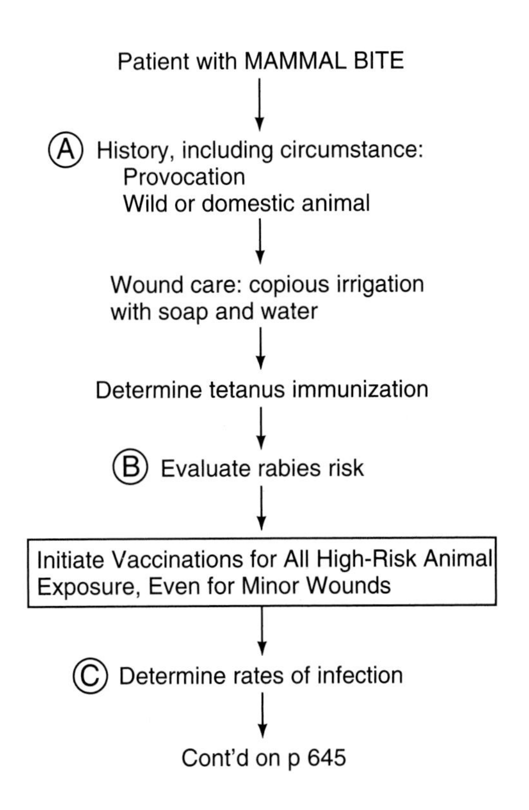
Patient with MAMMAL BITE
A History, including circumstance:
Provocation
Wild or domestic animal
Wound care: copious irrigation
with soap and water
Determine tetanus immunization
B Evaluate rabies risk
Initiate Vaccinations for All High-Risk Animal
Exposure, Even for Minor Wounds
C Determine rates of infection
Cont'd on p 645

D. Many bite injuries result in crush injury to tissue and may result in penetrating injuries. Nonviable tissue must be removed, and all puncture-type injuries must be explored for possible retained foreign body or substance and to inspect underlying structure such as muscle fascia and tendon. Injuries to hands resulting from a closed-fist punch to a mouth that causes a laceration over the joint should be treated as a human bite.

E Lacerations from bite injuries should be repaired in the typical fashion with approximation of viable tissue. Those bites that are at high risk for infection will have to be considered for management with delayed primary closure where the wound is essentially left open for 48–72 hours and then repaired. The cosmetic outcome and the functionality of the injured area must be considered (box and Table 2).

Essentials of Bite Care

Presentation
- Perform ABCs.
- Examine wound with attention to vascular and neurologic examinations.
- Elevate wound above level of heart, if possible.
- Take history, including circumstances of injury and information on animal (species of animal, wild or domestic, in captivity or not, etc.).
- Determine whether patient has a predisposing history for infection (diabetes, immunocompromise, etc.)
- Perform x-ray.

Wound Care
- Irrigate and clean wound.
- Use soap and water for rabies-prone wounds.
- Debride nonviable tissue, explore for foreign bodies or retained material.

Discharge
- Administer tetanus prophylaxis and prophylactic antibiotics, depending on specific of injury.
- Administer rabies prophylaxis if indicated.
- Follow-up within 36 hours.

Table 2 **Recommendations for Wound Closure and Antibiotics**

Species	Suturing	Prophylactic Antibiotics
Dog	All (± hands and feet)	High risk only*
Cat	Face only	All
Rodent	Yes (rarely needed)	No
Monkey	No	Yes
Human bites		
Hand	No	Yes
Other locations	Yes	Not necessary unless other high-risk concerns*
Self-Inflicted		
Mucosa	Yes	No
Through	Yes	Yes

*Hand wounds; deep punctures; heavy contamination; significant tissue destruction; >12 hours old; joint, tendon, or bone involvement; patients with diabetes, peripheral vascular disease, or corticosteroid use.
From Weber EJ. Mammalian bites. In Marx JA, Hockeberger RS, Walls RM, eds. Rosen's Emergency Medicine: Concepts and Clinical Practice, 5th ed. St. Louis: Mosby, 2002:774.

F. Prophylactic antibiotics may be indicated depending on the species of animal, the extent of tissue damage, and the comorbidities of the patient (Table 3).

Table 3 **Suggested Regimens for Prophylactic Antibiotics in Bite Wounds**

Species	Nonallergic Patient	Penicillin-Allergic Patient
Dog, most other animals	Dicloxacillin	Erythromycin
Cat	Cephalexin Cefuroxime Amoxicillin-clavulanate Dicloxacillin + penicillin	TMP-SMX Levofloxacin* Azithromycin TMP-SMX†
Dog, cat (patient without spleen, alcoholic, or lung disease) *[C. canimorsus]*	Penicillin Amoxicillin-clavulanate	Clindamycin Erythromycin Azithromycin or clarithromycin
Human (CFIs),‡ monkey	Cefuroxime Cefaclor Amoxicillin-clavulanate Ampicillin + first-generation cephalosporin Ampicillin + dicloxacillin	Levofloxacin* TMP-SMX†
Human: not CFI	Dicloxacillin or cephalexin	Erythromycin
Human: through and through	Penicillin	Clindamycin

*Includes levofloxacin, moxifloxacin, aparfloxacin. Quinolones not approved for children and pregnant women.
†Sulfonamides should not be given to pregnant women.
‡Anaerobic coverage not necessary unless established infection; 50% of human mouth anaerobes resistant to penicillin. CFI, closed-fist injury; TMP-SMX, trimethoprim-sulfamethoxazole.
From Weber, EJ. Mammalian bites. In Marx JA, Hockeberger RS, Walls RM, eds. Rosen's Emergency Medicine: Concepts and Clinical Practice, 5th ed. St. Louis: Mosby, 2002:774.

References

Brook I. Microbiology and management of human and animal bite wound infections. Prim Care 2003;30(1):25–39, v.

Freer L. Bites and injuries inflicted by wild animals. In Auerbach P, ed. Wilderness Medicine, 4th ed. St. Louis: Mosby, 2001:979–1001.

Freer L. North American wild mammalian injuries. Emerg Med Clin North Am 2004;22(2):445–473, ix.

Turner TW. Evidence-based emergency medicine/systematic review abstract. Do mammalian bites require antibiotic prophylaxis? Ann Emerg Med 2004;44(3):274–276.

Weber. EJ. Mammalian bites. In Marx JA, Hockeberger RS, Walls RM, eds. Rosen's Emergency Medicine: Concepts and Clinical Practice, 5th ed. St. Louis: Mosby, 2002.

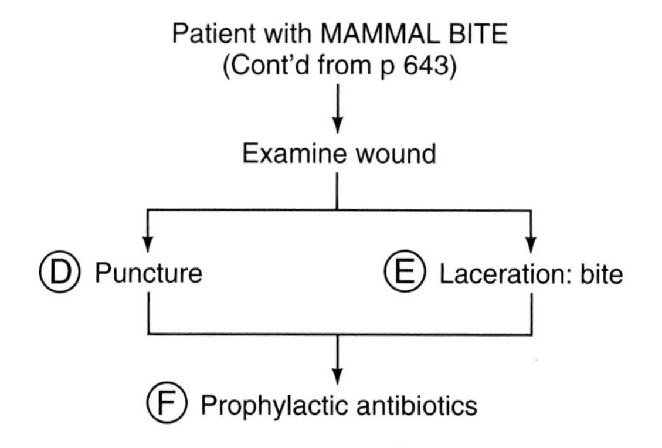
Patient with MAMMAL BITE
(Cont'd from p 643)
Examine wound
D Puncture
E Laceration: bite
F Prophylactic antibiotics

SNAKE VENOM POISONING

Richard D. Zane, MD, FAAEM

Globally, venomous snake bites are responsible for more than 100,000 deaths, with the majority occurring in Brazil, India, Southeast Asia, and certain parts of Africa. In the United States, approximately 50,000 snake bites are reported annually, with 8000 resulting from venomous snakes and leading to 10–15 deaths per year; the total number of snake bites is probably significantly more than that reported. The majority of all venomous snake bites in the United States are caused by pit vipers (rattlesnakes, cottonmouth, copperhead), coral snakes, and cobras. All venomous snake bites should be initially treated as a life-threatening event and require extremely careful management. The key factors influencing the treatment of the patient and the manifestation of pathology are the properties of the particular venom and the patients' response to envenomation. Although most venoms are complex toxins with many components and pathologic consequences, the majority of the manifestations are neurotoxic, hematotoxic, or a combination of the two. The presentation of envenomation can vary considerably, and a patient's comorbidities (vascular disease, diabetes, etc.) can have great influence on his or her ability to cope with the toxin.

A. In the United States the diagnosis of venomous snake bite is primarily determined by a history of a bite with or without the development of symptoms. A snake bite may appear as one, two, or multiple puncture wounds or small lacerations. Initial management, usually prehospital, is directed at limiting the spread or absorption of the venom by limiting the movement of the bitten extremity, by calming the patient, and by immobilizing the extremity. Preventing superficial venous and lymphatic flow with a constricting band may be used as long as arterial flow is not compromised. New techniques with whole limb constriction have shown promise. If applied within the first 3–5 minutes of a bite, a sawyer extractor may be useful in limiting the extent of absorbed toxin, as may an ice pack applied to the bitten extremity. Ice bath immersion or application of ice directly to the wound is not recommended. If possible, attempts should be made by a professional to identify the type of snake. If a patient has brought the snake with him or her, do not try to identify the snake unless you are specifically trained in venomous snake handling. Snakes are still capable of biting and causing severe injury even after they are dead.

B. By the time a victim of a venomous snake bite seeks care, there may have been sufficient time for serious consequences of envenomation to have occurred, and all patients should be treated as potentially critically ill with impending cardiovascular collapse. They should be placed on a cardiac monitor and should receive supplemental oxygen, IV fluids, and a careful and detailed physical examination. If the bite has occurred within 30 minutes of arrival, a constricting band may be useful. All patients should have a complete blood count (CBC), electrolyte analysis, coagulation studies, and an ECG performed.

The grade of envenomation is established by evaluating local wound findings, the presence of a coagulopathy, and the severity of systemic symptoms.

Grade 0. Suspected snake bite with no evidence of envenomation with no or minimal pain, <1 inch of erythema, and no systemic or laboratory abnormalities within 12 hours of the bite.

Grade I. Suspected snake bite, minimal evidence of envenomation, moderate pain, 1–5 inches of erythema, and no systemic or laboratory abnormalities within 12 hours of the bite.

Grade II. Suspected snake bite, moderate evidence of envenomation, severe pain, spreading erythema, petechiae, and systemic symptoms.

Grade III. Suspected snake bite, severe envenomation, spreading or generalized erythema, edema, ecchymoses and petechiae, severe systemic symptoms, and hemodynamic instability. Patient may initially present with mild symptoms and progress rapidly.

Grade IV. Suspected bite, very severe envenomation, usually a larger snake, sudden severe pain, systemic symptoms, hemodynamic collapse, or death. The grade of envenomation is important because it determines whether antivenin is initially used and the amount used.

C. Several cases of delayed worsening of the envenomation have been reported. Observe patients for 12 hours with the bitten part elevated above heart level. The grade of envenomation should be changed if local or systemic symptoms signs appear or worsen.

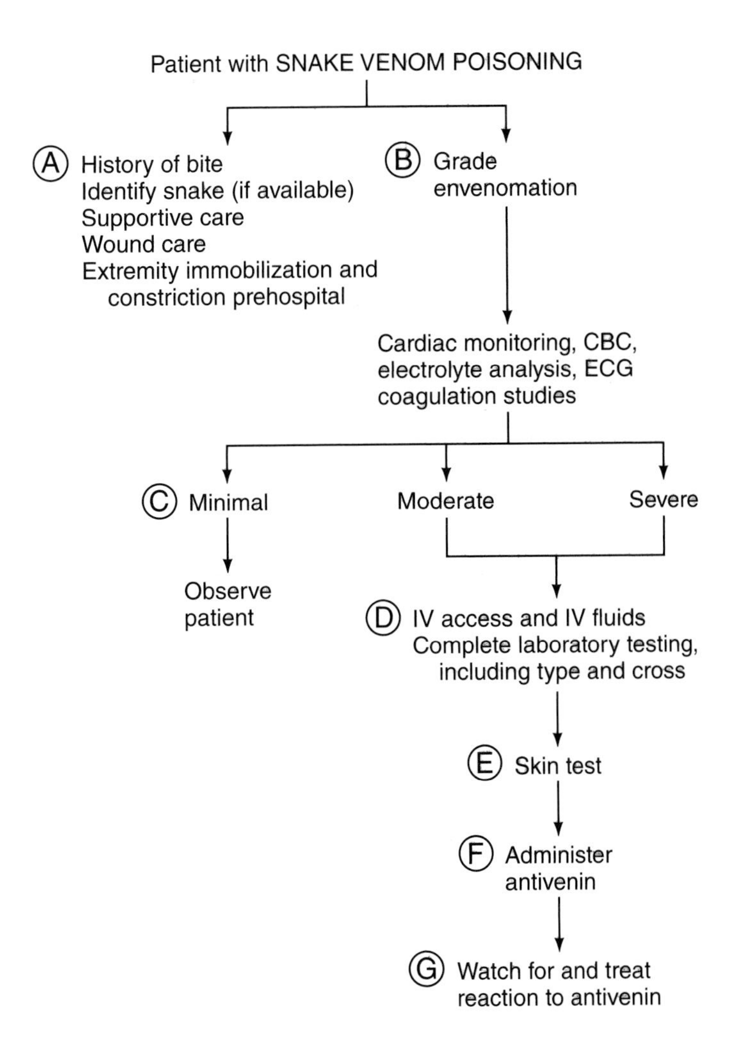

D. Most deaths from snake bites are caused by the patient's failure to seek medical attention or the physician's failure to recognize the severity of the envenomation. If antivenin is not immediately available, give a rapid crystalloid infusion to maintain blood pressure and reduce heart rate. If bleeding is apparent, replace platelets or coagulation factors by infusing platelets or fresh frozen plasma until antivenin can be infused. After rapid evaluation of the patient, treat with antivenin. Call poison control.

E. Use skin test only when the decision to administer antivenin has been made. Administer antivenin (Crotalidae) polyvalent to patients with moderate or severe envenomations who demonstrate worsening of local or systemic findings. The skin test consists of 0.02 ml of a 1:10 dilution of the skin test material provided with the antivenin in one shoulder and 0.02 ml of normal saline (control) in the other shoulder. A positive skin test consists of a wheal and flare 10 mm at the site of injection. Strong reactions to the skin test indicate a high probability of a severe reaction to antivenin infusion.

F. Antivenin administration consists of infusion of 5–10 vials in 250–500 ml of dextrose and water over 1–2 hours, except as noted in E. The initial infusion should be slow (60 ml/hr or 1 ml/min) in case an allergic reaction develops. If no reaction develops, the infusion rate can be increased to complete the infusion in 1–2 hours.

G. Up to 25% of patients develop some degree of reaction to antivenin infusion. If a reaction develops, stop the antivenin infusion immediately. Reactions take many forms, ranging from local erythema and itching to anaphylaxis. Give epinephrine, along with H_1 and H_2 receptor blockers, to control the acute reaction. At this point, consult with a regional poison control center or medical toxicologist. The benefits of continued antivenin infusion must be compared with the risks of restarting the infusion. In general, the antivenin can be restarted after diluting the antivenin and infusing it more slowly.

References

German BT. Pressure-immobilization bandages delay toxicity in a porcine model of eastern coral snake (Micrurus fulvius fulvius) envenomation. Ann Emerg Med 2005;45(6):603–608.

Gold BS. North American snake envenomation: diagnosis, treatment, and management. Emerg Med Clin North Am 2004;22(2):423–443, ix.

Otten EJ, Blomkalns AL. Venomous animal injuries. In Marx JA, Hockberger RS, Walls RM, et al, eds. Rosen's Emergency Medicine: Concepts and Clinical Practice, 5th ed. St. Louis: Mosby, 2002.

HYPOTHERMIA

Richard D. Zane, MD, FAEEM

The most common presentation of hypothermia is accidental. A few deaths each year from hypothermia are attributed to homicide and suicide. By definition, hypothermia is a core temperature <35° C, yet patients with the same core temperature may manifest signs and symptoms of hypothermia very differently. The most important variables influencing the outcome of patients with hypothermia are age, comorbidities, duration of cold exposure, nutritional status, medication use, or intoxicant use. Accidental hypothermia usually occurs when the normal compensatory mechanisms to heat loss are overwhelmed by exposure. When a patient has impaired compensatory mechanisms, hypothermia is more severe and likely to be fatal.

Initial therapy is directed at treating the underlying cause of the hypothermia and passive and active rewarming. It is important to recognize that hypothermia may be a manifestation of severe systemic disease, such as sepsis, stroke, cardiovascular accident, acute coronary syndrome, or myxedema coma.

A. All patients with symptomatic hypothermia should receive warm humidified supplemental oxygen; be placed on a cardiac monitor; receive IV access and administration of warm IV fluids (patients with symptomatic hypothermia are typically dehydrated); receive an ECG and laboratory studies, including a CBC, electrolytes, coagulation studies, and liver function studies; and have continuous temperature measurement. Patients with a failure to protect their airway or failure to oxygenate or ventilate may be safely intubated. ABG analysis is highly inaccurate in patients with hypothermia and should not guide management or therapy.

B. The initial cardiac response to hypothermia is tachycardia followed by bradycardia. Patients with a stable cardiac rhythm (including sinus bradycardia) and stable vital signs may undergo passive rewarming with blankets to prevent further heat loss. Noninvasive internal modalities may be used (warmed, humidified oxygen and warmed IV fluids), or warming blankets may be helpful.

C. Patients with cardiovascular instability need to be rapidly rewarmed using a combination of methods. Core warming (warming the heart before the extremities) must be used. Gastric/bladder/colon lavage, peritoneal lavage with warmed dialysate, or chest tube thoracostomy with warm saline irrigation should be considered in severe cases. Patients with severe hypothermia should receive extracorporeal blood warming with partial cardiopulmonary bypass if available. Continue warmed O_2, IV fluids, and blankets. For ventricular fibrillation or asystole, follow Advanced Cardiac Life Support guidelines. The hypothermic myocardium is often refractory to atropine, pacing, and defibrillation.

D. Prolonged resuscitation until the patient is actively rewarmed is typically indicated with the caveat that it will be impossible to fully restore patients to normal body temperature during cardiac arrest.

E. All patients with hemodynamic instability and hypothermia require intensive care unit (ICU) admission and should be observed for a minimum of 24 hours on a cardiac monitor once rewarming is complete and the patient is asymptomatic.

References

Danzl D, Pozos R. Accidental hypothermia. N Engl J Med 1994;331:1756.

Danzy D. Accidental hypothermia. In Marx JA, Hockeberger RS, Walls RM, eds. Rosen's Emergency Medicine: Concepts and Clinical Practice. 5th ed. St. Louis: Mosby, 2002.

Ulrich AS. Hypothermia and localized cold injuries. Emerg Med Clin North Am 2004;22(2):281–298.

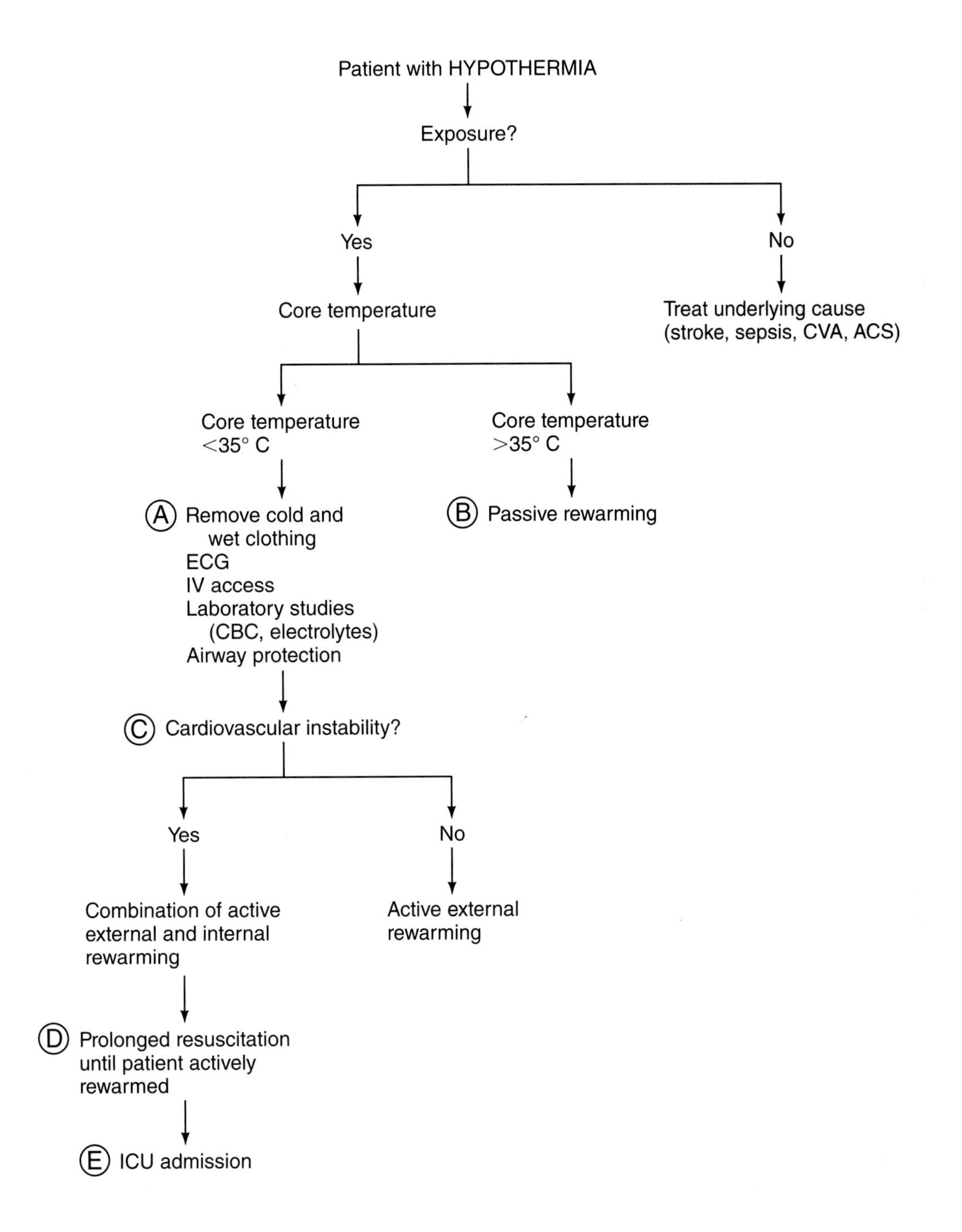
Patient with HYPOTHERMIA
Exposure?
Yes
No
Core temperature
Treat underlying cause (stroke, sepsis, CVA, ACS)
Core temperature <35° C
Core temperature >35° C
(A) Remove cold and wet clothing
ECG
IV access
Laboratory studies (CBC, electrolytes)
Airway protection
(B) Passive rewarming
(C) Cardiovascular instability?
Yes
No
Combination of active external and internal rewarming
Active external rewarming
(D) Prolonged resuscitation until patient actively rewarmed
(E) ICU admission

SUBMERSION

Richard D. Zane, MD, FAEEM

Drowning is death from suffocation as a result of submersion in a fluid, whereas near-drowning implies survival, at least temporarily, after such suffocation. In the United States, drowning accounts for approximately 5000 deaths, >10,000 hospital admissions, and > 30,000 emergency department (ED) visits per year. Drowning is typically in the top-five causes of traumatic death for all age groups and is a leading cause of death for children and adolescents. The backyard swimming pool is the most common cause of drowning for those < 5 years, and the bathtub is the most common household cause of drowning.

Submersion is usually accompanied by panic and breath holding. After a short period, patients will develop severe air hunger and some degree of hypoxia and hypercarbia, resulting in an involuntary gasp causing aspiration. This is usually followed by laryngospasm, more aspiration, and death. Of victims, 10%–15% succumb to asphyxia while submerged without evidence of aspiration, probably because of laryngospasm.

Morbidity and mortality are multifactorial and a consequence of the duration of submersion, the temperature of the water, the age and comorbidities of the victim, and the salinity and contamination of the water. Patients who are awake and conscious or have minimal alteration of consciousness on arrival have very good outcomes. The degree of neurologic impairment at presentation directly correlates to outcome.

A. Some victims of near-drowning do not aspirate water, have limited laryngospasm or breath holding, and regain effective ventilation before permanent damage occurs. These patients may appear sleepy or groggy or completely alert. Despite appearing stable, these patients may be severely hypoxic or become so quickly. Cervical spine (C-spine) precautions should be continued if neck injury is possible, and these patients should be transported with supplemental O_2 to the nearest ED.

B. The fundamental goal for initial resuscitation of the apneic near-drowning victim is to restore Pao_2 to normal as rapidly as possible. The victim should be extricated from the water as quickly as possible. If the victim is apneic and mouth-to-mouth ventilation in the water is possible, this should be initiated when the rescuer reaches the victim. Because chest compressions are not typically feasible in the water, they should be initiated when the victim can be removed. C-spine precaution should be followed during extrication if a fall or diving injury is suspected. The single most important factor related to a normal recovery is the prevention of irreversible hypoxia. This usually means that the first responder must know cardiopulmonary resuscitation (CPR) and be able to use it when necessary.

C. If the patient who is initially apneic has a palpable pulse, the rescuer should continue providing assisted ventilation and activate the emergency medical system by asking another person to call 911 (or other local emergency number). The rescuer should continue assessing the victim's airway to ensure its patency. If necessary, the rescuer may use a Heimlich maneuver to clear the airway (with the awareness that gastric contents may be aspirated during this maneuver). The Heimlich maneuver should not be used in an attempt to empty the stomach. The patient who is apneic should be intubated by paramedic personnel as soon as possible and transported to the nearest ED.

D. The patient who is apneic and pulseless should receive CPR according to American Cardiac Life Support (ACLS) guidelines while C-spine precautions are maintained. The rescuer should have a bystander call 911. The patient should be intubated by paramedic personnel as soon as possible and transported with CPR and ACLS in progress to the nearest ED.

(Continued on page 652)

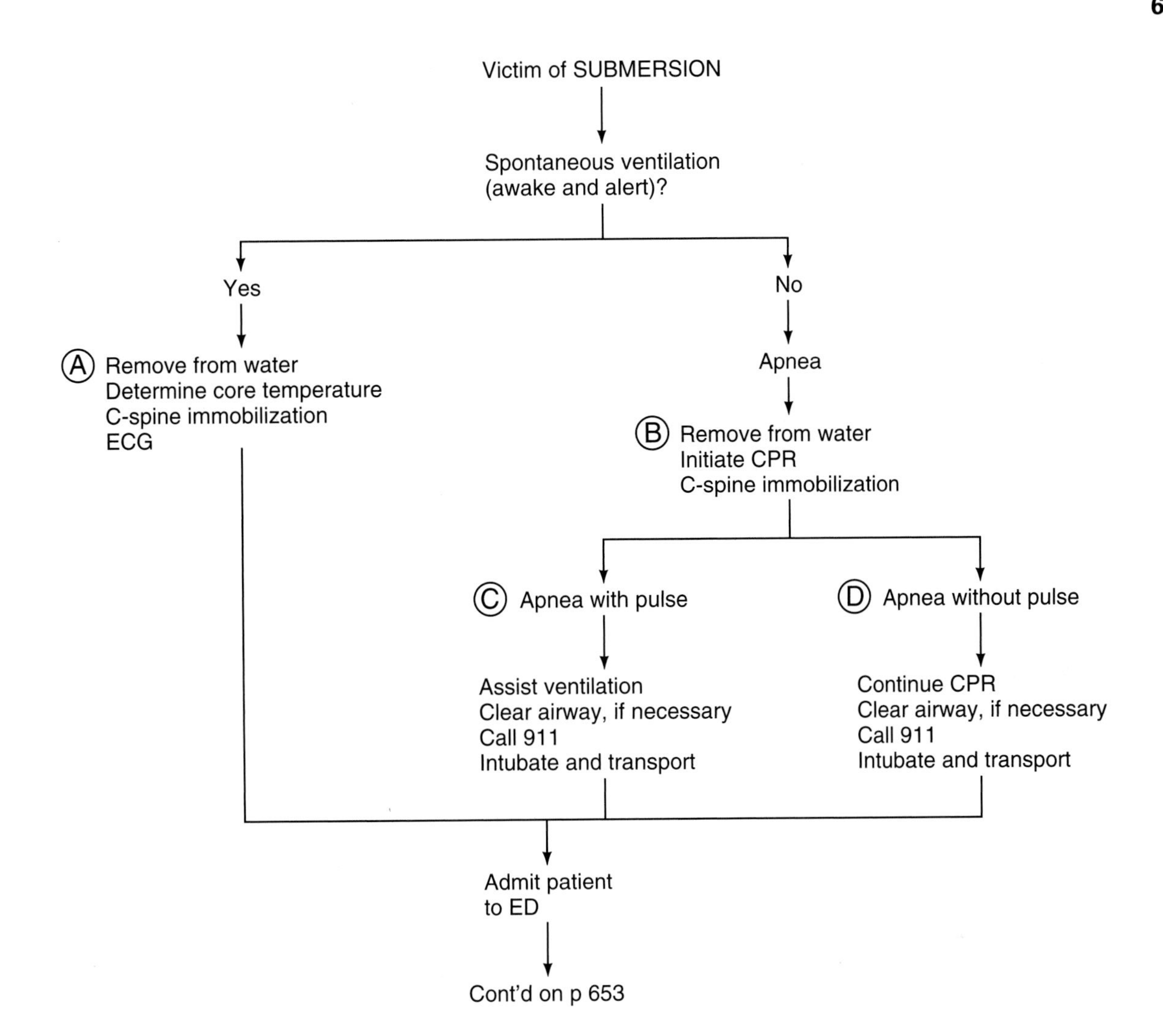
Victim of SUBMERSION
Spontaneous ventilation
(awake and alert)?
Yes
No
Apnea
(A) Remove from water
Determine core temperature
C-spine immobilization
ECG
(B) Remove from water
Initiate CPR
C-spine immobilization
(C) Apnea with pulse
(D) Apnea without pulse
Assist ventilation
Clear airway, if necessary
Call 911
Intubate and transport
Continue CPR
Clear airway, if necessary
Call 911
Intubate and transport
Admit patient
to ED
Cont'd on p 653

E. In the ED the patient who is alert yet hypoxic should be treated aggressively. If the patient is alert or able to be aroused, the physician may try to use a mask for continuous positive alveolar pressure (CPAP) first. If CPAP is not readily available or cannot be implemented because of altered consciousness, the patient should be intubated. The patient's oxygenation may then be augmented with positive end-expiratory pressure (PEEP). All intubated patients should have a gastric tube placed to decompress the stomach. Patients with altered consciousness should not have stomach decompression until intubation has been confirmed; those with normal consciousness typically do not need decompression. If present, treat hypothermia, bronchospasm, and acidosis. Admit these patients to the intensive care unit (ICU). If the near-drowning patient presents with shock, consider alternative causes of shock, such as major associated trauma, stroke, acute myocardial infarction, diabetes, and the like.

F. The near-drowning patient who is spontaneously breathing is extremely fortunate and will have a normal Pao_2, $Paco_2$, and pH. Check the C-spine for injuries. If the patient is normothermic and exhibits no other abnormalities, including bronchospasm or altered consciousness, he or she may be released to a strong social support system with strict precautionary advice. Treat the patient who is nonhypoxic and hypothermic for hypothermia (see I). Admit patients exhibiting bronchospasm or acidosis for observation. All pediatric patients should have a social services evaluation to determine whether child abuse or lack of supervision was a factor in the drowning.

G. The initially apneic patient with an intact circulation will likely be hypoxic on arrival at the ED. If not yet intubated by prehospital personnel, intubate the patient on arrival. Occasionally, patients begin breathing spontaneously during the initial prehospital resuscitation and present without hypoxia. In this situation, they should be treated as in F. Intubated hypoxic patients benefit from PEEP. This can dramatically improve the ventilation/perfusion mismatch. Place an orogastric (OG) tube to aspirate gastric contents. If present, treat bronchospasm and acidosis (inhaled β_2-adrenergic agonists and sodium bicarbonate). Examine the patient for C-spine injuries, and obtain chest film. Treat hypothermia (see I). Admit these patients to the ICU.

H. The apneic and pulseless patient who arrives without previous intubation should be intubated on arrival. CPR and ACLS should be continued.

I. In the patient with hypothermia, continue CPR until the core temperature is >32° C. In the severely hypothermic patient (core temperature <32° C), implement active core rewarming to prevent the phenomena of "afterdrop," which can occur when active external rewarming (e.g., warm immersion) used alone leads to reperfusion of cold peripheral tissues and subsequent cooling of the previously sequestered warm-core blood. Active core rewarming can include heated humidified O_2, heated peritoneal lavage, and cardiopulmonary bypass. Other methods include gastric and colonic irrigation, thoracostomy with pleural and mediastinal irrigation, and hemodialysis. Each of these techniques carries inherent risks and complications. Truncal active external rewarming may be added to augment core rewarming. For the patient with mild to moderate hypothermia (core temperature 32°–37° C), passive external rewarming is appropriate. This includes the removal of wet clothing and prevention of further heat loss by applying blankets. The efficacy of ACLS medications is controversial in hypothermia. Bretylium has been reported to be effective in ventricular fibrillation. The efficacy of atropine in hypothermia-induced bradycardia is doubtful. The combination of hypoxia and hypothermia can lead to a marked decrease in tissue O_2 delivery. Although hypothermia may be protective via diminished metabolic rate, it is more often lethal.

J. In the ICU, ventilatory management should be aggressive, including PEEP, frequent suctioning, and frequent monitoring of the ventilation/perfusion shunt. Acidosis and cardiac arrhythmias should also be treated aggressively. Although controversial, consider intracranial pressure (ICP) monitoring, pulmonary artery pressure monitoring, and barbiturate coma. These treatments contain risks and have questionable benefit. Ensure that no C-spine injury exists (if this is not already done). Treat hypothermia (see I). Treat bronchospasm and acidosis if present. Monitor electrolytes and fluid status closely. Steroids, barbiturates, and induced hypothermia have not been shown to improve survival. Address psychosocial issues with the family.

References

Feldhous KM. Submersion. In Marx JA, Hockberger RS, Walls RM, et al, eds. Rosen's Emergency Medicine: Concepts and Clinical Practice, 5th ed. St. Louis: Mosby, 2002:2050.

Kallas HJ. Drowning and near-drowning. In Behrman RE. Nelson Textbook of Pediatrics, 17th ed. Philadelphia: Saunders, 2004:321.

Olshaker JS. Submersion. Emerg Med Clin North Am 2004;22(2): 357–367, viii.

Zuckerbraun NS, Saladino RA. Pediat drowning: current management strategies for immediate care. Clin Pediatr Emerg Med 2005;6(1).

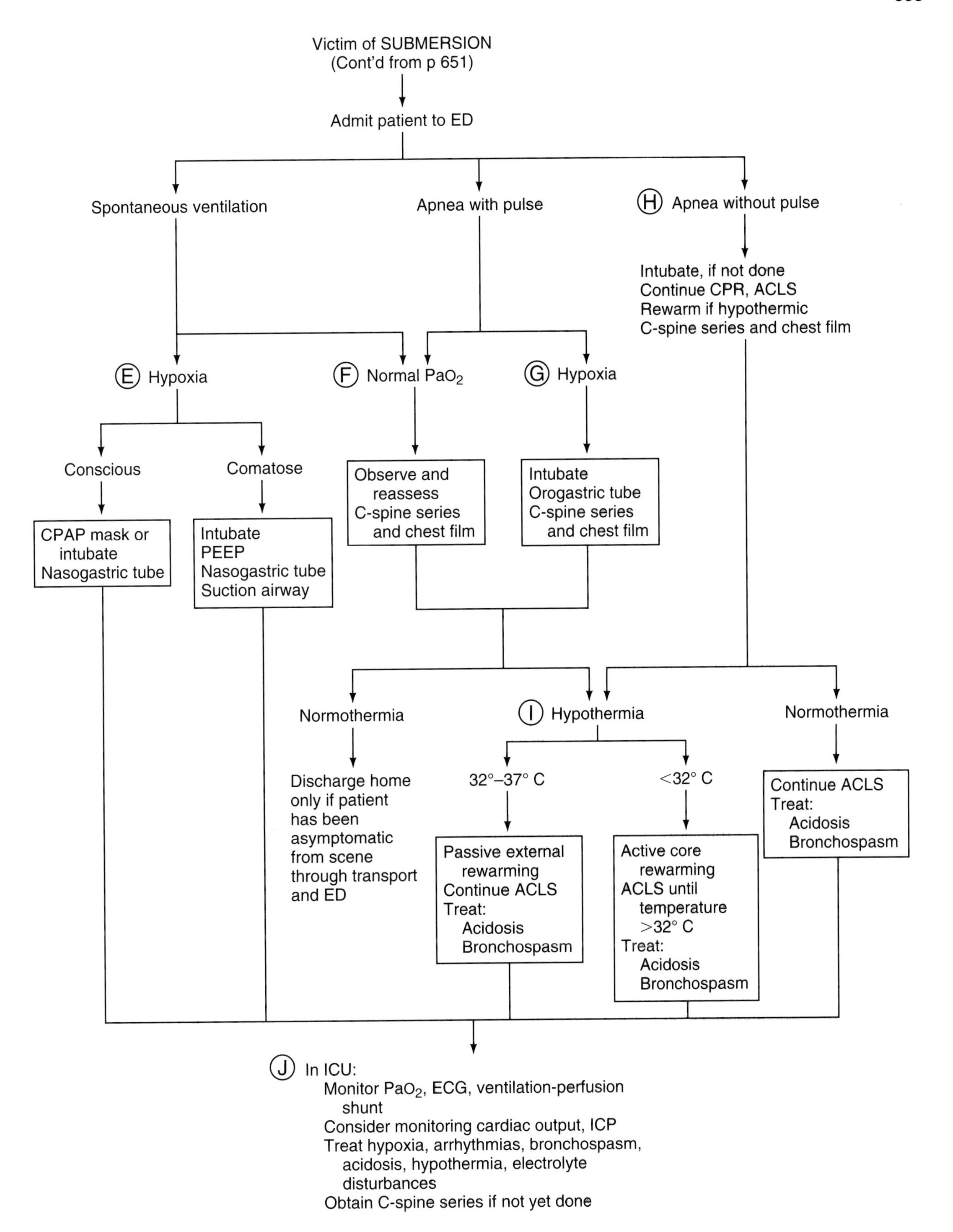
Victim of SUBMERSION
(Cont'd from p 651)
Admit patient to ED
Spontaneous ventilation
Apnea with pulse
H Apnea without pulse
Intubate, if not done
Continue CPR, ACLS
Rewarm if hypothermic
C-spine series and chest film
E Hypoxia
F Normal PaO_2
G Hypoxia
Conscious
Comatose
CPAP mask or intubate
Nasogastric tube
Intubate
PEEP
Nasogastric tube
Suction airway
Observe and reassess
C-spine series and chest film
Intubate
Orogastric tube
C-spine series and chest film
Normothermia
I Hypothermia
Normothermia
Discharge home only if patient has been asymptomatic from scene through transport and ED
32°–37° C
<32° C
Continue ACLS
Treat:
Acidosis
Bronchospasm
Passive external rewarming
Continue ACLS
Treat:
Acidosis
Bronchospasm
Active core rewarming
ACLS until temperature >32° C
Treat:
Acidosis
Bronchospasm
J In ICU:
Monitor PaO_2, ECG, ventilation-perfusion shunt
Consider monitoring cardiac output, ICP
Treat hypoxia, arrhythmias, bronchospasm, acidosis, hypothermia, electrolyte disturbances
Obtain C-spine series if not yet done

Behavioral Medicine

John A. Fromson, MD
Section Editor

ALCOHOLISM

John A. Fromson, MD; Michael E. Scott, MD; and Myra L. Muramoto, MD

Patients with alcohol problems rarely present with a chief complaint of problem drinking. More commonly they exhibit various complications of alcohol abuse. Some are psychological in nature (fatigue, anxiety, depression, insomnia, deteriorating relationships, domestic violence, and impaired work performance); others are somatic (palpitations, weakness, gastric upset, headaches). Emergency department physicians commonly encounter patients who are acutely intoxicated and brought in by police because of assaultive behavior, public intoxication, or driving under the influence of alcohol (DUI) or driving while intoxicated (DWI). Anxiety and depressive mood disorders are the most commonly occurring psychiatric disorders with alcohol dependence. Alcoholism is the primary diagnosis in 25% of suicides. It is also a significant contributor to birth defects, including fetal alcohol syndrome. The physician must maintain a *high index of suspicion* to avoid missing this common diagnosis. Consider alcohol-related problems in nearly every patient. This includes special populations, such as patients who are physicians. Nearly every state has distinct programs designed to guide and monitor recovery.

A. History is the key to a diagnosis of alcohol or drug abuse or dependence; however, patients often distort the history and minimize the problem. Denial is a strong defense in all those who abuse alcohol or drugs. Compounding denial are the recent studies that cite moderate alcohol consumption with decreased risk of heart disease, myocardial infarction, stroke, and cognitive decline. Thus, it often is necessary to interview family members to obtain an accurate drinking history and symptoms of abuse or dependence. Review patients' alcohol and drug use history in detail. Look for problems in social (divorce, job loss, family arguments, use in other family members), legal (DUI, DWI), and medical (gastritis, peptic ulcer, hepatitis, anemia) areas of the patient's life. It is important to identify negative consequences that suggest loss of control and support a diagnosis of dependence. Compulsive use and preoccupation with drinking complete the criteria for dependence or addiction. The mnemonic *CPR* (compulsivity, preoccupation, relapse) is useful for recalling the essential features of dependence. Also review the family history because alcoholism shows strong family trends. Physiologic dependence often is present but not required for the diagnosis of alcohol dependence.

B. Physical examination should be detailed and thorough. Patients with cirrhosis, ascites, edema, rhinophyma, peripheral neuropathy, and jaundice characterize end-stage alcoholism. These patients usually have been drinking uncontrollably for >10 years. Physical complications of alcohol are late findings and may not be evident early in the disease. Increased rates of oral, pharyngeal, laryngeal, esophageal, and liver cancers are seen with chronic alcohol use.

C. Laboratory screening can be informative. Look for elevations in aspartate aminotransferase (AST), alanine aminotransferase (ALT), and gamma glutamyltransferase (GGT). Typically, the AST is greater than the ALT. The GGT is a more sensitive indicator of alcohol-induced liver damage. The CBC often shows elevated mean corpuscular volume and mean corpuscular hemoglobin with prolonged regular use of alcohol. Hypercholesterolemia and hyperlipidemia often are present. Blood alcohol level of >300 mg/dl in an alert patient indicates significant tolerance.

D. Using the data thus far collected, the physician can usually make a diagnosis of alcohol abuse, dependence, or polysubstance dependence. The DSM-IV-TR lists the criteria for substance dependence and substance abuse. Seven criteria are included for a diagnosis of substance dependence, three of the seven criteria being required for a formal diagnosis. In addition, there are the categories of with and without physiologic dependence. There are also specifiers to further clarify the exact course of the illness. Four criteria are diagnostic for substance abuse. Only one of these criteria need be present for the formal diagnosis.

E. Dual diagnosis refers to substance abuse or dependence *plus* another major psychiatric diagnosis such as depression, bipolar disorder, schizophrenia, or anxiety disorder. These patients can be extremely difficult to diagnose and treat because substance abuse often causes or mimics many psychiatric syndromes. Conversely, there is a significant amount of comorbidity with depressive and anxiety disorders in patients who are alcohol dependent. Psychiatric consultation is suggested. Successful treatment of alcohol problems requires identification and treatment of all other comorbid psychiatric problems.

F. Individualize treatment to the particular patient's needs. Merely telling the patient to quit drinking is futile and potentially dangerous. Consultation with an experienced psychiatrist or addictionist is strongly recommended. Referral to Alcoholics Anonymous (AA) or another support group is an excellent place to begin

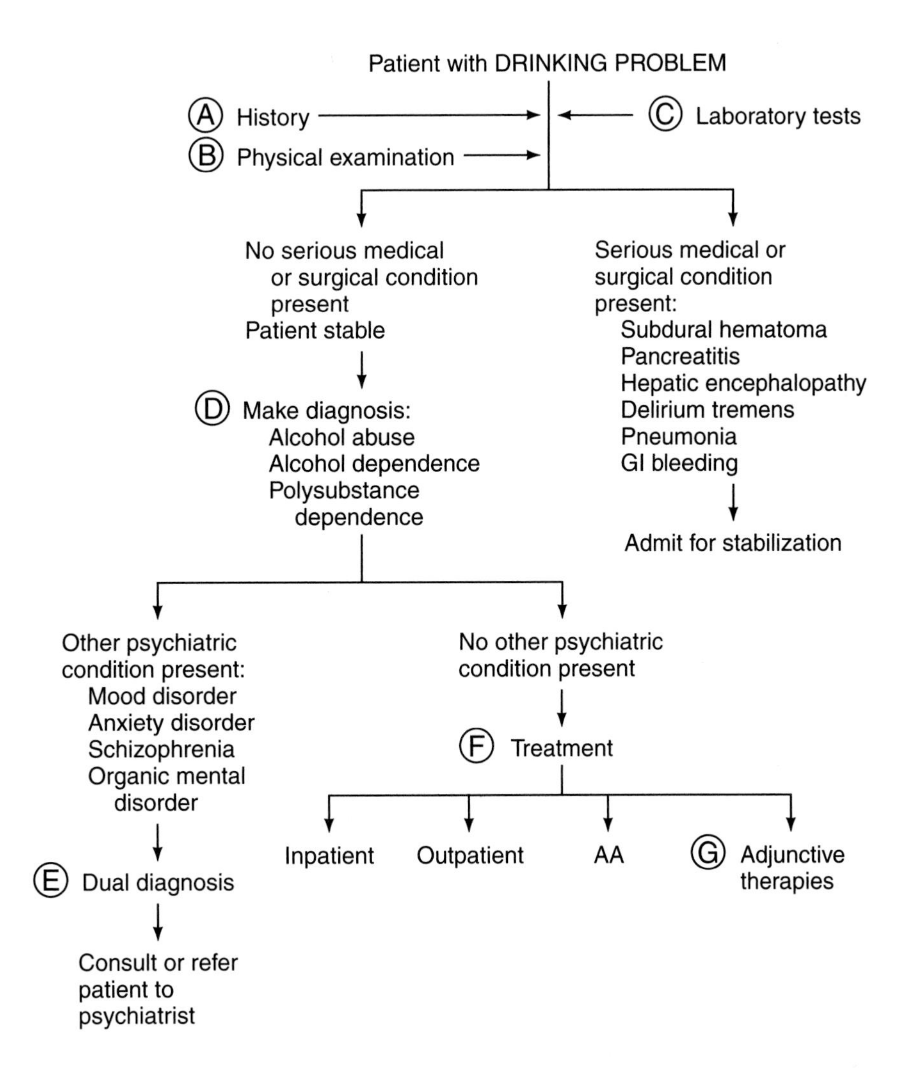

but may not be enough for patients with advanced disease or comorbid psychiatric disorders.

G. The use of pharmacologic agents, such as naltrexone, acamprosate, and disulfiram, may be useful adjunctive therapies to decrease craving, prolong sobriety, and increase time to relapse.

References

American Psychiatric Association. Diagnostic and Statistical Manual of Mental Disorders—Text Revision, 4th ed. Washington, DC: American Psychiatric Association, 2000.

Berger K, Ajani UA, Kase CS, et al. Light-to-moderate alcohol consumption and the risk of stroke among U.S. male physicians. N Engl J Med 1999;341:1557–1564.

Hays JT, Spickard WA Jr. Alcoholism: early diagnosis and intervention. J Gen Intern Med 1987;2:420.

Hines LM, Stampfer MJ, Ma J. Genetic variation in alcohol dehydrogenase and the beneficial effect of moderate alcohol consumption on myocardial infarction. N Engl J Med 2001;344:549–555.

Horgan C. Substance abuse: the nation's number one health problem. Princeton, NJ: Robert Wood Johnson Foundation, 2001.

Leape LL, Fromson JA. Problem doctors: is there a system-level solution? Ann Intern Med 2006;144:107–155.

Mason BJ. Treatment of alcohol dependent outpatients with acamprosate: a clinical review. J Clin Psychiatry 2001;62(Suppl 20):42–48.

Meyers JK, Weissman MM, Tischler GL, et al. Six-month prevalence of psychiatric disorders in three communities 1980–1982. Arch Gen Psychiatry 1984;41(10):959–967.

Milhorn JT Jr. The diagnosis of alcoholism. Am Fam Physician 1988;37:175.

Mukamal KJ, Conigrave KM, Mittleman MA, et al. Roles of drinking pattern and type of alcohol consumed in coronary heart disease in men. N Engl J Med 2003;348:109–118.

Practice guideline for the treatment of patients with substance use disorders, ed 2. Am J Psychiatry 2006;163:8.

Ringborg U. Alcohol and risk of cancer. Alcohol Clin Exp Res 1998; 22(7 Suppl):323S–328S.

Schorling JB, Buchsbaum D. Screening for alcohol and drug abuse. Med Clin North Am 1997;81:845.

Smith DE (special editor). Addiction medicine (special issue). West J Med 1990;152:502.

Stampfer MJ, Kang JH, Chen J, et al. Effects of moderate alcohol consumption on cognitive function in women. N Engl J Med 2005; 352:245–253.

ANXIETY

John A. Fromson, MD, and Eric M. Reiman, MD

A. Everyday stressors such as illness, injury, and loss can produce anxiety in patients and their families. Compassion, patience, and understanding can reduce feelings of helplessness and social isolation and increase patients' confidence and self-esteem. A benzodiazepine may be prescribed if patients understand that it is a temporary measure of no more than a few days' or weeks' duration and if they have no history of a psychoactive substance use disorder.

B. Organic factors can produce symptoms of anxiety. They include cardiovasculature (e.g., hypertension, arrhythmias), dietary (e.g., caffeine), physiologic or iatrogenic-induced delirium, substance related (e.g., cocaine, drug withdrawal syndromes, stimulants, bronchodilators), hematologic (e.g., anemias), immunologic (e.g., systemic lupus erythematosus), metabolic (e.g., hyperadrenalism, hyperthyroidism/hypothyroidism, menopause), neurologic (e.g., encephalopathies, intracranial mass lesions, seizure disorders), respiratory (e.g., asthma, pneumonia, chronic obstructive pulmonary disease), and secreting tumors (e.g., carcinoid, pheochromocytoma). In addition, patients may often experience anxiety during the initial stages of dementia (these patients may have a paradoxical response to sedative-hypnotics with increased anxiety and memory impairment). Therefore, it is critical to diagnose or rule out an organic etiology to the symptoms of anxiety. However, the presence of a nonpsychiatric medical disorder does not always exclude the possibility of a concurrent anxiety disorder.

C. Anxiety is a feature of many psychiatric disorders. These include, but are not limited to, attention-deficit and disruptive behavior disorders, childhood or adolescent separation anxiety, schizophrenia and other psychotic disorders, mood disorders (e.g., depression and bipolar disorders), and adjustment disorders. Diagnose and treat the underlying problem.

D. In addition to generalized anxiety disorder, the DSM-IV-TR identifies other anxiety disorders including panic, phobic, obsessive, acute, and posttraumatic stress disorders.

Panic disorder is characterized by frequent panic attacks, at least some of which occur at unexpected times. Panic attacks are sudden episodes of severe apprehension or fear associated with at least four of the following symptoms: choking sensations, shortness of breath or smothering sensations, palpitations or tachycardia, chest discomfort, dizziness, trembling or shaking, numbness or tingling, hot flashes or chills, sweating, nausea or abdominal distress, feelings of unreality, a fear of dying, and a fear of going crazy or losing control. Look for abrupt onset (maximal intensity within 10 minutes of onset) and short duration (typically, 2–30 minutes). Many patients see cardiologists or emergency physicians seeking a medical explanation of the problem. Indeed, they account for >30% of patients with atypical or nonanginal chest pain. Compared to controls, patients diagnosed with panic disorder may have a higher prevalence of asthma, labile hypertension, mitral valve prolapse, and migraine headaches. Several medications can block anxiety attacks. These include selective serotonin reuptake inhibitors (SSRIs), such as paroxetine, and tricyclic antidepressants, such as imipramine (start low, go slow, warn the patient of an exacerbation in symptoms early in treatment); monoamine oxidase inhibitors (MAOIs), such as phenelzine (provide a list of dietary and medication restrictions); and benzodiazepines, such as clonazepam or lorazepam (use standing doses to prevent attacks, warn patients about withdrawal symptoms and the related need for slow discontinuation, and avoid in patients with a history of a psychoactive substance use disorder). Recent evidence suggests that cognitive-behavioral therapy can prevent anxiety attacks as effectively as medication in patients with panic disorder. This standardized, short-term treatment should be administered by a well-trained professional; it is designed to help patients identify and revise the habit of responding to normally innocuous physical sensations as dangerous. Once the panic attacks are addressed, patients who have panic disorder with agoraphobia are encouraged to confront and learn to overcome their fears through repeated, frequent, intense exposures to the feared situations.

E. Phobias, irrational fears that are recognized by the individual as excessive, are extremely common. Agoraphobia is an irrational fear of situations from which it may be difficult or embarrassing to escape. Always consider the possibility of panic attacks in patients with this disorder. Social phobia is an excessive fear of being scrutinized in performance or social situations. Distinguish individuals who have the circumscribed type of social phobia (those who fear one particular performance situation, such as public speaking) from those who have generalized social phobia (excessively shy individuals who fear a variety of performance and social situations). Specific phobia is an irrational fear of particular objects or situations (e.g., animals,

(Continued on page 660)

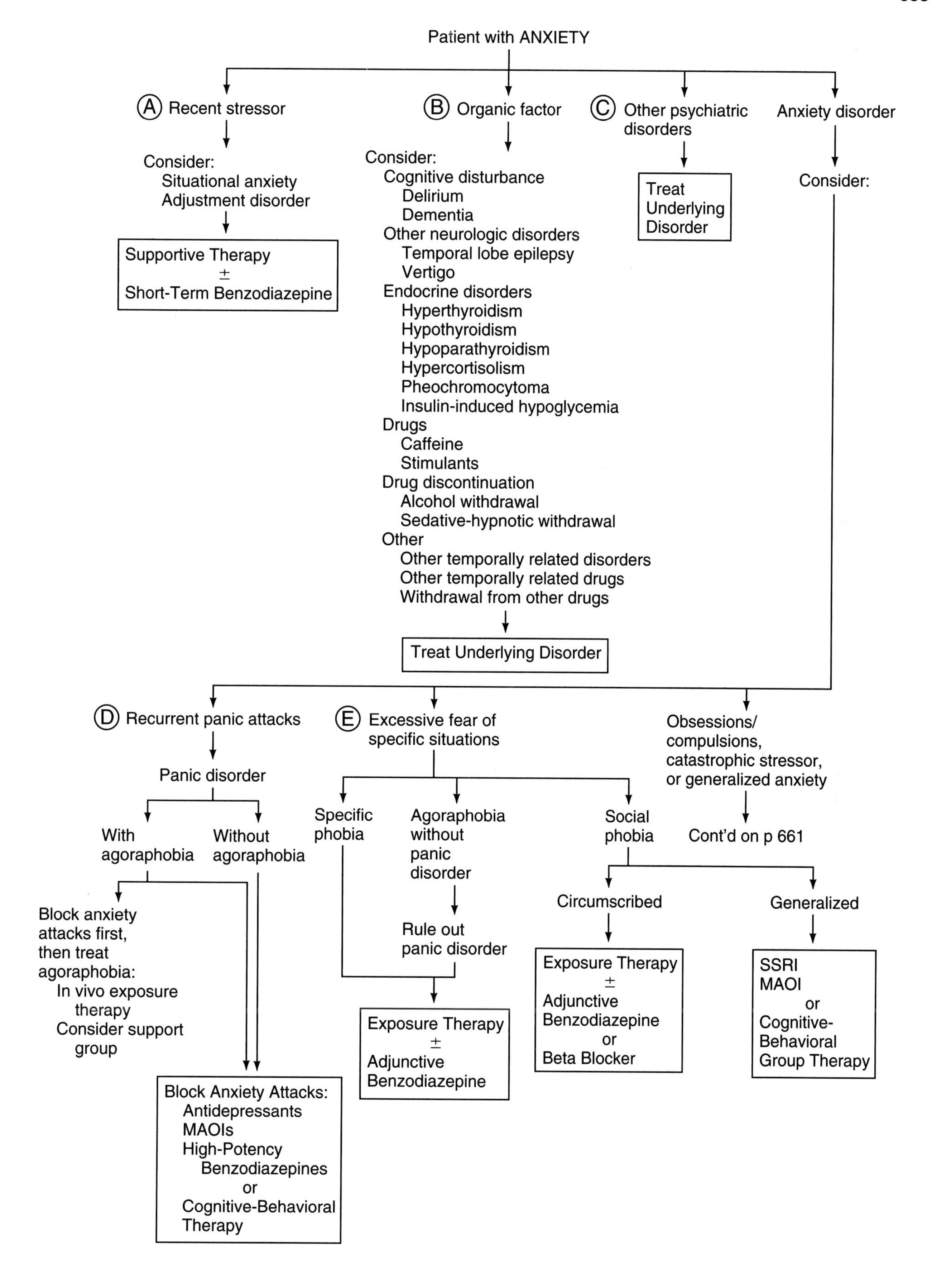
Patient with ANXIETY
(A) Recent stressor
Consider:
Situational anxiety
Adjustment disorder
Supportive Therapy
±
Short-Term Benzodiazepine
(B) Organic factor
Consider:
Cognitive disturbance
Delirium
Dementia
Other neurologic disorders
Temporal lobe epilepsy
Vertigo
Endocrine disorders
Hyperthyroidism
Hypothyroidism
Hypoparathyroidism
Hypercortisolism
Pheochromocytoma
Insulin-induced hypoglycemia
Drugs
Caffeine
Stimulants
Drug discontinuation
Alcohol withdrawal
Sedative-hypnotic withdrawal
Other
Other temporally related disorders
Other temporally related drugs
Withdrawal from other drugs
Treat Underlying Disorder
(C) Other psychiatric disorders
Treat Underlying Disorder
Anxiety disorder
Consider:
(D) Recurrent panic attacks
Panic disorder
With agoraphobia
Without agoraphobia
Block anxiety attacks first, then treat agoraphobia:
In vivo exposure therapy
Consider support group
Block Anxiety Attacks:
Antidepressants
MAOIs
High-Potency Benzodiazepines
or
Cognitive-Behavioral Therapy
(E) Excessive fear of specific situations
Specific phobia
Agoraphobia without panic disorder
Rule out panic disorder
Exposure Therapy
±
Adjunctive Benzodiazepine
Social phobia
Circumscribed
Exposure Therapy
±
Adjunctive Benzodiazepine
or
Beta Blocker
Generalized
SSRI
MAOI
or
Cognitive-Behavioral Group Therapy
Obsessions/ compulsions, catastrophic stressor, or generalized anxiety
Cont'd on p 661

enclosed places, heights). Exposure therapy encourages patients to gradually confront and learn to overcome the feared object, activity, or situation; frequency, duration, and intensity of exposures are directly related to outcome. Prescribe a benzodiazepine if patients understand that it is a temporary measure and if there is no history of a psychoactive substance use disorder. Circumscribed social phobia may respond to adjunctive use of a beta blocker or a benzodiazepine. Beta blockers can be administered prophylactically minutes before exposure to a perceived noxious stimuli, such as a public speaking engagement, and may be less sedating than benzodiazepines. However, when taken regularly this class of drug may induce depression. The best established treatments for the generalized type of social phobia include SSRIs, MAOIs, standing doses of the high-potency benzodiazepine clonazepam, and cognitive-behavioral group therapy.

F. Obsessions are recurrent, intrusive, unwanted ideas that insistently enter the mind; they are distressing and typically recognized as senseless by the individual. Compulsions are repetitive, ritualistic behaviors typically performed to neutralize an obsession and reduce distress; most of these individuals recognize that their behaviors are unreasonable and excessive. The Yale-Brown Obsessive Compulsive Scale Symptom Checklist may help identify additional obsessions and compulsions in these patients. Many patients benefit from a trial of an SSRI or the non-SSRI clomipramine (often at higher dosages than that used to treat other disorders); behavioral therapy (e.g., a structured, short-term protocol that involves repeated exposure to the obsession-eliciting situation together with a mandate to suppress anxiety-reducing compulsions); or a combination of the two. Some patients benefit from participation in a support group. Rarely, stereotactic surgery may be considered. Bilateral anterior cingulotomy is performed in patients with extremely disabling symptoms that are unresponsive to the arsenal of more conventional treatments.

G. Consider acute stress disorder (lasting <1 month) or posttraumatic stress disorder (PTSD; lasting >1 month) in individuals who have been exposed to traumatic events associated with a threat of injury or death to self or others and feelings of intense fear, helplessness, or horror (e.g., rape, accidental or natural disasters, military combat). Symptoms include reexperiences of the traumatic event (e.g., recurrent thoughts, nightmares, flashbacks, and distress in response to reminders of the event); avoidance behaviors (e.g., avoidance of thoughts, feelings, or situations associated with the event); restrictions in emotion and interpersonal relationships; and increased arousal (e.g., insomnia, irritability, or hypervigilance). These patients may also manifest profound feelings of guilt associated with having survived a trauma when others may have perished. Consider individual or group psychotherapy to increase self-esteem, decrease social isolation, and support coping resources; SSRIs, other antidepressants of PTSD or MAOIs to reduce symptoms or associated depression; and referral for participation in a structured program of behavioral therapy, one that involves frequent imagined exposures to the stressor.

H. Generalized anxiety disorder is a diagnosis of exclusion. Ask, "Have you worried excessively about everyday matters (e.g., work, school, family, and finances) most of the day more days than not for at least 6 months?" Consider the other disorders in the decision tree (e.g., panic disorder, major depression) first. Consider an antidepressant such as venlafaxine or imipramine first and the nonbenzodiazepine anxiolytic buspirone second; use benzodiazepines sparingly, especially in patients who are elderly or with cognitive impairment or a psychoactive substance use disorder; and discontinue medications that fail to work. Although nonmedication treatments do not yet have established value, interventions are being studied that target the hallmark feature of worry.

References

American Psychiatric Association. Diagnostic and Statistical Manual of Mental Disorders, 4th ed. Text Revision. Washington, DC: American Psychiatric Association, 2000.

Barlow DH. Anxiety and Its Disorders: The Nature and Treatment of Anxiety and Panic. New York: Guilford Press, 1988.

Davies SJ, Ghahramani P, Jackson PR, et al. Association of panic disorder and panic attacks with hypertension. Am J Med 1999;107:310.

Hyman SE, Arana GW. Handbook of Psychiatric Drug Therapy, 3rd ed. Boston: Little, Brown, 1995.

Reiman EM. Anxiety. In Gelenberg AJ, Bassuk EL, eds. Practitioner's Guide to Psychoactive Drugs, 4th ed. New York: Plenum, 1997.

Rosenbaum JF. The drug treatment of anxiety. N Engl J Med 1982;306:401–404.

Roth WT, Yalom D. Treating Anxiety Disorders. Boston: Jossey-Bass, 1996.

Zaubler TS, Katon W. Panic disorder and medical comorbidity: a review of the medical and psychiatric literature. Bull Menninger Clin 1996;60(2):A13.

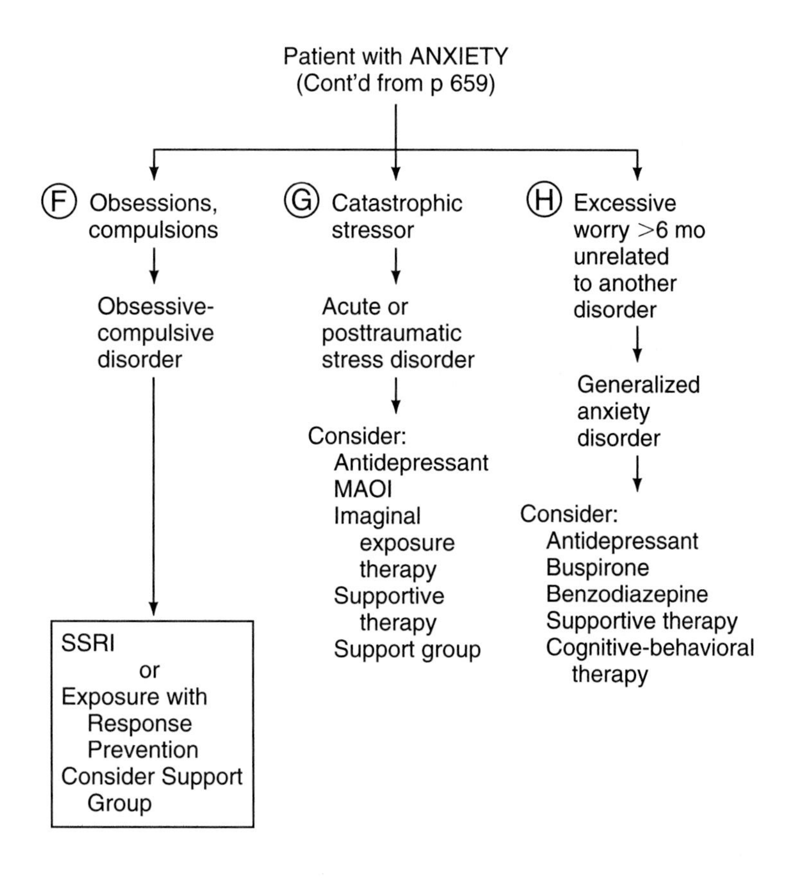
Patient with ANXIETY
(Cont'd from p 659)
F Obsessions, compulsions
Obsessive-compulsive disorder
SSRI
or
Exposure with Response Prevention
Consider Support Group
G Catastrophic stressor
Acute or posttraumatic stress disorder
Consider:
Antidepressant
MAOI
Imaginal exposure therapy
Supportive therapy
Support group
H Excessive worry >6 mo unrelated to another disorder
Generalized anxiety disorder
Consider:
Antidepressant
Buspirone
Benzodiazepine
Supportive therapy
Cognitive-behavioral therapy

DEPRESSION

John A. Fromson, MD, and Iris R. Bell, MD, PhD

Depression occurs in children, adolescents, adults, and the elderly. It is found in all ethnic groups, has high prevalence, and is a significant cause of disability worldwide. Following hypertension, it is the most commonly encountered chronic illness in general medical practice. It can be an emotion, a specific disease entity, or a symptom of another mental or medical illness such as schizophrenia or thyroid dysfunction. It can also be iatrogenically induced by medications such as glucocorticoids, narcotics, and benzodiazepines.

Dysphoria, a milder form of major depression, occurs in 5% of the general population, with women and persons aged 25–44 years most at risk. The full syndrome of major depression carries significant morbidity and mortality in terms of suicide risk and poorer outcome of concomitant medical disorders. Many patients with depression present first to the primary care physician with somatic concerns and seek a medical diagnosis or treatment for anxiety or "nerves," which often leads to overlooking the proper diagnosis and delaying treatment.

A. Depression is a clinical syndrome without a specific laboratory test to confirm the diagnosis; comprehensive clinical assessments provide the main data.

B. Criteria for diagnosis of major depression include having at least five of nine symptoms present daily or almost daily during the same 2-week period and indicative of a change from previous functioning. Symptoms are (1) depressed mood, (2) markedly reduced interest or pleasure in activities, (3) significant weight loss or gain or decrease or increase in appetite, (4) insomnia or hypersomnia, (5) psychomotor agitation or retardation, (6) fatigue or low energy, (7) feelings of worthlessness or inordinate guilt, (8) difficulty concentrating or indecisiveness, and (9) recurrent thoughts of death or suicide or a suicide attempt. Broad differential diagnosis must include organic mood disorder, depressed, and a major depression.

C. A screening battery of laboratory tests helps rule out specific organic causes. In combination with the history and physical examination, findings may suggest more specific laboratory studies (see D). Specialized tests that are sensitive, but not specific, to major depression include the dexamethasone suppression test, the thyrotropin-releasing hormone stimulation test, and polysomnography.

D. Differential diagnosis for organic causes includes substance abuse or dependence and use of certain prescription drugs. The latter group includes antihypertensives, hormones, analgesics, anticancer drugs, tiparkinsonian drugs, antianxiety and hypnotic drugs, and GI drugs; endocrine and metabolic disorders (especially thyroid and adrenal); nutritional deficiencies (vitamin B_1, niacin, folate, vitamin B_{12}); and heavy metal toxicity (e.g., lead). Depression in alcoholics may resolve with abstinence. Depressive symptoms follow stroke in up to 60% of cases within 2 years. Treatment of underlying medical problems may lead to resolution of depression; if not, standard antidepressant treatment strategies often are effective.

E. Initial antidepressant regimens, especially in patients whose illness is medically complex, often involve selective serotonin reuptake inhibitors (SSRIs; e.g., fluoxetine, sertraline, paroxetine). Secondary amine tricyclics such as nortriptyline and desipramine are an important alternative, especially for comorbid chronic pain. These may have less anticholinergic side effects and therefore are better tolerated than amitriptyline or doxepin. If SSRIs and tricyclics fail or are contraindicated, other choices include bupropion, nefazodone, venlafaxine, or monoamine oxidase inhibitors (MAOIs; phenelzine, tranylcypromine). Low-dose trazodone (note priapism as a possible side effect in males) is sometimes used for insomnia, in combination with activating agents such as fluoxetine. Choose medication to specific target symptoms (e.g., agitation versus psychomotor retardation) and address side effect profile. Watch for drug interactions with fluoxetine and MAOIs. MAOIs necessitate a tyramine-free diet. Amphetamine-based stimulants may mobilize patients who are apathetic and medically ill, but their long-term efficacy for major depression is uncertain.

F. Up to 50% of patients who are unipolar depressed with partial or no response to antidepressant therapy may respond more fully to the addition of lithium. More controversial augmentation strategies include buspirone supplementation (especially in agitated depression), thyroid supplementation, combination therapy of fluoxetine with a tricyclic, and combination therapy of an MAOI with a tricyclic; the last two approaches involve a significant risk of drug interactions.

G. Growing evidence suggests that bright-light therapy may suffice in some cases of winter depression; more standard somatic therapies also are effective.

H. Recent studies have shown the need for a combination of antidepressant and antipsychotic drugs rather than single-agent therapy to treat psychotic depression.

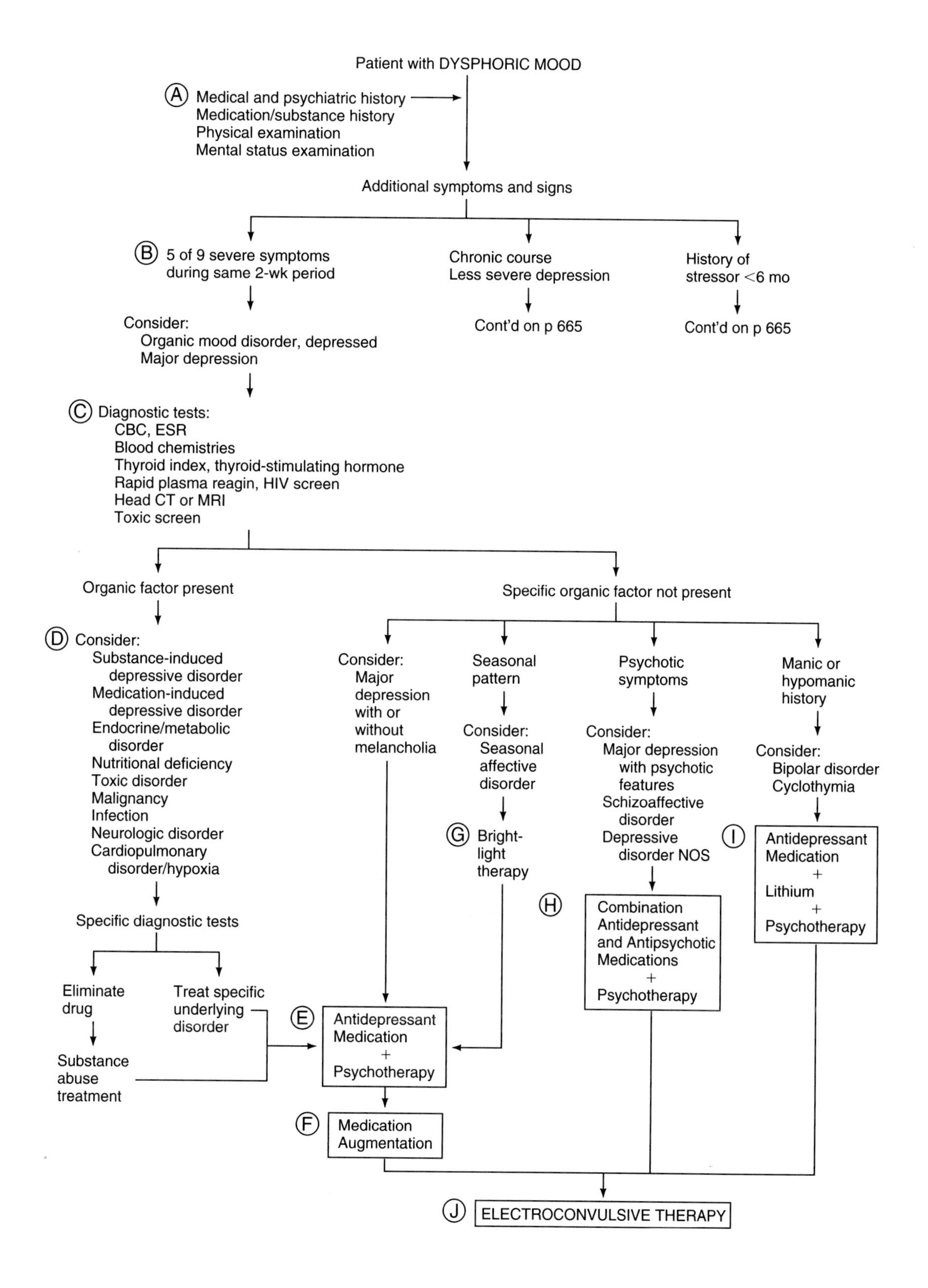

I. Patients who are bipolar may switch into manic episodes during treatment with antidepressant medications alone. This may necessitate concomitant coverage with lithium or another mood-stabilizing agent (e.g., divalproex, carbamazepine). Anecdotal evidence suggests possible usefulness of bupropion in treating bipolar depression.

J. Electroconvulsive therapy is the most effective treatment for major depression, especially for the subtype with psychotic features. It is the treatment of choice for acute suicidality, severe cachexia and dehydration secondary to poor intake, many medically complex major depressions, and antidepressant medication failures.

(Continued on page 664)

K. A chronic course of at least 2 years and a less severe depressive picture suggest a dysthymic disorder, which can co-occur with major depression. Dysphoria or fluctuating mood instability is also characteristic of a range of chronic personality disorders that vary in responsiveness to psychotherapeutic interventions.

L. An identifiable stressor, maladaptive symptoms lasting <6 months, and a generally less severe depressive picture suggest an adjustment disorder with depressed mood, which usually resolves with time and supportive psychotherapy.

References

Brown SA, Inaba RK, Gillin JC, et al. Alcoholism and affective disorder: clinical course of depressive symptoms. Am J Psychiatry 1995;152:45.
Charney DS, Miller HL, Licinio J, et al. Treatment of depression. In Schatzberg AF, Nemeroff CB, eds. Textbook of Psychopharmacology. Washington, DC: American Psychiatric Press, 1995:575.
Cole S, Raju M. Making the diagnosis of depression in the primary care setting. Am J Med 1996;101:10S.
Fava GA, Grandi S, Zielezny M, et al. Four-year outcome for cognitive behavioral treatment of residual symptoms in major depression. Am J Psychiatry 1996;153:945.
Kleinman S. Culture and depression. N Engl J Med 2004;351: 951–953.
Klerman GL, Weissman MM. The course, morbidity, and costs of depression. Arch Gen Psychiatry 1992;49:831.
McCoy DM. Treatment considerations for depression in patients with significant medical comorbidity. J Fam Practice 1996;43 (6 Suppl):S35.
Nierenberg AA. Treatment choice after one antidepressant fails: a survey of Northeastern psychiatrists. J Clin Psychiatry 1991;52:383.
Wells KB, Sturm R, Sherbourne CD, et al. Caring for Depression. Cambridge, MA: Harvard University Press, 1996.
Whooley MA, Simon GE. Primary care: managing depression in medical outpatients. N Engl J Med 2000;343:1942–1950.

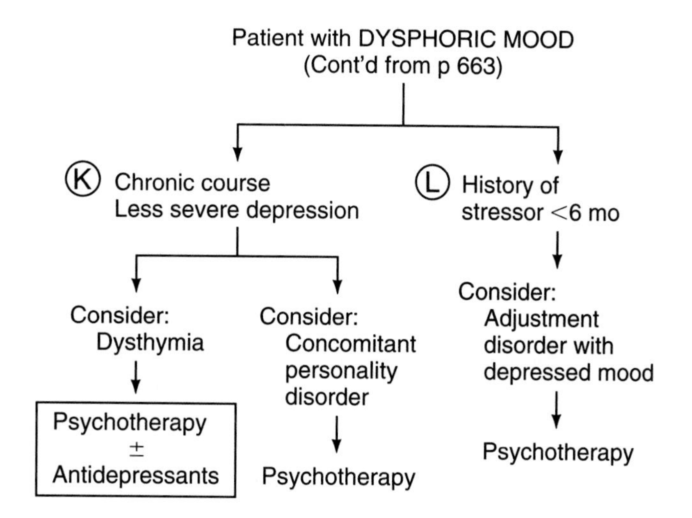
Patient with DYSPHORIC MOOD
(Cont'd from p 663)
K Chronic course
Less severe depression
L History of
stressor <6 mo
Consider:
Dysthymia
Consider:
Concomitant
personality
disorder
Consider:
Adjustment
disorder with
depressed mood
Psychotherapy
±
Antidepressants
Psychotherapy
Psychotherapy

EMOTIONAL DISORDERS WITH SOMATIC EXPRESSION

John A. Fromson, MD, and John Misiaszek, MD

Patients with emotionally based somatic complaints are largely unaware of their emotional conflicts. Often labeled as "crocks," they receive poor and fragmented treatment, although their tendency to express their emotional conflicts through somatizing behavior does not immunize them against bona fide physical illness. Furthermore, many physical disorders such as thyroid disease, multiple sclerosis, and temporal lobe epilepsy may initially or primarily present as an emotional disorder, causing delays in diagnosis and treatment. Physicians can reduce the physical, emotional, and iatrogenic morbidity of patients who somatize their psychic distress. This can be accomplished by providing consistency and support through exploring contributing psychosocial factors, explaining negative test results, and providing reassurance while minimizing invasive procedures and redundant evaluations. Patients who somatize are emotionally impaired; rejection serves only to heighten their impairment.

A. The medical history should include a review for similar, previously undiagnosed disorders in the patient and family members. Often the somatizing coping behavior has been modeled or reinforced earlier in life. Trauma experienced during early emotional development may result in more severe somatoform expression such as a factitious disorder. Personal or family history also may suggest a proclivity for one of the major psychiatric disorders.

B. Patients with acute or chronic psychoses may have bizarre somatic complaints (e.g., they may say that an alien force has turned their intestines inside out). Their overall thought disturbance is readily manifest in their report. It is sometimes difficult to differentiate between the complaint as a delusion or a symbolic and personalized interpretation of a genuine physical discomfort. Patients with psychotic depression or monodelusional disorders (e.g., delusions of parasitosis) may have more focused or fixed somatic concerns that may or may not diminish when treated with high-potency antipsychotics such as haloperidol or pimozide.

C. Although patients who are delirious or cognitively impaired may misperceive or fabricate somatic symptoms, their primary psychiatric problem is differentiated from "functional psychosis" by the presence of periodic or persistent confusion and disorientation. Antipsychotic medication may decrease the somatic delusions and behavioral difficulties, but treatment of the underlying disorder may be curative.

D. Depression may be masked by a complaint of headache or generalized fatigue. Vegetative signs of depression may be variably present, along with diminished self-esteem and a depressive affect; these often precede or coincide with somatic sensations. A primary depression must be distinguished from a secondary (or reactive) depression that is a result, not the cause, of a somatic problem.

E. Patients with a generalized anxiety disorder may present with a variety of somatic symptoms such as tachycardia, motor tension, or autonomic hyperactivity. Patients with panic attacks may fear cardiac or pulmonary disorders. A primary anxiety disorder needs to be differentiated from a secondary apprehension about a physical symptom.

F. A hypochondriacal reaction is distinguished from classical hypochondriasis in that it follows a clearly identified recent stressful event, is short-lived, and responds to reassurance. Examples include an individual who is concerned about minor chest discomfort after a cardiac-related death of a close friend, a medical student who has a phobia about the "disease of the day," and a luncheon crowd's hysteria in response to the erroneous report of a victim of food poisoning in their midst.

G. Conversion disorder is likely if there is loss or alteration in physical function after a stressful event. The resultant psychic conflict is not readily apparent to the individual or evaluator. The diagnosis also requires that the physical problem cannot be explained by a known physical disorder. "La belle indifference," an inappropriate lack of concern for the perceptions by others of one's disability, has been widely overstated as a characteristic symptom and is of little diagnostic value. Use caution when assigning a diagnosis of conversion disorder. Studies show that 13%–30% of patients so diagnosed later develop physical problems that could have explained their original physical complaint.

(Continued on page 668)

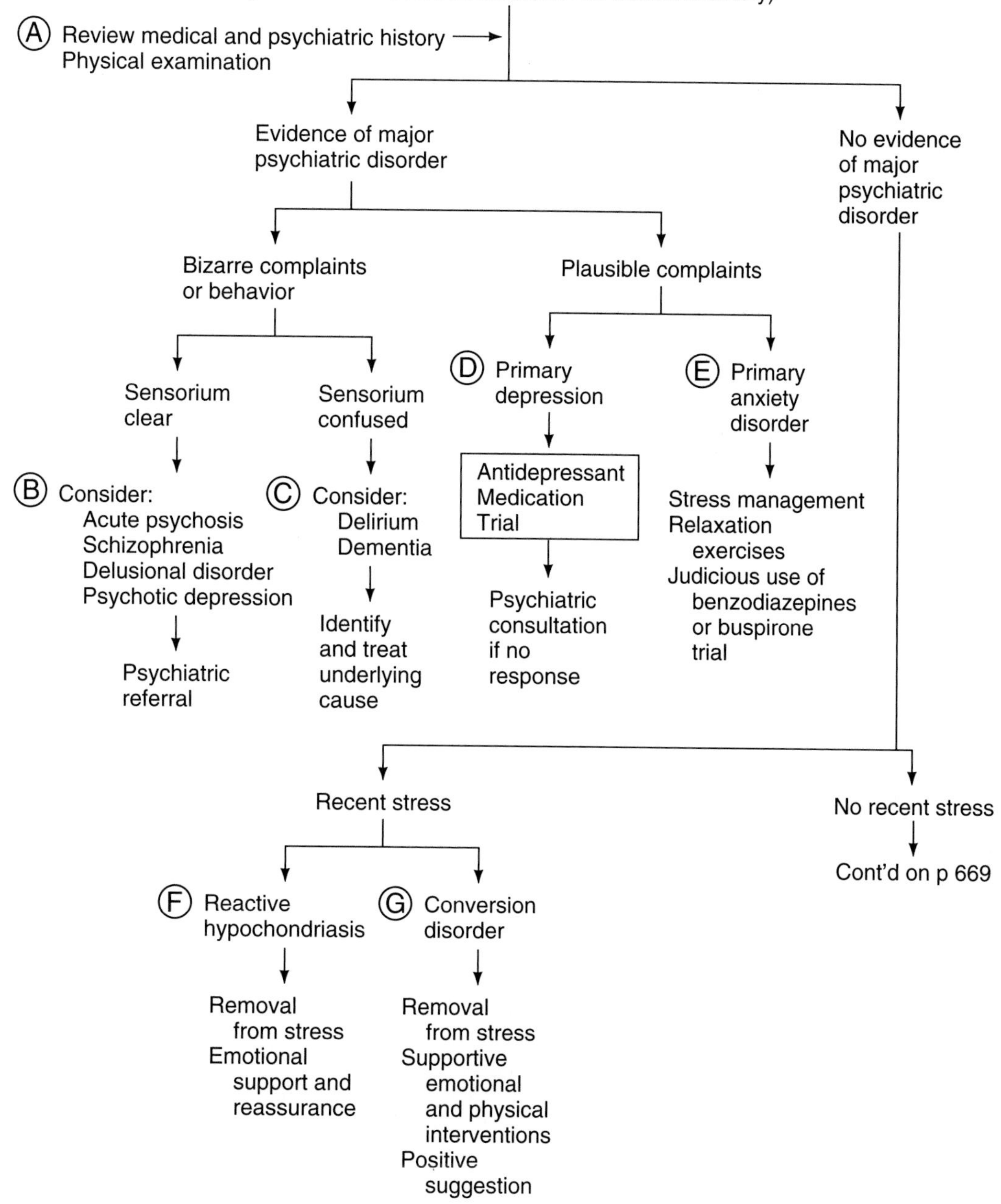
Patient with EMOTIONALLY BASED SOMATIC COMPLAINTS
(Previous or Recent Evaluations Are Noncontributory)
(A) Review medical and psychiatric history
Physical examination
Evidence of major psychiatric disorder
No evidence of major psychiatric disorder
Bizarre complaints or behavior
Plausible complaints
Sensorium clear
Sensorium confused
(D) Primary depression
(E) Primary anxiety disorder
(B) Consider:
Acute psychosis
Schizophrenia
Delusional disorder
Psychotic depression
(C) Consider:
Delirium
Dementia
Antidepressant Medication Trial
Stress management
Relaxation exercises
Judicious use of benzodiazepines or buspirone trial
Psychiatric referral
Identify and treat underlying cause
Psychiatric consultation if no response
Recent stress
No recent stress
Cont'd on p 669
(F) Reactive hypochondriasis
(G) Conversion disorder
Removal from stress
Emotional support and reassurance
Removal from stress
Supportive emotional and physical interventions
Positive suggestion

H. Conscious deceit is subdivided into malingering when secondary gain is apparent and factitious disorder when reasons for the deceit are not understood by the patient or the physician. For example, a military draft inductee who feigns a disorder to avoid conscription is malingering, whereas patients with factitious disorders (e.g., Munchausen syndrome) have complex, convoluted reasons for faking somatic disorders, are angry and emotionally traumatized, have unsettled lives, and displace hostility onto others. They are difficult patients to treat both medically and psychiatrically; confrontation in the absence of a comprehensive medical psychiatric treatment plan rarely works and risks escalating maladaptive behavior.

I. Hypochondriasis is the misinterpretation of physical signs or sensations as serious disease. Patients typically are fearful, do not respond readily to support and reassurance, return for further evaluation and treatment, or seek other physicians. These patients have been described as hostile, masochistic, and demanding individuals who deny their needs for dependence; less commonly, they are described as individuals who are clinging, passive, and overly dependent in their relationship with their doctor. Related terms are *somatization disorder,* in which patients develop multiple "review of systems" complaints as an early life-coping mechanism, and *somatoform pain disorder,* when pain is the specific hypochondriacal concern.

J. The absence of a physical finding or inability to establish a physical diagnosis by itself is insufficient for a diagnosis of a major psychiatric or somatoform disorder. These diagnoses can be made only when the associated psychiatric characteristics are present and when the dysfunction and somatic problems are a consequence of such characteristics. Because life stress or misfortune is found in most medical patients and nonpatients alike, take care not to magnify such occurrences when there is no obvious connection to the physical impairment.

References

Allen LA, Woolfolk RL, Escobar JI, et al. Cognitive-behavioral therapy for somatization disorder: a randomized controlled trial. Arch Intern Med 2006;166(14):1512–1518.

Barsky AJ. Hypochondriasis: Medical management and psychiatric treatment. Psychosomatics 1996;37:48.

Barsky AJ, Stern TA, Greenberg DB, et al. Functional somatic symptoms and somatoform disorders. In Stern TA, ed. Massachusetts General Hospital Handbook of General Hospital Psychiatry, 5th ed. St Louis: Mosby, 2004:269.

Gerdes TT, Noyes R Jr, Kathal RG, et al. Physician recognition of hypochondriacal patients. Gen Hosp Psychiatr 1996;18:106.

Lipsitt DR, Starcevic V, Franz CP. Psychotherapy and pharmacotherapy in the treatment of somatoform disorders. Psychiatr Ann 2006;36: 341–348.

Stephenson DT, Price JR. Medically unexplained physical symptoms in emergency medicine. Emerg Med J 2006;23(8):595–600.

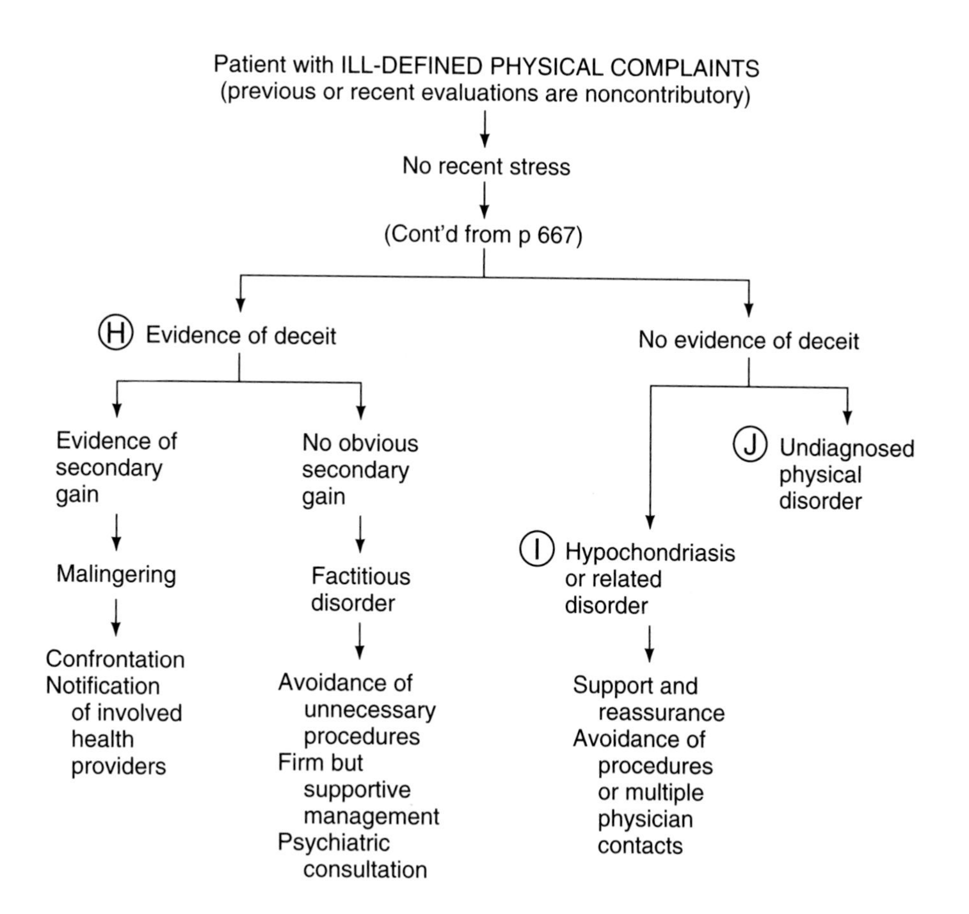
Patient with ILL-DEFINED PHYSICAL COMPLAINTS
(previous or recent evaluations are noncontributory)
No recent stress
(Cont'd from p 667)
(H) Evidence of deceit
No evidence of deceit
Evidence of secondary gain
No obvious secondary gain
(J) Undiagnosed physical disorder
(I) Hypochondriasis or related disorder
Malingering
Factitious disorder
Confrontation
Notification of involved health providers
Avoidance of unnecessary procedures
Firm but supportive management
Psychiatric consultation
Support and reassurance
Avoidance of procedures or multiple physician contacts

GRIEF

John A. Fromson, MD, and Gail L. Schwartz, MD

A. Normal grief responses vary. The process of grieving may be seen as occurring in three stages: initial shock or numbing, acute mourning, and a period of resolution or recovery. A lack of perceived social support is one predictor of difficulty in recovery. Those seen as grieving most intensely early in the bereavement may have a poorer outcome after 1 year than those with a relative absence of mourning. There is little evidence to support the efficacy of treatment for people experiencing uncomplicated bereavement.

B. Neurovegetative symptoms of depression are common in bereavement. Sleep disturbance may last for up to 1 year. Appetite usually returns within 4 months after the loss. However, motor retardation, ruminative guilt, and a feeling of worthlessness are not typical symptoms of bereavement and suggest the need for psychiatric evaluation and treatment.

C. Symptoms of complicated grief are distinct from symptoms of bereavement-related depression and anxiety. Persistent symptoms of anxiety and depression warrant a more detailed psychiatric evaluation. Patients who are clinically depressed are most often treated with a combination of antidepressant medication and psychotherapy.

D. More than 40% of bereaved spouses have at least one type of anxiety disorder during the first year of bereavement. A history of anxiety disorder is a strong predictor of its presenting during bereavement. Anxiety symptoms include somatic distress, obsessions and compulsions, phobias, and panic attacks.

E. Antidepressants are useful in the treatment of most anxiety disorders and may be preferred to benzodiazepines because of the lack of dependence potential.

F. A history of an addictive disorder is a strong predictor of substance abuse during grieving. Because there is a significant risk of morbidity and mortality with substance abuse, it is imperative that a careful history be taken and that bothersome symptoms of anxiety and sleeplessness be treated nonpharmacologically or with medications that have minimal addiction potential.

G. In normal grief the intensity of the emotional pain gradually decreases; significant resolution occurs by 1 year. Theories of attachment behavior have been used to explain the difficulties that complicate the grieving process for some people (Table 1).

H. It is suggested that expressive psychotherapy is most appropriate for conflicted grief syndromes, cognitive treatment may be particularly useful for dependent grief syndrome, and treatments developed specifically for persons with posttraumatic stress disorder may be most useful for those who have had a sudden, unexpected loss.

Table 1 **Pathologic Grief Syndromes**

Dependent	A stable sense of self depends on presence of the lost person
Unexpected loss	A posttraumatic stress syndrome with hyperreactivity, intrusive memories, and nightmares alternating with affect constriction and numbing
Conflicted	Ambivalence toward the lost person is unacceptable, and the grieving person turns the negative feelings on himself or herself

References

Boelen Paul A, van den Bout J. Complicated grief, depression, and anxiety as distinct postloss syndromes: a confirmatory factor analysis study. Am J Psychiatry 2005;162:2175.

Clayton PJ. Bereavement and depression. J Clin Psychiatry 1990; 51(Suppl):34.

Crow HE. How to help patients understand and conquer grief: avoiding depression in the midst of sadness. Postgrad Med 1991;89:117.

Kim K, Jacobs S. Pathologic grief and its relationship to other psychiatric disorders. J Affect Disord 1991;21:257.

Middleton W. Bereavement. Psychiatr Clin North Am 1987;10:329.

Rosenzweig A, Prigerson H, Miller MD, et al. Bereavement and late-life depression: grief and its complications in the elderly. Annu Rev Med 1997;48:421.

Rynearson EK. Psychotherapy of pathologic grief. Psychiatr Clin North Am 1987;10:487.

Zisook S. Anxiety and bereavement. Psychiatr Med 1990;8:83.

Zisook S, Schuchter SR, Sledge PA, et al. The spectrum of depressive phenomena after spousal bereavement. J Clin Psychiatry 1994;55(Suppl):29.

Patient Has Experienced SIGNIFICANT LOSS

History →

- (A) Normal grief
- (B) Depressed mood → Assess symptoms
  - (C) Clinical depression → Antidepressants, Psychotherapy
  - Normal grief
- (D) Anxiety → Assess symptoms
  - Normal grief
  - Anxiety disorders → (E) Pharmacotherapy, Behavioral Therapy
- (F) Psychoactive drug use → Assess use → Addictive disorder → Limit prescriptions; Education, Alcoholics Anonymous
- Unresolved grief → Relationship history → (G) Pathologic grief syndrome → (H) Psychotherapy

PSYCHOSIS

John A. Fromson, MD, and Alan J. Gelenberg, MD

A psychotic episode is typified by deranged thinking, speech, and behavior, often manifesting as hallucinations (false sensory impressions: visual, auditory, olfactory, gustatory, tactile), delusions (false fixed beliefs), difficulty distinguishing reality from fantasy, disorganized thinking, and strange and inappropriate behavior.

A. When confronted with a patient who is acutely psychotic, the first task is to ensure the safety of the patient and others against injury or possible death. A calm, low-stimulus environment with nonthreatening behavior by staff is essential. Physical force should not be threatened unless overwhelming force is available. The patient should not be left alone, and an examining physician should be accompanied by at least one other person. Some patients may need to be restrained chemically and/or physically. Patients should be questioned about any thoughts of suicide or injuring others, which must be taken extremely seriously, especially if the hallucinations are auditory and are of a command type.

B. A medical history is essential in the evaluation of a patient who is psychotic. Given the patient's mental status, the most valuable information will probably come from others who know him or her. Inquire about the time course of the emerging bizarre behavior and possible relation to any preexisting or acute medical conditions, recent-onset physical symptoms, exposure to infectious or toxic agents, medication use, drug abuse, recent surgery, or physical or psychological trauma.

C. Possible medical causes of acute psychotic behavior should be considered and ruled out immediately. Despite the difficulties, perform as complete a physical examination as possible, including pupils and, to the extent possible, fundi. Examine carefully the patient's entire body for evidence of trauma, substance abuse, or any other medical condition. Staring or stereotypic motor behavior may suggest a drug-induced or seizure-related state, and obtaining an electroencephalogram may be advisable.

D. Address such readily treatable (and potentially hazardous) conditions as hypoglycemia by such means as immediate drawing of blood followed by IV injection of a concentrated dextrose solution.

E. If the history (usually from others), a careful physical examination, and indicated laboratory tests fail to reveal any organic causes of psychosis, consider a psychiatric differential diagnosis.

(Continued on page 674)

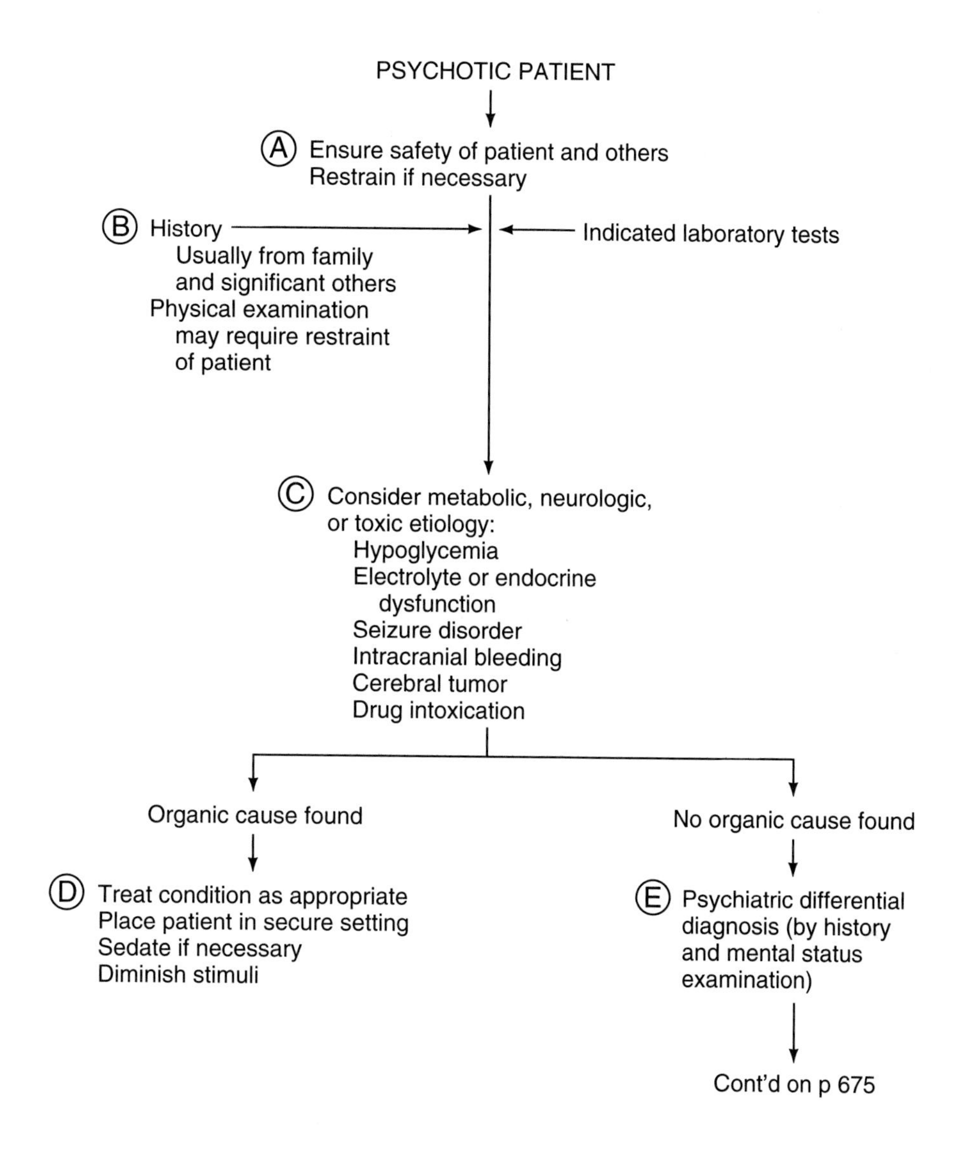
PSYCHOTIC PATIENT
(A) Ensure safety of patient and others
Restrain if necessary
(B) History
Usually from family
and significant others
Physical examination
may require restraint
of patient
Indicated laboratory tests
(C) Consider metabolic, neurologic,
or toxic etiology:
Hypoglycemia
Electrolyte or endocrine
dysfunction
Seizure disorder
Intracranial bleeding
Cerebral tumor
Drug intoxication
Organic cause found
No organic cause found
(D) Treat condition as appropriate
Place patient in secure setting
Sedate if necessary
Diminish stimuli
(E) Psychiatric differential
diagnosis (by history
and mental status
examination)
Cont'd on p 675

F. Schizophrenia is a lifelong chronic condition marked by acute psychotic episodes interspersed with periods of less disturbed but still abnormal behavior. Between episodes, people with schizophrenia often show poor motivation, social awkwardness, and isolation. Acute schizophrenic episodes are typically treated with antipsychotic agents, which usually are maintained at lower dosages to mitigate the likelihood and severity of future episodes. Now, more patients with schizophrenia are taking newer-generation antipsychotic drugs such as clozapine (Clozaril), risperidone (Risperdal), olanzapine (Zyprexa), and quetiapine (Seroquel). It is unclear whether these drugs are as able as traditional antipsychotic medications to suppress acutely emergent psychotic behavior. Moreover, to date, newer agents do not come in parenteral form. Use benzodiazepine sedation as needed as an adjunct to antipsychotic drugs during acute episodes, especially when the patient presents as a danger to self and others.

G. Mania often presents as an acute psychosis. A history typically reveals past episodes of mania or major depression. A mental status examination shows the patient to have grandiose ideas and be highly excited, emotionally labile, overtalkative, pressured in speech, and hypersexual. Acute treatment consists of antipsychotic drugs as needed, often with adjunctive lithium. Divalproex (Depakote) increasingly is being used to suppress acute symptoms of mania. Lithium is the mainstay therapy for most patients who are bipolar (manic-depressive). The mood stabilizer olanzapine (Zyprexa) is also effective in preventing manic and mixed-episode relapse/recurrence in patients acutely stabilized with olanzapine and lithium cotreatment. Both agents are comparable in preventing depression relapse/recurrence. Carbamazepine (Tegretol and others) and newer anticonvulsants (notably gabapentin [Neurontin] and lamotrigine [Lamictal]) are coming into use also. Electroconvulsive therapy (ECT) usually is effective for patients who fail to benefit or cannot tolerate these medications. Benzodiazepines can be used adjunctively to control an acute episode.

H. Psychotic depression may become manifest either as a recurrent mood disorder itself or as an episode in the course of a bipolar illness. Delusions and hallucinations commonly manifest such depressive themes as guilt and punishment. Effective treatments include ECT and combined antipsychotic and antidepressant drugs. Clozapine and possibly other new antipsychotics may be especially helpful in treating psychotic depression. Guard against suicide, an omnipresent hazard in these patients. In March 2004 the U.S. Food and Drug Administration warned physicians and patients regarding increased risk of suicide with 10 newer antidepressant drugs. However, available data do not indicate a significant increase in risk of suicide or serious suicide attempt after starting treatment with these newer antidepressant drugs.

I. Delusional (paranoid) disorder is a chronic condition characterized by a fixed and focused delusional system in the midst of otherwise-intact thinking. It often is refractory to biologic and psychologic treatments.

J. Patients with dementia often manifest psychotic behaviors that can complicate long-term management. Rule out acute medical conditions, and, if possible, handle disruptive behaviors through behavioral and environmental means. If this is not possible, low dosages of antipsychotic drugs may assist management.

References

American Psychiatric Association. Treatment of Psychiatric Disorders: A Task Force of the American Psychiatric Association. Washington, DC: American Psychiatric Association, 1989:1485, 1655, 1725.

Gelenberg AJ, Keith SJ. Psychosis. In Gelenberg AJ, Bassak EL, eds. The Practitioner's Guide to Psychoactive Drugs, 4th ed. New York: Plenum, 1997.

Kaplan HI, Sadock BJ, eds. Comprehensive Textbook of Psychiatry, 6th ed. Baltimore: Williams & Wilkins, 1994.

Practice guideline for the psychiatric evaluation of adults, 2nd ed. Am J Psychiatry 2006;163(6 Suppl):3–36

Simon GE, Savarino J, Operskalski B, et al. Suicide risk during antidepressant treatment. Am J Psychiatry 2006;163:41.

Tohen M, Greil W, Calabrese JR, et al. Olanzapine versus lithium in the maintenance treatment of bipolar disorder: a 12-month, randomized, double-blind, controlled clinical trial. Am J Psychiatry 2005;162:1281.

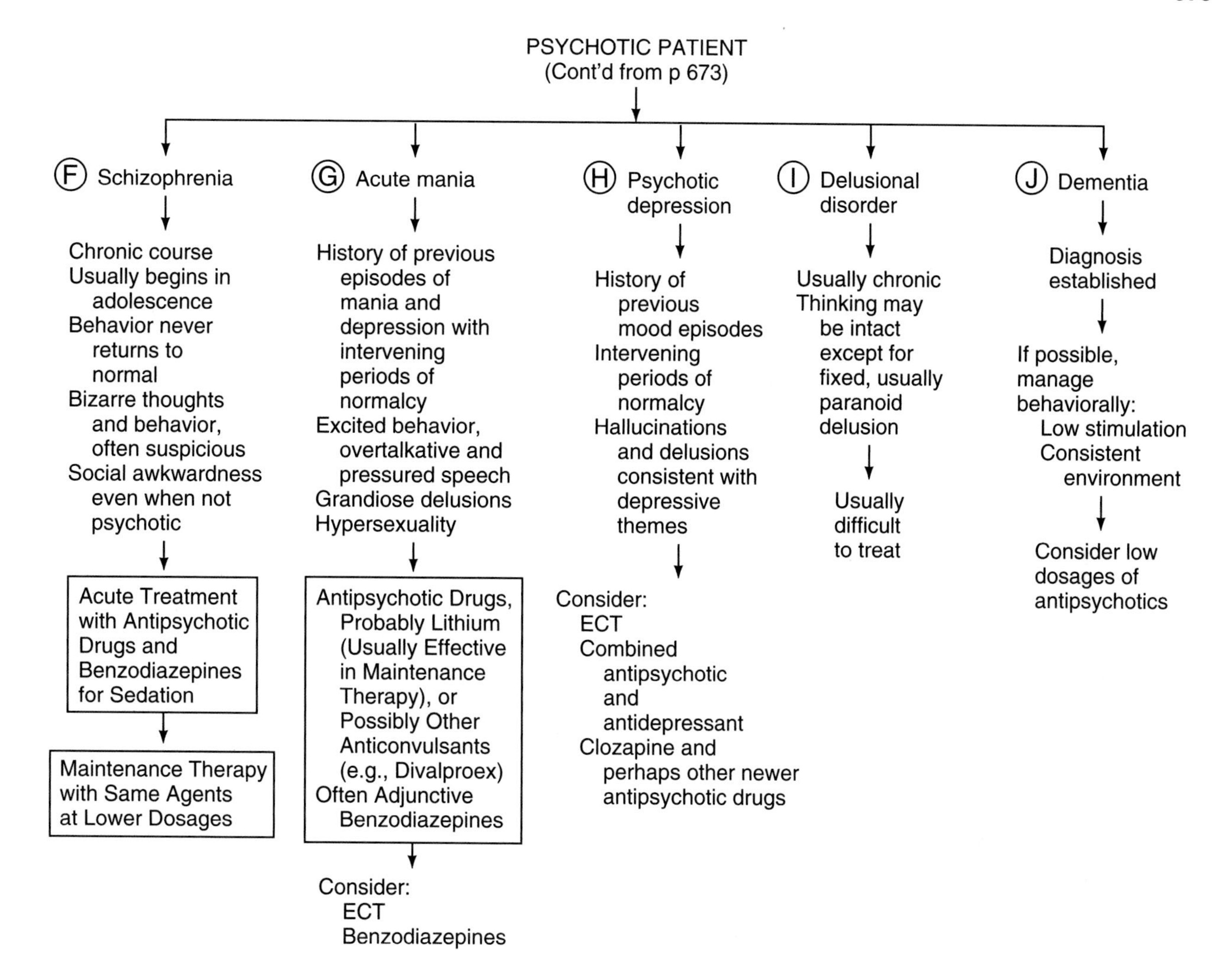
PSYCHOTIC PATIENT
(Cont'd from p 673)
F Schizophrenia
Chronic course
Usually begins in adolescence
Behavior never returns to normal
Bizarre thoughts and behavior, often suspicious
Social awkwardness even when not psychotic
Acute Treatment with Antipsychotic Drugs and Benzodiazepines for Sedation
Maintenance Therapy with Same Agents at Lower Dosages
G Acute mania
History of previous episodes of mania and depression with intervening periods of normalcy
Excited behavior, overtalkative and pressured speech
Grandiose delusions
Hypersexuality
Antipsychotic Drugs, Probably Lithium (Usually Effective in Maintenance Therapy), or Possibly Other Anticonvulsants (e.g., Divalproex)
Often Adjunctive Benzodiazepines
Consider:
ECT
Benzodiazepines
H Psychotic depression
History of previous mood episodes
Intervening periods of normalcy
Hallucinations and delusions consistent with depressive themes
Consider:
ECT
Combined antipsychotic and antidepressant
Clozapine and perhaps other newer antipsychotic drugs
I Delusional disorder
Usually chronic
Thinking may be intact except for fixed, usually paranoid delusion
Usually difficult to treat
J Dementia
Diagnosis established
If possible, manage behaviorally:
Low stimulation
Consistent environment
Consider low dosages of antipsychotics

SMOKING CESSATION

Harry L. Greene II, MD, FACP

The U.S. Surgeon General has determined that the leading preventable cause of death and disability in the United States is cigarette smoking. Annually, 3 million deaths worldwide are attributed to smoking. This toll is expected to reach 10 million by 2025. Although 75% of all adults visit a physician at least once a year, smokers visit more often because of increased illness. The first step in smoking cessation is to identify the smoker by simply asking, "Do you smoke?" Although a few smokers may be evasive about their smoking, most admit it, and surveys show that 80% say they would like to quit. It is estimated that there are 46 million people continuing to smoke as a result of addiction.

A. Congratulate patients who are nonsmokers. Encourage patients who have quit to maintain their cessation. Counsel preteens and teens about peer pressure, targeted advertising, and the fallacy of smoking as a way to appear more grown up. Work is being done currently to develop and test nicotine vaccines that, if efficacious, could be used to vaccinate teenagers at risk for initiation of smoking. Additional work is being conducted to determine the pharmacogenetics of those at greatest risk.

B. Inform smokers of the adverse health consequences of smoking and the benefits of stopping, emphasize the damage or disease already present, motivate them to consider quitting, and give firm and unequivocal advice to quit. Use guided questions such as, "Are you aware of the effects of smoking on your health?" Make the patient aware of any physical findings that are present and related to smoking in an effort to personalize the effects of smoking. Mention the benefits of quitting now, including lower risk of cancer, sudden death, or myocardial infarction (MI) and longer active life (at any age). Many smokers are fatalistic and unaware of the reversibility of smoking-related disease and risk. Make a statement such as, "As your physician, I must advise you that smoking is bad for your health."

C. One can sense whether a patient is contemplating quitting by his or her responses to questions such as, "How do you feel about being a smoker? What reasons do you have to quit? Were you able to stop smoking in the past? How did you do it that time? What caused you to start again? If you had that chance again, what would you do differently?" The purpose of these questions is to allow insight, build confidence, problem solve, and begin a plan for a new successful cessation attempt. Then a critical series of questions can be posed: "Have you thought about stopping? Do you think you can stop now? How will you do it? May I help you quit?"

D. At this point, some patients do not show adequate motivation or are unwilling to discuss or plan a cessation attempt. These people often lack the confidence that they can be successful and are unwilling to risk their self-esteem if they fail. Some investigators believe that these patients should sign a waiver stating they have been informed of the risks and for the moment are choosing to smoke against the physician's advice. They can be given a brochure to read, and the subject can be broached again on subsequent visits. Watch for a possible critical incident (e.g., acute illness; MI in patient, friend, or relative; cancer; pregnancy; death of a valued person) as a time when contemplation can be changed to action.

E. Patients who are ambivalent often are unwilling to choose a quit date or sign a contract to quit but may be willing to do other things. A smoking diary can help document when, where, what they were doing, with whom, and the value of the cigarette from 1 (crucial) to 5 (not very important). The diary helps build awareness. It can be accompanied by tapering (i.e., eliminating the not-very-important cigarettes). Other techniques include switching to cigarettes with lower tar and nicotine content and smoking fewer cigarettes each day. These measures are mainly directed at building confidence for a successful cessation attempt. Until patients are ready to change, it is better not to court failure. Awareness that newer pharmacologic agents are available may help to convince a person who is ambivalent to try quitting.

F. For patients ready to quit, a quit date should be set and a contract signed. These can be preprinted or simply written in the chart. The contract can serve as an additional reminder if it is on duplicate paper with a chart copy and another copy placed in a prominent location selected by the patient (e.g., refrigerator, mirror). Some patients may keep a smoking diary for a few days to increase awareness of when, where, and why they smoke. Once the quit date is chosen, develop an action plan with the patient to determine who will be the support people at home and at work and how weight gain will be handled (increased exercise, low-calorie diet, use of bupropion or nicotine replacement therapy [NRT]). As the lungs return to normal, patients often begin to cough; it is worth emphasizing this in a positive light (i.e., cleansing of the lungs). Tell patients to use a cough suppressant only as a last resort to help them sleep. Those patients who choose varenicline (Chantix) should start the medication 1 week before their actual quit date so that they will be taking a full dose when they stop using cigarettes.

(Continued on page 678)

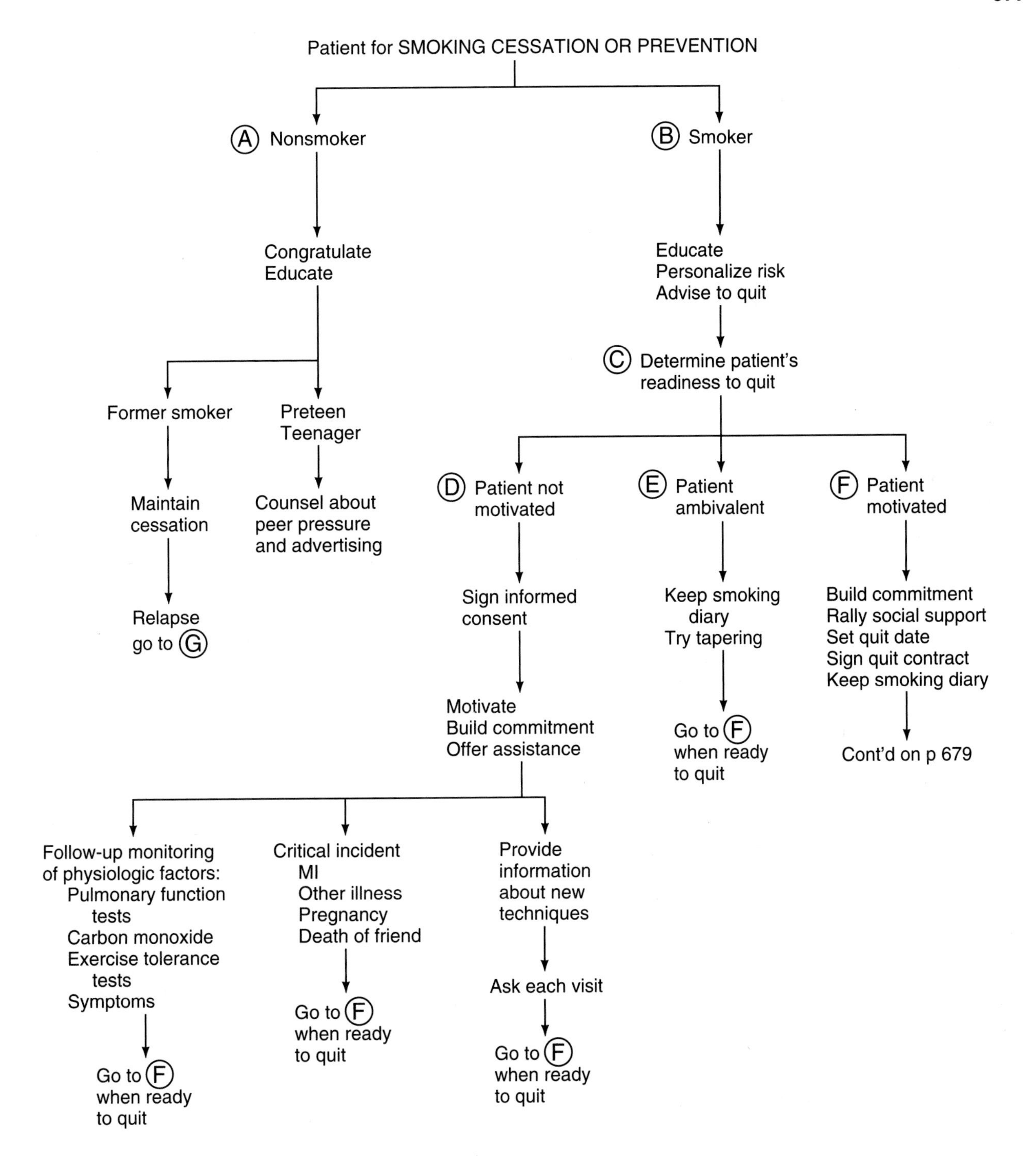
Patient for SMOKING CESSATION OR PREVENTION
(A) Nonsmoker
(B) Smoker
Congratulate
Educate
Educate
Personalize risk
Advise to quit
(C) Determine patient's readiness to quit
Former smoker
Preteen
Teenager
Maintain cessation
Counsel about peer pressure and advertising
Relapse go to (G)
(D) Patient not motivated
(E) Patient ambivalent
(F) Patient motivated
Sign informed consent
Keep smoking diary
Try tapering
Build commitment
Rally social support
Set quit date
Sign quit contract
Keep smoking diary
Motivate
Build commitment
Offer assistance
Go to (F) when ready to quit
Cont'd on p 679
Follow-up monitoring of physiologic factors:
Pulmonary function tests
Carbon monoxide
Exercise tolerance tests
Symptoms
Critical incident
MI
Other illness
Pregnancy
Death of friend
Provide information about new techniques
Ask each visit
Go to (F) when ready to quit
Go to (F) when ready to quit
Go to (F) when ready to quit

G. The decision to use NRT is based on whether the patient is heavily addicted to nicotine. This can be ascertained by historical data or the response to two questions: "Do you smoke within 30 minutes after rising in the morning?" and "Do you smoke more than 25 cigarettes a day?" One can also use the historical information of a previous attempt at quitting that was aborted because of withdrawal signs or symptoms. These patients may do better with NRT.

H1. For the individual who is nicotine dependent, one should offer both pharmacologic and psychologic intervention and discuss the options so patients can select the best choice for them. We suggest one continuous medication (patch) and one acute medication (inhaler, lozenge, or gum). The latter allows an acute dose that simulates the acute pulse of nicotine desired during acute craving. If varenicline is selected, neither an acute or chronic NRT medication is warranted because its mode of action is through nicotine blockade. Varenicline must be started 1 week before the quit date with an adjustment up to full dose. The choice of NRT should be approached as a menu of opportunities by the physician and patient. The agents available include nicotine polacrilex gum, nicotine-containing dermal patches, nasal spray, oral inhalers, nicotine-containing lozenges/microtabs, and psychoactive agents such as bupropion and varenicline. Clonidine and nortriptyline are now considered second-line agents because of frequent adverse effects. Some patients cannot chew gum because of dental work or temporomandibular joint problems or because they have tried the gum before and lack confidence in it. For these patients transdermal patches may be indicated. Other patients may be smoking a small number of cigarettes each day or may prefer not to use nicotine replacement; for these patients a trial of cessation without replacement therapy may be appropriate, or bupropion or varenicline alone may be added. All of these agents have been shown to increase the likelihood of success by from 1.5–3 times that of placebo. A minority of individuals may be smoking a small number of cigarettes a day or may wish to go "cold turkey" on their own. For those patients who are insistent and display confidence, a trial of cessation without NRT may be warranted. Careful follow-up should be used with this group.

For patients who are heavily addicted and choose to use gum, offer nicotine (Nicorette) gum, now available in multiple flavors and much more palatable than the early products. This can be done on a timed schedule and gradually tapered after the psychological aspects of addiction have abated. Many people who are unsuccessful in stopping do not use enough Nicorette gum or may use it incorrectly. For all patients beginning cessation, maintain close follow-up or contact over the first several days or weeks. This can be accomplished by a call from a staff member or by having patients call in with a report of how they are doing. The purpose of this is to identify slips (brief relapses) early and plan how to manage them and start the cessation attempt again. One slip is not a failure, and most patients who are successful have had to deal with three or four relapses. The details of relapse are important, and if acute craving is the cause, an acute NRT agent such as nasal spray, a lozenge, gum, or an inhaler may be added.

H2. Once the choice of medical therapy is made, one should consider a choice about counseling that has been shown to be a crucial part of care. The approaches include individual (you as the clinician or a member of your staff) or a cessation counselor, group (as with a cancer society or lung association group, hospital, or health care plan group), via phone as provided again by pharmaceutical manufacturers, health plans, and so on. Internet support has become available, but its efficacy is untested. Success in quitting correlates with more social support, with each additional means of psychological support raising the likelihood of success.

I. For successful patients, praise and support should be part of the maintenance plan.

J. For those who relapse, analyzing the cause for the relapse is helpful in designing subsequent therapy; starting again at F makes sense. Two forms of Nicorette are available, 2 or 4 mg. Depending on the patient's overall pack-year history and smoking pattern, an initial 2-mg dose helps taper craving for the nicotine in the cigarettes. David Sachs of Stanford suggests that a rule of 4s be followed with an eventual taper (i.e., 1 pack per day [ppd], 12 pieces Nicorette/day; 1.5 ppd, 16 pieces/day; 2 ppd, 20 pieces/day). He also suggests a chew, stop, and park regimen for the user (i.e., chew slowly until a tingle is felt, stop chewing and park the medication between cheek and gum, restart chewing when the tingle is gone, and stop when the tingle returns).

K. All future physician visits should include follow-up questions on cessation with reinforcement and praise for continued success.

L. For individuals who are addicted and for whom the transdermal nicotine patches are appropriate, the first dose is determined by amount of smoking and patient size.

M. Those weighing <105 pounds or smoking <20 cigarettes per day or who have frequent angina attacks should be considered for a 14-mg starting dose. Those who do not tolerate the 21-mg patch because of excess nicotine symptoms may do better on the lower dosage. The 14-mg dose is continued for at least 1 month.

(Continued on page 680)

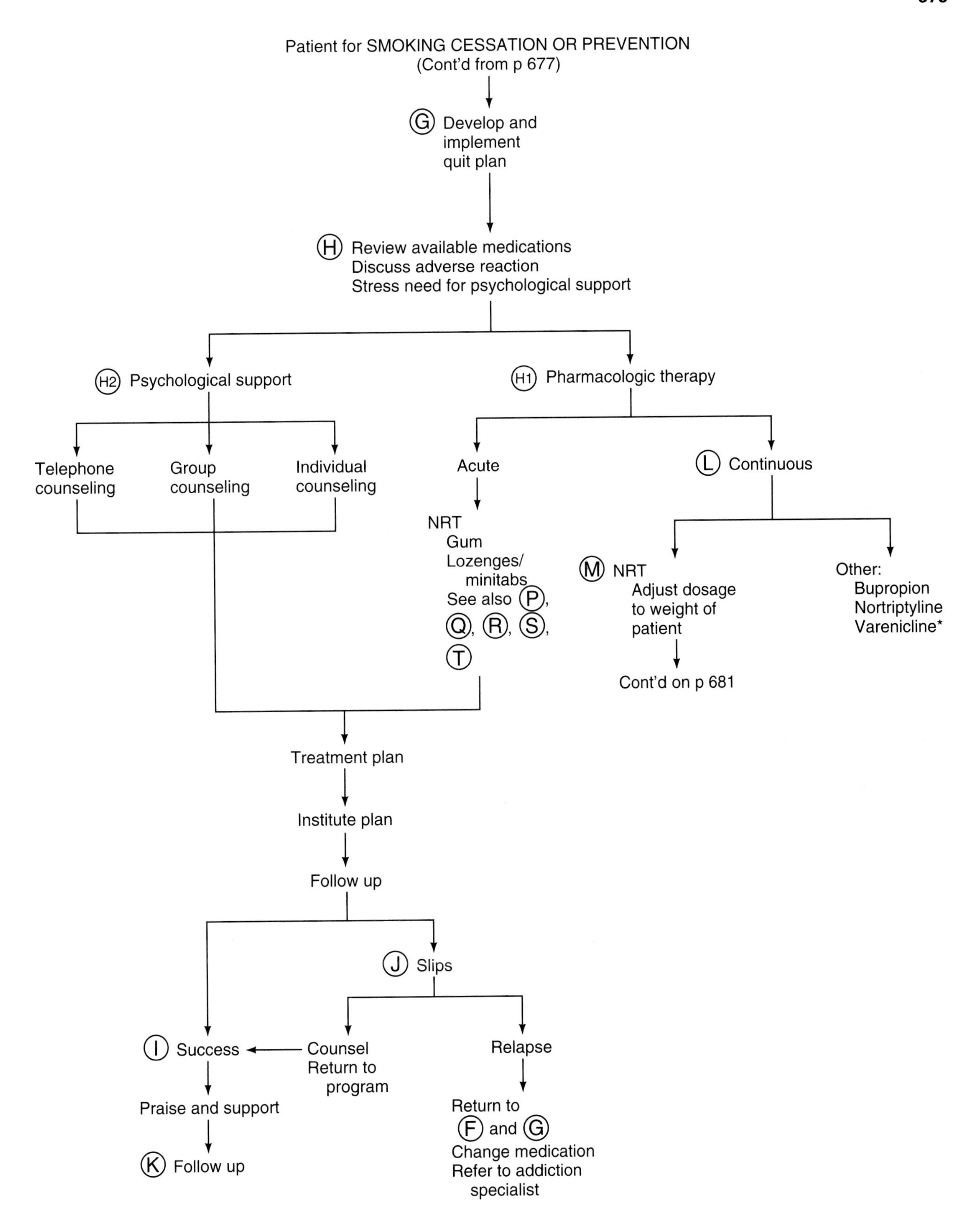

*Should be used alone; monitor closely for depression or suicidal ideation. See FDA Alert 2/1/2008.

N. Most smokers who are heavily addicted (with the exceptions noted in M) should begin with the 21-mg transdermal patch. This is continued for 1 month. Patients often report vivid, altered, or increased dreaming while using the 21-mg patch. Erythema develops beneath the patch in most patients. Patches should be moved to a new location each day. The manufacturer's instructions should be carefully followed. The patient must not smoke while using patches because this can lead to nicotine toxicity, increased angina, or MI. A small percentage of patients develop severe skin reactions (1%–3%) at the patch site. These patients should be managed using gum, inhaler, nasal spray, and/or bupropion or varenicline. After the initial dosage, the dose should be tapered, as suggested by the manufacturer.

O. Continue close follow-up and support as outlined in I and K. The patient who relapses while using patches should have the failure analyzed and if from acute craving, have an acute agent added to the last patch dose at which the relapse occurred.

P. Nasal spray delivers an earlier peak of nicotine than gum, inhaler, lozenges, or patches. The dose is one squirt per nostril with both nostrils being treated. The dosing schedule is two per hour. The spray may be used in conjunction with the patch for treatment of acute craving. Spray may be chosen by those smokers who need the "rush" effect of lighting up.

Q. Nicotine inhalers became available in the late 1990s and still require a prescription to be dispensed. The inhaler adds the physical benefit of "handling behavior" like handling a cigarette. It provides the patient with a mechanism that he or she controls to adjust dosing. Most of the nicotine absorbed from the inhaler is taken in through the oral mucosa, the esophagus, and stomach, with only a small amount being absorbed via the lungs. Used alone, it doubles quit rates over placebo and gives higher rates when coupled with the patch.

R. Bupropion (Wellbutrin, Zyban) has been shown to produce 20%–23% 1-year cessation rates when first used at a dosage of 150 mg twice a day. It is currently available in sustained-release form, which has decreased the seizure risk while enhancing efficacy. Cessation rates varied from 20% to nearly 45% with doses of 100–300 mg/day for 7 weeks. Bupropion can help reduce cigarette use in those attempting to taper daily use and gives additional efficacy when coupled with NRT. It may have a special role in those patients who are recently recovering from MI because, unlike NRT, it has no acute cardiac side effects. It seems to blunt the risk of weight gain with smoking cessation and has a Class B designation for use in pregnancy. Its side effects include xerostomia, headaches, and insomnia. It should not be used in those with a history of or predisposition to seizures.

S. Nortriptyline has been listed as a second-line therapy by the Agency for Healthcare Research and Quality. It has been used for smoking cessation in patients both with and without depression. When used with the "patch," it enhanced cessation rates over transdermal systems alone.

T. Varenicline (Chantix) is a new pharmacologic agent that binds with high affinity and selectivity at the alpha4beta2 neuronal nicotine acetylcholine receptor, thus producing agonist activity. The recommended dosage begins 1 week before the quit date with 0.5 mg orally for days 1–3. Then 0.5 mg is given orally twice a day for days 4–7 and then 1 mg orally from day 8 to completion of therapy. The initial course of treatment is for 12 weeks; for those who remain abstinent, therapy should be continued for another 12 weeks. Recent warnings have appeared regarding mood swings, depression, suicidal ideation, and attempted and completed suicides in those taking varenicline, thus prompting close psychological monitoring of these patients while receiving treatment.

References

Aubin HJ. Tolerability and safety of sustained release bupropion in the management of smoking cessation. Drugs 2002;62(Suppl 2):45–52.

Bartecchi CE, MacKenzie TD, Schrier RW. The human costs of tobacco use. N Engl J Med 1994;330:907.

Benowitz NL. Treating tobacco addiction: nicotine or no nicotine? N Engl J Med 1997;337:1230.

Bronson DL, Flynn BS, Solomon LJ, et al. Smoking cessation counseling during periodic health examinations. Arch Intern Med 1989;149:1653.

Coates TJ, Cummings SR. Behavior modification. In Kassirer JP, Greene HL II, eds. Current Therapy in Adult Medicine, 4th ed. St Louis: Mosby, 1997:26.

DeNelsky GY. Smoking cessation: strategies that work. Cleve Clin J Med 1990;57:416.

Frishman WH, Mittas W, Kupersmith A, et al. Nicotine and non-nicotine smoking cessation pharmacotherapies. Cardiol Rev 2006;14:57–73.

Greene HL II. Smoking cessation. In Kassirer JP, Greene HL II, eds. Current Therapy in Adult Medicine, 4th ed. St Louis: Mosby, 1997:35.

Guise BJ, Goldstein MG, Clark MM, et al. Behavior change: the example of smoking. In Noble J, Greene HL, Levenson W, eds. Primary Care Medicine. St. Louis: Mosby, 1996:1650.

Henningfield JE, Fant RV, Buchalter AR, et al. Pharmacotherapy of nicotine dependence. Ca Cancer J Clin 2005;55:281–299.

Hughes JR. Does smoking reduction increase future cessation and decrease disease risk? Nicotine and Tobacco Research 2006;739–749.

Hurt RD, Sachs DP, Glover ED, et al. Comparison of sustained-release bupropion and placebo for smoking cessation. N Engl J Med 1997;337:1230–1231

Joseph AM, Norman SM, Ferry LH, et al. The safety of transdermal nicotine as an aid to smoking cessation in patients with cardiac disease. N Engl J Med 1996;335:1792.

Ockene JK, Kristeller J, Goldberg R, et al. Increasing the efficacy of physician-delivered smoking interventions: a randomized clinical trial. J Gen Intern Med 1991;6:1.

Rigotti NA. Treatment of tobacco use and dependence. N Engl J Med 2002;346:506.

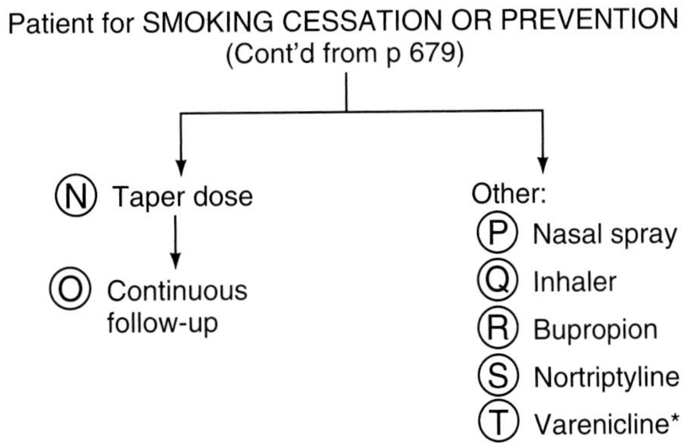

Patient for SMOKING CESSATION OR PREVENTION
(Cont'd from p 679)

- (N) Taper dose
  - (O) Continuous follow-up
- Other:
  - (P) Nasal spray
  - (Q) Inhaler
  - (R) Bupropion
  - (S) Nortriptyline
  - (T) Varenicline*

*Should be used alone; monitor closely for depression or suicidal ideation. See FDA Alert 2/1/2008.

SUICIDAL PATIENT

John A. Fromson, MD, and Rebecca L. Potter, MD

Most people who are suicidal communicate their self-destructive intentions to those around them, including their physicians. As many as two thirds of those who commit suicide have seen a doctor in the weeks to months before their death. Medical students and primary care physicians should therefore know how to evaluate the patient who is suicidal. Does a patient look or feel depressed and talk of "not being able to go on," giving up, and losing interest in activities? If so, a more detailed assessment of suicidal risk is in order. Factors to consider in a comprehensive suicide risk assessment include age, gender, social and cultural issues, psychiatric diagnosis, prevention strategies, treatment setting, and type of treatment.

A. Psychiatric disorders associated with an increased risk of suicidal ideation and attempt include depression, bipolar disorder, alcohol or drug abuse, panic attacks, and panic disorders. Factors associated with high acute suicide risk in patients with affective disorders include an agitated state and severe manifestations of anxiety, panic attacks, global insomnia, and anhedonia.

B. The following psychosocial factors place people at an increased risk of committing suicide: single, divorced, widowed, or separated marital status; unemployment; decreased social supports; humiliating life events (e.g., the recent loss of a job or an important relationship); a chronic medical illness; or a family history of suicide. A previous suicide attempt is a predictor of future completed suicide.

C. Do not ignore or minimize references to suicide, such as taking risks, talking of guilt over past events, talking of "ending it all," making a will, or giving away prized possessions. Ask patients directly whether they are suicidal and if so what plan they have; assess their understanding of the lethality of the plan. Do they have the means to carry out the plan? Have there been earlier attempts? Determine patients' mood, changes in appetite and sleep, the presence of hallucinations or delusions, and quality of speech. Patients with "command" hallucinations to commit suicide are at particularly high risk. A physical examination and laboratory studies to consider contributory or concomitant physical illness are necessary.

D. If the patient has serious immediate suicidal intent, consider psychiatric consultation and voluntary or involuntary hospitalization. If the risk is not as imminent, establish and make available a therapeutic relationship. Forming a no-suicide contract, scheduling frequent appointments, and providing reassurance and hope for the future are important. Allow the patient to ventilate feelings and help him or her problem solve, communicating empathy and caring. Treat any underlying psychiatric or medical disorder.

References

Blumenthal SJ. Suicide: a guide to risk factors, assessment, and treatment of suicidal patients. Med Clin North Am 1988;72:937.

Busch KA, Fawcett J, Jacobs DG. Clinical correlates of inpatient suicide. J Clin Psychiatry 2003;64:14–19.

Fawcett J, Clark DC, Busch KA. Assessing and treating the patient at risk for suicide. Psychiatr Annals 1993;23:244.

Fawcett J, Sheftner WA, Fogg L, et al. Time-related predictors of suicide in major affective disorder. Am J Psychiatry 1990;146:1189.

Hall RC, Platt DE, Hall RC. Suicide risk assessment: a review of risk factors in 100 patients who made severe suicide attempts: evaluation of suicide risk in a time of managed care. Psychosomatics 1999;40:18.

Hirschfeld JM, Russell JM. Assessment and treatment of suicidal patients. N Engl J Med 1997;337:910.

Malone KM, Szanto K, Corbitt EM, et al. Clinical assessment versus research methods in the assessment of suicidal behavior. Am J Psychiatry 1995;152:1601.

Roy A. Suicide. In Kaplan HI, Sadock BJ, eds. Comprehensive Textbook of Psychiatry, 6th ed. Baltimore: Williams & Wilkins, 1995.

Simon RI. Suicide risk: assessing the unpredictable. In Simon RI, Hales RE. The American Psychiatric Publishing Textbook of Suicide Assessment and Management. Washington, DC: American Psychiatric Publishing, 2006.

Weissman MM, Kierman GL, Markowitz JS, et al. Suicidal ideation and suicide attempts in panic disorder and attacks. N Engl J Med 1989;321:1209.

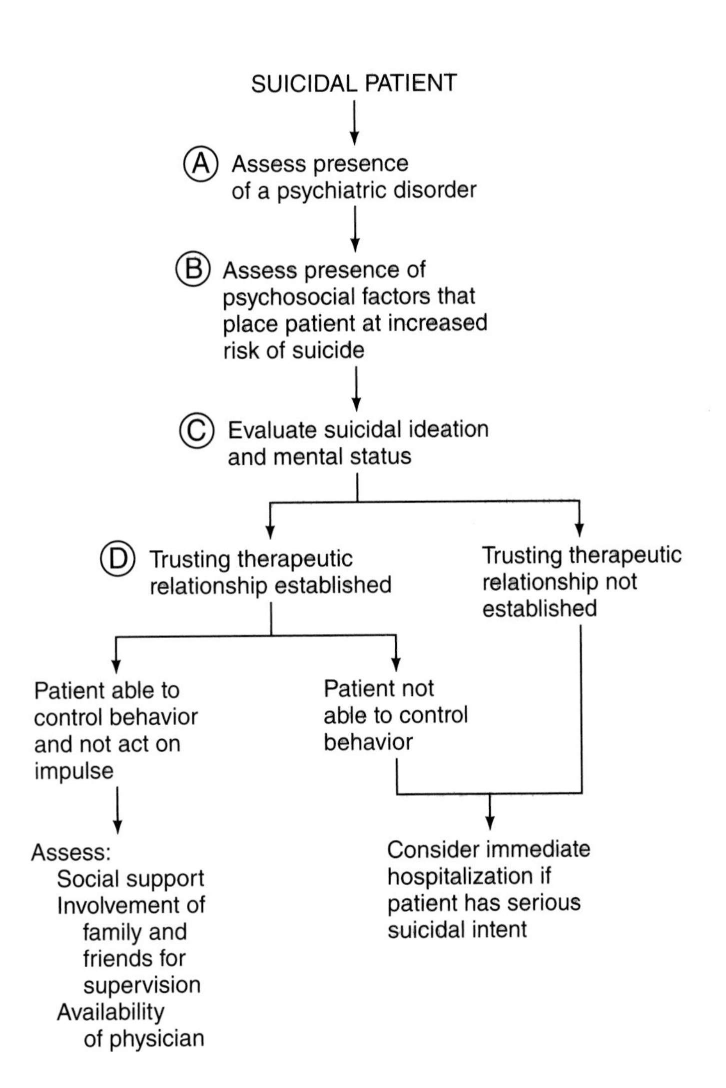
SUICIDAL PATIENT
(A) Assess presence of a psychiatric disorder
(B) Assess presence of psychosocial factors that place patient at increased risk of suicide
(C) Evaluate suicidal ideation and mental status
(D) Trusting therapeutic relationship established
Trusting therapeutic relationship not established
Patient able to control behavior and not act on impulse
Patient not able to control behavior
Assess:
Social support
Involvement of family and friends for supervision
Availability of physician
Consider immediate hospitalization if patient has serious suicidal intent

PHARMACOLOGY

Michael D. Katz, PharmD
Section Editor

ACUTE ANTICOAGULATION

Michael D. Katz, PharmD

Thromboembolic disorders and medical procedures that may require anticoagulation therapy include proximal deep venous thrombosis (DVT), pulmonary embolism (PE), atrial fibrillation with embolism, acute myocardial infarction, acute coronary syndrome, and placement of mechanical heart valves. In situations of apparent thromboembolic disorders (as opposed to prophylaxis) that are potentially life threatening (e.g., PE with shock), initiate heparin therapy before performing diagnostic tests.

A. Diagnostic tests vary in sensitivity and specificity. In patients with PE, a high degree of clinical suspicion may necessitate therapy even when the helical CT scan or ventilation-perfusion scan is inconclusive or negative.
B. Contraindications to heparin are relative: The risks must be weighed against the potential benefits. In most cases, patients with previous hypersensitivity or heparin-induced thrombocytopenia; active bleeding; intracranial hemorrhage; GI bleeding; hemophilia; thrombocytopenia; severe hypertension; or recent surgery of the brain, spinal cord, or eye should not receive heparin therapy. In patients with PE in whom there are contraindications to heparin therapy, consider placement of an inferior vena cava (IVC) filter.
C. In patients with massive PE or those with hemodynamic compromise, consider thrombolytic therapy with urokinase or tissue plasminogen activator (TPA). However, clinical trials have shown no clear advantage of thrombolytic therapy over heparin in most patients with venous thromboembolism.

(Continued on page 688)

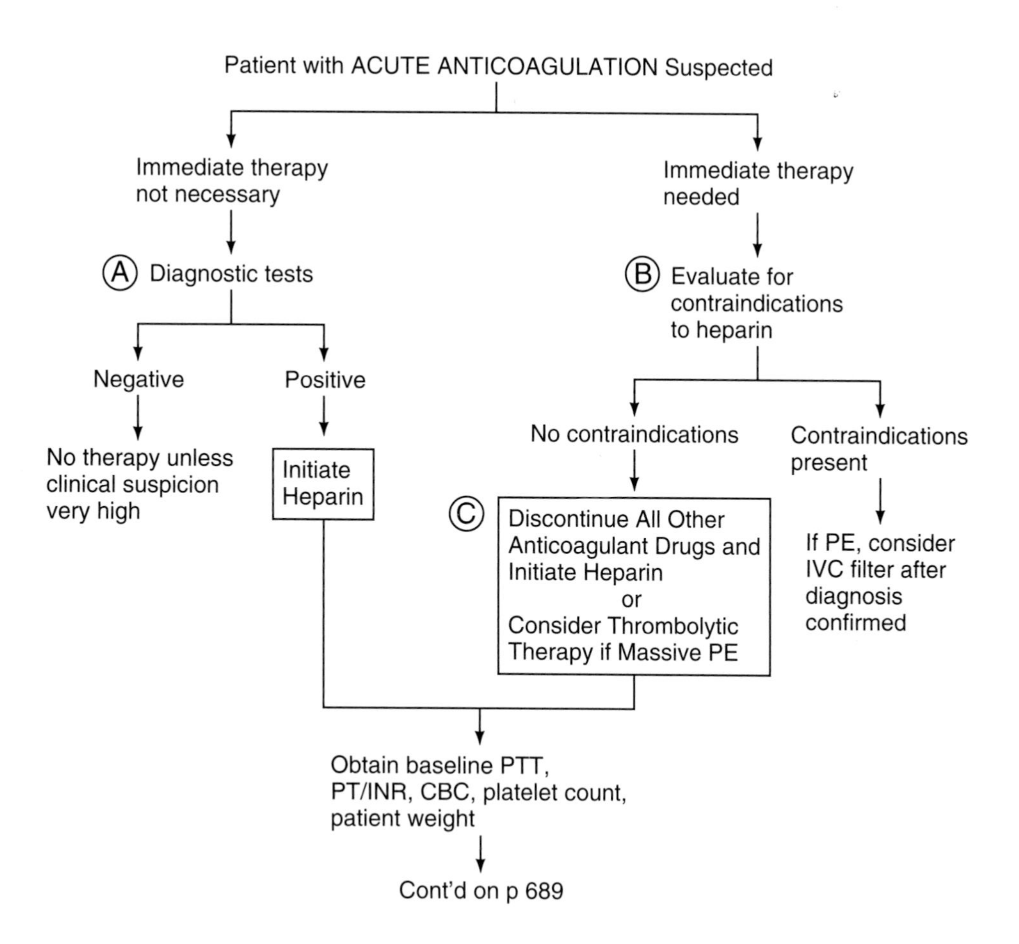

Patient with ACUTE ANTICOAGULATION Suspected
Immediate therapy not necessary
Immediate therapy needed
(A) Diagnostic tests
(B) Evaluate for contraindications to heparin
Negative
Positive
No therapy unless clinical suspicion very high
Initiate Heparin
No contraindications
Contraindications present
(C)
Discontinue All Other Anticoagulant Drugs and Initiate Heparin
or
Consider Thrombolytic Therapy if Massive PE
If PE, consider IVC filter after diagnosis confirmed
Obtain baseline PTT, PT/INR, CBC, platelet count, patient weight
Cont'd on p 689

D. Several studies show that a weight-based approach to administering heparin achieves more rapid anticoagulation without increased risk of bleeding. Many institutions have developed heparin-dosing protocols to facilitate the appropriate use of heparin. However, use of such protocols does not obviate the need for close clinical and laboratory monitoring by the physician. Check partial thromboplastin time (PTT) no sooner than 6 hours after any bolus; PTT checked sooner may be falsely elevated. The PTT target for heparin therapy must be based on values derived by individual laboratories. Many laboratories now standardize the PTT assay based on heparin levels. The PTT-based dose changes must be based on local laboratory standards, and published protocol can serve only as a guide.

E. A variety of low molecular weight heparin (LMWH) products such as enoxaparin have been marketed. These agents appear to be at least as effective as unfractionated heparin (UFH), do not require PTT monitoring, and can be administered by intermittent SC injection. However, these products are much more expensive than UFH and offer no particular advantage in the patient who is hospitalized. Several studies show that LMWH can be administered safely to outpatients with DVT or PE. A patient who is medically stable and has the appropriate home environment and insurance coverage may be discharged on LMWH (e.g., enoxaparin 1 mg/kg SC q12h or 1.5 mg/kg q24h). Such therapy is continued until the level of long-term anticoagulation (warfarin) is therapeutic.

F. If long-term anticoagulation is indicated and there are no contraindications to warfarin, initiate warfarin as soon as the PTT is therapeutic. The initial warfarin dose should be the same as the expected maintenance dose. There is no pharmacologic rationale for, and there is no outcome evidence supporting, the use of warfarin "loading" doses. Continue heparin therapy for at least 4 days after the initiation of warfarin. Earlier increases in the prothrombin time/International Normalized Ratio (PT/INR) result primarily from depletion of factor VII. Patients are not truly anticoagulated until significant depletion of factors II and X has occurred.

References

Buller HR, Agnelli G, Hull RD, et al. Antithrombotic therapy for venous thromboembolic disease: The Seventh ACCP Conference on Antithrombotic and Thrombolytic Therapy. Chest 2004;126:401–428.

Hirsh J, Raschke R. Heparin and low-molecular-weight heparin: The Seventh ACCP Conference on Antithrombotic and Thrombolytic Therapy. Chest 2004;126:188S–203S.

Raschke RA, Reilly BM, Guidry JR, et al. The weight-based heparin dosing nomogram compared with a "standard care" nomogram. A randomized controlled trial. Ann Intern Med 1993;119:874.

Spinler SA, Wittkowsky AK, Nutescu EA, et al. Anticoagulation monitoring. Part 2: unfractionated heparin and low-molecular-weight heparin. Ann Pharmacother 2005;39:1275–1285.

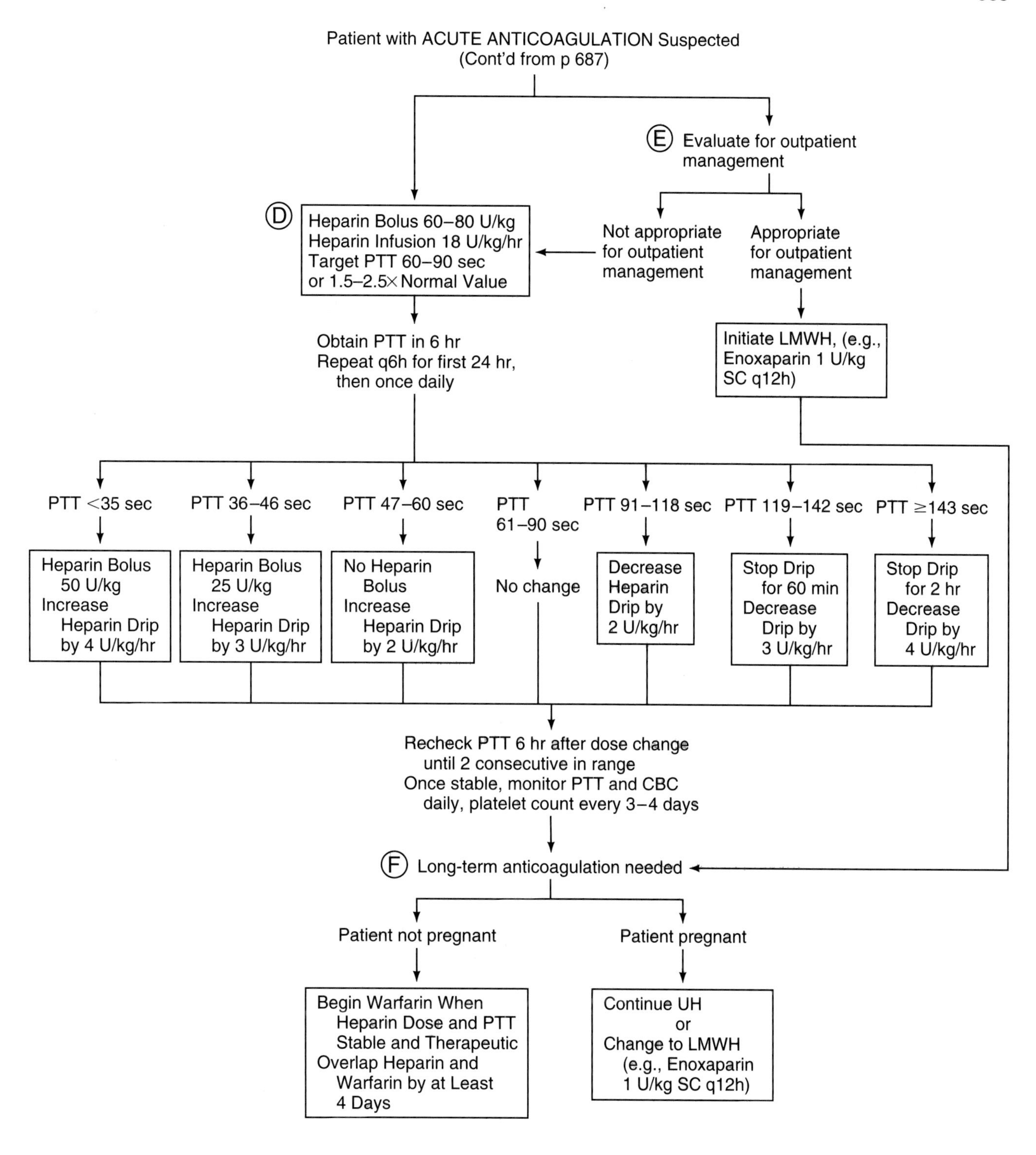
Patient with ACUTE ANTICOAGULATION Suspected
(Cont'd from p 687)
E Evaluate for outpatient management
D
Heparin Bolus 60–80 U/kg
Heparin Infusion 18 U/kg/hr
Target PTT 60–90 sec
or 1.5–2.5× Normal Value
Not appropriate for outpatient management
Appropriate for outpatient management
Initiate LMWH, (e.g., Enoxaparin 1 U/kg SC q12h)
Obtain PTT in 6 hr
Repeat q6h for first 24 hr, then once daily
PTT <35 sec
PTT 36–46 sec
PTT 47–60 sec
PTT 61–90 sec
PTT 91–118 sec
PTT 119–142 sec
PTT ≥143 sec
Heparin Bolus 50 U/kg
Increase Heparin Drip by 4 U/kg/hr
Heparin Bolus 25 U/kg
Increase Heparin Drip by 3 U/kg/hr
No Heparin Bolus
Increase Heparin Drip by 2 U/kg/hr
No change
Decrease Heparin Drip by 2 U/kg/hr
Stop Drip for 60 min
Decrease Drip by 3 U/kg/hr
Stop Drip for 2 hr
Decrease Drip by 4 U/kg/hr
Recheck PTT 6 hr after dose change until 2 consecutive in range
Once stable, monitor PTT and CBC daily, platelet count every 3–4 days
F Long-term anticoagulation needed
Patient not pregnant
Patient pregnant
Begin Warfarin When Heparin Dose and PTT Stable and Therapeutic
Overlap Heparin and Warfarin by at Least 4 Days
Continue UH
or
Change to LMWH
(e.g., Enoxaparin 1 U/kg SC q12h)

LONG-TERM ANTICOAGULATION

Michael D. Katz, PharmD

A. Contraindications to long-term anticoagulant therapy include those listed for acute anticoagulation (p 686); in addition, long-term anticoagulant therapy is contraindicated in those patients who are severely debilitated and malnourished, those who fall or undergo significant trauma, those with alcoholism, and those who are unlikely to understand or comply with therapy. As always, the risk-benefit ratio must be considered. Pregnancy is an absolute contraindication to warfarin. Women of childbearing age who receive warfarin must be using an effective contraceptive method.

B. Patients with recurrent thromboembolism on warfarin therapy should first be evaluated for compliance and adequacy of anticoagulation. If low-intensity anticoagulation was used, consider high-intensity therapy. Alternatively, consider subcutaneous low molecular weight heparin (LMWH) therapy. In patients with frequent recurrences of thromboembolism, consider the presence of malignancy or other hypercoagulable state (activated protein C deficiency, prothrombin mutation, etc.).

C. The average dose of warfarin required to achieve the target INR in adult patients is 5 mg. However, individual patient dose requirements vary widely, and there is no objective method that allows accurate prediction of the therapeutic dose in a given patient. The initial dose should be the expected therapeutic maintenance dose. Giving an initial loading dose is not rational given the pharmacology of warfarin and will not cause a more rapid achievement of therapeutic levels of anticoagulation. An initial 10-mg regimen can be useful in predicting subsequent dose requirements but should be administered only in the context of a formal dosing nomogram. Elderly patients usually require lower dosages of warfarin.

D. The level of anticoagulation during warfarin therapy is determined by the INR. This calculated value corrects for the widely varying thromboplastin reagents used to determine the prothrombin time (PT). Warfarin therapy cannot be safely or effectively managed without use of the INR. For most clinical indications, the target INR is 2.5 (range 2–3). For patients with most types of mechanical prosthetic heart valves or those who failed lower-intensity anticoagulation, a target INR of 3 (range 2.5–3.5) is desired. These INR ranges serve as clinical guidelines, not absolute values. The target INR for a specific patient is based on the risk of bleeding, age, and concomitant drug therapy.

E. Warfarin therapy must be closely monitored. Frequent monitoring is needed as therapy is titrated; less frequent visits are needed as the patient becomes stable. Initially, outpatients should be evaluated at weeks 1, 2, and 4. If the INR remains in the target range, the patient may be monitored every 4–8 weeks. Studies have shown that outcomes are consistently improved if patients are monitored by an anticoagulation clinic. All patients who are given warfarin must receive education and counseling regarding the underlying thromboembolic disorder, how to take the warfarin, possible side effects, and significant drug interactions. This information must be reviewed at each patient encounter.

(Continued on page 692)

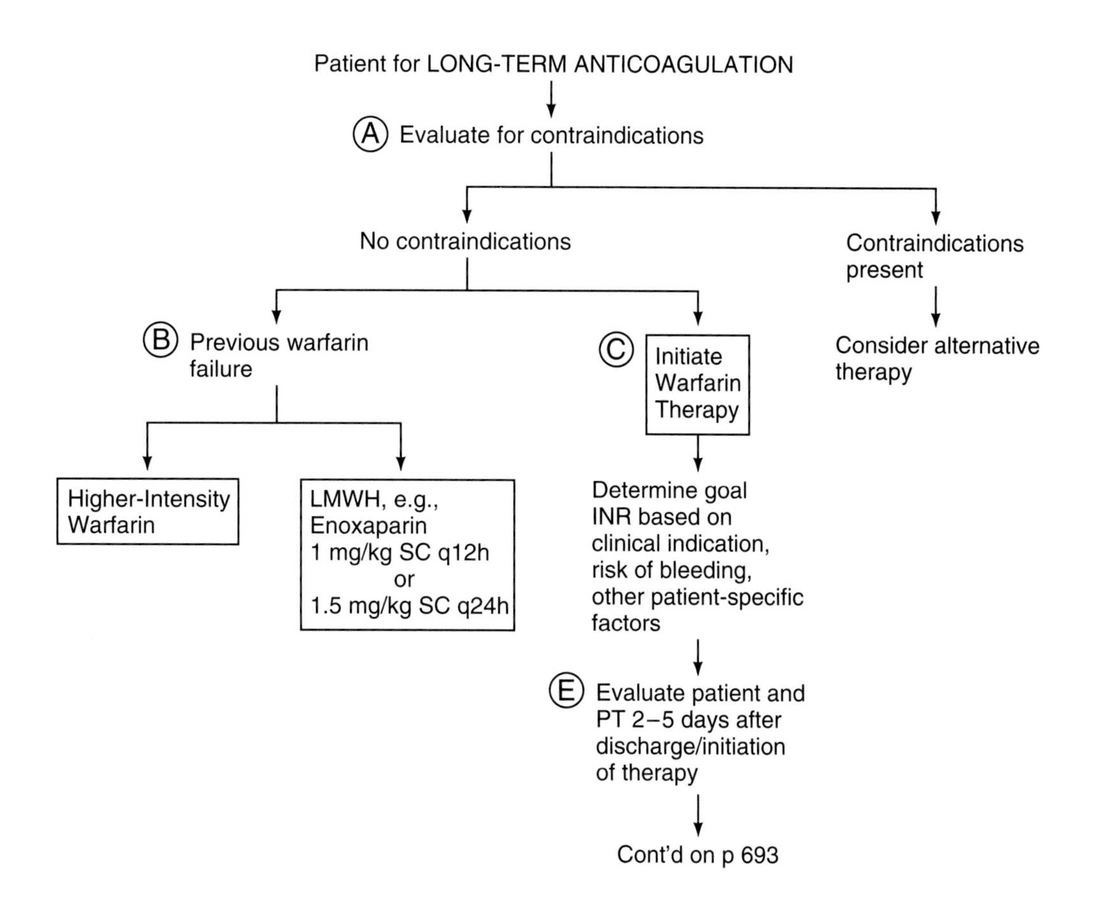
Patient for LONG-TERM ANTICOAGULATION
(A) Evaluate for contraindications
No contraindications
Contraindications present
Consider alternative therapy
(B) Previous warfarin failure
(C) Initiate Warfarin Therapy
Higher-Intensity Warfarin
LMWH, e.g., Enoxaparin 1 mg/kg SC q12h or 1.5 mg/kg SC q24h
Determine goal INR based on clinical indication, risk of bleeding, other patient-specific factors
(E) Evaluate patient and PT 2–5 days after discharge/initiation of therapy
Cont'd on p 693

F. If the INR is not in the target range, evaluate the patient for noncompliance, drug interactions, or a change in cardiac or hepatic function. Many drugs, including over-the-counter products, vitamins, and herbal/alternative agents, have significant interactions with warfarin. Any new drug should be initiated with great caution. If a correctable factor is identified and removed, the patient may continue taking the previous warfarin dose. In a patient who was previously stable with a minor fluctuation in INR and no change in clinical status, the warfarin dose may be continued and the INR should be rechecked in 1 week. Note that large changes in dose are not recommended and the change in INR will not be proportional to the change in dose. Patients with a very high INR (e.g., >6–10) should be assessed for bleeding complications. In the absence of bleeding, holding the warfarin dose may be the best approach. The INR can be reduced quickly by administering vitamin K 2.5 mg PO or 0.5–1 mg SC without causing warfarin resistance. Larger doses of vitamin K will cause prolonged resistance to subsequent warfarin therapy and should be avoided.

G. The duration of anticoagulant therapy is determined by the underlying disease and risk of recurrent thromboembolism. For patients with a first deep venous thrombosis (DVT) or pulmonary embolism (PE), 3–6 months of therapy may be adequate, especially if an underlying cause can be identified and removed. However, in patients with recurrent DVT or PE, atrial fibrillation with embolism or mechanical valves will require long-term therapy.

H. Bleeding complications may occur with a therapeutic or elevated INR. The risk of future anticoagulation must be weighed against the risk of future bleeding episodes. The management of warfarin-associated bleeding generally consists of holding the drug and administering vitamin K, fresh frozen plasma, or both. Full reversal of anticoagulation may not be desired in patients with mechanical heart valves. Administration of large doses of vitamin K (>5 mg SC/IV) will cause resistance to future warfarin therapy for several weeks. In patients who develop GI bleeding or hematuria with a therapeutic INR, a GI or urinary tract lesion may be present.

References

Ansell J, Hirsh J, Poller L, et al. The pharmacology and management of the vitamin K antagonists: the Seventh ACCP Conference on Antithrombotic and Thrombolytic Therapy. Chest 2004;126:204–233.

Ansell JE, Oertel LB, Wittkowsky AK. Managing Oral Anticoagulation Therapy. Gaithersburg, MD: Aspen, 1997.

Eckhoff CD, DiDomenico RJ, Shapiro NL. Initiating warfarin therapy: 5 mg versus 10 mg. Ann Pharmacother 2004;38:2115–2121.

Levine MN, Raskob G, Beyth RJ, et al. Hemorrhagic complications of anticoagulant treatment and thrombolytic therapy: the Seventh ACCP Conference on Antithrombotic and Thrombolytic Therapy. Chest 2004;126:287–310.

Spinler SA, Nutescu EA, Smythe MA, Wittkowsky AK. Anticoagulation monitoring part 1: warfarin and parenteral direct thrombin inhibitors. Ann Pharmacother 2005;39:1049–1055.

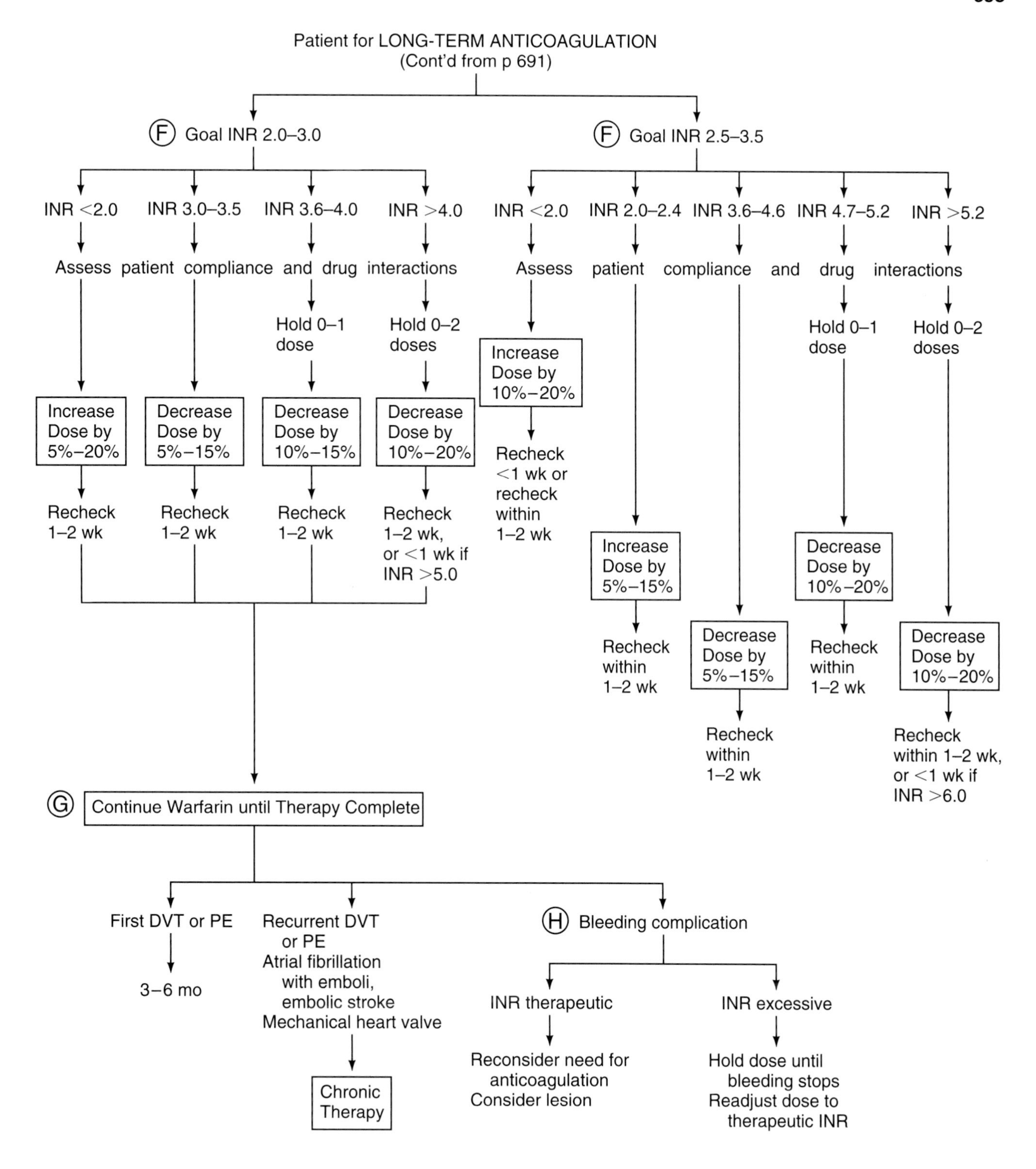
Patient for LONG-TERM ANTICOAGULATION
(Cont'd from p 691)
F Goal INR 2.0–3.0
F Goal INR 2.5–3.5
INR <2.0
INR 3.0–3.5
INR 3.6–4.0
INR >4.0
Assess patient compliance and drug interactions
Hold 0–1 dose
Hold 0–2 doses
Increase Dose by 5%–20%
Decrease Dose by 5%–15%
Decrease Dose by 10%–15%
Decrease Dose by 10%–20%
Recheck 1–2 wk
Recheck 1–2 wk
Recheck 1–2 wk
Recheck 1–2 wk, or <1 wk if INR >5.0
INR <2.0
INR 2.0–2.4
INR 3.6–4.6
INR 4.7–5.2
INR >5.2
Assess patient compliance and drug interactions
Increase Dose by 10%–20%
Recheck <1 wk or recheck within 1–2 wk
Hold 0–1 dose
Hold 0–2 doses
Increase Dose by 5%–15%
Recheck within 1–2 wk
Decrease Dose by 5%–15%
Recheck within 1–2 wk
Decrease Dose by 10%–20%
Recheck within 1–2 wk
Decrease Dose by 10%–20%
Recheck within 1–2 wk, or <1 wk if INR >6.0
G Continue Warfarin until Therapy Complete
First DVT or PE
3–6 mo
Recurrent DVT or PE
Atrial fibrillation with emboli, embolic stroke
Mechanical heart valve
Chronic Therapy
H Bleeding complication
INR therapeutic
Reconsider need for anticoagulation
Consider lesion
INR excessive
Hold dose until bleeding stops
Readjust dose to therapeutic INR

ANAPHYLAXIS

Michael D. Katz, PharmD

The common signs and symptoms of anaphylaxis include an aura, rhinitis, cough, pruritus, urticaria, laryngeal edema, generalized edema, decreased sensorium, shock, bronchospasm, GI cramps, and vomiting. Rarely, patients may develop heart failure, pulmonary edema, and DIC. Other conditions such as vasovagal reactions, hyperventilation, globus hystericus, and hereditary angioedema may mimic aspects of anaphylaxis and should be ruled out before initiating aggressive therapy.

A. Anaphylaxis is associated with a variety of factors, including foods, drugs, insect bites and stings, latex, semen, and exercise. More than one third of cases have no identifiable cause. Drugs associated with anaphylaxis include β-lactam antibiotics, sulfonamides, anesthetics, chymopapain, protamine, dextran, vaccines, and iodinated radiocontrast media. In any patient with anaphylaxis, obtain a complete exposure history, including any previous reactions.

B. Local reactions usually consist of redness, swelling, and pain at the site of injection. Systemic signs and symptoms may develop rapidly. Measures to slow absorption of the antigen from the injection site, such as application of ice or use of a venous (not arterial) occluding tourniquet, may be useful in the field until the patient reaches medical attention.

C. Base the initial management of anaphylaxis on support of airway, breathing, and circulation. Place all patients in the Trendelenburg position and give supplemental oxygen. In patients with cardiac or respiratory arrest or serious arrhythmias, initiate Basic and Advanced Cardiac Life Support measures.

D. Epinephrine is the mainstay of therapy for anaphylaxis; no other drug has proved as effective. Epinephrine reverses the effects of the mediators of anaphylaxis and may reduce the further release of these mediators. In most adults, give 0.3–0.5 ml of 1:1000 solution by SC injection (in children, 0.01 ml/kg). However, if the patient is in shock, give epinephrine through a central vein or instill into the endotracheal tube. If the desired response is not achieved and no adverse effects occur, repeat epinephrine in 10 minutes. Monitor elderly patients, especially those with underlying cardiac disease, very closely.

(Continued on page 696)

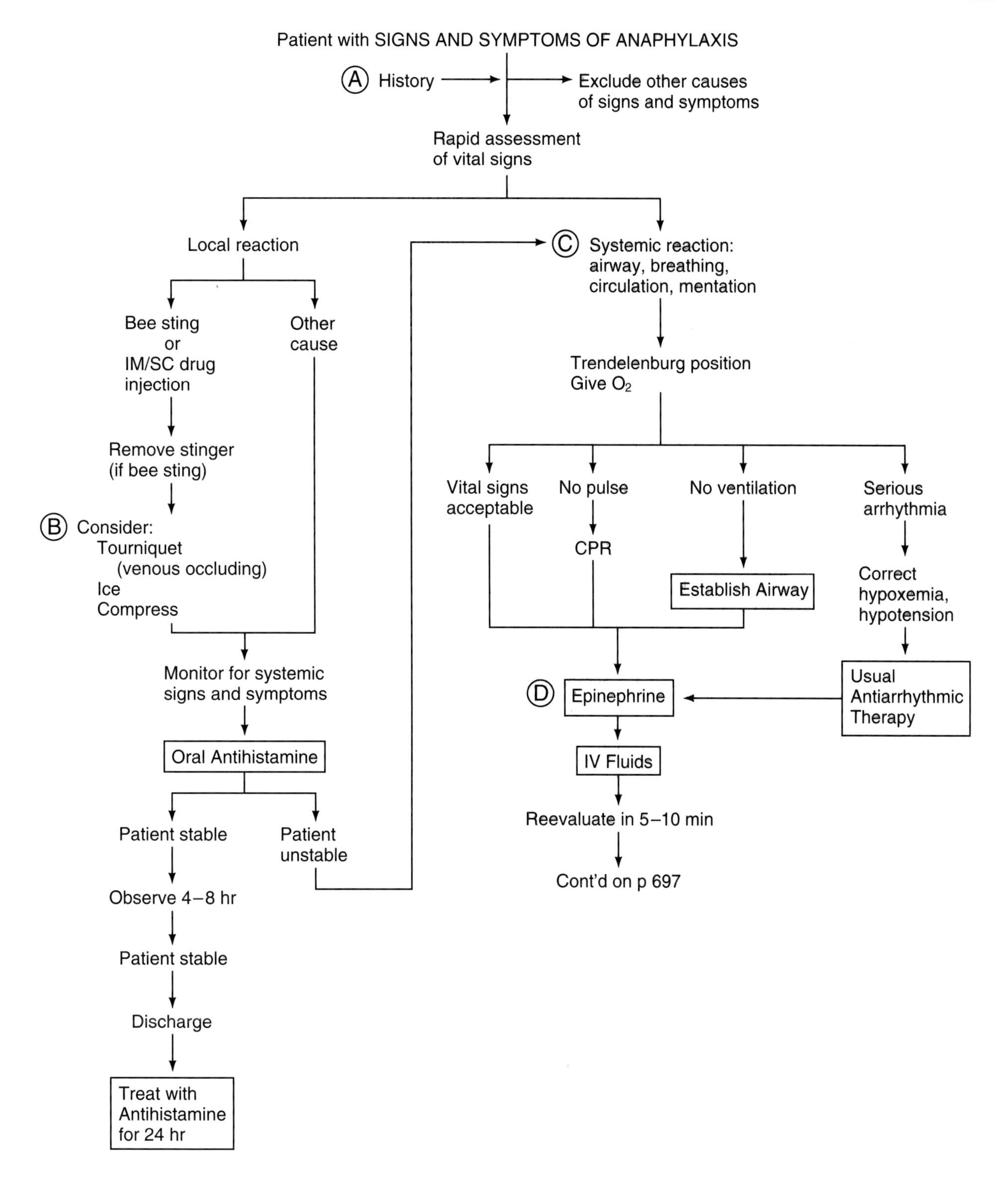
Patient with SIGNS AND SYMPTOMS OF ANAPHYLAXIS
(A) History
Exclude other causes of signs and symptoms
Rapid assessment of vital signs
Local reaction
Bee sting or IM/SC drug injection
Other cause
Remove stinger (if bee sting)
(B) Consider: Tourniquet (venous occluding) Ice Compress
Monitor for systemic signs and symptoms
Oral Antihistamine
Patient stable
Patient unstable
Observe 4–8 hr
Patient stable
Discharge
Treat with Antihistamine for 24 hr
(C) Systemic reaction: airway, breathing, circulation, mentation
Trendelenburg position Give O2
Vital signs acceptable
No pulse
No ventilation
Serious arrhythmia
CPR
Establish Airway
Correct hypoxemia, hypotension
Usual Antiarrhythmic Therapy
(D) Epinephrine
IV Fluids
Reevaluate in 5–10 min
Cont'd on p 697

E. In patients with severe bronchospasm, epinephrine and inhaled β_2 agonists (e.g., albuterol) are the most effective treatment. There is no evidence that IV theophylline is effective in the treatment of acute, severe bronchospasm, and it may increase the risk of cardiac arrhythmias. Early administration of an IV corticosteroid should be considered because these agents have a delayed onset of action. Methylprednisolone at IV dosages of 50–125 mg every 6 hours has been used. In less severe cases, oral prednisone may be appropriate.

F. Antihistamines serve as second-line therapy when a prolonged course is expected. H_1 blocking agents such as diphenhydramine or hydroxyzine may be especially useful in treating pruritus. In patients with a prolonged or refractory course, the addition of the H_2 blockers, such as ranitidine 50 mg IV or 150 mg PO, may be helpful.

G. Instruct all patients with anaphylaxis in ways to avoid future exposure to the inciting agent. The cause of the episode, if known, should be documented clearly in the patient's medical record, especially in drug-induced anaphylaxis. Because existing therapy with beta blockers or angiotensin-converting enzyme (ACE) inhibitors could worsen anaphylaxis, those agents should be discontinued, if possible.

H. In some instances specific preventive therapy may be indicated. Consider patients with bee-sting allergy who cannot easily avoid future exposures for desensitization. In patients with frequently recurrent idiopathic anaphylaxis, prophylactic therapy with corticosteroids and antihistamines has proved effective. Autoinjectors containing epinephrine also may be used by the patient at risk for another serious reaction.

References

Lieberman PL, Kemp SF, Oppenheimer J, et al. The diagnosis and management of anaphylaxis: an updated practice parameter. J Allergy Clin Immunol 2005;115:S483–523.

Neugut AI, Ghatak AT, Miller RL. Anaphylaxis in the United States: an investigation into its epidemiology. Arch Intern Med 2001;161:15–21.

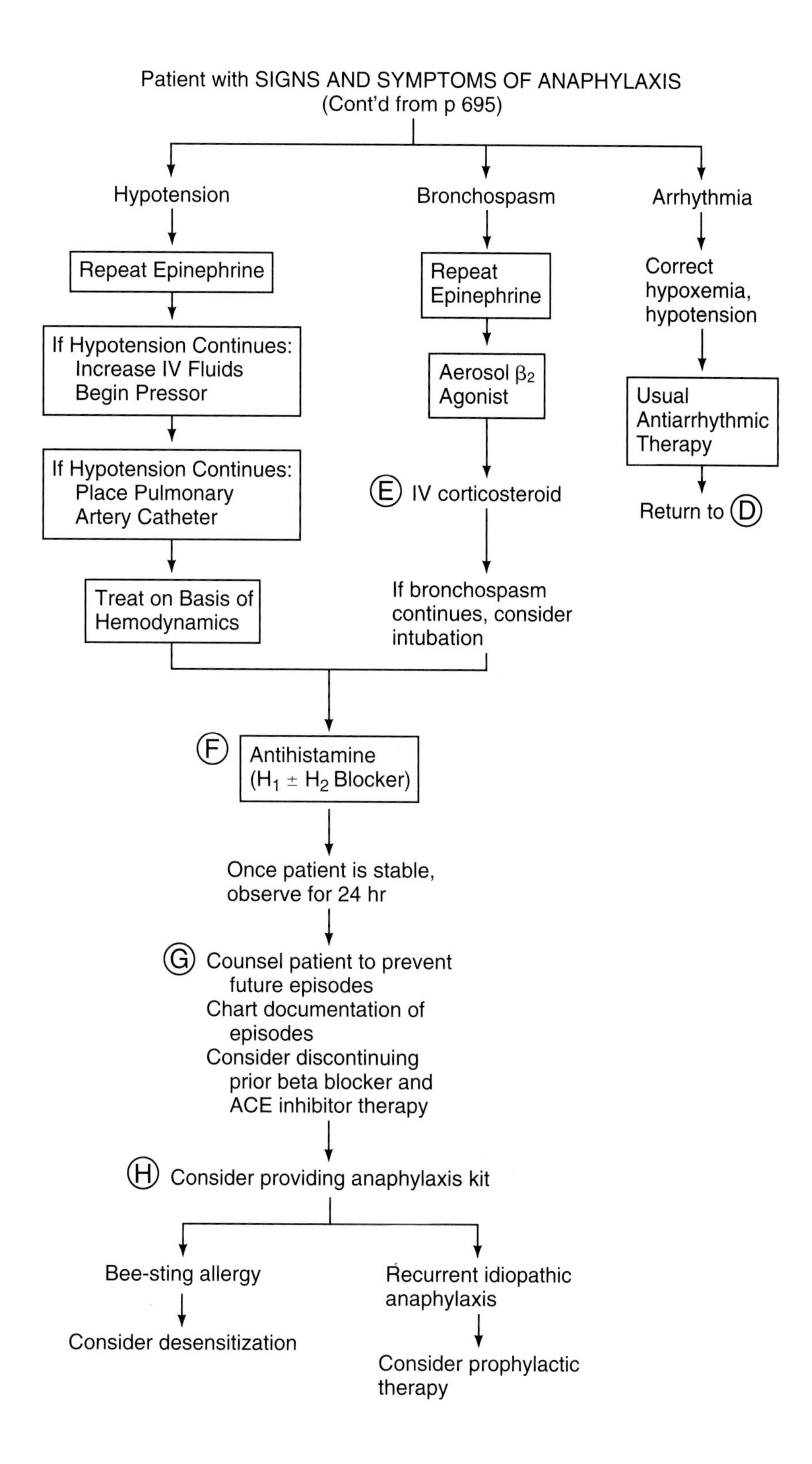
Patient with SIGNS AND SYMPTOMS OF ANAPHYLAXIS
(Cont'd from p 695)
Hypotension
Bronchospasm
Arrhythmia
Repeat Epinephrine
If Hypotension Continues: Increase IV Fluids Begin Pressor
If Hypotension Continues: Place Pulmonary Artery Catheter
Treat on Basis of Hemodynamics
Repeat Epinephrine
Aerosol β_2 Agonist
E IV corticosteroid
If bronchospasm continues, consider intubation
Correct hypoxemia, hypotension
Usual Antiarrhythmic Therapy
Return to D
F Antihistamine ($H_1 \pm H_2$ Blocker)
Once patient is stable, observe for 24 hr
G Counsel patient to prevent future episodes
Chart documentation of episodes
Consider discontinuing prior beta blocker and ACE inhibitor therapy
H Consider providing anaphylaxis kit
Bee-sting allergy
Consider desensitization
Recurrent idiopathic anaphylaxis
Consider prophylactic therapy

EVALUATION OF ADVERSE DRUG REACTIONS

Michael D. Katz, PharmD

A. An adverse drug reaction (ADR) is any unexpected, unintended, undesired, or excessive response to a drug or medication that (1) requires discontinuing the medication; (2) requires changing the medication; (3) requires modifying the dosage; (4) necessitates hospital admission; (5) prolongs stay in a health care facility; (6) necessitates supportive treatment; (7) significantly complicates diagnosis; (8) negatively affects prognosis; or (9) results in temporary or permanent harm, disability, or death. The concept of medication misadventures includes medication errors and ADRs.

ADRs are far more common than many clinicians believe. A recent meta-analysis of 39 prospective studies concluded that serious ADRs occur in 6.7% of hospitalized patients, with a fatality rate of 0.32%. Annually, 2.2 million hospitalized patients experience serious ADRs, with 106,000 deaths per year, making ADRs the fourth leading cause of death in the United States. The elderly are especially prone to ADRs. Approximately 5% of hospitalizations result from an ADR. It is estimated that 11% of hospitalized patients experience an ADR, with 2.1% of those considered serious. Many ADRs are preventable.

B. Evaluate any patient receiving a pharmacologically active substance (including diagnostic agents and alternative products) who has any adverse event for a possible ADR. Medication errors, including improper prescribing, dispensing, or administration of a drug, are one possible cause of ADRs. Standard drug information resources can help define the adverse effect profile of a given agent. However, information regarding newly marketed agents may be difficult to obtain.

C. Establishing a temporal association is often the most difficult part of the evaluation. Most ADRs manifest within the first day or two of treatment and most by the second week of therapy. The temporal relationship is drug, patient, and reaction specific. To establish a clear-cut temporal relationship, compare the time of onset of the reaction with that expected based on previous reported reaction or the known or proposed pathophysiologic mechanism. If the reaction has not been seen with the suspected drug, compare similar agents or drugs within the same class. Take into account patient specificity (e.g., type I hypersensitivity reactions may be immediate in nature in a patient who was previously exposed or delayed 5–10 days in a patient who has never been exposed).

D. Discontinue all potential offending agents, if possible. However, the decision to discontinue agents depends on the severity of the reaction, the effectiveness of the agent, the need for continued therapy, and the availability of therapeutic alternatives. If an alternative agent is used, choose one that is unlikely to cause the same ADR.

E. Like the onset of a reaction, resolution varies according to the specific nature of the reaction and the patient. Be aware that some adverse reactions, such as ototoxicity from aminoglycosides or nephrotoxicity from amphotericin B, may resolve only after long periods or may have permanent sequelae.

F. Rechallenge should not be undertaken unless the benefits outweigh the risks and should not be used merely to confirm the association between the ADR and the suspected drug. Be aware that there may be a different manifestation of the adverse reaction on rechallenge, particularly in cases of allergic reactions. These changes may be in the temporal relationship or in the severity of the reaction.

G. A variety of protocols are available to formally assess the probability and severity of an ADR. Unless the cause of the reaction is common and unambiguous, it may be helpful to apply one of these assessment protocols to the patient situation.

H. The U.S. Food and Drug Administration (FDA) MedWatch program is a voluntary system to report adverse events and products problems. The FDA is especially interested in serious or unusual reactions, reactions to new drugs, and reactions to herbal and other alternative medicine products. MedWatch reports can be submitted by fax (1-800-FDA-0178), by mail, or on-line (www.fda.gov/medwatch/). Vaccine-related ADRs should be reported to the Vaccine Adverse Event Reporting System (VAERS) at 1-800-822-7967.

References

American Society of Health-System Pharmacists. ASHP Guidelines on adverse drug reaction reporting and monitoring. Am J Health-Syst Pharm 1995;52:417–419.

Ayaji FO, Sun H, Perry J. Adverse drug reactions: a review of relevant factors. J Clin Pharmacol 2000;40:1093–1101.

Lazarou J, Pomeranz BH, Corey PN. Incidence of adverse drug reactions in hospitalized patients: a meta-analysis of prospective studies. JAMA 1998;279:1200.

Naranjo CA, Busto U, Sellers EM, et al. A method for estimating the probability of adverse drug reactions. Clin Pharmacol Ther 1981;30:239.

Thurmann PA. Methods and systems to detect adverse drug reactions in hospitals. Drug Saf 2001;24:961–968.

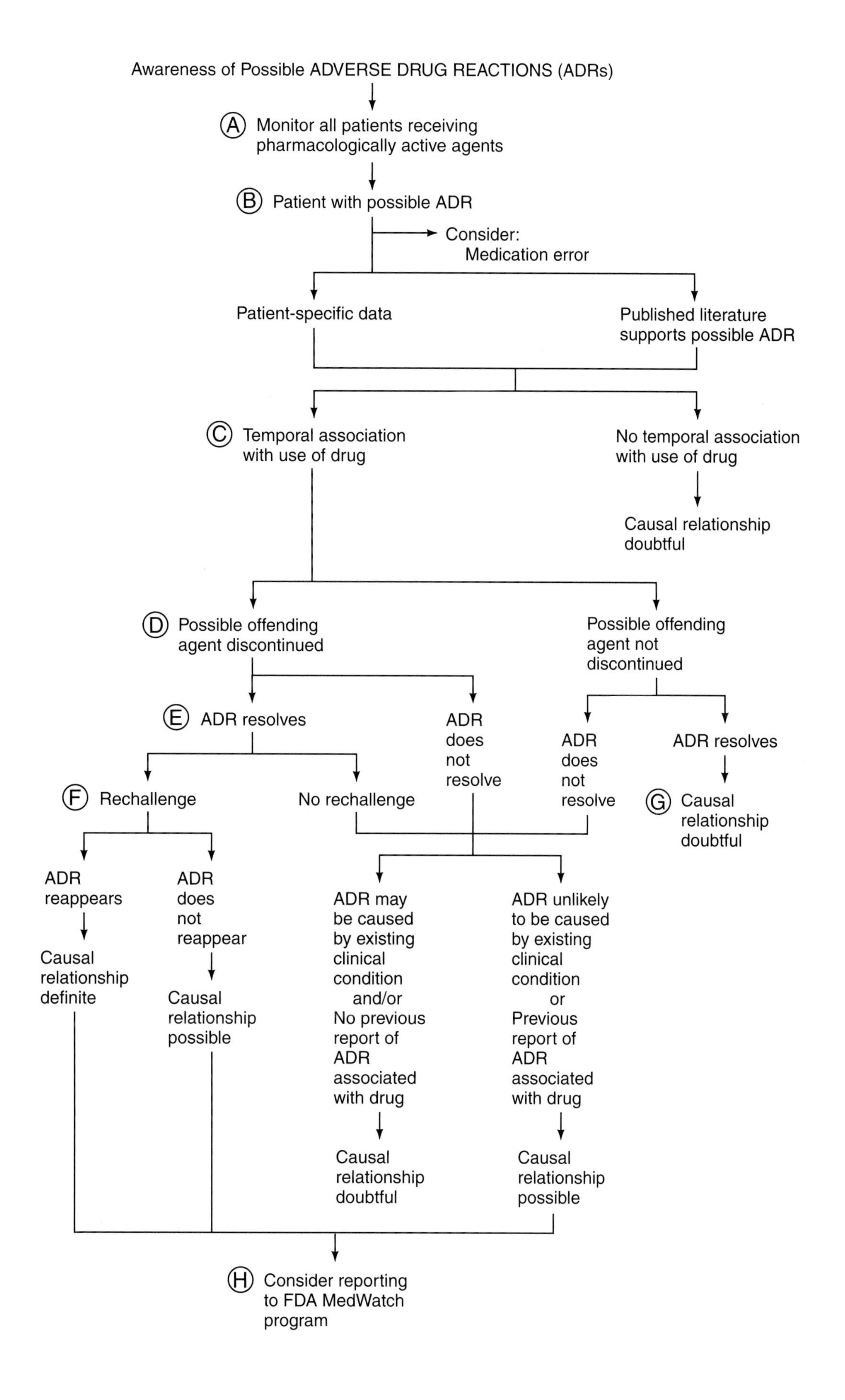
Awareness of Possible ADVERSE DRUG REACTIONS (ADRs)
(A) Monitor all patients receiving pharmacologically active agents
(B) Patient with possible ADR
Consider: Medication error
Patient-specific data
Published literature supports possible ADR
(C) Temporal association with use of drug
No temporal association with use of drug
Causal relationship doubtful
(D) Possible offending agent discontinued
Possible offending agent not discontinued
(E) ADR resolves
ADR does not resolve
ADR does not resolve
ADR resolves
(F) Rechallenge
No rechallenge
(G) Causal relationship doubtful
ADR reappears
ADR does not reappear
Causal relationship definite
Causal relationship possible
ADR may be caused by existing clinical condition and/or No previous report of ADR associated with drug
ADR unlikely to be caused by existing clinical condition or Previous report of ADR associated with drug
Causal relationship doubtful
Causal relationship possible
(H) Consider reporting to FDA MedWatch program

ANTIMICROBIAL PROPHYLAXIS IN SURGICAL PATIENTS

Brian L. Erstad, PharmD

A. A commonly used classification system categorizes surgical procedures as *clean, clean-contaminated, contaminated,* or *dirty,* based on predicted postoperative site infection rates; rates of infection are generally <2% for *clean* and about 40% for *dirty* procedures. However, infection rates for the same operation may vary at different institutions; physician- and institution-specific rates should be recorded and used in the consideration of prophylaxis. Other factors predictive of postoperative infection, including risks within particular categories, are described elsewhere (see Mangram et al.). In addition to the antimicrobials listed in the decision tree, mechanical bowel cleansing (e.g., oral polyethylene glycol solution, sodium phosphate with or without bisacodyl) is routinely used the day before elective colorectal surgery. For penetrating abdominal trauma, prophylaxis is indicated because the exact site and extent of injury cannot be determined until surgery. Treatment, not prophylaxis, is needed for *dirty* surgical procedures. Although guidelines usually state that treatment is also needed for *contaminated* procedures (e.g., colon injury with delayed surgery), prophylaxis may suffice in selected cases (e.g., minor break in technique with prompt lavage). Local antimicrobial prophylaxis with irrigations, impregnated beads or cement, and bonded grafts may provide protection equivalent to IV prophylaxis in some types of surgery, but well-designed trials are needed before recommendations can be made with confidence.

B. Do not base the decision to use antimicrobial prophylaxis solely on postoperative wound infection rates. Total hip replacement is classified as a *clean* operative procedure according to most criteria, but a postoperative infection of the prosthesis may be catastrophic. Hence, a clinically significant decrease in the incidence of an unacceptable complication may be sufficient justification for prophylaxis.

C. Cefazolin is the standard with which other antimicrobials (e.g., cefuroxime) should be compared for *clean* surgical procedures. Cefazolin is inexpensive, has a moderately long half-life, has a spectrum against most predominant pathogens, and has demonstrated activity in clinical trials. Clindamycin or vancomycin may be used instead of cefazolin in patients with β-lactam allergies. Additionally, vancomycin may be used for surgery involving prosthetic materials or devices (including total hip replacement) *if* a high rate of methicillin-resistant *Staphylococcus aureus* or *epidermidis* infection has been documented, but its use is not indicated for routine prophylaxis, given the concern of vancomycin-resistant bacteria.

D. Antimicrobials with aerobic and anaerobic activity (e.g., cefoxitin, cefotetan, cefazolin plus metronidazole; gentamicin plus clindamycin) are indicated for prophylaxis when mixed pathogens are common (i.e., clean-contaminated procedures). In colorectal surgery it is unclear whether IV antimicrobials with combined aerobic/anaerobic activity provide benefits beyond mechanical cleansing and oral antimicrobial prophylaxis, but the IV agent is often added.

Give IV antimicrobials within 60 minutes (120 minutes for vancomycin or ciprofloxacin) of the first incision to ensure adequate concentrations. Additional doses of the antimicrobial may be needed during extended procedures, depending on its pharmacokinetic properties (e.g., a second dose of cefazolin should be given 4 hours and cefoxitin should be given 2 hours from the start of an operation). With the possible exceptions of cardiothoracic procedures, there is little benefit from antimicrobial administration beyond 24 hours from the first surgical incision (unless treatment, not prophylaxis, is indicated). Recommended dosages are listed in Table 1.

Table 1 **Drug Dosages for Surgical Antimicrobial Prophylaxis in Adults***

Drug	Dosage
Cefazolin	1–2 g IV
Cefoxitin	1–2 g IV
Vancomycin	1 g IV
Clindamycin	600–900 mg IV
Gentamicin	1.5–2 mg/kg IV (use an adjusted weight if more than 30% above ideal body weight)
Ciprofloxacin	400 mg IV
Erythromycin	1 g PO × 3 doses†
Neomycin	1 g PO × 3 doses†

*Use the larger doses for patients who are obese and patients with substantial blood loss during surgery.
†Give at 1 PM, 2 PM, and 11 PM the day before surgery.

References

American Society of Health-System Pharmacists. ASHP therapeutic guidelines on antimicrobial prophylaxis in surgery. Am J Health-Syst Pharm 1999;56:1839.

Bratzler DW, Houck PM. Antimicrobial prophylaxis for surgery: an advisory statement from the National Surgical Infection Prevention Project. Clin Infect Dis 2004;38:1706.

Mangram AJ, Horan TC, Pearson ML, et al. Guideline for prevention of surgical site infection, 1999. Infect Control Hosp Epidemiol 1999;20:247.

National Nosocomial Infections Surveillance System. National Nosocomial Infections Surveillance (NNIS) report, data summary from October 1986–April 1996, issued May 1996. Am J Infect Control 1996;24:380.

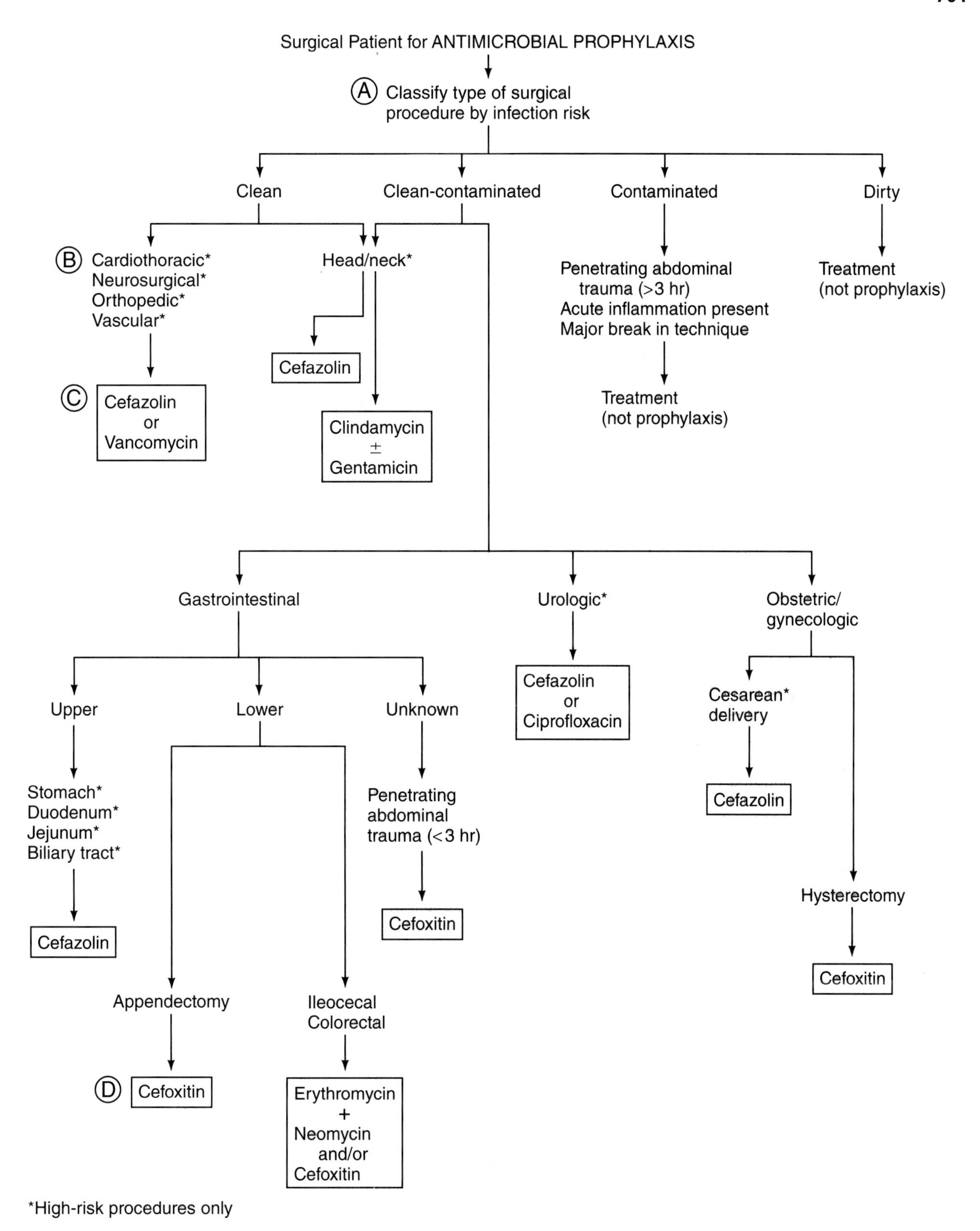
Surgical Patient for ANTIMICROBIAL PROPHYLAXIS
(A) Classify type of surgical procedure by infection risk
Clean
Clean-contaminated
Contaminated
Dirty
(B) Cardiothoracic*
Neurosurgical*
Orthopedic*
Vascular*
(C) Cefazolin or Vancomycin
Head/neck*
Cefazolin
Clindamycin ± Gentamicin
Penetrating abdominal trauma (>3 hr)
Acute inflammation present
Major break in technique
Treatment (not prophylaxis)
Treatment (not prophylaxis)
Gastrointestinal
Urologic*
Obstetric/gynecologic
Upper
Lower
Unknown
Cefazolin or Ciprofloxacin
Cesarean* delivery
Cefazolin
Stomach*
Duodenum*
Jejunum*
Biliary tract*
Cefazolin
Penetrating abdominal trauma (<3 hr)
Cefoxitin
Hysterectomy
Cefoxitin
Appendectomy
(D) Cefoxitin
Ileocecal
Colorectal
Erythromycin + Neomycin and/or Cefoxitin
*High-risk procedures only

CHOOSING APPROPRIATE ANTIMICROBIAL THERAPY

Michael D. Katz, PharmD

The choice of appropriate antimicrobial therapy should be based on several factors, including pathogens being treated, the antimicrobial spectrum, and a variety of patient-specific factors. Antibiotic choices should be based on a sound rationale.

A. Empiric therapy is based on a presumptive diagnosis of infection or clinical syndrome. Especially in the hospital setting, empiric therapy is broad in spectrum, designed to cover the most likely pathogens in the specific patient. Before initiating empiric therapy, obtain appropriate specimens for culture and sensitivity. Empiric therapy is indicated when the infection is potentially rapidly life-threatening (sepsis, pneumonia) or causes significant morbidity (urinary tract infection, severe dysentery). Therapy should be based on available evidence-based guidelines rather than drug manufacturer marketing and advertising.

B. The most likely pathogens at a site of infection may be based on normal flora at that site; tropism of certain pathogens for various tissues or organs; and patient-specific factors such as previous antimicrobial therapy, nosocomial versus community-acquired infection, and patient immune status. Not every possible pathogen requires coverage—just those that are most likely. Emergence of drug resistance in common bacterial pathogens such as *Streptococcus pneumoniae, Staphylococcus aureus,* and *Enterococcus* and spread of these organisms to the community has made antibiotic decision making more complex. The clinician must know current local resistance patterns of common pathogens and factors driving increased resistance. The use of certain drugs, such as vancomycin and linezolid, should be based on strict guidelines to reduce the development and spread of resistance.

C. Patient-specific factors include history of previous adverse reactions to antimicrobials, patient age, pregnancy or lactation, concomitant drugs, excretory organ function, immune status, and site of infection. For patients who are very ill, IV administration is preferable to ensure adequate drug concentrations at the site of infection.

D. Combination therapy is indicated when broad-spectrum coverage is desired (sepsis), in polymicrobial infections (intraperitoneal abscesses), to prevent the emergence of resistance (tuberculosis), or to provide antimicrobial synergy (streptococcal endocarditis, β-lactam/aminoglycoside for *Pseudomonas aeruginosa* infections, amphotericin/5-flucytosine for cryptococcal meningitis).

E. The cost of drug therapy is based not only on the drug cost but on the cost of administration, supplies, and monitoring. If all else is equal, choose the least expensive regimen. However, therapeutic efficacy is of primary importance.

F. Definitive therapy occurs when a microbiologic and a clinical diagnosis are confirmed. Definitive therapy is narrow in spectrum and generally requires only one drug. If the patient was previously receiving empiric therapy, determine the need for continued treatment.

G. Susceptibility data are useful in determining definitive therapy, but there are pitfalls. If the reported susceptibilities do not fit usual patterns for that organism, the reliability of the information is suspect. If minimal inhibitory concentrations (MICs) are present, in general, any drug in the sensitive MIC range will be effective. Some forms of antibiotic resistance may not be detected by standard laboratory methodology.

H. Even with positive cultures, broad-spectrum therapy may be indicated, especially in patients who are immunosuppressed. Base the choice of antimicrobial regimen on clinical judgment and laboratory data.

I. A variety of drug-specific factors must be considered. Certain agents do not penetrate well into certain tissues (e.g., aminoglycosides in CNS infections, vancomycin in pulmonary infections). If a relatively new antimicrobial is considered, there should be clinical trials documenting efficacy compared with the conventional regimen for that infection. Consider drug toxicity; reserve more toxic drugs (aminoglycosides, amphotericin B) for patients at higher risk.

J. If the patient is not critically ill and has adequate GI tract function, give oral antimicrobials as soon as possible. However, in some cases, long-term or home IV antimicrobial therapy is indicated if oral agents are not available for the specific infection.

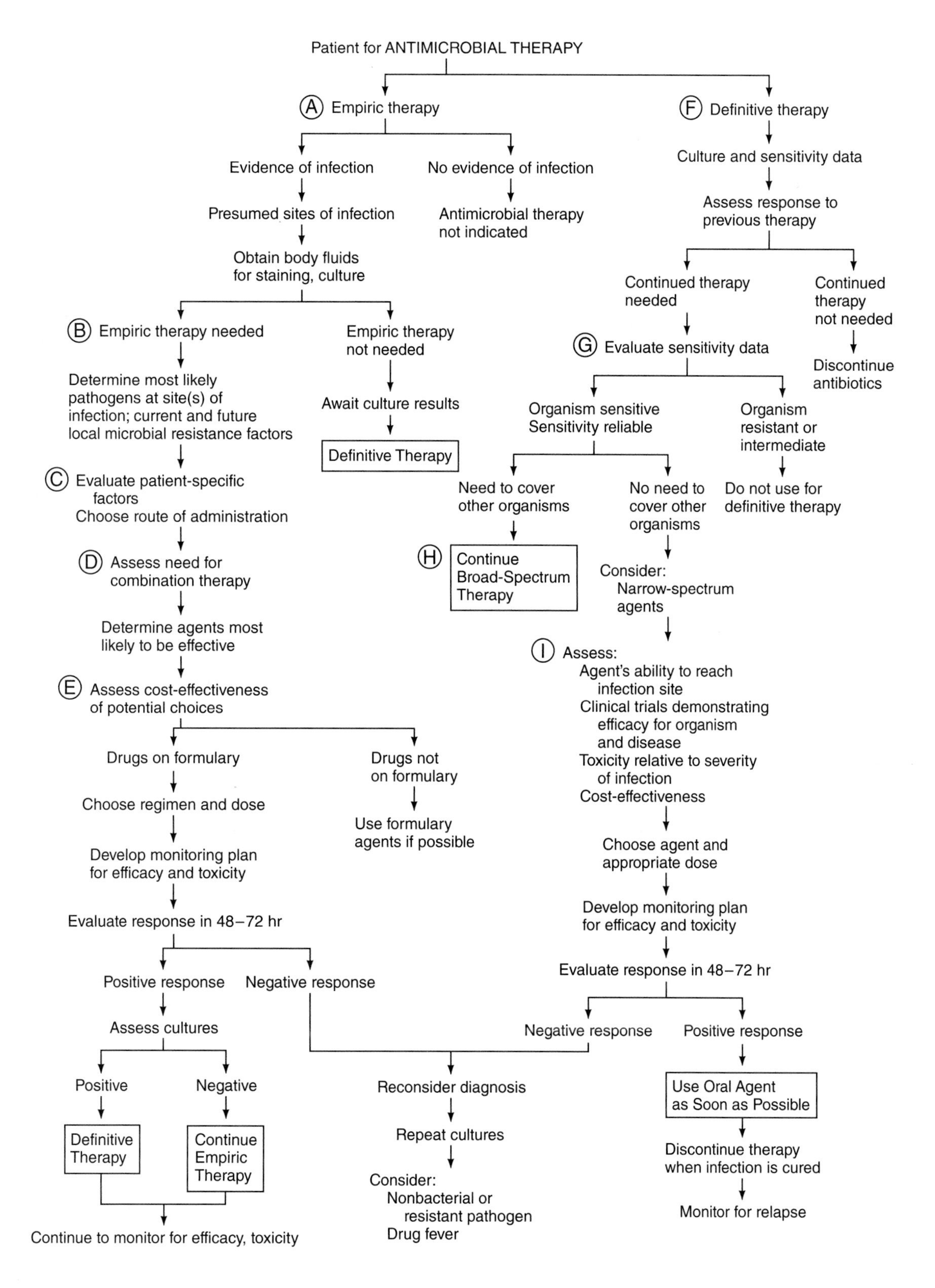

References

Avorn J, Solomon DH. Cultural and economic factors that (mis)shape antibiotic use: the nonpharmacologic basis of therapeutics. Ann Intern Med 2000;133:128–135.

Burgess DS, Abate BJ. Antimicrobial regimen selection. In DiPiro JT, Talbert RL, Yee CG, et al, eds. Pharmacotherapy: A Pathophysiologic Approach, 6th ed. New York: McGraw-Hill, 2005:1909–1919.

Centers for Disease Control and Prevention. Antibiotic/antimicrobial resistance. Available at www.cdc.gov/drugresistance/publications.htm. Accessed March 23, 2006.

Choice of antibacterial drugs. Treat Guidel Med Lett 2004;2:13–26.

Infectious Diseases Society of America Standards. Practice guidelines and statements. Available at www.idsociety.org/Content/Navigation-Menu/Practice_Guidelines/Standards_Practice_Guidelines_Statements/Standards,_Practice_Guidelines,_and_Statements.htm. Accessed August 23, 2006.

USE AND MONITORING OF AMINOGLYCOSIDE ANTIBIOTICS

Brian L. Erstad, PharmD

Gentamicin (G), tobramycin (T), and amikacin (A) are members of a class of antiinfectives known as the aminoglycosides. They are injectable antimicrobials primarily used for their excellent activity against gram-negative rod aerobic bacteria, with a few important exceptions (e.g., *Stenotrophomonas maltophilia*). These agents tend to have similar spectra, although tobramycin may be useful for *Pseudomonas aeruginosa* in institutions with gentamicin-resistant strains, and gentamicin may be useful in combination with penicillins or vancomycin for synergism when treating serious enterococcal or staphylococcal infections. Some infectious disease experts also recommend the addition of an aminoglycoside to β-lactam therapy for serious infections caused by organisms such as *P. aeruginosa,* although there is little evidence of improved efficacy with the combination, assuming the organism is susceptible to the β-lactam.

A. Although the loading dose of an aminoglycoside can be calculated on the basis of body weight, subsequent maintenance doses need to be calculated with consideration of the patient's extracellular volume status and renal function. Equations and computer programs have been developed for dosing the aminoglycosides, but once-daily regimens involve less complicated dosing calculations and are probably less labor intensive than traditional dosing methods yet have similar efficacy in most populations. However, some groups have not been well studied (e.g., pregnant women), and others (e.g., geriatric patients) may be more prone to toxicity with once-daily dosing.

B. One interaction between aminoglycosides and penicillins deserves special mention. Aminoglycoside concentrations may be lowered in vivo and in vitro by concomitant administration of penicillins. Although the significance of this interaction depends on a number of factors (e.g., specific antimicrobials, dosing regimens), it is best to minimize the potential for this interaction by scheduling these agents as far apart as possible.

C. Remember to monitor the patient and not just the serum aminoglycoside levels. Potential nephrotoxicity and ototoxicity concerns have led to use of aminoglycoside assays at many hospitals. When used appropriately, these assays can be valuable monitoring tools. However, they are not a substitute for clinical evaluation. Aminoglycoside levels may be in the therapeutic range, but the patient may not be clinically improving, which may require a change or reevaluation of therapy. Aminoglycoside levels may not be needed for expected therapy <5 days in patients with stable renal function and fluid balance. When aminoglycoside levels are needed, diligent attention to their collection and analysis is crucial. Aminoglycoside doses may be skipped or given at unexpected times. Blood may be drawn from a line containing the aminoglycoside or not drawn at all. The draw may not be at the proper time. If the level is ordered and drawn correctly, the specimen may not be properly stored before analysis.

D. The definitions of the pharmacokinetic terms *peak* and *trough* have not been standardized in the medical literature. In this chapter peak level refers to the blood concentration of an aminoglycoside drawn 30 minutes after a 30-minute infusion. The trough level is the concentration 30 minutes before a dose of the aminoglycoside. For once-daily dosing, some investigators recommend a single level drawn 6–14 hours after the dose is administered, with subsequent adjustment by nomogram (see Nicolau et al.). As a more straightforward alternative (with similar assumptions about the peak level), the clinician can draw a single trough level that should be < 0.5 mg/L with once-daily dosing. With once-daily dosing, the primary concern is related to unexpected aminoglycoside accumulation that should be reflected in an elevated trough concentration. A pharmacokinetic consultation would be in order if this accumulation is found.

(Continued on page 706)

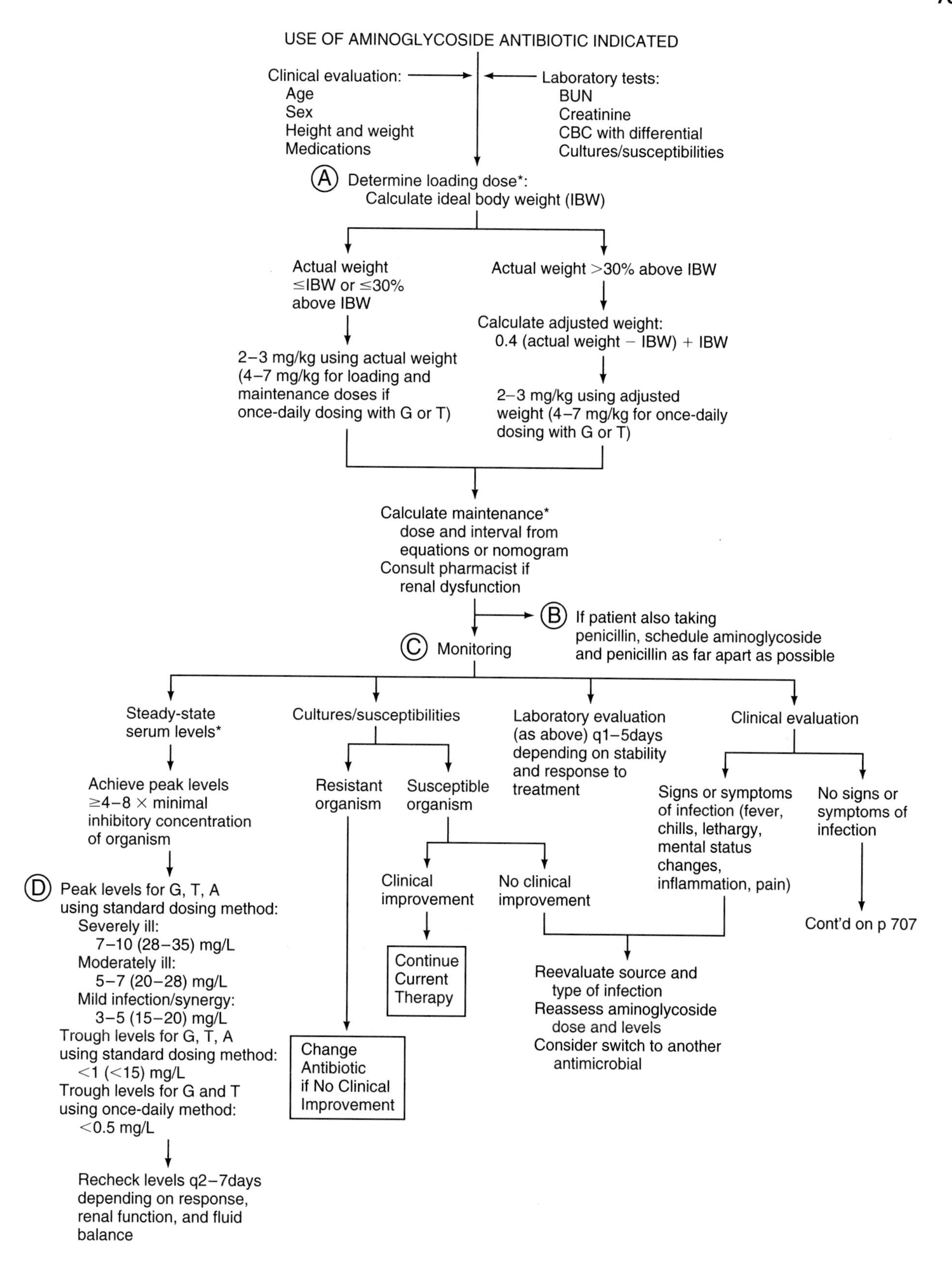
USE OF AMINOGLYCOSIDE ANTIBIOTIC INDICATED
Clinical evaluation:
Age
Sex
Height and weight
Medications
Laboratory tests:
BUN
Creatinine
CBC with differential
Cultures/susceptibilities
(A) Determine loading dose*:
Calculate ideal body weight (IBW)
Actual weight ≤IBW or ≤30% above IBW
2–3 mg/kg using actual weight (4–7 mg/kg for loading and maintenance doses if once-daily dosing with G or T)
Actual weight >30% above IBW
Calculate adjusted weight:
0.4 (actual weight − IBW) + IBW
2–3 mg/kg using adjusted weight (4–7 mg/kg for once-daily dosing with G or T)
Calculate maintenance* dose and interval from equations or nomogram
Consult pharmacist if renal dysfunction
(B) If patient also taking penicillin, schedule aminoglycoside and penicillin as far apart as possible
(C) Monitoring
Steady-state serum levels*
Achieve peak levels ≥4–8 × minimal inhibitory concentration of organism
(D) Peak levels for G, T, A using standard dosing method:
Severely ill:
7–10 (28–35) mg/L
Moderately ill:
5–7 (20–28) mg/L
Mild infection/synergy:
3–5 (15–20) mg/L
Trough levels for G, T, A using standard dosing method:
<1 (<15) mg/L
Trough levels for G and T using once-daily method:
<0.5 mg/L
Recheck levels q2–7days depending on response, renal function, and fluid balance
Cultures/susceptibilities
Resistant organism
Change Antibiotic if No Clinical Improvement
Susceptible organism
Clinical improvement
Continue Current Therapy
No clinical improvement
Laboratory evaluation (as above) q1–5days depending on stability and response to treatment
Clinical evaluation
Signs or symptoms of infection (fever, chills, lethargy, mental status changes, inflammation, pain)
Reevaluate source and type of infection
Reassess aminoglycoside dose and levels
Consider switch to another antimicrobial
No signs or symptoms of infection
Cont'd on p 707

*Use higher end of dosing range for patients who are critically ill and lower end for synergy.

E. The introduction of antimicrobials with enhanced gram-negative activity has allowed the clinician more choices for treating such infections. However, when the aminoglycosides are used for resistant organisms or for synergy against gram-positive cocci, proper monitoring of patients is necessary to reduce the incidence of nephrotoxicity and ototoxicity. It is thought that the nephrotoxicity associated with aminoglycosides primarily is related to multiple daily doses given for prolonged periods (i.e., area under the concentration time curve). Other factors associated with aminoglycoside toxicity include liver disease, shock, congestive heart failure, and the age and sex of the patient (higher in the elderly and females). Because nephrotoxicity and ototoxicity are most likely to occur in patients who receive aminoglycosides for prolonged periods, the duration of therapy should be limited to the shortest period of time necessary to clear the infection.

F. The optimal duration of aminoglycoside therapy has not been well studied. In general, extended courses (weeks) are necessary for more severe infections such as osteomyelitis caused by gram-negative bacteria that are resistant to other antimicrobials. Uncomplicated wound or urinary tract infections often resolve after 3–5 days of taking the aminoglycosides. Consider the site, severity, and clinical response in deciding when to discontinue therapy.

References

Barletta JF, Johnson SB, Nix DE, et al. Population pharmacokinetics of aminoglycosides in critically ill trauma patients on once-daily regimens. J Trauma 2000;49:869.

Bliziotis IA, Samonis G, Vardakas KZ, et al. Effect of aminoglycoside and β-lactam combination therapy versus β-lactam monotherapy on the emergence of antimicrobial resistance: a meta-analysis of randomized, controlled trials. Clin Infect Dis 2005;41:149.

Henderson JL, Polk RE, Kline BJ. In vitro interaction of gentamicin, tobramycin, and netilmicin by carbenicillin, azlocillin, or mezlocillin. Am J Hosp Pharm 1981;38:1167.

Nicolau DP, Freeman CD, Belliveau PP, et al. Experience with a once-daily aminoglycoside program administered to 2,184 adult patients. Antimicrob Agents Chemother 1995;39:650.

Prins JM, Weverling GJ, De Blok K, et al. Validation and nephrotoxicity of a simplified once-daily aminoglycoside dosing schedule and guidelines for monitoring therapy. Antimicrob Agents Chemother 1996;40:2494.

Rybak MJ, Abate BJ, Kang L, et al. Prospective evaluation of the effect of an aminoglycoside dosing regimen on rates of observed nephrotoxicity and ototoxicity. Antimicrob Agents Chemother 1999;43:1549.

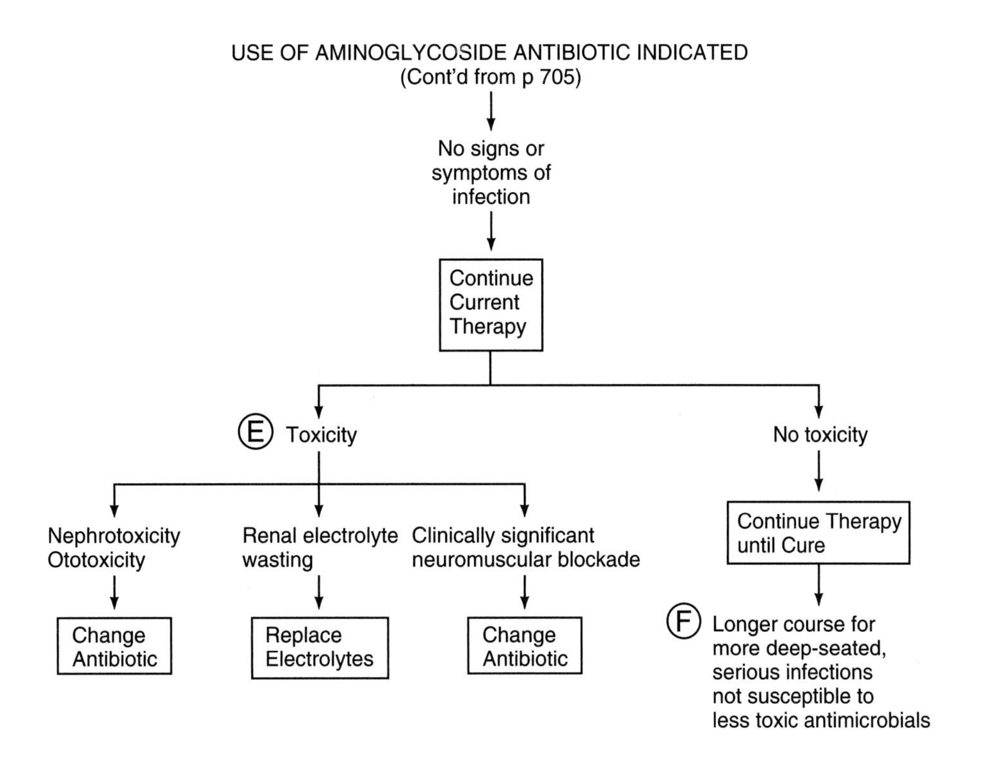
USE OF AMINOGLYCOSIDE ANTIBIOTIC INDICATED
(Cont'd from p 705)
No signs or symptoms of infection
Continue Current Therapy
E Toxicity
No toxicity
Nephrotoxicity Ototoxicity
Renal electrolyte wasting
Clinically significant neuromuscular blockade
Continue Therapy until Cure
Change Antibiotic
Replace Electrolytes
Change Antibiotic
F Longer course for more deep-seated, serious infections not susceptible to less toxic antimicrobials

USE AND EVALUATION OF SERUM DRUG LEVELS

Jason M. Rominski, PharmD; Kathryn R. Matthias, PharmD; and Brian L. Erstad, PharmD

A. Certain medications have a narrow therapeutic index (NTI), meaning there is a narrow range for a serum drug level (SDL) that will provide a therapeutic effect with minimal risk of toxicity. Examples of NTI medications include carbamazepine, digoxin, phenytoin, procainamide, quinidine, theophylline, lithium, cyclosporine, and the aminoglycoside antibiotics (see the chapter Use and Monitoring of Aminoglycoside Antibiotics). SDL assays can be useful when there is a known correlation between the SDL and pharmacologic effect of the drug. The availability of an SDL assay from the laboratory does not necessarily mean there is utility in measuring an SDL in a given patient. Some drugs may be monitored by SDL only under certain circumstances (e.g., aspirin in Kawasaki's syndrome). Prior to obtaining an SDL, it is important to consider the need for the drug and SDL while including an evaluation of the clinical goals, the outcomes that will be measured to assess these goals, and the risk of toxicity based on the drug dose and length of therapy. The availability of less toxic alternative agents with similar therapeutic efficacy should be considered. SDL assays are a tool to monitoring therapeutic outcomes, but the SDL is not in itself an outcome.

B. Proper therapeutic drug monitoring (TDM) requires obtaining SDLs at appropriate times for a particular drug therapy to maximize efficacy and minimize toxicity.

C. The use of pharmacokinetic calculations or nomograms often is helpful in developing a patient-specific drug-dosing regimen based on SDLs. Patient-specific parameters such as weight, height, age, sex, and renal and hepatic function should be obtained because these factors can affect an SDL and the response to drug therapy.

D. Most therapeutic or reference ranges of NTI drugs are based on a trough blood level, usually defined as an SDL obtained ≤30 minutes before the next scheduled dose of the drug. Drawing an SDL too early may cause an erroneously high level to be reported, resulting in misinterpretation of the data and potentially inappropriate changes in therapy. This can be especially problematic if the blood is drawn during the infusion or distribution phase of the drug (e.g., digoxin). The distribution phase is the period in which the drug in plasma is equilibrating with extravascular fluid and tissues into which the drug will distribute.

E. It is important that a patient's response to the medication be considered rather than just the reported SDL. SDLs are tools to supplement clinical response while achievement of desired therapeutic outcomes is the primary measure.

F. Changing a drug-dosing regimen on the basis of an SDL should be carefully considered. All benefits and risks of a dosage change need to be taken into account. For example, when a theophylline level has been reported correctly as 19 μg/ml (therapeutic 10–20 μg/ml) but the patient has not experienced clinical benefit, it is probably more prudent to add an additional therapy or switch to an alternative agent rather than to obtain a higher SDL. Additionally, possible drug interactions and the patient's compliance with the drug schedule should be considered prior to any dosage adjustments based on an SDL.

(Continued on page 710)

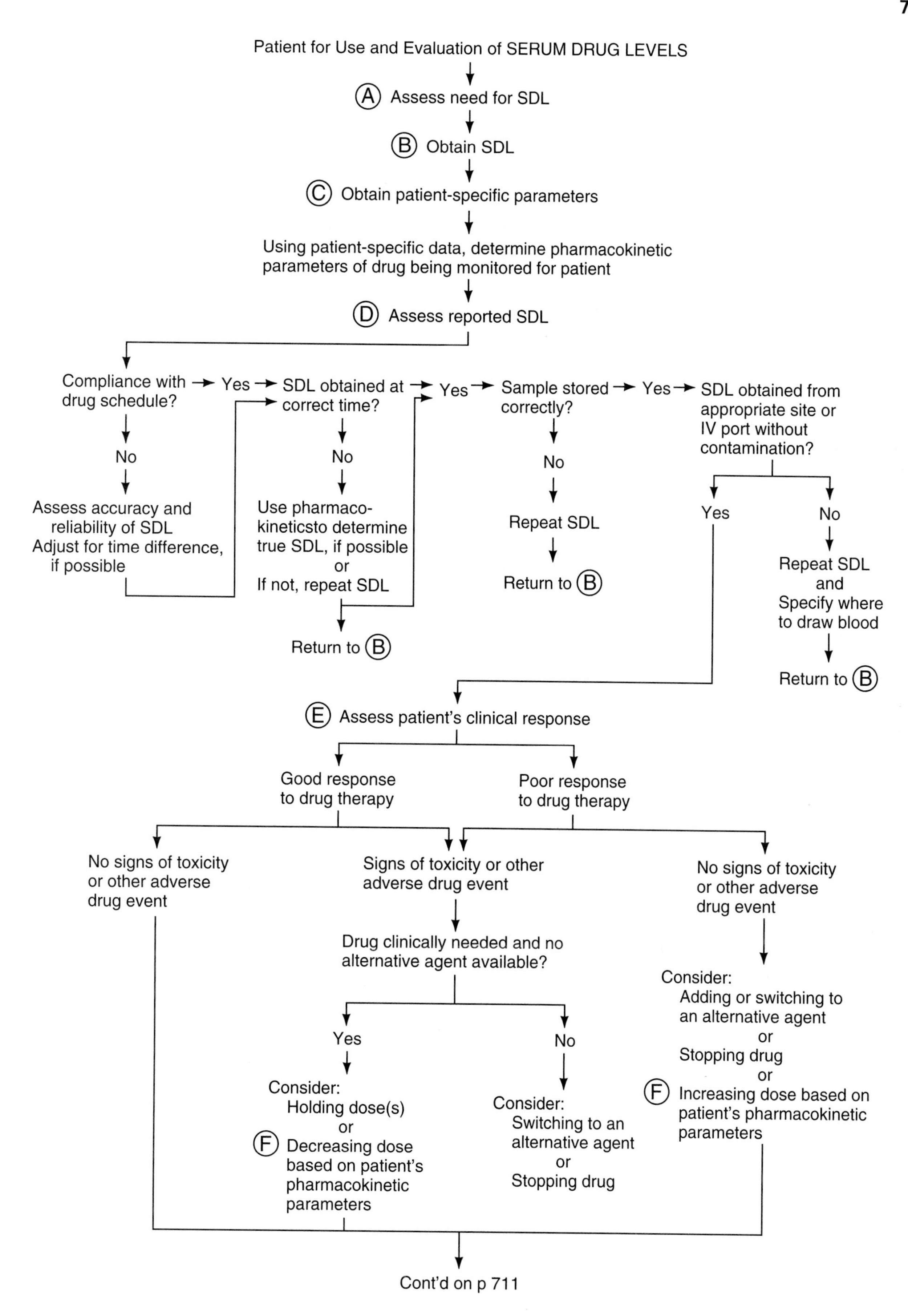

Cont'd on p 711

G. An SDL is often more useful when the patient's blood is drawn after steady state (SS) has been achieved. SS is when the rate of the drug administered is equal to the rate of drug elimination in drugs that have linear kinetics. Drawing blood and determining an SDL before the drug has reached SS may result in a lower-than-expected level than will occur at SS. SS is achieved after four to five half-lives of the drug and is independent of the number of doses given. Therefore, to calculate when a drug will reach SS, the clinician must first estimate the half-life of the drug for the particular patient (including effects of renal and liver dysfunction). If a loading dose of the drug was given, a higher-than-expected SDL may be seen prior to SS.

H. Certain total (protein-bound and free-drug) concentration SDL measurements for highly protein-bound agents such as phenytoin and salicylates should be evaluated based on several factors, including the patient's serum albumin level, renal function, coadministration of certain other agents, and any other factor that may alter the degree of protein-binding prior to dosage adjustments.

References

Holford NHG. Pharmacokinetics and pharmacodynamics: rational dosing and the time course of drug action. In Katzung BG, ed. Basic and Clinical Pharmacology, 9th ed. New York: McGraw-Hill, 2004: 35–50.

McCormack JP, Brown G. Rational use of drug concentration measurements. In Murphy JE, ed. Clinical Pharmacokinetics, 3rd ed. Bethesda, MD: American Society of Health-System Pharmacists, 2005:15–21.

Touw DJ, Neef C, Thomson AH, et al. Cost-effectiveness of therapeutic drug monitoring: a systemic review. Ther Drug Monit 2005;27(1): 10–17.

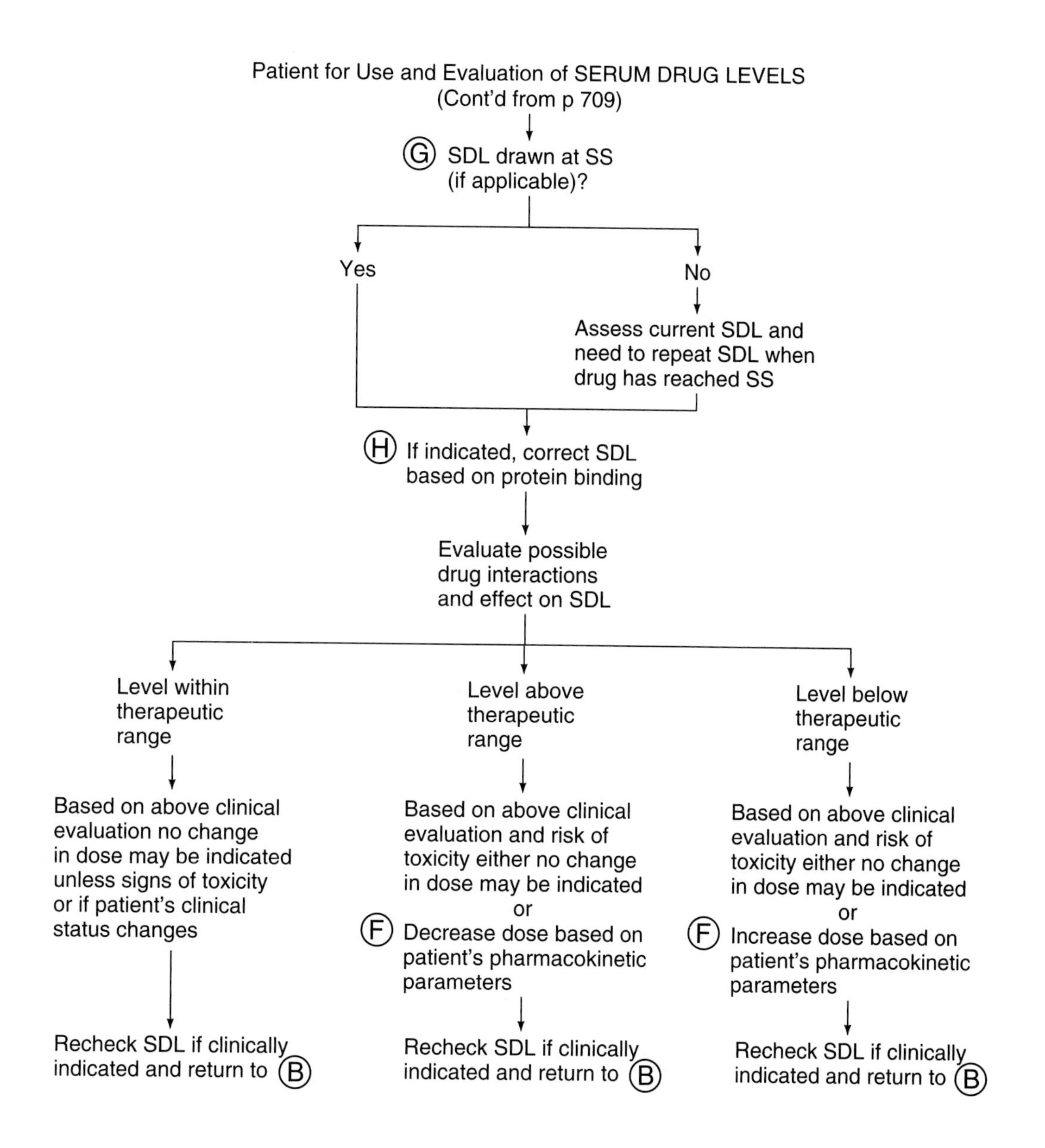
Patient for Use and Evaluation of SERUM DRUG LEVELS
(Cont'd from p 709)
G SDL drawn at SS
(if applicable)?
Yes
No
Assess current SDL and
need to repeat SDL when
drug has reached SS
H If indicated, correct SDL
based on protein binding
Evaluate possible
drug interactions
and effect on SDL
Level within
therapeutic
range
Level above
therapeutic
range
Level below
therapeutic
range
Based on above clinical
evaluation no change
in dose may be indicated
unless signs of toxicity
or if patient's clinical
status changes
Based on above clinical
evaluation and risk of
toxicity either no change
in dose may be indicated
or
F Decrease dose based on
patient's pharmacokinetic
parameters
Based on above clinical
evaluation and risk of
toxicity either no change
in dose may be indicated
or
F Increase dose based on
patient's pharmacokinetic
parameters
Recheck SDL if clinically
indicated and return to B
Recheck SDL if clinically
indicated and return to B
Recheck SDL if clinically
indicated and return to B

USE AND EVALUATION OF VANCOMYCIN SERUM DRUG LEVEL

Jason M. Rominski, PharmD, and Kathryn R. Matthias, PharmD

A. Vancomycin is a glycopeptide antibiotic introduced in the 1950s for gram-positive bacterial infections. Although once referred to as "Mississippi mud" for its muddy consistency (fermentation broth impurities), improved purification methods have changed both the appearance and adverse event profile of this drug. With its improved safety profile and the increasing incidence of multi–drug-resistant organisms, vancomycin use in both empiric and organism-specific treatment has increased. When using vancomycin empirically, it is important to consider the probable organism, local susceptibility patterns, and nationally recognized guidelines. After the need for vancomycin therapy has been determined, the need for vancomycin serum drug level (VSDL) monitoring must be decided. Although many clinicians still maintain the importance of monitoring vancomycin VSDLs, it is important to consider clinical outcomes when determining the need for VSDL monitoring. Relatively healthy patients requiring short-term therapy may not require a VSDL, whereas VSDL monitoring may be indicated in patients with renal insufficiency requiring long-term therapy and those who have unstable renal function or those with difficult-to-treat infections.

B. VSDL monitoring commonly consists of trough levels and occasionally peak levels. The utility of peak levels is controversial; however, peak levels are obtained 30–90 minutes after the end of an infusion. Trough VSDLs are obtained within 60 minutes prior to the next dose. It is recommended that VSDLs be obtained after the drug has reached steady state. Patient-specific parameters such as renal function, age, weight, site of infection, comorbidities, and route of administration should be included in VSDL evaluations (see Use and Evaluation of Serum Drug Levels for more details).

C. A patient's clinical response to vancomycin therapy is more important than whether a VSDL is within a standard therapeutic range (see Use and Evaluation of Serum Drug Levels for more details).

D. If a patient's abnormal WBC count, temperature, imaging studies, and other indicators of infection are not resolving within a reasonable time period, vancomycin therapy may need to be intensified or it may not be adequate antimicrobial coverage for the infection. Other clinical causes of these parameters should be considered.

E. Alternatively, if signs and symptoms of vancomycin toxicity are evident, such as leukopenia, thrombocytopenia, ototoxicity, or nephrotoxicity, an alternative antimicrobial should be considered. Other reported adverse effects such as myalgias, "red man's" syndrome, hypotension, and thrombophlebitis can generally be avoided by administering vancomycin through a central venous catheter over ≥60 minutes depending on the dose.

F. If multiple VSDLs are obtained and a pharmacokinetic evaluation is desired, consider consulting a clinical pharmacy specialist. Many patients may not require more than one VSDL depending on the duration of therapy. Short-term therapy is not likely to require VSDL monitoring unless renal function is impaired. Patients with fluctuating renal function or an unstable clinical course may require more frequent VSDL monitoring. Patients receiving continuous renal replacement therapy (CRRT), hemodialysis, or other renal alteration therapies should be evaluated individually.

(Continued on page 714)

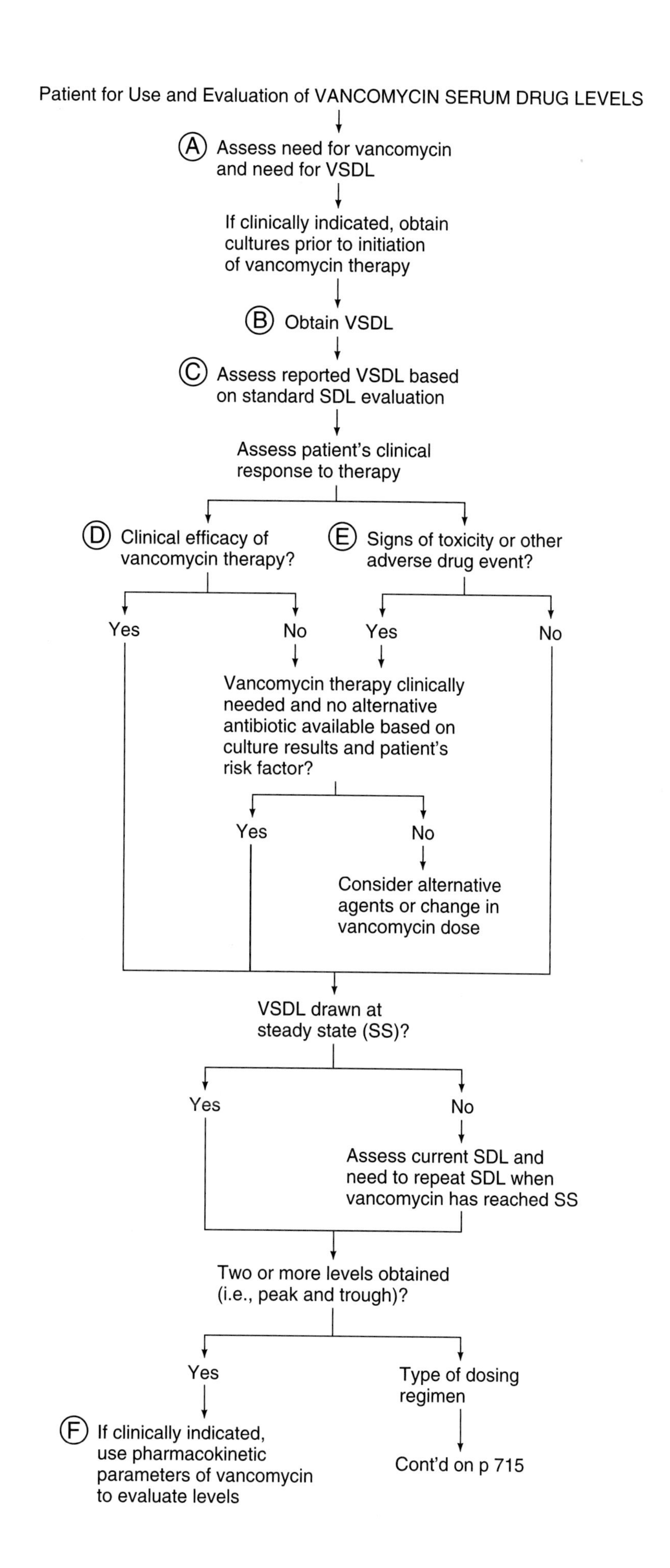
Patient for Use and Evaluation of VANCOMYCIN SERUM DRUG LEVELS
(A) Assess need for vancomycin and need for VSDL
If clinically indicated, obtain cultures prior to initiation of vancomycin therapy
(B) Obtain VSDL
(C) Assess reported VSDL based on standard SDL evaluation
Assess patient's clinical response to therapy
(D) Clinical efficacy of vancomycin therapy?
(E) Signs of toxicity or other adverse drug event?
Yes
No
Yes
No
Vancomycin therapy clinically needed and no alternative antibiotic available based on culture results and patient's risk factor?
Yes
No
Consider alternative agents or change in vancomycin dose
VSDL drawn at steady state (SS)?
Yes
No
Assess current SDL and need to repeat SDL when vancomycin has reached SS
Two or more levels obtained (i.e., peak and trough)?
Yes
Type of dosing regimen
(F) If clinically indicated, use pharmacokinetic parameters of vancomycin to evaluate levels
Cont'd on p 715

G. Dosage adjustments can be made by changing dose, frequency of administration, or both. Increasing the dose can increase peak concentrations and increase the time the concentration is above a desired trough level. Increasing the frequency of administration can have less of an effect on peak levels (at steady state) and can increase trough levels. The method of increasing dose frequency is generally more appropriate with vancomycin because it exhibits time-dependent killing rather than concentration-dependent killing.

H. Evaluation of a patient's VSDL should include clinical status, culture results, and the predicted penetration of the drug to the site of infection. The trough VSDL range for the majority of infections is traditionally reported as 5–15 μg/ml. Recently, clinical practice trends have used a trough VSDL target of 15–20 μg/ml for infections at sites with relatively poor vancomycin penetration such as the lungs and bones. Peak VSDL targets once aimed for 30–40 μg/ml; however, these ranges were empiric and there are limited data in the literature to support this practice.

I. Continuous infusions of vancomycin can maintain a relatively constant level of drug in the blood, which is theoretically advantageous with an agent that exhibits time-dependent killing. Lung, cerebrospinal fluid, and bone tend to be poorly penetrated by vancomycin, and levels achieved will be considerably less than the reported VSDL. If the site of infection is a difficult-to-penetrate tissue, random VSDLs should target the upper end of the desired range. Although SDLs can be relatively constant over a 24-hour period, the exposure to the drug is normally less than that of intermittent dosing regimens.

References

American Thoracic Society; Infectious Diseases Society of America. Guidelines for the management of adults with hospital-acquired, ventilator-associated, and healthcare-associated pneumonia. Am J Respir Crit Care Med 2005;171:388–416.

Baddour LM, Wilson WR, Bayer AS, et al. Infective endocarditis. Circulation 2005;111:e394–434.

Darko W, Medicis JJ, Smith A, et al. Mississippi mud no more: cost-effectiveness of pharmacokinetic dosage adjustment of vancomycin to prevent nephrotoxicity. Pharmacotherapy 2003;23(5):643–650.

Kitzis MD, Goldstein FW. Monitoring of vancomycin serum levels for the treatment of staphylococcal infections. Clin Microbiol Infect 2006;12(1):92–95.

Tunkel AR, Hartman BJ, Kaplan SL, et al. Practice guidelines for the management of bacterial meningitis. Clin Infect Dis 2004;39:1267–1284.

Vuagnat A, Stern R, Lotthe A, et al. High-dose vancomycin for osteomyelitis: continuous vs. intermittent infusions. J Clin Pharm Ther 2004;29(4):351–357.

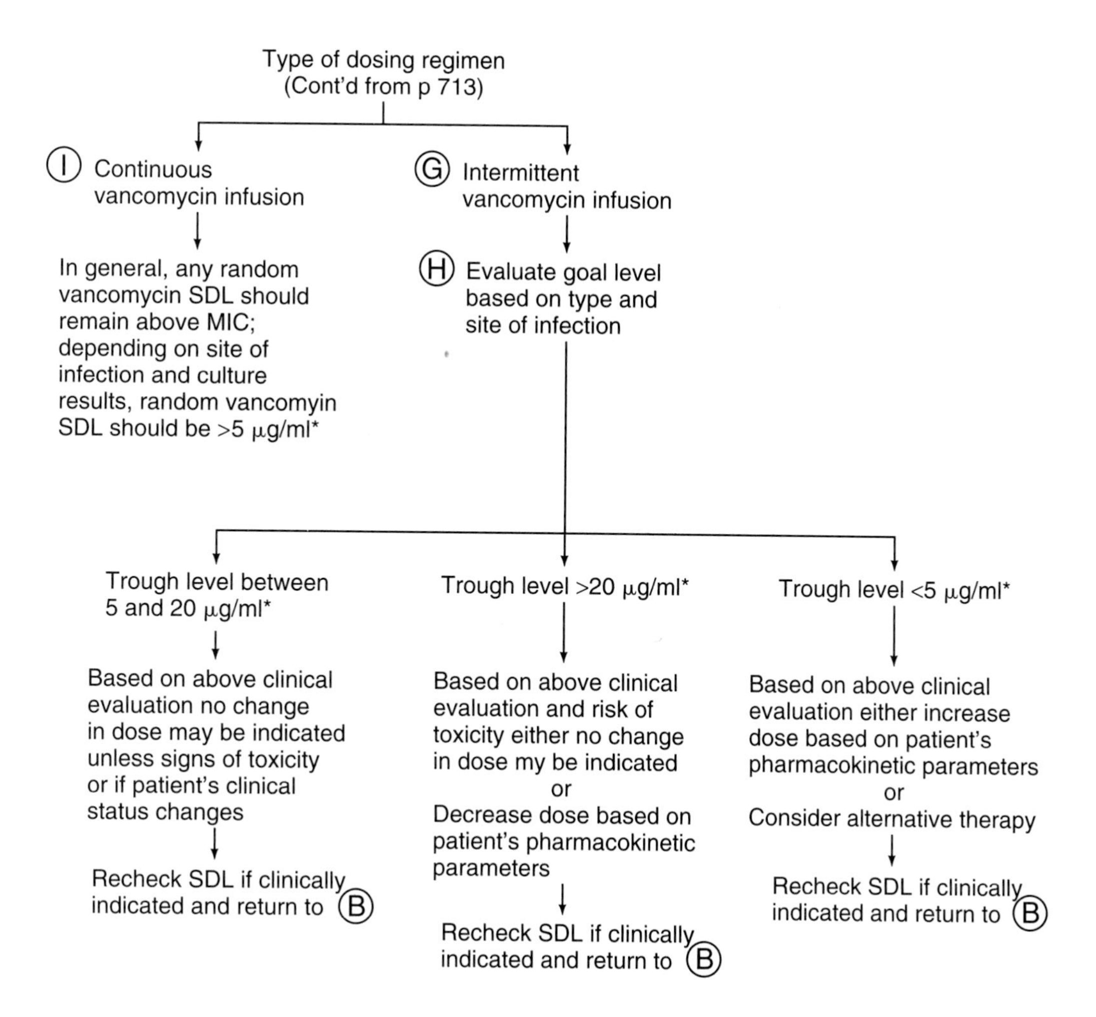

* Recommended goal trough vancomycin SDL is subject to change.
Recent reports in the literature suggest that higher trough SDLs may be indicated in certain clinical situations.

INDEX